Occupational Lung Disorders

Non numerentur auctoritates sed ponderentur.
(Do not count the number of authorities but weigh their truth.)
Thomas Aquinas

An ... 'advantage arising from the more attentive examination of morbid structure is, that we shall be able to distinguish between changes which may have some considerable resemblance to each other, and which have been generally confounded'.

Another ... 'advantage still from observing attentively morbid structure is, that theories taken up hastily about diseases will be occasionally corrected. The human mind is prone to form opinions upon every subject which is presented to it, but from a natural indolence is frequently averse to inquire into the circumstances which can alone form sufficient ground for them.'

Matthew Baillie, MD, FRS, in Preface
to *The Morbid Anatomy of Some of the
Most Important Parts of the Human Body*
London, Bulmer, 1st edn, 1793

Occupational Lung Disorders

Third edition

W. Raymond Parkes OBE MD (L'pool) FRCP FFOM DIH

Formerly:
Medical Boarding Centre (Respiratory Diseases), Department of Health and Social Security,
London; Honorary Clinical Lecturer, Professorial Unit (Thoracic Medicine), National Heart and
Lung Institute, London

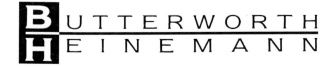

Butterworth-Heinemann Ltd
Linacre House, Jordan Hill, Oxford OX2 8DP

 A member of the Reed Elsevier group

OXFORD   LONDON   BOSTON
MUNICH   NEW DELHI   SINGAPORE   SYDNEY
TOKYO   TORONTO   WELLINGTON

First published 1974
Second edition 1982
Third edition 1994

British Library Cataloguing in Publication Data
A catalogue record for this book is available from the British Library

Library of Congress Cataloguing in Publication Data
A catalogue record for this book is available from the Library of Congress

ISBN 0 7506 1403 X

Composition by Scribe Design, Gillingham, Kent
Printed in Great Britain by BAS Printers, Over Wallop, Hants and bound by Hartnolls, Bodmin, Cornwall

Contents

Preface

A few years ago it was apparent that the second edition of this book (1982) needed to be brought up to date. Unfortunately, for a variety of reasons (some frustrating) this has taken longer than intended or anticipated. However, the delay, though having some inevitable drawbacks, has not been without advantage for it allowed more time for assimilation of the substantial changes and some of the shifts of emphasis that have occurred in the speciality since then. Like the earlier editions, the aim of the third, though developed further, is, in essence, an exercise in clinico-pathological correlation; that is, description and discussion of pathogenesis, pathology, physiology and clinical features (including imaging) of occupational pulmonary disorders which, it is hoped, are reasonably comprehensively represented. 'Pathogenesis', in this context, embraces, as previously, the identity and sources of agents in the workplace environment – not those in the general environment – that have potentially deleterious respiratory effects. While acknowledging that occupational and environmental respiratory disorders share some common ground, I believe that they are more conveniently and rationally treated as separate, even though closely collaborating, disciplines.

The complexity and speed of advances in knowledge in almost all aspects of the subject have resulted in a vastly increasing accumulation of publications – journals, monographs and textbooks – as well as in its further expansion into related auxillary sciences. Indeed, Max Planck's words as long ago as 1894, though referring to the world of physics, are amazingly relevant: 'The times are long gone when the general and the special can normally be cultivated in a single individual. Already today a gigantic intellect would be needed in that respect . . . and the miracle of such an intellect can only appear greater in the future'; or, in Pope's few words, 'So vast is Science, so narrow human wit'. With reflections such as these in mind and an awareness of my own limitations, I sought the collaboration of distinguished experts in the field to rewrite or revise 18 of the 25 chapters that now form the book. I am most grateful to them for the willingness and generosity of their responses for, without their contributions, the book would have foundered.

Although there are comprehensive texts that deal specifically with the basic principles of pulmonary morphology, cytology and immunology, these topics, formerly confined to one chapter, are now described in more detail in separate chapters. The reason for doing this is their relevance, in a variety of important ways, to the genesis and pathology of disease caused by occupational air-borne agents. The question of personal susceptibility – or resistance – to the development of such disease and the different factors that are likely to determine it are, therefore, given more emphasis than previously, notably in Chapters 1, 3, 4 and 15. The clinical differentiation of occupational and non-occupational pulmonary disease is also considered in more detail in Chapter 6, perhaps some may think, too much; nonetheless, I believe this to be worthwhile. Melville Arnott's remarks at the Inaugural Meeting of the Section of Occupational Medicine at the Royal Society of Medicine in 1964 are, in this respect, as apt today as then:

> 'One sees in occupational medicine an important and vital opportunity of bringing to bear upon problems of disease the resources of all the relevant divisions of medicine – and at one time or another they are all relevant . . . The physician, by tradition, has to make a total assessment of the patient.'

It is salutary for all who practise in this important, but relatively narrow, division of Medicine to recall these words from time to time.

I had considered deleting the chapter on 'Elements of geology and geochemistry' of the earlier editions (which, one reviewer of the second, thought 'may be somewhat unusual') as being, perhaps, too detailed in the setting of an essentially medical text and transferring part of its matter, where relevant, to other chapters. But, having noted that some uncertainty and confusion as to which minerals and their variants have pathogenic potential and which not, and in what occupational conditions they may or may not be found, are still to be seen in the medical literature; and that, at times, there is an unfortunate readiness to indict minerals that are in fact blameless as causal factors in disease with which they may happen to be associated, I have retained and rewritten this chapter as Appendix I. Similarly, Appendices IV and V, originally short sections in the Appendix of the previous editions, are also rewritten in greater detail.

In view of the substantial decline in the prevalence of silicosis and coal pneumoconiosis (both now uncommon) in the past 40 years and of a steady decrease in that of asbestosis and beryllium disease in more recent years, it may be argued that the chapters dealing with these disorders could now be shorter than previously. However, each, revised and mostly rewritten, is still described in some detail because all these diseases (those due to asbestos in particular) are still present in the community and new cases appear with variable frequency, often after occupational exposure has ceased. A consequence of their sporadic and sometimes unexpected occurrence is that clinicians may not always recognize the diagnosis in isolated cases. An awareness and a reasonably detailed knowledge of these disorders, therefore, should help to prevent this happening. In addition, accounts of their differing pathogenesis and pathology are a valuable foundation for understanding both aspects of a variety of other work-related pulmonary diseases. By contrast, occupational asthma and some types of extrinsic allergic alveolitis have become increasingly more important. All specific disorders, and groups of like disorders, are now considered in separate chapters which have been largely rewritten and brought up to date; other chapters are entirely new.

When the first edition was being prepared there was a need to re-emphasize the importance of taking a detailed occupational history in all patients with known or suspected pulmonary disease together with careful evaluation of the relevance of any possible hazard it reveals. Although, in principle, this is now taken for granted, there has of late been a growing tendency, when certain types of occupational exposure are identified, to accept these too readily and uncritically as the explanation of the patient's disease. The erroneous diagnosis that may ensue can prevent or delay necessary therapeutic measures. Whereas in the past an inadequate history often caused an occupational disease to be overlooked, sometimes for years, there is now a converse risk of such disease being wrongly diagnosed because of incorrect interpretation of the true significance of facts revealed by more detailed histories; or because a history, or its reprise, may at times be conducted in the hope of discovering exposure to some specific hazardous agent which will explain the patient's disease. Such mistaken procedures may, in part, be influenced by a widely current minimalist ('no threshold') interpretation of the significance of any potentially hazardous agent in the workplace together with an undue willingness to accept extrapolation of the results of unrealistic experiments on animals as validly applicable to human beings. The danger implicit in such thinking has been well-stated by Duncan (1986): 'There lies behind this whole attitude an assumption that if only we go on digging we shall eventually find some causal relation to satisfy our intellectual curiosity.' Plain common sense – or, as Chesterton preferred, uncommon sense – and an informed mind with a firm hold on the objective world and consequent alertness to a pervasive, contemporary, 'postmodernist' subjectivism, which holds that truth is something to be constructed and not something to be discovered (Charlton, 1993), are the best fortification against such intellectual pitfalls and their dangers. The process of critically evaluating relevancy in an occupational history is, in principle, really no different from that of a medical history which, of course, demands the same intellectual rigour. The words of Oderwald and Sebus (1991), incidentally, are worth considering in this context: 'Even proper history taking may, by adopting one guiding principle rather than another, follow a "wrong" path. It must be stressed that the chosen path must be followed to find out it is wrong.' The necessity of a well-disciplined approach to history-taking overall is, therefore, once again emphasized in this edition.

In order to identify and study substances in industry which might be responsible for pulmonary disease and to evaluate the effects of those known to cause disease a voluntary scheme for surveillance of work-related and occupational respiratory disease (SWORD) involving chest and occupational physicians was established in the UK by the British Thoracic Society, The Society of Occupational Medicine and the Health and Safety Executive in January 1989 (Meredith, Taylor and McDonald, 1991). The resulting 'database' of this and similar schemes will undoubtedly increase precision of knowledge and reduce harmful, sometimes wilful, speculations about causal or dose–response relationships of such substances.

Not surprisingly, multiple authorship reveals some differences of opinion between individual contributors (including myself) on certain topics. Such differences, though few, are important and, for the most part, I have left them to stand unaltered. For the reader should have the means to understand the reasoning behind opposing views on controversial topics and to weigh conjecture against acceptable demonstrable fact. To that end sufficient evidence and references are provided for their respective strengths and validity to be evaluated.

The previous editions were criticized by some reviewers for not giving more detailed consideration to the principles of industrial hygiene and the control and assessment of the occupational environment. This was intentional, because, although it is true that responsibility for prevention of disease lies with the occupational physician as well as with the hygienist and safety engineer, to describe such specialized, non-medical principles in sufficient detail to be of value to the novice would greatly increase the size of an already substantial volume. There are excellent comprehensive books, some of which are listed in Chapter 3, which are specifically concerned with principles, methods and standards of assessment and control of the work environment. Similarly, the topic of compensation is not addressed because the modes of definition and the laws of compensation differ widely from one country to another and even, in some instances, within the same country (for example, the USA), as do criteria for, and methods of, assessing respiratory disability for compensation purposes.

Every effort has been made to correct errors and inaccuracies of the second edition, and to forestall new ones in this – I hope, with success.

I am indebted to many experts for invaluable and unstinting advice and criticism during the preparation of the chapters of which I am sole author. They are listed in the Acknowledgements but I must make particular mention here of Professor Bryan Corrin, Dr Kevin Browne and Mr David Highley who, over a prolonged period, critically read numerous pages of typescript with great forbearance, and responded most generously to many questions.

Finally, it is a great pleasure to record, with gratitude, the encouragement and stimulation I have received over the years from Professor Lynne Reid since I contemplated the first edition of the book.

W. Raymond Parkes

References

Arnott, M. (1965) Inaugural Meeting, Section of Occupational Medicine Royal Society of Medicine, October, 1964. *Proc. R. Soc. Med.* **58**, 3–4

Charlton, B.G. (1993) Editorial: Medicine and post-modernity. *J. R. Soc. Med.* **85**, 497–499

Duncan, K.P. (1986) A professional duty to inform. *Br. J. Ind. Med.* **43**, 793–794

Meredith, S.K., Taylor, V.M. and McDonald, J.C. (1991) Occupational respiratory disease in the United Kingdom 1989: a report to the British Thoracic Society and the Society of Occupational Medicine by the SWORD project group. *Br. J. Ind. Med.* **48**, 292–298

Oderwald, A.K. and Sebus, J.H. (1991) The physician and Sherlock Holmes. *J. R. Soc. Med.* **84**, 151–152

Planck, M. (1894) Antrittsrede zur Aufnahme in die Akademie vom 28, Juni 1894. *Physikalische Abhandlungen* **3**, 4

Contributors

Peter M. Bretland MD MSc FRCR
Formerly: Consultant Radiologist, Whittington
Hospital, London, UK
Honorary Senior Lecturer, University College
Hospital, London, UK
Visiting Senior Lecturer, Chinese University of
Hong Kong

Kevin Browne MA MSc MB BS MFOM
Formerly: Department of Occupational Medicine,
Royal Brompton National Heart and Lung
Hospital, London, UK
Medical Adviser to Cape plc

David M. Denison PhD FRCP
Head of Medical Audit, Royal Brompton National
Heart and Lung Hospitals
Emeritus Professor of Clinical Physiology,
National Heart and Lung Institute, London,
UK

John Ernsting CB OBE PhD FFOM FRCP
Professor, Royal Air Force Consultant Adviser in
Aviation Medicine
Formerly Air Vice-Marshal and Commandant,
RAF Institute of Aviation Medicine, Farnborough,
UK

J. Malcolm Harrington CBE MSc MD FRCP FFOM
Professor and Director, Institute of Occupational
Health, University of Birmingham, UK

Patricia L. Haslam PhD MRCPath
Head of Cell Biology Group, Department of
Cardiothoracic Surgery, National Heart and Lung
Institute, London, UK

A.G. Heppleston DSc MD FRCP FRCPath
Emeritus Professor of Pathology, University of
Newcastle upon Tyne, Northumberland, UK

J.A.C. Hopkirk BA MB FRCP
Consultant Physician, King Edward VII Hospital,
Midhurst, UK

Robert N. Jones MD
Professor of Medicine, Section of Environmental
Medicine, Tulane University Medical Center, New
Orleans, USA

W. Jones Williams MD FRCP FRCPath
Emeritus Professor in Pathology, Department of
Medicine, University of Wales College of
Medicine, South Wales, UK

Leonard S. Levy MSc PhD FFOM(Hon)
Senior Lecturer in Industrial Toxicology, Institute
of Occupational Health, University of
Birmingham, Birmingham, UK

W.K.C. Morgan MD FRCP(Ed) FRCP(C) FACP
Professor of Medicine, University of Western
Ontario
Chief, Chest Diseases Unit, University Hospital,
London, Ontario, Canada

A.J. Newman Taylor OBE MSc(OccMed) FRCP FFOM
Professor and Director, National Heart and Lung
Institute, London, UK

W. Raymond Parkes OBE MD(L'pool) FRCP FFOM DIH
Formerly: Medical Boarding Centre (Respiratory
Diseases), Department of Health and Social
Security, London
Honorary Clinical Lecturer, Professorial Unit
(Thoracic Medicine), National Heart and Lung
Institute, London, UK

Ramsay R. Pearson MD
Formerly Head of Undersea Medicine, Institute of
Naval Medicine, Gosport, UK

C.A.C. Pickering FRCP FFOM DIH
Consultant Chest Physician, North West Lung
Centre, Wythenshawe Hospital, Manchester, UK

Katherine M. Venables MD MRCP
Senior Lecturer, Department of Occupational and
Environmental Medicine, National Heart and
Lung Institute, London, UK

H.A. Waldron PhD MD MRCP FFOM
Consultant Physician, Department of Occupational
Health, St Mary's Hospital, London, UK

Hans Weill MD
Professor of Medicine, Schlieder Foundation
Professor of Pulmonary Medicine, Tulane
University Medical Center, New Orleans, USA

Mark Woodhead BSc DM MRCP
Consultant Physician in General and Respiratory
Medicine, Manchester Royal Infirmary,
Manchester, UK

Acknowledgements

I am indebted to various experts, medical and non-medical, for their valuable criticism and advice while I was preparing my chapters.

Medical

Dr Kevin Browne; Dr D.J. Buchanan, Director of Research and Scientific Services, British Coal Corporation, Burton-on-Trent; Professor Bryan Corrin, National Heart and Lung Institute, London; Dr J.E. Earis, Fazakerley Hospital, Liverpool; Dr Morris Greenberg, London; Dr Keith Horsfield, King Edward VII Hospital, Midhurst; and Mr Terry Buckley, London Chest Hospital for preparing photomicrographs for Chapter 15.

Some contributors also wish to express their gratitude for assistance. Dr Patricia L. Haslam (Chapter 4): to Joanna Harwood for invaluable help with her typescript and to Dr David Hughes and Mr Phillip Townsend for help with the graphic figures. Dr K.M. Venables (Chapter 8): for helpful discussions with Dr Kevin Browne and Professors A.J. Newman Taylor and J.C. McDonald. Professors Hans Weill and Robert Jones (Chapters 12 and 16): to Drs Bruce Chase, Clark Cooper, Andrew Churg and Janet Hughes.

Non-medical

Mr John Addison, Chemistry and Mineralogy Group, Institute of Occupational Medicine, Edinburgh; Dr I.A.S. Edwards, Northern Carbon Research Laboratory, University of Newcastle upon Tyne; Mr D.E. Highley, MIGeol, British Geological Survey, Keyworth, Nottingham; Dr Alan A. Hodgson, FGS, Crowthorne, Berkshire; Mr G. Kowalczyk, Toxicology Unit, British Coal Corporation, Doncaster; Mr R.J. Merriman, British Geological Survey, Keyworth, Nottingham; Professor Harry Marsh, Northern Carbon Research Laboratory, University of Newcastle upon Tyne; Dr J.W. Patrick, Director, Carbon Research Group, Department of Chemical Engineering, Loughborough University of Technology; Drs Fraser Wigley and J. Williamson, Royal College of Science, Technology and Medicine, London; and Mr A.F.G. Woodley, Technical Strategy Unit, Technical Services and Research Executive, British Coal Corporation, Burton on Trent.

In my dual capacity of editor and co-author of this edition I am most grateful to Butterworth-Heinemann's staff for continued help and guidance. In particular: Sue Deeley during the greater part of the gestation of this edition; Cathie Staves for ever-present advice and support, particularly in the preparation of the illustrations; Deena Burgess, Editorial Manager; and Chris Jarvis, Production Manager. I am also thankful to Jane Sugarman for painstaking subeditorial work.

Lastly, my heart-felt thanks to my wife for her immense patience and tolerance throughout a third and unexpectedly prolonged and unwelcome period of domestic and social disruption, as well as for typing, yet again, all my manuscript material.

Glossary

Definitions of some terms used

alveolar lipoproteinosis this is predominantly lipidosis with comparatively little alteration in total protein. This term is, therefore, preferable to 'alveolar proteinosis'. According to Heppleston, when the disorder is caused by silica there is no chemical bonding of phospholipid and protein and the presence of lipid and protein in surfactant is artefactual. He emphasizes that 'lipo-proteinosis' should be hyphenated to make this clear (see Chapter 5). Elsewhere in the book the hyphen is omitted.

ceiling limit the concentration of agents (such as certain gases), which have an immediate or toxic effect, that should not be exceeded at any time

circadian rhythm the rhythm that varies at intervals in a day and by which some process increases or decreases at certain times – as exhibited by respiratory function which is minimal in the early hours of the day and maximal in the afternoon. Accordingly, a variation in peak expiratory flow greater than 15 per cent is deemed necessary to be taken as evidence of occupational asthma

coal pneumoconiosis this is the term used throughout the book for the structural changes caused by the composite dust, coal, and associated coal-mine dust. Some authorities, however, prefer to retain 'coal workers' pneumoconiosis' in the belief that this term is descriptively more accurate (see Chapter 13, page 349).

cumulative exposure the product of the concentration of air-borne particles (dust, fume) expressed in mg/ml^3 or of the number of fibres per millilitre or millions of particles per cubic foot (m.p.p.c.f.) in the workplace air and duration of exposure to the dust in months or years

dose-reponse relationship the proportion of individuals who develop a defined disorder in relation to the dose of the noxious agent believed to be responsible for the disorder

fibre/ml year unit of cumulative exposure to dusts – product of average level in fibres/ml to which subject is exposed × no. of years worked at this average level

Fourier transformation synthesis of a repetitive complex waveform from a series of sine or cosine terms of different wavelength and phase

half-life (radioactivity) ($T_{1/2}$) the time required for the number of active nuclei (or their activity) of a radioactive nuclide to decay to half its initial value

half-life (biological) ($t_{1/2}$) the time taken for the content in a biological system of a marked substance to fall to half its original value, assuming that the rate of removal is exponential

maximum allowable concentration (MAC) the level of maximum exposure to dust or fume which is not to be exceeded at any time. Equivalent to the maximum concentration over a working lifetime during which no disease or ill-health occurs

precessing this refers to the spinning motion of the magnetic axis of an atom or molecule, at an angle to its normal alignment in an external magnetic field, under the resonance conditions produced by an applied alternating magnetic field at right angles to it

refractory a material that has the capability of withstanding high temperatures without losing its chemical identity or becoming deformed in the conditions of use

short-term exposure limit the concentration of agents having a short-term cumulative effect (for example, sensitizing substances) averaged over a period of 10 minutes; it applies to any 10-minute period throughout a working shift (HSE)

threshold limit value (TLV) this standard, introduced by the American Conference of Governmental Industrial Hygienists, is defined as the concentration of a potentially hazardous air-borne aerosol to which workers can be exposed repeatedly without developing pulmonary disease. There are three categories that are applicable to the time required for the effects of disease to become apparent: *ceiling limit, short-term exposure limit* and *time-weighted average*

time-weighted average the concentration, which should not be exceeded during an 8-hour working day, of materials (such as coal-mine and asbestos dust) that can exert a cumulative effect over a prolonged period

Abbreviations

ACE	angiotensin-converting enzyme
AMDGF	alveolar macrophage-derived growth factor (now referred to as PDGF)
ANA	anti-nuclear antibodies
α_1–AT	α_1–antitrypsin
BAL	bronchoalveolar lavage
BALT	bronchus-associated lymphoid tissue
BEI	back-scattered electron imaging
CAE	centriacinar emphysema
CFA	cryptogenic fibrosing alveolitis; equivalent to IDIPF
CFRP	carbon fibre reinforced plastic
COPD	chronic obstructive pulmonary disease
CREST	initial letters of variant features of systemic sclerosis (calcinosis, Raynaud's phenomenon, oesophageal dysfunction, sclerodactyly and telangiectasia
CT	computed tomography
CTD	connective tissue disorder
DAE	distal acinar emphysema
DCS	decompression sickness
DHSS	Department of Health and Social Security (UK) – now known as the DSS
DIP	desquamative interstitial pneumonia
DIPF	diffuse interstitial pulmonary fibrosis
EAA	extrinsic allergic alveolitis
EDXA	energy-dispersive X-ray analysis
ELISA	enzyme-linked immunosorbent assay
ESR	erythrocyte sedimentation rate
FFD	focus–film distance
f/ml	fibres/ml
HLA	human leucocyte antigen
HRCT	high-resolution computed tomography
HSE	Health and Safety Executive (UK)
IARC	International Agency for Research on Cancer
IBD	inflammatory bowel disease
IDIPF	idiopathic diffuse interstitial pulmonary fibrosis; equivalent to CFA
Ig	immunoglobulin
IL	interleukin
ILO	International Labour Office
IRS	infrared spectrophotometry
LT	lymphocyte transformation
MAC	maximal allowable concentration
MFF	macrophage fibrogenic factor
MHC	major histocompatibility complex
MIF	(macrophage) migration inhibition factor
MMMF	man-made (synthetic) mineral fibre
m.p.p.c.f.	million particles per cubic foot
MRI	magnetic resonance imaging
NAA	neutron activation analysis
PAE	panacinar emphysema
PAF	platelet-activating factor
PAHs	polyaromatic hydrocarbons
PDGF	platelet-derived growth factor (previously referred to as AMDGF)
PG	prostaglandin
PMF	progressive massive fibrosis
PMR	proportional mortality ratio
PPD	purified protein derivative
p.p.m.	parts per million
RAST	radioallergosorbent test
RF	rheumatoid factor
RV	residual volume
SAED	selected area electron diffraction
SCUBA	self-contained underwater breathing apparatus

SEI	secondary electron imaging	TLC	total lung capacity
SEM	scanning electron microscopy	TLV	threshold limit value
SIMS	secondary ion mass spectrometry	TGF	tumour growth factor
SLE	systemic lupus erythematosus	TNF	tumour necrosis factor
SMR	standardized mortality ratio		
SS	systemic sclerosis	UDS	unit density spheres
		UIP	usual interstitial pneumonia
TEM	transmission electron microscopy	XRF	X-ray fluorescence

Some general physical units used and their equivalents

Quantity	Symbol	Unit	Abbreviation	Equivalent
acceleration				
linear	a	metre/second squared	m/s^2	3.281 $foot/s^2$
gravitational	**g**	gravitational constant	–	9.81 m/s^2
				32.2 $foot/s^2$
applied ratio	**G**	applied acceleration (**g**)	–	–
area	A	square metre	m^2	10.76 $foot^2$
		square centimetre	cm^2	$1.0 \times 10^{-4}\ m^2$
		square millimetre	mm^2	$1.0 \times 10^{-6}\ m^2$
density	ρ	kilogram per cubic metre	kg/m^3	
		gram per cubic centimetre	g/cm^3	$1.0 \times 10^{-3}\ kg/m^3$
directional subscripts with respect to body	x	anteroposterior		
	y	lateral		
	z	craniocaudal		
frequency	f	hertz (events per second for continuous periodic phenomena in general)	Hz	s^{-1}
length	l	centimetre	cm	$1.0 \times 10^{-2}\ m$
				0.954 inches
		millimetre	mm	$1.0 \times 10^{-3}\ m$
		micrometre	μm	$1.0 \times 10^{-6}\ m$
		nanometre	nm	$1.0 \times 10^{-9}\ m$
mass	m	kilogram	kg	2.205 lb
		gram	g	0.001 kg
		microgram	μg	$1.0 \times 10^{-6}\ g$
				$1.0 \times 10^{-9}\ kg$
pressure (physiology)	P	pascal	Pa	$kg/m/s^2$
		bar	bar	0.021 $lbf/foot^2$
				$1.0 \times 10^5\ Pa$
				14.504 lbf/in^2
		millibar	mbar	$1.0 \times 10^2\ Pa$
				$1.0 \times 10^3\ bar$
		millimetre of water	mmH_2O	9.807 Pa
		centimetre of water	cmH_2O	98.07 Pa

millimetre of mercury	mmHg (Torr)		133.322 Pa 0.019 lbf/in²
pound force per square inch	lbf/in² (psi)		6894.74 Pa 68.948 mbar 51.715 mmHg (Torr)
atmosphere (standard)	atm		101.325 kPa 1013.25 mbar 760 mmHg (Torr) 14.696 lbf/in² (psi)
time	t		
torr	–	≈1 mmHg	– ≈133 Pa

Measurements in respiratory physiology

Gas flow

FEF_{50}	forced expiratory flow at 50% of the FVC
$MEF_{25, 50, 75}$	maximum expiratory flow at 25, 50 and 75 per cent of forced vital capacity
MEFR	maximum expiratory flow rate
MMEF	maximum mid-expiratory flow at 50 per cent of forced vital capacity
MMFR	maximum mid-half flow rate
PEFR	peak expiratory flow rate

Gas exchange

$A–aPO_2$	alveolar–arterial difference of PO_2
$a–vPO_2$	arteriovenous difference of PO_2
D_L	diffusing capacity of lung
D_{LCO}	diffusing capacity of lung for carbon monoxide
K_{CO}	gas transfer coefficient for carbon monoxide (K = Krogh constant)
$\dot{Q}$	flow of blood in unit time
T_L	gas transfer factor for lung
T_{LCO}	gas transfer factor for carbon monoxide in lung

Pulmonary volumes

FEV_1	forced expiratory volume in 1 second
FRC	functional residual capacity
FVC	forced vital capacity
RV	residual volume
TLC	total lung capacity
TV	tidal volume
V_A	alveolar volume, single-breath dilution
VC	vital capacity

Pressures

P	pressure
$PaCO_2$	arterial partial carbon dioxide pressure (arterial carbon dioxide tension)
PaO_2	arterial partial oxygen pressure (arterial oxygen tension)
PAO_2	alveolar oxygen tension
PO_2	pressure (or tension) of oxygen
PV	pressure–volume relationship

Ventilation

MVV	maximum voluntary ventilation
$\dot{V}$	ventilation
$\dot{V}_A$	alveolar ventilation

1

Morphology of the respiratory tract

W. Raymond Parkes

The airways from the nares to the alveoli are separated into upper and lower respiratory tracts for convenience of anatomical description although they are structurally and functionally one.

> *Upper respiratory tract*
>   Naso- and oropharynx
> *Lower respiratory tract*
>   Tracheobronchial, gas-conducting airways
>   Gas-exchanging acini

Unfortunately, this convention has encouraged the physiology and pathology of the two regions to be considered largely in isolation. But, as might be expected, there is a close interrelationship between the two in health and disease, the importance of which is as relevant to the subject of this book as to pulmonary disease in general.

This chapter summarizes in brief the elements of morphology that influence or determine the fate of inhaled exogenous matter in the lungs, and their responses to it.

Upper respiratory tract

The upper respiratory tract extends from the external nares to the junction of the larynx and trachea. The two nasal passages are separated by the median septum, posterior to which they open into the nasopharynx. In the majority of individuals the septum is asymmetrical in greater or lesser degree, and deformity of the nasal bones posteriorly due to inequality of growth is common. These anomalies may contribute to nasal obstruction in one or both airways (Rhys Evans, 1987). The nasopharynx extends to the end of the soft palate, and the oropharynx from the palate to the larynx (Figure 1.1).

The nasal airways in adults vary in length from 10 to 14 cm and in width from 1 to 3 mm, although the cross-section is large. The width varies because patency of these airways normally alternates from one side to the other ('nasal cycle') at 2- to 4-hourly intervals (Proctor, 1986). Their lateral walls, into which the ostia of the paranasal sinuses open, are dominated by the convoluted turbinate bones. Pronounced deviation of the septum obstructs the airway on the side of the deviation, and consequential compensatory hypertrophy of the turbinates on the opposite side may result in obstruction of both airways and block the ostia of the sinuses, so fostering chronic infection.

During swallowing, communication between the nasopharynx and oropharynx is occluded by the soft palate, and the laryngeal aperture (glottis) is closed by backward and downward tilting of the epiglottis, thereby, under normal conditions, preventing aspiration of food or other materials into the lower respiratory tract.

The anterior one-third of the nasal airways is lined by squamous epithelium, and the posterior two-thirds and the upper part of the nasopharynx by ciliated, mucus-secreting, pseudostratified, columnar epithelium (similar to the lining of the airways of the lower respiratory tract) which propels deposited material towards the oropharynx (see 'The chief cells of the airways', later).

Nasopharyngeal tonsils on the roof of the nasopharynx (termed 'adenoids' when enlarged), palatine tonsils in the palatoglossal folds, tubal and lingual tonsils and smaller aggregates of lymphoid tissue encircling the wall of the pharynx (Waldeyer's ring) constitute part of the 'mucosa-associated

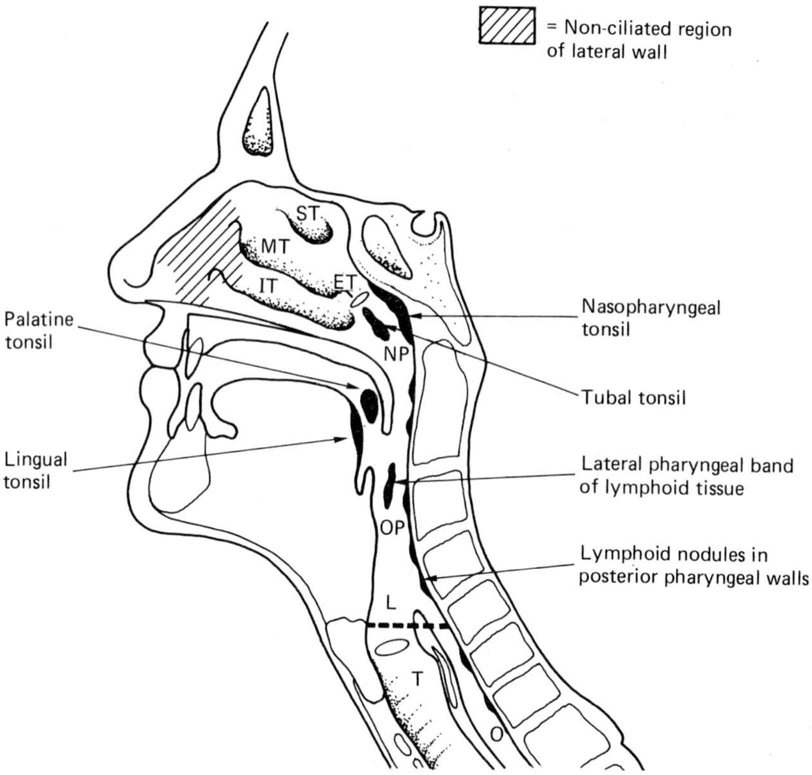

Figure 1.1 Simplified diagram of parasagittal section of the head showing relationships of the nasal cavity, nasopharynx (NP), oropharynx (OP), larynx (L) and distribution of lymphoid tissue (Waldeyer's ring). ST, MT and IT = superior, middle and inferior turbinates. ET = eustachian tube opening. Dotted line marks lower limit of the upper respiratory tract; below are the larynx (L), trachea (T) anteriorly and oesophagus (O) posteriorly

lymphoid tissue' (Beasley, 1987) (Figure 1.1). Unlike lymph nodes these structures are not encapsulated and have no afferent lymphatic vessels. Together with the bronchus-associated lymphoid tissue (BALT) (see page 11) they constitute an immunological defence of the respiratory tract. They enlarge in response to antigenic stimulation. Immunological factors involved are discussed in Chapter 4 (under 'Non-specific (innate) immune defences: Nasopharyngeal region').

Thus, anatomical anomalies and transient or chronic pathological states, such as chronic suppuration, in the nose or nasopharynx will affect the normal balance of oronasal breathing and, therefore, the efficiency of filtration, warming and humidifying of inhaled air which is essential for normal ciliary function and clearance of the airways of the lower respiratory tract. This may have an important bearing on the development of both occupational and non-occupational pulmonary disease.

Both acute and chronic irritation or inflammation in the upper respiratory tract may cause important functional changes in the nose and intrapulmonary airways via nasonasal and nasobronchial or laryngobronchial reflexes (see Chapters 3 and 6). The parasympathetic reflex arc in the nose consists of

afferent fibres from the mucosa in the maxillary branch of the trigeminal nerve passing to the medulla from which efferent fibres return via the sphenopalatine ganglion to the mucosa. Sympathetic efferent fibres course from the superior cervical ganglion to the mucosa. The lower respiratory tract connections are referred to later.

Lower respiratory tract

This extends from the laryngotracheal junction to the distal alveoli.

Tracheobronchial gas-conducting airways

These purely conductive airways – that is, airways without alveoli – arise by successive branching from

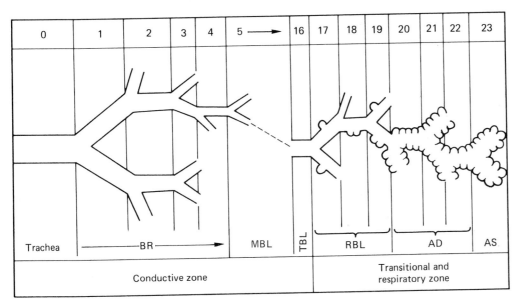

Figure 1.2 Conducting airways and respiratory unit (not to scale) as represented by Weibel's idealized system of generations branching from the trachea by symmetrical dichotomy. Numbers of generations are shown at the top. BR = bronchi, MBL = membranous bronchioles, TBL = terminal bronchiole, RBL = respiratory bronchioles, AD = alveolar ducts, AS = alveolar sacs. (Modified, with permission, from Weibel, 1963)

the parent trunk, the *trachea*. The main and lower lobe bronchi lie outside the lungs but all other bronchi are intrapulmonary. Two classes of these bronchi are distinguishable: *large bronchi*, in the walls of which cartilaginous plates are so abundant that any cross-section includes cartilage; and *small bronchi*, in which these plates are small or absent in some cross-sections and, distally, become progressively fewer with the result that the walls of the airways may be apposed in abnormal conditions. The airways distal to the last plate of cartilage are the *bronchioles* – membranous (non-respiratory) and respiratory. The *terminal bronchioles*, the last of the alveoli-free conducting airways, supply the pulmonary acini. The internal diameter of membranous bronchioles, proceeding distally from the first to the terminal bronchioles, ranges approximately from between 1.60 and 2.0 mm to 0.60 mm respectively (Olson, Dart and Filley, 1970; Horsfield, 1986), although the larger dimensions may include some distal small bronchi (Thurlbeck, 1976).

The division of lobar bronchi supplies 19 *bronchopulmonary* segments which are the smallest pulmonary units capable of being distinguished and dissected (Horsfield, 1974). Each segment is imperfectly subdivided into *lobules* which are incompletely outlined by fibrous septa. The pathways of conducting airways fall into two broad categories: *axial pathways* which run from the hilum to the distal alveoli adjacent to the pleural surface, and *lateral pathways* which arise at any point along the

length of the axial pathway. An axial pathway is the longest in the bronchopulmonary segment, although in some segments it is poorly developed, while in others there are two equally dominant branches. From the bronchi to the pleural region, therefore, there is considerable variation both in the length and in the number of branches of the pathways.

The anatomy of the airways is commonly represented as an idealized system of *generations*, beginning at the trachea as generation 0 and ending at the alveoli furthest from the hilum as generation 23 (Weibel, 1963) (Figure 1.2). This is a simplified dimensional model which expresses the airways in an average way as a bifurcating system in which each succeeding branch gives rise to two daughter airways of similar length and diameter (*symmetrical dichotomy*), and all pathways from the trachea to the periphery are identical. The concept can be applied equally to symmetrical and asymmetrical trees. However, although used extensively for physiological calculations and convenient for some clinical descriptions (for example, in bronchoscopy and bronchography), this model does not correspond to the anatomical facts just described and which are evident on bronchography. In reality, therefore, the branching of airways, though mostly dichotomous, is strongly *asymmetrical* in regard to angle, diameter and length of daughter branches, and to the different levels at which smaller, or 'lateral', branches join larger branches of the tree (Figure 1.3). Proceeding from the trachea to respiratory bronchioles, a lateral pathway can be as short as eight generations while

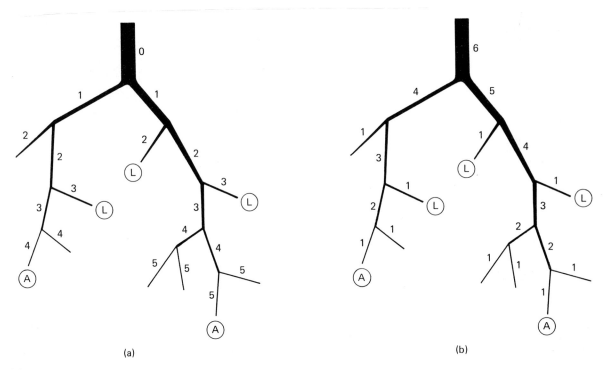

(a)   (b)

Figure 1.3 Methods of counting airways' branches. The diagram illustrates asymmetrical dichotomy. (a) Counting *generations* downwards by Weibel's method; (b) counting *orders* upwards by Horsfield's method. A = axial pathway, L = lateral pathways

an axial pathway includes every generation – a difference of 8 to 22 cm (Horsfield and Cumming, 1968).

It is clear, then, that a symmetrical model in which unlike branches are similarly classified or numbered does not describe these conditions; for example, generation 11 includes alveolar ducts, respiratory and terminal bronchioles, and bronchi up to 3 mm in diameter (Horsfield, 1974). Thus, it is more informative, anatomically, to count 'up' the tree by *orders* from the periphery, the most peripheral branches being order 1 and the trachea being the highest order. In this system, two order 1 branches meet to form an order 2 branch (also regarded as the parent branch) and so on to the trachea. When two daughter branches of different order join together the parent branch is one order higher than the greater of the two daughters. The larger the difference between the orders of the two daughter branches, the greater is the degree of asymmetry (Horsfield, 1986) (Figure 1.3). Varying branching angles (which are increased at the periphery) and differences in dimensions of daughter airways are functionally important in that they affect the patterns and degree of turbulence of airflow at bifurcations in the form of secondary rotations of the stream, and the partition of inspiratory flow between two daughter branches (see Chapter 3).

The advantage of Horsfield's order model of the conducting airways is that it corresponds closely to their anatomy and enables the varying asymmetry of branching patterns and pathway dimensions (see next section) to be understood and related to airflow behaviour and deposition of inhaled particles. It also allows better comparison to be made between asymmetrical trees and equivalent branches of those trees (Horsfield et al., 1987).

Gas-exchanging acini

Terminal bronchioles, as stated earlier, supply the acini. The *acinus* is defined as a complex of alveolated airways distal to the terminal bronchioles beginning with the first *respiratory bronchiole* (sometimes known as the *transitional bronchiole*). Acini vary in size and shape but are usually 0.5 to 1.0 cm in diameter, and, in general, there are three to five acini in each lobule. Each terminal bronchiole, as a rule, gives rise to three generations of respiratory bronchioles which, proceeding distally, have an increasing number of shallow alveoli partly covering their walls. After the last respiratory bronchiole there are a variable number of *alveolar ducts* which are completely surrounded by alveoli and end in *alveolar sacs* and *alveoli* (Figure 1.4).

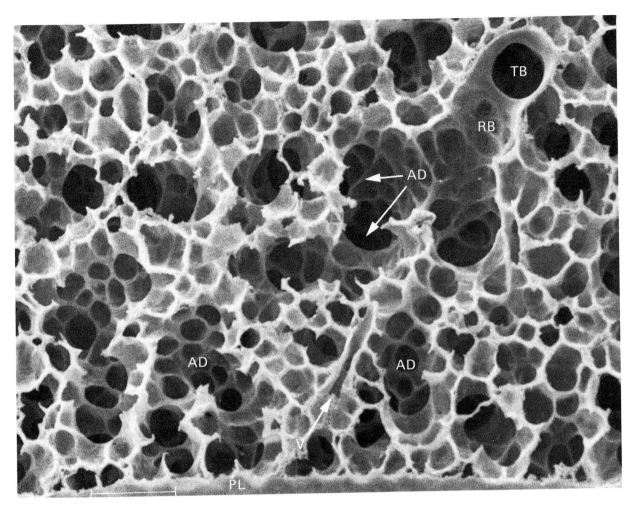

Figure 1.4 This shows detail of acinar airways. The wall of the alveolar ducts (AD) is formed by a network of coarse bundles of fibres around the alveolar mouths which represent the acinar extension of the axial fibre system from terminal (TB) and respiratory (RB) bronchioles. The peripheral system of fibres is represented by pleura (PL) and a small septum with a branch of the pulmonary vein (arrow). Perfusion-fixed rabbit's lung. Scale 200 μm. (Reproduced with permission from Weibel, 1985)

The intracinar airways branch by irregular dichotomy (exceptionally by trichotomy) for an average of nine generations (range 6 to 12) and their mean path lengths (from the first respiratory bronchioles to the alveolar sacs) differ as much as 5 to 12 mm according to the generation at which they end, with a mean of 8.25 mm for all acini (Haefeli-Bleuer and Weibel, 1988); their branching angles are greater than those of the conducting airways (Horsfield, 1986). The length of the longitudinal pathways is physiologically important because gas-exchanging units, the alveoli, are arranged serially along their paths. Considering these branches as generations, their internal diameters fall from approximately 0.50 mm to 0.27 mm between generations 0 (first respiratory bronchioles) and 10, although the outer diameters (including the sleeve

of alveoli) remain constant at about 0.70 mm. The difference between the inner and outer diameters, therefore, indicates the mean depth of the alveolar sleeve, which increases towards the periphery where the size of alveoli increases and clusters are more numerous (Haefeli-Bleuer and Weibel, 1988) (Table 1.1).

Between terminal and respiratory bronchioles and neighbouring alveoli there are small accessory communications up to 30 μm in diameter (Lambert's canals) in which dust particles and dust-containing macrophages may be found (Lambert, 1955). In addition, there are similar intersegmental communications, 80 to 150 μm in diameter, also bearing alveoli, between some adjacent respiratory bronchioles, and most numerous in the lower lobes (Figure 1.5) (Andersen and Jespersen, 1980). These

Table 1.1 Dimensions of intra-acinar airway segments

Generation	Length (mm) Mean	Inner diameter (mm) Mean	Outer diameter (mm) Mean
0	–	0.50	0.74
1	1.33	0.50	0.69
2	1.12	0.49	0.69
3	0.93	0.40	0.70
4	0.83	0.38	0.71
5	0.67	0.36	0.68
6	0.69	0.34	0.69
7	0.72	0.31	0.71
8	0.69	0.30	0.72
9	0.67	0.29	0.68
10	0.64	0.27	0.63
11	0.78	0.33	0.76
12	–	–	–
Mean	0.73	0.32	0.70

Generation 0 = first respiratory (transitional) bronchiole.
Average longitudinal path-lengths of all acini = 8.25 ± 1.41 mm.
Adapted, with permission, from Haefeli-Bleuer and Weibel (1988).

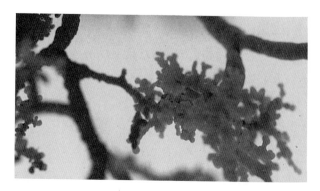

Figure 1.5 Intersegmental communication, 100 μm in diameter, between two adjacent respiratory bronchioles from a lower lobe. Note that it bears alveoli. Resin cast of human lung. (Courtesy of Dr J.B. Andersen)

channels provide the major route through which collateral ventilation can occur and may also affect the distribution of inhaled particles within the acini (see Chapter 3). Occasional openings (pores of Kohn) between alveoli in the same and contiguous acini are also thought to facilitate collateral ventilation but, if they do, this will be minimal because, at physiological transpulmonary pressures, the pores are very small (no more than 2.2 μm), and most are closed by surfactant (Delaunois, 1989). Collateral ventilation is probably negligible in normal human lungs but is increased when airways are obstructed by disease, such as obliterative bronchiolitis, or by increased resistance in proximal airways in emphysema with consequent reduction in collateral resistance (Delaunois, 1989). But such ventilatory shunting is impeded if these communicating channels – in particular, the intersegmental respiratory bronchioles – are closed by fibrosis (Berzon et al., 1986).

The fibrous skeleton of the lungs

Weibel and Gil (1977) described the form and extent of the connective tissue system of closely associated collagen and elastin fibres that forms the framework of the lungs, and which is held under tension by the negative intrapleural pressure normally exerted on the pulmonary pleura (see Chapter 5, 'Connective tissue frame-

work'). It comprises three anatomically distinct, though continuous, systems as a 'fibrous continuum'.

1. *The peripheral connective tissue system* envelops the lung as a continuous layer beneath the pulmonary pleura, with extensions into the interlobar and interlobular fissures and septa. These are associated with branches of pulmonary veins and lymphatic vessels. The innermost extension blends with the connective tissue elements of the alveolar walls, and has a strong elastic component.
2. *The axial connective tissue system* originates at the hilum and radiates into the pulmonary parenchyma around and along the airways to the centre of the acini, where it forms a fibrous lattice in the walls of alveolar ducts and suspends the alveoli in a three-dimensional network of fibres.
3. *The parenchymatous connective tissue system* consists of the fine fibres in the alveolar walls. It connects the peripheral and the axial systems, and, thereby, tethers the hilum to the pleura (see Figure 1.4).

The continuity of these interconnected systems is essential to the integrity of the lungs. During inspiration the peripheral system is drawn outwards and away from the axial system, thereby widening the intervening space and stretching the parenchymatous system (see Chapter 2, 'The bronchoalveolar system'). Various types of disease disrupt this integrity and the normal anisotropic tension within the continuum. For example, in diffuse interstitial pulmonary fibrosis there is an irregular or patchy excess (or condensation) of connective tissue; in emphysema, there is patchy destruction with the result that residual fibres can no longer be held under tension and so retract, forming airspaces of increased size (see Chapter 9).

Variability of airways' morphology and geometry

The adult trachea averages 10 to 12 cm in length and 1.6 to 1.8 cm in diameter, although there is considerable individual variation with age, sex and race (Weibel, 1963; Horsfield and Cumming, 1968); its diameter in females is approximately three-quarters of that in males (Pritchard, Jeffries and Black, 1988).

Asymmetrical patterns of branching differ in individual subjects. Genetic factors are known to influence the branching patterns of larger branches of the pulmonary arteries (Hislop and Reid, 1973) and it is likely that airways are similarly affected because they tend to branch in unison with the arteries. Horsfield (1980) has suggested that, although branching patterns and ratios are determined before birth, diameter and length ratios may adapt after birth to give maximal functional efficiency. In fact, there is evidence that all orders, or generations, of airways apparently grow in length and diameter in proportion to body height although the larger airways grow proportionally more rapidly than the smaller (Phalen et al., 1988), and differences in growth rates between males and females probably cause differences in the calibre of their airways (Pritchard, Jeffries and Black, 1988). Morphometric measurement of casts of the upper airways (generations 1 to 8) has demonstrated substantial variability in the lengths, diameters and branching angles within the same generations in the lungs of different adult males down to generations 7 and 8. Such intersubject differences – which can be large and, as mentioned earlier, affect patterns of airflow – increase with increasing generation number especially in the angles of branching, and are likely to cause significant diversity in the deposition of inhaled particles (Nikiforov and Schlesinger, 1985).

The total number of alveoli in the lungs is positively correlated with body height but the relationship is fairly weak because, although some 85 per cent of alveoli are formed after birth to produce the adult number of about 300×10^6, the process appears to be complete at about 18 months – certainly within 5 years, long before bodily growth ceases (Zeltner and Burri, 1987). Thereafter, pulmonary volume increases by alveolar expansion. The lungs of boys contain more alveoli (and probably more respiratory bronchioles) and are larger than those of girls of similar height. There is also a wide scatter in the total number of alveoli in the growing lung which is in keeping with the observation that the total number of alveoli is very variable

in adults (Thurlbeck, 1982). Thus, the total number of alveoli, which is genetically controlled, can be related only partially to height (Angus and Thurlbeck, 1972). Furthermore, there is substantial variability in the average diameters of airspaces in normal individuals with similar heights and lung volumes (Matsuba and Thurlbeck, 1971; Lapp et al., 1975); alveolar size also shows gradients in both vertical and horizontal directions in the lung (Forrest, 1980).

There is suggestive evidence that retarded bodily growth (underweight) in infancy may be associated with impaired growth of the lungs at this critical period of life (Barker, 1991).

Growth of the lungs may be impaired by the sequelae of severe infections – especially adenoviral – of the lower respiratory tract in infancy or childhood (see Chapter 9).

Thus, the morphology of the tracheobronchial tree is, in part, determined genetically and, in part, acquired. All the various ensuing differences in pulmonary structure between individuals who are, nonetheless, physiologically normal have an important effect on the mode and amount of deposition of aerosols – particles, mists and vapours (see Chapter 3). Together with other factors, discussed in Chapter 15, they influence to what degree an individual is susceptible or resistant to developing disease.

The chief cells of the airways

The surface of the airways is lined throughout by an uninterrupted sheet of epithelial cells. In the trachea and bronchi this consists of *ciliated, pseudostratified, columnar cells* interspersed by *mucus-secreting ('goblet') cells* and *basal stem cells* on a basement membrane (Figure 1.6). Below the basement membrane, in the submucosa, are the mucous glands whose ducts are continuous with the surface epithelium; they are present from the larynx to the last of the small bronchi but are not found in the bronchioles. The mucus-secreting cells of the mucous glands greatly outnumber the goblet cells, and goblet cells are sparse in normal membranous bronchioles. Hypersecretion of mucus by the glands characterizes chronic bronchitis (see Chapter 9).

In the membranous bronchioles, surface epithelial cells assume cuboidal form but are still ciliated down to, and including, the junctions of terminal and first respiratory bronchioles where they cease.

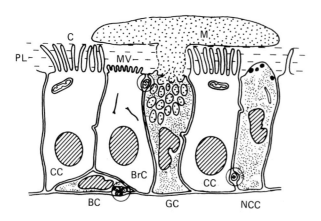

Figure 1.6 Diagrammatic representation of surface epithelium of gas-conducting airways showing basal (BC), mucous or goblet (GC), ciliated (CC), non-ciliated (NCC), brush (BrC) cells and nerve cells with irritant receptors (enclosed by circles). Mucus-secreting cells are sparse in membranous bronchioles less than 1 mm in diameter. Cilia are believed to beat in a low viscosity, or *periciliary*, layer (PL) of surfactant with the secreted mucus being moved only by their tips. M = mucus; C = cilia; MV = microvilli. (Redrawn from his original diagram by kind permission of Dr P.K. Jeffery)

They are interspersed with *Clara* (non-ciliated bronchiolar) *cells* which possess stem cell multipotentiality and probably secrete a neutrophil elastase inhibitor, antileukoprotease (see Figure 14.9 and Chapter 9). Goblet cells become progressively fewer and Clara cells progressively more numerous down to the respiratory bronchioles, but in inflammatory conditions the latter are transformed into goblet cells (Evans, Cabral-Anderson and Freeman, 1978). Those parts of the walls of the respiratory bronchioles in which there are no alveoli are lined by non-ciliated cuboidal cells but goblet cells and Clara cells are absent.

Thus, ciliated epithelium lines the nasal passage and sinuses and the airways of the lower respiratory tract. The epithelial cells form and maintain a thin layer of mucus which traps inhaled particulate matter, absorbs chemicals and is continuously moved backwards from the nasopharynx and upwards from the peripheral airways to the trachea by ciliary action (the so-called *mucociliary escalator*). Transportation of these materials by this means is dependent upon the functional integrity and efficiency of the 'escalator'.

The cilia beat continuously in co-ordinated manner in a two-layered fluid system which consists of a watery, low-viscosity, sol phase extending from the cell surfaces to the tips of the cilia when fully extended, and an overlying layer of mucus which they propel towards the oropharynx whence it is swallowed (Figure 1.6). High viscosity and elastic properties are conferred on the mucus by its chief structural component, glycoproteins. For normal efficient transport of mucus the cilia must beat sequentially in co-ordination (Wilson and Cole, 1988). Because the surface area of the small peripheral airways is vastly greater than that of the trachea – about 79 cm² at the level of the terminal bronchioles and 2.0 cm² at the trachea (Horsfield, 1974) – it follows that mucus must be cleared at increasing speed in the larger airways and trachea to prevent the lung being overwhelmed and drowned in accumulated mucus. It has been estimated that the approximate velocities of clearance in the small bronchi and trachea are 0.06 cm/min and 1.4 cm/min respectively (Morrow, Gibb and Gazioglu, 1967).

Thus, it is evident that malfunction of any of the component parts of the mucociliary escalator causes a greater or lesser degree of impaired clearance of mucus and transportation of entrapped particulate matter. Ciliary dysfunction (dyskinesia) in which beating of the cilia is absent or slowed, disorganized and inco-ordinated is an important factor. *Primary ciliary dyskinesia* is a rare genetic disorder but *secondary dyskinesia* appears to be fairly common. It may be caused by the effects of bacterial and viral infections and smoking; by alteration in the rheological properties of the mucus such as may occur with changes in humidity and temperature in the airways, and with hypersecretion of mucus; and, possibly, by changes in the depth and viscosity of the periciliary fluid (Wilson and Cole, 1988).

But clearance rates differ among normal individuals and are, to a large degree, genetically determined (Camner, Philipson and Friberg, 1972; Bohning et al., 1975; Brownstein, 1987), a fact which undoubtedly affects individual vulnerability or resistance to disease caused by inhaled particles (see Chapter 3).

Macrophages, lymphocytes and plasma cells are found in the submucosa and the peribronchial and peribronchiolar connective tissue sheaths.

The alveolar region

Epithelial cells line the alveolar walls, or septa, and between these cells and the walls of the capillaries and the pleura is the *interstitium* – supportive connective tissue framework (see page 6).

The alveolar epithelium

This consists of type I and type II cells or pneumocytes (Figure 1.7).

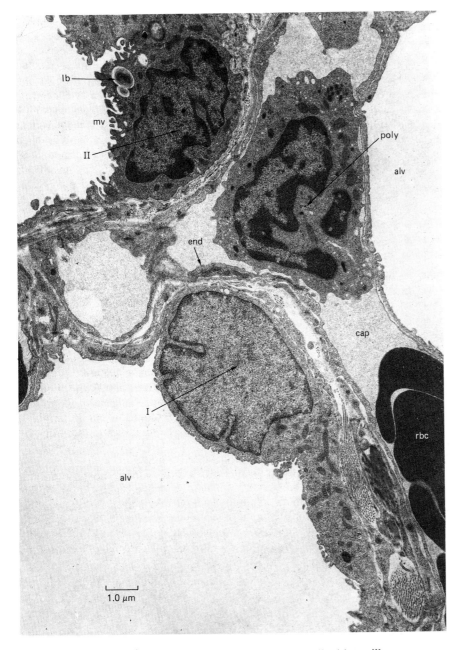

Figure 1.7 Electron micrograph of part of an alveolar wall with capillary demonstrating: type I cell with cytoplasmic extensions (EPI); type II cell (EPII) with microvilli (mv) and lamellar bodies (lb); endothelial cell (end) lining the capillary (cap) which contains red blood cells (rbc) and a granulocyte (poly). Part of a cytoplasmic extension of a fibroblast (fi) and fibres of collagen (co) and elastin (el) are seen in the interstitium (int). (Courtesy of Professor Lynne Reid)

Type I pneumocytes

Each cell extends from its nuclear region to cover a large area of alveolar wall with attenuated cytoplasm which contains few organelles. This cytoplasmic plate is seldom more than 2 µm thick and is invisible by light microscopy. In places the cell membrane is invaginated to form pinocytic vesicles capable of ingesting macromolecules and minute particles which may be present in alveolar spaces, affording their transfer (Figure 1.8) to the interstitium (Corrin, 1970). Translocation of asbestos fibrils and small particles of quartz can occur in this way (Brody et al., 1981, 1982) (see Chapter 3). These cells, which are highly vulnerable to damage by noxious agents, form tight junctions

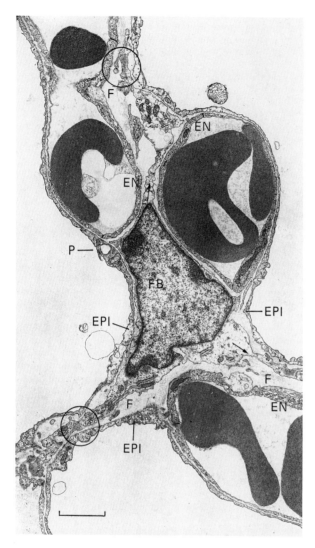

Figure 1.8 Septal fibroblast (FB) ramifies with slim extensions (arrows) into interstitial spaces between capillary endothelium (EN) and alveolar epithelium (EPI), following the fibre strands (F). Circles: cytoplasmic areas with condensed filaments spanning the interstitial space cross-wise. The close proximity of alveolar epithelium and capillary endothelium is clearly shown. Pinocytic vesicles (PV) can be seen in the cytoplasm of the type I cell to the left (EPI). Bar = 2 μm. (Reproduced, with permission, from Weibel, 1985)

('terminal bars') with each other and with type II cells. In places, however, gaps in the basal lamina between cells form alveolar pores through which macrophages may pass (Takaro, Gaddy and Parra, 1982).

Type II (secretory) pneumocytes

These are cuboidal and compact and more numerous than type I cells. Their free surface is covered by short microvilli and their cytoplasm richly endowed with a variety of organelles – in particular, osmophilic lamellar bodies which secrete surfactant phospholipids and complement proteins (Kikkawa et al., 1975; Strunk, Eidlen and Mason, 1988). They are the stem cells from which type I cells differentiate and are replaced after injury. If injury is prolonged, type II cells multiply but do not differentiate, thereby completely lining the alveolar wall with cuboidal epithelium which is visible by light microscopy. They do not appear to possess phagocytic properties.

Surfactant (see also page 53)

This is a highly stable surface-active agent which covers as a film the cells of the alveoli, alveolar sacs and ducts, and respiratory and terminal bronchioles. Its surface tension rises when it is stretched but falls almost to zero when compressed, a remarkable property which prevents the lungs collapsing when their transpulmonary pressure is reduced (as in expiration) and enables alveoli of different sizes to remain patent at the same transpulmonary pressure. Its chief component is the phospholipid dipalmitoyl phosphatidylcholine, together with three groups of associated proteins (Possmayer, 1988). Recent evidence indicates that it plays an important immunoregulatory role in normal lungs (Wilsher, Hughes and Haslam, 1988) and may influence their reaction to inhaled mineral particles (see Chapter 4, 'Non-specific (innate) immune defences: Respiratory bronchioles and alveoli' and Chapter 5, 'Lipidosis'). Spent surfactant appears to be disposed of by alveolar macrophages and in the sputum via the mucociliary escalator.

Blood vessels

Arteries and veins

Pulmonary arteries accompany and branch with the airways in their successive divisions down to the acinus and also send other shoots into the lungs. The arterial branch that enters the acinus accompanies the respiratory bronchiole and is, therefore, usually seen at its centre (Figure 1.9). From this branch a network of capillaries is formed in the alveolar walls which then conjoin to connect with the *pulmonary veins* at the periphery of the acinus. The fibrous framework of the lung supports the blood vessels. Pulmonary arteries are accompanied by the axial fibre system from the hilum to the centre of the

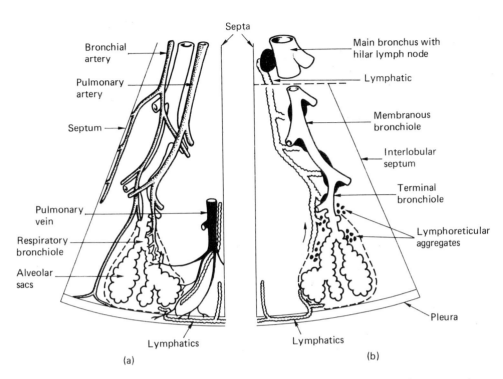

Figure 1.9 Simplified diagram of a lobule showing the relationships of membranous and respiratory bronchioles and alveolar sacs to blood vessels (A) and to lymphatics and lymphoid tissue (B). Note that veins, unlike arteries, run separately from the airways. (Acini are enclosed by dotted lines)

acinus; and the veins are associated with the peripheral fibre system between units of airway running first along interlobular septa and then accompanying the axial system around the airways to the hilum. The network of capillaries is intimately interwoven by fine strands of the septal fibre system (Weibel, 1979).

Bronchial arteries supply the walls of the airways and pulmonary vessels, lymph nodes, interlobular septa and the pulmonary pleura (Figure 1.9). They are systemic vessels and take no part in gas exchange. The bronchial circulation has been thoroughly reviewed by Deffebach et al. (1987). It is of interest that bronchial arteries supply tuberculous and other granulomatous lesions, and pneumoconiotic masses.

Lymphoid tissue

The lymphatic system in the lungs consists of lymph nodes, bronchus-associated lymphoid tissue, lymphoreticular aggregates and lymphatic vessels (Figure 1.9).

Lymph nodes

Typical encapsulated nodes occur at the hila, in connective tissue around bronchi for three or four generations and, infrequently, more peripherally in the lung and pulmonary pleura (Trapnell, 1964).

Bronchus-associated lymphoid tissue (BALT)

This was described by Bienenstock, Johnston and Perey (1973a,b) although its existence had been known for over a century yet strangely ignored (Burdon-Sanderson, 1870; Klein, 1875). It consists of follicular lymphoid nodules in the bronchi and the bronchioles, especially at their bifurcations where inhaled antigens may impact in greatest concentration; it is analogous to the lymphoid system of the naso- and hypopharynx (see Figure 1.1). Like Peyer's patches of the intestine ('gut-associated lymphoid tissue'), some of these nodules are present at birth but most appear later under the stimulus of antigenic activity and, thus, increase in size and number with age (Bienenstock and Beyfus,

1984) (see Chapter 4, 'Non-specific (innate) immune defences: Tracheobronchial region').

Lymphoreticular aggregates

These are small collections of lymphocytes and occasional plasma and eosinophil cells in a delicate net of connective tissue. They are scattered widely in the lungs near the bronchi, in interlobular septa and in the pulmonary pleura but are found especially between terminal and respiratory bronchioles and accompanying arterioles where the lymphatic vessels commence (Figure 1.9). Absent at birth, they are engendered by subsequent environmental and antigenic stimuli, and are present almost universally at 5 years of age (Emery and Dinsdale, 1973). Macklin (1955) regarded these aggregates as 'diminutive tonsils' in which dust and bacteria accumulate in large quantity. He considered them to be 'disastrous' rather than helpful in the defence of the lungs against these agents – surely an unfortunate misapprehension.

Altogether the lymph nodes, lymphoid tissue in the upper and lower respiratory tracts and intestine, and lymphoreticular aggregates form a common immune system.

Lymphatic vessels

These vessels, equipped with valves, arise as capillaries from lymphoreticular aggregates in the vicinity of respiratory and other bronchioles, and in proximity to BALT nodules, but not from alveolar walls. They are found in interlobular, pleural, peribronchial and perivascular connective tissue (Figure 1.9). Lymph flows into them from the alveolar interstitium driven by subatmospheric pressure during respiration. The direction of flow in these vessels at the periphery is outwards to the pulmonary pleura and, more proximally, inwards to the hilum. But both pleural and pulmonary vessels drain into the hilar, tracheal and mediastinal lymph nodes and thence into the systemic circulation via the thoracic duct and the great veins of the neck.

The importance of this organized and widely distributed lymphatic system to the defence of the lungs against 'all comers' is evident. It generates local mucosal immunity and systemic immune responses, which are discussed in Chapter 4; the lymphatic vessels are an ancillary route for clearance of foreign material from the alveolar region to the lymph nodes (see Chapter 3).

Nerve supply

The larynx is supplied by the vagus nerve and the lungs, by the vagus and by sympathetic nerves via the pulmonary plexus. Afferents form the nose (trigeminal nerve) and larynx from reflex arcs through the brain stem with efferent vagal parasympathetic and sympathetic fibres which supply the smooth muscle of the intrapulmonary airways down to the bronchioles. There are three types of sensory receptors in the lungs: slowly and rapidly adapting stretch receptors in the airways, and C fibre endings in the airways and the parenchyma.

Free pulmonary cells

These can be grouped into two important overlapping categories: cells of the interstitium and cells of the defence system (Weibel, 1985).

The cells of the interstitium

The alveolar interstitium is formed by the epithelial and endothelial basement membranes and the intervening connective tissues. In many places it is extremely thin, so the two membranes lie in such close proximity as to be virtually fused, thus facilitating rapid gas exchange between alveolar air and capillary blood (see Figures 1.7 and 1.8); like type I epithelial cells, capillary endothelial cells contain pinocytic vesicles. The interstitium contains a matrix of collagen, reticulin and elastic fibres and fibronectin supported in a milieu of ground substance (see Chapter 5, 'Connective tissue framework'), and also fibroblasts, myofibroblasts, and macrophages and their monocytic precursors, some lymphocytes and plasma cells, unmyelinated nerve axons and nerve endings, and interstitial fluid. It is continuous with the most bulky peribronchiolar connective tissue towards the centre of the acinus and that of the interlobular septa and pleura.

Fibroblasts

These cells, which make up the majority of interstitial cells, are present wherever there are connective tissue fibres. They elaborate collagen and elastin for the synthesis and maintenance of the fibres (see Chapter 5 for detailed discussion). Their cytoplasm

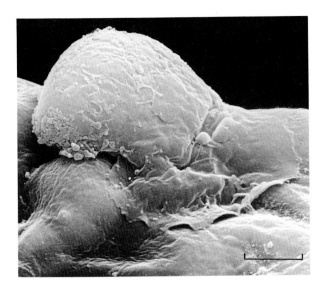

Figure 1.10 Scanning electron micrograph of human alveolar macrophage on alveolar epithelial surface. Thin advancing cytoplasmic lamella appears partly attached to epithelium. Bar = 5 μm. (From Weibel, 1963)

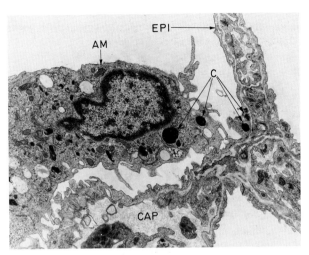

Figure 1.12 Alveolar macrophage containing inhaled carbon particles which are also present in the cytoplasm of a type I cell en route to the interstitium. AM, alveolar macrophage; EPI, type I pneumocyte; C, carbon particles; CAP, capillary. (EM magnification ×14 000.) (Reproduced from Bowden (1976) by courtesy of Dr D.H. Bowden and the Editor of *Environmental Health Perspectives*)

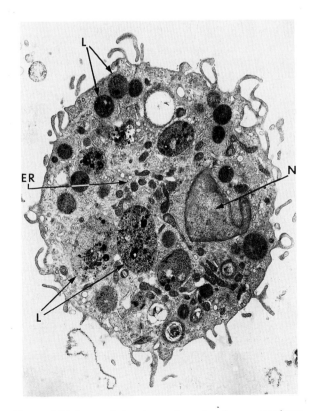

Figure 1.11 Internal structure of an alveolar macrophage from lung lavage fluid. Arrows indicate lysosomes (L), phagolysosomes (PL) and endoplasmic reticulum (ER) in the cytoplasm, and the nucleus (N). EM magnification ×6800. (Courtesy of Ann Dewar)

forms tenuous extensions along the fibres, and contains mitochondria, large Golgi complexes and prominent, rough (that is, ribosome-studded) endoplasmic reticulum (see Figure 1.8). Some cells also contain myofilaments and possess contractile properties (Kapanci et al., 1974). These so-called *myofibroblasts* are cytologically distinct from, but in some circumstances may differentiate into, smooth muscle cells (Judd, Finnegan and Curran, 1974; Weibel, 1985). Their function is uncertain but abnormal development of bundles of smooth muscle cells is a feature of some forms of diffuse intrapulmonary fibrosis (see Chapter 15).

Macrophages

Macrophages are present throughout the lungs and perform a crucial function in defence against the incursion of particulate matter and pathogens in inspired air. Apart from being actively phagocytic and migratory, they are secretory and immunoregulatory cells which produce a bewildering array of enzymes and mediators, and, among other activities, dissolve metallic particles generally regarded as insoluble (see Chapter 3) and control fibrogenesis and fibrinolysis (see Chapter 5). They are haemopoietic in origin, being recruited into the interstitium as monocytes which differentiate into interstitial and alveolar macrophages (Adamson and Bowden, 1980; Bowden and Adamson, 1980).

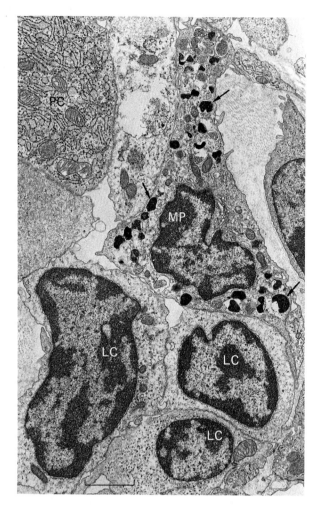

Figure 1.13 Interstitial macrophage (MP) from human lung containing heterogeneous dark material in phagolysosomes or residual bodies (arrows) is closely associated with free lymphocytes (LC) and a plasma cell (PC). Bar = 2 μm. (Reproduced, with permission, from Weibel, 1985)

Normal alveolar macrophages have a ruffled surface with prominent pseudopodal extensions and a few filopodia (Figure 1.10). Although there is considerable difference in the size of normal cells the majority (about 70 per cent) range from 14 to 19 μm in diameter with extremes of 9 to 40 μm in a minority (Fels and Cohn, 1986). Danel et al. (1983) found that the mean maximum diameter of alveolar macrophages harvested by bronchoalveolar lavage (BAL) from normal individuals, non-smokers and smokers alike, was 15 μm. There are many enzyme-rich lysosomes and phagosomal vacuoles in their cytoplasm which contain extracellular solutes and particles (Figures 1.11, 1.12 and see Figure 4.2). Wallace, Gillooly and Lamb (1992) have shown that

smokers have more alveolar macrophages than non-smokers when the number of cells is expressed quantitatively with respect to the underlying architecture of the lungs in terms of unit volume and unit surface area, although the relative increase is less than BAL studies have indicated.

Pulmonary macrophages fall into two main categories according to their location.

1. On the walls of the alveoli and alveolar ducts as *alveolar macrophages* loosely attached within the lining film to the epithelial surface (Figure 1.10). These cells, which often contain exogenous particles, tend to accumulate in the central region of the acinus and to migrate to the bronchioles and, thus, to the mucociliary escalator of the conducting airways.
2. In the interstitium as *interstitial macrophages*, which are equal to or greater in number than alveolar macrophages. They have characteristic antigenic features not shared by other mononuclear phagocytes (Kobzik et al., 1986) and are increased in the active lesions of injured lungs (Figure 1.13).

It is the interstitial and not the alveolar macrophages that are in close contact with other cells in the interstitium (Brain, 1988); their activation by fibrogenic dusts appears to cause a greater fibrotic response, due to direct stimulation by fibroblasts, than similar activation of macrophages confined to the alveoli (Bowden, Hedgecock and Adamson, 1989). They are present in the connective tissue of bronchial walls (so that some cells reach the mucociliary surface directly through the bronchial epithelium), perivascular and peribronchial sheaths, interlobular septa and subpleural layers (Weibel, 1985). Furthermore, macrophages are often grouped with lymphocytes and plasma cells in the vicinity of small lymphatic vessels (Figure 1.13); those that contain exogenous particles apparently migrate from alveoli and are transported to the tracheobronchial lymph nodes in these vessels (Corry, Kulkarni and Lipscomb, 1984; Harmsen et al., 1985) (see also Chapter 3). Therefore, it is likely that macrophages from both locations play an important part in stimulating immune cell proliferation in these nodes (see Chapter 4, 'Alveolar macrophages' and Chapter 5, 'Cell populations' for more detailed discussion).

Mast cells

Under normal conditions mast cells are present in small numbers in alveolar walls – about 2 per cent of surface epithelial cells (Fox, Bull and Guz, 1981) – and in larger numbers in airways' epithelium and in perivascular and subpleural connective tissue.

They produce a variety of important mediators (including histamine, serotonin and heparin) and are a feature of some types of pulmonary fibrosis, especially in thickened alveolar walls when they often present unusual morphological appearances (Kawanami et al., 1979). Intraepithelial mast cells are increased in smokers' lungs compared with those of non-smokers' (Lamb and Lumsden, 1982). These cells are discussed further in Chapters 4 and 20.

Cells of the defence system

Lymphocytes

These small round cells have a compact nucleus and a thin rim of encircling cytoplasm. They fall into two main groups: thymus-dependent cells (*T lymphocytes*) concerned with cell-mediated immunity and lymphoid tissue-dependent cells (*B lymphocytes*), responsible for humoral immunity. Interaction between T and B lymphocytes and other cells, notably macrophages, plasma cells and fibroblasts, are complex and important both in the defence of the lungs and in the pathogenesis of various forms of disease. (See Chapter 4 for detailed discussion.)

Lymphocytes are present along the conducting airways, especially in the vicinity of BALT nodules and bifurcations where inhaled noxious agents impact. They are most numerous in the larger bronchi but become progressively fewer distally to the bronchioles; they are rarely found in the parenchyma except in lymphoreticular aggregates near the apex of the acinus.

The fact that lymphocytes and macrophages are, as just stated, frequently seen in close proximity to lymphatics (Figure 1.13) undoubtedly reflects their immunological collaboration.

Plasma cells

These cells are formed by transformation of B lymphocytes. They are the chief source of circulating antibodies and also produce other proteins. In the normal lung they occur in the same locations as lymphocytes and also in close association with the acini and ducts of small bronchial glands; similarly, they are rare in the parenchyma.

Granulocytes

Neutrophils and eosinophils are normally present in small numbers in the walls of the conducting airways but rarely, if at all, in the interstitium of alveolar septa, although, of course, they circulate in the capillary blood. Under abnormal conditions, neutrophils, being actively amoeboid, readily migrate through the endothelium into the interstitium stimulated by chemotactic factors from macrophages and lymphocytes to produce the characteristics of inflammation. Certain of these enzymes may disrupt the integrity of the lung by attacking its supporting connective tissue (see Chapter 9). Eosinophils are actively involved in complement-dependent reactions and are greatly increased in number in allergic disorders (see Chapter 4).

The pleura

The membranes of both pleural layers – *pulmonary* (or visceral) and *parietal* – are separated throughout (apart from their fusion at the hilum) by a minimal film of fluid and are lined by a complete layer of flat mesothelial cells. These cells, mesenchymal in origin and embryologically identical with those covering the peritoneal and pericardial surfaces, are furnished with microvilli which are more numerous on the pulmonary than the parietal pleura and towards the lung bases (Whitaker, Papadimitriou and Walters, 1982). Isolated mesothelial cells apparently function as macrophages and, in some circumstances, are transformed into fibroblasts, potentialities of importance when the pleura is injured (Bakalos, Constantakis and Tsicricas, 1974; Domagala and Koss, 1981). The multipotentiality which these cells possess figures especially in the pathogenesis of mesothelial tumours (see Chapter 13).

Multiple stomata, which connect with underlying lymphatic vessels, are present in the parietal pleura mainly on the lower mediastinal, intercostal and diaphragmatic surfaces (Whitaker, Papadimitriou and Walters, 1982). Cells and particulate matter escape from the pleural space through these openings. By contrast, there are no stomata in the pulmonary pleura.

The mesothelium of both pleural layers lies on a continuous basement membrane beneath which, in sequence, are collagen fibres and a discontinuous elastic lamina, blood and lymphatic vessels; in the pulmonary pleura there is an additional internal elastic lamina which blends with the walls of peripheral alveoli (the peripheral connective tissue system). It is improbable, therefore, that particulate matter can pass outwards from alveoli through an intact pulmonary pleura into the pleural space.

Blood and lymphatic vessels

The pulmonary pleura is supplied both by bronchial arteries and by pulmonary veins, and its subpleural lymphatics join those of the lung, draining ultimately into the hilar lymph nodes. The parietal pleura receives its arterial supply from posterior intercostal, internal thoracic, superior intercostal and musculophrenic arteries, and its veins join the systemic system. Lymphatic vessels anterior to the midaxillary line drain into anterior intercostal, internal mammary and parasternal lymph nodes, and posterior to the line into the thoracic duct via posterior intercostal or prevertebral nodes. Lymph from the diaphragm flows posteriorly into the thoracic duct and anteriorly to the anterior diaphragmatic and parasternal nodes.

References

Adamson, I.Y.R. and Bowden, D.H. (1980) Role of monocytes and interstitial cells in the generation of alveolar macrophages. II. Kinetic studies after carbon loading. *Lab. Invest.* **42**, 518–524

Andersen, J.B. and Jespersen, N. (1980) Demonstration of intersegmental respiratory bronchioles in normal human lungs. *Eur. J. Respir. Dis.* **61**, 337–341

Angus, G.E. and Thurlbeck, W.M. (1972) Number of alveoli in the human lung. *J. Appl. Physiol.* **32**, 483–485

Bakalos, D., Constantakis, N. and Tsicricas, T. (1974) Distinction of mononuclear macrophages from mesothelial cells in pleural and peritoneal effusions. *Acta Cytol.* **18**, 20–22

Barker, D.J.P. (1991) The intrauterine origins of cardio-vascular and obstructive lung disease in adult life. *J. R. Coll. Phys. Lond.* **25**, 129–133

Beasley, P. (1987) Anatomy of the pharynx and oesophagus. In *Scott-Brown's Otolaryngology*, vol. 1 (ed. David Wright), Butterworths, London, pp. 245–283

Berzon, D.M., Menkes, H., Dannenberg, A.M., Gertner, A., Terry, P., Plump, D. and Bromberger-Barnea, B. (1986) Interstitial fibrosis and collateral ventilation. *J. Appl. Physiol.* **61**, 300–303

Bienenstock, J. and Beyfus, D. (1984) Gut- and bronchus-associated lymphoid tissue. *Am. J. Anat.* **170**, 437–445

Bienenstock, J., Johnston, N. and Perey, D.Y.E. (1973a) Bronchial lymphoid tissue. I. Morphological characteristics. *Lab. Invest.* **28**, 686–692

Bienenstock, J., Johnston, N. and Perey, D.Y.E. (1973b) Bronchial lymphoid tissue. II. Functional characteristics. *Lab. Invest.* **28**, 693–698

Bohning, D.E., Albert, R.E., Lippman, M. and Foster, W.M. (1975) Tracheobronchial particle deposition and clearance. *Archs Environ. Health* **30**, 457–462

Bowden, D.H. (1976) The pulmonary macrophage. *Environ. Health Persp.* **16**, 55–60

Bowden, D.H. and Adamson, I.Y.R. (1980) Role of monocytes and interstitial cells in the generation of alveolar macrophages. 1. Kinetic studies of normal mice. *Lab. Invest.* **42**, 511–513

Bowden, D.H., Hedgecock, C. and Adamson, I.Y.R. (1989) Silica-induced pulmonary fibrosis involves the reaction of particles with interstitial rather than alveolar macrophages. *J. Pathol.* **158**, 73–80

Brain, J.D. (1988) Lung macrophages: how many kinds are there? What do they do? *Am. Rev. Respir. Dis.* **137**, 507–509

Brody, A.R., Hill, L.H. Jr, and O'Connor, R.W. (1981) Chrysotile asbestos inhalation in rats: deposition pattern and reaction of alveolar epithelium and pulmonary macrophages. *Am. Rev. Respir. Dis.* **123**, 670–679

Brody, A.R., Roe, M.W., Evans, J.N. and Davis, G.S. (1982) Deposition and translocation of inhaled silica in rats. *Lab. Invest.* **47**, 533–542

Brownstein, D.G. (1987) Tracheal mucociliary transport in laboratory mice: evidence of genetic polymorphism. *Expl Lung Res.* **13**, 185–191

Burdon-Sanderson, J. (1870) Recent researches on tuberculosis. *Edin. Med. J.* **15**, 385

Camner, P., Philipson, K. and Friberg, L. (1972) Tracheobronchial clearance in twins. *Archs Environ. Health* **24**, 82–87

Corrin, B. (1970) Phagocytic potential of pulmonary alveolar epithelium with particular reference to surfactant metabolism. *Thorax* **25**, 110–115

Corry, D., Kulkarni, P. and Lipscomb, M.F. (1984) The migration of bronchoalveolar macrophages into hilar lymph nodes. *Am. J. Pathol.* **115**, 321–328

Danel, C., Dewar, A., Corrin, B., Turner-Warwick, M. and Chrétien, J. (1983) Ultrastructural changes in bronchoalveolar lavage cells in sarcoidosis and comparison with tissue granuloma. *Am. J. Pathol.* **112**, 7–17

Deffebach, M.E., Charan, N.B., Lakshminarayan, S. and Butler, J. (1987) The bronchial circulation. Small, but a vital attribute of the lung. *Am. Rev. Respir. Dis.* **135**, 463–481

Delaunois, L. (1989) Anatomy and physiology of collateral respiratory pathways. *Eur. Respir. J.* **2**, 893–904

Domagala, W. and Koss, L.G. (1981) Configurations of surfaces of cells in effusions by scanning electron microscopy. In *Advances in Clinical Cytology* (eds L.G. Koss and D.V. Coleman), Butterworths, London, pp. 270–313

Emery, J.L. and Dinsdale, F. (1973) The post-natal development of lymphoreticular aggregates and lymph nodes in infants' lungs. *J. Clin. Pathol.* **26**, 539–545

Evans, M.J., Cabral-Anderson, L.J. and Freeman, G. (1978) Role of the Clara cells in renewal of bronchiolar epithelium. *Lab. Invest.* **38**, 648–655

Fels, A.O.S. and Cohn, Z.A. (1986) The alveolar macrophage. *J. Appl. Physiol.* **60**, 353–369

Forrest, J.B. (1980) Lung airspace size and alveolar septal intersections. *Mikroskopie* **37**, suppl., 265–267

Fox, B., Bull, T.B. and Guz, A. (1981) Mast cells in the human alveolar wall. An electron microscopic study. *J. Clin. Pathol.* **34**, 1333–1342

Haefeli-Bleuer, B. and Weibel, E.W. (1988) Morphometry of the human pulmonary acinus. *Anat. Rec.* **220**, 401–414

Harmsen, A.G., Muggenburg, B.A., Snipes, M.B. and Bice, D.E. (1985) The role of macrophages in particle translocation from lungs to lymph nodes. *Science* **230**, 1277–1280

Hislop, A. and Reid, L.M. (1973) The similarity of the pulmonary artery branching system in siblings. *Forensic Sci.* **2**, 37–52

Horsfield, K. (1974) The relation between structure and function of the lung. *Br. J. Dis. Chest* **68**, 145–160

Horsfield, K. (1980) Are diameter, length and branching ratios meaningful in the lung? *J. Theor. Biol.* **87**, 773–784

Horsfield, K. (1986) Morphometry of airways. In *Handbook of Physiology*, section 3, *The Respiratory System*, vol. III, part 1 (ed. Alfred P. Fishman), American Physiology Society, Bethesda, MD, pp. 75–88

Horsfield, K. and Cumming, G. (1968) Morphology of the bronchial tree in man. *J. Appl. Physiol.* **24**, 373–383

Horsfield, K., Gordon, W.I., Kemp, W. and Phillips, S. (1987) Growth of the bronchial tree in man. *Thorax* **42**, 383–388

Judd, P.A., Finnegan, P. and Curran, R.C. (1974) Pulmonary sarcoidosis: a clinico-pathological study. *J. Pathol.* **115**, 191–198

Kapanci, Y., Assimacopoulos, A., Irle, C., Zwahlen, A. and Gabbiani, G. (1974) Contractile interstitial cells in pulmonary septae. *J. Cell Biol.* **60**, 375–392

Kawanami, O., Ferrans, V.J., Fulmer, J.D. and Crystal, R.G. (1979) Ultrastructure of pulmonary mast cells in patients with fibrotic lung disorders. *Lab. Invest.* **40**, 717–734

Kikkawa, Y., Yoneda, K., Smith, F., Packard, B. and Suzuki, K. (1975) The type II epithelial cells of the lung. II. Chemical composition and phospholipid synthesis. *Lab. Invest.* **32**, 295–302

Klein, E. (1875) The anatomy of the lymphatic system. In *The Lung*, Smith, Elder and Co., London

Kobzik, L., Hancock, W., O'Hara, C., Todd, R. and Godleski, J. (1986) Antigenic profile of human lung interstitial and alveolar macrophages. *Lab. Invest.* **54**, 32A

Lamb, D. and Lumsden, A. (1982) Intra-epithelial mast cells in human airway epithelium: evidence for smoking-induced changes in their frequency. *Thorax* **37**, 334–342

Lambert, M.W. (1955) Accessory bronchiolo-alveolar communications. *J. Pathol. Baceriol.* **70**, 311–314

Lapp, N.L., Hankinson, J.L., Amandus, H. and Palmes, E.D. (1975) Variability in the size of airspaces in normal human lungs as estimated by aerosols. *Thorax* **30**, 293–299

Macklin, C.C. (1955) Pulmonary sumps, dust accumulations, alveolar fluid and lymph vessels. *Acta Anat.* **23**, 1–33

Matsuba, K. and Thurlbeck, W.M. (1971) The number and dimension of small airways in non-emphysematous lungs. *Am. Rev. Respir. Dis.* **104**, 516–524

Morrow, P.E., Gibb, E.R. and Gazioglu, K.M. (1967) A study of particulate clearance from human lungs. *Am. Rev. Respir. Dis.* **96**, 1209–1221

Nikiforov, A.I. and Schlesinger, R.B. (1985) Morphometric variability of the human upper bronchial tree. *Respir. Physiol.* **59**, 289–299

Olson, D.E., Dart, G.A. and Filley, G.F. (1970) Pressure drop and fluid flow regime of air inspired into the human lung. *J. Appl. Physiol.* **28**, 482–494

Phalen, R.F., Oldham, M.J., Kleinman, M.T. and Crocker, T.T. (1988) Tracheobronchial deposition predictions for infants, children and adolescents. *Ann. Occup. Hyg.* **32**, suppl. 1, *Inhaled Particles VI*, 11–21

Possmayer, F. (1988) A proposed nomenclature for pulmonary surfactant-associated proteins. *Am. Rev. Respir. Dis.* **138**, 990–998

Pritchard, J.N., Jeffries, S.J. and Black, A. (1988) Regional deposition of 2.5 to 5.0 µm polystyrene microspheres inhaled by women. *Ann. Occup. Hyg.* **32** suppl. 1, *Inhaled Particles VI*, 939–946

Proctor, D.F. (1986) Form and function of the upper airways and larynx. In *Handbook of Physiology*, section 3, *The Respiratory System*, vol. III (ed. Alfred P. Fishman), American Physiology Society, Bethesda, MD, pp. 63–73

Rhys Evans, P.H. (1987) Anatomy of the nose and para-nasal sinuses. In *Scott-Brown's Otolaryngology*, vol. 1 (ed. David Wright), Butterworths, London, pp. 138–161

Strunk, R.C., Eidlen, D.M. and Mason, R.J. (1988) Pulmonary alveolar type II epithelial cells synthesize and secrete proteins of the classical and alternative complement pathways. *J. Clin. Invest.* **81**, 1419–1426

Takaro, T., Gaddy, L.R. and Parra, S. (1982) Thin alveolar epithelial partitions across connective tissue gaps in the alveolar wall of the human lung. Ultrastructural observations. *Am. Rev. Respir. Dis.* **126**, 326–331

Thurlbeck, W.M. (1976) *Major Problems in Pathology*, vol. 5, *Chronic Airflow Obstruction in Lung Disease* (ed. James L. Bennington), W.B. Saunders, Philadelphia, London, Toronto, p. 48

Thurlbeck, W.M. (1982) Postnatal human lung growth. *Thorax* **37**, 564–571

Trapnell, D.H. (1964) Recognition and incidence of intrapulmonary lymph nodes. *Thorax* **19**, 44–50

Wallace, W.A.H., Gillooly, M. and Lamb, D. (1992) Intra-alveolar macrophage numbers in current smokers and non-smokers: a morphometric study of tissue sections. *Thorax* **47**, 437–440

Weibel, E.R. (1963) *Morphometry of the Lungs*. Academic Press, New York

Weibel, E.R. (1979) Looking into the lungs: what can it tell us? *Am. J. Roentgenol.* **133**, 1021–1031

Weibel, E.R. (1985) Lung cell biology. In *Handbook of Physiology*, section 3, *The Respiratory System*, vol. I, part 1 (ed. Alfred P. Fishman), American Physiology Society, Bethesda, MD, pp. 47–91

Weibel, E.R. and Gil, J. (1977) Structure–function relationships at the alveolar level. In *Bioengineering Aspect of the Lung* (ed. J.B. West), Marcel Dekker, New York, Basel, pp. 44–53

Whitaker, D., Papadimitriou, J.M. and Walters, M.N.-I. (1982) The mesothelium and its reactions: a review. *CRC Crit. Rev. Toxicol.* **10**, 81–144

Wilsher, M.L., Hughes, D.A. and Haslam, P.L. (1988) Immunoregulatory properties of pulmonary surfactant: effect of lung lining fluid on proliferation of human blood lymphocytes. *Thorax* **43**, 354–359

Wilson, R. and Cole, P.J. (1988) The effect of bacterial products on ciliary function. *Am. Rev. Respir. Dis.* **138** S49–S53

Zeltner, T.B. and Burri, P.H. (1987) The postnatal development and growth of the human lung. II. Morphology. *Respir. Physiol.* **67**, 269–282

2

Physiological principles

D.M. Denison

This chapter concerns both the mode of working and the failings of lungs. To highlight these properties, the chapter makes an oblique start by describing a model lung that does not work at all.

Thinking about the lung

Why make a model lung?

In order to understand why systems present in nature are successful, it helps to make mental models of systems that do not exist. Some facts are needed to start with. At rest, an adult person consumes 250 ml oxygen/minute; blood can carry up to 200 ml oxygen/litre and respiring tissues can extract the top quarter – 50 ml/min – so that they require a blood flow of 5 litres/min to meet basal metabolic needs. On heavy exercise, oxygen uptake rises fifteenfold, but working tissues can extract the top three-quarters of the oxygen in blood, so cardiac output only needs to rise fivefold, that is, to 25 litres/min.

What determines lung size?

Curiously, the surface area of the lung is related to the size of the red cell. Red cells need one-third of a second to fill up with or be emptied of oxygen. The same is true of whole blood with carbon dioxide. Therefore, in heavy exercise, blood must spend one-third of a second in the pulmonary capillaries to complete gas exchange. Less time would be insufficient and more time would be wasteful

because the blood's task is complete in this time. If blood is flowing at 25 litres/min, 140 ml will flow in one-third of a second, so the pulmonary capillary blood volume in heavy exercise must be 140 ml. If the capillary diameter is 5 μm, a capillary length of 7000 km is needed to accommodate 140 ml, and the surface area of that length is 110 m², slightly larger than a tennis court.

Does the capillary diameter have to be 5 μm? Why is it smaller than the red cell (7 μm)? Does the red cell need to be that big or even to exist at all? The answers to these questions lie in the red cell content. Haemoglobin is the most studied and best understood macromolecule, consisting of four monomers. Each of these has a molecular weight of 16 000 and is designed as an elaborate nest to carry a very small egg, that is, one oxygen molecule (molecular weight of 32). The function of the nest is to keep the oxygen at arm's length away from the iron that has attracted it and to keep the iron dry and hidden from other components of the plasma. To carry 200 ml oxygen in a litre of blood requires 6×10^{21} monomers of haemoglobin. If they were simply suspended in plasma they would greatly increase its colloid osmotic pressure, and somewhat increase its viscosity. The monomers would very rapidly be wasted through the renal trap-door and be expensive to replace; also these monomers would attract oxygen avidly but would not release it subsequently.

The packing of haemoglobin monomers into red cells overcomes these difficulties and provides an environment that permits grouping together and the easy loss of oxygen. However, the larger the red cell, the longer it takes to exchange gas. Almost all mammals, regardless of their size or their metabolic rate per kilogram have selected red cells of 5 to 7 μm in diameter. Erythrocytes are generally slightly larger than the capillaries they travel through, so that they can be massaged as they roll on their own membranes through the narrower vessels. This brings fresh haemoglobin to the surface and significantly accelerates gas exchange.

Another reason for the size of red cells concerns the resistance of capillaries. Each time there is a halving of the diameters of a system of branching tubes of fixed volume (for example, 140 ml), the surface area of the system is doubled and the diffusion path length is halved (both benefits), but the length is quadrupled and the perfusion and pump power needed to maintain a given flow rise 64-fold (the costs). These effects are substantial, even for subtle variations in capillary diameter.

It seems to be obligatory to have something in the order of 7000 km of capillaries for a model of the human lung. How should it be arranged? As a single thread, or as several threads in parallel, and if so how many? The single thread option is impossible. It would have a very high resistance and would need blood to travel 7000 km in one-third of a second. Dividing the thread into a series of parallel tubes greatly reduces the resistance to perfusion, but increases the complexity of the arterial and venous systems at each end. The first need is that each element should be short enough so that the pressure required for perfusion is less than the colloid osmotic pressure of blood (25 mmHg), otherwise the arterial end of the capillary would drown. For tubing of this diameter, the critical length is about 1 mm.

A discoid lung

The model lung is nearly complete. We can divide the 7000 km into 1-mm lengths, arrange them side by side and serve them with dichotomously branching arterial and venous trees. To minimize the lengths and resistances of these trees the capillaries could be grouped as a disc (10 metres in diameter) around a central main pulmonary artery and vein. Owing to its corrugated surface, the apparent area would be rather less than 110 m^2 – about 80 m^2, the true size of a tennis court. It is not unthinkable for such a structure to exist in nature. It resembles the giant Victoria water lily leaf, which grows to a diameter of several metres from a minute bud in 3 months. How would this model lung work? Would it survive for 70 years?

Unroll the disc in a city park. The underside consists of a dense layer of capillaries with a mean diameter of 5 μm; the topside is a 1-μm thick layer of epithelium exposed to air, winds and dust. At first it would be an excellent oxygenator. Blood would leave it with an oxygen tension (P_{O_2}) very close to that of ambient air. On an average Spring day (air temperature 20°C, relative humidity 50 per cent, barometric press 760 mmHg), the air would have a water vapour pressure of 10 mmHg. Arterial P_{O_2} would be close to 21 per cent of the remaining

750 mmHg (that is, 157 mmHg). However, due to the naturally high and variable airflows over the surface, 'alveolar' and, thus, arterial P_{CO_2} would be very low and uncontrolled. This is a serious disadvantage because the prime function of the lung is to regulate brain pH by controlling arterial P_{CO_2} (at 40 mmHg). There would also be a continuous, substantial and unregulatable loss of water vapour and considerable cooling of blood.

Quite quickly dust and organisms would fall on the moist surface and be held there by surface tension. The organisms would multiply. The dust and the microbes would obstruct gas exchange and irritate the surface. In addition, any noxious gases in the air would be passively absorbed. This lung is not built to detect them and, even if it were, could do little or nothing about them. It has few defences. The vessels beneath occluded areas could sense obstructed gas exchange by changes in local P_{O_2} or P_{CO_2} and divert blood elsewhere, but it would not be long before most of the surface was covered. Then arterial P_{O_2} would fall and arterial P_{CO_2} rise.

Macrophages could come out and patrol the exposed surface, ingesting particles smaller than themselves, but they would have to be present in vast numbers to keep the surface clean, obstructing gas exchange as they did so. Also they would have to return with their trophies to the blood stream or face a very long walk indeed before they could drop off the edge of the disc. In the meantime the disc would be subject to various insults: earwigs would come and nibble, wasps would sting and children would use the disc as a trampoline.

Hanging the disc on a line would get over some of the effects of dust but would require high perfusion pressures and, therefore, a great deal of work to perfuse the top of the disc; considerable arterial constriction and even more perfusion would then be required to avoid drowning the bottom of the disc.

It can then be seen that the flat disc is not a good design: the model has to be folded to work successfully but folding introduces its own disadvantages.

A folded lung

Folding the lung greatly shortens the lengths of the pulmonary arterial and venous trees, reducing their resistances and the commensurate work of perfusion. It also conserves water vapour, prevents evaporative cooling and stops unwanted ventilation of the surface. However, offsetting this, the lung now has to be ventilated actively and continuously. Breath-holds longer than about 1 minute cannot be tolerated easily. The more detailed the folding the harder it becomes to ventilate the lung, because the air passages become smaller which increases their resistance to airflow. They also become more difficult to stretch, because surface forces rise as tubes and cul-de-sacs get smaller. Making a model lung is not easy but thinking about it has revealed some fundamental flaws that are neatly avoided in the real lung.

The real lung

The real lung has a surface area the size of a tennis court, produced from about a tenth of a kilogram of connective tissue, invaded and expanded many-fold by branching air-, blood- and lymph-filled trees.

The bronchoalveolar tree

The air-filled tree has a volume which can be rapidly varied from a minimum of about 1.5 to a maximum of about 6 litres. A fourfold increase in volume implies changes of about 60 per cent in length and 250 per cent in surface area. The early part of the tree – the first 2 or 3 per cent – branches more or less dichotomously through some 23 diminishing generations and ensures easy access of air to the remainder. If the early bronchial part was made to exact dimensions by the finest craftsmanship, but from hypodermic steel, it would not work. Such an arrangement would invade the lung as a rigid endoskeleton preventing any volume change at all. The bronchial tree has to be extensible. However, making it out of some lightly folded tubing which could expand with ease would only permit a single breath in, because floppy tubing buckles as it is squeezed, preventing expiration. The trachea and bronchi are reinforced with rings and spirals of cartilage to keep them open, and a dense mesh of longitudinal elastic fibres running from the larynx to the pleura (the 'fibrous skeleton') to ensure that they do not buckle but retract in an orderly way on expiration (see Chapter 1, page 6).

As we age, these elastic fibres weaken, and the small airways become more compliant than the alveoli they serve. As this progresses, airways close off earlier and earlier in expiration, so that *residual volume* (the volume of air remaining in the lungs after maximal expiration) rises with age. Some inhaled agents, notably cigarette smoke, accelerate this process, which is the main functional component of emphysema. Other agents scar the lung, generating fibres which limit lung expansion and keep airways open unnaturally. Such lungs are small

and difficult to inflate. They also empty with unusual completeness and ease.

The airways lead to an exchange surface usually visualized as closely packed clusters of hollow grapes or alveoli. Some anatomists regard them as uniformly bulbous tubes which extend their lengths, but not their diameters, as the body ages. Normal alveoli at full inflation are about one-third of a millimetre in diameter. Moist tubes of this diameter are very difficult to stretch due to surface forces. A powerful sufactant reduces surface tension in the alveoli and small airways manyfold, but residual surface tensions still provide a large part of the opposition to stretching of the lung. Some inhaled agents destroy the surfactant and so make the lung abnormally stiff.

The vascular trees

The pulmonary arterial and venous trees serve the distal third of the bronchial tree and the exchange surface, so they only need to branch some 17 times, but they have to follow the same route, and be as extensible as the air-filled tree, to avoid interference with one another occurring through changes in volume of the lung. Because the vascular trees are perfused at positive pressures they do not need as much reinforcement and longitudinal elasticity as the air-filled tree. The bronchial arterial tree normally serves the proximal two-thirds of the airways, which has a small surface area covered by columnar cells, so it takes little part in gas exchange. The bronchial veins normally return one-third of bronchial blood flow to the hilum and two-thirds to the pulmonary venous tree. The latter forms part of the anatomical shunt of the lung.

The lymphatic tree

The outer centimetre or so of the lung is drained by lymphatic tubes that course over the surface. The internal remainder is drained by lymphatics that follow the blood vessels and bronchi to the hila (see Chapter 1).

The exchange surface

The exchange surface can be treated as a sheet of blood, 5 μm thick, and 100 m² in area, covered on both sides by a 1 μm thick epithelium exposed to a pulsatile stream of air. The epithelial surfaces are held apart by minute pillars occupying 5 per cent of the available 'floor space'.

At rest, red cells take about 1 second to pass through the capillary sheet of the lung. As they only require one-third of a second to exchange gas, there is plenty of time in hand. The healthy lung maintains alveolar, and therefore arterial $P\text{CO}_2$ close to 40 mmHg regardless of the quantity or quality of the venous blood offered to it. At sea level this permits an alveolar $P\text{O}_2$ ($P\text{AO}_2$) of about 100 mmHg and arterial $P\text{O}_2$ ($P\text{aO}_2$) of about 10 mmHg lower. Consequently, blood leaves the normal lung fully saturated with oxygen. This is true even in extreme exertion when blood flow has increased fivefold and blood volume has expanded some 65 per cent. Red cells take one-third of a second on their capillary run just completing gas exchange in time. Even at rest, systemic tissues impose a cardiac output on the lung. Thus, as alveolar capillaries are stolen by disease, blood travels faster and faster through the remaining vessels. Crudely, when half the capillaries are gone, erythrocytes travel through the remainder twice as fast; when two-thirds of the vessels have gone, red cells are on the verge of leaving the lung incompletely filled with oxygen. The slightest exertion will send them through too fast and they will fail to saturate.

At one time it was imagined that oxygen and carbon monoxide diffusing from the alveolar interior to the blood perfusing its wall had to negotiate two barriers. First, they had to struggle through the alveolar epithelium, and then they had to fight their way through the red cell interior to find an unoccupied seat on the haemoglobin train. Nowadays, it is believed that the alveolar lining is an easily negotiated barrier but train seats are hard to find.

When agents damage alveolar membranes they destroy pulmonary capillaries and introduce new difficulties. Platforms become scarce and trains go through at increasing speed. The time available for loading oxygen on haemoglobin in red cells shortens and becomes limiting. Blood leaves the lung blue because it is unfilled. Using arguments similar to earlier ones, it is quite easy to predict how blood will behave as it flows through such lungs at rest and on exercise.

The ventilatory pump

The deeply folded lung has to be ventilated actively. Its prime purpose is to dilute metabolically produced carbon dioxide eighteenfold to maintain $P\text{aCO}_2$ of 40 mmHg, and so preserve brain pH. As the body produces about 220 ml carbon dioxide/min

at rest and up to 5 litres/min in heavy exercise, alveolar ventilation must range from 4 to at least 100 litres/min. This is achieved by displacing the surrounding 'chest wall' inwards and outwards through the equivalent cumulative volumes. It consists of the thoracoabdominal wall, the diaphragm and the abdominal contents. The pelvic bowl is its only rigid part. The abdominal contents are treated as incomprehensible. Therefore, if the abdominal wall were made of steel, no part of the respiratory apparatus could move; the rib-cage would be glued to it through the lower ribs, and the diaphragm would be unable to shift. The diaphragm generates two-thirds of the vital capacity, and the bucket-handle motion of the ribs produces the other third. The abdominal wall allows the ribs to rise and the diaphragm to fall. Converting the rib-cage into a rigid structure would be less embarrassing, because the abdomen, and therefore the diaphragm, could still develop two-thirds of the vital capacity. In fact, the rib-cage contains many joints that have to move in harmony, and disabling a few is sufficient to immobilize a large part of the cage (see Chapter 6, page 140).

There are also perils if either part of the wall is unduly floppy. For example, in the early stages of high spinal injury, in which the diaphragm is the only important respiratory muscle to retain power, the vital capacity does not fall to the unexpected two-thirds of 4.5 litres (3000 ml), but to 300 ml. This is because, as the diaphragm and abdominal wall achieve an outward displacement of 3000 ml, the flaccid rib-cage is drawn inward through some 2700 ml. When spastic paralysis supervenes, this paradoxical motion reduces and the vital capacity rises towards 3 litres. Similarly, when the abdominal wall is flaccid it cannot push the diaphragm back. Such patients cannot breathe easily in upright postures without elastic support for the abdomen. When they lie down, gravity acting on the semi-fluid contents of the abdomen has the same elastic effect.

The link mechanism

The moist inner lining of the chest wall is attached to the moist outer surface of the lung by surface tension. The strength of this linkage is commonly illustrated by the difficulty in attempting to separate two moist sheets of plate glass. In the plate glass example, the surface forces at first act to minimize the air–water interface at the periphery. When the top sheet eventually lifts, the water–glass interface reduces rapidly with little further increase in the air–water interface and the top sheet breaks away. This is a poor model of the pleural space. Air is not normally present, gases are dissolved in the liquid and the highly corrugated surfaces, which are perfused with gas-containing liquids, are highly permeable to liquids and gases. Forces must be acting to prevent the evolution of gases and liquids in the pleural space. Colloid osmotic pressures in blood, and active lymphatic drainage, resorb non-colloidal liquid. Metabolic consumption of dissolved oxygen, and the production of a lower volume of much more soluble carbon dioxide concentrate raise the P_{N_2} of pleural liquid forcing it to diffuse into the surrounding pleura, so keeping the space free of gas.

Pleural pressure

Pleural pressure is yet another 'as-if' concept, in this case employed to understand the mechanical properties of the lung. The lung behaves as if it hangs from whichever part of the chest wall happens to be uppermost at the time, and rests on the part that is lowest. The best guides to the pressures in pleural liquid suggest that there is a negative pressure of a few centimetres of water at the uppermost interface, and positive pressure of a few centimetres of water at the lowest surface. The pressure gradient down the pleural surface is about 0.3 cmH$_2$O/cm descent, that is, the liquid is not behaving as a continuous sheet of water would, but the lung is behaving as a bag of foam with a density of about 0.3 g/cm^3, collapsing under its own weight.

When the lung is stretched by expanding the chest wall, all the pressures become more negative. When the lung is squashed by compressing the chest wall, all the pressures become more positive. In addition, for reasons that are not entirely clear, there is a fall in pleural pressure from the costal to the mediastinal surface. It may be related to the smaller radii of curvature of the latter. It is one of the factors promoting the movement of lymph to the hila.

Clearly, pleural pressure varies widely from the top to the bottom of the lung, and from its costal to its mediastinal surface, so it cannot have a single value. However, for convenience, the pressure that can be measured in the middle third of the lumen of the relaxed oesophagus is taken as representative, and is commonly labelled *pleural pressure*. It is estimated by sensing the pressure in a small and floppy balloon at the tip of a fine oesophageal catheter. The balloon is deliberately long, thin and almost empty, with a capacity of 2 ml. It is filled with 0.5 ml air which hunts for the most negative pressure surrounding the balloon. This is the pressure transmitted to the perforated tip of the catheter and recorded by the manometer as 'pleural pressure'.

Oesophageal balloon studies and straight observations from animal and human surgery indicate that the longitudinal elastic fibres and surface tension of the bronchoalveolar tree cause the unstretched lung to collapse until the airways close off at the true residual volume of the lung. If perfusion takes place at this time, gas will be resorbed, and the lung will become airless (*absorption atelectasis*). However, the rib-cage has a natural tendency to spring outwards to a position close to maximal inspiration. When the lung and the relaxed rib-cage are glued together by suface tension, they come to a resting position at which the inward recoil of the lung is balanced by the outward recoil of the rib-cage. This is the so-called *functional residual capacity* (FRC) of the lung. At this position the healthy lung is about half-full. Compressing the rib-cage can empty the lung to about one-quarter of its capacity before closure of the airways occurs. Expanding the lung to a pleural pressure of about 30 cmH$_2$O will fill it. Greater negative pressure does not allow very much more air in; healthy lungs burst at about –75 cmH$_2$O.

Compliance

The relationship between the gas content of the lung and the pleural pressure surrounding it is known as the *pressure–volume (PV) curve* of the lung. The slope of this curve (that is, dV/dP) is the compliance or stretchability of the lung. Because the *PV* curve is sigmoid it cannot have a single value. For convenience the slope at functional residual capacity – that is, when the lung is half-full and the slope is maximal – is taken as the compliance of the lung. On the whole, pathologically large lungs are floppy (highly compliant) and pathologically small lungs are stiff (poorly compliant). Once this is realized, there is no diagnostic value in measuring compliance.

Effects of gravity on lung mechanics

All alveoli are made from the same materials, to the same plan. In a weightless world they would have the same volume. However, normally, as mentioned earlier, the lung hangs from the uppermost part of the rib-cage, so stretching the uppermost alveoli, and it rests on the lowest part of the rib-cage, compressing the lowest alveoli. These effects are continuous from the top to the bottom of the lung. There is, therefore, a vertical gradient of alveolar size. At rest, at FRC, the upper alveoli are already close to total capacity and the lower alveoli are close to residual volume. The same is true of the smaller airways. On inspiration, air travels more easily at first to the open spaces of the upper lung, but it soon fills up. By then the lower spaces are opening up. Eventually, the bulk of the inspirate fills the lower parts (Hoppin and Hildenbrandt, 1977).

Gravity also affects blood flow. Pulmonary capillary pressure cannot exceed 25 mmHg without drowning alveoli, so pulmonary arterial pressure is low, so low, in fact that, at rest, blood barely reaches the top of the lung, which is poorly perfused as well as poorly ventilated. The hydrostatic head of blood at the bottom of the lung is sufficient to distend vessels locally, lowering vascular resistance and encouraging flow. Consequently, the bases of young and healthy lungs are well ventilated and richly perfused. With age, and the consequent loss of elastic tissue, the airways at the bases tend to close, and then, the rich blood flow favours absorption atelectasis (West and Wagner, 1977).

Gravity appears to affect the distribution of some lung disease. Because human lungs are shaped like a beehive, and they spend much time hanging from the narrow apex of the hive, apical alveoli are particularly overstretched. This stress concentration is especially marked in people with long thin lungs. Similar effects are seen at the sharp upper margins of the lower lobes. In these regions, close to the pleura, alveoli rupture easily, and air escapes to collect as subpleural blebs. They may be the sources of spontaneous pneumothoraces, and certainly commonly accompany them. However, some investigators believe that air from sites of stress concentration is pumped towards the hila along periarterial sheaths, ascends the mediastinum and breaks through the particularly thin parietal pleura by the medial surface of the apex.

It is thought that stress concentration and poor blood flow account for the distribution of tuberculosis which is most common in the apices of human lungs, the dorsal regions of the lungs of cattle and the phrenic zones of the lungs of bats (West, 1979). Gravity obviously affects the deposition of large particles, biases the distribution of contaminant dusts or gases that are inhaled early or late in inspiration (see Chapter 3), and influences the accumulation of blood-borne particles, extravasations and dissolved agents such as bleomycin (see Chapter 15).

The effects of disease on lung mechanics

In general, loss of elastic tissue makes the lung easier to stretch and the airways more ready to close. Fibrosis has the opposite effects. When loss of elastic tissue only affects part of the lung, that part tends to expand because it is easily stretched, and is difficult to empty because its airways close off prematurely. As a result, the remainder of the lung does not get as much ventilation, and is difficult to fill. Some clinicians describe this situation inaccurately as the bullous part compressing the normal part of the lung. There are no positive pressures and, so, no compression – simply incomplete transmission of inflation pressures to the healthy part of the lung. When fibrosis is localized to part of the lung, it opposes local inflation, but transmits excessive inflation stresses to the healthy part, causing compensatory stretching. It is quite common to get a combination of emphysema and fibrosis. In such cases the lungs have deceptively normal volumes and, for what they are worth, 'compliances', but both processes destroy the pulmonary vascular bed and oppose local inflation. In these lungs damage can be much worse than implied from the lung volume, lung compliance or FEV_1/FVC ratio.

How does the lung keep dry?

There is plenty of evidence that there are large holes in the postcapillary venules of the lung, and it is surprising to find that it is not flooded all of the time. It used to be thought that the circulation was intact, and that the fluid that leaked across the colloidal osmotic pressure barrier, or was carried through defects along with colloid, was simply pumped away by the lymphatics. It is now believed that surfactant plays an important role in keeping the lung dry. It can act in two ways: first, by reducing the surface tension within alveoli, it decreases the drag that tension exerts on fluid within vessels; secondly, and more attractively, Hills (1981) has suggested that the surfactant lines the margins of defects in the circulation forming hydrophobic coronets which oppose the transit of water, much as rainproofing prevents dampness passing through a macintosh. Once water has flooded into an alveolus, an all-or-nothing situation is set up. As the water enters it reduces the radius of curvature of the air–water interface and surface tension rises pulling water in more quickly until the stable diameter of the airways is reached. It is not easy for an alveolus to remain half-drowned.

Arterial oxygen and carbon dioxide tensions

The principal function of the lung is to produce systemic arterial blood of acceptable quality; that is, with a $P\text{CO}_2$ of 40 mmHg and a $P\text{O}_2$ of 100 mmHg whatever levels of exertion and cardiac output exist at the time. It is best to begin with the arterial carbon dioxide tension ($Pa\text{CO}_2$). It reflects the ratio of alveolar ventilation to carbon dioxide production.

Alveolar ventilation

This is a concept, rather than a volume that can be easily measured. It is expressed by the volume of inspired air, or gas, that appears to be diluting the carbon dioxide excreted into the lung. In order to explain why the $Pa\text{CO}_2$ has to be interpreted with caution, it is necessary to describe the notions of anatomical dead space, physiological dead space, ventilation–perfusion inequality, time constraints in pulmonary capillaries, anatomical shunt, hypoxic pulmonary vasoconstriction and physiological shunt.

Anatomical dead space

The simplest model of the lung consists of a single bloodless tubular airway leading to a single richly perfused alveolus or balloon. In this model it is imagined that no gas exchange occurs in the airway and that composition of gas in the balloon is uniform but different from that in the airway due to respiratory gas exchange. The volume of the tubular airway is the anatomical, or series, dead space of the system, because it is determined by anatomy and empties in series with alveolar gas. It supposes that there is a sharp boundary between the gas in the tube and the gas in the balloon.

In the real lung, things are different. There are many alveoli at the ends of a complex system of branching tubes, and the alveoli are not treated equally. The total cross-sectional area of the airways increases dramatically as the alveoli are approached. Consequently, in-coming air slows down markedly and diffusion becomes the dominant exchange mechanism well before the alveoli are reached. So there are no sharp boundaries in the real lung and there are several ways of estimating its notional dead space volume. The simplest is to assume that alveolar gas has a single composition which can be estimated from the composition of end-tidal air or arterial blood, and then to collect all of the expirate, mix it up, determine its carbon dioxide content and calculate what volume of inspirate must have diluted the alveolar gas to produce the observed composition of the mixture. Most methods suggest that the anatomical dead space of an adult lung under resting conditions is about 200 ml, but it increases considerably if deeper breaths are taken.

Physiological dead space

The real lung consists of many compartments that are not ventilated evenly. As a result the composition of mixed expired air is biased by the larger volumes of gas with low carbon dioxide tensions, coming from the better ventilated alveoli. This means that more gas is expired from alveoli than would be required to excrete the same amount of carbon dioxide if alveolar $P\text{CO}_2$ ($P\text{CO}_2$) was uniform. In fact, the true average $P\text{CO}_2$ value of gas residing in alveoli cannot be measured for precisely this reason, that is, it is not possible to sample equal volumes of gas from all alveoli. The excess expirate, which reflects the unevenness or inefficiency of ventilation, is the *parallel* dead space of the lung – so-called because it empties at the same time as the conceptually ideal alveolar ventilation. Together with the anatomical dead space, it forms the physiological or functional dead space of the lung. It is another 'as-if' quantity in that the lung functions as if it had a dead space of this volume.

Ventilation–perfusion inequality

Very similar arguments apply to blood leaving alveoli. Blood flow varies from one alveolus to the next. The composition of mixed pulmonary venous blood will be biased by the greater quantities coming from the over-perfused spaces, so it will have a higher $P\text{CO}_2$ and a lower $P\text{O}_2$ than the mean of the gases residing in the alveoli. Again, from this viewpoint the mean alveolar gas composition cannot be determined because it is not possible to sample equal volumes of blood from all alveoli. For these reasons we are obliged to assess the lung by looking at two imperfect reflections of mean alveolar gas: expired air and systemic arterial blood. The differences in their gas tensions are created in part by the unevenness of alveolar ventilation and perfusion. These inequalities are magnified by disease and compounded by other factors which introduce differences between the composition of mixed pulmonary venous blood that cannot be sampled, and mixed atrial or systemic arterial blood that can.

Time constraints in pulmonary capillaries

Red cells need one-third of a second to pick up oxygen and to exchange carbon dioxide. In healthy lungs, even on heavy exertion, they have this time in hand. Some diseases destroy pulmonary capillaries, obliging blood to travel faster through the remaining bed. In these circumstances blood can leave the capillaries before gas exchange is complete, even though the histology of the alveolus it is hurrying through is normal. This draws attention to the hidden weakness of histological slides. Time is missing from the picture that they present. Lack of equilibration time is one reason why patients desaturate arterial blood on exertion, and others have arterial blood that is desaturated at rest.

Anatomical shunt

Some systemic venous blood bypasses alveoli altogether, through the interatrial or interventricular septa, the thebesian veins, the bronchial drainage into the pulmonary veins or arteriovenous anastomoses in the lung. In healthy people the bypass constitutes about 5 per cent of cardiac output. It is 'as-if' 19 parts of pulmonary end-capillary blood were mixed with 1 part of systemic mixed venous blood.

This fraction is commonly estimated by asking the patient to breathe pure oxygen for a while until the concentration of nitrogen in expired air has fallen to less than 1 per cent. Then a sample of systemic arterial blood is drawn and its P_{O_2} measured. It is supposed that all the alveoli that can be ventilated will contain very little nitrogen, normal amounts of carbon dioxide and water vapour, and that the rest will be oxygen. For example, if the barometric pressure is 760 mmHg, alveolar pressure will be the same, water vapour pressure will be 47 mmHg, $P_{A_{CO_2}}$ will be 40 mmHg, and $P_{A_{O_2}}$ will be close to $760 - 87 = 673$ mmHg. Each 1 per cent of resting mixed venous blood, which is added to pulmonary capillary blood equilibrated to alveolar gas of that composition, will lower the P_{O_2} by 20 mmHg. Consequently, assuming a 5 per cent anatomical shunt, we expect a systemic $P_{a_{O_2}}$ some 100 mmHg lower, that is, close to 570 mmHg. This is the value normally seen. It is very sensitive to exertion, which lowers mixed venous P_{O_2} ($P_{\bar{v}_{O_2}}$). However, there is an important fallacy in this approach which arises from hypoxic pulmonary vasoconstriction.

Hypoxic pulmonary vasoconstriction

Pulmonary arteries and anterioles are peculiar in that they constrict if ambient P_{O_2} is low. This is an important protective reflex which operates at a microscopic level, diverting blood away from poorly ventilated alveoli, so matching perfusion to ventilation. It has disadvantages. If many parts of the lung are hypoxic, as in high altitude exposure or advanced obstructive lung disease, vasoconstriction is widespread resulting in pulmonary hypertension and right heart failure. Also, in obstructive lung disease, breathing pure oxygen raises $P_{A_{O_2}}$, restoring blood flow to poorly ventilated spaces. The blood going through such regions cannot get rid of

carbon dioxide, so that $P_{a_{CO_2}}$ rises. This mechanism contributes substantially to the hypercapnia seen in patients with obstructive lung disease, who are given oxygen to breathe. It also opens up blood flow to alveolar vessels, and may lead to underestimates of anatomical shunts.

Physiological shunt

Due to the uneveness of blood flow to alveoli, there is an additional discrepancy between the composition of mean alveolar gas and systemic arterial blood. The pulmonary venous blood is biased by the flow from over-perfused alveoli, so its P_{CO_2} is higher than that of mean alveolar gas. This excess can be expressed as the *percentage* of systemic venous blood that would have to be mixed with end-capillary blood to produce blood of systemic arterial gas composition. It sums the effects of the anatomical shunt and the inequalities of perfusion, and is known as the physiological shunt of the lung.

Interpretation of arterial blood gas tensions

All of these factors complicate the interpretation of arterial blood gas tensions. Conventions have been established along the following lines: $P_{a_{CO_2}}$ is taken to equal mean resident $P_{A_{CO_2}}$, unless there is a substantial anatomical shunt. If it is more than a few millimetres of mercury above 40 mmHg, it is assumed that alveolar hypoventilation is present. (Note that it is normal for $P_{A_{CO_2}}$ to rise by several millimetres of mercury during sleep.) If $P_{A_{CO_2}}$ is more than a few millimetres of mercury less than 40 mmHg, it is supposed that alveolar hyperventilation is present. $P_{a_{CO_2}}$ is then used to calculate $P_{A_{CO_2}}$, from the alveolar air equation. This has a simple form, for rough and ready use:

$$P_{A_{O_2}} = P_{I_{O_2}}* - (P_{A_{CO_2}})/R$$

where $P_{I_{O_2}}*$ is the P_{O_2} of warm moist inspirate, and R is the respiratory exchange ratio, taken to be 0.8, in the absence of better information. The more accurate form of the equation, which should be used whenever the inspirate is not air, or the barometric pressure is much less than 760 mmHg is:

$$P_{A_{O_2}} = P_{I_{O_2}}* - P_{A_{CO_2}} [F_{I_{O_2}} + (1 - F_{I_{O_2}})/R]$$

where $F_{I_{O_2}}$ is the fractional concentration of oxygen in dry inspirate.

Whichever way it is calculated, the ideal $P_{A_{O_2}}$ is then compared with the measured arterial value ($P_{a_{O_2}}$) to determine the $P_{A_{O_2}}$ gradient. Normally, it is about 11 mmHg of which 5 mmHg are attributed to anatomical shunt (on air), 5 mmHg are assigned to ventilation–perfusion inequality, and a nominal 1 mmHg represents the contribution of diffusion barriers and time constraints in pulmonary capillaries. In disease, the alveolar–arterial gradient widens from many causes. The contribution of anatomical shunt is estimated from prolonged oxygen breathing using the rule of thumb that each 1 per cent of shunt widens the gradient by 20 mmHg. If the actual Pao_2 is less than 100 mmHg, this rule cannot be used, and the shunt has to be measured by simultaneous sampling of pulmonary and systemic arterial bloods. The contribution of ventilation–perfusion inequality should reduce on exertion. By contrast, exertion widens the contributions due to anatomical shunt, diffusion barriers and time constraints in capillaries.

Threats and defences

Threats

The deeply folded lung protects its exchange surface from simple fall-out of irritants and pathogens but its minute tubular airways are much more prone to blockage. The exchange surface is a virtually passive structure which permits the equilibration of any gas that reaches it. This is the basis of chemical warfare, carbon monoxide poisoning and inhalational anaesthesia. If gases are very soluble they are resorbed by the moist and richly perfused mucosae of the nose and trachea and may, as with perfumes, never reach the lung at all. Other gases of moderate solubility arrive at the alveoli almost undiluted, and cross into the blood stream at rates determined by their solubility in blood and tissue water. Insoluble gases are exposed to the aerial surface of the alveoli, but cross the barrier much more slowly. If the gases are truly inert, as helium or nitrogen are, they may do no harm to the lung at all. But if, as with sulphur hexafluoride or carbon tetrafluoride, they are very soluble in fat and highly insoluble in water, they may dissolve in the surfactant lining, stripping it away and causing a foamy oedema. Oxygen is a much more complex and dangerous molecule than previously thought. A few hours' exposure of alveoli to a partial pressure of half an atmosphere is sufficient to produce some damage to surfactant and, probably, to cause other oxygen radical damage to the lung. Many of these gases have no, or little, affect on the airways and arrive at alveoli unannounced.

Irritant gases inflame the airways from the nares down. As with particles, the gases can be sensed and avoided. The external nares are arranged to force inspirate to accelerate and turn a right angle on entry, causing gross particles that have bypassed the filter of nasal hair to crash into the mucosa and stay there. As the inspirate passes over the mucosa it is warmed and wetted to 37°C and 47 mmHg water pressure. However cold and dry the inspirate, it is rare for it to get further than the first few generations of airways without being completely warmed and wetted. At each bifurcation, as the air stream changes direction and slows down, finer and finer particles are embedded in carinae. Their arrival stimulates mucosal receptors, initiates coughing and accelerates mucociliary escalators. Only the smaller particles, of 10 µm or less aerodynamic diameter, reach the alveoli (see Chapter 3). Here, patrolling macrophages sense their presence, more probably by chemical than by physical signals, engulf them and transport them to hilar lymph nodes or to the mucociliary escalators. Excited macrophages and injured alveolar surfaces also excite the influx of further inflammatory cells (see Chapter 4). In addition, inflamed airways can shut off, protecting distal alveoli, and the larynx can shut, protecting the lung as a whole. Also, the owner can breath-hold, walk away from unpleasant stimuli or use protective apparatus. All these are benefits of the folded lung.

Common tests of lung function

Introduction

Three tests are used routinely to assess the functional state of the lung: spirometry, lung volume measurement and gas transfer.

Spirometry

The first test, spirometry, measures the rate and extent to which air can be moved in and out of the lung. The details are straightforward. Patients are sat upright with legs uncrossed, so as not to squash the abdomen and push up the diaphragm. They are asked to fill their lungs at leisure until they cannot get another teaspoonful in. Then, and only then, are they asked to breathe out as fast and completely as possible and when they are completely 'empty', to inspire swiftly until they are completely 'full' again. Air movements are recorded by a spirometer. The record that results is the maximal flow–volume loop of the lung (Figure 2.1). It is highly reproducible and very informative. It has several features of enduring

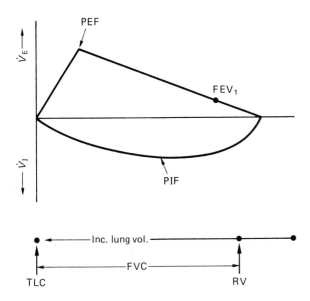

Figure 2.1 The maximal flow–volume loop of a normal lung $\dot{V}_\mathrm{E}$ is the axis for expiratory flow and $\dot{V}_\mathrm{I}$ is the corresponding axis for inspiration

significance. There is a linear rise to peak expiratory flow (PEF) which is reached about one-tenth of the way through expiration. Then there is a substantially slower linear fall to residual volume (RV). The total volume expired is the *forced vital capacity* (FVC). The volume expired in the first second is about three-quarters of the FVC, that is, the *forced expiratory volume in one second* (FEV_1). On inspiration, there is a smoothly curved return via peak inspiratory flow (PIF) to *total lung capacity* (TLC). *Peak inspiratory flow* is about three-quarters of the *peak expiratory flow*.

The maximal flow–volume loop has these features because peak expiratory pressure takes a brief time to develop and is then held constant, but as the lung empties the airways collapse progressively (hence the linear fall), closing off completely as residual volume is reached. On inspiration, the collapsed airways open up almost immediately to the smooth development and then reduction of inspiratory pressure. Many cottage industries are devoted to over-interpretation of this signal. However, analysed with caution, it remains a powerful description of the ventilatory properties of the lung.

Absolute lung volumes

The second type of test determines absolute lung volumes. This can be done in three ways, giving different answers. The *first method* is radiological: patients are given ample time to fill their lungs completely, and then posteroanterior (PA) and lateral radiographs of the chest are taken. A feature common to both views (for example, the crest of the aortic arch) is taken as a reference point, and PA and lateral diameters of the rib-cage's interior are calculated for a series of horizontal planar slices from the apex to the base of the lung. The volumes of the heart, spinal mass and subphrenic space are calculated similarly and subtracted. If peformed properly, this method determines the displacement volume of the lung (blood, gas, tissue and exudates), with an accuracy of ±3 per cent (Rodenstein et al., 1985). The *second method* of measuring lung size is through whole-body plethysmography: patients are asked to blow into a manometer while sitting in a rigid sealed box. The manometer measures the pressure developed in alveolar gas. A spirometer attached to the box measures the reduction in the patients' lung size as they compress their alveolar gas. The rest is down to Boyle's law. The procedure is used to determine the compressible gas volume of the chest which is smaller than the displacement volume of the lung because it does not include the volumes of the blood tissue and exudate. The *third method* of estimating lung volume depends on gas dilution. An insoluble gas such as helium is introduced into the lung for a known time and then expired. Its new concentration is proportionately reduced by the helium-free gas with which it is mixed in the lung. This method measures the accessible gas volume of the lung which is less than the compressible gas volume because it does not reach isolated or poorly ventilated spaces.

Gas transfer

The third type of common, non-invasive test of overall lung function requires the patient to inhale a mixture of oxygen, helium and carbon monoxide. The helium behaves as just described, measuring the volume of gas to which the carbon monoxide has access. The carbon monoxide is absorbed to an extent determined by local microvascular blood volume. The test is known as the (rebreathing or single-breath) *transfer test of the lung for carbon monoxide* (T_LCO). When the result is divided by the helium dilution volume (V_A), a measure of pulmonary capillary blood volume per litre of accessible gas is obtained (K_CO).

Common patterns of disease

The results of these three tests are sufficient to summarize the functional state of most lungs. After the results have been normalized for predicted influences of age, sex, height and race, they can be presented graphically as in Figure 2.2, which shows a rectangle scaled in units or predicted TLC on its

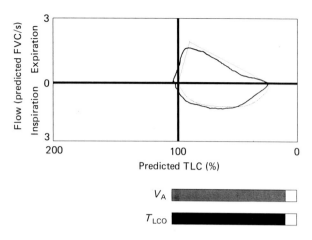

Figure 2.2 Normal lung function: the dotted line indicates the predicted flow–volume loop

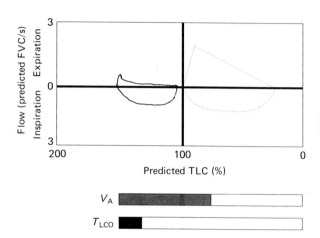

Figure 2.3 Emphysema: the dotted line indicates the predicted flow–volume loop

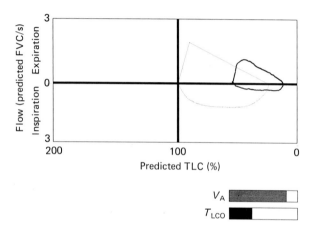

Figure 2.4 Fibrotic lung disease: the dotted line indicates the predicted flow–volume loop

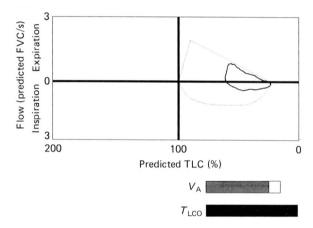

Figure 2.5 External compression: the dotted line indicates the predicted flow–volume loop

abscissa and predicted FVC/second on its ordinate. When TLC is known, the flow–volume loop can be placed on this frame and the results of the gas transfer test can be represented as appropriately scaled bars. In healthy lungs, helium reaches some 87 per cent TLC in 10 seconds. This is shown as the shaded part of the upper bar, V_A. The unshaded part of the bar is the shortfall of V_A on TLC, the inaccessible gas volume of the lung. The T_{LCO} is shown as the shaded lower bar. When it is normal it has the same length as the shaded bar above. Seven basic variants of this pattern are seen in chest disease. With very little practice they can be recognized with ease (Denison, DuBois and Sawicka, 1983).

Destruction without fibrosis

In emphysema, which damages the longitudinal elastic fibres of the airways and destroys alveolar walls, the lungs are easily stretched and have to be

held at high volumes to keep the airways open – hence the high TLC (Figure 2.3). On expiration the airways collapse immediately, emitting a brief pulse of air. Thereafter, expiration is very slow so that FEV_1 is a low percentage of FVC. The airways close off completely at a high RV. On inspiration, the floppy airways open up and inspiration occurs relatively easily. However, many airspaces are barely ventilated at all, so that there is a large shortfall of V_A on TLC. Because many capillaries have been lost along with alveolar walls, K_{CO} is low.

Destruction with fibrosis

When the lung is internally fibrosed, the scars make the lung difficult to stretch, destroy alveolar walls and keep airways open unnaturally, so a flattened inspiratory limb is associated with a low TLC, a domed expiratory limb, a low RV, a small shortfall of V_A on TLC and a low K_{CO} (Figure 2.4).

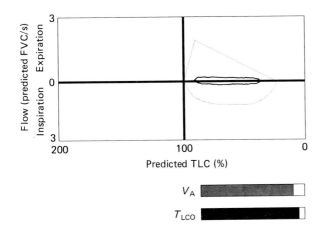

Figure 2.6 Tracheal stenosis: the dotted line indicates the predicted flow–volume loop

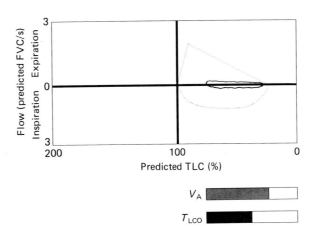

Figure 2.7 Tracheal stenosis after pneumonia: the dotted line indicates the predicted flow–volume loop

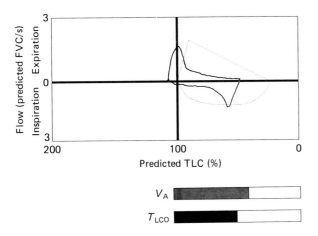

Figure 2.8 Stenosis of one main bronchus: the dotted line indicates the predicted flow–volume loop

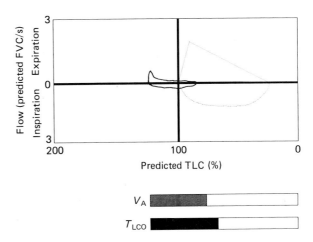

Figure 2.9 Asthma: the dotted line indicates the predicted flow–volume loop

External compression

A flattened inspiratory limb is also seen in phrenic palsy, and other defects of the chest wall, where there is insufficient power to expand the lung to a normal TLC. Because there is no airways' or alveolar damage, RV and the shortfall of V_A on TLC are normal and the lung is over stuffed with blood for its size, so that the K_{CO} is high (Figure 2.5).

Tracheal obstruction

Patients who present with isolated stenoses of the trachea show marked reductions in expiratory and inspiratory flow (Figure 2.6). Sometimes they are too obstructed to be able to reach TLC or RV. However, once the transfer test gas gets past the stenosis it finds normal airways and alveoli, quickly invades most of the lung and finds a normal or even slightly

raised capillary blood volume. If the stenosis is associated with alveolar damage, for example, after prolonged intubation following pneumonia, the flow–volume loop of rigid obstruction is associated with a low V_A and K_{CO} (Figure 2.7). Lesions of the upper (extrathoracic) trachea commonly interfere with inspiration more than expiration, because that part of the trachea narrows on breathing in, so a flattened inspiratory limb to the flow–volume loop should always raise that possibility.

Obstruction of a main bronchus

When a lesion narrows one main bronchus but not the other, the obstructed lung fills and empties more slowly than its partner, and the pair of lungs generates a characteristic composite flow–volume loop (Figure 2.8).

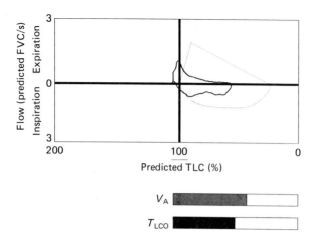

Figure 2.10 Chronic bronchitis: the dotted line indicates the predicted flow–volume loop

Acute inflammation of the bronchial tree

In asthma, airways are oedematous, constricted by muscle and obstructed by exudate, so their lumina seal prematurely. Once more the lung has to be held at a high lung volume to breathe at all (Figure 2.9), but there is no damage to elastic fibres, so it is not stretched as easily as in emphysema. Inspiration is obstructed by the airways, which do not open readily with a consequent large shortfall of V_A on TLC. However, the alveoli beyond are undamaged. The inspiratory effort draws more blood into the lungs, the obstructed spaces divert blood to the ventilated parts and the inflamed airways also adsorb more carbon monoxide, so that K_{CO} is high. This effect persists when the other abnormalities fade away and a high K_{CO} is a good pointer to unsuspected asthma in remission.

Chronic inflammation of the bronchial tree

In bronchitis, there is oedema of the airways and exudates with some damage to airways' elasticity and to alveolar walls: the pattern is, therefore, intermediate between that of emphysema and that of asthma (Figure 2.10).

Interpretation

These variants allow functional sense to be made of most chest disorders. Mixed patterns suggest unsuspected components, for example, an unannounced lobectomy or the scarring of bronchiectasis or cystic fibrosis in obstructive lung disease. Routine lung function tests are not diagnostic; they simply summarize functional states and are best reported in that way. There are other more specialized tests that may sometimes be helpful in establishing mechanisms or severities.

Other tests of lung function

Compliance and regional mechanics

The measurement of compliance by oesophageal manometry has been described already, but it is of interest to note that regional compliance can be estimated from computed tomography (CT) scans. The same is true of regional vital capacity (VC), TLC, RV and tissue volume. These measures have a volume resolution of about 1 per cent total lung capacity (Millar and Denison, 1990). In the absence of CT scanning facilities, much the same information can be obtained down to the lobar level, if the major and minor fissures can be seen on conventional posteroanterior and lateral radiographs, taken first at full inspiration and then again at full expiration.

Closing volumes

If the beginning or end of an inspirate is marked with an insoluble gas, such as helium, continuous analysis of the following expirate reveals the contribution of early and late inspirate to each of its aliquots. Commonly, a sharp change in marker concentration is seen part-way through expiration as dependent or pathologically floppy airways close off. The lung gas volume at which this jump occurs is called the 'closing volume'. It rises in many obstructive diseases, but its measurement has not found much favour in routine practice because it is only reproducible in highly trained respiratory gymnasts.

Effective pulmonary blood flow

If a mixture of an insoluble and a soluble gas is inspired and then slowly expired or rapidly rebreathed, the divergent fates of the two gases can be followed almost continuously for many seconds. The rate of reabsorption of the soluble gas is a measure of effective pulmonary blood flow, which is that part of right heart output that takes part in respired gas exchange. The test can be conducted at the mouth, or during fibreoptic bronchoscopy where it can be resolved to subsegmental level. The results are useful for research purposes, for mapping regional blood flow and ventilation, and for following the course of disease in patients with end-stage circulatory involvement. They may also be helpful in intensive care decisions but they do not contribute much to routine management.

Exercise tests

These are uncomfortable for the patient, often carried out in circumstances that deny them the opportunity for a shower afterwards, commonly require costly equipment, and usually occupy two highly trained technicians for about half an hour. Often they provide many graphs and numbers but give no information of additional value. If a patient's routine lung function tests are abnormal at rest, they are going to be abnormal on exertion. Exercise tests are usually done to detect exercise-induced asthma, hyperventilation or desaturation of arterial blood on exertion. Exercise-related asthma is induced by evaporative cooling of hyperreactive airways. Nowadays this can be invoked more quickly, selectively and cheaply by asking the patient to undergo isocapnic hyperventilation of cold dry air. Liability to hyperventilation is more readily detected by asking the patient to undergo hypocapnic hyperventilation and discovering whether this reproduces the symptoms or not. Exercise-induced desaturation of arterial blood is reasonably well related to whole-lung carbon monoxide transfer. If this is already low on routine tests, nothing more is to be learnt by watching blood desaturate on exertion. Exercise tests are found to be invaluable in distinguishing circulatory from ventilatory causes for unexplained dyspnoea, and for establishing a baseline aerobic capacity for disability assessments.

Sleep studies of respiratory function

These are being done much more frequently now than hitherto. They are based on two observations. Some patients, particularly those who are overweight, may be perfectly normal when seen in the laboratory during the day, but they tend to snore, close off their upper airways and desaturate at night. Other patients with established hypoxaemia or hypercapnia, or both, during the day, lose some of their respiratory drive and become more desaturated and hypercapnic at night. These tests are a proper part of the investigation of many patients with chronic lung disease whether or not it is of occupational origin.

Respiratory muscles

At present there is also much more interest in the respiratory muscles, and whether or not they are weak or easily fatigued. There is some evidence that chronically stressed respiratory muscles fatigue more readily and contribute to respiratory failure. There is also clear evidence that some myopathies have previously unsuspected respiratory muscle components, which may be relevant to the investigation of myopathies caused by occupational factors.

Airways' reactivity and reversibility

Tests of airways' reactivity and reversibility are very useful. Some airways react excessively to standard irritant stimuli. They are labelled hyperreactive airways and are believed to overreact to irritants generally. Other airways have acquired overreactive sensivity to specific irritants and only exhibit this when challenged appropriately. Such challenge tests are helpful in identifying occupational causes for asthma. Once the airways have responded, it is important to determine the reversibility of their reaction in order to access prognosis and decide on therapy. All these tests are done by recording maximal spirometry before and after challenge and therapy (see Chapter 21, 'Investigations: inhalation testing').

Mucociliary clearance and ciliary motility

Some inhaled agents damage the mucociliary escalator. This can be assessed in two ways. The first distributes a radio-isotope-labelled aerosol in the depths of the lungs and records subsequent scans to map centripetal progress of deposited material towards the throat. The second takes a biopsy of the nasal or tracheobronchial mucosa and records ciliary motility directly, before and after exposure to the agent under suspicion.

Pulmonary circulation

In late-stage disease, pulmonary vascular resistance rises, pulmonary hypertension becomes obvious and right heart failure likely. The appearance is associated with progressively poorer prognoses, which may be especially important in investigations for compensation. There is no substitute for proper invasive examination by right heart catheterization, with a formal measurement of pulmonary vascular resistance and reversibility. It is not sufficient to measure pulmonary arterial pressure. Many studies have shown that pulmonary vascular resistance is the stricter index of damage, and that it must be remeasured after administration of a pulmonary vasodilator to obtain a correct estimate of its reversible component.

Regional lung function

This phrase is interpreted in two ways. For some it is simply a measure of the dispersal of functional attributes, measured at the mouth. The best example of this is the multiple inert gas tracer technique of Wagner and West (1980). They ask patients to breathe quietly following the intravenous infusion of saline equilibrated with six inert gases of widely varing blood/gas partition coefficients. From the degree to which each of these is retained or excreted on first passage through the lung, they can, for example, produce a 50-compartment model of the distribution of ventilation and blood flow, which is very informative but contains no geographical information. The alternative is geographically distributed information of the sort obtained by radio-isotope scans or endobronchial spirometry. The latter is uncomfortable for patients but obtains data on units of clearly defined anatomy, which is helpful to surgeons. The former are less invasive and more comfortable but have unimpressive spatial resolution. Until recently, CT scans had high spatial resolution for the distribution of vital capacity but not for quiet ventilation or any degree of perfusion. However, the advent of high-speed CT scans with acquisition times of around 50 milliseconds has transformed this, and it is reasonable to suppose that they will be one of the best ways of assessing the geographical distribution of ventilation and perfusion in future patients. Magnetic resonance imaging is of some value in defining pulmonary perfusion, but almost valueless in defining ventilation (see Chapter 7). The whole topic of gas exchange in the lung is analysed in detail by Hlastala and Robertson (1989), and more generally by Chang and Paiva (1989).

Limitations of lung function tests

Width of the normal range

The values of lung function tests in healthy people are markedly determined by their age, height, race and sex. But, even when these influences are accounted for, there is a large residual variation,

such that the range of normality about a regression line already weighted for these four factors is about ±15 per cent. This means, for example, that most people have to halve or double the functional characteristics of about one-seventh of their alveoli or airways before any diffuse damage can be recognized by routine tests. Those people already lying at the healthier extreme of the normal range would have to suffer twice that much damage before a functional deficit appeared. So it is not surprising that chest radiographs often show considerable changes in functionally 'normal' lungs.

Intrasubject variability

For these reasons, it is argued that such tests are better at determining trends. To find out whether this was true, Yeo et al. (1993) calculated their reproducibility in a group of highly motivated healthy young adults. Routine tests were performed on 60 to 160 occasions in each of 20 people aged 20 to 28 years at onset, over periods spanning 1 to 12 years. This is the age range over which variation in lung function with age is least marked, and so ought to give the best view of reproducibility. All of the tests were conducted, on the same apparatus, at the same time of day, in the same upright sitting posture. The best of three results each day was recorded. The first five sets of data were considered as training runs and excluded from the analysis.

Coefficients of variation were calculated for each set of results. They were lowest for the FVC, the TLC and the accessible gas volume of the lung. All of these had a variability of ±3.5 per cent. The variation in total carbon monoxide transfer (T_{LCO}) and specific transfer (K_{CO}) were ±5 per cent and 6 per cent respectively. FRC, which depends on a psyche-based decision of the resting place of the chest wall, was more variable (±7.5 per cent), and RV, which is vulnerable to the absolute volume errors of whole-body plethysmography, was even more variable (±14 per cent). Variability reduced with time over the first 30 sets of tests for each parameter, which suggests that there are some long-term training effects at play. Variabilities within each individual were greater over 10 than over 5 consecutive tests. As this implied non-random distribution of results with time, the authors examined directly the resolution of consecutive runs of tests and concluded that a 5 per cent change in function would be missed in two-thirds of the subjects but a 10 per cent change would be detected in all. Because these observations were made on highly motivated young adults, who had already done several tests before and in whom variability ought to be minimal, they suggest that it would be naïve to attach consequence to functional changes of less than ±10 per cent, when monitoring the progress of disease.

Independence of sense of well-being

Another factor to consider is the poor association of functional change with the sense of physical well-being. In another study by Bellfield-Smith et al. which is summarized in Search and Denison (1988), 176 people who were aged 30 years or older felt they were unfit and wanted to do something to set that right. They were put on a reasonably strenuous exercise programme for 1 year. At the end of that time, many, who previously could barely stagger across a room with a glass of something, were jogging long distances, and some were running half-marathons. Almost all of them felt considerably better. Their lives had been transformed from sluggishness to quite vigorous activity. Yet their lung function tests, their aerobic capacities, their ventilation on exertion and their pulse rates hardly changed at all. There is no doubt that these conventional tests were not detecting very real changes in lifestyle and sense of well-being.

Dependence on patient co-operation

All routine lung function tests require patients to make maximal manoeuvres. It may not always be to their comfort or advantage to do so. This introduces further unreliability into the results of routine tests. The best way to minimize this is by ensuring that the results of tests at one sitting are highly reproducible, generally to less than ± 5 per cent.

Lack of information on state of the pulmonary circulation

Routine tests are non-invasive and heavily biased towards the ventilatory side of the lung. None of them gives direct and unfiltered information about defects of the pulmonary circulation, even though such damage is often the final common path to end-stage disease.

Summary

Routine lung function tests have evolved by convenience rather than by reason. They are quite variable even within an individual, and they give a lop-sided view of the functional state of the lung. But a huge literature has accumulated on the changes they do show in various diseases. They describe functional states; with the exception of specific challenge tests, they cannot establish causes. Considerable functional changes have to occur before limits of normality are transgressed. It is unwise to attach meaning to any change if less than ±10 per cent in an individual patient.

The functional investigation of occupational lung disease

With these reservations in mind, routine tests still have a definite place in the study and management of occupational lung disease. It is important to distinguish the two fields. In research, many measurements can be justified, for example, to establish mechanisms that are not necessary when caring for an individual patient. In the care of a patient, it is wasteful and sometimes wrong to make any measurement unless it has the potential to alter management. The first set of routine tests is made not so much to sharpen a diagnosis, but to determine a baseline state against which subsequent results can be assessed. Later results are used to refine prognosis, adjust drug levels, establish levels of disability and evaluate people for surgery.

There is no doubt that specific challenge tests are useful in identifying causal allergens in occupational asthma and allergic alveolitis. Functional assessments of disability are slightly harder to defend. The wide discrepancy between the results of exercise tests and the sense of well-being suggests that they should be used with caution. Also, especially because determination is such an important factor, it is not easy to extrapolate from aerobic capacities to the demands of specific tasks in industry, even if their oxygen costs are known. The best test of whether a person can do a task is the task itself.

It may be helpful to illustrate this by a single example. A First Division mid-field footballer was injured in the chest in a motoring accident. Subsequently, by fiercely determined training, he returned to his team. But his game had suffered and he was eventually transferred to a Second Division team. He was still young, and still by normal standards superfit, but his loss of potential earnings was great. He sued for damages, but the Insurers correctly observed that routine lung function and exercise tests were all within or slightly better than the normal range. However, two things were in his favour. Studies by us on other top athletes showed that they commonly had results substantially better than normal. By their standards he had dropped. Secondly, a CT scan of his chest, several years after the injury, showed the damaged side of his rib-cage achieved considerably less outward displacement than the undamaged side. In healthy people, the outward displacements of the two sides agree within ±1 per cent. This would limit the maximal voluntary ventilation necessary for mid-field play. He eventually won his appeal.

Physiological tests can be used with much greater precision in research on mechanisms and epidemiology. If the range of normality for an age-, sex-, race- and height-weighted prediction were ±15 per cent, then roughly speaking the standard error of the mean for a group of 100 subjects would be ±1.5 per cent and for 1000 subjects it would be 0.5 per cent. Changes over time within the two groups could be resolved to about 0.5 per cent and 0.2 per cent respectively. Changes between one part of the lung and another can be resolved to about ±2 per cent.

Conclusions

The lung is a complicated organ adapted to operate in non-industrial surroundings. Although it is equipped with devices to sense and deal with many natural threats, it has limited means for sensing and protecting itself against unnatural hazards. Most lung function tests are crude attempts to summarize its elaborate distributed behaviour by a few imperfect lumped parameters. Their results have a wide range of normality, and are quite variable within individuals, so they have to be interpreted with care and used as expressions of functional state only. They can be employed with more precision in research on mechanisms and epidemiology.

References

Chang, H.K. and Paiva, M. (eds) (1989) *Respiratory Physiology: An Analytic Approach.* Marcel Dekker, New York, p. 868

Denison, D.M., DuBois, R. and Sawicka, E. (1983) Does the lung work? 6. Pictures in the mind. *Br. J. Dis. Chest* **77**, 35–50

Hills, B.A. (1981) What is the true role of surfactant in the lung? *Thorax* **36**, 1–4

Hlastala, M.P. and Robertson, H.T. (1989) Quantification of ventilation–perfusion heterogeneity. In *Respiratory Physiology: An Analytic Approach* (eds H.K. Chang and M. Paiva), Marcel Dekker, New York

Hoppin, F.G. and Hildebrandt, J. (1977) Mechanical properties of the lung. In *Bioengineering Aspects of the Lung* (ed. J.B. West), Marcel Dekker, New York

Millar, A.B. and Denison, D.M. (1990) Vertical gradients of lung density in patients with fibrosing alveolitis or emphysema. *Thorax* **45**, 602–605

Nunn, J. (1987) *Applied Respiratory Physiology*, Butterworths, London, p. 582

Rodenstein, D.O., Sopwith, T.A., Stanescu, D.C. and Denison, D.M. (1985) Re-evaluation of the radiological method for measurement of total lung capacity. *Bull. Eur. Physiopathol. Resp.* **21**, 521–525

Search, G. and Denison, D.M. (1988) *Getting in Shape*, pp. 1–144. London: New English Library

West, J.B. (ed.) (1979) Stresses. In *Regional Differences in the Lung*, pp. 281–323. New York: Academic Press

West, J.B. and Wagner, P.D. (1977) Pulmonary gas exchange. In *Bioengineering Aspects of the Lung* (ed. J.B. West), Marcel Dekker, New York

West, J.B. and Wagner, P.D. (1980) Ventilation–perfusion relationships. In *Pulmonary Gas Exchange*, vol. 12 (ed. J.B. West), Academic Press, San Francisco, pp. 219–262

Yeo, C.T., Bush, A., Ward, S., Cramer, D. and Denison, D.M. (1993) Uses and abuses of routine lung function tests. *Thorax* in press

3

Aerosols: their deposition and clearance

W. Raymond Parkes

The association of the inhalation of air-borne particles with respiratory disease involves consideration of their interrelationship. First, however, in order to appreciate the mechanisms of deposition, it is necessary to have some understanding of the properties and behaviour of particles. A definition of pneumoconiosis is also appropriate here.

Pneumoconiosis may be defined as the non-neoplastic reaction of the lungs to inhaled mineral or organic dust and the resultant alteration in their structure but excluding asthma, bronchitis and emphysema.

Table 3.1 Comparison of particle sizes

Material	Dimension range
Sand grains	200–2000 µm diam.
Cement dusts	4–10 µm diam.
Pollens	10–100 µm diam.
Fungal spores	{ 2–100 µm length { 0.5–7 µm diam.
Actinomycete spores	0.6–2.5 µm length
Rock dusts	1–10 µm diam.
Tobacco smoke	0.1–1.0 µm diam.
Fumes	0.1–0.4 µm
Viruses	28 nm–0.2 µm diam.

Definition and characteristics of aerosols

An *aerosol*, by analogy with a hydrosol (a colloidal sol in liquid), is a two-phase system consisting of a discontinuous phase of individual particles in a continuous gaseous phase – most commonly air.

Dusts are solid aerosols caused by mechanical disintegration of rocks, minerals and other materials from such impulsive forces as drilling, blasting, crushing, grinding, milling, sawing and polishing, or by the agitation or breakdown of organic materials such as cotton fibres, pollens and fungal spores. Dusts, therefore, may be inorganic or organic.

Fumes are solid aerosols formed by combustion, sublimation and condensation of minute particles from the gaseous state; they are most frequently generated by vaporization of a metal, with subsequent oxidation of the vapour and condensation of the oxide. The particles are very small, ranging from 0.1 to 0.4 µm.

Smokes are solid aerosol products of combustion processes.

Vapours are the gaseous, molecularly dispersed form of substances which normally exist in the solid or liquid state, and, as such, are distinct from aerosols.

Mists are liquid aerosols formed by disintegration of a bulk liquid and condensation of the resulting vapour as droplets around appropriate nuclei. While air-borne, droplets quickly evaporate, leaving the nuclei which are much smaller – about 2 to 3 µm or less.

Table 3.1 gives an indication of approximate size ranges of the different types of particles for comparison.

Properties of particles

The majority of particles are not spherical but of irregular shape and, according to their composition, exist either individually or as aggregations. Particles which approximate to a sphere (for example, bituminous coal, some clays and some spores) are referred to as *compact*, and those whose length substantially exceeds their diameter, as *fibrous*. The United States Occupational Safety and Health Administration (1974) defined a *fibre* as having a length to diameter ratio (so-called *aspect ratio*) of 5:1 or more, but a notional aspect ratio of 3:1 – derived from a convenient 'cut-off' size for counting particles in dust sampling instruments (Holmes, 1965) – has been widely adopted by pathologists and research workers. This is unfortunate because the mineralogical definition specifies an aspect ratio of 10:1 or greater as one of the essential criteria of the fibrous habit. These differences have led to confusion and misunderstanding in interpretation of the pathogenesis of disease in human beings and in experimental animals. This important matter is discussed in more detail in Appendix I (page 856).

Apart from experimental conditions, aerosols hardly ever consist of particles of similar size and shape (monodisperse) but have a wide variety of sizes and shapes (heterodisperse). The two most important factors which determine the deposition of a given aerosol are mean diameter and distribution of particle diameter. In the case of spherical particles the definition of diameter is clear but for particles of irregular shape (the overwhelming majority) the concept of aerodynamic diameter is employed.

All particles when air-borne have a tendency to settle under the influence of gravity. The gravitational force exerted on a particle is equal to its mass multiplied by acceleration due to gravity. Opposing this, for a particle in motion, is the force due to the viscosity of air which exactly balances the mass of a particle when it has accelerated to its terminal rate of fall – an effect that is greater for large than for small particles. The *terminal (settling) velocity* of a particle due to gravity is roughly proportional to its density and the square of its diameter. The terminal velocity – *free-falling speed* – is an important determinant of the aerodynamic behaviour of particles in the airways and is related to their size, shape, surface characteristics and density. It is not their *apparent* size that decides the manner in which particles behave, but their aerodynamic properties. Thus, *aerodynamic diameter*, which incorporates both particle density and frictional drag, denotes the *diameter of a unit density sphere which has the same terminal velocity as the particle in question*. The aerodynamic diameter of such particles can be measured by aerosol spectrometry (Timbrell, 1972). For compact particles, or aggregates, 1 to 40 µm in diameter the velocity of fall is determined by Stoke's law of air resistance, but for other particles a 'shape factor' is required (see Appendix II). Even within this size range the behaviour of a particle in the airways of the lungs is not wholly governed by its aerodynamic diameter: particles of extreme shape (fibres, plates, chain aggregates) and particles of extremely low density are more likely to entangle themselves with the epithelium of airways' walls than the respective aerodynamic diameters would indicate. The orientation of irregularly shaped particles – mica plates, for example – in the air stream influences their settling velocity, which can differ widely depending upon their axis of symmetry, and appears to explain how unexpectedly large particles may be found in the periphery of the lung (Tomb and Corn, 1973).

Particles smaller than 1 µm diameter are referred to as '*submicron*' particles. They are apt to remain air-borne for long periods of time and, hence, may present a special hazard if their concentration is sufficiently high.

Other factors that can influence deposition are absorption of water by hygroscopic particles (such as a variety of salts and sulphuric acid) in the near-saturated air of the lungs, evaporation and agglomeration, all of which may cause substantial alteration in the size of particles with time. Radioactive gases (such as radon daughters) in the ambient air may become attached to dust particles, and so the pattern of their deposition becomes that of the dust particles (see Appendix I, 'Ionizing radiation from rocks').

Mechanisms of deposition

Deposition and retention of particles, of course, are not the same. Retention is the difference between the amount of aerosol deposited and the amount cleared.

Particles inhaled into the respiratory tract closely follow the movement of the air in which they are suspended, and the depth to which they penetrate into the lung depends not only upon their physical characteristics (size, density, shape and aerodynamic properties) but also upon the volume of each respiration. Once a particle comes in contact with the wall of an airway or alveolus it cannot again become air-borne, and is then said to be *deposited*. Because the majority of inhaled particles less than 1 µm diameter are expelled in exhaled air (Figure 3.1), their concentration in the inhaled air must be high to enable some of them to be deposited in the lungs. The total number of particles exhaled differs from the total number inhaled during steady breathing by the number deposited in the dead space airways during inhalation and exhalation, and the number retained in the alveolar regions. This applies to repeated breaths and not to a single breath.

Percentage deposition for compact particles of different diameters throughout the airways beyond the glottis during steady breathing is shown in Figure 3.2. Although the curves are derived from

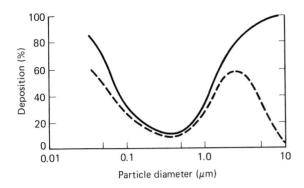

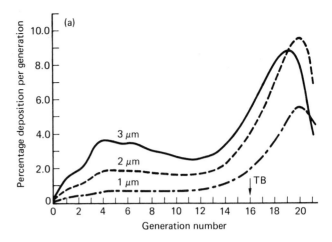

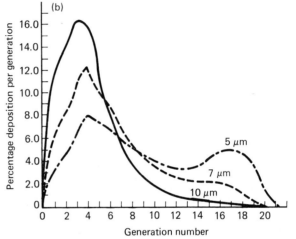

Figure 3.1 Deposition curves of compact particles during mouth breathing. The dotted curve represents particle deposition in the alveolar region of the respiratory tract (alveolar deposition); maximum deposition is seen to lie in the 2 μm to 5 μm range. The continuous curve represents deposition throughout the respiratory tract from nose to alveoli (total deposition). (Reproduced, with permission, from Muir, 1972)

Figure 3.2 Graphs showing the calculated percentage deposition of compact particles for airway generations 0 to 21 using Weibel's symmetrical model (see text). Average inspiratory flow rate = 500 cm³/s; tidal volume = 700 cm³; breathing frequency = 15.8 breaths/m. (a) Particles 1, 2 and 3 μm in diameter; (b) particles 5, 7 and 10 μm in diameter. For both the density is 2.5 g/cm³. Aerodynamic diameters from 1.6 to 16 μm. TB = terminal bronchioles. (Reproduced, with permission, from Gerrity et al., 1979)

calculations using Weibel's model of symmetrical generations (see Chapter 1), the results are in reasonable agreement with experimental results (Gerrity et al., 1979); in fact, similar peaks of deposition in the larger airways and alveoli are found using an asymmetrical model which corresponds more closely to normal anatomy, although the peak in the terminal bronchioles and alveoli is somewhat greater (Gerrity, Garrard and Yeates, 1981).

There are five different ways by which solid particles are deposited: (1) inertial impaction, (2) gravitational sedimentation, (3) interception, (4) electrostatic precipitation and (5) diffusion.

Inertial impaction

The passage of air through the airways of the upper and lower respiratory tracts is subjected to many changes in direction. With each change, particles tend to follow the trajectory of their original paths and, thus, are liable to impinge on the walls of the airways (Figure 3.3a). In these circumstances deposition is determined by the density × diameter² of particles, by the diameter and change of direction of airways and by the velocity of airflow in the airways. It is, in the main, larger compact particles (between 3 and 20 μm) that suffer impaction at the bifurcations of larger airways, assisted by turbulence at these sites. To a lesser degree fibres are also affected (see 'Interception').

Maximal deposition by impaction occurs in, or close to, segmental or subsegmental bronchi (Agnew, Pavia and Clarke, 1984).

Gravitational sedimentation

This applies particularly to the smaller airways (bronchi and bronchioles) and alveoli where, because flow velocity is low, the effect of gravity predominates. It is governed by the aerodynamic properties of particles according to Stoke's law, their concentration and their 'residence time' in the lung (Figure 3.3b). It ceases to operate for particles equivalent to 'unit density' spheres (UDS) of about 0.5 μm diameter or less, when diffusion assumes greater importance.

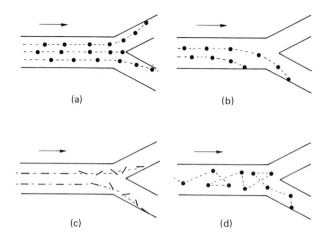

Figure 3.3 Diagrammatic representation of the movement of aerosol particles in the airways, caused by their different modes of deposition across the air stream: (a) inertial impaction; (b) gravitational sedimentation; (c) interception; (d) diffusion

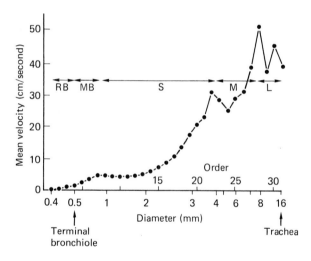

Figure 3.4 Mean velocity of airflow in airways of each *order* for a tracheal flow rate of 100 ml/second. The slight peak in airways of 0.8 mm diameter is probably an artefact due to the joining of two sets of data from which the curve was constructed. L, M, S = large, medium, small bronchi; MB = membranous bronchioles; RB = respiratory bronchioles. (Reproduced, with permission, from Horsfield, 1974)

At this point it is worth noting (Figure 3.4) that the mean velocity of airflow in the trachea and main bronchi is relatively constant and is only slightly lower in the medium bronchi; proceeding down the small airways, however, it falls abruptly and considerably at first and, then, much more slowly towards the periphery (Horsfield, 1974).

The settling velocity of fibrous particles is, in general, determined more by the square of their diameter and less by their length and shape. Sedimentation of fibres occurs mainly in larger airways and this limits the diameter of fibres that can penetrate to small airways to less than about 3 μm (Timbrell, 1970). Thus, deposition of fibres in the small airways is determined by their length and shape rather than by their settling velocities – that is, interception.

Although pollen particles are generally thought to be too large to reach the peripheral airways, a small percentage of those that are 20 to 30 μm do (Driessen and Quanjer, 1991).

Particles of cigarette smoke as they leave the cigarette are 0.1 to 1.0 μm (mean 0.4 μm) diameter and, as such, would suffer negligible deposition in the airways. However, like most hygroscopic particles, on encountering the almost 100 per cent humidity of air in the airways, they double their size within 5 seconds and are then subject to deposition on airways' walls (Ferron, 1977); a particle of 0.4 μm diameter, for example, will grow to 1.1 μm (Davies, 1974).

Interception

This chiefly affects particles of fibrous habit and, to some extent, those of irregular shape in which length and shape – aerodynamic diameter – are rather more important than settling velocity.

The lower the aspect ratio of a fibrous particle, the more its behaviour resembles that of a compact particle; but the higher that ratio (that is, the longer the fibre), the less likely it is to behave in this way. Hence, short fibres (less than 5 μm in length) reach the pulmonary parenchyma more readily than long fibres. Long fibres of less than 3.5 μm diameter are carried axially in the air stream, tending to avoid impaction and sedimentation in larger airways but, when their trajectory brings them into close proximity with the airflow surfaces, they are intercepted by collision with the walls of terminal and respiratory bronchioles particularly at bifurcations (Figure 3.3c). This explains the fact that amphibole asbestos and other straight fibres up to about 200 μm long may be found in the periphery of the lungs. In the lungs of shipyard workers, for example, Churg (1990) observed that amosite fibres with the greatest lengths and highest aspect ratios were found more in those regions with the longest airways' path-lengths, that is, the regions of the lungs where asbestosis occurs (see Chapter 14). Nevertheless, although deposition is closely related to fibre diameter, increased length of fibre also tends to increase deposition, in some degree, both by impaction and by sedimentation in larger airways (Burke and Esmen, 1978), owing to the fact that the aerodynamic drag of longer fibres, as well as their increased settling velocity, affects their orientation in the airways.

The influence of the shape of fibres on deposition by interception is about twice as great for straight stiff fibres in ordered orientation as it is for irregular (curled) fibres, such as chrysotile asbestos in random orientation, which are intercepted higher up the airways (Harris and Timbrell, 1977) – a point of considerable importance (see Chapter 14).

Longer and thicker fibres may be deposited in the periphery of the lungs of infants and very young children than in those of adults because their incompletely developed airways are, temporarily, wider and shorter (Timbrell, 1982; Horsfield et al., 1987) (see Chapter 1).

Electrostatic precipitation

This is often considered to be of little significance in human subjects. However, deposition of electrically charged particles is increased in the respiratory tract in the absence of an external field applied to the chest, although the effect is usually small. But recently fractured mineral dust (for example, sand and rock) may be highly charged (Lippman, Yeates and Albert, 1980). Rats subjected to inhalation of charged asbestos (chrysotile) fibres for 1 year had significantly more dust retained in their lungs and more pulmonary fibrosis than those similarly treated with non-charged fibres. These findings suggest that, likewise, highly charged fibres in the ambient air of the workplace are more likely to be deposited in human lungs (Davis et al., 1988), the magnitude of the electrostatic effect being, apparently, proportional to their length (Vincent, 1985).

Diffusion

Particles equivalent to 1 μm UDS diameter and less are constantly propelled in random directions by bombardment of gas molecules – that is, brownian motion (Figure 3.3d). Under the influence of diffusion a 1-μm UDS moves 13 μm in 1 second. This random displacement varies with the square root of time and increases as particle size increases, independent of density (Brain and Valberg, 1979). Diffusion is an important cause of deposition of particles less than 0.5 μm in diameter and especially those less than 0.1 μm in diameter in the small airways and alveoli in which air velocity is very low and surface area high. But turbulent diffusion of particles in this size range may cause significant deposition in a large airway such as the trachea (Hamill, 1979).

Influence of anatomical factors, respiratory patterns and reflexes on deposition

Upper respiratory tract

Events in the nasopharynx have an important influence on those in the tracheobronchial airways and alveoli. Breathing through the nose filters particles from the air much more efficiently than breathing through the mouth. Nasal airflow is turbulent even during quiet breathing but is increasingly so with rising rates of ventilation. Inspired air, which enters the anterior nares almost vertically, is deflected posteriorly 80 to 90 degrees by the nasal vault to flow horizontally until it impinges on the posterior wall of the nasopharynx whence it turns sharply downwards 80 to 90 degrees. Impaction of particles caused by these two abrupt changes in direction and by the resultant turbulence of the airflow is virtually complete for particles greater than 5 to 6 μm in diameter. The likelihood of impaction is directly proportional to the linear velocity of nasal airflow (Proctor, 1986). Furthermore, deposition of particles under 5 μm in diameter may increase during transit as they become larger due to humidification. By contrast, deposition by sedimentation is of minor importance although it occurs to some degree in the posterior nares where airflow velocity is substantially reduced. However, diffusion of minute particles may also occur in this region.

If resistance to nasal airflow rises, the workload of nasal breathing increases, demanding higher ventilation rates which, in turn, result in a change from nasal to mouth breathing. But even when the ventilatory rate is high, under normal conditions, some air still flows through the nose (Proctor, 1986). The nasal minute volume is smaller at all respiratory minute volumes and the oral minute volume correspondingly higher during mouth breathing compared to normal nasal breathing (Niinimaa et al., 1981). Nasal resistance is increased during heavy exertion, by congestion of the mucosa, by disease and by low ambient temperature (Salman et al., 1971), but it also differs widely among apparently normal subjects (Proctor, 1977) due, possibly, to variations in anatomy (see Chapter 1). The point at which the change from predominantly nasal to oral breathing occurs also varies between individuals, so that some switch to mouth (oronasal) breathing more readily than others, and some are habitual mouth breathers owing to chronic abnormality of their nasal airways. The proportion of habitual mouth breathers among healthy adults is about 13 per cent (Niinimaa et al., 1981). Oronasal breathing greatly increases the number of particles capable of reaching the lower respiratory tract, and it is interesting that, as long ago as 1935, Lehman suggested a relationship between the incidence of silicosis in miners and the efficiency of nasal filtration.

Artificial total obstruction of the nasal airways for 96 hours causes significantly increased resistance to tracheobronchial airflow (Wylie et al., 1976), and partial obstruction caused by nasal pathology increases pulmonary resistance during breathing through the nose or mouth. Thus, a reflex relationship between the nose and bronchomotor tone has been postulated (Ogura, 1970). Irritant stimuli applied to the nasal mucosa can elicit either bronchodilator or bronchoconstrictor reflexes, and there seems to be no consistent pattern as to which response will occur with a given stimulus (Widdicombe, 1986). Stimulation of the larynx, however, invariably evokes a powerful bronchoconstrictor effect; where irritants in the nose have caused bronchoconstriction, it is possible that they may also have reached, and stimulated, the larynx (Widdicombe, 1986). Nevertheless, the case for a nasal bronchoconstrictor reflex appears to be supported by these, among other, observations.

1. Unilateral irritation of the nasopharynx applied on the side of previous resection of the maxillary division of the fifth cranial nerve for trigeminal neuralgia has no effect on tracheobronchial resistance but, when applied to the opposite intact side, significant increase in resistance occurs. Administration of atropine prior to nasal irritation abolishes the pulmonary response (Kaufman and Wright, 1969; Kaufman, Chen and Wright, 1970).
2. Cold stimuli to the nasal mucosa cause bronchoconstriction in normal individuals (Widdicombe, 1986).
3. Strong stimulation (pepper) of the nasal mucosa in human subjects with laryngectomy (and, thus, absence of the laryngobronchial reflex) induces a statistically significant increase in airways' resistance (Konno et al., 1983).
4. Increased tracheobronchial resistance reverts to normal after surgical correction of associated nasal pathology in most cases (Ogura, 1970).

However, because a bronchodilator response may also occur, it is likely that different afferent pathways are involved.

Thus, differences in structure (such as anatomical anomalies) and the absence, or the presence and severity, of pathology in the nasopharynx have an important influence upon the degree to which oronasal breathing occurs and the proportion of particles that reaches, and is distributed within, the lungs in different individuals (see next section).

Lower respiratory tract

Deposition of particles varies greatly from subject to subject, whether they be smokers or non-smokers with or without chronic obstructive pulmonary disease (Lippman, Yeates and Albert, 1980). Factors that determine this variability are the following.

Nasal conductance

These are differences, which have just been discussed, in the efficiency of nasal conductance and, thus, in the predominance of nasal of oronasal breathing in the same individual and between individuals.

Patterns of ventilation

The tidal volumes of each respiration and the respiratory rate profoundly influence the behaviour of particles in the airways. The greater the tidal volume, the deeper the mass flow of transporting air penetrates into the lungs, whereas with increasing frequency of respiration the deposition of compact particles decreases (Muir and Davies, 1967). Both tidal volume and respiratory frequency (the product of which is the *minute volume*) are increased by exercise and, as the minute volume and, consequently, the flow velocity rise, the air stream becomes increasingly turbulent and deposition is enhanced, especially for particles in the 1 to 3 μm range (Dennis, 1971). During exercise, minute volumes may reach 120 l/min and high flow velocities in the large airways increase inertial impaction. In short, the increase in minute volume that accompanies heavy physical effort results in greater deposition of particles by impaction in large airways, and sedimentation and diffusion in smaller airways, than occurs when the subject is at rest or performing light work. Thus, variations in minute volume determine percentage deposition of particles rather than variations of respiratory rate (Dennis, 1971).

The lower zones of the lungs are ventilated more than the upper when breathing from functional residual capacity (FRC) but, at lung volumes approaching residual volume (RV), ventilation of the upper zones is greater than the lower (Milic-Emili, Henderson and Kaneko, 1968). During quiet respiration, compact particles 3.5 μm in diameter have been shown to be deposited preferentially in the upper rather than the lower zones compared with smaller (1.1 μm diameter) particles which are deposited more in the lower zones; the penetrance of 3.5-μm particles beyond the mucociliary escalator is greater in all zones, but particularly the apical (Pityn et al., 1989). Deposition of 'submicron' particles (0.7 μm diameter) at rest is similar and almost entirely alveolar, but, during the hyperventilation of moderately heavy exertion, regional alveolar distribution changes from being predominantly in the lower zone to more even dispersal in the upper and lower zones, although still with some greater affinity for the lower; tracheobronchial distribution increases in all zones, but especially in the upper (Morgan et al., 1984). These findings may be significant in the pathogenesis of disease associated with the inhalation of particles, vapours or fumes (Pityn et al., 1989).

In the presence of airflow obstruction, deposition is increased in the more central airways and is substantially reduced at the periphery (Lippman, Albert and Petersen, 1971; Dolovich et al., 1976; Pavia, Bateman and Clarke, 1980). In fact, the depth of deposition correlates positively with forced expiratory volume in 1 second (FEV$_1$) so that, as FEV$_1$ falls, peripheral deposition decreases (Pavia et al., 1977; Garrard et al., 1981). Thus, bronchoconstriction, even of mild degree, reduces regional alveolar deposition which becomes progressively less as bronchoconstriction increases, although there are large differences between individuals (Svartengren, Philipson and Camner, 1989).

The anatomy of airways and alveoli

The diameter, branching angles and inclination of airways and the number and size of alveoli, all of which vary between individuals, are particularly important (see Chapter 1). Differences in the angles of branching and in the diameters of daughter airways influence, respectively, the patterns and degree of turbulence and secondary rotatory flow at bifurcations and the partition of inspiratory flow between two daughter branches (Horsfield, 1986). The pronounced variability of total deposition of compact particles in the airways and alveoli which have been observed between subjects breathing aerosols of the same size, whether under similar breathing conditions or spontaneously, is most probably attributable to these differences in airways' geometry (Heyder et al., 1982; Svartengren, Philipson and Camner, 1989). Intersegmental communications between adjacent bronchioles may also affect the distribution and deposition of particles within the acini (see Chapter 1, 'Gas-exchanging acini' and Figure 1.5). Deposition of fibrous particles (asbestos), however, is influenced more by the length and bifurcation of airways than by their branching angles or whether daughter airways arise from major or minor branches (Pinkerton et al., 1986).

Total deposition of particles is the same for men as for women but tracheobronchial deposition is greater, and alveolar deposition smaller, in women than in men. This difference is explained by the fact that, as noted in Chapter 1, the diameter of the female trachea is smaller than that of the male, and that the size of bronchial airways is computed to be dependent upon tracheal size in approximately linear fashion. This results in, among other effects, significant differences in flow velocity for given flow volumes (Pritchard, Jefferies and Black, 1988).

Smoking and zonal distribution

The reversal of the usual base-to-apex gradient of alveolar deposition, referred to earlier, is enhanced in smokers (Morgan et al., 1984). A postmortem study has shown that the number of cigarettes smoked over the years (pack-years) appears to have a greater effect on the long-term retention of particles in the upper than in the lower lobes, and that particles in the upper lobes are larger than those in the lower (Churg and Wiggs, 1987).

Gravitational acceleration

Increasing gravitational acceleration (**G**) causes an almost linear increase in total deposition of 2.0 μm compact particles, mainly by sedimentation, from about 20 per cent at 0 **G** to about 45 per cent at 2 **G** (Hoffman and Billingham, 1975). A similar trend undoubtedly exists for particles of other sizes and, although distribution of deposition was not estimated, it is likely that this also altered. (**G** is the unit of the ratio of an applied acceleration to the gravitational constant, *g* (32.2 feet/s^2, 9.81 m/s^2).)

Elimination of particles

Efficient clearance of particulate matter from the whole of the respiratory tract is essential for its health, and the mechanisms by which this is achieved can be impaired by a number of disparate causes.

Upper respiratory tract

Mucociliary clearance

The mucociliary apparatus moves surface material forwards from the anterior end of the turbinate bones to the non-ciliated region (see Figure 1.1) but otherwise transports it posteriorly to the nasopharynx whence it is swallowed. The average rate of clearance, which depends on interaction between cilia and mucus, varies widely between individuals – even healthy young adults – due, possibly, to differences in physiochemical properties of the secretions (Proctor, 1982). It is prolonged by systemic dehydration (Proctor, 1982) and by purulent secretions which reduce the frequency of ciliary beat (secondary dyskinesia) by releasing bacterial products and host factors such as neutrophil elastase (Smallman, Hill and Stockley, 1984; Wilson, Roberts and Cole, 1985; Wilson et al., 1986).

Thus, chronic nasal infection not only impairs mucociliary clearance but is also likely to impose frequent or habitual oral or oronasal breathing.

Lower respiratory tract

Cough

The reflex forced expiration of coughing expels mucus (especially when it is increased in amount) and deposited material from the trachea and airways probably as far as the small bronchi, and possibly beyond. It is less efficient when the viscosity of mucus is increased. During coughing (when airflow velocity can be up to three-quarters of the speed of sound) larger bronchi are subjected to transient dynamic collapse due to high intrathoracic pressure. As a consequence, there is limitation of flow in lobar bronchi and redistribution and deposition of mucus and particles from smaller to larger airways. However, the average clearance time of particles from the lungs of normal subjects is increased for some hours after coughing, due, apparently, to delayed mucociliary flow in the central airways although transport of mucus from the periphery into these airways is normal. Delayed clearance may also be the result of damage to the mucociliary system in the central airways, but, in subjects with mucus hypersecretion, cough effectively removes particles deposited in the central airways (Foster et al., 1988).

Cough can occur either in association with excess production of mucus, leading to productive cough, or with an increase in the sensitivity of the cough reflex, possibly resulting in non-productive cough (Choudry and Fuller, 1992).

Cough nerve receptors are most numerous at the bifurcations of the trachea and larger airways where impaction of particles is likely to occur, the afferent fibres being conveyed in the vagus nerve to the medulla.

Mucociliary clearance

Particles deposited in the airways are transported out of the lungs – especially the more central airways – within hours by mucociliary action, but elimination of those deposited in the acinar region takes days or months. The mucociliary apparatus has been referred to already in Chapter 1. Normal long-term clearance of compact particles by this route occurs in two stages. In human non-smokers, the shorter of these (which is probably due to movement of particle-carrying macrophages from alveoli to the ciliated airways) has a half-time period of about 30 days, and the longer some 300 or more days, although there is considerable variation in the rate of clearance between different subjects (Bohning, Atkins and Cohn, 1982; Bailey, Fry and James, 1985). Consequently, there is substantial intersubject variation in the degree of *retention* of particles in the lung which, in fact, appears to be characteristic for the individual (Bailey, Fry and James, 1985).

In the case of fibrous particles (such as amphibole asbestos and other non-friable fibres) deposition is closely related to their diameter but clearance is greatly influenced by their length. The ability of alveolar macrophages to engulf fibres completely and transport them successfully is limited by the size of these cells, the mean maximum diameter of which is about 15 μm (see Chapter 1, 'Free pulmonary cells: Macrophages') so that phagocytosis of long fibres by single macrophages is incomplete; although other macrophages come to their aid, these are equally unsuccessful (see Figures 3.5 and 14.8 to 14.10). Thus, the clearance of very short fibres is virtually complete but that of long fibres decreases inversely with their length (Timbrell, 1982). Fibres short enough to be engulfed by macrophages are conveyed by them from the acini to the ciliated epithelium or to the BALT system. But the failure of complete phagocytosis of long fibres interferes with their transportation to the ciliary escalator and, consequently, with their clearance by this route. This situation is exemplified by an experiment in rats in which the length distribution of inhaled anthophyllite fibres recovered from the lungs by bronchopulmonary lavage and those remaining in the lungs following lavage were measured sequentially (using light microscopy) over a period of 205 days. Fibres shorter than 5 μm were cleared from the lungs via the airways more efficiently than longer fibres but fibres in excess of 50 μm in length were not removed by this route. Although fibres about 200 μm long were present in all the lungs examined, the longest recovered by lavage after fibres deposited in the airways had been cleared was about 100 μm and this decreased to 60 or 70 μm after 205 days (Morgan, Talbot and Holmes, 1978). This difference in efficiency of clearance of fibres according to their length has been confirmed by the results of other experiments (Morgan, 1980; Davis, 1989). Incomplete phagocytosis of long fibres appears to be an essential factor in the fibrogenesis

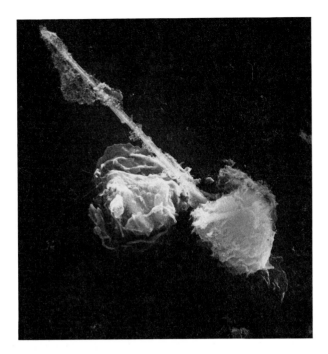

Figure 3.5 Scanning electron micrograph showing attempted phagocytosis of crocidolite fibre by several alveolar macrophages in vitro. The cell at the upper end of the fibre is dead. EM magnification × 1440. (Reproduced, with permission, from Miller, Handfield and Kagan, 1978)

of asbestosis (see Chapter 14, 'The pathogenesis of asbestosis: Fibre dimensions').

In human subjects, the clearance rates of fibres, like those of compact particles, exhibit substantial intersubject variation (Timbrell, 1982).

Factors affecting mucociliary clearance rates

Constitutional factors

As noted in Chapter 1, the overall pattern of tracheobronchial clearance in an individual subject is characteristic and constitutionally determined, clearance rates in constitutionally similar individuals, such as monozygotic twins, being virtually identical (Camner, Philipson and Friberg, 1972; Bohning et al., 1975). Clearance is faster in 21- to 37-year-old individuals than in those aged over 50 (Pavia, Bateman and Clarke, 1980). Furthermore, different rates of clearance between individuals are related more to the size of their lungs than to variations in deposition; indeed, because of differences in lung

volume, clearance is significantly slower in males than in females (Garrard, Gerrity and Yeates, 1986).

In normal individuals the frequency of ciliary beat in the nasal airways, trachea and lobar bronchi is similar; in subsegmental airways, however, it is substantially slower. No doubt this reflects the necessity for an increased speed of clearance in the larger airways to prevent excessive accumulation of secreted mucus in the lungs (see Chapter 1). However, the rates of mucociliary clearance and ciliary beat frequency are not necessarily the same; for example, the chemical composition and viscoelastic properties of mucus differ in the small and central airways. For these and other reasons, a relationship between nasal and tracheobronchial clearance rates may be less evident and more difficult to establish than is the case for ciliary beat frequency (Rutland, Griffin and Cole, 1982).

Sleep

The clearance rate in the lungs of normal human subjects is considerably reduced during sleep. This appears to be a sleep-related effect, and not due to diurnal variation, that is likely to be of significance in individuals with chronic bronchitis or asthma in whom production of sputum is prominent in the early morning on waking (Bateman, Pavia and Clarke, 1978). It is also likely to be relevant to the clearance of inhaled or aspirated material.

Smoking

Clearance from the larger airways is impaired by smoking (Bohning et al., 1975). The slow phase of long-term clearance is increasingly prolonged with every 'pack-year' of smoking, though this may take a few years, from starting smoking, to become apparent (Bohning, Atkins and Cohn, 1982). Disorientation of ciliary action in smokers appears to be common (Sleigh, Blake and Liron, 1988).

Airflow obstruction

In the presence of chronic airflow obstruction, particles are, as stated earlier, deposited more centrally than in normal subjects but long-term clearance is substantially impaired whether or not there is associated emphysema (Bohning, Atkins and Cohn, 1982), and is erratic due, apparently, to lack of control in the mucociliary system (Yeates, Gerrity and Garrard, 1982).

In asthmatic subjects, mucociliary transport is depressed in the tracheal, bronchial and small airways but can be greatly improved by β-adrenergic drugs (Foster, Langenback and Bergofsky,

1982); in the absence of treatment, however, this impairment may persist for some days after they are symptom-free (Pavia, Bateman and Clarke, 1980). Sputum sol from patients with acute asthma has been shown to inhibit human bronchial cilia in a dose-dependent fashion (Dulfano and Luk, 1982), an effect that ceases when the patient improves.

Alteration in the quantity and viscosity of the mucus layer in the airways also contributes to reduced clearance.

Chronic bronchial sepsis

As mentioned in Chapter 1, this plays an important role in delaying mucociliary clearance due, probably, to factors derived both from the host and from bacteria which compromise ciliated epithelium (Wilson and Cole, 1988). Sol of purulent sputum contains products, including neutrophil elastase, capable of damaging ciliary epithelium. Consequent impairment of clearance allows these products to remain in the airways, thus compounding the damage (Greenstone and Cole, 1985) and diminishing elimination of deposited particles. Indeed, tracheobronchial clearance is much reduced in patients with bronchiectasis compared with normal subjects and, to a similar degree, to that found in patients with chronic obstructive lung disease without bronchiectasis (Currie et al., 1987). This topic is also referred to in Chapter 6.

Alcohol

Ingestion of alcohol in 'social drinking' quantity immediately after inhaling a monodisperse aerosol of 8.1 μm aerodynamic diameter increases the variability of clearance, although the magnitude of the changes differs considerably between individuals (Venizelos, Gerrity and Yeates, 1981).

Other

Clearance rates are increased by exercise, hyperventilation and adrenergic drugs, and decreased by the administration of atropine.

Acinar clearance

Particles, either in the free state or within alveolar macrophages, reach the ciliated epithelium aided, possibly, by changes in surfactant tension between inspiration and expiration (see Chapter 1). Macrophages and the mucociliary system probably

work in co-operation (Brain, 1988), the macrophages being largely responsible for the shorter phase of the long-term clearance of particles (Bohning, Atkins and Cohn, 1982). If, however, the dust burden is heavy, the capacity of macrophages to ingest particles is overwhelmed to a greater or lesser degree, and so, although many particles still appear to be eliminated via the mucociliary escalator, the likelihood of others crossing the alveolar epithelial 'barrier' increases (Adamson and Bowden, 1982). These particles penetrate into the interstitium either in the free state due to pinocytosis by intact type I cells (Barry et al., 1983) or by incorporation of both free and intracellular particles into the interstitium when type I cells have been damaged and eroded by the accumulation of particles and before these cells can regenerate (Heppleston and Young, 1973) (see Chapter 1). Animal experiments suggest that alveolar macrophages containing inert compact particles migrate from alveoli to hilar lymph nodes via the interstitium (Corry, Kulkarni and Lipscomb, 1984; Harmsen et al., 1985); other evidence, however, using particles of similar type, indicates that most are translocated in the free state (Lehnert, Valdez and Bomalaski, 1988) – in which case some are likely to be engulfed by interstitial macrophages. Species difference (guinea-pigs, dogs and rats) in translocation pathways of alveolar macrophages might account for the discrepancy. Thus, although this matter has not been fully clarified, it seems possible that both processes occur in varying degree. Either way, whether intra- or extracellular, particles are transported into the BALT system and, according to their nature, may play a role in inducing pulmonary immunity; some may reach the systemic circulation by this route.

There is experimental evidence that human and animal alveolar macrophages can dissolve inorganic particles, including those of such metals as manganese and arsenic (Lundborg et al., 1985; Marafante et al., 1987), a capacity that would be expected to contribute materially to alveolar clearance.

Migratory macrophages of both intra- and extravascular origin can also convey exogenous and endogenous particulate matter and macromolecules from other parts of the body to the bronchial tree for clearance (Cordingly and Nicol, 1967). This process could well be important in the pathogenesis of some forms of cryptogenic fibrosing alveolitis (idiopathic diffuse interstitial fibrosis).

The dynamics of regional accumulation of particles in the lungs cannot be measured in human subjects. Nevertheless, using a mathematical model of regional retention of continuously inhaled particles in Weibel's 23 generation model of the lung (see Chapter 1) with various assumptions, Gerrity, Garrard and Yeates (1983) deduced that the major effect of long-term inhalation of toxic particles is at

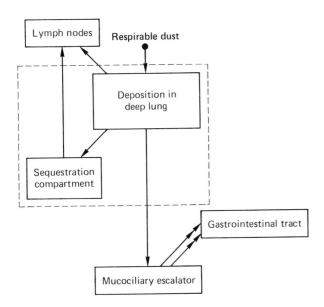

Figure 3.6 Schematic diagram for describing the kinetics of deposition, clearance, redistribution and storage of inhaled mineral particles. (Reproduced, with permission, from Vincent and Donaldson, 1990)

the level of the respiratory bronchioles. This appears to be supported by a report that particle counts in the lungs of dust-exposed individuals showed the number of particles per unit area to be greater in distal respiratory bronchioles than in membranous bronchioles (Churg and Wright, 1988).

However, simple kinetic models of deposition and clearance offered in the past do not account adequately for a steady, linear accumulation of dust in the lungs and lymph nodes which is observed with prolonged chronic (that is, repeated), but not short, exposures to dust; it is substantially more rapid and does not level off as these models predict. This is explained by the suggestion that, after an initial stage of clearance during the early period of exposure, and as the burden of dust in the lungs increases, some particles are transported to locations from which they cannot be properly cleared, for example, epithelial cells, macrophages in alveolar spaces, the alveolar interstitium, areas of parenchymal fibrosis and lung-associated lymph nodes (collectively, a *sequestration compartment*) (Figure 3.6). This model, a mathematical concept derived from inhalation experiments in animals, implies that the longer a particle – compact or fibrous – remains in the lungs the less likely it is to be cleared. Impaired transportation of particles from the 'deep lung' becomes significant only when its burden of dust exceeds a certain threshold value. This threshold is lower for toxic dusts, such as

quartz, than for non-toxic dusts, such as titanium dioxide (Vincent et al., 1985, 1987; Vincent and Donaldson, 1990). Accumulation of quartz in this way is, probably, important in the progression of silicosis and in the pathogenesis of coal and some other carbonaceous pneumoconioses (see Chapter 13, 'The effect of quartz'). Overloading of alveolar macrophages by particles as a result of heavy exposure appears to impair their mobility and, thus, their ability to clear these particles from the lungs (Morrow, 1988; Lehnert et al., 1990). Furthermore, the presence of fibrosis, both in human and in animal lungs, is associated with reduced clearance of long and also shorter fibres that is more pronounced in areas of fibrosis than in normal lung (Morgan and Holmes, 1980; Timbrell, 1982; Roggli, George and Brody, 1987) and the clearance of compact particles appears to be similarly affected (Bohning, Atkins and Cohn, 1982). Some implications of these observations are discussed in Chapter 15.

Mermelstein et al. (1992) reported that 'overloading' of the lungs of rats with concentrations of dusts by long-term inhalation resulted in decreased alveolar clearance, a disproportionate increase in retention of particles and a slight to moderate degree of fibrosis preceded by an inflammatory response. They noted that, with this technique, some fibrosis was associated with titanium dioxide and carbon black dusts (see Chapters 11 and 13). By using various mathematical assumptions, the authors proposed that their results suggest that current limits of exposure for specific dusts over a 40-hour working week are too high (see 'Control standards'). However, apart from the fact that these findings and conclusions need validation, extrapolation of such grossly abnormal physiological conditions in animals to the lungs of workers exposed to dusty environments appears unreal. The appearance of alveolar macrophages in rats subjected to such conditions suggests an analogy with the forced feeding of Strasbourg geese. Indeed, any relatively non-toxic or 'inert' dust, if inhaled in 'sufficiently large quantities' by experimental animals, can elicit a short-term inflammatory response (Vincent and Donaldson, 1990).

Conclusion

The variability of structure and function in the upper and lower respiratory tracts have an important influence on the quantity and the distribution of inhaled particles that reach, and are retained, in the lungs, and, thus, upon the probability as to whether disease will or will not develop – that is, individual susceptibility or resistance. The multiplicity and diversity of factors involved are large and should ever be in mind in the clinical appraisal of lung disease in workers and ex-workers.

The provision of clean air

This large and important subject is not discussed in this book because, on the one hand, its methodology is of limited interest to clinicians and pathologists and, on the other, it demands particular expert knowledge. The information can be found in a variety of works on occupational health and safety, for example: Cotes and Steel (1987), Chapters 1, 2 and 3; *Encyclopaedia of Occupational Health and Safety* (Parmeggiani, 1983); Hammad, Corn and Dharmarajan (1981); the UK Health and Safety Commission (1989); *Patty's Industrial Hygiene and Toxicology* (Clayton and Clayton, 1978); and the World Health Organization (WHO) Technical Report Series published periodically. However, the principles involved can be summarized briefly.

The working environment

This includes the identification, quantification and analysis of potentially hazardous substances (gases, fumes, vapours or dusts) in the workplace air by sampling the general air and that within the workers' 'breathing zone' with sampling instruments and strategies appropriate to the industry.

Protection of personnel

This means the elimination or tight control of the harmful substance. It can be achieved by enclosure of the hazard-producing process, remote control systems, local and general exhaust ventilation, and personal protection apparatus (for example, specialized respirators), or by a combination of any or all these.

Control standards

These consist of the upper limits of concentration of individual substances in the workplace air to which it is considered safe for workers to be exposed. They are derived from data from epidemiological and statistical studies of working populations, dose–response relationships (namely, the proportion of

workers who develop a particular abnormality related to the dose of the noxious substance that is believed to be its cause) and clinical experience associated with the substance in question. The purpose of the standards is to keep contamination of the air at a minimum level either over a short period (hours) or long period (usually 40 hours/week) according to the substance involved.

In the UK the principles are currently referred to as: (1) *occupational exposure limits*, a term that embraces erstwhile *maximum exposure limits* or *maximum allowable concentration* (MAC), both short and long term, the latter corresponding to threshold limit values (TLVs); (2) *occupational exposure standards*. TLVs are the standard employed, and regularly reviewed, by the US Occupational Health and Safety Administration and, in modified form, by the UK Health and Safety Executive (1992), published annually. The only international standards are those of the World Health Organization.

Codes of practice in the workplace

The subject is outside the scope of this work; the interested reader should consult that by Cotes and Steel (1987).

References

Adamson, I.Y.R. and Bowden, D.H. (1982) Effects of irradiation on macrophage response and transport of particles across the alveolar epithelium. *Am. J. Pathol.* **106**, 40–46

Agnew, J.E., Pavia, D. and Clarke, S.W. (1984) Aerosol particle impaction in the conducting airways. *Physics Med. Biol.* **29**, 767—777

American Conference of Governmental Industrial Hygienists. Committee on Threshold Limit Values (annual) *Threshold Limit Values of Airborne Contaminants.* Cincinnati, Ohio

Bailey, M.R., Fry, F.A. and James, A.C. (1985) Long-term retention of particles in the human respiratory tract. *J. Aerosol Sci.* **16**, 295–305

Barry, B.E., Wong, K.C., Brody, A.R. and Crapo, J.D. (1983) Reaction of rat lungs to inhaled chrysotile asbestos. *Expl. Lung Res.* **5**, 1–21

Bateman, J.R.M., Pavia, D. and Clarke, S.W. (1978) The retention of lung secretions during the night in normal subjects. *Clin. Sci. Mol. Med.* **55**, 523–527

Bohning, D.E., Atkins, H.L. and Cohn, S.H. (1982) Long-term particle clearance in man: normal and impaired. *Ann. Occup. Hyg.* **26**, 259–271

Bohning, D.E., Albert, R.E., Lippman, M. and Foster, W.M. (1975) Tracheobronchial particle deposition and clearances. *Archs Environ. Health* **30**, 457–462

Brain, J.D. (1988) Lung macrophages: how many kinds are there? What do they do? *Am. Rev. Respir. Dis.* **137**, 507–509

Brain, J.D. and Valberg, P.A. (1979) Deposition of aerosol in the respiratory tract. *Am. Rev. Respir. Dis.* **120**, 1325–1373

Burke, W.A. and Esmen, N. (1978) The inertial behaviour of fibres. *Am. Ind. Hyg. Assoc. J.* **39**, 400–405

Camner, P., Philipson, K. and Friberg, L. (1972) Tracheobronchial clearance in twins. *Archs Environ. Health* **24**, 82–87

Choudry, N.B. and Fuller, R.W. (1992) Sensitivity of the cough reflex in patients with chronic cough. *Eur. Respir. J.* **5**, 296–300

Churg, A. (1990) The distribution of amosite asbestos in the periphery of the normal human lung. *Br. J. Ind. Med.* **47**, 677–681

Churg, A. and Wiggs, B. (1987) Types, numbers, sizes and distribution of mineral particles in the lungs of urban male cigarette smokers. *Environ. Res.* **42**, 121–129

Churg, A. and Wright, J.L. (1988) Mineral particles in airway walls in the lungs of long-term chrysotile miners. *Ann. Occup. Hyg.* **32**, suppl. 1, 173–180

Clayton, G.D. and Clayton, F.E. (Eds) (1978) *Patty's Industrial Hygiene and Toxicology*, 3rd edn, vol. 1, John Wiley, New York

Cordingly, J.L. and Nicol, T. (1967) The lung: an excretory route for macromolecules and particles. *J. Physiol.* **190**, 7P

Corry, D., Kulkarni, P. and Lipscomb, M.F. (1984) The migration of bronchoalveolar macrophages into hilar lymph nodes. *Am. J. Pathol.* **115**, 321–328

Cotes, J.E. and Steel, J. (1987) Chapters 1, 2 and 3 in *Work-related Lung Disorders*, Blackwell Scientific, Oxford, London, Edinburgh (pp. 1–22; 23–48; 49–60)

Currie, D.C., Pavia, D., Agnew, J.E., Lopez-Vidriero, M.T., Diamond, P.D., Cole, P.J. and Clarke, S.W. (1987) Impaired tracheobronchial clearance in bronchiectasis. *Thorax* **42**, 126–130

Davies, C.N. (1974) Deposition of inhaled particles in man. *Chem. Ind.* June, 441–444

Davis, J.M.G. (1989) Mineral fibre carcinogenesis: experimental data relating to the importance of fibre type, size, deposition, dissolution and migration. In *Non-occupational Exposure to Mineral Fibres*, IARC Scientific Publications, no. 90 (eds. J. Bignon, J. Peto and R. Saracci), International Agency for Research on Cancer, Lyon, pp. 33–45

Davis, J.M.G., Bolton, R.E., Douglas, A.N., Jones, A.D. and Smith, T. (1988) Effects of electrostatic charge on the pathogenicity of chrysotile asbestos. *Br. J. Ind. Med.* **45**, 292–299

Dennis, W.L. (1971) The effect of breathing rate on the deposition of particles in the human respiratory system. In *Inhaled Particles III*, vol. 1 (ed. W.H. Walton), Unwin Brothers, Old Woking, Surrey, pp. 91–102

Driessen, M.N.B.M. and Quanjer, P.H. (1991) Pollen deposition in intrathoracic airways. *Eur. Respir. J.* **4**, 359–363

Dolovich, M.B., Sanchis, J., Rossman, C. and Newhouse, M.T. (1976) Aerosol penetrance: a sensitive index of peripheral airways obstruction. *J. Appl. Physiol.* **40**, 468–471

Dulfano, M.J. and Luk, C.K. (1982) Sputum and ciliary inhibition in asthma. *Thorax* **37**, 646–651

Ferron, G.A. (1977) The size of soluble aerosol particles as a function of the humidity of the air. Application to the human respiratory tract. *J. Aerosol. Sci.* **8**, 251–267

Foster, W.M., Langenback, E.G. and Bergofsky, E.H. (1982) Lung mucociliary function in man: interdependence of bronchial and tracheal mucus transport velocities with lung clearance in bronchial asthma and healthy subjects. *Ann. Occup. Hyg.* **26**, 227–244

Foster, W.M., Langenback, E.G., Smaldone, G.C., Bergofsky, E.H. and Bohning, D.E. (1988) Flow limitation on expiration induces central particle deposition and disrupts effective flow of airway mucus. *Ann. Occup. Hyg.* **32**, suppl. 1, 101–111

Garrard, C.S., Gerrity, T.R. and Yeates, D.B. (1986) The relationships of aerosols deposition, lung size, and the rate of mucociliary clearance. *Archs Environ. Health* **41**, 11–15

Garrard, C.S., Gerrity, T.R., Schreiner, J.F. and Yeates, D.B. (1981) Analysis of aerosol deposition in the healthy human lung. *Archs Environ. Health* **36**, 184–193

Gerrity, T.R., Garrard, C.S. and Yeates, D.B. (1981) Theoretic analysis of sites of aerosol deposition in human lung. *Chest* **80**, suppl., 898–901

Gerrity, T.R., Garrard, C.S. and Yeates, D.B. (1983) A mathematical model of particle retention in the air-spaces of human lungs. *Br. J. Ind. Med.* **40**, 121–130

Gerrity, T.R., Lee, S.P., Hass, F.J., Marinelli, A., Werner, P. and Lourenço, R.V. (1979) Calculated deposition of inhaled particles in the airway generations of normal subjects. *J. Appl. Physiol.* **47**, 867–873

Greenstone, M. and Cole, P.J. (1985) Ciliary function in health and disease. *Br. J. Dis. Chest.* **79**, 9–26

Hamill, P. (1979) Particle deposition due to turbulent diffusion in the upper respiratory system. *Health Physics* **36**, 355–369

Hammad, Y., Corn, M. and Dharmarajan, V. (1981) Environmental characterization. In *Occupational Lung Disease: Research Approaches and Methods*, vol. 18, *Lung Biopsy in Health and Disease* (eds. H. Weill and M. Turner-Warwick), Marcel Dekker, New York, Basel, pp. 291–371

Harmsen, A.G., Muggenberg, B.A., Snipes, M.B. and Bice, D.E. (1985) The role of macrophages in particle translocation from lungs to lymph nodes. *Science* **230**, 1277–1280

Harris, R.L. Jr and Timbrell, V. (1977) The influence of fibre shape in lung deposition – mathematical estimates. In *Inhaled Particles IV* (Ed. W.H. Walton), Pergamon, Oxford, New York, Toronto, Sydney, pp. 75–88

Health and Safety Commission (1989) *Control of substances hazardous to health; regulations and approved codes of practice*, Health and Safety Executive, London

Health and Safety Executive (1986) *Occupational Exposure Limits, Guidance Notes EH.* HSE, London

Health and Safety Executive (1992) *Occupational Exposure Limits: Guidance Notes.* HMSO, London

Heppleston, A.G. and Young, A.E. (1973) Uptake of inert particulate matter by alveolar cells: an ultrastructural study. *J. Pathol.* **111**, 159–164

Heyder, J., Gebhart, J., Stahlhofen, W. and Stuck, B. (1982) Biological variability of particle deposition in the human respiratory tract during controlled and spontaneous mouth-breathing. *Ann. Occup. Hyg.* **26**, 137–147

Hoffman, R.A. and Billingham, J. (1975) Effect of altered G levels on deposition of particulates in the human respiratory tract. *J. Appl. Physiol.* **38**, 955–960

Holmes, S. (1965) Development in dust sampling and counting techniques in the asbestos industry. *Ann. NY Acad. Sci.* **132**, 288–297

Horsfield, K. (1974) The relation between structure and function in the airways of the lung. *Br. J. Dis. Chest* **68**, 145–160

Horsfield, K. (1986) Morphometry of airways. In *Handbook of Physiology*, section 3, *The Respiratory System*. vol. III, part 1 (Ed. Alfred P. Fishman), American Physiological Society, Bethesda, MD, pp. 75–88

Horsfield, K., Gordon, W.I., Kemp, W. and Phillips, S. (1987) Growth of the bronchial tree in man. *Thorax* **42**, 383–388

Kaufman, J. and Wright, G.W. (1969) The effect of nasal and nasopharyngeal irritation on airway resistance in man. *Am. Rev. Respir. Dis.* **100**, 626–630

Kaufman, J., Chen, J.C. and Wright, G.W. (1970) The effect of trigeminal resection on reflex bronchoconstriction after nasal and nasopharyngeal irritation in man. *Am. Rev. Respir. Dis.* **101**, 768–769

Konno, A., Togawa, K., Itasaka, Y. and Hoshino, T. (1983) Computer analysis of changes in pulmonary resistance induced by nasal stimulation in man. *Eur. J. Respir. Dis.* **64**, suppl. 128, 97–104

Lehman, G. (1935) The dust filtering efficiency of the human nose and its significance in the causation of silicosis. *J. Ind. Hyg.* **17**, 37–40

Lehnert, B.E., Valdez, Y.E. and Bomalaski, S.H. (1988) Analysis of particles in the lung free cell, tracheobronchial lymph nodal, and pleural space compartments following their deposition in the lung as related to lung clearance mechanisms. *Ann. Occup. Hyg.* **32**, suppl. 1, *Inhaled Particles VI*, pp. 125–140

Lehnert, B.E., Ortiz, J.B., London, J.E., Valdez, Y.E., Cline, A.F., Sebring, R.J. and Tietjen, G.L. (1990) Migratory behaviors of alveolar macrophages during alveolar clearance of light to heavy burdens of particles. *Expl Lung Res.* **16**, 451–479

Lippman, M., Albert, R.E. and Peterson, P.T. Jr (1971) The regional deposition of inhaled aerosols in man. In *Inhaled Particles III*, vol. 1 (ed. W.H. Walton), Unwin Brothers, Old Woking, Surrey, pp. 105–120

Lippman, M., Yeates, D.B. and Albert, R.E. (1980) Deposition, retention and clearance of inhaled particles. *Br. J. Ind. Med.* **37**, 337–362

Lundberg, M., Eklund, A., Lind, B. and Camner, P. (1985) Dissolution of metals by human and rabbit alveolar macrophages. *Br. J. Ind. Med.* **42**, 642–645

Marafante, E., Lundberg, M., Vahter, M. and Camner, P. (1987) Dissolution of two arsenic compounds by rabbit alveolar macrophages *in vitro. Fundam. Appl. Toxicol.* **8**, 382–389

Mermelstein, R., Klipper, R.W., Morrow, P.E. and Muhle, H. (1992) Lung overload, dosimetry of lung fibrosis and their implications on the respiratory dust standard. Abstracts of Proceedings, Seventh International Symposium on Inhaled Particles, Edinburgh, Sept. 1991

Milic-Emili, J., Henderson, J.A.M. and Kaneko, H. (1968) Regional distribution of pulmonary ventilation. In *Form and Function in the Human Lung* (eds G. Cumming and L.B. Hunt), Livingstone, London, pp. 66–75

Miller, K., Handfield, R.I.M. and Kagan, E. (1978) The effect of different mineral dusts in the mechanism of phagocytosis: a scanning electron microscope study. *Environ. Res.* **15**, 139–154

Morgan, A. (1980) Effect of length on the clearance of fibres from the lung and on body formation. In *Biological Effects of Mineral Fibres* (ed. J.C. Wagner), IARC Scientific Publications 30, Lyon, pp. 329–335

Morgan, A. and Holmes, A. (1980) Concentrations of coated and uncoated asbestos fibres in human lungs. *Br. J. Ind. Med.* **37**, 25–32

Morgan, A., Talbot, R.J. and Holmes, A. (1978) Significance of fibre length in the clearance of asbestos fibres from the lung. *Br. J. Ind. Med.* **35**, 146–153

Morgan, W.K.C., Ahmad, D., Chamberlain, M.J., Clague, H.W., Pearson, M.G. and Vinitski, S. (1984) The effect of exercise on the deposition of an inhaled aerosol. *Respir. Physiol.* **56**, 327–338

Morrow, P.E. (1988) Possible mechanisms to explain dust overloading of the lungs. *Fundam. Appl. Toxicol.* **10**, 369–384

Muir, D.C.F. (1972) *Clinical Aspects of Inhaled Particles.* Heinemann, London

Muir, D.C.F. and Davies, C.N. (1967) The deposition of 0.5 μm diameter aerosols in the lungs of man. *Ann. Occup. Hyg.* **3**, 161–173

Niinimaa, V., Cole, P., Mintz, S. and Shephard, R.J. (1981) Oronasal distribution of respiratory airflow. *Respir. Physiol.* **43**, 69–75

Ogura, J.H. (1970) Physiologic relationships of the upper and lower airways. *Ann. Otol. Rhinol. Laryngol.* **79**, 495–498

Parmeggiani, L. (Ed.) (1983) *Encyclopaedia of Occupational Health and Safety*, 3rd edn, International Labour Office, Geneva

Pavia, D., Bateman, J.R.M. and Clarke, S.W. (1980) Deposition and clearance of inhaled particles. *Bull. Eur. Physiopathol. Respir.* **16**, 335–366

Pavia, D., Thompson, M.L., Clarke, S.W. and Shannon, H.S. (1977) Effect of lung function and mode of inhalation on penetration of aerosol into the human lung. *Thorax* **32**, 144–197

Pinkerton, K.E., Plopper, C.G., Mercer, R.R., Roggli, V.R., Patra, A.L., Brody, A.R. and Crapo, J.D. (1986) Airway branching patterns influence asbestos fibre location and the extent of tissue injury in the pulmonary parenchyma. *Lab. Invest.* **55**, 688–695

Pityn, P., Chamberlain, M.J., Fraser, T.M., King, M. and Morgan, W.K.C. (1989) The topography of particle deposition in the human lung. *Respir. Physiol.* **78**, 19–29

Pritchard, J.N., Jefferies, S.J. and Black, A. (1988) Regional deposition of 2.5 to 5.0 μm polystyrene microspheres inhaled by women. *Ann. Occup. Hyg.* **32**, suppl. 1, 939–946

Proctor, D. (1977) The upper airways. I. Nasal physiology and defence of the lungs. *Am. Rev. Respir. Dis.* **115**, 97–129

Proctor, D. (1982) The mucociliary system. In *The Nose, Upper Airway Physiology and the Atmospheric Environment* (eds D. Proctor and I.I. Anderson), Elsevier, Amsterdam, pp. 245–278

Proctor, D.F. (1986) Form and function of the upper airways and larynx. In *Handbook of Physiology*, section 3, *The Respiratory System*, vol. III (ed. Alfred P. Fishman), American Physiological Society, Bethesda, MD, pp. 63–73

Roggli, V.L., George, M.H. and Brody, A.R. (1987) Clearance and dimensional changes of crocidolite asbestos fibres isolated from lungs of rats following short-term exposure. *Envir. Res.* **42**, 94–105

Rutland, J., Griffin, W.M. and Cole, P.J. (1982) Human ciliary beat frequency in epithelium from intrathoracic and extrathoracic airways. *Am. Rev. Respir. Dis.* **125**, 100–105

Salman, S., Proctor, D.F., Swift, D.L. and Evering, S.A. (1971) Nasal resistance: description of a method and effect of temperature and humidity changes. *Ann. Otolaryngol.* **80**, 736–743

Sleigh, M.A., Blake, J.R. and Liron, N. (1988) The propulsion of mucus by cilia. *Am. Rev. Respir. Dis.* **137**, 726–741

Smallman, L.A., Hill, S.L. and Stockley, R.A. (1984) Reduction of ciliary beat frequencies *in vitro* by sputum from patients with bronchiectasis: a serine proteinase effect. *Thorax* **39**, 663–667

Svartengren, M., Philipson, K. and Camner, P. (1989) Individual difference in regional deposition of 6-μm particles in humans with induced bronchoconstriction. *Expl Lung Res.* **15**, 139–149

Timbrell, V. (1970) The inhalation of fibres. In *Pneumoconiosis*, Proceedings of the International Conference, Johannesburg, 1969 (ed. H.A. Shapiro), Oxford University Press, London and Capetown, pp. 3–9

Timbrell, V. (1972) An aerosol spectrometer and its applications. In *Assessment of Airborne Particles* (eds T.T. Mercer, P.E. Morrow and W. Stober), Thomas, Springfield, IL, pp. 290–330

Timbrell, V. (1982) Deposition and retention of fibres in the human lung. *Ann. Occup. Hyg.* **26**, 347–369

Tomb, T.F. and Corn, M. (1973) Comparison of equivalent spherical volume and aerodynamic diameter for irregularly shaped particles. *Am. Ind. Hyg. Assoc. J.* **34**, 13–24

United States Occupational Safety and Health Administration (1974) *Field Memorandum* No. 74-92. Dept of Labor, Washington DC

Venizelos, P.C., Gerrity, T.R. and Yeates, D.B. (1981) Response of human mucociliary clearance to acute alcohol administration. *Archs Environ. Health* **36**, 194–201

Vincent, J.H. (1985) On the practical significance of electrostatic lung depositiaon of isometric and fibrous aerosols. *J. Aerosol Sci.* **16**, 511–519

Vincent, J.H. and Donaldson, K. (1990) A dosimetric approach for relating the biological response of the lung to the accumulation of inhaled mineral dust. *Br. J. Ind. Med.* **47**, 302–307

Vincent, J.H., Johnston, A.M., Jones, A.D., Bolton, R.E. and Addison, J. (1985) Kinetics of deposition and clearance of inhaled mineral dusts during chronic exposure. *Br. J. Ind. Med.* **42**, 707–715

Vincent, J.H., Jones, A.D., Johnston, A.M., McMillan, C., Bolton, R.E. and Cowie, H. (1987) Accumulation of inhaled mineral dust in the lung and associated lymph nodes: implications for exposure and dose in occupational lung disease. *Ann. Occup. Hyg.* **31**, 375–393

Widdicombe, J.G. (1986) Reflexes from the upper respiratory tract. In *Handbook of Physiology*, section 3, *The Respiratory System*, vol. III, art. 1. (ed. Alfred P. Fishman), American Physiological Society, Bethesda, MD, pp. 363–394

Wilson, R. and Cole, P.J. (1988) The effect of bacterial products on ciliary function. *Am. Rev. Respir. Dis.* **138**, S49–S53

Wilson, R., Roberts, D. and Cole, P.J. (1985) Effect of bacterial products on human ciliary function *in vitro*. *Thorax* **40**, 125–131

Wilson, R., Sykes, D.A., Currie, D. and Cole, P.J. (1986) Beat frequency of cilia from sites of purulent infection. *Thorax* **41**, 453–458

Wylie, J.W., Kern, E.B., O'Brien, P.C. and Hyatt, R.E. (1976) Alteration of pulmonary function associated with artificial nasal obstruction. *Surg. Forum* **27**, 535–537

Yeates, D.B., Gerrity, T.R. and Garrard, C.S. (1982) Characteristics of tracheobronchial deposition and clearance in man. *Ann. Occup. Hyg.* **26**, 245–257

4

Basic immunology and immunopathology

Patricia L. Haslam

Introduction

The purpose of this chapter is to provide a broad overview of the mechanisms used by the body to defend itself against invasion by foreign materials.

The chapter will focus on the immune defences available in the respiratory system, because most agents associated with occupational lung diseases gain access via the inhalation route. The respiratory immune defences are extremely diverse, because the epithelial surfaces of the lungs and airways probably encounter a greater daily load of environmental agents than any other internal organ system, apart from the gut.

Efficient, 'first-line', non-specific, immune defence barriers are present within the respiratory tract ensuring that most inhaled agents are rapidly cleared from the lungs and airways without, or with only transient, ill effects to the host. These 'first-line' defences are part of the 'natural' or 'innate' defences of the immune system which, unlike specific immune responses, are available at all times without the need for previous sensitization to specific antigenic components in the foreign materials. They include physical barriers such as the nasal hairs, the secretions that line the respiratory tract, the mucociliary escalator and alveolar macrophages that protect the alveolar surfaces through their phagocytic and microbicidal properties (see Chapter 1). These non-specific defences are usually sufficient to protect the host under normal circumstances; however, in many occupational lung diseases, there is evidence that the non-specific defence barriers have been breached and that the 'second-line' specific (or 'acquired') immune defence mechanisms that guard the tissues and other internal regions have been activated. These defences are mediated by specialized antigen-presenting cells and lymphocytes. They are also induced when foreign antigens gain access to, and interact with, these cells in an appropriate manner (see under 'Specific (acquired) immune defences'). The involvement of

specific immune responses in lung diseases is indicated by the presence of increased numbers of lymphocytes and plasma cells within the tissue lesions. When these reactions persist, inflammatory mediators released by the activated antigen-presenting cells and lymphocytes can induce chronic inflammation and the evidence suggests that such *immune hypersensitivity* reactions may contribute to the pathogenesis of many chronic lung diseases. Due to the complexity of the respiratory immune defences, there are many possible reasons why 'immune hypersensitivity' reactions might arise and the precise mechanisms appear to differ in different lung diseases. A detailed review of knowledge on pathogenic mechanisms in each occupational lung disease is given in the relevant chapters. The aim of this chapter is to provide an introduction to basic immunology and immunopathology.

Immunology has been one of the most rapidly expanding of the biomedical sciences and the reader requiring more detailed knowledge of this vast subject is advised to refer to specialist text books (Weir, 1986; Johnstone and Thorpe, 1987; Daniele, 1988; Dale and Foreman, 1989; Davey, 1989; Roitt, Brostoff and Male, 1989; Miller, Turk and Nicklin, 1992).

Factors that can influence the host response to inhaled agents

There are various factors that need to be taken into account to understand why certain dusts can escape the normal immune defences and stimulate immune hypersensitivity reactions in the lungs or airways:

1. Properties of the agent.
2. Host factors.
3. Secondary factors that can influence host immune response.
4. Atopic status.
5. Genetic susceptibility.

Properties of the agent

The physical properties of the agents themselves can influence their depth of penetration and persistence in the respiratory tract (see Chapter 3). They may, for example, be capable of damaging the first-line, non-specific, immune defence mechanisms if they are toxic to host cells, or can cause sublethal injury that may interfere with cell functions without causing cell death. Alternatively, agents may be capable of interfering with the functioning of enzymes or other biologically active molecules in the respiratory secretions. The rates of clearance of inhaled particles are also influenced by their biophysical properties, such as size and shape; and their biochemical properties, such as solubility, ability to bind to host components and resistance to biodegradation.

Host factors

Host factors also have a bearing on the effects of inhaled agents. For example, innate or acquired defects in the host's non-specific immune defences can lead to inefficient clearance of inhaled agents, which may result in hypersensitivity reactions due to the prolonged stimulation of specific immunological responses. Defects in specific immune defence, either hyperreactivity in effector mechanisms or hyporeactivity in regulatory mechanisms, can also predispose to local immune hypersensitivity. In some diseases, including occupational lung diseases related to fibrogenic dusts, immune responses can be demonstrated against host tissue components ('autoimmune responses'), indicating that, for unknown reasons, host mechanisms that maintain immunological tolerance have been surmounted.

Secondary factors that can influence host immune responses

Apart from host factors, secondary factors, such as smoking or infection which damage the respiratory tract, can increase susceptibility to occupational lung diseases by interfering with clearance mechanisms. Smoking also interferes with the functions of many

cells that participate in immune and inflammatory responses, including alveolar macrophages, lymphocytes and natural killer cells (see under 'Immunopathology'). Heavy exposure to dust can also increase susceptibility to infections and in some situations, for example, the massive fibrotic response in patients with silicosis and pulmonary tuberculosis, the immune response to the infective agent may influence the response to the dust. These effects of smoking and infection in occupational lung diseases are described in greater detail in the relevant chapters.

Atopic status

Some individuals are predisposed to respond to organic antigens by producing specific antibodies of the IgE immunoglobulin class, also termed 'reaginic' antibodies. These subjects develop positive 'immediate' skin reactions when prick tested with such antigens: this is known as *atopy*. They are also prone to develop allergic diseases such as hay fever, rhinitis, urticaria and asthma when they are exposed to the sensitizing antigen. This aspect of immune response can cause disease in workers exposed to organic dusts of various kinds, and is also implicated in some types of occupational asthma (see under 'Immunopathology' and see also Chapter 21).

Genetic susceptibility

The major advances in molecular biology have shown that the development of specific immune responses is regulated by the *genotype* of the individual (see 'Genetic control of immune responses') providing one explanation for the considerable variation in immunological responsiveness between individuals. It is most probable that this information on the genetic control of immunological responses will lead to a greater understanding of the genetic factors associated with susceptibility to occupational lung diseases (see Chapter 15).

Non-specific (innate) immune defences

The maintenance of health depends on the ability of the host to achieve rapid elimination of the invading agent, and the 'first-line' non-specific (innate) immune defence barriers of the respiratory tract clear most inhaled agents before they ever reach the subepithelial tissues or other internal regions. These defences operate without any requirement for prior contact with, or specific sensitization to, the foreign invader.

The non-specific defence mechanisms progressively encountered in the respiratory tract are those described in the following subsections.

Nasopharyngeal region

The first defensive barriers encountered by inhaled agents are found in the nasopharyngeal region where particles can become trapped in the nasal hairs, the nasal secretions or saliva. Clearance of particles is then aided by mechanical propulsion mechanisms such as coughing, sneezing and swallowing. The respiratory secretions also contain bactericidal substances, for example, the enzyme lysozyme, a muraminidase optimally active at acid pH, which is capable of splitting the peptidoglycan wall of susceptible bacteria. Gram-positive bacteria have an exposed peptidoglycan wall and are especially sensitive to the action of lysozyme; Gram-negative bacteria are more resistant because their peptidoglycan wall is covered with an outer lipid bilayer. By contrast, mycobacteria have a compound cell wall and are extremely resistant to degradation. The main sources of lysozyme are phagocytic cells, such as macrophages and polymorphonuclear leucocytes, which have abundant stores of this, and other enzymes, in their cytoplasm within organelles known as lysosomes. The respiratory secretions also contain iron-binding proteins, including lactoferrin and transferrin which restrict the availability of free iron required for bacterial growth.

Tracheobronchial region

Microbial and other particles that escape the nasopharyngeal barriers and reach the tracheobronchial region are readily entrapped in the highly viscous mucus secretion which lines this region. This fluid consists of a complex mixture of mucus macromolecules which form a 'gel' layer on the surface of a continuous 'sol' phase adjacent to the epithelial cells. Particles are cleared by the continuous upward propulsion of the mucoid fluid which is induced by the wave-like beating of ciliated epithelial cells – the *mucociliary escalator*. These cells are abundant throughout the trachea and bronchi, but they become progressively sparser in the smaller airways

and are absent from the more peripheral bronchioles. They, and the 'mucociliary escalator', are discussed in Chapter 1 (under 'The chief cells of the airways').

Apart from mechanical clearance mechanisms, as for the other respiratory secretions, mucus also contains bacteriostatic substances such as lysozyme and lactoferrin and a variety of other molecules, including interferons, complement components and immunoglobulins, which contribute either to non-specific or specific host defence mechanisms.

Defective clearance from the tracheobronchial region can be the consequence of abnormalities in mucus production or damage to ciliated epithelial cells. Some types of damage to the epithelium can also result in increased permeability across the tight junctions between the epithelial cells, allowing easier access of foreign antigens to the many lymphocytes that are dispersed in the loose connective tissue of the lamina propria beneath the basement membrane of the bronchial epithelium, where they can more readily stimulate the specific immune system of the host and induce inflammatory reactions. Bronchial inflammation is a notable feature of the pathogenesis of asthma and bronchitis, both of which can occur as a consequence of exposure to certain occupational or environmental agents.

In a number of species, including the rat and rabbit, there is evidence that some of the lymphocytes in the walls of the large bronchi are organized into lymphoid aggregates in the lamina propria covered by a specialized squamous epithelium, which consists of cells devoid of cilia. These specialized lymphoid regions – *bronchus-associated lymphoid tissue* (BALT) – occur mainly near bifurcations of the bronchi (Bienenstock, Johnston and Percy, 1973; Bienenstock, 1984) (see Chapter 1, 'Lymphoid tissue'). The distinctive squamous epithelial cells which cover the BALT contain many plasmalemmal vesicles and they are involved in the selective transport of antigens from the bronchial lumen to the immunocompetent cells within BALT (Fournier et al., 1977). Because inhaled particles tend to be impacted near bifurcations of the bronchi, the position of BALT in these regions presumably facilitates antigen uptake. BALT shows many similarities to the specialized 'gut-associated lymphoid tissue' (GALT), namely the Peyer's patches in the ileal mucosa. These patches are covered by specialized 'M cells' ('microfold cells') which transport antigens across the surface epithelium from the gut into the subepithelial lymphoid tissue. Organized BALT structures are very difficult to detect in man and in a number of other species, but many lymphocytes and plasma cells are present, distributed diffusely and in loose collections, in the tissues beneath the basement membrane of the bronchial epithelium, and differentiation into lymphoid follicles can occur. Evidence of areas equivalent to the specialized epithelium of BALT is also very limited in human bronchial epithelium, but Holt et al. (1989) have recently reported that numerous 'dendritic' cells can be demonstrated in the basal zones of the bronchial epithelium, and it is conceivable that these play a role in antigen transport and in presentation of antigens to the subepithelial lymphocytes (see 'Antigen-presenting cells'). Lymphocytes are also present in the bronchial epithelium, and immunocytochemical studies indicate that there is a predominance of T-suppressor or T-cytotoxic cells in these locations (Fournier et al., 1989). By contrast, T-helper cells, which are involved in inducing specific immune reactions, are the predominant subtype of T lymphocytes in subepithelial locations in the bronchi (Azzawi et al., 1990). Many B lymphocytes and plasma cells are also present in subepithelial locations in the bronchi and these cells are thought to play an important role in local production of immunoglobulins, including IgA molecules that can bind to an additional fragment, termed *secretory piece*, synthesized by mucosal epithelial cells, to form 'secretory IgA', which is a specialized form of IgA found in the respiratory secretions (see under 'Specific (acquired) immune defences' – 'Lymphocytes and their subpopulations').

Respiratory bronchioles and alveoli

The terminal airspaces of the lungs, as for the remainder of the airways, are lined with fluid, but the composition is distinct from that of mucus. The major components of the fluid are the phospholipids and specialized apoproteins of the *pulmonary surfactant system*, which are produced by the type II alveolar epithelial lining cells. The main function of the pulmonary surfactant system is to form a surface-active film over the airspaces, which is capable of varying the surface tension at the air–liquid interface sufficiently to counteract the surface pressure that would otherwise cause the airways to fill with liquid and the alveoli to collapse at end-expiration. The main surface active component is dipalmitoyl phosphatidylcholine. However, the surfactant film also plays a role in host defence by entrapping and aiding clearance of particles that reach the alveoli, because it meets and merges with the film of mucus being transported on the mucociliary escalator.

Surfactant also has biological properties that aid host defence, although these have been investigated relatively little. It appears to enhance non-specific immune defences by exerting a chemotactic effect on macrophages, which may aid the recruitment of these cells to the airspaces (Zeligs, Nerurkar and Bellanti, 1977; Schwartz and Christman, 1979). It

also has opsonic properties which can aid the adherence of particles to macrophages, enhancing phagocytosis (Juers et al., 1976; O'Neill, Lesperance and Klass, 1984). In addition, it increases the ability of macrophages to kill bacteria by providing an additional source of lipid to generate toxic products of lipid peroxidation within the phagolysosomes (Juers et al., 1976).

By contrast with its ability to enhance non-specific immune defences, surfactant appears to play an important role in suppressing the development of specific immune responses in the airspaces of normal lungs. This is suggested by the evidence that normal pulmonary surfactant from all species so far investigated suppresses T-lymphocyte responses to antigens, mitogens and alloantigens (Ansfield et al., 1979; Ansfield and Benson, 1980; Wilsher, Hughes and Haslam, 1988a, 1988b; Wilsher, Parker and Haslam, 1990). The importance of such an immuno-suppressive mechanism in vivo is that it will help to prevent the constant development of specific immune and inflammatory reactions to inhaled antigens in the airspaces where there would be a risk of injury to the delicate gas-exchanging structures of the lungs. A number of observations suggest that compositional changes in pulmonary surfactant may favour the development of chronic inflammation. In the chronic inflammatory lung disease, cryptogenic fibrosing alveolitis (synonym: idiopathic diffuse interstitial pulmonary fibrosis), many patients have reduced proportions of phosphatidylglycerol and increased proportions of sphingomyelin in lung lavage fluids (Robinson et al., 1988; Hughes and Haslam, 1989) which return to normal, in parallel with falling inflammatory cell counts, in patients responding to corticosteroids (Hughes and Haslam, 1989). Reductions in phosphatidylglycerol have also been reported in the bleomycin model of pulmonary fibrosis (Thrall et al., 1987). It is not yet known whether similar compositional changes occur in pulmonary fibrosis associated with exposure to asbestos and other inorganic dusts, although it is well recognized that patients with silicosis can develop alveolar lipoproteinosis (Beuchner and Ansari, 1969; Heppleston, Fletcher and Wyatt, 1974; Dethloff et al., 1985) (see Chapter 5, under 'Lipidosis').

Another important non-specific defence barrier in the terminal airspaces, which helps to restrict the development of specific immune responses, is the structure of the alveolar epithelium. The junctions between the alveolar epithelial cells are tighter, and there appears to be less capacity for particles to traverse the epithelium, than in the conducting airways. However, changes in permeability can be induced by a wide variety of toxic substances (Boucher and Ranga, 1988) and, thus, increase access of particles to the interstitial tissues. They are then more likely to stimulate the specific immune system because recent evidence suggests that *the* most potent antigen-presenting cell types (Weissler et al., 1986) *and functional lymphocytes* (Kaltreider and Salmon, 1973; Kirby et al., 1985; Weissler et al., 1987) *in the lungs are found in interstitial locations*.

Finally, the terminal airspaces are the main sites where alveolar macrophages reside. They are the main 'free' cell type in the lung lining fluid, although studies using the technique of bronchoalveolar lavage have indicated that the lining fluid of normal lungs can also contain up to 20 per cent of lymphocytes, which are mainly T lymphocytes with phenotypes similar to those in normal blood (Semenzato et al., 1986) (see under 'Specific (acquired) immune defences: Antigen-presenting cells'). However, despite the fact that alveolar macrophages are potential antigen-presenting cells and that they encounter numerous inhaled potential antigens each day, they do not appear constantly to stimulate the lymphocytes that reside in the fluids to mount specific immune reactions. This would clearly be disadvantageous to the host because it would lead to a constant state of immune hyperreactivity near to the delicate alveolar epithelium. This appears to be due partly to the fact that normal alveolar macrophages have poor antigen-presenting function and partly to the fact that the responses of the lymphocytes that reside in the airspaces appear to be down-regulated (Kaltreider and Salmon, 1973; Robinson, Pinkston and Crystal, 1984; Kirby et al., 1985), possibly, in part, as a result of the immuno-suppressive action of pulmonary surfactant components. Because specific immune responses are down-regulated in the airspaces, innate immune functions appear to be the main functions of alveolar macrophages in normal lungs. They can move freely over the epithelial surfaces by extending pseudopodia and they are the 'sentry' cells that aid host defences through their potent phagocytic and microbicidal functions. However, like other cells of the monocyte/macrophage lineage, alveolar macrophages have the capacity to perform numerous other functions when appropriately stimulated; in certain disorders, they appear to contribute in specific as well as in non-specific immune responses. They also have the capacity to produce a wide range of inflammatory mediators and regulators, and there is much evidence that persistent stimulation of alveolar macrophages, maintaining their activation over an abnormally prolonged period, may play a key role in the pathogenesis of many chronic inflammatory lung diseases, including those related to occupational agents (see 'Immunopathology').

Alveolar macrophages

The morphology and locations of the alveolar macrophages are described in Chapter 1 ('Free

pulmonary cells'). Their main function in normal pulmonary immune defence is to maintain alveolar sterility by phagocytosing and degrading microbes and particles that reach the terminal airspaces. Although these are innate immune functions which do not require specific recognition of foreign antigens, specialized surface receptors are present on the surface membranes of macrophages (and other phagocytes) which enable them to recognize and bind with a number of ligands on particles or microbes, facilitating their phagocytic uptake. The body also possesses mechanisms to enhance phagocytosis, which involve coating the particles or microbes with a variety of opsonic molecules present in body fluids. These provide additional ligands to aid attachment to cell surface receptors. Receptor binding also activates the events that transport the bound agents into the phagocytes where killing and digestion take place within intra-cytoplasmic vacuoles (phagosomes) without causing harm to the cell.

Opsonins

The major opsonins present in lung-lining fluid, which can coat particles and microbes preparing them for phagocytosis, include immunoglobulins, in particular IgG and IgA, complement components, surfactant phospholipids and glycoproteins such as *fibronectin* (see Chapter 5, 'Basal conditions'). Coating with immunoglobulin can occur either non-specifically or by binding with specific antibodies, which may be present in the body fluids if the individual has previously encountered the agent and mounted a specific immune response. The complement system provides an important source of additional opsonins, which can be generated if the bound antibody is of an immunoglobulin class (for example, IgG1 or IgG3) which can activate the complement system via the classical pathway (Figure 4.1a). A fragment of the third component of complement, C3b, is a potent opsonin that can bind to the surfaces of microbes, particles, immune complexes or cell membranes by forming covalent bonds with exposed hydroxyl or amino groups. Many bacteria, viruses, fungi and parasites are capable of activating the complement system directly, thus non-specifically generating the opsonin C3b without the need for immunoglobulin. This usually occurs via the *alternative pathway of complement activation* (Figure 4.1a), although some agents, for example retroviruses, can activate

Figure 4.1 (a) Classical and alternative pathways of complement activation. (b) Terminal lytic sequence of complement activation

(a)

Classical pathway (activated by immune complexes or other classical pathway activators)

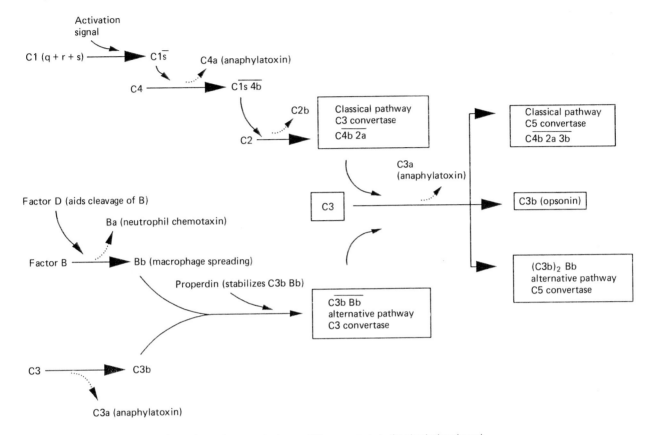

Alternative pathway (activated by alternative pathway activators or C3b generated via the classical pathway)

(b)

Lytic pathway

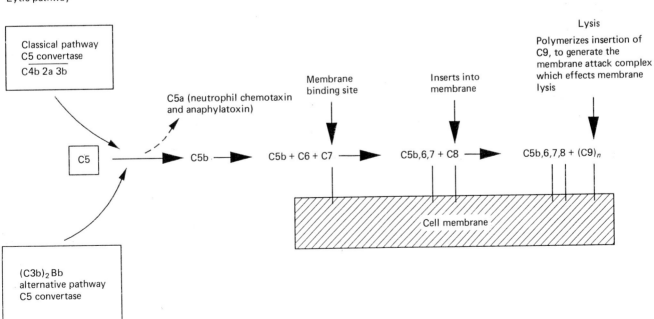

complement via the classical pathway (Kolb, 1988). Many other particles including asbestos fibres (Wilson, Gaumer and Salvaggio, 1977) can also activate the alternative pathway of complement directly.

Opsonins can enhance phagocytosis because receptors are present on the surface membranes of phagocytic cells that can recognize and bind with specific groupings on the opsonins. It is presumed that receptors are present for all known opsonins, but the best characterized are the receptors for the Fc region of immunoglobulin molecules and the receptors for complement components (Ross, Walport and Hogg, 1989; Sibille and Reynolds, 1990). A brief review of these receptors follows.

Fc receptors

Phagocytes constitutively express receptors for the Fc region of immunoglobulin molecules, which play a major role in the recognition, binding and phagocytosis of particles or microbes which have become coated (opsonized) with immunoglobulin molecules. Some agents, for example staphylococci, can bind IgG directly (Verbrugh et al., 1982), whereas others may become coated through immune complex formation with specific antibodies directed against antigenic components on the microbes or particles. 'Natural antibodies' which recognize common carbohydrate structures shared between bacteria are also present in body fluids and participate in the opsonic process.

Fc receptors for three immunoglobulin classes – IgG, IgA and IgE – have been demonstrated on human monocytes and macrophages and these are termed 'Fcγ, Fcα and Fcε receptors', respectively. Fc receptors for IgG predominate and have been most fully investigated (Rossman and Douglas, 1988; Ross, Walport and Hogg, 1989; Sibille and Reynolds, 1990). Fc receptors for all four subclasses of IgG (IgG1, IgG2, IgG3 and IgG4) have been detected on human monocytes and macrophages (Huber et al., 1971; Alexander et al., 1975), and also on human alveolar macrophages (Naegel, Young and Reynolds, 1984), but there are more binding sites for IgG1 and IgG3 than for IgG2 and IgG4 (Naegel, Young and Reynolds, 1984). IgG2 and IgG4 are also less efficient opsonins because they bind with lower affinity to Fc receptors, and IgG4 also fails to activate complement thus failing to generate additional opsonins in the form of C3b (Ross, Walport and Hogg, 1989). The change that occurs in the Fc region of IgG molecules following their interaction with antigens to form immune complexes (or their aggregation by heating) markedly increases the avidity of their binding to Fc receptors. Free (monomeric) IgG can also bind to Fc receptors but, unlike the case for immune-

complex-bound IgG, the binding is of low avidity and can be readily reversed by washing the phagocytes (Knutson, Kijlstra and Van Es, 1977).

Three structurally distinct Fcγ receptors – Fcγ-R1, Fcγ-R2 and Fcγ-R3 – consisting of glycoproteins of molecular weights between 42×10^6 and 72×10^6 daltons, have been identified on human macrophages (Ross, Walport and Hogg, 1989) and all three forms are present on alveolar macrophages (Levy et al., 1988). However, human monocytes express only Fcγ-R1 and Fcγ-R2 (Ross, Walport and Hogg, 1989). The three types of Fcγ receptors are also found on neutrophils, and some are found on non-phagocytic cells including Fcγ-R2 on eosinophils and platelets and Fcγ-R3 on natural killer cells (Ross, Walport and Hogg, 1989).

Although Fc receptors for IgG are the most common, it is now recognized that monocytes and macrophages, including human alveolar macrophages, can also express Fcε receptors for IgE (Melewicz et al., 1982; Spiegelberg et al., 1983) and Fcα receptors for IgA (Gauldie, Richards and Lamontagne, 1983; Sibille et al., 1989). Binding of IgE-containing immune complexes to Fcε receptors in vitro has been shown to induce macrophages to release arachidonic acid metabolites, including leukotriene C_4 which is one of the mediators implicated in the pathogenesis of 'late' allergic reactions (see under 'Immunopathology') (Rankin et al., 1982; Rouzer et al., 1982); and alveolar macrophages from asthmatic subjects have been reported to express greater numbers of Fcε receptors than those from control subjects (Joseph et al., 1983). IgA is one of the major immunoglobulin classes in the respiratory lining fluids, but early studies failed to detect Fcα receptors on alveolar macrophages (Reynolds, Kazmierowski and Newhall, 1975; Reynolds et al., 1975). However, more recent evidence indicates that these cells can bind both monomeric and polymeric forms of IgA1 and IgA2 (Sibille et al., 1989), and that binding to Fcα receptors can mediate phagocytosis (Richards and Gauldie, 1985).

The body appears to have mechanisms to increase Fc receptor expression, presumably to enhance phagocytosis when necessary, because several products that are produced during the course of immune and inflammatory reactions can increase Fc receptor expression. These include interferon-γ, a lymphokine produced by activated T lymphocytes (Friedman et al., 1980; Guyre, Morganelli and Miller, 1983); fibronectin – a glycoprotein produced by many cell types including activated alveolar macrophages, which aids cellular attachment to the intracellular connective tissues (Bevilacqua et al., 1981); peptide products of bacteria (Rossman et al., 1982); and 1,25-dihydroxy-vitamin D_3, which is produced in increased amounts by alveolar macrophages in some situations (Maliszewski, Shen and Fanger, 1985).

Following binding to Fc receptors, phagocytosis of some types of particles may occur independently of other cell surface receptors (Griffin, Bianco and Silverstein, 1975), but in many cases Fc-receptor binding appears to act synergistically with other cell surface receptors, in particular complement receptors (Griffin, Bianco and Silverstein, 1975; Scornik, 1976).

Complement receptors

The majority of particles and microbes that become coated with immunoglobulin also become coated with C3b, because many immunoglobulins activate the complement system after they bind with antigen. Microbes and particles that can directly activate the complement system also become coated with C3b (Pangburn, 1983; Weinberg et al., 1984). Bound C3b can adhere to a *complement receptor*, termed 'CR1', which is present on the surface of phagocytes, including monocytes, macrophages and neutrophils, and also on some other cell types including eosinophils, B lymphocytes, T lymphocytes and erythrocytes. CR1 is a glycoprotein and there are four allotypic variants ranging in molecular weight from 160 000 to 260 000 daltons. Apart from its opsonic properties, bound C3b also amplifies complement activation by providing the site for assembly of the convertase enzyme that activates the alternative pathway of complement generating further fragments of C3b; it also promotes assembly of the C5 convertase enzyme that allows the lytic sequence of the complement system to proceed to completion (Figure 4.1b). The opsonic activity of C3b is relatively limited because it is very rapidly degraded by binding with the inhibitor factor H which acts as a pro-factor potentiating the enzymatic cleavage of C3b by the inhibitor factor I. However, this leaves an inactivated fragment, iC3b, bound to the particles which has potent opsonic properties, although it cannot continue to activate the complement system; iC3b binds with structurally distinct receptors, termed 'CR3', which are present in high density on monocytes, neutrophils, cytotoxic T cells, natural killer (NK) cells and eosinophils, and in low density on macrophages. The increased opsonic efficiency of iC3b relates to its longer half-life compared with C3b (approximately 30 minutes compared with seconds). Any iC3b remaining bound to CR1 receptors can be further degraded by factor I leaving a smaller bound fragment, C3dg, and this can be further degraded by proteolytic enzymes (for example, plasmin and neutrophil elastase) leaving a smaller bound fragment C3d. Both C3dg and C3d have a reduced binding affinity for CR1 and CR3 and, thus, have poor opsonic activity, but C3d can bind to a distinct receptor, CR2, which is present on lymphocytes.

Tissue macrophages frequently have low expression of CR1 and CR3 receptors compared with monocytes and neutrophils, but have higher expression of another receptor, CR4, which also binds iC3b (Myones et al., 1988). Similar to other macrophages, alveolar macrophages also express surface receptors for bound complement (Reynolds et al., 1975a; Daughday and Douglas, 1976; Warr and Martin, 1977), but less is known about the actual structural types.

Complement receptors differ from Fc receptors in that they are not constitutively expressed, but are stored in the cytoplasm until the cells are stimulated with products of inflammation such as interleukin-1 (see under 'Specific (acquired) immune defences') and C5a. They facilitate particle adherence to phagocytes but usually act synergistically with Fc and other receptors to mediate phagocytosis. The types, structure and functions of C3 receptors have been reviewed in detail by Ross, Walport and Hogg (1989), Kolb (1988) and Rossman and Douglas (1988).

Other receptors involved in phagocytosis

Monocytes and macrophages also express a number of other receptors involved in phagocytosis, including receptors for terminal sugar residues of polysaccharides and glycoproteins (mannosyl–fucosyl receptors) which aid the phagocytosis of bacteria and fungi and in the removal of effete cells and glycoproteins (Gordon and Mokoena, 1989).

Degradation and killing mechanisms

Following attachment of particles or microbes to macrophages, the events which complete the process of phagocytosis are activated. Pseudopodia are extended around the particle and the portion of the plasma membrane surrounding the particle is invaginated into the cell to form an intracellular vacuole. Small particles or fluids may also be taken into the cells by the process of pinocytosis which results in the incorporation of small plasmalemmal vesicles. Inside the cell, the vacuoles can fuse with lysosomes to form 'secondary lysosomes' or 'phagosomes' where digestive and killing processes take place. The lysosomes are of variable forms, but all contain stores of powerful degradative enzymes and toxic molecules that are used to degrade ingested substances and inactivate and kill micro-organisms. The presence of numerous lysosomes and vacuoles within the cytoplasm is a most notable feature of alveolar macrophages at ultrastructural level (Figure 4.2a).

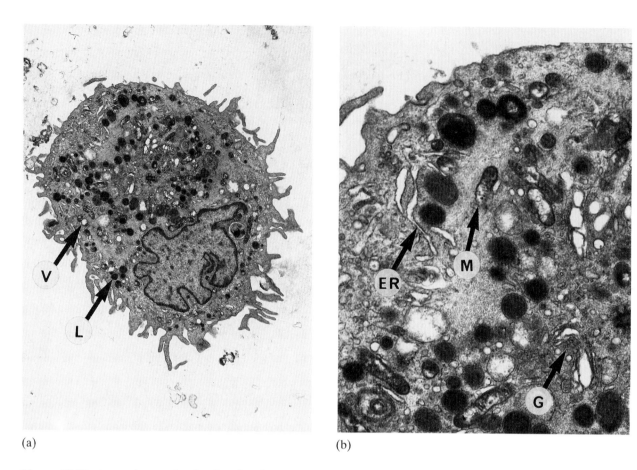

(a)   (b)

Figure 4.2 Electron micrographs showing the ultrastructural appearance of an alveolar macrophage: (a) low power appearance (magnification × 5000) showing the numerous lysosomes (L) and vacuoles (V) within the cytoplasm of the cell; (b) high power appearance of the cytoplasm of the same cell (magnification × 15 350) showing the Golgi apparatus (G), endoplasmic reticulum (ER) and mitochondria (M). (By courtesy of Ann Dewar)

The lysosomes contain a wide range of hydrolytic enzymes including acid hydrolases, lysozyme, lipoprotein lipase and neutral proteases such as collagenase and elastase that can degrade most phagocytosed materials. Macrophages also use oxygen-dependent metabolic pathways to generate highly toxic derivatives of molecular oxygen within the phagolysosomes that can kill micro-organisms. The pathways leading to release of oxidants are not as well worked out in monocytes and macrophages as they are in polymorphonuclear leucocytes, but they result in the release of highly reactive oxidizing agents including hydrogen peroxide, superoxide anion, hydroxyl radicals and singlet oxygen. Toxic oxygen metabolites are short lived but they can act on proteins, carbohydrates and lipids. They may also be involved in the cytotoxic mechanisms used by macrophages to mediate extracellular killing of tumour cells or cells expressing foreign antigens, for example virus-infected cells or allografts.

The functions of macrophages are not simply restricted to phagocytosis and degradation of particles and micro-organisms. They can produce and release into the extracellular milieu many other important products that aid in host defence. These include factors that can recruit neutrophils to the reaction site to aid phagocytosis of microbes, particles and damaged tissue cells, factors which can aid in healing by promoting wound repair, and many other factors (Table 4.1). However, excessive production of these factors can induce pathological reactions as described under 'Immunopathology'.

The high level of metabolic activity of alveolar macrophages is reflected at the ultrastructural level by their well-developed Golgi apparatus and endoplasmic reticulum, which are the organelles involved in the synthesis and transport of newly synthesized proteins, and by their pronounced mitochondria which are the organelles concerned with cell respiration (Figure 4.2b).

Table 4.1 Secretory products of macrophages

Enzymes
  Lysozyme
  Neutral proteases
    Collagenase
    Elastase
    Plasminogen activator
    Angiotensin-converting enzyme
  Lysosomal acid hydrolases
    Proteases
    Lipases
    Ribonucleases
    Phosphatases
    Glycosidases
    Sulphates
  Lipoprotein lipase
Enzyme inhibitors
  Antiproteases
    α_1-Antiprotease
    α_2-Macroglobulin
    Collagenase inhibitor
    Plasminogen activator inhibitors
    Plasma inhibitor
Bioactive lipids
  Cyclo-oxygenase products
    Prostaglandins (PG) E_2, $F_{2\alpha}$
    Prostacyclin (PGI)
    Thromboxane A_2 (TxA_2)
  Lipoxygenase products
    Leukotrienes B_4, C_4, D_4
    5-Hydroxyeicosatetraenoic acid
  Platelet-activating factor
Reactive oxygen intermediates
  Superoxide
  Hydrogen peroxide
  Hydroxyl radical
  Hypohalous acids
Antioxidants
  Glutathione
Reactive nitrogen intermediates
  Nitrites
  Nitrates

Nucleosides and their products
  Thymidine
  Uracil
  Uric acid
  Deoxycytidine
  Neopterin
Complement components and inhibitors
  C1, C4, C2, C3 and C5
  Factors B, D and properdin
  C1 inhibitor
  C3b inactivator and β-1H
Coagulation factors
  Factors V, VII, IX, X
  Plasminogen activator
Binding proteins
  Transferrin
  Ferritins
  Fibronectin
  Laminin
  Apolipoprotein E
  Avidin
Cytokine mediators and hormones
  IL1α and IL1β
  TNFα
  Interferon-α (INFα)
  IL6
  IL8 (neutrophil chemotactic factor)
  Colony stimulating factors:
    Granulocytes and macrophages (GM-CSF)
    Granulocytes (G-CSF)
    Macrophages (M-CSF)
  Fibroblast growth factor (insulin growth factor 1)
  'Platelet-derived growth factor'
  TGFβ
  1,25-Dihydroxyvitamin D_3
  β-Endorphin
  Adrenocorticotrophic hormone
Other inhibitors
  IL1 inhibitor
  Phospholipase inhibitor: lipomodulin

Specific (acquired) immune defences

Invertebrates and lower vertebrates utilize mainly innate mechanisms of immune defence, but human and other higher vertebrates have 'second-line' immune defence mechanisms which can be invoked if foreign agents breach the 'first-line' innate defences and gain access to the tissues and internal regions of the body. The *'second-line' defences* are mediated by antigen-presenting cells and lymphocytes and are stimulated as a specific response to molecular configurations on the foreign invader that are not present on the cells of the host. Agents capable of stimulating a specific immune response are termed 'antigens'. By contrast with innate immune defence mechanisms, which are constitutively available throughout the body, the 'second-line' defences are an *adaptive* response to appropriate antigenic stimulation and they are thus termed 'specific' or 'acquired immune defences'. Although the innate and specific immune defences are described in separate sections of this chapter for clarity, there is an important interplay between the two systems that enhances the overall efficiency of both. The ability of specific antibodies to act as opsonins enhancing the uptake of particles by phagocytes is one example, and many other examples will be apparent throughout this chapter.

The importance of the interplay between different components of immune responses cannot be over-emphasized. Numerous products are generated which have many different effects, some acting as mediators of immune and inflammatory reactions whilst others act as regulators; some have the potential to cause tissue damage whilst others are involved in the mechanisms of healing. Indeed, the events in an immune and inflammatory reaction site are often referred to as a 'soup' due to their complexity. It is not surprising that the final outcome of the reactions cannot, in all situations, be accurately predicted. Although basic immunological mechanisms are usually described separately for clarity, the reader must bear in mind that in real life they are inevitably subject to the influence of many other immune and inflammatory events in the same location.

Antigens

As implied above, a single foreign agent can have many molecular configurations in its structure which the host may recognize as foreign. Under appropriate conditions, the host may mount specific immune responses against each distinct configuration. Such molecular configurations are termed *antigenic determinants* or *epitopes*. It is clear that epitopes present on one particular agent may also form part of the structure of other agents and this explains why specific immune responses raised against one agent may give cross-reactions with other agents.

The ability of different molecular structures to act as antigens varies for many reasons. In the context of this brief chapter, it is probably sufficient to state that 'antigenic determinants' are usually polypeptides, glycoproteins or glycolipids, whereas pure lipids and nucleic acids are poor immunogens. In addition, molecules of high molecular weight are generally better antigens than those of low molecular weight. Low-molecular-weight substances, too small to be immunogenic, can, however, become immunogenic if they are capable of forming chemical complexes with larger molecules, such as body proteins, that can act as carriers. Low-molecular-weight substances complexed in this way are known as *haptens*. Haptenic interactions can have potentially adverse effects on the host, and good examples of this are the hypersensitivity reactions that can be induced by chemicals such as picryl chloride and formaldehyde, and by drugs such as aspirin, penicillin and sulphonamides. The mechanisms of immune tolerance, which prevent the host from mounting specific immune responses against its own body components, can also be bypassed if haptenic or other interactions occur which render changes to their structures. In some diseases, including inorganic dust diseases, there is an increased prevalence of immune responses to components of host tissues. These are termed *autoimmune responses* and they are discussed in more detail under 'Immunopathology'.

Antigen-presenting cells

Specific immune responses are mediated by two main classes of lymphocytes: B lymphocytes which mature in the bone marrow of mammals, and T lymphocytes which mature in the thymus. T lymphocytes require the help of specialized 'antigen-presenting cells' in order to recognize, bind with and respond to antigens. By contrast, B lymphocytes can bind with antigens in their native or 'free form'. However, only a small number of antigens termed *T-cell independent antigens* can induce B cells to produce all the signals that they require to complete their proliferation and maturation into antibody-producing cells. To respond to the majority of antigens, B lymphocytes also require the help of factors released from activated T-helper lymphocytes after their interaction with antigen-presenting cells (see the next section). These antigens are consequently termed *T-cell dependent antigens*.

Antigen receptors are present in the surface membranes of B lymphocytes which have almost the same immunoglobulin structure, and the same antigenic specificity, as that of the antibody effector molecules secreted by each B cell (see the next section). The specificity of different immunoglobulin molecules (antibodies or B-cell immunoglobulin receptors) for different antigens is determined by variable regions in the molecules which contain the *antigen-binding sites*, and each antigen-binding site is specific for a particular antigenic determinant.

The antigen receptors on T lymphocytes are very different from those on B lymphocytes. They can only recognize and bind with antigens that have become attached to, or incorporated by, cells in the body, and that are accessible at the surface of the cell in association with products of the genes of the *major histocompatibility complex* (MHC). The MHC products of different individuals differ due to allotypic differences between individuals, and only individuals of the same genotype, for example, identical twins, express exactly the same MHC molecules. T cells only recognize antigens in association with MHC molecules on cells of the same genotype as themselves; thus, T-cell responses are MHC restricted. There are two main groups of MHC molecules known as 'class I' and 'class II'.

T-helper lymphocytes, which aid the clonal expansion of T- and most B-lymphocyte populations, can only recognize and respond to antigens in association with class II MHC products on the surface of antigen-presenting cells. Only a limited range of host cells express class II MHC products, and they cannot all act as antigen-presenting cells. An antigen-presenting function requires not only that cells express class II products, but also that they are able to 'process' antigens and release *cytokine mediators* (in particular interleukin-1), which are required for the initial steps of T-helper cell activation. The main types of classic antigen-presenting cells in the body include Langerhan's cells, which are found in the skin lining the junction of the epidermis and dermis. These cells carry antigens from the skin into the draining lymph nodes. Within the paracortex of lymph nodes, antigen-presenting cells, termed 'inter-digitating dendritic cells', come into close contact with T-helper lymphocytes; 'interdigitating cells' are also found in the thymus. Blood monocytes and tissue macrophages can, in addition, be induced to express class II MHC molecules and function as antigen-presenting cells; however, alveolar macrophages are relatively inefficient (see later). B lymphocytes express class II MHC antigens and can present antigens to T-helper lymphocytes. The majority of other body cells do not express class II MHC antigens constitutively, but they are expressed on a high proportion of T lymphocytes following their activation. Many tissue cell types, including epithelial cells and endothelial cells, can also be induced to express these products by the cytokine interferon-γ which is produced by activated T cells (Geppert and Lipsky, 1987). It is thought that such tissue cells may play a role in amplifying localized cell-mediated hypersensitivity reactions, and in the pathogenesis of certain disorders where anti-tissue reactions are implicated. Thus, whereas primary specific immune responses rely on classic antigen-presenting cells, secondary immune responses can involve a much wider range of cell types that have acquired antigen-presenting capacity.

The structure of the antigen receptors on T lymphocytes is very different to those on B lympho-cytes. Each receptor consists of two polypeptide chains that contain the antigen-binding site; there are millions of different clones of T lymphocytes with antigen-binding sites selective for different antigenic determinants. In the most common form of T-cell receptor, the two polypeptide chains are α- and β-chains. Each chain has two regions, the outer having a variable amino acid sequence that deter-mines the antigenic specificity of the T cell. There is another subpopulation of T cells, which expresses a less common form of T-cell receptor having γ and δ polypeptide chains containing the antigen-binding site. Three other polypeptide chains, termed 'CD3' molecules are associated with each T-cell antigen receptor, and these are common to all T cells (see the next section). They are involved in the signal transduction steps which induce the activation of the T cells following antigen binding to the receptor.

Other molecules are also associated with the T-cell antigen receptors; these participate in the recog-nition and binding of T cells to MHC molecules. CD4 molecules on T-helper lymphocytes aid in binding these cells to class II MHC molecules on antigen-presenting cells. By contrast, T-cytotoxic lymphocytes express CD8 molecules which aid in binding to antigens in association with class I MHC molecules on the surface of the target cells (see next section and under 'Immune defences against tumour cells').

The MHC restriction of the T-cell response is one of the reasons why there are genetically determined differences between individuals in their immune responses to the same antigens.

The identity of the main antigen-presenting cell types in the lungs is still under investigation. Although alveolar macrophages express class II MHC products, and are present in large numbers in the airspaces of normal lungs, there have been many reports that normal human alveolar macrophages have poor antigen-presenting function (Holt, 1987). 'Macrophages' extracted from interstitial locations in lung tissue appear to be much more efficient antigen-presenting cells (Weissler et al., 1986). Strong expression of class II MHC products has also been reported on type II alveolar epithelial cells in patients with the fibrosing lung disease, cryptogenic fibrosing alveolitis; it has been suggested that such cells may play a role in stimulating the autoimmune reactions that occur in this disease (Kallenberg et al., 1987). Expression of class II MHC antigens has also been demonstrated on lung fibroblasts follow-ing their interaction with interferon-γ (Phipps et al., 1989) and on endothelial cells in the lungs of patients following heart–lung transplantation (Taylor, Rose and Yacoub, 1989).

Lymphocytes and their subpopulations

After binding of antigen to antigen receptors on lymphocytes, events take place which result in the proliferation, maturation and differentiation of the clone of lymphocytes committed to the elimination of that particular antigen. At birth, each clone contains only a small number of cells; and these lymphocytes are termed *naïve cells*. After contact with antigen, they undergo clonal expansion, matur-ation and differentiation to mount what is termed the *primary immune response* against the agent. When the agent has been eliminated, the effector cells involved in the response are suppressed, but some of the lymphocytes persist as long-lived 'memory cells' so that a greater number of committed lymphocytes is available to attack the agent if it is encountered a second time. This is known as 'immunological memory' and it explains why, in specific immunity, the *secondary immune response* to an agent is stronger than the primary one. (The cells involved in non-specific immune responses retain no memory of previous encounters, but their efficiency can be enhanced by products generated from coexisting specific immune response.)

Of the two main classes of lymphocytes, B lymphocytes produce the antibody mediators of the *humoral limb of specific immunity* and T lymphocytes mediate the *cellular limb of specific immunity*. T lymphocytes also play a major role in regulating both limbs of the specific immune response.

B lymphocytes

As explained in the previous section, the majority of antigens (T-dependent antigens) can only stimulate B lymphocytes to proliferate and mature into antibody-producing cells, with the help of regulatory molecules released from activated T-helper lymphocytes, although a few antigens (T-independent antigens) can drive B lymphocytes into proliferation and maturation without the help of T lymphocytes. A summary of the events that follow antigen binding to B lymphocytes is shown in Figure 4.3.

T-independent antigens are large polymeric molecules with repeating antigenic determinants in their structure which are able to cross-link adjacent antigen receptors on the surface membrane of the B cell. This cross-linking appears sufficient to activate the B cell to begin clonal expansion and complete its differentiation into mature antibody-secreting plasma cells without further help. Although there are *five main immunoglobulin classes of antibodies* (IgM, IgG, IgA, IgE and IgD), both the primary and the secondary immune responses to T-independent antigens are generally weaker than those for T-dependent antigens, and both are mainly limited to production of IgM antibodies. At high concentrations, some T-independent antigens can induce polyclonal activation of B cells stimulating B-cell clones that are not specific to the antigen. T-independent antigens are also frequently very resistant to degradation (Roitt, Brostoff and Male, 1989). It is interesting to reflect that, in asbestosis, there is evidence of polyclonal activation of B cells indicated by polyclonal increases in serum immunoglobulin levels, and the anti-nuclear antibodies that occur in the sera of these patients are of low titre and predominantly of the IgM class (Haslam, 1976). Examples of known T-independent antigens include bacterial lipopolysaccharide, polymeric bacterial flagellin and Epstein–Barr virus.

B-lymphocyte responses to T-dependent antigens are promoted by cytokine factors (see 'Cytokine mediators', later) released from activated T-helper lymphocytes (Figure 4.3). The cytokines derived from lymphocytes are frequently termed *lymphokines* and recombinant-DNA technology has made available pure preparations of several human lymphokines, so that it has been possible to assess their ability to replace T-helper cells in experiments of B-cell responses to antigens in vitro. B lymphocytes spend a short time in the blood and are found mainly in the lymphoid organs and bone marrow. In the lymphoid organs, they interact with T-helper lymphocytes and antigen-presenting cells, and all three cell types are required for the induction of T-dependent B-cell responses. The 'naïve' B cells bind via their antigen receptors with free antigen, or possibly with antigen fragments released from antigen-presenting cells, and this provides a 'priming' signal that activates the cells in readiness for proliferation. Lymphokines released from activated T-helper cells are then required to drive the B cells to complete their proliferation, maturation into plasma cells and secretion of immunoglobulins. The activation of T-helper lymphocytes occurs following binding of their antigen receptors to antigen in association with class II MHC molecules on the surface of antigen-presenting cells. This results in the release of a cytokine termed 'interleukin-1' (IL1) by the antigen-presenting cells which aids the activation of T-helper cells resulting in the release of at least 20 known lymphokine factors. The exact identity of the lymphokines that aid B-cell activation and differentiation in human beings is still under investigation, but current evidence suggests that the activation step involves B-cell growth factor$_{low}$ (BCGF$_{low}$) and interleukin-4 (IL4); that these two factors, interleukin-2 (IL2) and interferon-γ (IFNγ,) are involved in the proliferation step; and that all these factors and IL6 are involved in the differentiation to plasma cells. IL5 has also been shown to be involved in the proliferation and differentiation of B cells in a murine model. In addition, it has been shown that the cytokines, IL1 and *tumour necrosis factor* (TNFα) released by activated antigen-presenting cells, can enhance B-cell activation.

The primary immune response to T-dependent antigens, similar to that to T-independent antigens, mainly results in the production of IgM antibodies, but the secondary immune response is much stronger and molecules of other immunoglobulin classes, in particular IgG, are also generated. The mechanisms that determine which class of immunoglobulin is secreted by plasma cells (that is, IgM, IgG, IgA, IgE or IgD) are not well understood, but there is evidence that lymphokine factors may play a role. For example, recent observations suggest that IL4 can act as a differentiation factor

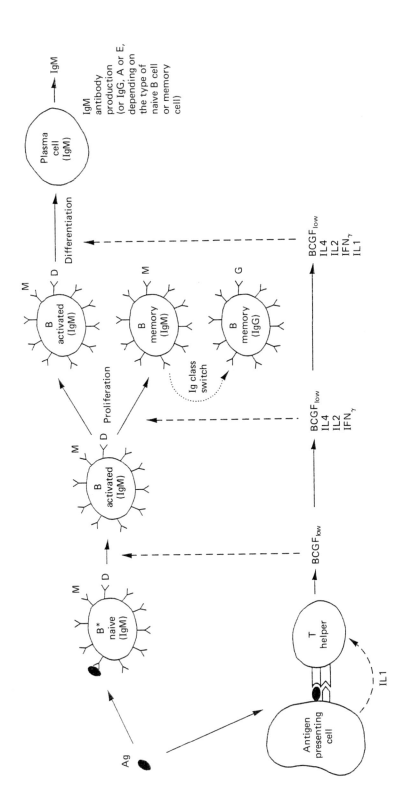

Figure 4.3 Events that follow binding of T-dependent antigens to B lymphocytes. * Naïve IgM B cells have IgM and IgD surface receptors for antigen; naïve IgG B cells have IgM, -D and -G surface receptors; naïve IgA cells have IgM, -D and -A surface receptors; and naïve IgE B cells have IgM, -D and -E surface receptors. B-memory cells have only one type of surface receptor (IgM, -G, -A or -E) and Ig receptors are not expressed on plasma cells

stimulating the production of IgE by B cells (Finkelman et al., 1986; Nomo et al., 1986). 'Naïve' B cells contain the genes for all the different immunoglobulin classes and they can express antigen receptors of more than one immunoglobulin type, although the majority express IgM and IgD. During the primary immune response, only mRNA for the first gene in the sequence, namely the heavy chain of IgM, is transcribed; thus, only IgM is secreted. The formation of memory B cells during the primary immune response appears, however, to involve a recombination event resulting in immunoglobulin class switching and the generation of many memory cells expressing IgG receptors, as well as those expressing IgM. This explains why the secondary response to antigen predominantly involves the production of IgG antibodies. Class switching to IgA and IgE memory cells can also occur (Davey, 1989).

The immunoglobulin antibodies generated as a result of B-lymphocyte activation are the effector molecules of the humoral limb of specific immunity. After release they can persist in the body fluids for weeks after the primary immune response, and for months or even years after the secondary immune response to antigen. They have no biological effect until they encounter, and bind with, the specific antigen; then, a number of changes take place in the structure of the Fc region of the antibody molecule which facilitate antigen removal. The binding of the 'activated' Fc region of the antibody to the Fc receptors on phagocytic cells is enhanced, thus aiding removal of the antigen by phagocytes. Cell-mediated cytotoxic responses are also aided by interaction between antibody-coated targets and the Fc receptors on cytotoxic cells, bringing the cytotoxic cells and the antibody-coated targets into close contact (see under 'Immune defences against tumour cells'). The Fc region of bound antibody can also activate the complement system via the 'classical pathway' enabling the terminal 'lytic sequence' of complement components to exert a lytic effect on antigen-bearing targets (see Figure 4.1b). Fragments of activated complement components can also act as inflammatory mediators recruiting inflammatory cells to the reaction site, so enhancing non-specific immune reactions. C5a has a strong chemotactic attraction for granulocytes; both C5a and C3a are anaphylatoxins capable of activating the degranulation of mast cells, thereby leading to the release of many other pro-inflammatory mediators (see under 'Immunopathology'). Another advantageous effect of antibodies is that their binding to infective agents, for example viruses, can neutralize infectivity by preventing the attachment of the agent to host cells. The phagocytic removal of small antigens is also aided by antibodies, because each antibody molecule has at least two binding sites for antigen and most agents express more than one antigenic determinant; consequently, aggregated immune complexes can form that are more readily phagocytosed.

Different classes and subclasses of immunoglobulins vary in their ability to mediate the above functions; individuals vary in their genetic predisposition to produce antibodies of different immunoglobulin classes and subclasses. This explains the increased susceptibility of some individuals to develop certain types of antibody-mediated immune hypersensitivity reactions, for example, type I IgE-mediated hypersensitivity (see under 'Immunopathology'). Table 4.2 shows the biological activities of the main immunoglobulin classes and subclasses in man.

The profile of immunoglobulin classes found in the respiratory secretions differs from that in the serum; whilst IgM, IgG and IgA are all found in relatively large amounts in serum, IgG and IgA are the predominant immunoglobulin classes in the mucosal secretions including those of the lungs, gut, salivary, lacrimal and mammary glands, and the urogenital tract. Furthermore, the structure of the IgA in the secretions is distinct from that of serum IgA, and this renders the molecules resistant to the effects of proteolytic enzymes that are frequently found in these locations. IgA accounts for 14 to 20 per cent of the total serum immunoglobulins and, in the serum, it mainly occurs in the form of a monomer (single molecules consisting of two immunoglobulin heavy chains and two light chains). However, secretory IgA exists mainly in the form of dimers consisting of two exactly similar IgA molecules joined by a 'J-chain' (synthesized by the same plasma cell), and bearing an additional 'secretory component'. The 'secretory piece' is synthesized by the mucosal epithelial cells, and is expressed as a receptor on their surfaces. The exposed receptor is able to bind with the dimers of IgA, linked by J-chain, released from the submucosal plasma cells; then the entire complex of IgA dimers, J-chain and secretory piece (secretory IgA) is internalized and transported within vesicles across the epithelial cells, then expelled by exocytosis into the luminal fluid. Evidence suggests that from 56 to 67 per cent of the plasma cells in the bronchial mucosa appear to be involved in IgA production, whilst 12 to 16 per cent appear to be involved in IgG production (Soutar, 1976).

There are two main subclasses of IgA: IgA1 and IgA2; whilst IgA1 is the predominant subclass in serum, IgA2 is the predominant subclass in the secretions. This is thought to be due to the fact that IgA1 is more susceptible to cleavage by bacterial proteases than IgA2. The most important function of secretory IgA appears to be in protecting the respiratory system against infections. It is able to agglutinate bacteria and inhibit their binding to mucosal surfaces; it also has a neutralizing effect

Table 4.2 Biological properties of the main immunoglobulin (Ig) classes and subclasses in human beings

	IgG	Serum IgA	Secretory IgA	IgM	IgD	IgE
Major characteristics	Most abundant Ig in serum and other body fluids. It is the major Ig produced in the secondary immune response	Represents 15–20 per cent of the total serum Ig pool	Most abundant Ig apart from IgG, in the respiratory secretions and in other seromucous secretions, e.g. gastrointestinal	The pentomeric form accounts for about 10 per cent of the serum Ig pool and it is present in very small accounts extravascularly. It is the major Ig produced in the primary immune response. The monomeric form is an antigen receptor on B lymphocytes	Mainly found in the form of an antigen receptor on B lymphocytes	Found in only trace amounts in normal serum but serum levels are raised in parasitic worm infections and in patients with atopic asthma. It is involved in type I allergic reactions by sensitizing human mast cells and basophils for anaphylaxis
Molecular weight (daltons)	150 000	160 000	385 000	900 000	184 000	188 000
Molecular form	Monomer	Monomer 80% Dimer 20%	Dimer + J chain + secretory piece	Pentamer in serum Monomer on B cells	Monomer	Monomer
Serum concentration (mg/ml)	8–16	1.5–4.0	Trace	0.6–2.0	Trace	Trace
Subclasses	IgG1–4	IgA1 and 2	Mainly IgA2	–	–	–
Biological properties						
Complement fixation (classical pathway)	Yes (mainly G1 and G3)	No	No	Yes	No	No
Crosses placenta	Yes (mainly G1, G3 and G4)	No	No	No	No	No
Binds to staphylococcal cell walls	Yes (mainly G1, G2 and G4)	No	No	No	No	No
Binds to Fc receptors on mast cells and basophils	No	No	No	No	No	Yes
Binds to Fc receptors on monocytes and macrophages	Yes (mainly G1 and G3)	?	?	Some?	No	Yes
Binds to Fc receptors on neutrophils	Yes (mainly G1 and G3)	Some?	?	Some?	No	No
Binds to Fc receptors on platelets	Yes (mainly G1 and G3)	No	No	No	No	No

against virus infections by inhibiting the binding of viruses to mucosal epithelial cells. It may also play a role as an opsonin, aiding the phagocytosis of micro-organisms and other particles; however, it is still uncertain whether IgA is a major opsonin because, until recently, it has proved difficult to detect Fc receptors for IgA on macrophages. IgA is also a poor activator of the classic pathway of complement and, even though it can activate complement by the alternative pathway, the levels of many complement components in the respiratory secretions appear to be extremely low. These observations suggest that the more important role of secretory IgA may be to help prevent antigens traversing the walls of the bronchi, gut and other mucosal surfaces, and gaining access to the submucosal lymphoid tissues, where they could stimulate specific immune reactions. In support of this, infants with IgA deficiency show an increased prevalence of allergic diseases and also have increased levels of circulating antibodies to milk and food proteins in their blood, indicating that higher than normal levels of these antigens have traversed the gut (Cunningham-Rundles et al., 1978). Because there are also large amounts of IgG in the respiratory secretions, and alveolar macrophages are known to express Fc receptors for IgG strongly, it is possible that IgG plays a more important role than IgA as an opsonin within the lungs.

Summary

B lymphocytes and their antibody products provide an efficient specific immune defence against free antigens that escape the first-line non-specific defence barriers. They play an important role in enhancing non-specific immune defence mechanisms in the location of the reaction site, and the persistence of the antibodies in body fluids means that they provide some degree of passive specific immunity which can act without delay when an antigen is encountered for a second time. Antibodies (for example, tetanus antitoxin) can also be used as a rapid means to immunize passively individuals who have not previously encountered the antigen.

T lymphocytes

Whereas B lymphocytes and their antibody products provide an efficient specific immune defence against free antigens, the effector responses of T lymphocytes are designed to combat antigens that have gained access to intracellular locations and are less accessible to antibody attack. T lymphocytes also release mediators that recruit inflammatory cells and aid clearance and tissue repair mechanisms at the reaction site; in addition, they play a key role in regulating immune responses.

There are many subpopulations of T lymphocytes with distinct functions. These subpopulations can be distinguished by the surface molecules they express, which can be identified using monoclonal antibodies. By international agreement, such cell surface markers expressed on lymphocytes (and other leucocytes) are now assigned *cluster designation* or 'CD' numbers as they are characterized (CD1, CD2 and so on), and a long list already exists. In relation to T lymphocytes, some markers, for example CD3, are present on all T lymphocytes, but others are expressed only during activation and maturation. There are two main subpopulations of T lymphocytes that can be distinguished by the expression of CD4 and CD8, respectively. In general, the CD4 population contains most of the T-helper cells that recognize and respond to antigens in association with class II MHC products on the surface of antigen-presenting cells. They also contain most of the lymphokine-producing cells that induce the activation and clonal expansion of different T-cell subsets (and of B lymphocytes). The expansion of T-cytotoxic and T-suppressor cells is thought to be induced by a subset of CD4 cells that expresses the CD45R marker. The CD4 population also contains most of the cells (sometimes termed 'delayed hypersensitivity' T cells) which release the lymphokine mediators of inflammation. By contrast with the CD4 population, the CD8 population recognizes antigens in association with class I MHC products. It contains most of the T-cytotoxic lymphocytes that mediate specific class I MHC-restricted cytotoxic responses against target cells bearing the antigen to which they are committed. It also contains most of the T-suppressor cells that function to down-regulate lymphocyte responses when the stimulating antigen has been eliminated. A diagram indicating the cellular interactions and cytokine mediators involved in the activation of the main functional subsets of T lymphocytes is shown in Figure 4.4 which is explained later.

Cytokine mediators

The soluble mediators released by antigen-presenting cells, lymphocytes, other leucocytes or tissue cells during immunological and inflammatory responses are collectively termed 'cytokines'. They have a wide range of biological functions and were initially given names which reflected their activities (for example, 'lymphocyte activating factor' and 'migration inhibition factor'). However, it is now realized that some cytokines can mediate more than one function, others have similar functions and

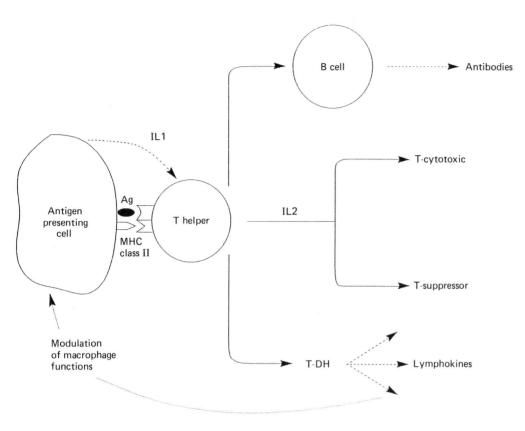

Figure 4.4 Cellular interactions and cytokine mediators involved in activation of the main functional subsets of T lymphocytes

some functions are mediated by the synergistic effect of two or more cytokines acting together. Although some functional terms are still retained, the cytokines that have been purified and cloned by genetic engineering techniques are now termed 'interleukins'. The terms 'lymphokines' and 'monokines' are also widely used to denote the mediators released by lymphocytes and cells of monocytic lineage, respectively.

Cytokines regulating lymphocyte subpopulations

The monokines and lymphokines involved in the proliferation and differentiation of T-lymphocyte subpopulations are indicated in Figure 4.4, and those involved in regulating B lymphocytes have already been described (see previous section). After the binding of a T-helper cell by its antigen receptors to processed antigen and to class II MHC molecules on an antigen-presenting cell, the T-helper cell undergoes activation and mRNA for the lymphokine interleukin-2, and for IL2 receptors, can be detected in its cytoplasm for as long as 24 to 40 hours after stimu-

lation. IL2 receptors are then expressed on the cell surface and IL2 is released. This binds to the IL2 receptors and activates the T-helper cell into proliferation. The IL2–IL2-receptor complex is rapidly internalized (within 30 minutes); therefore, detection of IL2 receptors provides a useful indication of recent T-helper cell activation. Receptors for transferrin are also transiently expressed on T-helper cells early after activation, because the cells require an increase in their uptake of free iron to complete the process of proliferation. Activated T-helper lymphocytes also release the lymphokine interferon-γ (IFNγ), which can enhance the activation of antigen-presenting cells by binding with the IFNγ receptors such cells express. This increases their oxygen uptake, enhances their phagocytic and killing function and their expression of class II MHC products which, as a consequence, enhances their antigen-presenting function. IFNγ also increases the production of the cytokine IL1 by antigen-presenting cells. This cytokine potentiates the activation and proliferation of T-helper cells by binding with IL1 receptors on their surface, which enhances their expression of IL2 receptors and release of IL2. Apart from its effects on CD4+ lymphocytes, IL2 from activated T-helper cells is also required to drive the proliferation of T-cytotoxic lymphocytes, which express receptors for IL2 after they have bound with antigen and class I MHC molecules on the surface of target cells. IL4 released from activated T-helper cells is another lymphokine that can promote T-cell proliferation, although it is less potent than IL2. IL4, however, appears to play an important role in promoting the proliferation and differentiation of B lymphocytes in response to T-dependent antigens (see previous section). Evidence in mice suggests that there are different subpopulations of activated CD4+ T-helper cells which secrete different lymphokines; one subpopulation termed 'TH-1' produces IL2, IFNγ, TNFβ (lymphotoxin), IL3 and granulocyte–macrophage-colony stimulating factor (GM-CSF), whereas another subpopulation termed 'TH-2' produces IL4, IL5, IL3 and GM-CSF. This suggests that different T-helper cells may aid the activation of different T- and B-lymphocyte populations dependent upon the lymphokine receptors the latter express.

The responses of T and B lymphocytes are regulated by T-suppressor lymphocytes that belong mainly to the CD8 population. The mechanisms that control T-suppressor lymphocytes are not well understood, but there is evidence that a subpopulation of CD4+ lymphocytes acts as T-suppressor/inducer cells. These inducer cells appear to recognize antigens on the surface of an antigen-presenting cell in a way that is genetically restricted, but the genes controlling this restriction are not fully identified. After antigen binding, the T-suppressor/inducer cells release a factor that activates the CD8+ T-suppressor lymphocytes. These release a suppressor factor that induces another cell (an *acceptor cell*) to release a non-specific immunosuppressive factor that acts on both T and B lymphocytes. There is another population of T lymphocytes that can block the action of T-suppressor lymphocytes. These *T-contrasuppressor* cells appear to act by protecting T-helper lymphocytes from the action of T-suppressor cells. It is thought that their role is to allow local immune responses to take place in the face of systemic suppression to the same antigen. Contrasuppressor cell activity appears to be important in the gut, and possibly at other mucosal sites, allowing potentially harmful antigens to be dealt with locally without inducing systemic reactions.

Cytokines involved in inflammation

Apart from their involvement in regulating the growth of lymphocytes, cytokines can recruit, stimulate and regulate the growth and activation of many inflammatory cell types including monocytes, neutrophils, eosinophils, mast cells and natural killer cells. It is now recognized that cytokines can also have important regulatory effects on the growth and

functions of tissue cells (which themselves probably serve as another important source of cytokine mediators). The inflammatory cells serve to strengthen the local attack against foreign invaders through their diverse functions in non-specific immune defence. They also aid the removal and repair of damaged tissue components and are a source of inhibitors that are important in regulating inflammation. However, in situations where a foreign agent is resistant to attack, prolonged antigenic stimulation can lead to chronic inflammation, which can have a harmful effect on host tissues. This is thought to be a major contributory factor in the pathogenesis of many lung diseases, including occupational diseases of the lungs, where immunopathogenic mechanisms appear to play an important role (see under 'Immunopathology').

Some of the better characterized cytokines, their cellular sources and functional effects are listed in Table 4.3.

The possible relevance of cytokines to the behaviour of fibroblasts in interstitial lung diseases and in pneumoconioses is discussed further on pages 77–79 and in Chapter 5.

Immune defences against tumour cells

The existence of immunological defence mechanisms against tumour cells has long been recognized and for many years it was thought that such mechanisms may play the major role in suppressing the development of malignancy in vivo. In 1970, Burnet proposed the theory of 'immunosurveillance' suggesting that T lymphocytes play a major role in detecting and eliminating these cells as they arise in the body due to mutational errors in dividing host cell populations (which theoretically might amount to millions of errors per day). It was proposed that this occurs because tumour cells express new antigenic determinants that the T cells recognize as foreign. In recent years, this conventional theory of 'immunosurveillance', involving specific immune recognition of tumour cells, has been brought into doubt for reasons explained later. Nevertheless, it is clear that non-specific immune defence mechanisms, as well as T lymphocytes, may play an important role in anti-tumour defence. Immunological principles are also employed in many promising new approaches to cancer therapy, and may be relevant to intrathoracic tumours associated with occupational hazards – in particular, malignant mesothelioma.

Table 4.3 List of the main interleukins that have been characterized indicating their main cellular sources and functional effects

Cytokine	$10^{-3} \times$ mol. wt (daltons)	Cellular sources	Main functions
IL1α	17	Monocytes, macrophages,	Activates and promotes the differentiation of T and B lymphocytes.
IL1β	17	dendritic cells, B cells, epithelial cells, endothelial cells, other tissue cells	Induces release of IL2 and IL6. Has stimulatory effects on fibroblasts and other tissue cells. Induces release of acute phase proteins from hepatocytes
IL2	14–16	T cells	Promotes the proliferation and/or activation of T cells, B cells, NK cells, monocytes and macrophages
IL3	14.6	T cells	Has effects on stem cells promoting growth, differentiation and activation of basophils, mast cells, macrophages, eosinophils and megakaryocytes
IL4	20	T cells, mast cells	Promotes growth and differentiation of B cells and enhances IgE and IgG production. Promotes growth of mast cells and enhances macrophage activation
IL5	50	T cells	Promotes growth of B cells and enhances IgA and IgM production. Promotes growth and differentiation of eosinophil precursors
IL6	22–29	T cells, fibroblasts, endothelial cells, epithelial cells, mono-cytes and macrophages	Stimulates Ig production by B cells. Promotes stem cell differentiation. Promotes IL2 production and differentiation of T-cytotoxic cells
IL7	25	Bone marrow	Induces proliferation of pre-B cells and thymocytes
IL8	10	Monocytes and macrophages	Chemotactic factor for neutrophils

T-cytotoxic lymphocytes

The T lymphocytes which mediate antigen-specific cytotoxic responses mainly belong to the CD8+ subset of T cells and 'T-cytotoxic' lymphocytes can only recognize and bind with antigens in association with class I MHC products on target cells of their own or identical genotype. Nearly all nucleated cell types express class I MHC products (HLA-A, -B, and -C antigens) and can, thus, become the target of T-cytotoxic responses if they undergo any change (for example, infection with viruses or intracellular pathogens, mutation or chemically induced alteration) which causes them to express new antigens that are recognized as foreign. However, the theory of 'immunosurveillance' – that tumour cells expressing new antigens frequently arise by mutation and become the target for T-cytotoxic cells – appears to be flawed for the following reasons. In particular, it has been demonstrated that the rate of spontaneous tumours in 'nude' mice which have no thymus glands and in neonatally thymectomized mice is no higher than in normal mice, even though these mice have defective T-cell function. Patients with acquired T-cell deficiency (for example, patients with AIDS or those on immunosuppressive therapy after organ transplantation) also show no increase in the most common cancers of the lungs, gut, breast and urinogenital tract. However, the increased incidence of Kaposi's sarcoma in AIDS patients and of cancers of the lymphoid system in transplant patients suggests that T-cell-mediated immunoregulation may be important in these particular instances. Experimental evidence suggests that the ability of tumours to stimulate a specific immune response in the host may relate to the manner in which the tumour is induced. Although neonatally thymectomized mice show no increase in spontaneous tumours, they do show an increased incidence of tumours induced by chemical carcinogens (such a methylcholanthrene and dibenzanthracene) and viruses (for example, the DNA viruses – polyoma and SV40). New antigens are frequently detectable on cells from these induced tumours, but not on cells from the spontaneously arising tumours. This suggests that T-cytotoxic lymphocytes are more likely to be involved in host protection against tumours induced by exposure to environmental agents. Numerous explanations have been proposed to explain how such immunogenic tumours might spread, including poor immunogenicity of the tumour cells, heterogeneity within the tumour cell population allowing selection of non-antigenic variants, shedding of tumour antigens, generation of T-suppressor lymphocytes, and the poor adhesion of tumour cells to other cell types that might interfere with their interaction with cytotoxic cells. The full extent to which viruses or carcinogens are involved in human tumours is unknown, but there are many examples of involvement of chemical carcinogens, including asbestos-related malignancies and lung cancer related to carcinogens, such as benzo[α]pyrene, in tobacco smoke. Human tumours where viruses are directly or indirectly implicated include hepatocellular carcinoma (hepatitis B virus); Burkitt's lymphoma, non-Hodgkin's lymphoma and nasopharyngeal carcinoma (Epstein–Barr virus); cervical carcinoma (human papilloma viruses 16 and 18); T-cell leukaemia (human T-cell lymphotropic virus, HTLV-1) and Kaposi's sarcoma (cytomegalovirus + human immunodeficiency virus, HIV).

The genes that control cell proliferation are normally repressed by regulator sequences of the genome in close proximity. It is thought that inappropriate activation of these genes occurs in malignant cells, either because viruses have acquired the genes from the host cell and transferred them to inappropriate positions in the genomes of other cells where they are not repressed, or because translocations have occurred in the host cells resulting in the genes occupying an aberrant location away from the influence of the regulator sequences. These genes are known as 'oncogenes' and viruses that can transfer them are known as *oncogenic* viruses. In some situations, malignancy appears to result from the activation of latent oncogenic RNA viruses, stimulated by some other factor, for example, radiation exposure or exposure to chemical carcinogens. Radiation-induced murine leukaemias are one example of this. There is evidence in mice that herpes viruses may also be capable of activating RNA tumour viruses. The possibility that similar associative mechanisms of tumour induction might occur in some occupational malignancies, possibly involving carcinogens in occupational dusts, smoking-related carcinogens and virus infections, has been the subject of speculation and is one potential area for future research.

Although many tumour cells may not be subject to regulation by T-cytotoxic lymphocytes because they do not express tumour-specific antigens, nevertheless there are ways in which these cells might be controlled by immunotherapy. Tumour cells are usually poorly differentiated cells, resembling embryonic cells, and they frequently bear surface molecules that are expressed during embryonic development (for example, carcinoembryonic antigen in the gut) but are normally repressed during adult life. Monoclonal antibodies can be raised against these neoantigens, and they are useful in tracing tumour cells in vivo. There is also considerable research aimed at linking such antibodies (and monoclonal antibodies to tumour-specific markers) with cytotoxic drugs, with the aim of selectively targeting highly toxic compounds to the tumour cells without harm to other host cells.

Natural killer cells, LAK cells and K cells

Many tumours apparently do not stimulate specific immune responses in the host, yet the incidence of cancer is generally highest early and late in life when the immune system is least efficient. Infiltrates of mononuclear cells, including lymphocytes and macrophages, are also frequently seen in histological sections of solid tumours. This suggests that immune mechanisms of some kind are involved in cancer regulation, even though the role of specifically sensitized T lymphocytes may be limited to those instances where tumours express tumour-specific antigens. Apart from T-cytotoxic lymphocytes, other cell types have been identified in the body that can mediate cytolytic or cytostatic effects against tumour cells; these include natural killer cells (NK cells), lymphokine-activated killer cells (LAK cells), killer cells (K cells) and macrophages. The tumoricidal functions of these cells are part of non-specific immune defences because they are capable of lysing tumour cells without the need for specific sensitization of the host.

Natural killer cells is the name given to a heterogeneous population of cells that are normally found mainly in the blood and spleen. They are able to mediate non-specific killing of a wide variety of tumour cell targets including those of autologous, allogeneic and xenogeneic derivation. They are also able non-specifically to lyse virus-infected cells and some normal cell types of bone marrow and thymic origin. This has led to the view that they may be involved in regulating haemopoietic cell populations as well as playing a role in the killing of tumour cells and virally infected cells. NK cells in the blood are mainly found among the 2 to 5 per cent of cells that have the morphology of 'large granular lymphocytes'. These cells are 'null' cells that do not express phenotypic pan-B-cell or pan-T-cell markers, but some express the CD8 marker and most express Fc receptors (CD16) and lymphocyte function antigens (LFA1) that aid cell adherence (CD11a and CD18). Killing by NK cells is not MHC restricted and the identity of the receptor molecules involved in their binding to target cells is not known. Following binding, NK cells release biologically active proteins that include 'perforin'. Perforin becomes inserted into the target cell membranes, opening up pores that allow the diffusion of sodium ions into the cell thus altering the osmotic pressure so that the target cell eventually bursts. The functional differentiation and activation of NK cells is enhanced by the lymphokines IL2 and IFNγ released from activated T lymphocytes, providing another example of interplay between non-specific and specific immunity. Other classes of interferons – IFNα released from activated monocytes and macrophages and IFNβ released from fibroblasts and other tissue cells during virus infection or following stimulation of such cells with various cytokines – can also enhance NK cell activity. Activated NK cells themselves also produce IFNα which, like other interferons, has anti-tumour as well as anti-viral effects.

When peripheral blood lymphocytes are incubated with the lymphokine IL2 in vitro for at least 48 hours, a population of cells termed 'lymphokine-activated killer cells' (LAK cells) is generated, which are thought possibly to develop from NK-cell precursors although they express CD3 markers and lack some of the markers characteristic of NK cells. LAK cells are more effective than NK cells in killing freshly isolated tumour cells, and they are less cytotoxic to normal cells. (Cultured tumour cell lines are mainly used to demonstrate NK cell function because they are more susceptible.) Clinical trials have shown that prolonged administration of IL2 to patients, with the aim of enhancing in vivo killer cell function, has little measurable effect on solid tumours. However, trials administering IL2 together with LAK cells (produced by in vitro incubation of autologous lymphocytes from the patient with IL2) have produced some regression of solid tumours including renal carcinomas and melanomas; it appears to be particularly effective in the prevention of metastases (Rosenberg, Lotz and Muul, 1985). There is also recent evidence that IL2 plus LAK-cell infusion may be of potential benefit in patients with pleural mesotheliomas (Manning et al., 1989a, b).

The large granular lymphocyte population also contains cells that mediate 'antibody-dependent cell-mediated cytotoxicity' (ADCC). These cells are often called 'K cells'. K cells combine with and induce the lysis of antibody-coated target cells and, although antibodies are the product of specific immune responses, K-cell activity is non-specific in that the cells bind to antibodies irrespective of their specificity. There is a very close correlation between K-cell and NK-cell activity in the same populations suggesting that there may be close overlap between these populations.

Although interferons (α, β and γ) are able to activate NK cells, clinical trials treating cancer patients with recombinant interferons (mainly IFNα) have had little more than anecdotal successes except in hairy-cell leukaemia. Because interferons have a very short half-life, it is thought that a more useful approach in the future may be to achieve more accurate targeting of interferons to tumour sites with the aid of monoclonal antibodies.

macrophage activators, for example, endotoxin, immune complexes or the lymphokine IFNγ. Virtually all newly isolated tumour cells or cultured cell lines appear to be susceptible to the cytolytic or cytostatic effects of activated macrophages. These effects are directed in a highly selected way at tumour cells and normal cells are not affected. The molecules involved in selective recognition are not known but cell-to-cell contact is required. The actual killing activity is thought to involve the release of lysozomal enzymes from macrophages which damage target cell membranes, release of oxygen metabolites such as hydrogen peroxide, and also release of the cytokine *tumour necrosis factor* (TNFα). As well as being released from activated macrophages (and monocytes), TNFα is also present on the surface of macrophages in membrane-bound form. Acting in synergy with other cytokines, in particular IL1 and IFNγ, it is able to induce necrosis in tumours; it also has a wide range of other effects, notably acting on endothelial cells to enhance adhesion of leucocytes inducing intravascular coagulation and tissue necrosis. It is thought that the local effect of TNF on the vasculature feeding tumours may aid its anti-tumour effects. T-cytotoxic lymphocytes also produce a slightly different form of TNF – TNFβ – which has 50 per cent homology with TNFα. This is often called *lymphotoxin*.

An in vivo role for macrophages in anti-tumour defence is suggested by the observation of more rapid development of ultraviolet-induced skin tumours in mice treated with substances that are damaging to macrophages and by the frequent finding of macrophages showing features of activation in tumour cell infiltrates. However, the in vivo efficiency of macrophage-mediated anti-tumour effects is likely to be influenced by many other factors, not least of these being the fact that activated macrophages can release prostaglandin E_2 (PGE$_2$) which can suppress lymphoproliferation and secretion of lymphokines that play a role in enhancing the tumoricidal activity of macrophages and other killer cells. IL1 and TNFα produced by activated macrophages have also been reported to act synergistically to enhance PGE$_2$ production by fibroblasts (Elias, 1988; Elias, Gustilo and Freundlich, 1988). These observations raise the question of whether indomethacin treatment might have advantageous effects in potentiating anti-tumour activity.

Macrophage-mediated cytotoxicity

Among their numerous functions in immune defence, macrophages also have tumoricidal activity. It can be demonstrated in vitro that they acquire tumoricidal activity after they have undergone stimulation with

Immunopathology

The normal protective immune responses described earlier are, in some circumstances, inappropriately deployed to excess and, as a result, the reactions designed to eliminate foreign agents can also cause 'spill-over' damage to the host's own tissue cells. Such excessive immune reactions are termed 'hypersensitivity' reactions and they are implicated in the pathogenesis of many chronic inflammatory diseases, including those of the lungs. These hypersensitivity reactions, together with their pathological effects, form the basis of the field of 'immunopathology', which also includes disorders associated with defective immunity.

There are many ways in which immune hypersensitivity reactions might arise, for example, inappropriate access of agents to sites where they can more readily stimulate specific immune reactions; abnormal persistence of agents because of their resistance to biodegradation or defective host clearance mechanisms; or congenital or acquired defects in host immune effector or regulatory mechanisms.

Over the years, it has proved convenient for descriptive purposes, to classify hypersensitivity reactions into various types; however, in practice more than one of these types is likely to occur together in the same individual and, thus, the disease entity is without doubt the expression of their combined effects. The most widely used classification is that of Coombs and Gell (1968), which is regularly updated as the mechanisms are more fully elucidated (Roitt, Brostoff and Male, 1989).

Classification of antibody and cell-mediated hypersensitivity reactions

The Coombs' and Gell classification describes four main types of hypersensitivity reactions: types I, II, III and IV. The first three types involve reactions induced by specific antibodies, and the fourth type involves cell-mediated hypersensitivity reactions induced by the products of specifically sensitized T lymphocytes and macrophages. It will be clear from the information given in the preceding sections of this chapter that these classic definitions of hypersensitivity are limited in some aspects, and that hypersensitivity might also arise due to aberrations of other immune responses not included in these definitions. This will also be apparent from the detailed information on pathogenic mechanisms given in the appropriate chapters on different occupational lung diseases.

Type I hypersensitivity

Type I hypersensitivity plays a role in the pathogenesis of the common 'allergic' disorders, such as hay fever, rhinitis and allergies to food, wasp or bee venom, and penicillin. It is also implicated in the pathogenesis of the acute 'anaphylactic' reactions that occur in extrinsic asthma and in some types of occupational asthma, in particular those related to toluene diisocyanate and trimellitic acid compounds. 'Immediate reactions' characteristic of type I hypersensitivity are induced following interaction between the antigens ('allergens') involved in these reactions and cytophilic antibodies, mainly of the IgE immunoglobulin class, which have the ability to bind to the surfaces of a number of cell types, in particular mast cells and basophils, by interacting with Fcε receptors expressed on the surfaces of these cells. Such IgE antibodies are also known as *reaginic antibodies*. Provided the antigens are large enough to cross-link adjacent molecules of IgE bound to the cell surfaces (that is, divalent or polyvalent, but not monovalent antigens), this induces changes in the surface membrane associated with the influx of Ca^{2+} ions into the cell, and these changes immediately stimulate the degranulation of the cells, with consequent release of pharmacologically active mediators which increase capillary permeability causing oedema, induce the contraction of smooth muscle and stimulate inflammation at the reaction site, giving rise to the acute symptoms. The granules within mast cells and basophils are specialized forms of lysosomes which contain stores of pre-formed mediators. These are released following degranulation, and include *histamine*, which can induce vasodilatation and stimulate smooth muscle contraction; *heparin*, which has anticoagulant effects and can inhibit complement activation by binding to C1q; *proteolytic enzymes* including mast cell tryptase, which can activate C3 directly; and *chemotactic factors* for neutrophils (NCF molecular weight 750 000) and for eosinophils (ECF-A molecular weight 380 to 2000). Apart from these pre-formed mediators, antigen binding to cell-bound IgE also incites the synthesis and release of newly formed mediators which are implicated in the 'late phase' reactions associated with type I hypersensitivity. These mediators are metabolites of arachidonic acid, which is generated through the activation of phospholipase A_2 in the cell membrane. Arachidonic acid metabolism can proceed via two separate pathways. In the *lipoxygenase pathway*, metabolism by the enzyme lipoxygenase leads to the synthesis of the leukotriene mediators of inflammation, LTC_4 and LTD_4 (once known as *slow-reacting substance of anaphylaxis* or SRS-A). These, like histamine, cause smooth muscle contraction and are powerful bronchoconstrictors, but they act at a slightly later stage in the inflammatory response. Another product, LTB_4, has potent chemotactic and chemokinetic effects for neutrophils, eosinophils and monocytes. In the second pathway of arachidonic acid metabolism, the *cyclo-oxygenase pathway*, the action of the enzyme cyclo-oxygenase results in the synthesis of prostaglandins and thromboxanes, in particular PGD_2 and thromboxane A_2; these newly synthesized mediators can induce bronchial smooth muscle contraction (mainly the prostaglandin F series), platelet aggregation (thromboxanes), and vasodilatation (mainly the prostaglandin E series) with oedema and mucus secretion.

Activated neutrophils can also contribute to mediator release by generating leukotrienes, mainly LTB_4; activated macrophages and eosinophils produce LTC_4 and LTD_4, as well as prostaglandins. Eosinophils are additionally involved in the inflammatory reactions initiated as a consequence of type I responses, and blood and tissue eosinophilia is a notable feature of the late-phase reactions. Similar to mast cells and basophils, eosinophils contain intracellular lysosomal granules, and cell activation prompts the release of the granule contents. These include toxic proteins (major basic protein and eosinophil cationic protein), which can damage the respiratory epithelium, enhancing permeability and facilitating further damage. Eosinophils have a high content of peroxidase enzymes which have the potential to cause tissue damage, and they can produce LTC_4 and LTD_4, as well as prostaglandins, which may contribute in mediating smooth muscle contraction and vasodilatation. They also release *platelet-activating factor* (PAF), which can induce platelet aggregation causing microthrombi and is a potent mediator being chemotactic for neutrophils, inducing smooth muscle contraction and having vasodilatory effects that increase vascular permeability. PAF is also released from activated neutrophils, macrophages and platelets. In addition, eosinophils release molecules that regulate inflammatory responses, including histaminase, which inactivates histamine, and aryl sulphatase, which inactivates LTC_3 and LTD_4, and eosinophils mediate direct cytotoxic responses that are of particular importance in host protection against parasitic infections with protozoa and worms, which are usually too large to be phagocytosed.

In the respiratory tract and gut where there is a propensity for allergic reactions to occur, mast cells are particularly abundant in subepithelial locations, and some are also detectable in the mucosal epithelium. Large numbers of mast cells are also present in the connective tissues around blood vessels, in the skin, in the peritoneum and in other connective tissues. Mast cell populations show heterogeneity both in morphology and functions, and whilst the majority of *connective tissue mast cells* can still be stained after formaldehyde fixation, the majority of those in mucosal tissues (*mucosal mast cells*) have granules that lose their staining properties after formaldehyde fixation. The mucosal type of mast cells can be demonstrated using other fixatives, for example, methanol. These differences reflect diversity in the type of proteoglycan in the granules which is mainly heparin in the connective tissue type of mast cells, but chondroitin sulphate in the mucosal type. The proliferation of mucosal mast cells is dependent on lymphokines, including IL3 and IL4, derived from activated T cells, but that of connective tissue mast cells is independent of T-cell factors. Both types of mast cells can produce arachidonic acid metabolites, but the mucosal type produce relatively more LTC_4 than PGD_2 while the connective tissue type produce relatively more prostaglandin. Evidence from studies in rats indicates that sodium cromoglycate and theophylline inhibit histamine release only from the connective tissue type of mast cells. Recent evidence suggests that the various types of mast cells and basophils develop from a common precursor and that their differentiation and maturation are dependent upon local factors, such as the lymphokines, which play a role in the maturation of mucosal mast cells. Mast cell degranulation can be provoked by a range of factors, apart from antigens, including lymphokines, the anaphylatoxins C3a and C5a, lectins present in certain plants, certain drugs, and mast cell activators such as calcium ionophore and Compound 48/80. All of these factors induce an increased flux of calcium ions into the mast cells. The clinical symptoms associated with type I allergic reactions are, presumably, influenced by the heterogeneity in mast cell functions, the tissue location, and the nature of the stimulating allergen.

The majority of the population (approximately 70 per cent) are 'non-atopic' individuals who do not produce high levels of IgE antibodies or exhibit positive immediate 'skin-prick test' reactions to common antigens which are normally innocuous. Such individuals are not susceptible to the common allergic disorders involving type I reactions. However, the remainder of the population do have an increased predisposition to produce antibodies of the IgE immunoglobulin class (atopy) and exhibit positive skin-prick test reactions to common antigens, and at least a third of these suffer from allergic diseases. Individuals showing positive immediate skin-prick test reactions to common antigens such as pollen, house dusts, animal fur, fungi and certain foods, are termed 'atopic' individuals. There is evidence that genetic factors may be involved in susceptibility to allergic diseases, possibly associated with a deregulation of the genes coding for IgE or some defect in the generation of T-suppressor lymphocytes which down-regulate IgE production. Individuals with IgE-related allergies, in general, have a higher frequency of HLA-B8 and HLA-DW3 than non-allergic individuals. Furthermore, ragweed allergy has been shown to be closely related to HLA-DW2 (present in more than 90 per cent of responders to ragweed allergen 5A).

Antihistamines are frequently employed to treat the common allergies, such as hay fever, whilst the more varied approaches required in treatment of asthma are discussed under 'Therapeutic approaches'. On the rare occasions when high levels of antigen meet with IgE antibody in the circulation, for example in penicillin allergy, anaphylactic shock can occur which can be sufficiently severe to result in death. Type I allergic reactions do not occur when an individual is exposed to allergen for the first time, but can occur on second or subsequent exposures when specific IgE antibody production has commenced and these antibodies have become bound to Fcε receptors on cell surfaces. Although IgE predominantly binds to the high affinity Fcε receptors on mast cells and basophils, a number of other cells express low affinity Fc receptors for IgE. These have been reported on eosinophils, platelets, T and B lymphocytes, monocytes and also on alveolar macrophages, but the importance of interactions with these low affinity Fcε receptors is not yet clear.

Type II hypersensitivity

Type II hypersensitivity reactions can occur when cells become coated with antibodies directed against components of the cells themselves, which are recognized as foreign, for example, components related to infection of the cells by viruses or other microbial agents; changes induced by drugs or drug attachment to cells; tumour cells expressing tumour-specific antigens; transplanted tissues expressing incompatible HLA antigens; transfused erythrocytes or platelets expressing antigens incompatible with those of the host; and host cells which, for unknown reasons, have undergone alterations causing them to stimulate 'autoimmune responses'. These reactions directed against infected cells or tumour cells are an important part of normal protected immunity, but when they occur to excess or are inappropriately invoked, as in the additional examples mentioned previously, damage to the host tissues can result and this is termed 'type II hypersensitivity'. The mechanisms by which the host attacks target cells coated with antibodies bound to cell-associated antigens are either cytolytic reactions mediated as a result of the complex activating the complement system (see 'Alveolar macrophages', under 'Non-specific (innate) immune defences') or *cytotoxic reactions* mediated by the cells of the non-specific immune system which can function in 'antibody-dependent cell-mediated cytotoxicity', in particular K cells, monocytes, macrophages, neutrophils and eosinophils (see under 'Immune defences against tumour cells'). The actual mechanisms involved in type II hypersensitivity vary according to the class of antibody involved which determines its biological activity, including its complement fixing ability and ability to bind to the Fc receptors on cytotoxic cells (see 'Lymphocytes and their subpopulations'). The larger IgM antibodies are also more likely to cause problems due to cell agglutination. For example, in blood transfusion reactions, antibodies to the ABO blood group antigens are usually IgM and the reactions involve erythrocyte agglutination, complement activation and intravascular haemolysis. Other erythrocyte antigens, including the rhesus D antigen, which is most commonly involved in haemolytic disease of the newborn, usually induce IgG antibodies and, as well as inducing complement activation, these antibodies often bind to Fc-receptor bearing cells.

Type II reactions are involved in a number of autoimmune diseases, such as autoimmune haemolytic anaemias, thrombocytopenias, Goodpasture's syndrome and myasthenia gravis, in which patients produce autoantibodies to relevant cells and structures of their own bodies. Many other disorders are associated with the production of autoantibodies. Autoantibodies to components of cell nuclei (*anti-nuclear antibodies*) and autoantibodies to immunoglobulins (*rheumatoid factors*) occur in increased frequency in interstitial fibrosing lung diseases, including those related to occupational exposure to fibrogenic dusts. There is, however, no evidence that such autoantibodies to intracellular and extracellular components participate in type II reactions. Autoantibodies to lymphocytes and neutrophils have been demonstrated in patients with systemic lupus erythematosus (who also produce autoantibodies to cell nuclear antigens and numerous other intracellular components), and anti-lymphocyte antibodies have also been detected in patients with the granulomatous lung disease sarcoidosis; however, the role of these anti-leucocyte antibodies in pathogenesis is unclear.

In conclusion, it is appropriate to consider the possibility that type II hypersensitivity reactions may be involved in pathogenesis in situations where antigens associated with host cell surfaces stimulate the production of specific antibodies, either because they are recognized as foreign or because they stimulate the production of autoantibodies. Type II reactions are also inevitably associated with features of inflammation, because inflammatory mediators are generated as a consequence of complement activation, and cytokines and other mediators (for example, leukotrienes and prostaglandins) are released from cytotoxic cells following their activation.

Type III hypersensitivity

Type III hypersensitivity reactions differ from type I and type II reactions, in that they involve combinations between antibodies and antigens free in the circulation or tissue spaces rather than attached to cell surfaces. These combinations result in the formation of immune complexes, which vary in their size and solubility depending upon the relative amount of antigen to antibody in the complex, their respective valencies (number of antigenic determinants per antigen molecule relative to the number of antigen-combining sites per antibody molecule) which influence the extent of cross-linking, and the immunoglobulin class and subclass of the antibody which influences its biological activity and, consequently, the rate of degradation and clearance of the immune complex (which depends on the rate of complement-mediated solubilization, the rate of clearance by phagocytes, and binding to CR1 receptors on erythrocytes that transport them to the liver for removal by the resident tissue macrophages). The formation of immune complexes is a normal part of host defence which occurs continuously, and under normal circumstances they are rapidly eliminated by phagocytic and other clearance mechanisms without causing any harm to the host. However, if circumstances arise where the rate of immune complex formation exceeds their rate of elimination, tissue damage can result due to trapping of circulating microaggregates in small capillaries, or deposition of larger aggregates within the tissues. The adverse reactions which occur when circulating immune complexes are trapped in capillaries are described as *serum-sickness-type* reactions because, prior to the use of antibiotics and vaccines, these reactions could occur in patients treated with antisera 'raised in horses' to treat diseases such as diphtheria. The reactions were the result of antibodies produced by the patient against the horse immunoglobulin in the antisera which, in situations of antigen excess, caused the formation of small immune complexes; these tended to become trapped in small capillary beds, particularly in the kidneys, joints, skin and sometimes in the capillaries of other organs including the heart and lungs, giving rise to classic symptoms of 'serum sickness'. Apart from mechanical trapping, it appears that the mechanisms of serum sickness can be attributed to fixation of complement by the immune complex deposits, resulting in the generation of chemotaxins, which attract neutrophils to the reaction site where they are thought to contribute to tissue damage by releasing proteolytic enzymes and oxidants.

Anaphylatoxins are also released as a consequence of complement activation, and can interact with mast cells and basophils in the locality to induce the release of vasoactive amines; these, in turn, can increase vascular permeability aiding the access of neutrophils to the tissues, where their products are more likely to cause damage because they are less accessible to the effects of serum inhibitors. Immune complexes can also activate platelets by binding to their Fc receptors, causing platelet aggregation, microthrombi formation and the further release of vasoactive mediators.

The immunoglobulin classes which are most efficient in complement fixation and, therefore, more likely to participate in type III reactions, are IgM, IgG1, IgG2 and IgG3. Serum-sickness-type reactions can occur in patients with hypersensitivity to penicillin or sulphonamides. They are also thought to be responsible for poststreptococcal glomerulonephritis and may explain the skin rashes and joint pains associated with other bacterial and viral infections. Increases in circulating immune complexes also occur in many autoimmune diseases and there is strong evidence that deposits of immune complexes containing DNA may contribute to the skin lesions and glomerulonephritis of serum sickness.

Patients with fibrosing alveolitis (diffuse interstitial pulmonary fibrosis, DIPF), either 'lone' cryptogenic fibrosing alveolitis or fibrosing alveolitis in association with 'autoimmune' connective tissue diseases, also frequently have increases in circulating immune complexes, especially at an early stage of disease (Dreisin et al., 1978; Haslam et al., 1979; Martinet, Haslam and Turner-Warwick, 1984). Immune complex deposits have also occasionally been reported in the lungs (Turner-Warwick, Haslam and Weeks, 1971; Dreisin et al., 1978), and it has been suggested that binding of immune complexes may induce the activation of alveolar macrophages associated with pathogenesis. However, the relevance of type III hypersensitivity mechanisms to the pathogenesis of these lung diseases is still unclear.

Apart from serum-sickness-type reactions, type III hypersensitivity reactions of a different form, known as *Arthus-type reactions*, can occur when high concentrations of antigen are introduced into the tissues of pre-sensitized individuals who already have appreciable levels of antibodies to the antigen in their blood, tissue fluids or local secretions. This type of reaction is classically demonstrated when antigen is injected into the dermis of the skin where it interacts with antibody, of a class that is able to fix complement, diffusing from the small blood vessels. An area of reddening and swelling develops a few hours after antigen injection (peaking at about 4 to 6 hours) and persists for approximately 24 to 48 hours. This reaction is the consequence of the deposition of complement fixing immune complexes in the walls of the small vessels, which induces the release of biologically active fragments of complement leading to the influx of granulocytes to the reaction site, intravascular clumping of platelets, increased vascular permeability and local oedema.

In some abnormal situations, it is believed that an Arthus-type reaction might occur in the lungs across the walls of the bronchi or alveoli. This is thought to be one of the mechanisms involved in the disease 'extrinsic allergic alveolitis' which occurs in some individuals exposed to organic dusts. These dusts are of many different kinds, for example, mouldy hay dust containing thermophilic actinomycetes, which are causally associated with farmers' lung disease, avian protein antigens, which are causally associated with pigeon breeders' and budgerigar fanciers' lung diseases, and many other occupational exposures. Type III reactions are considered to contribute to the acute reactions in these diseases, but the exact mechanisms are still unclear because many exposed individuals develop specific antibodies without exhibiting symptoms of disease. The evidence suggests that type IV cell-mediated hypersensitivity reactions (see the next section) also play a most important role in extrinsic allergic alveolitis. They appear to mediate the chronic granulomatous reactions that occur in the interstitial tissues of the lungs and bronchi. There is also evidence that release of mediators from T-dependent mast cells, which are increased in bronchoalveolar lavage (BAL) fluids at times of current or recent antigen exposure, might contribute to the acute phase responses by increasing local permeability and allowing easier access of inhaled antigens to subepithelial locations (Haslam et al., 1987). The pathogenic mechanisms in extrinsic allergic alveolitis are described in detail in Chapter 20.

Type IV hypersensitivity

Type IV hypersensitivity reactions differ from types I, II and III reactions in that they are not mediated by antibodies, but are mediated by cytokines released by activated antigen-presenting cells and sensitized lymphocytes, after their stimulation by specific antigens (see 'Cytokine mediators'). Consequently, type IV reactions are commonly known as *cell-mediated hypersensitivity reactions*. The classic example of a type IV reaction is the 'delayed-hypersensitivity' reaction which occurs in the skin following intradermal injection of 0.1 ml of an appropriate dilution (1:10 000, 1:1000 or 1:100) of purified protein derivative (PPD) extracted from *Mycobacterium tuberculosis*. Individuals already sensitized to *M. tuberculosis* develop an area of reddening and induration of the skin at the site of injection of the antigen but, unlike type III Arthus skin reactions, this takes a longer time to develop (12 hours or more, peaking at 24 to 48 hours) and can persist for several weeks. This is the reason why type IV reactions are called 'delayed hypersensitivity reactions'. Histologically, the reaction is characterized by dense infiltrates of T lymphocytes, with CD4+ cells outnumbering

CD8+ cells, and with some macrophages. T lymphocytes expressing HLA-DR can be detected, indicating that they have undergone activation, and HLA-DR is also expressed on the infiltrating macrophages indicating that they may play a role in antigen presentation. As the reaction progresses, the keratinocytes in the skin also begin to express HLA-DR, presumably as a response to the stimulating effect of IFNγ released by activated T lymphocytes, and they may then also contribute in antigen presentation to amplify the local immune reactions. The lymphocyte infiltrates are mainly perivascular, and the reaction persists until the antigen has been cleared. The time course, intensity and histological features of type IV reactions vary for reasons that relate partly to the location, and partly to the amount and nature of the antigen, which influences its potency and persistence; in some instances, it appears that variability in the host's T-suppressor cell function may also influence the strength of delayed reactions.

The normal role of T cells in specific immune defence is to regulate the proliferation and activation of T- and B-cell populations, to mediate specific cytotoxic responses against target cells bearing foreign antigens, and to produce the lymphokine mediators of delayed hypersensitivity which can recruit many types of inflammatory cells (including monocytes, mast cells or basophils, neutrophils and eosinophils) to the reaction site, and then induce their proliferation and activation to aid the elimination of the stimulating agent. Mediators released from the array of inflammatory cells then serve further to amplify the local inflammation. If these reactions are short-lived and the agent rapidly eliminated, the risk of 'spill-over' damage to the host is limited; however, if the antigenic stimulus persists and the reactions are prolonged, the consequences to the host can be serious.

Contact hypersensitivity skin reactions are an example of one of the clinically relevant forms of delayed hypersensitivity. They can be induced by a variety of chemicals, which are all haptens capable of binding to body proteins to form sensitizing antigens. These chemicals include nickel, chromium, potassium dichromate, picryl chloride, dinitrochlorobenzene, *p*-phenylenediamine in hair dyes, and plant poisons such as poison ivy. If these substances penetrate the epidermis of the skin, the resultant sensitizing antigens can interact with Langerhan's cells at the junction of the epidermis and dermis; these antigen-presenting cells then stimulate the delayed hypersensitivity reactions. The eczematous skin reactions characteristic of contact hypersensitivity are apparent after 24 to 48 hours, and the lesions are infiltrated with lymphocytes and monocytes. Basophils are also sometimes present, and the local keratinocytes become HLA-DR positive.

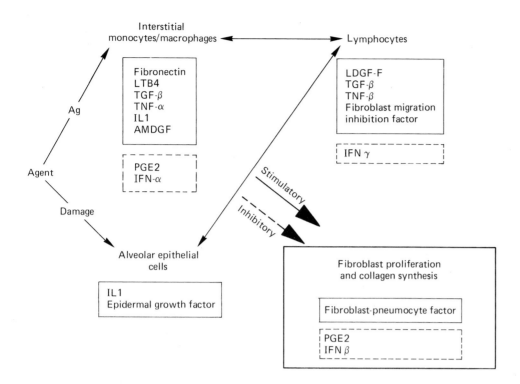

Figure 4.5 Factors produced by macrophages, T lymphocytes and epithelial cells which have effects on fibroblasts. LTB$_4$ = leukotriene B$_4$; TGFβ = transforming growth factor β; TNFα and -β = tumour necrosis factor α and β; IL1 = interleukin 1; AMDGF = alveolar macrophage-derived growth factor; PGE$_2$ = prostaglandin E$_2$; IFNα and γ = interferon α and γ; LDGF-F = lymphocyte-derived growth factor for fibroblasts

A different form of delayed-type hypersensitivity is associated with various chronic granulomatous diseases, including tuberculosis, 'tuberculoid'-type reactions in leprosy, schistosomiasis, sarcoidosis, chronic beryllium disease and extrinsic allergic alveolitis. Formation of 'epithelioid-type' granulomas in the involved tissues is a characteristic feature of these diseases. The granulomatous lesions are the result of delayed-type hypersensitivity reactions induced as a consequence of the presence of agents within macrophages which these cells find difficult to destroy. Because the agents are antigens, the macrophages can present them to T-helper lymphocytes, and incite their activation with the release of the lymphokine interleukin-2 (IL2), which drives the subsequent proliferation and differentiation of T-lymphocyte subpopulations. Lymphokine mediators of delayed hypersensitivity are then released, and these are the effectors of delayed-type hypersensitivity responses (see 'Cytokine mediators'). These mediators include factors that act on macrophages aiding the development of granulomas by attracting more monocytes and macrophages to the reaction site, causing their focal aggregation, and enhancing their activation and differentiation to form the core of cells that are found at the centre of the granulomas. In mature granulomas, this central core of cells

includes typical macrophages, macrophages that have formed multinucleate giant cells of the Langhans' type with a peripheral ring of nuclei, and 'epithelioid cells' that are characteristic of granulomas generated by immunological mechanisms. The origin of epithelioid cells is still unclear but they are thought to differentiate from macrophages as a result of stimulation by lymphokines, although the nature of the exact stimulus is still unknown. They show many similarities to macrophages, but ultrastructurally their cytoplasm can be seen to contain numerous translucent vesicles and very few phagolysosomes, indicating that they are more secretory than phagocytic in their functions. In some diseases, such as tuberculosis, the central core of the granuloma can also show a zone of necrosis due to cell death, but this is not a feature of all granulomatous diseases. The central core of the granuloma is surrounded by numerous T lymphocytes, which have been shown by immunocytochemical studies to be predominantly CD4+ (T-helper/inducer cells) in the central areas, but with an increasing proportion of CD8+ (T-suppressor/cytotoxic phenotype) towards the periphery. At the edge of the granuloma a protective border of fibroblasts forms, 'walling-off' the area of inflammation from the surrounding tissue. Collagen fibres may also be deposited. The amount of fibrosis that forms around the granulomas is a very variable feature, both between individual patients and between the different disorders. The mechanisms that regulate the fibrogenic reactions are still unclear, although it is known from in vitro studies that macrophages and T lymphocytes produce an array of factors which have effects on fibroblasts, some acting to enhance the fibrogenic response whilst others have inhibitory effects (Figure 4.5). The risk of development of widespread fibrosis is the most serious clinical complication of chronic granulomatous disorders because, although the cellular inflammatory reaction is often self-limiting or responsive to corticosteroids, fibrosis shows little, or only limited, response to most current therapeutic agents.

There is an even greater need to clarify the role played by immunological factors in the development of fibrosis (Figure 4.5) in certain non-granulomatous chronic lung diseases, where interstitial fibrosis is one of the main histological features and, as a consequence, the prognosis is often poor. These include cryptogenic fibrosing alveolitis, fibrosing alveolitis associated with systemic connective tissue disorders, and fibrogenic dust diseases, such as asbestosis. In these diseases, the main histological appearances are alveolar wall thickening and widespread interstitial fibrosis, accumulations of alveolar macrophages in the airspaces, and diffuse infiltrates of mononuclear cells (including lymphocytes) in the alveolar walls and septa.

Studies of cells washed from the lungs of patients with these diseases, using the technique of bronchoalveolar lavage, have focused attention on the role of macrophages and granulocytes in pathogenesis, because alveolar macrophages, together with increased numbers of neutrophils and eosinophils, are the main cell types washed from the terminal airspaces in these diseases (Klech and Hutter, 1990). The macrophages show many features of activation, and release a variety of factors which are thought to play a central role in fibrogenesis by stimulating the proliferation of fibroblasts and inducing collagen synthesis. These include fibronectin, which is a chemotactic factor for fibroblasts and is also able to act as a 'competence factor' priming fibroblasts in readiness for proliferation. The fibroblasts can then be driven into proliferation by *alveolar macrophage-derived growth factor* (AMDGF, Figure 4.5). Other factors produced by macrophages can then act to enhance fibroblast proliferation. These include IL1 and TNFα; however, although these factors have an enhancing effect when present independently, it has been shown that when both are present together they can induce an increase in intracellular levels of PGE_2 within fibroblasts, which has the effect of inhibiting fibroblast proliferation (Figure 4.5). TGFβ is another mediator which can, on the one

hand, induce fibroblast proliferation and collagen synthesis but, on the other hand, lead to an elevation in PGE_2. The macrophages are also thought to play a key role in recruiting neutrophils into the lungs, which are thought to promote tissue damage through their release of proteolytic enzymes and oxidants. It is clear, however, from the studies of lung biopsy samples that many lymphocytes are also present within the alveolar walls where they are, presumably, less accessible to sampling by bronchoalveolar lavage. Lymphocytes also have the capacity to produce a range of mediators that can affect fibroblasts (Figure 4.5).

Immunocytochemical studies of lung biopsies from patients with fibrosing alveolitis have demonstrated that the majority of the lymphocytes in the diffuse infiltrates are T cells, consisting of variable proportions of CD4+ and CD8+ cells, and that some express receptors for interleukin-2 indicating that they have undergone recent antigenic stimulation (Kradin et al., 1986; Haslam, 1990). The alveolar epithelial cells in the lungs of these patients also differ from those in normal lungs because they strongly express HLA-DR antigens, indicating that they may have acquired the capacity to function as antigen-presenting cells (Kallenberg et al., 1987; Haslam, 1990).

Epithelial cells and other tissue cell types, including fibroblasts, are now also known to be capable of releasing a variety of mediators with effects on fibroblasts (Figure 4.5); the most recent theories of pathogenesis propose that pathogenic mechanisms probably involve complex interactions between networks of cytokines released from a wide variety of cell types, including tissue as well as inflammatory cells. The role of T lymphocytes in the pathogenesis of the more fibrogenic lung diseases has been relatively little investigated, even though the observations on lung biopsies indicate that T-lymphocyte-mediated hypersensitivity reactions may make a contribution. More interest has previously centred on the role of B lymphocytes, because lymphoid follicles containing B lymphocytes that produce immunoglobulins were recognized many years ago to be present in lung biopsies of some patients with fibrosing alveolitis (see Chapter 15). It has been proposed that antibody-mediated reactions may contribute in the pathogenesis because elevated levels of immune complexes can be demonstrated in the serum of many patients at earlier stages of the disease (Dreisin et al., 1978; Haslam et al., 1979; Martinet, Haslam and Turner-Warwick, 1984) and in BAL fluids (Turner-Warwick et al., 1981). Immune complex deposits containing complement have occasionally been detected in the alveolar walls (Turner-Warwick, Haslam and Weeks, 1971), suggesting the involvement of type III hypersensitivity mechanisms. The antigens involved in immune complex formation are unknown, but autoantibodies to non-organ-specific antigens, in particular anti-nuclear antibodies and rheumatoid factors, can be detected in the serum of many patients, and there is speculation that they may play some role in the disease. Immune complexes can interact with Fc receptors on alveolar macrophages stimulating the release of a chemotactic factor for neutrophils; this is believed to be one of the mechanisms by which neutrophils are recruited to the lungs of patients with fibrosing alveolitis. It is thought that the neutrophils participate in local tissue destruction by releasing proteolytic enzymes, including collagenase and elastase, and through their release of oxidants, such as superoxide anion and hydrogen peroxide, which also have tissue-damaging potential. The recent observation that BAL levels of glutathione, a major antioxidant in epithelial lining fluid, are decreased markedly in cryptogenic fibrosing alveolitis (Cantin et al., 1989), suggests that the clinical role of oxidant–antioxidant imbalance at the alveolar epithelial surfaces should be investigated further in fibrosing lung diseases. This observation has also led to the suggestion that glutathione may be useful in therapy (Borok et al., 1991). Eosinophils increase in lavage fluids at a later stage of disease in patients with fibrosing alveolitis and they are an indicator of poor prognosis, being associated with progressive deterioration and failure to respond to cortico-steroids (Haslam et al., 1980; Rudd, Haslam and Turner-Warwick, 1981; Libby, 1987; Peterson, Monick and Hunninghake, 1987). Some patients with elevated counts of eosinophils in BAL do, however, respond favourably to cyclophosphamide (Turner-Warwick and Haslam, 1987). The stimulus for the influx of eosinophils is unknown, but eleva-tions in histamine have been demonstrated in BAL samples of these patients correlating with the eosinophil counts, suggesting that ECF-A (eosinophil chemotactic factor of anaphylaxis) from mast cells may be involved (Haslam et al., 1981b). Ultrastructural studies of lung biopsies from these patients have demonstrated that mast cells occur in increased numbers in sites of dense fibrosis, and show evidence of degranulation. Elevated numbers of mast cells have also been demonstrated in the fibrotic lesions in animal models of asbestosis (Wagner et al., 1984).

The role of lymphocytes in fibrosing lung disease is important to elucidate, because studies have shown that a minority of patients with cryptogenic fibrosing alveolitis who have elevated lymphocyte counts in BAL tend to be at an earlier stage of disease, and have a better chance of responding to corticosteroids (Haslam et al., 1980; Rudd, Haslam and Turner-Warwick, 1981; Watters et al., 1987). There is also evidence in pulmonary sarcoidosis that patients with higher pre-treatment BAL lymphocyte counts are more likely to achieve maintained radio-graphic clearing on steroids (Foley et al., 1989; Prior

et al., 1990). In relation to these observations, it is of interest that T lymphocytes can produce, among other factors, factors that can inhibit fibroblast growth and collagen synthesis (Figure 4.5). These include the lymphokine IFNγ (Elias, Jiminez and Freundlich, 1987); it has recently been shown that IFNγ occurs in higher levels in the serum of patients with pulmonary sarcoidosis who show a more favourable response to corticosteroids (Prior and Haslam, 1991). Furthermore, a recent clinical trial has indicated that recombinant IFNγ has a benefi-cial effect in the treatment of the connective tissue disease scleroderma (Kahan et al., 1989), which can occur in clinical association with fibrosing alveolitis. Recombinant IFNγ has also been shown to reduce fibrosis in the bleomycin model of pulmonary fibro-sis (Hyde et al., 1988). This raises the question as to whether recombinant IFNγ (or interferon-α or -β which also have inhibitory effects on fibroblasts) may provide another therapeutic approach for consideration in the treatment of fibrosing lung diseases, when patients fail to respond to conven-tional treatment with corticosteroids or cyclophos-phamide (see under 'Therapeutic approaches').

T lymphocytes from the blood of patients with scleroderma have been shown to be defective in production of IFNγ (Stolzenburg et al., 1988); it has been reported that IFNγ production by blood lymphocytes from some patients with sarcoidosis, cryptogenic fibrosing alveolitis and fibrosing alveoli-tis in association with scleroderma is also defective (Prior and Haslam, 1992). It is conceivable that patients who are less efficient in their production of IFNγ may be less well able to down-regulate fibro-sis. IFNγ is also a potent macrophage-activating factor, and, thus, patients with less efficient produc-tion of IFNγ may also be less well able to degrade phagocytosed agents.

Autoimmunity and occupational lung diseases

As mentioned in earlier sections, the immune and inflammatory disturbances in diffuse interstitial fibrosing lung diseases, and in several other chronic inflammatory diseases, include the production of 'autoantibodies' to components of the host's own tissues. In many diseases it is thought that the autoantibodies play no role in pathogenesis, but are merely epiphenomena that result from some alter-ation induced by the disease process; in other diseases they appear to be a main causal factor (type II hypersensitivity) or a contributory factor (type III hypersensitivity) in pathogenesis. Under normal circumstances, individuals do not mount immune reactions against components of their own body, even though these components are antigenic if they are injected into animals or genetically non-identical individuals (such as occurs in rhesus disease). This immunological non-responsiveness to self components is termed 'immunological tolerance' and is established during the neonatal period.

The mechanisms of induction of immunological tolerance are still under investigation, but one of the main mechanisms appears to be that clones of T lymphocytes bearing antigen receptors to self-antigens are destroyed during neonatal processing of T lymphocytes within the thymus gland. Clones of B lymphocytes expressing antigen receptors to self-antigens are still detectable in adults, but they are normally unresponsive in vivo. It is thought that this lack of response may be due to the clonal deletion of T-helper cells, which are required to aid the activation of self-reactive B cells. Another mechanism also appears to exist to maintain immune tolerance to persistent T-helper clones to self-antigens, and this involves the generation of T-suppressor lymphocytes which inhibit effector cells with receptors for self-antigens.

Autoimmune responses presumably occur as a consequence of breakdown in any one of the above mechanisms which maintain tolerance; tolerance can also be bypassed in a variety of ways. For example, bypass of tolerance can result from interactions between foreign agents (such as viruses or drugs) which can induce changes in the molecular structure of host components so that they are recognized as foreign. Antibodies produced against such altered components can frequently cross-react with antigenic determinants on the unaltered host molecules. In addition, autoimmune reactions can also be stimulated by the release of host antigens which are normally sequestered within cells and are not accessible to the cells of the immune system. Tolerance is not normally established to such intracellular components, and if high levels are released due to continuing tissue damage, this is another mechanism whereby autoimmune reactions might be stimulated. There is also recent evidence that certain cell types which do not normally express class II MHC (major histocompatibility complex) antigens, but which express them during the course of immunological reactions, may be capable of inducing reactions to self-antigens (Londei et al., 1984). Indeed, strong expression of class II MHC antigens has been demonstrated on alveolar epithelial cells in lung biopsies of patients with fibrosing alveolitis, and it has been suggested that this may have relevance to autoantibody production in this disorder (Kallenberg et al., 1987; Haslam, 1990).

Diseases associated with production of autoantibodies fall into two main groups: those involving the production of autoantibodies to antigens which are specific to a particular organ, that is, *organ-specific*

autoantibodies (such as autoantibodies against thyroglobulin in Hashimoto's thyroiditis) and those which involve production of autoantibodies to antigens common to many tissues – *non-organ-specific autoantibodies*. The latter frequently include autoantibodies to intracellular components such as cell nuclei, mitochondria or microsomes, as well as autoantibodies to immunoglobulins (rheumatoid factors). A classic disorder associated with the production of non-organ-specific autoantibodies is systemic lupus erythematosus (SLE); the evidence that immune complexes involving DNA may be involved in the glomerulonephritis of this disease has already been mentioned. The autoantibodies that have been reported in human lung diseases are mainly non-organ-specific and it is still not known what role, if any, they play in the pathogenesis of these diseases. The one exception is Goodpasture's syndrome, where the pulmonary haemorrhage and glomerulonephritis are thought to involve type II hypersensitivity reactions mediated by autoantibodies which cross-react with the pulmonary and glomerular basement membranes (see 'Type II hypersensitivity'). The fact that fibrosing alveolitis can occur in association with SLE has raised speculation that trapping of DNA-containing immune complexes in the fine capillary beds may occur in the lungs as well as in the kidneys, and may be involved in the pathogenesis of the lung disease; however, the evidence for this is still not well substantiated (see 'Type III hypersensitivity'). Table 4.4 lists the various lung diseases, including occupational lung diseases, that are associated with an increased frequency of autoantibodies, and indicates some of the autoantibodies involved.

Effects of smoking on immune responses

It has been recognized for many years that inhalation of tobacco smoke can induce numerical and functional changes in a variety of immune and inflammatory cells, detectable not only at a local level within the respiratory system, but also in peripheral blood populations. Thus, possible effects of smoking must be taken into account when considering the pathogenic mechanisms in any lung disease. Current knowledge on effects of smoking, gained from studies in animal models and in human beings, has been reviewed in detail by Holt (1987), to which readers are referred. There have been contradictory reports regarding some of the observations; therefore, this brief summary will focus only on the more consistent findings.

Table 4.4 Prevalence of antinuclear antibodies (ANA) and rheumatoid factor (RF) in some disorders of the lung

Disorder	ANA prevalence			RF prevalence		
	No. of patients	No. with ANA	Percentage with ANA*	No. of patients	No. with RF	Percentage with RF*
Pleuropulmonary SLE	30	30	100	18	7	39
Rheumatoid arthritis with FA	36	16	44	34	23	68
Systemic sclerosis with FA	14	10	71	14	0	0
CFA	97	33	34	97	14	14
Silicosis (sandblasting)	39	17	44	40	3	8
Asbestosis	75	19	25	75	17	23
Asbestos exposure (normal radiographs)	75	2	3	75	2	3
Coal pneumoconiosis	109	19	17	71	5	7
Extrinsic allergic alveolitis	54	2	4	57	3	5

* Healthy controls: ANA 3–9%; RF 3–10% (the prevalence of ANA and RF increases with age).
Data from Haslam (1976); Haslam and Turner-Warwick (1981); Turner-Warwick (1978).
SLE = systemic lupus erythematosus; CFA = cryptogenic fibrosing alveolitis; FA = fibrosing alveolitis.

Studies comparing the cell populations washed from the terminal airspaces of the lungs of healthy smoking and non-smoking volunteers, using the technique of bronchoalveolar lavage (BAL), have demonstrated that smoking induces a striking increase in the numbers of alveolar macrophages, which are five- to tenfold higher in smokers compared with non-smokers (Reynolds and Newball, 1974). Neutrophils are also present in greater numbers (approximately fourfold higher) in the BAL samples of smokers compared with non-smokers (Hunninghake and Crystal, 1983). Smoking does not, however, induce any increase in the numbers of lymphocytes in BAL samples (although when BAL cell counts are expressed as differential percentages, the percentages appear higher in non-smokers – up to 20 per cent, compared with counts of up to 10 per cent in smokers – due to the difference in the relative proportions of macrophages present in the samples). Numerical increases in neutrophils and monocytes are also demonstrable in the blood of smokers compared with non-smokers (Bridges, Wyatt and Rehm, 1985; Nielsen, 1985). By contrast with the findings in BAL, T-lymphocyte numbers are also frequently increased in the blood with CD4+ (helper/inducer) T cells predominating in light to moderate smokers (Ginns et al., 1982; Hughes et al., 1985), and CD8+ (suppressor/cytotoxic) T cells predominating in heavy smokers (Ginns et al., 1982; Miller et al., 1982). The light to moderate smokers also show impaired T-suppressor function to pokeweed mitogen-stimulated immunoglobulin production (Hughes et al., 1985). Natural killer cell function has also been reported to be significantly lower in the peripheral blood of smokers compared with non-smokers (Ferson et al., 1979; Hughes et al., 1985).

Although B-lymphocyte numbers are increased in the blood of smokers (Hughes et al., 1985), there have been many reports that serum levels of IgG, IgM and IgA are lower in smokers than in non-smokers (Onari et al., 1978; Ferson et al., 1979; Andersen et al., 1982) whereas smoking can induce striking elevations in serum levels of IgE (Burrows et al., 1981; Warren et al., 1982; Stein et al., 1983). Smoking related increases have also been reported in serum levels of IgD (Bahna, Heiner and Myhre, 1983). The effect of smoking on immunoglobulin production in the respiratory tract and lungs is less clear, but reduced levels of IgG and IgA have been reported in saliva (Jedrychowski, Adamczyk and Jaskolka, 1980), although levels in BAL fluids have generally been reported to be normal or elevated (Reynolds and Newball, 1974; Bell et al., 1981). There is, however, little information on whether smoking induces any alteration in the form of IgA present in the secretions (that is, whether it affects the production of 'secretory piece' and its attachment to the IgA dimers). The findings in BAL fluid do, nevertheless, present difficulties in interpretation, because the dilution factor due to the procedure cannot be accurately determined. Furthermore, there is convincing evidence that smoking increases epithelial permeability (Minty, Jordan and Jones, 1981). Thus, increases of immunoglobulin in BAL fluid are likely to be due partly to increased diffusion from plasma.

Despite these difficulties in interpreting the local findings, there is indirect evidence that strongly supports the serological evidence that smoking can suppress the production of IgG and IgA antibodies, but enhance the production of IgE antibodies. This includes evidence that smokers are much more likely than non-smokers to produce IgE antibodies, and develop symptoms of disease, when exposed to certain allergens associated with occupational asthma (Zetterström et al., 1981; Venables et al., 1985). By contrast, smokers exposed to antigens that can cause extrinsic allergic alveolitis have a much lower prevalence of precipitating IgG antibodies to these antigens in their serum than non-smokers; the prevalence of disease is also lower in smokers (Morgan et al., 1973; Andersen and Christensen, 1983; McSharry et al., 1984; Cormier, Belanger and Durand, 1985). Smokers also appear less susceptible to another granulomatous disease – pulmonary sarcoidosis (Douglas et al., 1986).

One possible mechanism which may be relevant to the reductions in antibody production in smokers is the observation that alveolar macrophages from smokers have been reported to express lower levels of class II MHC antigens, and to have lower antigen-presenting function compared with alveolar macrophages from non-smokers (Clerici et al., 1984). This raises the possibility that smoking may also reduce class II expression by more efficient antigen-presenting cells, such as macrophages in interstitial locations within the lungs. The levels of lymphoproliferative responses to antigens and mitogens are also known to decrease as the numbers of macrophages relative to lymphocytes are increased in functional assays (McCombs et al., 1982; Ettensohn and Roberts, 1983; Twomey, Laughter and Brown, 1983). This suggests that smoking-related increases in alveolar macrophages and blood monocytes may also contribute to the reductions in antibody production in smokers. The explanation for the enhancing effect of smoking on IgE responses is not known, but it has been speculated that this might be due to smoking-related suppression of a T-cell subpopulation which normally down-regulates IgE responses.

Smoking also has a wide variety of other effects, apart from those just mentioned, and alveolar macrophages have been extensively studied. Those from smokers show many morphological features of 'activation' including increases in endoplasmic reticulum and phagolysosomes, and smoking-related inclusions can also be demonstrated in the cytoplasm, such as kaolin particles, which are present in tobacco from some geographical locations, for example, from Virginia (Pratt et al., 1971). The cells have an increased content of lysosomal enzymes (Harris et al., 1975), the enzyme lysozyme is present in increased amounts in the BAL fluids of smokers (Harris et al., 1975), and there is also evidence of transient increases in elastase derived from macrophages and neutrophils in BAL fluids (Janoff, Raju and Dearing, 1983). Elevations in fibronectin (Villiger et al., 1981) and in some complement components (Robertson et al., 1976) in BAL fluids of smokers may also be a consequence of enhanced macrophage activation.

Alveolar macrophages from smokers also release greater amounts of oxidants, in particular hydrogen peroxide and superoxide anion (Razma et al., 1984). It is believed that oxidant-induced damage may be responsible for the functional deficiency in protease inhibitors which has been reported in the BAL fluids of smokers (Gadek, Felb and Crystal, 1979; Carp et al., 1982). Although smoking enhances many functions of alveolar macrophages, it appears to depress certain other functions. These include depressed phagocytic function mediated by opsonic attachment to surface C3b receptors (Shimada, 1982), which appears to be due to a smoking-related decrease in the C3b receptors (Warr and Martin, 1977); and decreased production of arachidonic acid metabolites, in particular prostaglandins and LTB_4 (Laviolette et al., 1986). Increased activation of alveolar macrophages, in respect of increased release of enzymes and oxidants, is thought to be a main contributory factor in smoking-induced tissue damage. In relation to smoking-released increases in epithelial permeability, it is also of interest that increased numbers of mast cells are present in the airways' epithelium of smokers (Lamb and Lumsden, 1982), and increases of histamine have been reported in the sputum (Leitch, Lumb and Kay, 1981).

Bronchoalveolar lavage in investigation of occupational lung diseases

Since its introduction into clinical investigation in the 1970s, the technique of small-volume, segmental bronchoalveolar lavage (BAL), via the fibreoptic bronchoscope, has generated considerable information on inflammatory cells and other components washed from the airspaces of the lungs of patients with a wide range of diffuse lung diseases. Apart from making an important contribution to studies of pathogenic mechanisms, some of the information generated by BAL has proved of value as an aid to differential diagnosis of these diseases and, as a consequence, BAL is now widely included as part of routine clinical investigation.

BAL is a minimally invasive procedure, which involves only a simple addition to routine fibreoptic bronchoscopy (Figure 4.6). It is important to follow a standardized procedure and, although there are minor differences of detail, most centres use a standardized introduction volume of lavage fluid (sterile physiological saline, maximum of 300 ml, employing 50- or 60-ml introduction aliquots or minimum of 100 ml, employing 20-ml introduction aliquots) and also use a standardized site for lavage

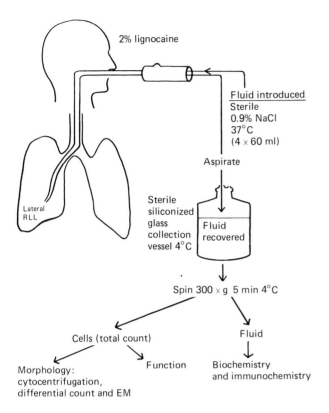

2% lignocaine

Fluid introduced
Sterile
0.9% NaCl
37°C
(4 × 60 ml)

Aspirate

Lateral
RLL

Sterile
siliconized
glass
collection
vessel 4°C

Fluid
recovered

Spin 300 × g 5 min 4°C

Cells (total count)   Fluid

Morphology: Function   Biochemistry
cytocentrifugation,   and immunochemistry
differential count and EM

Figure 4.6 Diagram indicating the procedure of bronchoalveolar lavage. RLL = right lung, lateral segment of lower lobe

(usually the right middle lobe or the lateral segment of the right lower lobe) (Klech and Pohl, 1989; BAL Co-operative Group Steering Committee, 1990). Due to its safety, BAL has the advantage that it can be included early in clinical investigation prior to deciding whether to proceed to more invasive biopsy procedures. Although lung biopsy has the advantage that it provides information on appearances in situ in interstitial as well as in intra-alveolar locations, and it can identify well-characterized pathognomonic features, BAL is a useful complementary method because it provides information on pooled inflammatory cells and other components washed from the airspaces of a relatively large segment of the lungs, which can be advantageous if the disease is patchy. It is important to emphasize that, even though, on some occasions, BAL can identify specific features that can indicate the diagnosis and avoid the need to proceed to biopsy, the form of data generated by BAL is very different from that obtained by biopsy, and specialist knowledge is required for interpretation – as with most investigatory procedures.

The samples obtained by BAL contain a wide range of components, including immune and inflammatory cells, and a wide variety of soluble extracel-lular components, including proteins derived from the serum, enzymes, enzyme inhibitors and lipids, and many other components. On occasions, additional components may also be present, for example, inorganic dust particles or micro-organisms, indicating a specific exposure or infection. In normal volunteers or patients with radiologically normal lungs, the main cell types in BAL are alveolar macrophages and a few lymphocytes, but other cell types are uncommon. The reported average total cell count for normal, healthy, non-smoking young adults is 0.1×10^6 cells/ml and for normal smokers is higher at 0.4×10^6 cells/ml (Reynolds and Newball, 1974; Hunninghake et al., 1979). There is, however, a wide variation around these average figures. The higher total cell counts in smokers are mainly due to an increase in alveolar macrophage numbers (Reynolds and Newball, 1974). This difference between smokers and non-smokers is detectable but is less in patients with interstitial lung disease, presumably due to superimposed disease-related inflammatory cell increases (see later).

Although total BAL cell counts can give an indication of overall cellularity, the interpretation is difficult because it is not technically possible to standardize both the lavage fluid introduction and recovery volumes. In practice, the differential percentage counts of the cell types in BAL have proved of greater value in routine clinical investigation. *Normal ranges* from figures in the literature (Reynolds and Newball, 1974; Klech and Pohl, 1989; BAL Co-operative Group Steering Committee, 1990) are:

1. Macrophages ≥ 80 per cent in non-smokers, ≥ 90 per cent in smokers.
2. Lymphocytes ≤ 20 per cent in non-smokers, ≤ 10 per cent in smokers.
3. Neutrophils ≤ 4 per cent (very occasionally higher in older or very heavy smokers).
4. Eosinophils ≤ 3 per cent.
5. Mast cells ≤ 0.5 per cent.

Ciliated or squamous epithelial cells from the bronchi may also be present but usually do not exceed 5 per cent of the total cells. When epithelial cells exceed 5 per cent this suggests the presence of bronchial inflammation, which needs to be taken into account when interpreting the lavage result (Haslam, 1984). In patients with chronic, diffuse lung diseases, the differential percentage counts of BAL cells can aid differential diagnosis, because different types of inflammatory cells predominate in BAL in the different disorders which can either support the provisional diagnosis or suggest an alternative when considered in the full clinical context. Although useful, the trends of difference in BAL cell counts are not sufficient by themselves to establish a diagnosis due to the overlap which occurs

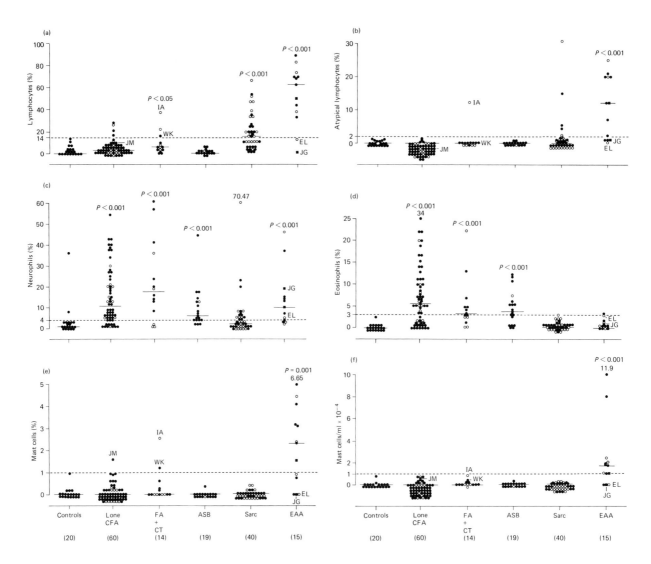

Figure 4.7 Differential percentage counts of cell types in bronchoalveolar lavage samples from patients with interstitial lung diseases. CFA = cryptogenic fibrosing alveolitis; FA + CT = fibrosing alveolitis in association with systemic connective tissue diseases; ASB = asbestosis; Sarc = sarcoidosis; EAA = extrinsic allergic alveolitis; EL,JG = patients with EAA who had ceased exposure several years before lavage, unlike the remaining patients in the group who had current or recent exposure. ○ = Untreated non-smokers; ● = untreated current or ex-smokers; ■ = current or ex-smokers being treated with prednisolone

between the disorders, and to the variability between individuals (Figure 4.7).

Neutrophils are the inflammatory cell type most often increased in disorders in which interstitial fibrosis is a predominant feature of the pathology, such as the inorganic dust diseases asbestosis and silicosis (Bignon et al., 1978; Gellert et al., 1985a; Haslam et al., 1987; Rom et al., 1987; Wallaert et al., 1990), and diseases of unknown cause such as cryptogenic fibrosing alveolitis (CFA) and fibrosing alveolitis associated with systemic connective tissue diseases such as rheumatoid arthritis and sclero-derma (Reynolds et al., 1977; Weinberger et al.,

1978; Haslam et al., 1980; Garcia et al., 1986; Wallaert et al., 1986). Patients with these disorders also frequently have increased eosinophils in lavage (Haslam, Dewar and Turner-Warwick, 1982; Gellert et al., 1985b; Haslam et al., 1987; Hällgren et al., 1989). The finding of increased eosinophils in associ-ation with neutrophil increases in BAL, in the absence of any evidence of allergy or peripheral blood eosinophilia, is a strong indication of the diagnosis of a diffuse interstitial lung disorder because, apart from this, high counts of BAL eosinophils have only been reported in cases of cryptogenic pulmonary eosinophilia, Churg–Strauss syndrome, amiodarone-induced pneumonitis and allergic bronchopulmonary aspergillosis (Velay et al., 1987); slight increases have also been reported in patients with asthma (Velay et al., 1987). The finding of lone increases in neutrophils in BAL is of less value in differential diagnosis because increases in neutrophils can occur for many reasons, for example, in heavy smokers possibly as an indication of infection, in bacterial pneumonias, in asthma, in patients with granulomatous lung diseases when there is extensive radiographic shadowing on the chest radiographs, and in the occupational lung disease extrinsic allergic alveolitis as part of the acute, and subacute, response after recent antigen exposure (Haslam et al., 1981a, 1987; Roth et al., 1981; Lin, Haslam and Turner-Warwick, 1985; Klech and Hutter, 1990).

By contrast with the diffuse interstitial fibrosing lung diseases, lymphocytes are the inflammatory cell type most commonly increased in granulomatous lung diseases, such as the organic dust disease extrinsic allergic alveolitis, the inorganic dust disease beryllium disease, and in non-occupational granulomatous lung diseases such as tuberculosis and sarcoidosis (Reynolds et al., 1977; Weinberger et al., 1978; Haslam, 1984; Daniele et al., 1985; Klech and Hutter, 1990). The counts of BAL lymphocytes tend to be higher in patients with extrinsic allergic alveolitis (often $\geqslant$ 60 per cent) than in the other granulomatous lung diseases (where counts are usually $\leqslant$ 40 per cent). However, there is a wide variation in different patients and lymphocyte counts alone are insufficient to differentiate reliably between the disorders. The diagnosis of extrinsic allergic alveolitis can, however, be strongly indicated by the demonstration of increases in mast cells (counts up to 6 per cent) as well as striking increases in lymphocytes at times of current or recent antigen exposure (Haslam et al., 1987; see Chapter 20, 'Immunological mechanisms'). *Elevated mast cell counts of this order are very rare in other interstitial lung diseases.* The diagnosis of beryllium disease can be aided by the demonstration of specifically sensitized lymphocytes among the BAL cells which can be stimulated into proliferation via the addition of beryllium salts (Epstein et al., 1982; Cullen et al., 1987; Rossman et al., 1988; Saltini et al., 1989; see also Chapter 17, 'BAL lymphocytes').

It is now recognized that slight to moderate increases in lymphocytes can also occur in patients with diffuse interstitial pulmonary fibrosing lung disease if it is detected at a very early stage. For example, increases in BAL lymphocytes have been reported in a minority of patients with CFA at an early corticosteroid-responsive stage (Haslam et al., 1980; Rudd, Haslam and Turner-Warwick, 1981; Watters et al., 1987) and in patients with systemic connective tissue diseases as an early indication of pulmonary involvement (Wallaert et al., 1986).

Increases in BAL lymphocytes have also been reported prior to the development of symptoms in workers exposed to asbestos or silica (Christman et al., 1985; Gellert et al, 1985a). It is important to be aware that increases in BAL lymphocytes can also occur in many workers exposed to organic dust who show no evidence of symptoms of extrinsic allergic alveolitis (Leatherman et al., 1984; Cormier, Belanger and Laviolette, 1986). The prognostic value of these early changes is not yet known with any certainty.

Although the diagnostic value of BAL cell counts has limitations, a number of other appearances can be detected in BAL samples which can be of greater help in differential diagnosis by identifying and including some of the rarer lung diseases. These include the disease alveolar lipoproteinosis which can be indicated by the presence of large lipoprotein aggregates in BAL samples, the disease histiocytosis X which can be indicated by the demonstration of elevated numbers of histiocytosis X cells among the BAL macrophages, using electron microscopy to identify the unusual X bodies in the cytoplasm of the cells, and the disease pulmonary haemosiderosis resulting from occult bleeding, which is indicated by using Perl's iron stain to demonstrate that the alveolar macrophages in the BAL samples are heavily laden with ferric iron (Haslam, 1984; Daniele et al., 1985; Klech and Hutter, 1990). In recent years, BAL has proved of considerable value to identify pulmonary opportunistic infections in patients with AIDS or following organ transplantation (Klech and Hutter, 1990).

BAL is also a sensitive method to detect inorganic particles relating to a wide range of occupational and environmental exposures (Bignon et al., 1978; De Vuyst et al., 1982, 1986a, b, 1987a, b; Davison et al., 1983; Christman et al., 1985; Johnson et al., 1986; Chiappino et al., 1988; Sebastien et al., 1988). Although the presence of particles in BAL samples does not establish the diagnosis of occupational lung disease because they relate to exposure rather than to disease, their demonstration in a patient with chronic lung disease of indeterminate cause means that this diagnosis must be seriously considered and the occupational exposure carefully checked. In patients where there is no known history of exposure, techniques of mineralogical analysis, employing electron microscopes fitted with energy-dispersive X-ray spectroscopy systems, can be used to identify the particles (Johnson et al., 1986). The presence of ferruginous bodies lying among the BAL cells can be readily detected in the cytocentrifuge preparations used for routine differential BAL cell counting, and the presence of unusual particles within the cytoplasm of alveolar macrophages can also be readily detected in the routine cytocentrifuge preparations at the level of light microscopy (Haslam, 1984; Johnson et al.,

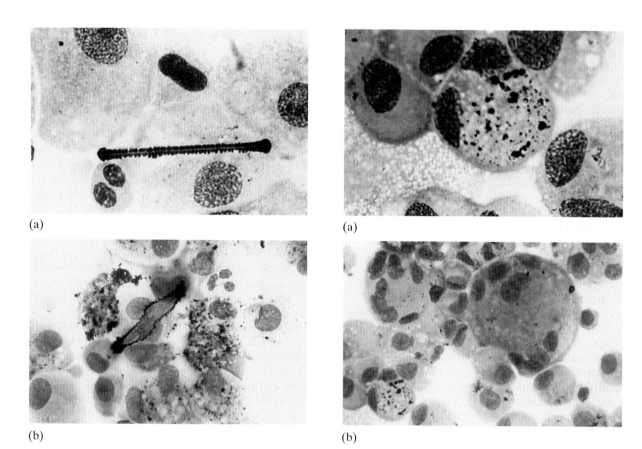

(a)

(b)

(a)

(b)

Figure 4.8 Example of (a) a typical ferruginous body ('asbestos-body') in the cytocentrifuge preparation of a BAL sample from a patient with asbestosis (magnification × 750); (b) a typical ferruginous body ('talc-body') in the cytocentrifuge preparation of a BAL sample from a patient with talc pneumoconiosis (magnification × 750)

Figure 4.9 Example of (a) particles of high refractive index in the cytoplasm of an alveolar macrophage in the cytocentrifuge preparation of a BAL sample from a patient exposed to hard metal dust; (b) 'giant' forms of macrophages in the same cytocentrifuge preparation indicating the possible diagnosis of giant-cell interstitial pneumonia, which was subsequently confirmed by lung biopsy (magnification × 405)

1986). In the author's experience, particles are invariably detectable in the BAL samples of patients with known exposure to a wide range of inorganic dusts at the level of both light and electron microscopy (Johnson et al., 1986).

Examples of ferruginous bodies in BAL samples from patients with asbestosis and talc pneumoconiosis are shown in Figure 4.8. Ferruginous bodies have been reported in BAL samples from controls without occupational exposure (De Vuyst et al., 1987b), but their detection appears to require the screening of much larger volumes of lavage fluid than used to prepare conventional cytocentrifuge preparations. Uncoated fibres, too small to form ferruginous bodies, are not readily detectable by light microscopy and need to be identified by electron microscopy. However, the current evidence suggests that quantification of asbestos bodies, rather than the total of coated and uncoated fibres

in BAL, gives a more specific discrimination between patients with and without interstitial lung disease (De Vuyst et al., 1982, 1987b; Gellert et al., 1986), although still lacking consistent reliability, due to differences among individuals (see also Chapter 15).

Figure 4.9a shows an example of bright particles (that is, particles with a higher refractive index and, thus, brighter than the surrounding cellular material seen by plane white light using maximum contrast), indicative of the presence of mineral matter in the cytoplasm of an alveolar macrophage from a patient exposed to hard metal dust. Energy dispersive X-ray microanalysis demonstrated that these particles were mainly tungsten (Davison et al., 1983; Johnson et al., 1986). This patient also had unusual 'giant' forms of macrophages among the BAL cells (Figure 4.9b) indicating that the diagnosis of giant cell interstitial pneumonia relating to hard metal exposure should be considered; this diagnosis was subsequently confirmed by open lung biopsy (Davison et al., 1983). The presence of particles of varying degrees of luminosity, or 'brightness', as distinct from birefringence, is also a notable feature in patients exposed to crystalline silica, aluminium (De Vuyst et al., 1986a) and chromium–cobalt–molybdenum alloys used in dentistry (De Vuyst et al., 1986b). (The refractive index and birefringence of minerals are discussed briefly in Appendix IV). Particles in the alveolar macrophages of smokers can be readily discriminated by the experienced observer and identified by energy-dispersive X-ray microanalysis. When using X-ray microprobe analytical techniques, it is essential to establish background levels by studying controls without known exposure, because it has been found that levels of certain elements such as silicon and titanium in exposed individuals can be difficult to distinguish from the high background levels (Johnson et al., 1986).

There is relatively little information in the literature on the clinical value of quantifying the numbers of asbestos bodies, total fibre burden or quantification of other particles in BAL samples of patients with occupational lung diseases, but De Vuyst et al. (1982) have shown that asbestos body counts in BAL (sodium hypochloride extracts on 0.45 µm micropore filters counted by light microscopy) correlate with the type of disease, being higher in asbestos-exposed patients with interstitial disease than in those with benign pleural disease or malignant mesothelioma. It has also been shown (Sebastien et al., 1988) that BAL concentrations of ferruginous bodies are positively correlated with the lung parenchymal concentrations studied from material obtained by open lung biopsy or autopsy. These workers found that a BAL containing more than one asbestos body/ml is highly predictive of a lung tissue concentration exceeding 1000 asbestos bodies/g. Individual susceptibility of human beings to the development of occupational lung disease may be influenced by many factors, including individual differences in the rate of clearance and degradation of different types of particles (see Chapters 3 and 15). BAL offers the opportunity to study patients prospectively to address this question, and this has not been possible in the studies to date which have mainly relied on autopsy or lung biopsy material.

Apart from studies of cells and particles, BAL offers the opportunity to study many acellular components obtained from the airspaces of the lungs, including the phospholipids and apoproteins which make up the pulmonary surfactant system, immunoglobulins and other components which can diffuse from serum, and enzymes, cytokines and other components secreted from living cells or released from dead or dying cells within the diseased lungs. In interstitial lung diseases, including occupational lung diseases, there are many types of activated inflammatory cells, and increases in many cell products have been reported in the BAL fluids. These include increases in chemotactic factors which attract granulocytes and other cells to the lungs (Hunninghake et al., 1981), increases in mediators such as histamine, products of arachidonic acid metabolism and fragments of complement activation (such as C5a) which can have effects on vascular permeability (Haslam et al., 1981; Robbins, Gadek, Crystal, 1981; Fireman et al., 1989), and increases in albumin indicating that lung permeability has been increased (Haslam et al., 1981; Baughman et al., 1983). A wide range of other components has been identified in cell-free BAL fluids, including factors such as fibronectin and alveolar macrophage-derived growth factor which can stimulate fibroblast proliferation and collagen synthesis (Bitterman et al., 1986; Elias et al., 1990; Kovacs, 1991), but the clinical value of measuring such components is still unclear. This is largely because the quantification of components in solution in BAL fluids poses particular difficulties owing to the fact that it is not possible to standardize the lavage technique to avoid the variable dilution due to the lavage procedure, nor is there any accepted method of determining the dilution factor accurately. This question has been the subject of much discussion (Klech and Pohl, 1989), and readers requiring detailed information on the vast amount of research data relating to acellular components in BAL, and to the products and functions of activated BAL cells, are referred to the extensive literature on the subject which is beyond the scope of this chapter.

A summary of some of the main diagnostic trends that can be gleaned from differential counts of BAL cells and observations of particles in cytocentrifuge preparations in some of the main groups of interstitial lung disorders is shown in Table 4.5.

Genetic control of immune responses

Many of the conventionally held theories on immunopathogenesis will soon need to be updated as we gain a better understanding of disease susceptibility, due to major recent advances in molecular genetics. These are elucidating the genes that control immune responses and they are also demonstrating that allotypic variation in these genes is

Table 4.5   Profiles (underlined) of BAL cell types that can aid the differential diagnosis of the main groups of interstitial lung diseases

Patients	Number	Ferruginous bodies	Eosinophils >3%*	Neutrophils >4%*	Lymphocytes >14%*	>28%*	Atypical lymphocytes >2%*	Mast cells >1%*	Total with increases (any cell) type) (%)
					Percentage of patients with				
Lone CFA	60	0	**68**	**77**	7	0	0	**2**	83
Asbestosis	19	**100**	47	**63**	0	0	0	0	74
Sarcoidosis	40	0	0	**33**	**55**	**15**	**13**	0	60
Extrinsic allergic alveolitis	11	0	0	**64**	**91**	**73**	**73**	**64**	100
'Controls' with normal lungs (smokers)	20	0	0	**10**	0	0	0	0	10

Data from Haslam (1984).
CFA = cryptogenic fibrosing alveolitis.
*BAL cell percentage count.

associated with differences in immunological responsiveness between individuals.

MHC-linked genes

The genes that control the ability of immunocompetent cells to respond to antigens are closely linked with the MHC genes which regulate the expression of the surface MHC products that aid antigen recognition by T lymphocytes. These MHC products are also known as histocompatibility locus antigens (HLA antigens) because they are the main antigenic determinants on cells that are recognized as foreign and can stimulate graft rejection, or graft versus host reactions between allogeneic individuals. The human MHC genes are found on chromosome 6 and the MHC locus consists of three consecutive regions: first the class II region, followed by the class III region, and then the class I region. Within each region, there are subregions containing genes which code the expression of different products (Figure 4.10). There are many allelic forms of these genes which play a central role in determining differences in immune responsiveness between individuals. As previously explained (see 'Antigen-presenting cells'), the products of the class II genes play an essential role in aiding the presentation of antigens to T-helper lymphocytes. The class II region is also called the 'D region' of the human HLA genes, and three subregions have been identified known as the DP, DQ and DR loci. The genes at these loci in different individuals are of different allelic forms determined by genetic differences. The

alleles are designated by letters and numbers, DR2, DR3, DR4, and so on. It has been shown in mice that a change in a single allele in the 'IA' or 'IE' regions, which is equivalent to the human 'D region', is sufficient to change a strain from a high immune responder to a low responder, or vice versa for a given antigen. This probably occurs because the 'goodness-of-fit' or 'affinity' between the antigen and MHC product or the affinity between these and the antigen receptors on the T cells, or both, is likely to be influenced by the allelic form of the MHC product. Individuals with high binding affinity are likely to generate stronger immune responses than those with low binding affinity to the same antigen.

Allotypic differences between individuals also influence the efficiency of T-cytotoxic responses, which are directed against antigens in association with class I MHC products on target cells. The class I MHC genes consist of three subregions B, C and A. Different individuals can express different allelic forms at each of these loci (for example, B4, B6 and so on) and this can influence the affinity between antigen and class I MHC products on target cells and their 'goodness-of-fit' with the antigen receptors on T-cytotoxic cells.

As mentioned earlier (see 'Cytokine mediators'), the responses of T-suppressor lymphocytes also appear to be genetically restricted, but the actual genes have not been identified. The term 'I–J' region has been proposed to designate this region in the mouse, pending further information.

The class III region of the MHC complex incorporates the genes that are involved in the production of some of the components of the complement system (C2, factor B, C4a and C4b). In different

Major gene loci:

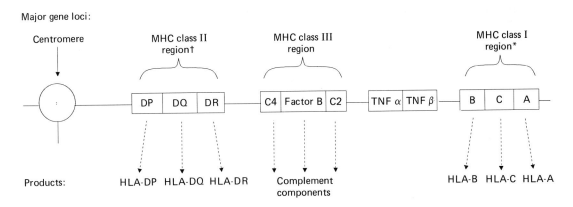

Figure 4.10 The relative location of the human major histocompatibility (MHC) genes on the short arm of chromosome 6. *Class I products are constitutively expressed on most nucleated cells and on platelets. †Class II products are constitutively expressed only on selected cell types, including monocytes/macrophages, dendritic cells and B lymphocyte

individuals, these components exhibit polymorphism indicating that there are different allelic forms of the class III genes. The genes encoding other components of the complement system are not associated with the MHC complex, but at least seven of these components also exhibit polymorphism (McLean and Winkelstein, 1984). In most instances, the polymorphism does not have any demonstrable effect on the overall function of the complement system assessed by haemolysis, but it has been shown that one of the common forms of C3 – 'C3-Fast' – is a more efficient opsonin than another common form of C3 – 'C3-Slow'. Genetically based deficiencies in production or dysfunction of complement components or their inhibitors do, however, appear to play a role in some human diseases, notably in systemic lupus erythematosus, some other 'autoimmune' diseases of the collagen vascular tissues, glomerulonephritis, recurrent infections, and in certain rarer diseases such as hereditary angioedema.

The importance of genetic factors in susceptibility to immunological diseases is further indicated by an association between the products of different allotypes of class I and class II genes (HLA types) and a variety of diseases, in particular autoimmune diseases, where immunological mechanisms appear to be involved in pathogenesis. A list of diseases where the relative risk of development is higher in individuals with particular HLA types is shown in Table 4.6. The question of whether there are any HLA associations with the development of occupational lung diseases remains uncertain because, while some observers have reported trends of association with certain disorders, for example, asbestosis and extrinsic allergic alveolitis, these have

not been consistently established and figures for relative risk are not available.

Table 4.6 Examples of human diseases where the relative risk of development is higher in individuals of certain HLA types

Disease	HLA type	Relative risk*
Haemochromatosis	A3	8.2–9.0
Ankylosing spondylitis	B27	87.4–87.8
Reiter's disease	B27	35.9–37.0
Beçhet's disease	B5	10.1
Subacute thyroiditis	B35	13.7
Myasthenia gravis	B8	3.4–4.4
Coeliac disease	B8	8.6
Chronic active hepatitis	B8	9.2
Dermatitis herpetiformis	B8	8.7
Psoriasis	CW6	13.3
Multiple sclerosis	DR2	3.8–4.8
Goodpasture's syndrome	DR2	13.1
Tuberculoid leprosy	DR2	8.1
Myasthenia gravis	DR3	3.0
Coeliac disease	DR3	10.8–73.0
Chronic active hepatitis	DR3	4.6–13.9
Dermatitis herpetiformis	DR3	10.8–56.4
Sjögren's syndrome	DR3	9.7
Addison's disease	DR3	6.3–8.8
Graves' disease	DR3	3.7–5.5
Systemic lupus erythematosus	DR3	5.8
Insulin-dependent diabetes	DR3/4	3.3–14.3
Rheumatoid arthritis	DR4	4.0–5.8
Hashimoto's thyroiditis	DR5	3.2
Pernicious anaemia	DR5	5.4

* Increased risk of individuals of the denoted HLA type developing the disease relative to individuals without that HLA type.

Immunoglobulin genes

There is an extreme diversity of antibodies within any given individual and the genes controlling production of these immunoglobulins are not part of the MHC complex. The genes coding production of the heavy chains of human immunoglobulin molecules, which determine the class (or isotype) of immunoglobulin, are found on chromosome 14. There are two identical heavy chains in each immunoglobulin molecule, and also two identical light chains. The light chains are of two forms, λ or κ, which can occur on immunoglobulins of all classes, and the genes for these are present on chromosomes 22 and 2, respectively. The vast (idiotypic) diversity in the structure of antibody molecules of all classes within a given individual is determined by variable regions of the molecules in the portions which contain the antigen-binding sites (*Fab regions*). Two Fab regions are present on each immunoglobulin molecule, and each antigen-binding site consists of a part of the variable region of one of the light chains and a part of the variable region of one of the heavy chains of each molecule. A description of the genetic events involved in the operation of antibody diversity within and between individuals is beyond the scope of this chapter. However, many mechanisms appear to be involved including isotypic variation in the germ-line, allotypic variation, somatic recombination events and somatic mutations.

Non-MHC-linked immune response genes

It is clear that the overall immune responsiveness of any individual is under polygenic control. Although MHC-linked genes are important in controlling some aspects of immune response, in particular T-cell recognition of, and binding to, antigens, other responses are controlled by other genes, for example, those regulating macrophage function, production of cytokines and production of numerous cell surface receptors. Evidence of this has been obtained in animal models, from investigations of genetic immunodeficiency states, and from the products of gene cloning experiments which have enabled many of the factors involved in immune responses to be purified and characterized. Due to the important role of macrophages in many aspects of non-specific and specific immunity, it is of interest that, in mice, resistance or susceptibility to infection by *Leishmania donovani*, *Salmonella typhimurium* and *Mycobacterium bovis* appears to map to a gene located on chromosome 1, which is

linked with macrophage function. The efficiency of antigen processing by macrophages also appears to be influenced by allotypic differences in non-MHC-linked genes, and lower levels of immune response appear to be associated with more efficient degradation of antigens within the lysosomes of macrophages, probably due to genetic differences in the rates and levels of production of hydrolytic enzymes and other substances involved in degradative mechanisms.

Therapeutic approaches

In the current state of knowledge, the exact mechanisms involved in *initiating* the tissue-damaging reactions in most inflammatory disorders are poorly understood, even in those associated with known aetiological agents, so the selection of therapeutic approaches on a purely scientific basis has not been feasible. When the agent is known, management policy is likely to include measures aimed at eliminating the agent, such as using appropriate antimicrobial drugs to combat infections, or using measures aimed at avoiding or reducing exposure in the case of occupational dusts or environmental contaminants. However, because much of the tissue damage is thought to be the consequence of the persistence of immune and inflammatory reactions, a wide variety of drugs is also employed to arrest or alleviate the effects of these reactions. Many of the drugs in conventional use were initially selected by serendipity and their use has continued on the basis of clinical trials showing at least some efficacy. However, there are numerous chronic inflammatory diseases where only a minority of patients show any response to current drugs, and many occupational diseases of the lungs have come to be regarded as untreatable. The newer developments arising from continuing research efforts to identify more effective therapeutic approaches are, therefore, most important.

Conventional approaches

Owing to the fact that immune and inflammatory reactions are the consequence of interactions between a vast array of cell types and their diverse products, there are many points in these networks where intervention with drugs is possible. Conventional drugs include those that can interfere in antigen processing and presentation to suppress the proliferation and functional maturation of T or B lymphocytes; others that can suppress mediator release from inflammatory cells; and others that can interfere with or reverse the effects of these mediators on target cells. Some drugs are relatively selective in their effects whilst others have broad effects spanning more than one of the above functions.

The group of drugs most widely used to treat chronic inflammatory diseases is the corticosteroids, in particular synthetic analogues of the naturally occurring glucocorticoid, hydrocortisone. The natural corticosteroids are hormones secreted by the adrenal cortex and are classified into two main groups: glucocorticoids and mineralocorticoids. Their respective physiological effects are well known: regulation of water and electrolyte balance in the latter; a potent effect on carbohydrate and protein metabolism; and anti-inflammatory action by the former. There is, however, overlap in the spectrum of functional activity between these two main groups, and some synthetic analogues offer advantages over others in terms of having a longer biological half-life and lower mineralocorticoid activity. The risk of side effects associated with prolonged systemic treatment with corticosteroids due to the fact that they can cause fluid imbalance and imbalance in carbohydrate, protein and lipid metabolism, and also to the hazard of abrupt cessation of therapy, does not need reiteration. Given awareness of these risks and of the necessity of careful monitoring of patients during treatment, there are numerous advantageous anti-inflammatory effects. These can act both early and late in inflammation, irrespective of the initiating stimuli, and the main effects include: reducing vasodilatation and lowering fluid exudation from blood vessels; decreasing the influx of neutrophils from blood vessels into sites of inflammation (despite the fact that they appear to enhance the release of neutrophils from the bone marrow and induce a circulatory leucocytosis); decreasing the influx of monocytes into sites of inflammation (and also decreasing the release of monocytes from the bone marrow); decreasing the proliferative responses of lymphocytes to mitogens and antigens; decreasing the activation of macrophages and, consequently, their efficiency in killing micro-organisms; and reducing the synthesis of collagen and proteoglycans by fibroblasts. Many of these effects are presumed to be the consequence of a corticosteroid-induced reduction in the synthesis or release of a range of inflammatory mediators including interleukin-1, interleukin-2, interferons, arachidonic acid metabolites (prostaglandins and leukotrienes), platelet-activating factor, bradykinin and histamine.

The exact mechanism of action of corticosteroids is not known but the biological effects of glucocorticoids are known to be caused by the binding of these hormones to intracellular steroid receptors which are found within the cytoplasm of most cells. After receptor binding, the complex moves into the nucleus where it interacts with control sites on 'steroid-sensitive genes' either to increase or to decrease the rate of transcription of the gene. This is indicated by an increased or decreased production of mRNA within the cell. A number of specific proteins are generated as a consequence of increased transcription, and these are thought to be mainly responsible for the anti-inflammatory effects of steroids. A family of proteins termed 'lipocortins' are thought to be especially relevant, and a cell membrane-bound form of one of these proteins appears to be involved in the regulation of phospholipase A_2 activity. There are a number of other terms used for molecules within the lipocortin family including 'macrocortin' and 'lipomodulin'. Research is currently in progress to determine whether pure preparations of lipocortins might have potential as a future therapeutic alternative to corticosteroids avoiding the side effects of conventional therapy.

Apart from corticosteroids, other drugs with immunosuppressive properties are also commonly used to treat disorders associated with immunopathological mechanisms. *Cyclophosphamide* is one of the most frequently used of these 'immunosuppressive drugs'. It is an alkylating agent which has anti-mitotic properties due to the fact that its biologically active metabolites (produced in the liver) can substitute chemical groupings into DNA molecules, disrupting DNA replication and mRNA transcription. In most situations, it is a strong inhibitor of antibody production and can cause depletion of B cells. However, it has diverse effects on T cells, and only appears capable of suppressing T-cell function if given during the proliferative phase of T-cell responses.

By contrast, it has been found in experimental models that many forms of delayed-type hypersensitivity can be *enhanced* by cyclophosphamide treatment, and that this may occur due to an inhibitory effect of cyclophosphamide on the subpopulations of B cells and T cells which mediate suppressor function. Due to this effect, it has also been demonstrated that cyclophosphamide can reverse immunological tolerance induced by T-suppressor cells. The mechanism of action of this drug on suppressor cells is unknown, but it does not appear to depend upon an effect on DNA because it can affect cells prior to proliferation. There is also evidence in animal models that, through its effect on suppressor cells, cyclophosphamide can also enhance T-cytotoxic responses against immunogenic tumours. Cyclophosphamide is also one of the drugs that has been used with moderate success to treat patients with the fibrosing lung disease cryptogenic fibrosing alveolitis, and patients with fibrosing alveolitis occurring in association with collagen vascular diseases (Turner-Warwick and Haslam, 1987; Johnson et al., 1989). Whether the beneficial effects in these diseases are due to the suppressive effect of this drug on antibody formation, or due to enhancement of T-cell activity through its inhibitory effect on suppressor cells, is not known. It is also unknown whether this drug might be of any value in the treatment of patients with asbestosis who have lesions resembling those of cryptogenic fibrosing alveolitis.

Azathioprine is another immunosuppressive drug in current use. It is an analogue of the purine base guanine, and it interferes with nucleic acid biosynthesis. It has been shown to suppress antibody production, and it also inhibits T-cell proliferation and enhances skin graft survival in animal models. It is, therefore, frequently used as a part of immunosuppressive regimens in patients after organ transplantation. The heavy immunosuppression in such patients is, however, associated with an increased risk of opportunistic infections, including cytomegalovirus, *Pneumocystis carinii* and *Candida albicans*, and there is also an increased risk of lymphomas, especially B-cell lymphomas related to reactivation of Epstein–Barr virus.

There are many other agents with immunosuppressive properties, including many of the drugs used in cancer chemotherapy but, as yet, these are not widely used in the treatment of chronic inflammatory diseases.

The difficulty with many immunosuppressive drugs is that their effects are directed against proliferative cells of all types rather than having a selective effect on immune or inflammatory cells. Inevitably, this increases the risk of side effects and research efforts are directed towards identifying more selective immunomodulatory agents (see next section).

Prolonged treatment with systemic preparations of corticosteroids or immunosuppressive drugs, or both, is mainly restricted, due to the risk of side effects, to chronic progressive diseases where there is a high risk of irreversible tissue damage. In allergic diseases, such as asthma, where the clinical symptoms are often acute and episodic, different therapeutic approaches are employed (except in the patients who develop chronic disease). Conventional anti-asthma drugs include those that inhibit the release of mediators involved in either the immediate or late allergic reactions that occur in this disease, and others which prevent or reverse some of the effects of these mediators on the target tissues. In the former category, the drug sodium cromoglycate is an effective prophylactic drug which prevents both immediate and late allergic reactions if delivered by inhalation onto the bronchial mucosa prior to antigen challenge. It can inhibit both classic IgE- and also IgG-mediated immediate reactions, and immediate and late reactions induced by nonspecific stimuli, such as exercise or direct exposure to cold air. It can also inhibit the reactions induced by unknown stimuli (in 'non-atopic' [or 'cryptogenic'] asthma). Sodium cromoglycate was developed from the chromone, khellin, isolated from the plant *Amni visnaga*. Its main effect appears to be due to the fact that it prevents the release of histamine and other mediators, including neutrophil chemotactic factor, from mast cells by inhibiting their degranulation. This, in turn, prevents the subsequent inflammatory events which follow mast cell degranulation. Whilst the current evidence indicates that mast cells are involved in immediate allergic reactions, the mechanism by which cromoglycate suppresses late reactions is less certain. It has been suggested that this may be due to an effect of the drug on the neurophysiological mechanisms that appear to be involved in asthma.

Other drugs, used prophylactically in the treatment of asthma, include theophylline and isoprenaline inhalants, and these drugs are also able to reduce histamine release from mast cells through their ability to increase intracellular levels of cyclic AMP. Apart from the prophylactic drugs, other drugs are used to treat patients poststimulation. β_2-Adrenoceptor agonists (for example, salbutamol and isoprenaline) are potent mast cell stabilizers and they are of further value due to their ability to cause relaxation of respiratory smooth muscle as well as vasodilatation. They exert their effects by binding with β_2-adrenoceptors which are localized to many different cells in the airways, including mast cells. Inhalant preparations of corticosteroids can also reduce late reactions but have little effect on immediate reactions. It is thought that they act by reducing the bronchial inflammatory cell infiltrates associated with pathogenesis. Drugs that inhibit the synthesis of the prostaglandins can also abort late but not immediate reactions when given to patients with asthma prior to challenge. Prostaglandins are produced by many cell types, including mast cells and macrophages, and they can aid infiltration of inflammatory cells to tissue sites through their vasodilator effects. They can also enhance the effects of other vasoactive agents, including histamine and bradykinin.

There are many drugs that can inhibit prostaglandin biosynthesis and, collectively, they are termed 'non-steroidal anti-inflammatory drugs'. They include aspirin, indomethacin, phenylbutazone, ibuprofen, paracetamol and many others. The different drugs vary in the potency of their anti-inflammatory effects and they also have variable analgesic and anti-pyretic actions. The most potent anti-inflammatory drugs have proved particularly effective in the treatment of rheumatoid arthritis. Other non-steroidal drugs with anti-inflammatory effects are also used in the treatment of arthritis, including penicillamine, chloroquine and gold, but the mechanisms by which these drugs exert their effects are less clear.

More recent developments

In the search for more selective immunomodulatory agents, cyclosporin A is an immunosuppressive drug of particular interest, which is used to prevent graft rejection in patients following organ transplantation. With increasing knowledge of its mechanism of action, there is now interest in the possible wider applications of this drug in a variety of chronic inflammatory disorders, including some that affect the lung (Martinet et al., 1988; Alton, Johnson and Turner-Warwick, 1989; Fukazawa et al., 1990; Hammond and Bateman, 1990). Cyclosporin A is a cyclic undecapeptide from the fungus *Trichoderma polysporum*. It acts selectively on T lymphocytes early in their activation, inhibiting their proliferation by arresting the cells in their resting state (G_0) or early growth (G_1) phase of the cell cycle. It has been demonstrated that the release of interleukin-2, and that of other lymphokines, is suppressed. However, although the drug suppresses the induction of T-cell responses, it has no effect on the functioning of effector T cells once these have formed. Probably for this reason, it is more effective in suppressing primary than secondary immune responses. It can, however, inhibit some types of delayed hypersensitivity (skin reactions to tuberculin) in fully sensitized animals, and it can reverse the symptoms in some animal models of autoimmune diseases even when administered after the onset of the disease. This is probably because it interferes with the continuing activation and recruitment of effector cells during the course of the disease. Cyclosporin A has been shown to be capable of suppressing disease in the NZB/NZW F1 strain of mouse which spontaneously develops an autoimmune disease resembling systemic lupus erythematosus in man.

Many fibrosing lung diseases, including those related to fibrogenic dusts, show features of autoimmunity and can occur in association with autoimmune diseases including SLE. This raises the question of whether cyclosporin A might be of potential therapeutic benefit in such diseases. The success of cyclosporin A in the field of organ transplantation also means that transplantation is an option that can now be considered more widely in patients with end-stage lung diseases, including those relating to occupational agents.

Another developing domain of especial interest in relation to more selective immunomodulating approaches is that of cytokine research. Recombinant DNA technology has enabled the production of purified preparations of several human cytokines, including interleukin-2 and interferon-α, -β and -γ in sufficient quantities for them to be used in therapy. Current trials of such cytokines have mainly been directed towards cancer therapy, and there have also been a number of phase I trials of interferons (mainly IFNα) in patients with a variety of virus diseases. The results using intramuscular injections of pure cytokines have so far proved disappointing, except in IFNα treatment of hairy-cell leukaemia; however, cytokines have a very short half-life and it is believed that, when introduced by the peripheral route, they may not reach their target site in sufficient quantity to exert any notable effect. The aims of current research are, therefore, to develop novel approaches to target cytokines more accurately to the desired target site in high quantities. An approach already in development is the use of monoclonal antibodies directed to selective antigenic determinants on the target cells (for example, to tumour-specific antigens or to other specific cell surface markers), as carrier molecules to aid drug delivery.

Apart from the direct use of cytokines as therapeutic agents, another approach, when deficient immune function is suspected, is to employ cytokine preparations to activate the patient's own immune cells in vitro prior to reintroducing them into the patient. An example of this approach is the therapeutic use of lymphokine-activated killer cells, combined with interleukin-2 therapy, in the treatment of some cancers. Preliminary evidence suggests that this approach may be of potential value in mesothelioma.

A more recent development is the evidence that monoclonal antibodies directed towards cytokines themselves may be of potential therapeutic value in the treatment of patients with chronic inflammatory diseases. Most interesting preliminary results have been obtained, demonstrating the potential value of this approach, using antibodies to tumour necrosis factor in a variety of models (Tracy et al., 1988; Piguet et al., 1989, 1990).

These new developments with regard to immunomodulatory agents, together with other new approaches aimed at suppressing damage due to the release of enzymes and oxidants from activated inflammatory cells, for example, glutathione therapy (Borok et al., 1991), should be followed with interest in the hope that they may identify much needed new approaches to the treatment of chronic occupational lung diseases.

References

Alexander, M.D., Andres, J.A., Leslie, R.G.Q. and Wood, N.J. (1975) The binding of human and guinea pig IgG subclasses to homologous macrophage and monocyte Fc-receptors. *Immunology* **35**, 115–123

Alton, E.W., Johnson, M., and Turner-Warwick, M. (1989) Advanced cryptogenic fibrosing alveolitis: preliminary report on treatment with cyclosporin A. *Respir. Med.* **83**, 277–279

Andersen, P. and Christensen, K.M. (1983) Serum antibodies to pigeon antigens in smokers and non-smokers. *Acta Med. Scand.* **213**, 191–193

Andersen, P., Pedersen, D.F., Bach, B. and Bonde, G.J. (1982) Serum antibodies and immunoglobulins in smokers and non-smokers. *Clin. Expl. Immunol.* **47**, 467–473

Ansfield, M.J. and Benson, B.J. (1980) Identification of the immunosuppressive components of canine pulmonary surface active material. *J. Immunol.* **125**, 1093–1098

Ansfield, M.J., Kaltreider, H.B., Benson, B.J. and Caldwell, J.L. (1979) Immunosuppressive activity of canine pulmonary surface active material. *J. Immunol.* **122**, 1062–1066

Azzawi, M., Bradley, B., Jeffery, P.K., Frew, A.J., Wardlaw, A.J., Knowles, G., Assoufi, B., Collins, J.V., Durham, S. and Kay, A.B. (1990) Identification of activated T-lymphocytes and eosinophils in bronchial biopsies in stable atopic asthma. *Am. Rev. Respir. Dis.* **142**, 1407–1413

Bahna, S.L., Heiner, D.C. and Myhre, B.A. (1983) Changes in serum IgD in cigarette smokers. *Clin. Expl. Immunol.* **51**, 624–630

BAL Co-operative Group Steering Committee. (1990) Bronchoalveolar lavage constituents in healthy individuals, idiopathic pulmonary fibrosis, and selected comparison groups. *Am. Rev. Respir. Dis.* **141** (suppl.), S169–S202

Baughman, R.P., Bosken, C.H., Loudon, R.C., Hurtubise, P. and Wesseler, T. (1983) Quantitation of bronchoalveolar lavage with methylene blue. *Am. Rev. Respir. Dis.* **128**, 266–270

Bell, D.Y., Haseman, J.A., Spock, A., McLennan, G. and Hook, G.E.R. (1981) Plasma proteins of the bronchoalveolar surface of the lungs of smokers and non-smokers. *Am. Rev. Respir. Dis.* **124**, 72–79

Beuchner, H. and Ansari, A. (1969) Acute silica-proteinosis: a new pathologic variant of acute silicosis in sandblasters, characterized by histologic features resembling alveolar proteinosis. *Dis. Chest* **55**, 274–284

Bevilacqua, M.P., Amrani, D., Mosesson, M.W. and Bianco, C. (1981) Receptors for cold-insoluble globulin (plasma fibronectin) on human monocytes. *J. Expl. Med.* **153**, 42–60

Bienenstock, J. (1984) Bronchus-associated lymphoid tissue. In: *Immunology of the Lung and Upper Respiratory Tract* (ed. J. Bienenstock), McGraw-Hill, New York, pp. 96–118

Bienenstock, J., Johnston, N. and Perey, D.Y.W. (1973) Bronchial lymphoid tissue. 1. Morphologic characteristics. *Lab. Invest.* **28**, 686–692

Bignon, J., Atassi, K., Jaurand, M.C., Geslin, P. and Solle, R. (1978) Cellular and protein content analysis of bronchoalveolar lavage fluid from patients with idiopathic pulmonary fibrosis and asbestosis. *Am. Rev. Respir. Dis.* **117**, 56

Bignon, J., Sebastien, P., Gaudichet, A. and Bientz, M. (1978) Analysis of mineral particles recovered by bronchoalveolar lavage for the diagnosis of dust related lung disease. (abstract) *Am. Rev. Respir. Dis.* **117**, 218

Bitterman, P.B., Wewers, M.D., Rennard, S.I., Adelberg, S. and Crystal, R.G. (1986) Modulation of alveolar macrophage-driven fibroblast proliferation by alternative macrophage mediators. *J. Clin. Invest.* **77**, 700–708

Borok, Z., Buhl, R., Grimes, G.J., Bokser, A.D., Hubbard, R.C., Holroyd, K.J., Roum, J.H., Czerski, D.B., Cantin, A.M. and Crystal, R.G. (1991) Effect of glutathione aerosol on oxidant–antioxidant imbalance in idiopathic pulmonary fibrosis. *Lancet* **338**, 215–226

Boucher, R.C. and Ranga, V. (1988) Fate and handling of antigens by the lung. (1988) In: *Immunology and Immunologic Diseases of the Lung* (ed. R.P. Daniele), Blackwell Scientific, Boston, pp. 55–78

Bridges, R.B., Wyatt, R.J. and Rehm, S.R. (1985) Effect of smoking on peripheral blood leukocytes. *Eur. J. Respir. Dis.* **139**, 24–33

Burnet, F.M. (1970) The concept of immunological surveillance. *Progr. Expl. Tumor Res.* **13**, 1–27

Burrows, B., Halonen, M., Barbee, R.A. and Lebowitz, M.D. (1981) The relationship of serum immunoglobulin E to cigarette smoking. *Am. Rev. Respir. Dis.* **124**, 523–525

Cantin, A.M., Hubbard R.C. and Crystal, R.G. (1989) Glutathione deficiency in the epithelial lining fluid of the lower respiratory tract in idiopathic pulmonary fibrosis. *Am. Rev. Respir. Dis.* **139**, 370–372

Carp, H., Miller, F., Hoidal, J.R. and Janoff, A. (1982) Potential mechanisms of emphysema: alpha 1-proteinase inhibitor recovered from lungs of cigarette smokers contains oxidised methionine and has decreased elastase inhibitory activity. *Proc. Natl Acad. Sci. USA* **79**, 2041–2045

Chiappino, G., Friedrichs, K.H., Rivolta, G. and Forni, A. (1988) Alveolar fiber load in asbestos workers and in subjects with no occupational asbestos exposure: An electron microscopy study. *Am. J. Ind. Med.* **14**, 37–46

Christman, J.W., Emerson, R.J., Graham, W.G.B. and Davis, G.S. (1985) Mineral dust and cell recovery from the bronchoalveolar lavage of healthy Vermont granite workers. *Am. Rev. Respir. Dis.* **132**, 393–399

Clerici, N., Reboiras, S., Fierro, C. and Leyva-Cobian, F. (1984) Expression of Ia like (HLA-DR) antigens on human alveolar macrophages. *Clin. Expl. Immunol.* **58**, 388–394

Coombs, R.R.A. and Gell, P.G.H. (1968) Classification of allergic reactions responsible for clinical hypersensitivity and disease. In: *Clinical Aspects of Immunology* (eds R.R.A.. Coombs and P.G.H. Gell), Blackwell Scientific, Oxford, pp. 575–596

Cormier, Y., Belanger, J. and Durand, P. (1985) Factors influencing the development of serum precipitins to farmer's lung antigen in Quebec dairy farmers. *Thorax* **40**, 138–143

Cormier, Y., Belanger, J. and Laviolette, M. (1985) Persistent bronchoalveolar lymphocytosis in asymptomatic farmers. *Am. Rev. Respir. Dis.* **133**, 843–847

Cullen, M.R., Kominsky, J.R., Rossman, M.D., Cherniack, M.G., Rankin, J.A., Balmes, J.R., Kern, J.A., Daniele, R.P., Palmer, L., Naegel, G.P., McManus, K. and Cruz, R. (1987) Chronic beryllium disease in a precious metal refinery. *Am. Rev. Respir. Dis.* **135**, 201–208

Cunningham-Rundles, C., Brandeis, W.E., Good, R.A. and Day, N.K. (1978) Milk precipitin, circulating immune complexes and IgA deficiency. *Proc. Natl Acad. Sci. USA.* **75**, 3387–3391

Dale, M.M. and Foreman, J.C. (1988) *Textbook of Immunopharmacology*, 2nd Ed. Blackwell Scientific, Oxford

Daniele, R.P. (ed.) (1988) *Immunology and Immunologic Diseases of the Lung.* Blackwell Scientific, Boston

Daniele, R.P., Elias, J.A., Epstein, P.E. and Rossman, M.D. (1985) Bronchoalveolar lavage: role in the pathogenesis, diagnosis and management of interstitial lung disease. *Ann. Intern. Med.* **102**, 93–108

Daughday, C.C. and Douglas, S.D. (1976) Membrane receptors on rabbit and human pulmonary alveolar macrophages. *J. Reticuloendoth. Soc.* **19**, 37–45

Davey, B. (1989) *Immunology: A Foundation Text.* Open University Press, Milton Keynes

Davison, A.G., Haslam, P.L., Corrin, B., Coutts, I.I., Dewar, A., Riding, W.D., Studdy, P.R. and Newman-Taylor, A.J. (1983)

Interstitial lung disease in hard metal workers: bronchoalveolar lavage, ultrastructural and analytical findings and results of bronchial provocation tests. *Thorax* **38**, 119–128

De Vuyst, P., Jedwab, J., Dumortier, P., Vandermoten, G., Van de Weyer, R. and Yernault, J.C. (1982) Asbestos bodies in bronchoalveolar lavage. *Am. Rev. Respir. Dis.* **126**, 972–976

De Vuyst, P., Dumortier, P., Richaert, F., Van de Weyer, R., Olenclud, C. and Yernault, J.C. (1986a) Occupational lung fibrosis in an aluminium polisher. *Eur. J. Respir. Dis.* **68**, 131–140

De Vuyst, P., Van de Weyer, R., De Coster, A., Marchandise, F.X., Dumortier, P., Ketelbant, P., Jedwab, J. and Yernault, J.C. (1986b) Dental technicians pneumonconiosis. A report of two cases. *Am. Rev. Respir. Dis.* **133**, 316–320

De Vuyst, P., Dumortier, P., Leophonte, P., Van de Weyer, R. and Yernault, J.C. (1987a) Mineralogical analysis of bronchoalveolar lavage in talc pneumoconiosis. *Eur. J. Respir. Dis.* **70**, 150–156

De Vuyst, P., Dumortier, P., Moulin, E., Yourassowsky, N. and Yernault, J.C. (1987b) Diagnostic value of asbestos bodies in bronchoalveolar lavage fluid. *Am. Rev. Respir. Dis.* **136**, 1219–1224

Dethloff, L.A., Gilmore, L.B., Brody, A.R. and Hook, G.E.R. (1985) Induction of intra- and extra-cellular phospholipids in the lungs of rats exposed to silica. *Biochem. J.* **233**, 111–118

Douglas, J.G., Middleton, W.G., Gaddie, J., Petrie, G.R., Choo-Kang, Y.F.J., Prescott, R.J. and Crompton, G.K. (1986) Sarcoidosis: a disorder commoner in non-smokers? *Thorax* **41**, 787–789

Dreisin, R.B., Schwarz, M.I., Theofilopoulos, A.N. and Stanford, R.E. (1978) Circulating immune complexes in the idiopathic interstitial pneumonias. *N. Engl. J. Med.* **298**, 353–357

Elias, J.A. (1988) Tumor necrosis factor interacts with interleukin-1 and interferons to inhibit fibroblast proliferation via fibroblast prostaglandin-dependent and -independent mechanisms. *Am. Rev. Respir. Dis.* **138**, 652–658

Elias, J.A., Gustilo, K. and Freundlich, B. (1988) Human alveolar macrophage and blood monocyte inhibition of fibroblast proliferation : evidence for synergy between interleukin-1 and tumor necrosis factor. *Am. Rev. Respir. Dis.* **138**, 1595–1603

Elias, J.A., Jiminez, S.A. and Freundlich, B. (1987) Recombinant gamma, alpha and beta interferon regulation of human lung fibroblast proliferation. *Am. Rev. Respir. Dis.* **135**, 62–65

Elias, J.A., Freundlich, B., Kern, J.A. and Rosenbloom, J. (1990) Cytokine networks in the regulation of inflammation and fibrosis in the lung. *Chest* **97**, 1439–1445

Epstein, P.E., Dauber, J.H., Rossman, M.D. and Daniele, R.P. (1982) Bronchoalveolar lavage in a patient with chronic berylliosis: evidence for hypersensitivity pneumonitis. *Ann. Intern. Med.* **97**, 213–216

Ettensohn, D.B. and Roberts, N.J, Jr (1983) Human alveolar macrophage support of lymphocyte response to mitogens and antigens. *Am. Rev. Respir. Dis.* **128**, 516–522

Ferson, M., Edwards, A., Lind, A., Milton, G.W. and Hersey, P. (1979) Low natural killer-cell activity and immunoglobulin levels associated with smoking in human subjects. *Int. J. Cancer* **23**, 603–609

Finkelman, F.D., Katona, I.M., Urban, J.F., Snapper, C.M., Ohara, J. and Paul, W.E. (1986) Suppression of in vivo polyclonal IgE responses by monoclonal antibody to the lymphokine B-cell stimulatory factor 1. *Proc. Natl Acad. Sci. USA* **83**, 9675–9678

Fireman, E., Ben Efraim, S., Greif, J., Alguetti, A., Ayalon, D. and Topilsky, M. (1989) Suppressive activity of alveolar macrophages and blood monocytes from interstitial lung diseases: role of released soluble factors. *Int. J. Immunopharmacol.* **11**, 751–760

Foley, N.M., Coral, A.P., Tung, K., Hudspith, B.N., James, D.G. and Johnson, N.McL. (1989) Bronchoalveolar lavage cell counts as a predictor of short term outcome in pulmonary sarcoidosis. *Thorax* **44**, 732–738

Fournier, M., Vail, F., Derenne, J.P. and Pariente, R. (1977) Bronchial lymphoepithelial nodules in the rat. Morphologic features, and uptake and transport of exogenous proteins. *Am. Rev. Respir. Dis.* **116**, 685–694

Fournier, M., Lebargy, F., Le Roy Ladurie, F., Lenormand, E. and Pariente, R. (1989) Intraepithelial T-lymphocyte subsets in the airways of normal subjects and of patients with chronic bronchitis. *Am. Rev. Respir. Dis.* **140**, 737–742

Friedman, W.H., Gressler, I., Bandu, M.T. and Aguet, M. (1980) Interferon enhances the expression of Fc receptors. *J. Immunol.* **124**, 2436–2441

Fukazawa, M., Kawano, M., Hisano, S., Ueda, K. and Matsuba, K. (1990) Efficacy of cyclosporin A for idiopathic pulmonary fibrosis. *Eur. J. Pediatr.* **149**, 441–442

Gadek, J., Felb, G.A. and Crystal, R.G. (1979) Cigarette smoking induces functional antiprotease deficiency in the lower respiratory tract of humans. *Science* **206**, 1315–1316

Garcia, J.G.N., Parhami, N., Killam, D., Garcia, P.L. and Keogh, B.A. (1986) Bronchoalveolar lavage fluid evaluation in rheumatoid arthritis. *Am. Rev. Respir. Dis.* **133**, 450–454

Gauldie, J., Richards, C. and Lamontagne, L. (1983) Fc receptors for IgA and other immunoglobulins on resident and activated alveolar macrophages. *Mol. Immunol.* **20**, 1029–1037

Gellert, A.R., Kitajewska, J.Y., Uthayakumar, S., Kirkham, J.B. and Rudd, R.M. (1986) Asbestos fibres in bronchoalveolar lavage fluid from asbestos workers: examination by electron microscopy. *Br. Med. J.* **43**, 170–176

Gellert, A.R., Langford, J.A., Uthayakumar, S. and Rudd, R.M. (1985a) Bronchoalveolar lavage and clearance of 99m-Tc-DTPA in asbestos workers without evidence of asbestosis. *Br. J. Dis. Chest* **79**, 251–257

Gellert, A.R., Langford, J.A., Winter, R.J.D., Uthayakumar, S., Sinha, G. and Rudd, R.M. (1985b) Asbestosis: assessment by bronchoalveolar lavage and measurement of pulmonary epithelial permeability. *Thorax* **40**, 508–514

Geppert, T.D. and Lipsky, P.E. (1987) Dissection of the antigen presenting function of tissue cells induced to express HLA-DR by gamma-interferon. *J. Rheumatol.* **14** (suppl 13), 59–62

Ginns, L.C., Goldenheim, P.D., Miller, L.G., Burton, R.C., Gillick, L., Colvin, R.B., Goldstein, G., Kung, P.C., Hurwitz, C. and Kazemi, H. (1982) T-lymphocyte subsets in smoking and lung cancer. *Am. Rev. Respir. Dis.* **126**, 265–269

Gordon, S. and Mokoena, T. (1989) Receptors for mannosyl structures on mononuclear phagocytes. In: *Human Monocytes* (eds M. Zembala and G.L. Asherson), Academic Press, London, pp. 141–150

Griffin, F.M., Bianco, C. and Silverstein, S.C. (1975) Characterization of the macrophage receptor for complement and demonstration of its functional independence from the receptor for the Fc portion of immunoglobulin G. *J. Expl. Med.* **141**, 1269

Guyre, P.M., Morganelli, P.M. and Miller, R. (1983) Recombinant immune interferon increases immunoglobulin G Fc receptors on cultured human mononuclear phagocytes. *J. Clin. Invest* **72**, 393–398

Hällgren, R., Bjermer, L., Lungren R. and Venge, P. (1989) The eosinophil component of the alveolitis in idiopathic pulmonary fibrosis. *Am. Rev. Respir. Dis.* **139**, 373–377

Hammond, J.M. and Bateman, E.D. (1990) Successful treatment

of life-threatening steroid-resistant pulmonary sarcoidosis with cyclosporin in a patient with systemic lupus erythematosus. Respir. *Med.* **84**, 77–79

Harris, J.O., Olsen, G.N., Castle, J.R. and Maloney, A.S. (1975) Comparison of proteolytic enzyme activity in pulmonary alveolar macrophages and blood leukocytes in smokers and non-smokers. *Am. Rev. Respir. Dis.* **111**, 579–586

Haslam, P.L., (1976) Antibody and lymphocyte responses to cell nucleii in human lung diseases. PhD Thesis, University of London

Haslam, P.L. (1984) Bronchoalveolar lavage. *Semin. Respir. Med.* **6**, 55–70

Haslam, P.L. (1990) Evaluation of alveolitis by studies of lung biopsies. *Lung* **168** (suppl.), 984–992

Haslam, P.L. and Turner-Warwick, M. (1981) Immunological reactions to autoantigens. In: *Scientific Foundations of Respiratory Medicine* (eds J.C. Scadding and G. Cumming), William Heinemann Medical Books, Oxford, pp. 451–472

Haslam, P.L., Dewar, A. and Turner-Warwick, M. (1982) Lavage eosinophils and histamine. In: *Cellular Biology of the Lung* (eds G. Cumming and G. Bonsignore), Plenum, New York, pp. 77–87

Haslam, P.L., Thompson, B., Mohammed, I., Townsend, P.J., Hodson, M.E., Holborow, E.J. and Turner-Warwick, M. (1979) Circulating immune complexes in patients with cryptogenic fibrosing alveolitis. *Clin. Expl. Immunol.* **37**, 381–390

Haslam, P.L., Turton, C.W.G., Lukoszek, A., Salsbury, A.J., Dewar, A., Collins, J.V. and Turner-Warwick, M. (1980) Bronchoalveolar lavage fluid cell counts in cryptogenic fibrosing alveolitis and their relation to therapy. *Thorax* **35**, 328–339

Haslam, P.L., Coutts, I.I., Watling, A.F., Cromwell, O., Du Bois, R.M., Townsend, P.J., Collins, J.V. and Turner-Warwick, M. (1981a) Bronchoalveolar lavage features associated with radiographic evidence of fibrosis in pulmonary sarcoidosis. In: *Proceedings of the IXth International Conference on Sarcoidosis* (eds J. Chrétien, J. Marsac and J.C. Saltiel), Pergamon Press, Paris, pp. 209–215

Haslam, P.L., Cromwell, O., Dewar, A. and Turner-Warwick, M. (1981b) Evidence of increased histamine levels in lung lavage fluids from patients with cryptogenic fibrosing alveolitis. *Clin. Expl. Immunol.* **44**, 587–593

Haslam, P.L., Dewar, A., Butchers, P., Primett, Z.S., Newman-Taylor, A. and Turner-Warwick, M. (1987) Mast cells, atypical lymphocytes and neutrophils in bronchoalveolar lavage in extrinsic allergic alveolitis. *Am. Rev. Respir. dis.* **135**, 35–47

Heppleston, A.G., Fletcher, K. and Wyatt, I. (1974) Changes in the composition of lung lipids and the 'turn-over' of dipalmitoyl lecithin in experimental alveolar lipo-proteinosis induced by inhaled quartz. *Br. J. Expl. Pathol.* **55**, 384–395

Holt, P.G. (1987) Immune and inflammatory function in cigarette smokers. *Thorax* **42**, 241-249

Holt, P.G., Schon-Hegrad, M.A., Philips, M.J. and McMenamin, P.G. (1989) Ia positive dendritic cells from a tightly meshed network within the human airway epithelium. *Clin. Expl. Allergy.* **19**, 597–601

Huber, H., Douglas, S.D., Nusbacher, J., Kochwa, S. and Rosenfield, R.E. (1971) IgG subclasses specificity of human monocyte receptor sites. *Nature* **229**, 419–420

Hughes, D.A. and Haslam, P.L. (1989) Changes in phosphatidylglycerol in bronchoalveolar lavage fluids from patients with cryptogenic fibrosing alveolitis. *Chest* **95**, 82–89

Hughes, D.A., Haslam, P.L., Townsend, P.J. and Turner-Warwick, M. (1985) Numerical and functional alterations in circulatory lymphocytes in cigarette smokers. *Clin. Expl. Immunol.* **61**, 459–466

Hunninghake, G.W. and Crystal, R.G. (1983) Cigarette smoking and lung destruction: accumulation of neutrophils in the lungs of cigarette smokers. *Am. Rev. Respir. Dis.* **128**, 833–838

Hunninghake, G.W., Gadek, J.E., Kawanami, O., Ferrans, V.J. and Crystal, R.G.. (1979) Inflammatory and immune processes in the human lung in health and disease: Evaluation by bronchoalveolar lavage. *Am. J. Pathol.* **97**, 149–198

Hunninghake, G.W., Gadek, J.E., Lawley, T.J. and Crystal, R.G. (1981) Mechanisms of neutrophil accumulation in the lungs of patients with idiopathic pulmonary fibrosis. *J. Clin. Invest.* **68**, 259–269

Hyde, D.M., Henderson, T.S., Giri, S.N., Tyler, N.K. and Stovall, M.Y. (1988) Effect of murine gamma interferon on the cellular responses to bleomycin in mice. *Exp. Lung Res.* **14**, 686–704

Janoff, A., Raju, L. and Dearing, R. (1983) Levels of elastase activity in bronchoalveolar lavage fluids of healthy smokers and non-smokers. *Am. Rev. Respir. Dis.* **127**, 540–544.

Jedrychowski, W., Adamczyk, B. and Jaskolka, E. (1980) Level of immunoglobulins G and A in saliva and serum in relation to tobacco smoking and respiratory tract symptoms. *Pneumonol. Pol.* **48**, 63–69

Johnson, M.A., Kwan, S., Snell, N.J.C., Nunn, A.J., Darbyshire, J.H. and Turner-Warwick, M. (1989) Randomised controlled trial comparing prednisolone alone with cyclophosphamide and low dose prednisolone in combination in cryptogenic fibrosing alveolitis. *Thorax* **44**, 280-288

Johnson, N.F., Haslam, P.L., Dewar, A., Newman-Taylor, A.J. and Turner-Warwick, M. (1986) Identification of inorganic dust particles in bronchoalveolar lavage macrophages by energy dispersive X-ray microanalysis. *Archs Environ. Hlth* **41**, 133–144.

Johnstone, A. and Thorpe, R. (1987) *Immunochemistry in Practice.* Blackwell Scientific, Oxford

Joseph, M., Tonnel, A.B., Torpier, G., Capron, A., Arnoux, B. and Benveniste, J. (1983) Involvement of immunoglobulin E in the secretory processes of alveolar macrophages from asthmatic patients. *J. Clin. Invest.* **71**, 221–230

Juers, J.A., Rogers, R.M., McCurdy, T.B. and Cook W.W. (1976) Enhancement of bactericidal capacity of alveolar macrophages by human alveolar lining material. *J. Clin. Invest.* **58**, 271–275

Kahan, A., Amor, B., Menkes, C.J. and Strauch, G. (1989) Recombinant interferon-gamma in the treatment of systemic sclerosis. *Am. J. Med.* **87**, 273–277

Kallenberg, C.G.M., Schilizzi, B.M., Beaumont, F., Poppema, S., De Leij, L. and The, T.H. (1987) Expression of class II MCH antigens on alveolar epithelium in fibrosing alveolitis. *Clin. Expl. Immunol.* **67**, 182–190

Kaltreider, H.B. and Salmon, S.E. (1973) Immunology of the lower respiratory tract: functional properties of bronchoalveolar lymphocytes obtained from the normal canine lung. *J. Clin. Invest.* **52**, 2211–2217

Kirby, J., Wood, A., Reader, J., Isted, K., Hynd, J., Hawkes, D., Hudson, L. and Pepper, J. (1985) Origin and immunological hyporeactivity of canine alveolar lymphocytes. *Immunology* **55**, 531–538

Klech, H. and Hutter, C. (eds) (1990) Clinical guidelines and indications for bronchoalveolar lavage (BAL): Report of the European Society of Pneumology Task Group on BAL. *Eur. Respir. J.* **3**, 937–974

Klech, H. and Pohl, W. (eds) (1989) Technical recommendations and guidelines for bronchoalveolar lavage (BAL): Report of the European Society of Pneumology Task Group on BAL. *Eur. Respir. J.* **2**, 561–585

Knutson, D.W., Kijlstra, A. and Van Es, LA. (1977) Association and disassociation of aggregated IgG from rat peritoneal macrophages. *J. Expl. Med.* **145**, 1368–1381

Kolb, W.P. (1988) The complement system of the lung. In: *Immunology and Immunologic Diseases of the Lung* (ed. R.P. Daniele), Blackwell Scientific, Boston, pp. 127–157

Kovacs, E.J. (1991) Fibrogenic cytokines: the role of immune mediators in the development of scar tissue. *Immunol. Today* **12**, 17–23

Kradin, R.L., Divertie, M.B., Colvin, R.B., Ramirez, J., Ryu, J., Carpenter, H.A. and Bhan, A.K. (1986) Usual interstitial pneumonitis is a T-cell alveolitis. *Clin. Immunol. Immunopathol.* **40**, 224–235

Lamb, D. and Lumsden, A. (1982) Intra-epithelial mast cells in human airway epithelium: evidence for smoking-induced changes in their frequency. *Thorax* **37**, 334–342

Laviolette, M., Coulombe, R., Picard, S., Braquet, P. and Borgeat, P. (1986) Decreased leukotriene B4 synthesis in smokers' alveolar macrophages in vitro. *J. Clin. Invest.* **77**, 54–60

Leatherman, J.W., Michael, A.F., Schwartz, B.A. and Hoidal, J.R. (1984) Lung T cells in hypersensitivity pneumonitis. *Ann. Intern. Med.* **100**, 390–392

Leitch, A.G., Lumb, E.M. and Kay, A.B. (1981) Mediators of hypersensitivity in the sputum of young symptomatic cigarette smokers. *Clin. Allergy* **11**, 257–262

Levy, P.C., Looney, R.J., Roberts, N.J., Frampton, N.W., Ryan, D.H. and Utell, M.J. (1988) Human alveolar macrophage antibody-dependent cellular-cytotoxicity (ADCC): Fc-gamma receptor 1 (Fc R1) dependence and inhibition by human surfactant (abstract). *Am. Rev. Respir. Dis.* **137**, 39

Libby, D.M. (1987) The eosinophil in idiopathic pulmonary fibrosis. *Chest* **92**, 7–8

Lin, Y.H., Haslam, P.L. and Turner-Warwick, M. (1985) Chronic pulmonary sarcoidosis: relationship between lung lavage cell counts, chest radiograph, and results of standard lung function tests. *Thorax* **40**, 501–507

Londei, M., Lamb, J.R., Bottazzo, G.F. and Feldman, M. (1984) Epithelial cells expressing aberrant MHC Class II determinants can present antigen to cloned human T-cells. *Nature* **312**, 639-641.

McCombs, C.C., Michalski, J.P., Westerfield, B.T. and Light, R.W. (1982) Human alveolar macrophages suppress the proliferative response of peripheral blood lymphocytes. *Chest* **82**, 266–271

McLean, R.H. and Winkelstein, J.A. (1984) Genetically determined variation in the complement system: Relationship to disease. *J. Pediatr.* **105**, 179–188

McSharry, C., Banham, S.W., Lynch, P.P. and Boyd, G. (1984) Antibody measurements in extrinsic allergic alveolitis. *Eur. J. Respir. Dis.* **65**, 259–265

Maliszewski, C.R., Shen, L. and Fanger, M.W. (1985) The expression of receptors for IgA on human monocytes and calcitriol-treated HL-60 cells. *J. Immunol.* **35**, 3878–3881

Manning, L.S., Bowman, R.V., Darby, S.B. and Robinson, B.W. (1989a) Lysis of human malignant mesothelioma cells by natural killer (NK) and lymphokine-activated killer (LAK) cells. *Am. Rev. Respir. Dis.* **39**, 1369–1374.

Manning, L.S., Bowman, R.V., Davis, M.R., Musk, A.W. and Robinson, B.W. (1989b) Indomethacin augments lymphokine-activated killer cell generation by patients with malignant mesothelioma. *Clin. Immunol. Immunopathol.* **53**, 68–77

Martinet, Y., Haslam, P.L. and Turner-Warwick, M. (1984) Clinical significance of circulating immune complexes in 'lone' cryptogenic fibrosing alveolitis and those with associated connective tissue disorders. *Clin. Allergy* **14**, 491–497

Martinet, Y., Pinkston, P., Saltini, C., Spurzem, J., Muller-Quernheim, J. and Crystal, R.G. (1988) Evaluation of the in vitro and in vivo effects of cyclosporine on the lung T-lymphocyte alveolitis of active pulmonary sarcoidosis. *Am. Rev. Respir. Dis.* **138**, 1242–1248

Melewicz, F.M., Kline, L.E., Cohen, A.B. and Spiegelberg, H.L. (1982) Characterization of Fc receptors for IgE on human alveolar macrophages. *Clin. Expl. Immunol.* **49**, 364–370

Miller, K., Turk, J. and Nicklin, S. (1992) *Principles and Practice of Immunotoxicology.* Blackwell Scientific, Oxford

Miller, L.G., Goldstein, G., Murphy, M. and Ginns, L.C. (1982) Reversible alterations in immunoregulatory T cells in smoking. Analysis by monoclonal antibodies and flow cytometry. *Chest* **82**, 526–529

Minty, B.D., Jordan, C. and Jones, J.G. (1981) Rapid improvement in abnormal epithelial permeability after stopping cigarettes. *Br. med J.* **282**, 1183–1187

Morgan, D.C., Smyth, J.T., Lister, R.W. and Pethybridge, R.J. (1973) Chest symptoms and farmers lung; a community survey. *Br. J. Ind. Med.* **30**, 259–261

Myones, B.L., Dalzell, J.G., Hogg, N. and Ross, G.D. (1988) Neutrophil and monocyte cell surface p150, 95 has iC3b-receptor (CR4) activity resembling CR3. *J. Clin. Invest.* **82**, 640–651

Naegel, G.P., Young, K.R., Jr and Reynolds, H.Y. (1984) Receptors for human IgG subclasses on human alveolar macrophages. *Am. Rev. Respir. Dis.* **129**, 413–418

Nielsen, H. (1985) A quantitative and qualitative study of blood monocytes in smokers. *Eur. J. Respir. Dis.* **66**, 327–332

Nomo, Y., Sideras, P., Naito, T., Bergstedt-Lindquist, S., Azuma, C., Severinson, E., Tanabe, T., Kinashi, T., Matsuda, F., Yaoita, Y. and Honjo, T. (1986) Cloning of cDNA encoding the murine IgG1 induction factor by a novel strategy using SP6 promoter. *Nature* **319**, 640–646

O'Neill, S.J., Lesperance, E. and Klass, D.J. (1984) Human lung lavage surfactant enhances staphylococcal phagocytosis by alveolar macrophages. *Am. Rev. Respir. Dis* **130**, 1177–1179

Onari, K., Seyama, A., Inamizu, T., Kodomari, N., Takaishi, M., Yorioka, N., Ikuta, T., Iwamato, K., Sadamoto, K., Katsube, M., Yamakido, M. and Nishimoto, Y. (1978) Immunological study on cigarette smokers. Part 1. Serum protein pattern in smokers. *Hiroshima J. Med. Sci.* **27**, 113–118

Pangburn, M.K. (1983) Activation of complement via the alternative pathway. *Fed. Proc.* **42**, 139–143

Peterson, M.W., Monick, M. and Hunninghake, G.W. (1987) Prognostic role of eosinophils in pulmonary fibrosis. *Chest* **92**, 51–56

Phipps, R.P., Penney, D.P., Keng, P., Quill, H., Paxhia, A., Derdak, S. and Felch, M.E. (1989) Characterization of two major populations of lung fibroblasts: distinguishing morphology and discordant display of Thy 1 and Class II MHC. *Am. J. Respir. Cell Mol. Biol.* **1**, 65–74

Piguet, P.F., Collart, M.A., Grau, G.E., Kapanci, Y. and Vassalli, P. (1989) Tumor necrosis factor/cachectin plays a key role in bleomycin-induced pneumopathy and fibrosis. *J. Expl. Med.* **170**, 655–663

Piguet, P.F., Collart, M.A., Grau, G.E., Sappino, A.P. and Cassalli, P. (1990) Requirement of tumour necrosis factor for development of silica-induced pulmonary fibrosis. *Nature* **344**, 245–247

Pratt, S.A., Smith, M.H., Ladman, A.J. and Finley, T.N. (1971) The ultrastructure of alveolar macrophages from human cigarette smokers and non-smokers. *Lab. Invest.* **24**, 331–338

Prior, C. and Haslam, P.L. (1991) Increased levels of serum interferon-gamma in pulmonary sarcoidosis and relationship with response to corticosteroid therapy. *Am. Rev. Respir. Dis* **143**, 53–60

Prior, C., Barbee, R.A., Evans, P.M., Townsend, P.J., Primett, Z.S., Fyhrquist. F., Grönhagen-Riska, C. and Haslam, P.L. (1990a) Lavage versus serum measurements of lysozyme, angiotensin converting enzyme and other inflammatory markers in pulmonary sarcoidosis. *Eur. Respir. J.* **3**, 1146–1154

Prior, C. and Haslam, P.L. (1992) In vivo and in vitro production of interferon-gamma in fibrosing interstitial lung diseases. *Clin. Expl. Immunol.* **88**, 280–287

Rankin, J.A., Hitchcock, M., Merrill, W.W., Bach, M.K., Brashler, R.J. and Askenase, P.W. (1982) IgE-dependent release of leukotriene C4 from alveolar macrophages. *Nature* **297**, 329–331

Razma, A.G., Lynch, J.P., III, Wilson, B.S., Ward, P.A. and Kunkel, S.L. (1984) Human alveolar macrophage activation and DR antigen expression in cigarette smokers. *Chest* **85**, 415–435

Reynolds, H.Y. and Newball, H.H. (1974) Analysis of proteins and respiratory cells obtained from human lung by bronchial lavage. *J. Lab. Clin. Med.* **84**, 559–573

Reynolds, H.Y., Kazmierowski, J.A. and Newball, H.H. (1975) Specificity of opsonic antibodies to enhance phagocytosis of *Pseudomonas aeruginosa* by human alveolar macrophages. *J. Clin. Invest.* **56**, 376–385

Reynolds, H.Y., Atkinson, J.P., Newball, H.H. and Frank, M.M. (1975) Receptors for immunoglobulin and complement on human alveolar macrophages. *J. Immunol.* **114**, 1813–1819

Reynolds, H.Y., Fulmer, J.D., Kazmierowski, J.A., Roberts, W.C., Frank, M.M. and Crystal. R.G. (1977) Analysis of cellular and protein content of bronchoalveolar lavage fluid from patients with idiopathic pulmonary fibrosis and chronic hypersensitivity pneumonitis. *J. Clin. Invest.* **59**, 165–175

Richards, C.D. and Gauldie, J. (1985) IgA-mediated phagocytosis by mouse alveolar macrophages. *Am. Rev. Respir. Dis.* **132**, 82–85

Robbins, R.A., Gadek, J.E. and Crystal, R.G. (1981) Potential role of the complement system in propagating the alveolitis of idiopathic pulmonary fibrosis (abstract). *Am. Rev. Respir. Dis.* **123**, 50

Robertson, J., Caldwell, J.R., Castle, J.R. and Waldman, R.H. (1976) Evidence for the presence of components of the alternative pathway of complement activation in respiratory secretions. *J. Immunol.* **117**, 900–904

Robinson, B., Pinkston, P. and Crystal, R.G. (1984) Natural killer cells are present in the normal human lung but are functionally inert. *J. Clin. Invest.* **74**, 942–950

Robinson, P.C., Watters, L.C., King, T.E. and Mason, R.J. (1988) Idiopathic pulmonary fibrosis. Abnormalities in bronchoalveolar lavage fluid phospholipids. *Am. Rev. Respir. Dis.* **137**, 585–591

Roitt, I.M., Brostoff, J. and Male, D.K. (1989) *Immunology*. Churchill Livingstone, Gower Medical, London

Rom, W.N., Bitterman, P.B., Rennard, S.I., Cantin, A. and Crystal, R.G. (1987) Characterization of the lower respiratory tract inflammation of non smoking individuals with interstitial lung disease associated with chronic inhalation of inorganic dusts. *Am. Rev. Respir. Dis* **136**, 1429–1434

Rosenberg, S.A., Lotz, M.T. and Muul, M.M. (1985) Observations on the systemic administration of autologous lymphokine activated killer cells and recombinant interleukin 2 to patients with metastatic cancer. *N. Engl. J. Med.* **313**, 1485–1492

Ross, G.D., Walport, M.J. and Hogg, N. (1989) Receptors for IgG Fc, and fixed C3. In: *Human Monocytes* (eds M. Zembala and G.L. Asherson), Academic Press, London, pp. 123–139

Rossman, M.D. and Douglas, S.D. (1988) The alveolar macrophage: receptors and effector cell function. In: *Immunology and Immunologic Diseases of the Lung* (ed. R.P. Daniele), Blackwell Scientific, Boston, pp. 167–183

Rossman, M.D., Cassizzi, A.M., Schreiber, A.D. and Daniele, R.P. (1982) Pulmonary defense mechanisms: modulation of Fc-receptor activity in alveolar macrophages and other phagocytic cells by N-formyl peptides. *Am. Rev. Respir. Dis.* **126**, 136–141

Rossman, M.D., Kern, J.A., Elias, J.A., Cullen, M.R., Epstein, P.E., Preuss, O.P., Markham, T.N. and Daniele, R.P. (1988) Proliferative response of bronchoalveolar lymphocytes to beryllium. *Ann. Intern. Med.* **108**, 687–693

Roth, C., Huchon, G.J., Arnoux, A., Stanislas-Lequern, G., Marsac, J.H. and Chrétien, J. (1981) Bronchoalveolar lavage cells in advanced pulmonary sarcoidosis. *Am. Rev. Respir. Dis.* **124**, 9–12

Rouzer, C.A., Scott, W.A., Hamill, A.L., Liu, F., Katz, D.H. and Cohn, Z.A. (1982) Secretion of leukotriene C and other arachidonic acid metabolites by macrophages challenged with immunoglobulin E immune complexes. *J. Expl. Med.* **156**, 1077–1086

Rudd, R.M., Haslam, P.L. and Turner-Warwick, M. (1981) Cryptogenic fibrosing alveolitis: Relationship of pulmonary physiology and bronchoalveolar lavage to response to treatment and prognosis. *Am. Rev. Respir. Dis.* **124**, 1–8

Saltini, C., Winestock, K., Kirby, M., Pinkston, P. and Crystal, R.G. (1989) Maintenance of alveolitis in patients with chronic beryllium disease by beryllium-specific helper T cells. *N. Engl. J. Med.* **320**, 1103–1109

Schwartz, L.W. and Christman, C.A. (1979) Alveolar macrophage migration: Influence of lung lining material and acute lung insult. *Am. Rev. Respir. Dis.* **120**, 429–439

Scornik, J.C. (1976) Complement dependent immunoglobulin G receptor function in lymphoid cells. *Science* **192**, 563–565

Sebastien, P., Armstrong, B., Monchaux, G. and Bignon, J. (1988) Asbestos bodies in bronchoalveolar lavage fluid and in lung parenchyma. *Am. Rev. Respir. Dis.* **137**, 75–78

Semenzato, G., Agostini, C., Zambello, R., Trentin, L., Chilosi, M., Pizzolo, G., Marcer, G. and Cipriani, A. (1986) Lung T-cells in hypersensitivity pneumonitis: phenotypic and functional analysis. *J. Immunol.* **137**, 1164–1172

Shimada, H. (1982) A study on functions of human pulmonary alveolar macrophages – effects of smoking. *Shikoku Acta Medika* **38**, 355–370

Sibille, Y., Chatelain, B., Staquet, P., Merrill, W.W., Delacroix, D.L. and Vaerman, J.P. (1989) Surface IgA and Fc-alpha receptors on human alveolar macrophages from normals and patients with sarcoidosis. *Am. Rev. Respir. Dis.* **139**, 292–297

Sibille, Y. and Reynolds, H.Y. (1990) State of the Art: Macrophages and polymorphonuclear neutrophils in lung defense and injury. *Am. Rev. Respir. Dis.* **141**, 471–501

Soutar, C. (1976) Distribution of plasma cells and other cells containing immunoglobulin in the respiratory tract of normal man and class of immunoglobulin contained therein. *Thorax* **31**, 158–166

Spiegelberg, H.L., Boltz-Nitulescu, G., Plummer, J.M. and Melewicz, F.M. (1983) Characterization of the IgE Fc receptors on monocytes and macrophages. *Fed. Proc.* **42**, 124–128

Stein, R., Evans, S., Milner, R., Rand, C. and Dolovich, J. (1983) Isotopic and enzymatic IgE assays in non-allergic subjects. *Allergy* **38**, 389–398

Stolzenburg, T., Binz, H., Fontana, A., Felder, M. and Wagenhäuser, FJ. (1988) Impaired mitogen-induced interferon-gamma production in rheumatoid arthritis and related diseases. *Scand. J. Immunol.* **27**, 73–81

Taylor, P.M., Rose, M.L. and Yacoub, M.H. (1989) Expression of MHC antigens in normal human lungs and transplanted lungs with obliterative bronchiolitis. *Transplantation* **48**, 506–510

Thrall, R.S., Sendsen, C.L., Shannon, T.H., Kennedy, C.A., Fredrick, D.S., Grunze, M.F. and Sulavik, SB. (1987) Correlation of changes in pulmonary surfactant phospholipids with compliance in bleomycin-induced pulmonary fibrosis in the rat. *Am. Rev. Respir. Dis.* **136**, 113–118

Tracy, K.J., Wei, H., Manogue, K.R., Fong, Y., Hesse, D.G., Nguyen, H.T., Kuo, G.C., Beutler, B., Cotran, R.S., Cerami, A. and Lowry, S.F. (1988) Cachectin/tumor necrosis factor induces cachexia, anemia, and inflammation. *J. Expl. Med.* **167**, 1211–1228

Turner-Warwick, M. (1978) *Immunology of the Lung.* Edward Arnold, London

Turner-Warwick, M. and Haslam, P.L. (1987) The value of serial bronchoalveolar lavage in assessing the clinical progress of patients with cryptogenic fibrosing alveolitis. *Am. Rev. Respir. Dis.* **135**, 26–34

Turner-Warwick, M., Haslam, P.L. and Weeks, J. (1971) Antibodies in some chronic fibrosing lung diseases. II. Immunofluorescent studies. *Clin. Allergy* **1**, 209–219

Turner-Warwick, M., Haslam, P.L., Lukoszek, A., Townsend, P.J., Allan, F., Du Bois, R.M., Turton, C.W.G. and Collins, J.V. (1981) Cells, enzymes and interstitial lung disease. *J. R. Coll. Phys. (Lond.)* **15**, 5–16

Twomey, J.J., Laughter, A. and Brown, M.F. (1983) A comparison of the regulatory effects of human monocytes, pulmonary alveolar macrophages (PAM's) and spleen macrophages upon lymphocyte responses. *Clin. Exp. Immunol.* **52**, 449–454

Velay, B., Pages, J., Cordier, J.F. and Brune, J. (1987) Hypereosinophilia in bronchoalveolar lavage. Diagnostic value and correlations with blood eosinophilia. *Rev. Mal. Respir.* **4**, 257–260

Venables, K.M., Topping, M.D., Howe, W., Luczynska, C.M., Hawkins, R. and Newman-Taylor, A.J. (1985) Interaction of smoking atopy in producing specific IgE antibody against a hapten protein conjugate. *Br. Med. J.* **290**, 201–206

Verbrugh, H.A., Hoidal, J.R., Nguyen, B.Y.T., Verhoef, J., Quie, P.G. and Peterson, P.K. (1982) Human alveolar macrophage cytophilic immunoglobulin G-mediated phagocytosis of protein A-positive staphylococci. *J. Clin. Invest.* **69**, 63–74

Villiger, B., Broekelmann, T., Kelley, D., Heymach, G.J.,III and McDonald, J.A. (1981) Bronchoalveolar fibronectin in smokers and non-smokers. *Am. Rev. Respir. Dis.* **124**, 652–654

Wagner, M.M., Edwards, R.E., Moncrieff, C.B. and Wagner, J.C. (1984) Mast cells and inhalation of asbestos in rats. *Thorax* **39**, 539–544

Wallaert, B., Hatron, P., Grosbois, J., Tonnel, A., Devulder, B. and Voisin, C. (1986) Subclinical pulmonary involvement in collagen-vascular diseases assessed by bronchoalveolar lavage. *Am. Rev. Respir. Dis.* **133**, 574–580

Wallaert, B., Lassalle, Ph, Fortin, F., Aerts, C., Bart, F., Fournier, E. and Voisin, C. (1990) Superoxide anion generation by alveolar inflammatory cells in simple pneumoconiosis and progressive massive fibrosis of non smoking coal workers. *Am. Rev. Respir. Dis.* **141**, 129–133

Warr, G.A. and Martin, R.R. (1977) Immune receptors of human alveolar macrophages: comparison between cigarette smokers and non-smokers. *J. Reticuloendoth. Soc.* **22**, 181–187

Warren, C.P.W., Holford-Stevens, W.M., Wong, C. and Manfreda, J. (1982) The relationship between smoking and total immunoglobulin E levels. *J. Allergy Clin. Immunol.* **69**, 370–375

Watters, L.C., Schwarz, M.I., Cherniack, R.M., Waldrom, J.A., Dunn, T.L., Stanford, R.E. and King, T.E. (1987) Idiopathic pulmonary fibrosis. Pretreatment bronchoalveolar lavage cellular constituents and their relationships with lung histopathology and clinical response to therapy. *Am. Rev. Respir. Dis.* **153**, 696–704

Weinberg, P.F., Matthay, M.A., Webster, R.O., Rokos, K.V., Goldstein, I.M. and Murray, J.F. (1984) Biologically active products of complement and acute lung injury in patients with the sepsis syndrome. *Am. Rev. Respir. Dis.* **130**, 791–796

Weinberger, S.E., Kelman, J.A., Elson, N.A., Young, R.C. Jr, Reynolds, H.Y., Fulmer, J.D. and Crystal, R.G. (1978) Bronchoalveolar lavage in interstitial lung disease. *Ann. intern. Med.* **89**, 459–466

Weir, D.M. (1986) *Handbook of Experimental Immunology*, 4th Ed. Blackwell Scientific, Oxford

Weir, D.M. (1988) *Immunology*, 6th Ed. Churchill Livingstone, Edinburgh

Weissler, J.C., Lyons, C.R., Lipscomb, M.F. and Toews, G.B. (1986) Interstitial macrophages from human lungs stimulate a mixed leukocyte reaction more efficiently than alveolar macrophages. *Am. Rev. Respir. Dis.* **133**, 473–477

Weissler, J.C., Nicod, L.P., Lipscomb, M.F. and Toews, G.B. (1987) NK cell function in human lung is compartmentalized. *Am. Rev. Respir. Dis.* **135**, 941–949

Wilsher, M.L., Hughes, D.A. and Haslam, P.L. (1988a) Immunoregulatory properties of pulmonary surfactant: effect of lung lining fluid on proliferation of human blood lymphocytes. *Thorax* **43**, 354–359

Wilsher, M.L., Hughes, D.A. and Haslam, P.L. (1988b) Immunoregulatory properties of pulmonary surfactant: influence of variations in the phospholipid profile. *Clin. Expl. Immunol.* **73**, 117–122

Wilsher, M.L., Parker, D.J. and Haslam, P.L. (1990) Immunosuppression by pulmonary surfactant: mechanisms of action. *Thorax* **45**, 3–8

Wilson, M.R., Gaumer, H.R. and Salvaggio, J.E. (1977) Activation of the alternate complement pathway and generation of chemotactic factors by asbestos. *J. Allergy Clin. Immunol.* **60**, 218–222

Zeligs, B.J., Nerurkar, L.S. and Bellanti, J.A. (1977) Maturation of the rabbit alveolar macrophage during animal development. 1. Perinatal influx into alveoli and ultrastructural differentiation. *Pediatr. Res.* **11**, 197–208

Zetterström, O., Osterman, K., Machado, L. and Johansson, S.G.O. (1981) Another smoking hazard: raised serum IgE concentration and increased risk of occupational allergy. *Br. Med. J.* **283**, 1215–1217

5

Pathogenesis of mineral pneumoconioses

A.G. Heppleston

Preliminary considerations

Inhaled dust represents one type of aerosol, that is, solid particles or liquid droplets small enough to form more or less stable suspensions in the atmosphere. Most occupational dust hazards are presented by minerals, which constitute naturally occurring, crystalline inorganic compounds or elements. The prime site of reaction to inhaled dust is the alveolar region of the lung, to reach which particles need to be of respirable size. The definitions of aerosols in general, their characteristics, aerodynamic behaviour in and clearance from the lungs are discussed in Chapter 3.

The development of tissue changes depends first on what Mavrogordato (1926) called the effective occupation of the lung by dust, that is, retention which represents the balance between the complex processes of deposition and clearance. Combined with quantity of dust, which embraces both the *intensity* and the *duration* of exposure (that is, the dose × time relationship), is its qualitative nature, which to a large extent determines the inception and the evolution of lesions. The present discussion proceeds from the stage at which dust begins to accumulate.

Structural maintenance

Basal conditions

Cell population

The cell population comprises four groups: *epithelial*, *phagocytic*, *endothelial* and *interstitial*. These are described in Chapter 1 but more detailed discussion of alveolar macrophages, the immunological functions of which are discussed in Chapter 4, is relevant in this chapter.

Alveolar macrophages are large cells with abundant cytoplasm and pseudopodia applied closely to the epithelium, but phagocytosis is only one of their functions. They contain many vesicles and membrane-bound lysosomes up to 2 μm diameter, whilst phagolysosomes may occur in different sizes and include fragments of lamellar bodies taken up after extrusion from type II cells. Mitochondria are small but readily identified. Alveolar macrophages from animals and human beings are regarded as part of the mononuclear phagocytic system and as being marrow-derived (Thomas et al., 1976). After depletion of monocytes by whole-body irradiation of mice, interstitial precursors appeared not only to maintain the normal level of alveolar macrophages but also to provide a reserve mechanism to handle a particle load (Bowden and Adamson, 1982). Although quantitative electron microscopy of normal rat lung revealed that the great majority of monocytes accumulated, not extravascularly in the interstitium, but within capillaries (Masse et al., 1977), and more macrophages occurred in blood vessels than in alveolar spaces of ruminant lung (Warner, Barry and Brain, 1986), the proliferative capacity of macrophages from the interstitium was greater than those from alveoli, thereby supporting the role of the former in maintenance of the lung macrophage population (Kobzik et al., 1988). The systemic emphasis has been challenged on evidence derived from mice rendered monocytopenic and then stimulated with carbon particles; the results pointed to dividing alveolar macrophages as the prime source of new cells (Evans, Shami and Martinez, 1986). Cell kinetics likewise suggested that, in normal rats, the population of alveolar macrophages was maintained by local proliferation rather than by vascular emigration (Shellito, Esparza and Armstrong, 1987).

However, macrophage populations are not homogeneous, whether between different sites or from the same location. This functional heterogeneity may be seen in respect of both alveolar and interstitial macrophages of rat lung (Holt, Warner and Papadimitriou, 1982; Chandler, Kennedy and Fulmer, 1986) as well as in human alveolar macrophages obtained by lavage (Gant and Hamblin, 1985). Replication of alveolar macrophages may prove to be a phenomenon of immature cells, whether in newly born animals or in adults, stimulated by irritants, or to be influenced by the microenvironment; nonetheless, the evidence pointing ultimately to their derivation from the marrow seems incontrovertible. Indeed, isoenzyme mapping led to the conclusion that alveolar macrophages originated from blood monocytes by tissue-specific stimulation (Radzun, Parwaresch and Kreipe, 1983). Under a dust burden there is no reason why all three compartments – haematogenous, interstitial and alveolar – should not contribute, but the balance may well be determined by the nature of the particles (see later).

Of the *total cell population* of the human lung, type I epithelium represents 8 per cent, type II 16 per cent, endothelium 30 per cent and interstitial cells (mostly fibroblasts) 37 per cent (Crapo et al., 1982). However, on a morphometric basis, the overall volume of type I exceeds that of type II epithelium and the difference in area covered is much greater. Alveolar macrophages vary in number, but their incidence in clean lung is considered to be 2 to 5 per cent of the total population. Cell proportions are remarkably similar in human, baboon and rat lungs, suggesting a structural homogeneity of cells in animals, despite vastly different total numbers of lung cells and a difference of over 200-fold in body weight. These observations afford a measure of confidence in the application of experimental findings to human pneumoconioses.

Connective tissue framework
(See Chapter 1, 'The fibrous skeleton of the lungs')

Collagen

This forms the major protein of human lung, contributing 10 to 20 per cent of the dry weight; it is weakly birefringent under polarized light and ultrastructurally exhibits cross-striations with characteristic periodicity. Collagen occurs as closely packed fibrils, with diameters as much as 100 nm, each of which is made up of rod-like molecules 300 nm in length and 3 nm in diameter. These molecules are composed of three polypeptide α-chains arranged as a right-handed triple helix. The chains contain about 1000 amino acids, notably glycine, proline and hydroxyproline, and are stabilized by inter- and intramolecular cross-links which involve lysine and hydroxylysine. The amino acid sequence determines the collagen type, of which 11 are considered to exist although only the first 5 are important in respect of the lung, where types I and III are the most abundant and normally occur in the ratio of approximately 2 : 1 (Laurent, 1986). Immunohistochemical procedures are employed to determine the distribution of collagen types within the lung. Type I collagen is thought to take up conventional connective tissue stains such as Masson trichrome or Van Gieson and it forms thick fibres which are presumably less compliant than those of type III (Rennard et al., 1982). Type II collagen is confined to cartilage, whilst type IV is found only in basement membranes and the same may apply to type V which is less well characterized (Table 5.1). In addition to collagen, basement membranes contain a glycoprotein known as *laminin*, which assists cellular attachment, and proteoglycans.

Table 5.1 The main types of collagen

Type	Structure	Occurrence
I	$[\alpha_1(I)]_2[\alpha_2(I)]$	Most connective tissues, except hyaline cartilage
II	$[\alpha_1(II)]_3$	Hyaline cartilage
III	$[\alpha_1(III)]_3$	As type I, largely
IV	$[\alpha_1(IV)]_2[\alpha_2(IV)]$ or $[\alpha_1(IV)]_3$	Basement membrane predominantly
V	$[\alpha_1(V)][\alpha_2(V)][\alpha_3(V)]$	Pericellular

α_1, α_2 and α_3 represent collagen chains in the triple helix.

Although serving to restrict expansion of the lung, especially at higher volumes, by virtue of its high tensile strength, collagen, according to Laurent (1986), may no longer be regarded simply as an almost inert interstitial supporting structure because its rates of synthesis and catabolism are believed to be considerable. However, Last and Reiser (1989), relying on sensitive biochemical techniques, were unable to detect turnover of mature extracellular lung collagen in normal rats or in animals rendered fibrotic by bleomycin; they suggested that other investigators might have been studying different pools of lung collagen.

Collagen is produced mainly by fibroblasts but also by epithelium and endothelium as well as by chondrocytes through a complex process (Figure 5.1), and degradation of extracellular collagen (chiefly types I and III) occurs via the agency of collagenases, which are relatively type specific and cause the triple helix to cleave at a particular site. Denaturation of polypeptides is completed either by

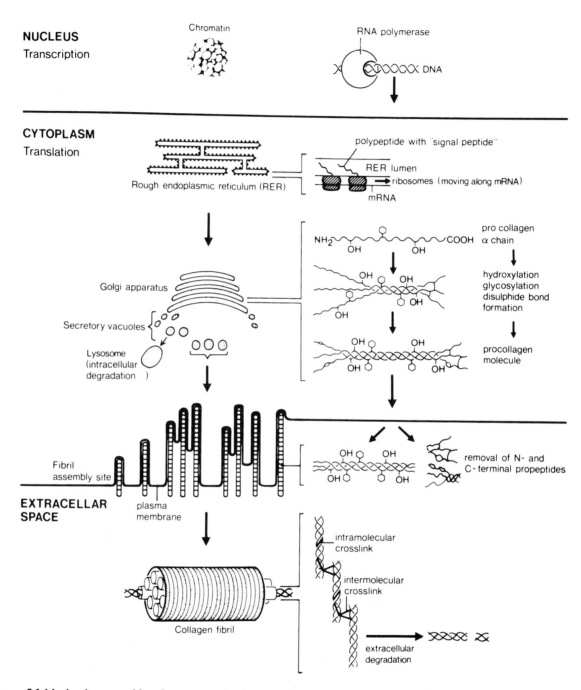

Figure 5.1 Mechanisms considered to operate in the synthesis and degradation of collagen. (Reproduced with permission from Laurent, 1986)

neutral proteases or through intracellular digestion by macrophages. The procollagen molecule may, however, be degraded rapidly within the cell of formation, that is, before secretion. Fibroblasts, macrophages and neutrophils are all capable of producing collagenases, which are formed as proenzymes requiring activation by other proteases and these can be inhibited by antiproteases (see also Chapter 4).

Reticulin

This is the descriptive term applied to fine-branched fibres which by light microscopy stain black after silver impregnation, but are isotropic under polarized light while exhibiting cross-striations electron microscopically. Although the chemical basis of the silver reaction is unclear, serological and immunohistological studies suggest that reticulin is a compound fibrous structure consisting of type III collagen, fibronectin and one or more non-collagenous glyco-proteins (Unsworth et al., 1982). *Fibronectin* is a further component of the extracellular matrix, antigenically similar to plasma fibronectin and secreted by alveolar macrophages. It is a glycoprotein which serves as an adhesive between cell surfaces and collagen; it is also a chemoattractant for human lung fibroblasts (Rennard et al., 1981). The so-called *ground substance* consists largely of proteoglycans in which the predominant disaccharide chains (glycos-aminoglycans) distinguish several types.

Elastic fibres

By light microscopy, these form a loose network in alveolar walls, but are denser in bronchioles, respiratory or otherwise, bronchi and pleura. Ultrastructurally the fibres occur as fenestrated sheets or as cylinders without striations and possess two components: elastin and microfibrils. *Elastin* is a hydrophobic protein which appears amorphous and chemically consists of cross-linked tropoelastin subunits of polypeptides containing little hydroxyproline but no hydroxylysine or carbohydrate. The *microfibrillar* element lies peripherally in the developed fibre and is composed of amino acids with carbohydrate side chains but no hydroxyproline or hydroxylysine; it may appear to exist as cylinders that are relatively diminished with fibre maturity (Rennard et al., 1982). Proteoglycans and collagens types III and VI are demonstrable by immunohistochemical procedures, as are nectins and plasma protease inhibitors. Conventionally, elastic tissue is considered to regulate parenchymal recoil on expiration, although the geodesically arranged smooth muscle fibres of bronchioles are probably more important in this connection.

Dust-laden states

The fundamental features of the pulmonary response to inhaled particles can be appreciated best in the light of the structural changes they induce, taking as reference points dusts that are compact and either silica-rich or silica-poor or that are fibrous in nature. Random histological sections fail to convey a precise idea of microanatomical changes, to grasp which the three-dimensional approach is necessary. This procedure requires blocks of tissue, at least 1 cm³ and taken from lung fixed in distension, to be sectioned in strict series.

Irrespective of the composition of the dust, the site at which simple lesions form is similar, namely in the region of respiratory bronchioles, the anatomy of which is described in Chapter 1.

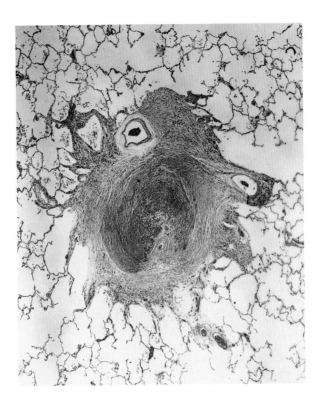

Figure 5.2 Small but mature silicotic nodule, exhibiting the three characteristic zones, lying in normal parenchyma. Magnification × 25; H&E

Silica-rich dust

Characteristic changes follow exposure to dusts containing 20 per cent or more of quartz, the common crystalline form of silicon dioxide, although a somewhat lower proportion may be effective.

Well-established silicotic nodules are hard and measure up to 5 or 6 mm in diameter; they are widely distributed but tend to be larger and more numerous in the upper zones of the lung. The depth of the grey colour depends on the content of carbon particles and a concentric pattern of connective tissue may be seen peripherally. Histologically, three zones may be distinguished (Figure 5.2). The central zone consists of one or more islets of whorled connective tissue that has become hyalinized; in the mid-zone, collagen fibres are concentrically arranged around the islets, whilst, peripherally, collagen and reticulin mingle irregularly with macrophages bearing silica and carbonaceous particles, the latter coming from the working or urban environment. Birefringence, however, is inconstant, probably on account of small particle size and the planes of silica surfaces (see Appendix IV). Microincineration and incident light reveal an ash pattern which differs in the three zones. Islets contain a variable amount of dispersed dust, the mid-zone is largely lacking in particles, whilst the

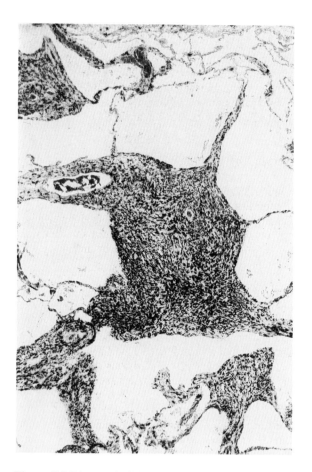

Figure 5.3 Discrete lesion in a coal worker's lung. Dust overshadows connective tissue; surrounding airspaces are enlarged and represent proximal acinar emphysema. Magnification × 35; H&E

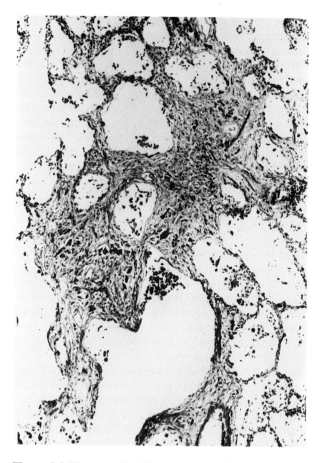

Figure 5.4 Circumscribed fibrotic lesion of asbestosis lying in relation to respiratory bronchioles with incipient cystic change. Terminal bronchiole (below) also shows mural fibrosis. Magnification × 35; H&E. (Reproduced with permission from Heppleston, 1979)

periphery appears as an enveloping halo; this distribution suggests that fibrous tissue is generated in the external zone and accumulates internally. In proportion to the quantity of siliceous dust, the developed nodule exhibits exuberant fibrosis, which has a peculiar arrangement and compresses respiratory bronchioles. Localized emphysema is not, therefore, an integral component, but if expansion ceases limited fibrous contraction may ensue resulting in a minor degree of irregular ('scar') emphysema (see Chapter 9).

Silica-poor dust

The best example is coal pneumoconiosis, although hematite miners acquire simple lesions of similar structure but different colour. In both cases the average proportion of quartz in the lungs lies in the region of 5 per cent or less, although somewhat

higher levels may exceptionally be encountered. Coal workers usually exhibit sharply defined black lesions up to 5 mm across with three to five occupying a lobule. Some lesions are palpable but they are never as firm as silicotic nodules. The larger ones possess a stellate outline and may have in their substance, or peripherally, enlarged airspaces reaching 2 to 3 mm in size (Figure 5.3). The most advanced lesions tend to merge and their initially discrete outlines are then obscured. As with silica, dust-laden phagocytes accumulate around respiratory bronchioles, notably the second order, their alveoli becoming consolidated so as to form a partial or complete cylindrical sleeve around them. Some such bronchioles undergo dilatation to produce the change decribed as proximal acinar emphysema. In many lesions connective tissue occurs as irregularly disposed reticulin fibres although collagen is sometimes seen. In simple coal pneumoconiosis there is no evidence of bronchiolar stenosis and destruction of alveolar walls is not a primary event. Incinerated preparations disclose an even ash pattern with few birefringent particles. Three features thus characterize the simple lesion of coal pneumoconiosis: a large proportion of dust, a relatively small fibrotic response and, in some cases, emphysema localized to the immediate vicinity of the dust aggregate which partially or wholly encloses the spaces. Differentiation of the lesion has been elaborated elsewhere (Heppleston, 1972) and its pathology is discussed further in Chapter 13.

Fibrous dust

The changes produced by fibrous dusts, among which asbestos figures prominently, differ from those caused by compact dusts in being unevenly distributed and possessing irregular outlines. Lower and posterior parts of the lung are often the main sites of disease with other areas escaping. Early lesions form small, grey, relatively circumscribed foci of induration, but, as the disease extends, the parenchyma is more diffusely affected in a patchy fashion, leading to fibrocystic features. Microanatomically, the changes begin in relation to respiratory bronchioles but are not well defined (Figure 5.4) and non-respiratory (membranous) bronchioles may become involved as the disease progresses, often communicating with cystic spaces via patent or obstructed orifices. Connective tissue occurs as reticulin or collagen and asbestos fibres, uncoated or coated (asbestos bodies), lie in fibrosed areas, while macrophages often aggregate in patent alveoli where fibres in both forms are also found free and intracellularly. The changes in airways and parenchyma induced by asbestos have recently been elaborated and compared with the effect of smoking (Heppleston, 1991). (The pathology of asbestosis is discussed in Chapter 14.)

Mast cells accumulate in relation to diverse fibrotic lesions and are believed to provide mediators, such as serotonin and histamine, for events comprising the inflammatory reaction; experimental asbestosis, whether from serpentine or amphiboles, conformed to this pattern (Wagner et al., 1984; Keith et al., 1987). The position is similar in human and experimental silicosis (Behrendt et al., 1990), but the precise role of mast cells in dust disease remains obscure (see Chapter 4, pages 73 and 85).

Inert dust

The collective name applied to these compact dusts indicates a minimal or absent capacity to induce fibrosis. They include oxides of titanium, tin and antimony together with the sulphate or carbonate of barium. Small discrete aggregations of dust-bearing macrophages develop in the usual location but reticulin fibres are scanty. The main impact of these dusts lies in their ability, by virtue of high atomic numbers, to produce a radiological 'snow-storm' appearance which requires differentiation. They have no deleterious effects, but barytes miners are liable to acquire silicosis from contamination by quartz present in associated rock strata (see Chapter 11).

Sequence of events

The silicotic nodule, as well as the simple lesions of coal pneumoconiosis and asbestosis, present a singularly quiescent appearance and their evolution is not easy to assess solely from human material, but a series of events is indicated by invoking the support of experimental evidence:

1. Inhaled compact particles are deposited widely if not evenly on the lining layer of respiratory parenchyma and their phagocytosis by macrophages is rapid. Fibrous particles tend to be thrown out of atmospheric suspension more proximally and most alight at divisions of the terminal or early respiratory bronchioles (see Chapter 3).
2. By cellular agency or in a free state, compact dusts aggregate in alveoli belonging to, or abutting on, respiratory bronchioles, notably those of the second and first orders. Fibrous dusts are already at these sites.
3. Depending on dust amount and toxicity, macrophages disintegrate and liberate their load.
4. Newly produced macrophages accumulate in the typical location to reingest particles.
5. Reticulin or collagen forms among the phagocytes.

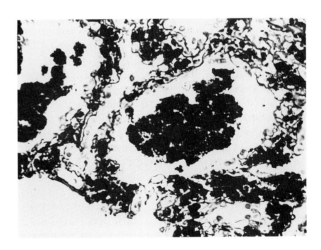

Figure 5.5 Macrophages laden with coal-mine dust lie within thickened alveolar walls and have also accumulated in shrunken alveoli. Magnification × 300; reticulin. (Reproduced with permission from Heppleston, 1947)

From human and experimental observations it appears that, at first, laden macrophages line alveolar walls whose type I pneumocytes are damaged, but then grow over the dust cells to give them an interstitial location (Figure 5.5). As more particles arrive, alveoli are gradually filled until eventually they are wholly consolidated and overtaken by connective tissue, mostly reticulin in coal workers but collagen in silicosis and, later, also in asbestosis. Because fresh dust continues to arrive over a prolonged period, these events overlap and the sequence is not readily perceived. To elucidate the interconnections requires the parallel deployment of in vitro techniques.

Dynamic aspects

Particle aggregation and translocation

Elimination of deposited particles by the bronchial or lymphatic routes is limited, because focal accumulations begin to form in both human and animal lungs after comparatively short exposure. The static impression conveyed by small or large dust lesions in conventional preparations was dispelled by an innocuous tracer technique, which permitted the movement of inhaled compact particles to be followed even though they reached the lung at widely separated times. Differential labelling was achieved by employing dusts such as coal, hematite and quartz which could be recognized in sections by their colour under a combination of transmitted and reflected light, together with incineration in the case of quartz (Heppleston, 1958, 1962).

Preferential settling or subsequent aggregation from widespread distal deposition may explain the occurrence of circumscribed lesions at particular sites within the lung. Initially deposition of poorly or highly siliceous dust was widespread although not always uniform; however, with the passage of time discrete intra-alveolar collections developed at the apex of the acinus, that is, in alveoli adjacent to the terminal bronchiole. Pre-existing coniotic lesions, whether from coal or quartz, modified the deposition pattern of hematite which now penetrated more distally in the acinus and was cleared more rapidly as compared with non-coniotic lungs. However, much of the second dust, accumulating around lesions formed by coal or quartz, remained and was gradually incorporated from their periphery (Figures 5.6 and 5.7) and, additionally, into the aggregates formed in lymphoid tissue, both within the lung and in the hilar nodes, the admixture extending to individual macrophages. This process became evident even during the second exposure and ultimately a more or less uniform mixing obtained at most sites and in most phagocytes (Heppleston, 1963).

An elegant experiment, already referred to in Chapter 3 ('Acinar clearance'), using microspheres labelled with red or green fluorescent dyes, established that intact macrophages conveyed inert material from alveoli, through the interstitium and along lymphatic vessels to the hilar nodes (Harmsen et al., 1985). For irritant compact or fibrous particles, however, the idea of passive conveyance within intact macrophages is hardly tenable and the cycle of cellular dissolution and reingestion seems inescapable. Dust transfer within the lung parenchyma and lymphoid system evidently combined exchange of particles between alveolar macrophages, as laden ones perished and fresh cells took up the liberated load of mineral, and carriage extracellularly on the lung lining layer in a proximal direction. New generations of macrophages were thus able to ingest particles from the first and second exposures to achieve the intimate mixture seen in cells and lesions. It should be emphasized that such incorporation occurred in fibrotic lesions from quartz as well as in non-fibrotic lesions from coal or hematite and, although in the former case the process was slower, penetration still occurred in severely fibrosed lymph nodes. The release–reingestion sequence has also been detected in miners who first worked in coal and subsequently in hematite-laden atmospheres (Policard, Collet and Martin, 1963), dusts that in the human being excite a mild fibrotic reaction. So long as macrophages are available, the persistence of quartz ensures continued fibrotic activity, *that is, the process becomes self-propagating in the absence of further exposure.* The arrival at the boundaries of established silicotic nodules of dusts such as coal or hematite, which at least in animals are themselves non-fibrogenic, might conceivably aggravate quartz fibrosis by this cyclical process, a view with which experimental evidence was consistent (Heppleston and Morris, 1965). It is thus possible to account for the progressive nature of silicotic fibrosis following cessation of exposure and its stimulation when complicated by accession of inert dust.

Short air-borne fibres tend to be deposited around the divisions of respiratory bronchioles, especially the more proximal ones (Brody et al., 1981), but wider fibres are less likely to penetrate so far. Macrophages are able to ingest the shorter fibres which may, therefore, be transported in the same way as compact particles. In either case fibrosis is promoted in the same location. Transfer of fibres from the interstitium to regional nodes is well attested (for example,

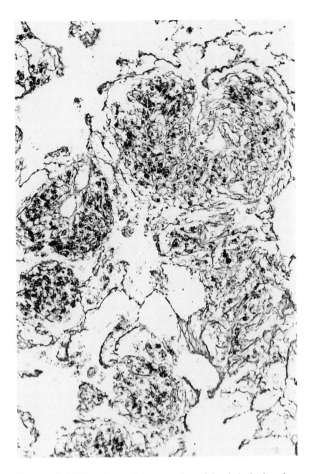

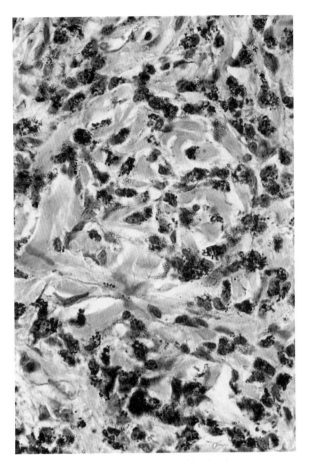

Figure 5.6 Silicotic nodules produced by inhalation in a rabbit. Hematite (black) inhaled later eventually came to lie in macrophages distributed throughout the lesions. Magnification × 160; reticulin

Figure 5.7 Hematite-laden macrophages (black) lie among the collagen fibres of a silicotic nodule in rabbit lung. The animal first inhaled quartz and, after an interval, hematite which subsequently penetrated to the centre of the fibrous nodule. Magnification × 500; H&E

Bignon et al., 1978), although negotiation of the route through the natural openings in lymphatic vessels is likely to restrict the process, and so also is distant migration of both compact and fibrous particles by blood or lymphatic conveyance.

Macrophage mobilization

The presence of dust augments the pulmonary demand for macrophages in two ways. A regular supply is required to ingest inhaled particles as they accumulate progressively, the need being greater with cytotoxic agents such as quartz, while prolonged provision of the *macrophage fibrogenic factor* (see page 113) depends on repeated uptake by new cells. To ensure that the population of macrophages is maintained at a level exceeding

normal requirements, local proliferation or systemic recruitment, or both, may be invoked.

The arguments of protagonists on each side, which have already been outlined, either do not refer primarily to particle disposal or rely on intra-tracheal bolus injection, which abolishes the natural reaction to air-borne dusts and, in the case or quartz or fibres, provokes an uncharacteristic acute response and, possibly, damage to type I epithelium. Macrophages dominate the scene when particles arrive slowly and in low concentration over a prolonged period from atmospheric suspension, as was reaffirmed both experimentally (Barry et al., 1983) and in human subjects (Voisin et al., 1985). Cell kinetics applied to murine lung after particle inhalation suggested that, for dusts of low toxicity such as coal, local division met the need for macrophages but, where toxicity was high, as with quartz, recruitment of marrow precursors was required. These recently formed cells of the monocytic line, identified by parallel ultrastructural observations on the response to inhaled particles of different types, did not remain long enough in the interstitium for mitosis to occur before emigrating into the alveoli (Brightwell and Heppleston, 1977). Cellular flux thus determined whether mitosis of macrophages was observed in the lung.

The functional activity of the mononuclear phagocytic system may be measured by the rate of clearance of pure carbon from the circulation, expressed as the 'phagocytic index' (prolonged elevation following administration of silica) and, also, of simple or complex lipids (Conning and Heppleston, 1966). In addition to functional stimulation it was necessary to demonstrate replenishment of macrophages by marrow monopoiesis. Quartz or titanium dioxide induced recruitment of phagocytes from the marrow and was attributed to the activity of breakdown products, notably lipid, from lung macrophages (Katsnelson and Privalova, 1984). Cell kinetic techniques were not, however, applied and the ability of alveolar macrophages to acquire large lipid burdens by uptake of type II cell secretion was overlooked. Lipid forms a prominent component of the response to silica (see later), mainly as dipalmitoyl lecithin. Using this endogenous material parenterally, the marrow monocytic series, identified functionally by behaviour towards particles, was examined kinetically (Civil and Heppleston, 1979). Compared with controls, marrow promonocytes of rats treated with lipid had an increased rate of entry into, and a reduced duration of, DNA synthesis along with a shortened cell cycle time, indicating augmented proliferation. Lipid feedback from lung to marrow via the circulation may, therefore, serve to recruit monocytic cells for the organ of need. The feedback is presumably proportional to the pulmonary stimulus and, hence, quiescence of lipidosis may be expected to be accompanied by subsidence of the macrophage response, as ultimately occurred under experimental conditions. It now appears that surfactant is processed by alveolar macrophages to release a stimulatory factor which maintains normal production of monocytes by the marrow (Sluiter et al., 1988). See Chapter 4, 'Respiratory bronchioles and alveoli'.

Monocytic emigration

The flux of cells through the vascular compartment is probably too rapid to detect monocytosis. To emerge as alveolar macrophages, monocytes have to traverse the capillary endothelium, the pulmonary interstitium and the attenuated type I epithelium; their outflow will be facilitated by co-operation of local mechanisms regulating capillary permeability and the production of chemotactic agents.

Endothelium, having labile intercellular junctions, offers an adaptable barrier, whereas the discontinuous interstitium permits cellular migration. Passage through basement membrane may be facilitated by the laminin component which in vitro assisted neutrophil attachment to and subsequent release from type IV collagen (Bryant et al., 1987); monocytes may behave similarly. The tight junctions of epithelium (see Chapter 1, 'The alveolar region') present an obstacle and its dissolution may, under normal circumstances, depend on enzymatic products of the emigrating cells; however, in the presence of an irritant such as silica, disruption of type I epithelium, evident ultrastructurally (Heppleston and Young, 1972), simplifies egress from the interstitium. The outflow of cells will be facilitated by increased permeability of capillaries, such as may be induced by E-type prostaglandins formed in alveolar macrophages after stimulation with materials that include particles. Phagocytosis was identified as the process through which these cells released prostaglandin (see Chapter 4, page 71 *et seq.* and Figure 4.5).

Chemoattractants comprise endogenous and exogenous products. Alveolar macrophages from monkeys exhibited directional migration towards lung lining material from the same species (Schwartz and Christman, 1979) and surfactant protein from rats encouraged similar activity (Hoffman et al., 1987). Proximal conveyance of the lining layer towards lymphatics originating in the vicinity of terminal bronchioles might account in part for selective concentration of dust cells at the apex of the acinus. Breakdown products of collagen may also be chemotactic for macrophages and degradation of lung collagen by macrophage collagenase could assist monocytic emigration in fibrotic states such as silicosis. Quartz inhalation induced a chemotactic property in normal guinea-pig alveolar macrophages, but non-dusted macrophages were ineffective (Miller, Calverley and Kagan, 1980). Moreover, both crocidolite and chrysotile asbestos inhaled by rats enhanced the release of an alveolar macrophage chemoattractant for homologous cells (Kagan, Oghiso and Hartmann, 1983). This activity is evidently complement derived and sustained, because inhaled asbestos augmented in a time-dependent fashion the normal transudation of serum complement onto the alveolar surface (Warheit et al., 1986), whilst chrysotile and crocidolite (as well as fibreglass) provoked chemotactic activity for alveolar macrophages in serum or lavaged lung proteins (Warheit et al., 1988). Fibronectin, deposited at sites of inflammation and wound healing, when cleaved by endogenous proteases, generated fragments which proved potent chemoattractants for blood monocytes

(Norris et al., 1982), a sequence that may be envisaged as part of the silicotic response. Chemotactic activity towards alveolar macrophages is not confined to the products of cell–particle interaction. An extract of *Escherichia coli* filtrates, especially the lipid fraction, had a powerful chemotactic effect on rabbit alveolar macrophages (Tainer, Turner and Lynn, 1975), thus raising the possibility that bacteria causing infections of the lung may operate similarly.

Cytotoxicity

The more obvious deleterious effects imposed on cells by particles are revealed by changes in membrane permeability and in metabolism, the former being recognized by dye penetration and the latter reflected by release of enzymes from lysosomes or cytosol. A prior requisite for these events is particle attachment to and reaction with both plasma and intracellular membranes, about which several theories exist, and to isolate these phenomena erythrocytes have been employed extensively.

Erythrolysis

In the case of particulate *quartz* simple electrostatic attraction may be excluded because both it and red cells carry negative surface charges. Haemolysis may, however, depend on the high affinity of silica for positively charged trimethylammonium groups on the membrane surface, because adsorption of these ions by the particles inhibited the reaction (Depasse, 1980). Moreover, silica toxicity to erythrocytes depended on their sialic acid content, sheep cells with a low level being much more susceptible than horse cells with a high level, and resistance being eliminated by neuraminidase. Compared with quartz (tetrahedrally co-ordinated), natural titanium dioxide (octahedrally co-ordinated and in the rutile phase) used as control in biological experiments was devoid of membranolytic activity (Nolan et al., 1987). (The possibility of differences in the biological effects of natural and synthetic titanium dioxide is discussed in Chapter 11.) Hydrogen donation by polymeric silicic acid was held to mediate silica toxicity through the formation of hydrogen-bonded complexes, particularly with phospholipids of cell membranes (Nash, Allison and Harington, 1966). Haemolysis was much

diminished by the polymer polyvinylpyridine-*N*-oxide (PNO) (Harington, Miller and Macnab, 1971), which was known to inhibit both experimental silicosis and cell damage in culture. PNO might establish hydrogen bonds preferentially with silicic acid, thereby preserving the integrity of biological membranes, but by accumulation on the quartz surface the polymer may present a simple barrier to interaction with red cell membranes (Nolan et al., 1981). However, hydrogen bonding may be less important than electrostatic interactions in determining biological activities (Wiessner et al., 1990). Aluminium and iron cations were able to inhibit quartz reactivity by binding to its negative surface centres, a phenomenon which may be important when miners are exposed to coal dust or contaminated silica. Large amounts of aluminium chloride, however, may induce lysis by vigorous shifts of pH. An alternative view attributed membrane damage by silica, not to lipid binding, but to abstraction of a protein component (Summerton et al., 1977). Yet another interpretation invoked adsorption by quartz particles of cell constituents such as red cell 'ghosts' or synthetic liposomes of dipalmitoyl lecithin (Jaurand, Renier and Bignon, 1980). However membrane damage is incurred, the effect is to increase permeability and permit alterations of intracellular electrolyte balance (especially Na^+ and K^+) with osmotic changes leading to rupture. It may be noted that, in vivo, the fibrogenic and membranolytic activities of quartz were dissociated according to particle size (Wiessner et al., 1989).

Disparities exist between the prevalence of pneumoconiosis in coal workers and the mineral content, especially quartz, of the air-borne dust, high progression being sometimes associated with low dust concentration or vice versa. Wide and unexplained colliery-associated variations occurred and were not explicable in terms of the quartz content of respirable dust, averaging 5 per cent and rarely exceeding 10 per cent. Only with higher levels of quartz exposure were unusual radiographic changes observed (see Heppleston, 1988a). Haemolysis by dust from low and high rank mines revealed disparities and did not identify a role for quartz, whilst correlation with toxicity was poor (Gormley et al., 1979).

Among *fibrous particles* amphiboles (see Appendix I) were comparatively inactive but chrysotile proved strongly haemolytic, the magnesium although not the silicon content of the latter bearing a linear relationship to the degree of lysis (Harington, Miller and Macnab, 1971). The activity of chrysotile was reduced by acid leaching which removed the outer layer of magnesium hydroxide (brucite), itself highly lytic (Morgan et al., 1977), whilst non-specific chelation of metal ions by ethylenediaminetetraacetate was also effective. Silica and glass do not, however, require magnesium for lysis. The negative charge imparted by the sialic acid component of membranes attracts the positively charged (apparently by Mg^{2+}) chrysotile fibre, the binding being thought to distort glycoprotein complexes and induce clustering of proteins, leading via ionic-sized gaps (as with silica) to osmotic disturbance and rupture (Brody, George and Hill, 1983). Furthermore, neuraminidase treatment of erythrocytes diminished their susceptibility to lysis by chrysotile. In the absence of hydrogen bonding, PNO exerted little protective effect, but the surface charges of serpentine or amphibole asbestos may be altered by contact with surfactant. An alternative view attributed lysis to extraction of membrane lipids by chrysotile (Depasse, 1982), its activity being inhibited by adsorption of dipalmitoyl lecithin (DPL) liposomes or red cell ghosts, although this explanation did not hold for amphiboles (Jaurand, Renier and Bignon, 1980).

Toxicity to phagocytes

Attachment of positively charged particles, such as chrysotile and aluminium, to alveolar macrophages is evidently mediated by negatively charged sialic acid residues on the plasma membrane, but surface sialic acid on macrophages appears to be sialidase resistant (Gallagher, George and Brody, 1987). However, this mechanism is not available for negatively charged particles such as silica and crocidolite; their binding sites on macrophages are unknown, although phospholipid or protein seem to be possibilities, as are cationic receptors for anionic particles such as amphiboles. Extracellular Ca^{2+} is considered to promote particle–cell binding through a trypsin-sensitive receptor on the pulmonary macrophage membrane (Parod and Brain, 1983).

Surface hydroxyl (silanol, -SiOH) groups, which readily form when *quartz* is hydrated, are thought to be the adsorption sites for membranes, possibly via their phospholipids, because high temperature converts silanol into siloxane (Si-O-Si) groups and renders the particles much less active biologically (Kriegseis et al., 1977). The configuration of silanol groups may provide an indication of toxicity (Kriegseis, Scharmann and Serafin, 1987), whilst the relative biological activities of different crystalline forms of silica and of TiO_2 could depend on atomic density combined with surface irregularities from which reactive oxygen atoms protrude (Wiessner et al., 1988). Macrophages take up particles by invagination of their surface membrane to form phagosomes, which soon fuse with lysosomes enclosing acid hydrolases. Phagolysosomes of quartz (Figure 5.8) at first retain their complement of enzymes but soon rupture to release them into the cytoplasm and

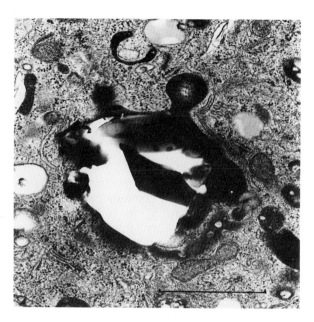

Figure 5.8 Alveolar macrophage lavaged from a rat after quartz inhalation. A lysosome (above) is in process of fusion with a phagosome containing quartz particles (below). Bar, 1 μm. (Courtesy of Professor Dr med. H. Behrendt)

then into the extracellular environment along with cytoplasmic lactate dehydrogenase (LDH); inert dusts lack such effects. Enzyme release affords an in vitro means of grading cytotoxicity quantitatively by using reduction of triphenyltetrazolium chloride (TTC) to assess dehydrogenase activity. In some hands tridymite and cristobalite proved more toxic than quartz or amorphous silica (Marks and Nagelschmidt, 1959), but equal toxicity has been ascribed to quartz and cristobalite (Klosterkötter and Robock, 1967). Quartz cannot, however, be considered a standard compound, because cytotoxicity and in vivo fibrogenicity are affected by source and enzyme assays do not always exhibit consistency (Beck et al., 1973; Robock and Klosterkötter, 1973; Le Bouffant et al., 1982). These differences may depend on surface contamination with amorphous silica or on incorporation of foreign ions such as aluminium, whose inhibitory effect in respect of both cytotoxicity and fibrogenicity probably reflects substitution for silicon ions in the silica lattice. In vivo, the toxicity of quartz to alveolar macrophages is likely to be reduced by coating with surfactant. The recognition that human macrophages are much more resistant to silica toxicity than cells of animal origin (Behrendt et al., 1987) complicates interpretations.

The noxiousness of respirable *coal-mine dusts*, judged by the TTC test, could not be correlated simply with their quartz or mineral contents (Seemayer and Manojlovic, 1979; Robock and

Reisner, 1982). Although submicroscopic foci with the electronic structure of silica may remain, much of the quartz from coal-mine dusts exhibits surface contamination (Kriegseis and Scharmann, 1982). In the hope of standardizing the target, natural sources of cells have been supplemented by phagocytic lines such as P388D$_1$ derived from a mouse macrophage tumour. Relying on this line, toxicity of coal-mine dusts was not defined solely by quartz content, some dusts being less harmful than TiO$_2$ that served as control (Gormley et al., 1979). It is now known that P388D$_1$ cells do not behave consistently (Donaldson, K., personal communication) and the same defect may apply to other artificially maintained cell lines. Results such as these cast doubt on the ability of in vitro tests of toxicity to predict the potential harmfulness of coal-mine dusts and also question a role for quartz in the genesis of coal pneumoconiosis.

The biochemical consequences of *asbestos* ingestion by macrophages vary with fibre type, acid phosphatase being released by chrysotile, as by silica, but not crocidolite or the rutile phase of TiO$_2$. Chrysotile, in contrast to silica, allowed selective escape of lysosomal enzymes in a dose-dependent manner, whilst non-lysosomal LDH rose but remained intracellular (Davies et al., 1974). The distinction between lysosomal and cytoplasmic enzyme release is not, however, sharply defined. Removal of magnesium hydroxide from the surface of chrysotile fibres affected the in vitro biochemical consequences inconsistently, while a non-homogeneous loss of magnesium from chrysotile occurred in fibres recovered from human lung or from alveolar macrophages after ingestion in vitro (Jaurand et al., 1977). Microsomal and lysosomal membranes of rat lung cells exhibited enhanced lipid peroxidation after treatment with crocidolite both in vitro and in vivo (Gulumian and Kilroe-Smith, 1987a; Jajte, Lao and Wiśniewska-Knypl, 1987), an effect inhibited by antioxidants (Gulumian and Kilroe-Smith, 1987b). Injection or inhalation of silica also stimulated lipid peroxidation along with lysosomal enzyme release, and these changes preceded the development of fibrosis (Jajte et al., 1988; Mendez et al., 1989), but whether such responses relate to fibrogenesis remains obscure. Membrane effects of asbestos fibres thus differ in some respects, not only from those of quartz, but also between the two main groups, and give some support to the view that surface properties may influence the biological outcome.

Attention has lately focused on the possible role of *reactive oxygen species* in cell toxicity by mineral particles and the hydroxyl radical may operate through lipid peroxidation. Alveolar macrophages from pneumoconiotic human subjects spontaneously released superoxide anion and hydrogen peroxide and, thus, could injure parenchymal cells (Rom et al., 1987). Generation of this anion by alveolar

macrophages became evident in coal workers, especially those affected by progressive massive fibrosis (Wallaert et al., 1990). Fibrous rather than compact dusts augmented release of the superoxide radical from alveolar macrophages of hamster and rat (Hansen and Mossman, 1987). Under the influence of superoxide in vitro, rat lung fibroblasts were stimulated to produce collagenous and non-collagenous proteins, but the pulmonary response to inhaled crocidolite also included a compensatory increase in the antioxidant enzyme superoxide dismutase (Mossman et al., 1989); the effect of superoxide may thus be counteracted in vivo. However, spontaneous release of superoxide was not increased in alveolar phagocytes from sheep given chrysotile or quartz intratracheally, although such cells might be primed to do so through other agencies (Cantin, Dubois and Bégin, 1988). Contradictory in vitro studies with bronchoalveolar-derived leucocytes from the rat indicated that reactive oxygen species were not a major element in tissue injury by pathogenic mineral dusts such as quartz and asbestos (Donaldson, Slight and Bolton, 1988), but may mediate detachment of type II cells (Donaldson et al., 1988). Reactive oxygen species may not, therefore, be concerned with either the inception or maintenance of dust-induced damage to parenchymal cells of the lung or with connective tissue destruction, but epithelial separation combined with protease degradation of the framework (Brown and Donaldson, 1988) may facilitate access of the macrophage fibrogenic factor to interstitial fibroblasts (see page 113).

Fibrogenesis

Silica

Forms of silicosis

Human and animal evidence established the existence of two forms of the disorder, one due to the action of dust alone and the other to the combination of dust with infection, that is, the discrete nodule and massive fibrosis. Early observations from several countries revealed tuberculosis as a common complication of silicosis and the part played by infection emerged from the immense postmortem experience of Simson and Strachan (1935) among gold miners in South Africa. Massive fibrosis may occur without histological or bacteriological evidence of tuberculosis, but participation of infection is not necessarily eliminated, because it could have died out or remained inconspicuous.

Moreover, viable bacilli may reside in human pulmonary scar tissue devoid of histological features of tuberculosis and the organism may sometimes be recovered from the lung or hilar nodes of atmospherically exposed rabbits in the absence of obvious disease. Activity of the mononuclear phagocytic system is stimulated by both quartz and tubercle bacilli (Conning and Heppleston, 1966) and, in combination, may so overtax the system that it fails to respond adequately to the infective component whose progression is accordingly facilitated. Subtoxic doses of silica are known to potentiate the growth of *Mycobacterium tuberculosis* in cultured macrophages.

Factors influencing fibrogenesis

Quantitative aspects at first relied on intratracheal injection because removal of inhaled dust proceeds during and after exposure, the severity of pulmonary fibrosis being directly related to the amount of quartz administered (Chvapil and Holusa, 1965). Inhalation of dust mixtures by rats led to definite fibrosis only when the air-borne and lung dusts contained 20 per cent or more quartz (Ross et al., 1962). Furthermore, for the classic silicotic reaction with massive fibrosis to occur, a quartz content generally exceeding 18 per cent was required (Nagelschmidt, 1960). For lower proportions, contact with target cells is evidently inadequate to provide an appropriate stimulus.

Particle size and surface area have both been implicated in silica fibrogenesis (King et al., 1953a). The rate of development and the severity of fibrosis were maximal for injected particles in the 1 to 2 μm range, smaller ones being less and larger ones the least active, although each size fraction dissolved with equal facility. Other studies laid more emphasis on particle size operating in conjunction with the degree of retention. The question has recently been reopened by the demonstration that, at constant surface area and with corresponding deposition and clearance, quartz particles measuring 5 to 11.2 μm were more fibrogenic that those of 1 μm (Wiessner et al., 1989).

The most striking property of silica to affect formation of connective tissue is its *physical form*. Administered by the intratracheal route, the same dose of similarly sized dust fractions of high purity revealed that the degree of fibrosis and its rate of development ascended from amorphous silica through quartz and then cristobalite to a maximum with tridymite, the solubility of all forms being similar (King et al., 1953b). Still greater divergences were found in the tissue response to high-pressure, high-temperature forms of silica (coesite and stishovite) with comparable surface area. Particles with irregular surfaces and protruding oxygen atoms, such as the crystalline forms of silica, exhibited greater fibrogenic activity than coesite and TiO_2 with their more regular outlines (Wiessner et al., 1988). The fibrogenic action of silica hence appears to depend on surface properties unconnected with solubility and surface area alone may not offer a sufficient explanation.

Theories of pathogenesis

The old idea that sharp, gritty particles exerted *mechanical irritation* on lung tissues was firmly discounted by Zenker's (1867) observation that rounded particles of iron oxide readily penetrated to the pulmonary interstitium after inhalation. Furthermore, hard particles of silicon carbide (carborundum) failed to elicit fibrosis when inhaled by guinea-pigs (Gardner, 1923).

A *piezoelectric effect* of quartz was believed to account for fibrogenesis as a result of crystal deformation in vivo (Evans and Zeit, 1949). Although application to fibrosis was never apparent, the theory failed to account for the absence of piezoelectric effect with tridymite which is strongly fibrogenic. Nevertheless, electrical disturbance may prove to be a factor in particle–membrane interactions, as the work of Kriegseis et al. (1977), Kriegseis, Scharmann and Serafin (1987), and Wiessner et al. (1990) pointed out, but even this may not be directly relevant to fibrogenesis (see later).

Silica solubility formed the basis of a hypothesis that long held sway and originated with observations on the response to colloidal silica, but the results of experiments on particle size and physical form, already quoted, militated against this interpretation. An *extended solubility theory* proposed that collagenous precursors adsorbed silicic acid which caused them to polymerize into mature fibres (Holt and Went, 1960), but this view likewise failed to dispose of earlier objections. These were amplified by experiments employing diffusion chambers, of a pore size small enough to retain particulate minerals but not their solutes, implanted subcutaneously or intraperitoneally. Fibrosis failed to develop around the chambers, even though all five test samples were fibrogenic on direct application (Heppleston, Ahlquist and Williams, 1961). Closer contact was required between silica and cells than diffusion chambers permitted. The theory did, however, lead to the introduction of compounds or elements thought to inhibit fibrogenesis by solubility depression, iron and particularly aluminium being best known. Compared with controls inhaling only quartz, fibrosis was much diminished in rabbits exposed to a mixture of quartz and metallic aluminium (Denny, Robson and Irwin, 1937, 1939), these findings being confirmed by observations employing various species and routes of administration (Policard et al., 1971). Soluble compounds of aluminium administered to rats as aerosols in the form of the hydroxide, hydroxychloride or chlor-hydroxyallantoinate salts achieved success prophylactically and some therapeutic benefit accrued, but quartz fibrogenesis resumed after withdrawal of treatment (Le Bouffant, Daniel and Martin, 1977). Substitution of silicon by aluminium in the surface lattice of quartz particles is considered to account for the inhibitory effect, which presumably is reversible. Aluminium lactate, a recently available inert and soluble compound given to sheep prophylactically by intrabronchial instillation, reduced quartz damage possibly through more rapid clearance of particles; therapeutically, by injection or inhalation, the lactate had less effect (Bégin et al., 1987; Dubois et al., 1988). Human trials of aluminium therapy or prophylaxis by inhalation in populations at risk from dust have, however, failed to confer indisputable benefit.

Resemblance between well-established tuberculous and silicotic lesions, combined with the capacity of tuberculous lipids to reproduce the histological features of the tubercle, suggested to Fallon (1937) that *phospholipid* might be responsible for genesis of silicotic changes, but the experiments were not controlled. The idea that silicotic nodules arise from the operation of lipid may now be dismissed, because, extracted from macrophages derived from silica-exposed rabbits or guinea-pigs, lipid given subcutaneously to other animals failed to induce a fibrotic response (Webster et al., 1967); lipid accumulation in the lungs of rats after inhalation of quartz was not followed by formation of typical silicotic nodules (Heppleston, Wright and Stewart, 1970).

The *membrane effect* of silica (see earlier) clearly forms the first line of cellular attack and is readily visualized by dye (trypan blue or eosin) penetration, which indicates pathological permeability, while retraction of processes and damage to organelles presage cell death. Under appropriate conditions of culture, the end-point is conclusive and light microscopy affords a quantitative estimate. Silica toxicity is delayed in the presence of serum, which enzymatic degradation removes after the formation of phagolysosomes.

Of the theories so far advanced, none takes account of the fact that phagocytosis of quartz particles precedes fibrogenesis. The nature of the connection was disclosed when the two processes were allowed to proceed independently, interactions obscured in vivo or organ culture being revealed by cell culture techniques. By this means the *macrophage fibrogenic factor* (MFF) was discovered and later elaborated (Heppleston and Styles, 1967; Heppleston, 1978). On the basis of a range of control procedures, several conclusions emerged. The macrophage/quartz extract repeatedly led to a highly significant elevation of hydroxyproline

formation by fibroblasts, but they did not respond to dissolved or particulate quartz applied directly. Simple damage to plasma membrane was unable to account for the stimulatory effect of quartz and, hence, an essential reaction occurred with other cell components. Pre-treatment of macrophages with PNO abolished the quartz effect, which may thus be attributed to the combination of an initial attack on cell membranes followed by an intracellular reaction leading to the formation or release of the MFF. In all experiments DNA levels in fibroblasts remained unaltered from control values, permitting the conclusion that augmented functional activity rather than proliferation was concerned. Titanium dioxide formed a control dust and, as in vivo, proved inactive. Because inhaled particles come into contact with alveolar macrophages, which exhibit functional differences from cells of peritoneal origin, they were subjected to the same procedures and likewise produced the MFF. The methodology also allowed immune mechanisms, humoral or cellular, to be excluded from participation.

Confirmatory observations came from several sources (Burrell and Anderson, 1973; Kilroe-Smith et al., 1973; Nourse et al., 1975; Aalto, Potila and Kulonen, 1976; Gritter, Adamson and King, 1986; Reiser and Gerriets, 1986; Sjöstrand and Rylander, 1987), the contributions inspired by Kulonen in Finland and recently summarized by Heppleston (1989a) being particularly important. The fibrogenic factor was considered to be released from, rather than synthesized in, macrophage lysosomes that had engulfed silica particles and to have a peptide structure. Translation of labelled collagen occurred from rough endoplasmic reticulum, through secretory vesicles to the extracellular fibrillary state. The MFF thus originates within cells and not simply as a surface event, while its target must be regarded as fibroblasts located in the interstitium and exposed by concomitant silica-induced damage to type I epithelium. Because human macrophages are much less susceptible to the toxic effect of quartz than cells of animal origin (Behrendt et al., 1987), generation of the MFF may be facilitated. Treated with quartz, human monocytes/macrophages preserved their lysosomal membranes but developed a vacuolar network, in which cellular products and particles lay and which opened onto surface pits (Behrendt and Seemayer, 1990). Channels thus became available for discharge of secretions, among which mediators such as the MFF could well be included, into the extracellular environment. Silica inhalation by rats led to increased levels in their lungs of type III procollagen mRNA followed by type I procollagen mRNA (Vuorio et al., 1989), thereby suggesting a step in the development of fibrosis.

The in vivo relevance of these findings was soon established by Kulonen and his colleagues, because rheumatoid synovium also released a fibrogenic factor from macrophages. Silica-treated monocytes and macrophages from human subjects reacted similarly. A particular protein fraction from silicotic rat lung stimulated proline incorporation into collagen by fibroblasts (Kulonen et al., 1982). The activity resided in a protein with a molecular weight of about 16 000, which was active at a concentration of 10^{-10} M in a dose-dependent manner; the purity of this protein was such that its amino acid composition was characterized (Aalto, Kulonen and Pikkarainen, 1989). Antisera prepared against the purified MFF neutralized its activity in vitro and in vivo. Biological as well as mineral agents thus provoke generation of the MFF, whose operation appears to have a wide relevance.

In parallel with enhanced collagen synthesis by fibroblasts, the Finnish workers found that silica also released and bound macrophage ribonuclease (RNase), so that is concentration in the medium became very low. The main target of macrophage RNase proved to be the nuclear RNA of fibroblasts, so by binding the enzyme silica suppressed its destructive activity and enhanced collagen processing to microsomal RNA with great augmentation of translational capacity. In purified forms, however, macrophage RNase and the direct fibrogenic factor appeared to be immunologically distinct.

Coal-mine dust

Despite the striking *structural differences* between the typical coal dust lesion and the silicotic nodule, participation of quartz still tends to dominate thinking on the genesis of connective tissue in coal pneumoconiosis. Human and animal studies directed to the relationship between dust composition and disease failed to sustain a particular *role for quartz* at the low concentrations customarily inhaled by coal workers (Heppleston, 1988a). Coal trimmers were exposed to dust virtually uncontaminated by minerals from adjacent strata, yet they developed disease identical with that of underground miners (Gough, 1940). Coal workers may acquire simple pneumoconiosis in the presence of very little quartz or even none, and exposure to hematite produced structurally similar though differently coloured lesions with low or undetectable proportions of quartz (Faulds and Nagelschmidt, 1962). Closely corresponding changes occurred in carbon electrode (Watson et al., 1959), carbon black (Miller and Ramsden, 1961) and graphite workers (Rüttner, Bovet and Aufdermaur, 1952), whose lungs were almost or entirely devoid of quartz. [The assumptions upon which it was deemed that quartz was absent, or 'almost' so, in these dusts, and recently reappraised, are discussed in Chapter 13,

'Pneumoconiosis associated with other carbonaceous materials' and 'The role of quartz'. (editor's note).] Nepheline, a mineral of the feldspathoid family containing no free silica, is reported to have induced a pneumoconiosis resembling that in coal workers, apart from colour, in one worker after 4 years' exposure and subsequent survival for 6 years (Barrie and Gosselin, 1960). Observations such as these certainly minimize and may even be considered to eliminate quartz in the usual low concentrations as an agent essential to the genesis of simple pneumoconiosis in coal workers. Furthermore, neither aluminium nor PNO exerted a permanent beneficial effect, prophylactic or therapeutic, on the reaction to coal-mine dusts with low quartz levels in experimental animals (Le Bouffant, Daniel and Martin, 1977; Weller, 1977).

The generally inconclusive behaviour of coal-mine dusts in respect of cytotoxicity (as described earlier) and the recognition of disparities in the prevalence of disease when related to both quartz and ash contents suggested that *assay of fibrogenicity* in vitro should be attempted by measurement of collagen formation using the two-phase technique (Heppleston, Kulonen and Potila, 1984). The quartz and ash composition of *native respirable mine dusts* bore no apparent relationship to collagen levels, and disparities again transpired in comparison with findings from epidemiology. Concentration appeared to be more important than composition in respect of both artificial mixtures and natural mine dusts (see Chapter 13 for further discussion).

The major *carbonaceous or silicate components* of air-borne or lung dust may well serve to isolate quartz particles rather than affect their surfaces, but the predominant constituents should not be considered merely as diluents because they evidently act as minor irritants. The simple coal dust lesion may, therefore, be regarded as a non-specific reaction leading, in some cases, to interference with local respiratory movements and circumscribed emphysema. For the latter, elastase activity does not appear to be concerned, because elastin fragmentation occurs in lesions with and without emphysema, whilst its development at a relatively late stage negates an initiatory role for local deficiency of α_1-antiprotease. Moreover, elevated elastase levels were not found in emphysematous human lung (Bull et al., 1988).

Evidence favouring a tuberculous element for generation of massive fibrosis in coal workers has recently been summarized (Heppleston, 1988a). Viral-induced synthesis of interferon by human and simian cells is inhibited by coal or asbestos, an effect which PNO limits or prevents (Hahon and Eckert, 1976; Hahon, 1983; Hahon and Booth, 1987). Interferon suppression by particles of these minerals could thus favour viral infection with secondary invasion by bacteria; if the latter included *M. tuberculosis* a connection with the genesis of PMF may be envisaged, but other organisms might lead to interstitial fibrosis. (See also Chapter 13, 'Pathogenesis'.)

Asbestos

Factors influencing fibrogenesis

Quantification of dust in lung specimens relies on digestion or low temperature ashing followed by counting and sizing, using either phase contrast microscopy (PCM) for routine purposes or electron microscopy (transmission (TEM) and scanning (SEM)) in research programmes. Prediction of TEM counts from PCM proved reasonably accurate in human material (Ashcroft and Heppleston, 1973) and Roggli, Pratt and Brody (1986) demonstrated a regular relationship between light microscopy and SEM determination of uncoated fibres from human lungs, the ratio to coated fibres being of the order of 10 or more. Characterization is accomplished by energy-dispersive analysis of X-rays (EDAX) or selected area electron diffraction (SAED) along with X-ray diffractometry. Reliance solely on coated fibres (asbestos bodies) is inadequate, because only uncoated fibres are regarded as being biologically active (Vorwald, Durkan and Pratt, 1951; McLemore et al., 1981) and may constitute the great majority of the total content. The fibrotic response is generally assumed to increase in proportion to the quantity of asbestos retained, but this view oversimplifies the relationship by ignoring the type of pathological change. Comparison of counts obtained by PCM and TEM with the grade of fibrosis revealed an overall parallel rise, but with wide ranges, until severe disease was encountered when all connection was lost as judged by fibre content between aerated lung, focal lesions, fibrocystic change and solid fibrosis occurring in individual lungs (Ashcroft and Heppleston, 1973). Aerated lung sometimes revealed fibre concentrations comparable to those of advanced fibrosis. From this evidence it appeared that in order to cause solid lesions intervention of a complicating element was required, which on the basis of earlier British and South African experience may be tuberculous infection (Smither, 1965; Webster, 1970). This likelihood is now much reduced in Britain. Quantification of mineral fibres still presents obstacles and pronounced disparities between different laboratories analysing the same lung material (Gylseth et al., 1985) have yet to be explained.

The irregular distribution of lesions caused by inhaled asbestos has not been explained satisfactorily. Experimental observations suggest that fibre deposition and aggregation, as well as the subsequent tissue reaction, may be affected by regional differences in length of airways and their number of subdivisions (Pinkerton et al., 1986; Pinkerton and Yu, 1989) (see Chapter 3). Gravitational effects in human disease have, however, been minimized and the roles of fibre length, surface area and mass emphasized, although individual variation has still to be invoked to account for inequalities of intrapulmonary distribution of fibres (Churg and Wiggs, 1989). Similar to previous authors, Churg (1990) found fibre concentration in normal lungs of amosite-exposed workers to be higher in the apical than in the basal regions. Compact and fibrous dusts, thus, show comparable retention patterns, but differ in distribution of the reaction to them, with asbestotic fibrosis predominating basally and the changes due to coal-mine dust or quartz affecting mainly upper zones. The disparity between concentration and size of fibres and the site of maximal lesions, apparently unrelated to anatomical or physiological factors, raises the question of intervention by secondary processes such as bacterial or viral infections.

All the main *forms of asbestos* proved fibrogenic, although not necessarily to the same degree, in human beings and in animals, amphiboles being more harmful to the former and chrysotile to rats. The distinction arose from observations that, although human exposures were mainly to chrysotile, amphibole predominated in the lung (Bignon et al., 1978; Wagner et al., 1982; Gylseth, Mowé and Wannag, 1983). By way of explanation, differences in deposition have been invoked, with the curled chrysotile fibres presenting a larger collision area, but the suggestion has also been made that chrysotile fibres, due to their susceptibility to chemical dissolution, undergo more effective clearance over the much longer lifespan of human subjects, in whom inception of the disease may, accordingly, be slower. Fibrotic and neoplastic potential might thus be more evident in rats, because chrysotile persists long enough over the animals' lifespan to exert its effects. The position is complicated by the tendency of chrysotile fibres to separate in vivo into constituent fibrils, so exposing a greater surface area and possibly initiating a more vigorous reaction, at least temporarily, relative to amphiboles. Taking surface area into account, the more common types of amphibole appeared to be equally fibrogenic (Timbrell et al., 1988). Moreover, the particularly deleterious effect of erionite fibres evidently depends on the existence of internal spaces, communicating with the exterior by means of minute pores, and thereby affording a very large internal surface area (Coffin et al., 1989).

Doubt concerning the pathogenicity of chrysotile arose because so few cases of mesothelioma occurred in a large cohort of miners and millers

(McDonald and McDonald, 1980). Moreover, a much higher proportion of tremolite to chrysotile was found in the lungs of miners and millers than in the ore, suggesting that during life chrysotile was removed but tremolite retained (Rowlands, Gibbs and McDonald, 1982). In cases of mesothelioma following exposure to chrysotile mine dust, the concentration ratio of tremolite compared with controls was much higher than the corresponding chrysotile ratio (Churg et al., 1984). Furthermore, tremolite may be blamed not only for neoplasia (Yazicioglu et al., 1980) but also for non-malignant pleural disease and pulmonary fibrosis (Baris et al., 1988). Inhalation of tremolite by rats led to pulmonary fibrosis and lung carcinoma with an occasional mesothelioma (Davis et al., 1985). The reason for the altered amphibole/chrysotile ratio in lung tissue as compared with the ore may, on the basis of animal experiment, apparently be attributed to preferential clearance of chrysotile by fibre fracture rather than by dissolution (Churg et al., 1989a). It is pertinent to note, however, that cases of mesothelioma in Japan have now been attributed solely to chrysotile (Morinaga et al., 1989) and a similar claim was made in respect of US railroad machinists (Mancuso, 1988). [This important question is discussed in Chapter 14, 'Diffuse malignant mesothelioma of pleura and peritoneum: The influence of fibre type'.]

The contention that *long as opposed to short fibres* are responsible for fibrosis emerged from early experimental observations (for example, Vorwald, Durkan and Pratt, 1951) and the distinction continues to be advanced in the genesis of asbestos-related disease. The crucial ranges generally assigned for fibrosis – and consequently for carcinoma which is now believed to be preceded by asbestosis in human subjects and animals – are more than or equal to $10\,\mu m$ in length and less than $0.3\,\mu m$ in diameter, with mesothelioma being attributed to fibres more than $5\,\mu m$ long and less than $0.25\,\mu m$ across. This view derived mainly from experimentation in vivo and in vitro. For instance, Davis et al. (1986), employing long and short amosite fibres by inhalation and injection in rats, concluded that, in contradistinction to long fibres, short ones failed to induce fibrosis in spite of greater retention and congregation of dust-laden macrophages in relation to respiratory air passages. Although these authors asserted that their ball-milled sample of amosite retained its crystalline structure and elemental composition, fibre comminution by this means has been shown to affect the structural and surface characteristics of fibres as well as the reaction with cell membranes (Langer et al., 1978; Spurny et al., 1980). Moreover, the ball-milled amosite used by Davis et al. (1986) contained only a minority of particles that could properly be classed as fibres and, as with coal or hematite, fibro-

sis would not be expected as readily in animals as in human beings. In this study more short fibres than long ones were recovered from the lung, but activity of the former could well have been restrained by the predominance of compact particles. When the effects of long and short chrysotile fibres were compared after inhalation by rats, the former led to much more severe fibrosis and more pulmonary neoplasms than the latter (Davis and Jones, 1988). These findings do not, however, establish long fibres as necessarily more pathogenic than short ones, which, although retained in greater quantity by the end of the exposure, subsequently disappeared from the lungs much more rapidly than did long fibres. More effective clearance or dissolution of short fibres, which were not, however, devoid of fibrogenic or neoplastic potential, suffices to account for the differences observed. Furthermore, the short-fibre chrysotile used by Platek et al. (1985) may well have been too low in dose (thereby facilitating clearance) and too altered in structure by ball-milling for pulmonary fibrosis to develop in exposed rats and monkeys. It is not surprising that Vorwald, Durkan and Pratt (1951) obtained little reaction from ball-milled chrysotile because 98.6 per cent of the dust was non-fibrous. Generally ignored is the tentative observation that short fibres of chrysotile ($5\,\mu m$ or less in length), even though ball-milled, appeared to be fibrogenic for rats after inhalation (Holt, Mills and Young, 1964), as did serpentine and amphibole fibres in guinea-pigs (Holt, Mills and Young, 1965). Support came from very brief exposure of rats to chrysotile or crocidolite, the great majority of fibres in the lung remaining less than about $7\,\mu m$ despite some increase in length with survival time (Roggli and Brody, 1984; Roggli, George and Brody, 1987).

Intratracheal injection of particles in fluid suspension interferes with the natural mechanisms of deposition, allowing the impaction of long fibres as a bolus in proximal conducting airways, whilst short fibres, being easier to disperse, are carried almost exclusively into the alveolar region. With long crocidolite fibres an acute inflammatory reaction including focal necrosis ensued in bronchi and bronchioles of mice, but short ones (separated by sedimentation) excited only a macrophage response in alveoli, a distinction held to incriminate long fibres in fibrogenesis (Adamson and Bowden, 1987a,b). However, granulomatous lesions of the airways thus induced are dissimilar in character and location to the changes following long-term inhalation by animals and human subjects. Moreover, the ready clearance of short fibres from the lung seriously detracts from this comparison of length and fibrogenic capacity. Intrapleural administration to rats of ball-milled crocidolite led to fewer mesotheliomas from short than from long fibres (in the ratio 1:2.4), but there was a selective loss of short fibres from the lesions

(Wagner, Griffiths and Hill, 1984); accordingly it may be argued that, had they been retained, short fibres would have contributed appreciably to mesothelioma development from the long fibre sample.

In vitro comparisons of fibre length and toxicity sometimes employed unreal targets in the form of cell lines derived from a human alveolar type II – such as tumour (A549) or Chinese hamster lung fibroblasts (V79/4) – whilst short fibres were often prepared by milling (Brown et al., 1978; Brown et al., 1986). Short chrysotile fibres proved more toxic than long ones to human alveolar macrophages in culture (Yeager et al., 1983), and Tilkes and Beck (1983) reaffirmed that short fibres can exhibit high toxicity in vitro. Furthermore, Goodglick and Kane (1990) found that in vitro cytotoxicity is exhibited by both short and long crocidolite fibres, operating through oxidant and surface iron-dependent mechanisms, and that in vivo short fibres are cytotoxic provided their removal from the peritoneum is prevented by repeated injections. Assessment of fibrogenicity (as contrasted with cytotoxicity) in vitro by means of the macrophage fibrogenic factor afforded additional evidence favouring a role for short fibres (Aalto and Heppleston, 1984).

Release of inflammatory mediators by macrophages may be facilitated by long fibres protruding from the cell surface, but that does not deny a role for short fibres even though these become completely ingested. Escape of such particles from laden macrophages as they perish affords opportunity for transfer to fresh cells and accordingly could enable mediators, including the MFF, to be released continuously. In vitro tests of cytotoxicity, as well as diffusion chamber experiments such as those of Bateman, Emerson and Cole (1982), suffer from lack of macrophage recruitment, absence of which may account for some of the emphasis on long fibres. Although often used to describe the cellular composition of an exudate, in the formation of which vascular permeability and chemoattractants are concerned, the term 'recruitment' more precisely connotes and should be reserved for the marrow response to a stimulus originating at a distance (Civil and Heppleston, 1979). Short-fibre amosite induced in the mouse peritoneum a much less intense inflammatory reaction than long fibres (Donaldson et al., 1989), both samples coming from the same sources as those used by Davis et al. (1986). It must be recollected that the ball-milled amosite had over 60 per cent of non-fibrous particles, which, being compact, would not be expected to excite a reaction as readily in small animals as in human subjects.

A recent attempt to assess the role of short fibres relied on the tumorigenic and fibrogenic potential of erionite (Wagner, 1990) which has been implicated as a potent agent for induction of human mesothelioma. Milled by disc and inhaled by rats, no

mesotheliomas occurred with particles equal to or less than 5 μm but those greater than 3 μm were highly effective. However, it must be noted that, at the end of the experiment, the number of long fibres per gram dried lung tissue was 2.4 times greater than in the case of short ones: a comparable experiment with crocidolite (in which long fibres were virtually non-pathogenic) gave an even higher ratio of 6.1. Furthermore, the shortened fibres of both erionite and crocidolite appeared by electron microscopy to contain many compact particles. Significantly, the comparative fibrogenicity to the lung of the different fibre lengths varied by only a single grade on an eight-point scale.

Crucial information still seems to be required in order to establish whether similar numbers of retained short and long fibres (or preferably an excess of short ones to compensate for lack of length), sized within narrow limits and clearly separated, differ in pathogenicity. Critical examination of the experimental evidence thus reveals that the overall conclusion implicating long fibres may not be wholly valid and against this conclusion human lung analyses stand in sharp contrast. After mixed exposures all fibre types were less than 0.5 μm diameter and 70 to 90 per cent had lengths less than 5 μm, whilst a proportion was less than 1 μm long (Sebastien et al., 1977; Pooley and Clark, 1979). Preponderance of short fibres was detected in lung parenchyma (mean 4.9 μm) and especially in alveoli (mean 3.3 μm), where amphibole exceeded chrysotile, and also in lymph nodes (mean 2.5 μm) where amphibole was concentrated (Bignon et al., 1978). Furthermore, amosite fibres recovered from the lung in cases of mesothelioma showed a marked preponderance of fibres of less than 8 μm with mean geometric lengths of 3.2 to 4.2 μm (Churg and Wiggs, 1987), confirming earlier findings for both amphiboles and serpentine (Churg and Wiggs, 1984, 1986; Churg et al., 1984). Yet another analysis of lungs from individuals affected by asbestosis or mesothelioma confirmed that chrysotile and tremolite had fibre lengths with geometric means of less than 3 μm or 5 μm allowing for geometric standard deviations (Churg and Wright, 1989). The great majority of fibres in bronchoalveolar lavage fluid from occupationally exposed subjects was less than 5 μm and the case for fibres longer than 5 μm alone carrying a biological risk was considered non-proven (Chiappino et al., 1988). Likewise, in the lungs of non-occupationally exposed subjects chrysotile and amphibole fibres had means of less than 2 μm (Chiappino et al., 1989).

Contrary to animal studies, fibre length of amphibole and chrysotile in human lungs did not increase with time since last exposure, and for both groups of fibres the mean geometric lengths remained less than 3 μm, still being short when standard deviations were taken into account (Churg and DePaoli,

1988a). Similar findings emerged from lung analyses on individuals with pleural plaques who resided near a chrysotile mining town (Churg and DePaoli, 1988b). Relating fibre size and degree of fibrosis, Churg et al. (1989b) obtained a positive correlation for tremolite and a lesser one for chrysotile concentrations; no correlation with fibrosis grade was found for chrysotile fibre size, surface area or mass, but in the case of tremolite these features were *negatively* correlated. A similar relationship held in human asbestosis caused by amosite, the grade of fibrosis increasing with fibre concentration but decreasing with length and other fibre size parameters (Churg et al., 1990). These authors concurred that short fibres may be more important in the genesis of pulmonary fibrosis than is commonly believed. This contention received reinforcement from observations on rats exposed to tremolite in which the cloud consisted of predominantly short fibres (Davis et al., 1985), whilst study of differential clearance between chrysotile and tremolite in guinea-pigs similarly employed fibres that could not be considered as long (Churg et al., 1989a).

Short fibres cannot, therefore, be dismissed as of little import to human beings and, with continued retention, they may behave in a manner similar to compact particles of coal-mine dust, that is, to initiate a relatively low-grade progressive fibrotic reaction, with the added potential for neoplastic change. To induce disease, long fibres with a high aspect ratio do not seem to form an indispensable condition and greater abundance of short fibres with lower aspect ratio may well compensate for lack of length, as appeared to be the case experimentally (Le Bouffant et al., 1985) and after human exposure (Churg et al., 1984; Churg and Wiggs, 1987). Retention of short fibres within viable alveolar macrophages may be seen as an essential component of the reaction to inhaled asbestos (Barry et al., 1983). Sufficient ground, thus, exists to challenge an exclusive role for long fibres in fibrogenesis as well as in carcinogenesis. [The alternative interpretation of the comparative significance of 'short' and 'long' fibres in fibrogenesis is discussed in Chapter 14, 'The pathogenesis of asbestosis: Fibre dimensions' and 'Malignant mesothelioma: Pathogenesis' (editor's note).]

Mechanisms of fibrogenesis

Membrane changes and release of enzymes fail to explain the means of fibrogenesis and attention had to be redirected to fibroblast participation. Their growth in suspension culture was maximal on long, narrow glass fibres to which they became attached. Linear extension apparently stimulated cell division and the phenomenon was described as *anchorage dependence* (Maroudas, 1973), but its role has never been established by cell kinetic techniques coupled

with measurement of collagen production.

This interpretation is, however, incomplete by taking no account of the *macrophage–fibroblast interaction*, evidence implicating which has, indeed, been obtained. Macrophage accumulation, even in the interstitium (Barry et al., 1983), is an early feature following asbestos inhalation. For instance, brief inhalation of chrysotile (77 per cent less than 5 μm long) by rats rapidly led to macrophage accumulation in alveoli and interstitium as well as to an increase in epithelial cells (type I exceeding type II) and interstitial fibrosis, the changes being localized to the vicinity of bifurcations in the acinus (Chang et al., 1988). Nuclear labelling with tritiated thymidine substantiated these findings by revealing proliferative activity in epithelial and interstitial cells of exposed rats (Brody and Overby, 1989), but whether as a direct result of cellular contact with fibres or via macrophage mediation remained undecided. Activation of the MFF occurred after treatment of macrophages with chrysotile and amphiboles (Aalto, Turakainen and Kulonen, 1979; Aalto and Heppleston, 1984). Glass fibres also proved stimulatory as did short fibres, whether of asbestos or glass; under certain conditions short amosite fibres were as potent as quartz, but collagen formation was not increased when the macrophage stage was omitted (Aalto and Heppleston, 1984). Although pulmonary fibrosis is commonly considered to be an unlikely consequence of human exposure to fibrous glass, it was fibrogenic to baboons on inhalation (Goldstein, Rendall and Webster, 1983). Perhaps the evidence of an increased risk from lung cancer in the past, although not of mesothelioma (Doll, 1987), implies some degree of preceding pulmonary fibrosis. By the diffusion chamber technique, chrysotile reacted with macrophages to cause surrounding fibrosis, which subsided as the reaction time lengthened (Bateman, Emerson and Cole, 1982). Silica was also active but only at the smallest dose, presumably by permitting better cell survival, but hematite had no effect and nor did minerals on their own. Further emphasis is thus given to the role of a diffusible factor from macrophages operating on fibroblasts, as well as to the importance of macrophage recruitment to sustain the response. Using monoclonal antibodies to distinguish circulating monocytes from mature alveolar macrophages obtained by lavage, both enhanced recruitment and in situ replication were implicated in the accumulation of mononuclear phagocytes in the lower respiratory tract of asbestos-exposed subjects (Spurzem et al., 1987).

Mesothelial cells in culture were able to replace macrophages in releasing the silica-provoked factor, which led to collagen synthesis by fibroblasts, and the medium of the silica-treated mesothelial cells reacted equally when applied to the same cell type (Aalto et al., 1981). Mesothelial cells thus acted as both initiator and effector in fibrogenesis and, assuming a corresponding response to asbestos, a connection arises with pleural fibrosis and possibly with the mesenchymal component of mesothelioma. Subsequent observations established that, in vitro, mesothelial cells of pleural origin possessed the ability to synthesize a range of connective tissue components including collagen and elastin (Rennard et al., 1984).

The fibroblast population

Macrophage or monocyte derived factor(s), which affect fibroblast proliferation in vitro, now appear to be established, but the direction of their influence is subject to variation (see Chapter 4).

Enhanced growth of fibroblasts was effected by human blood monocytes via mediators (De Lustro et al., 1983) or by a factor released from human alveolar macrophages after stimulation by particulate matter (Bitterman et al., 1982), which may include minerals (Bauman, Jetten and Brody, 1987). Regulation of fibroblast growth by this means has, however, exposed complexities notably in respect of prostaglandin interference. Bronchoalveolar lavage fluid from patients with idiopathic pulmonary fibrosis stimulated proliferation of human lung fibroblasts in vitro (Cantin, Boileau and Bégin, 1988) and fibroblasts from fibrotic lungs had a higher growth rate than control fibroblasts (Jordana et al., 1988). Production of growth factors for fibroblasts by alveolar macrophages derived from cases of interstitial fibrosis was largely suppressed by exposure to colchicine in vitro and raised a therapeutic possibility (Rennard et al., 1988).

Mineral particles also appear to be concerned in macrophage regulation of fibroblast proliferation. Having reacted with quartz instilled in vivo, guinea-pig alveolar macrophages inhibited or enhanced the growth of fibroblasts in culture according to whether the duration of treatment was short or long (Lugano et al., 1984). Under the influence of quartz or coal-mine dusts, human monocytes/macrophages released a growth factor for human fibroblasts in vitro (Seemayer, Braumann and Maly, 1987) and alveolar macrophages from coniotic subjects behaved similarly (Rom et al., 1987). As with silicosis, the primary cellular reaction in asbestosis is dominated by macrophages and production of a growth factor for fibroblasts was enhanced in rats by chrysotile, whereas the fibroblast growth inhibition factor released by blood monocytes was depressed, activities which coincided with the development of pulmonary fibrosis (Lemaire, Beaudoin and Dubois, 1986; Lemaire et al., 1986a). It may also be noted that pleural mesothelial cells produced, in culture, a soluble factor which promoted fibroblast replication, an effect which short fibre

amosite enhanced (Wiedemann, Lwebuga-Mukasa and Gee, 1985), thereby substantiating the observations with silica of Aalto et al. (1981).

Several agents that influence fibroblast proliferation have been identified and merit consideration in the particle context. The cytokine *interleukin-1* (IL1) represents two closely related polypeptides, derived from mammalian phagocytes among other cells, whose functions include activation of T lymphocytes and fibroblasts and also mediation of acute inflammatory responses (see Chapter 4, 'Cytokine mediators'). Recombinant IL1 stimulated fibroblast growth and synthesis of type I procollagen as well as collagenase and prostaglandin E_2 (PGE_2) (Postlethwaite et al., 1988), thus appearing to be distinct from and less specific than the MFF. However, IL1 alone did not prove a potent mitogen for fibroblasts (Singh, Adams and Bonin, 1988) and, mediated by human blood monocytes or alveolar macrophages, proliferation of lung fibroblasts was inhibited through intervention of IL1, an effect which indomethacin reversed and PGE_2 restored (Jordana, Newhouse and Gauldie, 1987). To complicate the issue further, silica or asbestos released from monocytes or macrophages an IL1-like product which encouraged fibroblast proliferation (Schmidt et al., 1984; Kampschmidt, Worthington and Mesecher, 1986; Oghiso and Kubota, 1986). Together with IL1, alveolar macrophages from cases of coal pneumoconiosis released another cytokine, *tumour necrosis factor* (TNF) (Lassalle et al., 1990). However, TNF, acting synergistically with IL1, was considered to inhibit lung fibroblast proliferation; enhanced secretion of TNF by alveolar macrophages treated with quartz or chrysotile (Dubois, Bissonnette and Rola-Pleszczynski, 1989) suggests that coal-mine dust may act similarly to limit the fibroblast population. By contrast, an elevated level of TNF, but not of IL1, in murine lung was thought to encourage focal accumulation of fibroblasts accompanied by collagen formation in locations where silica-laden macrophages aggregate (Piguet et al., 1990).

Platelet-derived growth factor (PDGF), now regarded as being the so-called alveolar macrophage-derived growth factor (AMDGF), is a glycoprotein released by macrophages, among other cell types, and possesses mitogenic and chemoattractant properties for mesenchymal cells (see Figure 4.5). Rat alveolar macrophages provoked by particulates, including chrysotile, secreted in vitro a PDGF-like growth factor for lung fibroblasts (Bauman et al., 1990) and inhaled chrysotile had a similar effect (Bonner and Brody, 1991). Observations on subjects with idiopathic pulmonary fibrosis detected PDGF-like proteins in biopsy specimens, though localized primarily to epithelial cells (Antoniades et al., 1990), and PDGF(B), but not *transforming growth factor-β* (TGFβ) (see Chapter 4, 'Type IV hypersensitivity'), may be increased in alveolar macrophages from this disease (Shaw et al., 1991). In contrast, production of the B chain of PDGF was depressed in monocytes from asbestos-exposed individuals and no clinical correlations emerged (Schwartz, Rosenstock and Clark, 1989). PDGF may be a growth factor for mesothelioma cells although not for normal mesothelial cells (Gerwin et al., 1987). The polypeptide TGFβ exhibits the peculiarity of counteracting the stimulatory effect of PDGF on lung fibroblasts (Kalter and Brody, 1991). Synthesis of surfactant-associated proteins may also be depressed by TGFβ, but stimulated by epidermal growth factor (Whitsett et al., 1987). *Fibroblast growth factor*, whose amino acid sequence is known, represents a further mitogen for mesenchymal cells produced by alveolar macrophages along with other cell types (Böhlen, 1989), but its involvement and that of TGFβ in gradual fibrogenesis by inhaled minerals has yet to be established.

Allied to proliferation of fibroblasts is the means by which they are directed to sites of need. Simple expansion seems too haphazard and a role for *chemoattractants towards fibroblasts* has been identified in culture. Fibronectin, which binds to collagen and originates from cells of the mononuclear phagocytic system, proved chemotactic for fibroblasts (Rennard et al., 1981; Sëppa et al., 1981), as did collagens of types I, II and III and collagen-derived peptides (Postlethwaite, Seyer and Kang, 1978) (see Figure 4.5). Degradation products of collagen may accordingly assist in the fibrotic process. Moreover, fibronectin evidently serves a dual purpose because, in fragmented form, it proves to be a potent chemoattractant for monocytes although not for neutrophils or lymphocytes (Norris et al., 1982), and so is able to bring together the two principal cells required for fibrogenesis.

Relevance in vivo

Findings on the behaviour of fibroblasts towards macrophage products, whether proliferative or chemotactic, depend on in vitro procedures, which are unlikely to be reproduced in vivo, where constraints imposed by closely apposed structures are liable to limit population increase or movement of connective tissue cells. Disentangling the interplay of multiple cytokines in the regulation of fibroblast proliferation presents a formidable problem, as recent reviews reveal (Kelley, 1990; Kovacs, 1991), and their participation in the slow evolution of fibrosis after inhalation of mineral particles is at present obscure. The position is aggravated by variations in proliferative capacity among human lung fibroblast lines (Elias, Rossman and Phillips, 1987), combined with the ability of macrophages and fibroblasts to degrade collagen in varying degree via a collagenase (Laub et al., 1982; Huybrechts-Godin, Peeters-Joris and Vaes, 1985), as

well as by the capacity of human alveolar macrophages to produce both collagenase and a collagenase inhibitor (Welgus et al., 1985). On the contrary, mineral generation of fibrosis by means of the MFF could readily proceed from indigenous lung fibroblasts with only restricted replication and no apparent need for migration of extrapulmonary fibroblasts. Additionally, the MFF has been shown to operate in vivo and has been characterized down to its amino acid composition (Aalto, Kulonen and Pikkarainen, 1989).

The immunological component

The general immunological aspects are considered in Chapter 4; particular features in respect of silica, coal and asbestos were outlined by Heppleston (1988b). The immunological theory of pathogenesis no longer enjoys its former popularity as a prime mechanism. The presence of humoral components in silicotic lesions does not necessarily imply production of an autoantigen or an adjuvant effect, because sequestration of serum proteins could alter their configuration non-immunologically so that they first stimulated formation of rheumatoid factor, then reacted with it and finally bound complement. Moreover, immunological phenomena, humoral or cellular, are inconstant in human pneumoconiosis, occurring secondarily to fibrosis whether induced by quartz, coal or asbestos.

A consequential role for immune reactions may, however, be envisaged. Antiserum to lung connective tissue incubated with macrophage supernatants and then applied to fibroblasts led to elevated collagen levels, but antibodies alone had no such effect (Lewis and Burrell, 1976); in this system antibodies had first to be stimulated by connective tissue. Denaturation of newly formed collagen in vivo might, with macrophage co-operation, continue the process. Serum anticollagen antibodies occur in rheumatoid arthritis and other chronic disorders associated with collagen breakdown, although antibodies in rheumatoid synovial fluid appear to be directed towards glycosaminoglycans rather than to collagen (Holborow et al., 1977); fibroblasts may, thereby, be stimulated into collagen synthesis. In vitro, fibroblast growth may, in part, be regulated by artificially activated rat or human blood lymphocytes whose inhibitory effect was abolished in the presence of chrysotile (Lemaire et al., 1986b), but whether such an effect occurs naturally is undetermined. IL1 release by alveolar macrophages treated with silica or asbestos (Oghiso and Kubota, 1986, 1987; Oghiso, 1987) may be regarded as an epiphenomenon occurring simultaneously with, or in consequence of, fibrogenesis and possibly contributing towards a cell-mediated response. Godelaine

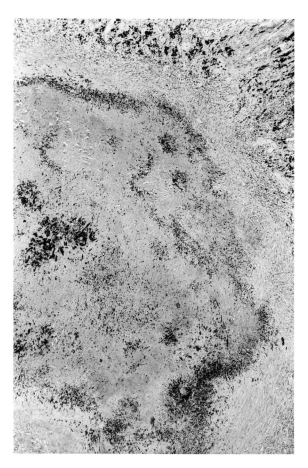

Figure 5.9 Rheumatoid nodule in a coal worker. Bands of dust lie in the connective tissue and represent previous inflammatory episodes, in which collagen and laden macrophages were destroyed, to be followed by further fibrosis. Magnification × 35; H&E

foreign proteins, are inhaled; the immune system then contributes to the primary response. According to one theory, byssinosis may be regarded as falling into this category (see Chapter 21, 'Antigen–antibody reaction').

Rheumatoid pneumoconiosis

To the general position respecting immunological involvement in pneumoconiosis, an exception has to be made where the rheumatoid diathesis obtrudes, notably in coal workers. Recognition of the syndrome in Welsh miners is to the credit of Caplan (1953), the statistical significance of his observations being established epidemiologically (Miall et al., 1953) and the pathological features being described by Gough, Rivers and Seal (1955). Rheumatoid nodules have also been encountered after exposure to other dusts, including silica and asbestos, but without the same epidemiological foundation. Massive lesions are produced by confluence of nodules, which are generally larger than simple coal dust lesions. An inflammatory reaction to necrotic collagen is thought to constitute one feature of rheumatoid disease and the collagen may be normal to the organ or produced pathologically; in pneumoconiosis, connective tissue may be derived from simple or complicated lesions. Repeated inflammatory episodes also destroy phagocytes and liberate their dust, whilst subsidence is accompanied by fibrosis, so explaining the layered appearance of dust and collagen (Figure 5.9) (see Chapter 13).

and Beaufay (1989) regarded IL1 release from macrophages exposed to quartz or chrysotile as being consistent with non-specific stimulation of the immune system such as could occur in silicotic or asbestotic individuals. Chronicity does not, however, necessarily depend on immune intervention because dust alone, and especially quartz, instigates by the reingestion cycle a self-propagating state. Individual susceptibility, as revealed by *histocompatibility antigens*, has not been shown to have any consistent bearing on the prevalence of pneumoconiosis. Although histocompatibility antigens HLA-A29 and HLA-B44 occurred in excess among silicotic subjects, no clinically useful parameters (including PMF) correlated with the presence of either antigen (Kreiss, Danilovs and Newman, 1989) (see Chapter 4, 'Major histocompatability-linked genes').

A different situation arises when particles of organic material, such as fungal spores or diverse

Lipidosis

Along with the non-lipid or fibrogenic response, mineral particles may excite excessive formation of lipid from stimulation of type II alveolar epithelial cells, although the extent of this reaction varies with mineral type.

Silica: alveolar lipo-proteinosis

The lipid effect in human beings is seen most clearly following exposure to high concentrations of quartz, usually in confined spaces over comparatively short periods of time. An accelerated form of silicosis then progresses to a fatal termination. It was encountered in men tunnelling through quartzite

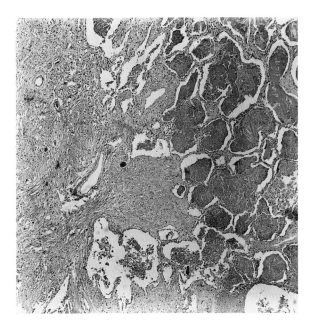

Figure 5.10 Human alveolar lipo-proteinosis following quartz exposure. At the top alveoli are filled with amorphous material and, below, fibrosis is irregularly disposed. Magnification × 40; H&E

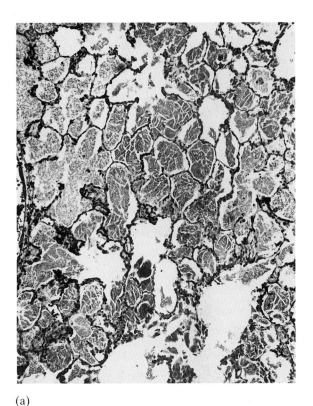

(a)

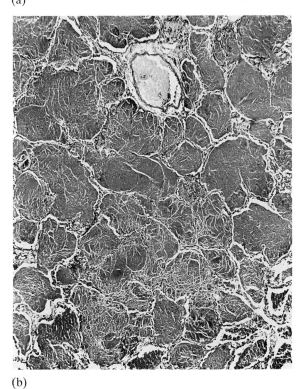

(b)

rock (as in the notorious Hawk's Nest incident in the USA) or as a result of sandblasting. The latter operation is proscribed in the UK and the EC, but US shipyards provided recent cases (Ziskind et al., 1976). Mycobacterial complications, especially from atypical varieties, proved to be common (see Chapter 12, 'Acute silicosis').

Irregular fibrosis affects the lungs with little to suggest true nodulation, but intervening tracts of parenchyma, as well as areas beyond, are consolidated by a pale greasy material. Histologically (Figure 5.10), fibrosis may be extensive, circumscribed or interstitial, while the eosinophilic, granular accumulation in non-fibrosed alveolar tissue contains neutral mucopolysaccharides (positive to the diastase–periodic acid–Schiff reaction) and lipid. Elemental silicon may be detected by energy-dispersive X-ray spectrometry.

Analysis of the disorder depends largely on the experimental approach. Specific pathogen-free rats, exposed to quartz inhalation and allowed prolonged survival thereafter, developed extensive and sometimes fatal pulmonary consolidation by amorphous material (Figure 5.11). Initially, it was accompanied by hyperplasia, hypertrophy (Figure 5.12) and enzyme hyperactivity of type II cells, along with vacuolated alveolar macrophages, but as the process evolved these cells disappeared, the epithelium reverted to a flattened form, while the

Figure 5.11 (a) Rat lung after prolonged quartz inhalation shows consolidation by granular material devoid of structure but without fibrosis of alveolar walls. Magnification × 100; H&E. (b) Spontaneous human alveolar lipo-proteinosis shows similar features. Magnification × 40; H&E

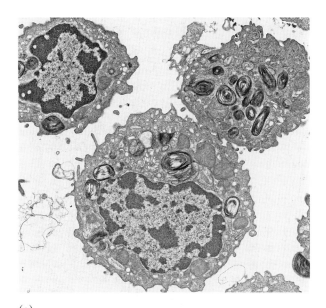

(a)

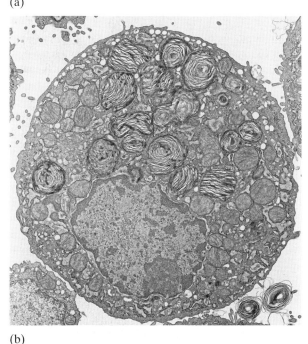

(b)

Figure 5.12 Type II cells isolated from rat lung: (a) control, (b) injected with quartz. Note hypertrophy of typical cells from treated animals along with increase in number and size of osmiophilic inclusions and dilated endoplasmic reticulum. Magnification × 6500. (Reproduced with permission from Miller and Hook, 1988)

alveolar content became granular and at all times lacked enzymatic activity. Fibrosis was minimal in degree and atypical in pattern, despite the presence of abundant quartz particles (Heppleston, Wright and Stewart, 1970).

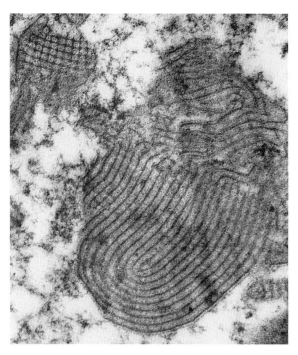

Figure 5.13 Alveolar material from long-surviving quartz-dusted rat reveals a quadratic lattice with a periodicity of about 45 nm. The lamellae represent the lattice-work sectioned longitudinally. Magnification × 45 000

Ultrastructurally, the alveolar material often assumed the form of quadratic lattices or lamellae characteristic of the liquid–crystalline phase of lipid–water systems (Figure 5.13); embedded in it were numerous and usually fragmented osmiophilic lamellar bodies extruded from type II cells, together with extracellular quartz particles (Heppleston and Young, 1972). Concomitantly, type I epithelium showed frequent defects to expose the alveolar interstitium. Phospholipid, mainly in the form of dipalmitoyl lecithin (DPL), was the principal contributor to the massive increase of total lipid (Heppleston, Fletcher and Wyatt, 1974). Unlike pulmonary fatty acids, those of the plasma were unchanged in both total and proportion following quartz inhalation, pointing to a local rather than a systemic origin for the pulmonary lipids. Metabolically, exposed animals had a threefold rate of DPL synthesis but only a twofold rate of decay, the imbalance accounting for phospholipid retention. Biophysical characterization of excised lungs and their extracts indicated the presence of a surface-active material (Heppleston, McDermott and Collins, 1975). The lipid response was not restricted to quartz-exposed pathogen-free rats but also affected conventional animals similarly treated

(Heppleston, 1986). Protein constitutes a minor component of the reaction and its attachment to lipid in lung surfactant is known to be non-specific and artefactually engendered (Shelley, L'Heureux and Balis, 1975). Pulmonary lipidosis induced by injection of crystalline silica may be divided into extra- and intracellular compartments, phospholipid increasing in the latter much more than in the former, although protein elevation was minor (Dethloff et al., 1986a, b). Hyperplasia and hypertrophy affected type II cells (Miller et al., 1987), as had been observed after inhalation of quartz by animals (Heppleston, Wright and Stewart, 1970) and by human subjects (Schuyler et al., 1980). Overall, these findings add weight to the belief that type II cells constitute the source of excess phospholipid under dust burdens (see 'Macrophage mobilization', page 107). Since type II epithelial cells are secretory and not actively phagocytic, their proliferation may depend on macrophage intervention rather than on simple contact with particles. Macrophage products augmented DNA synthesis by type II cells in vitro (Leslie et al., 1985), whilst in vivo macrophage accumulation in alveoli provoked by particles led to type II cell division (Shami, Evans and Martinez, 1986). In view of the close correspondence between the experimental and the human forms of the disorder, its appropriate designation is, thus, alveolar lipo-proteinosis.

The interaction of the lipid and fibrotic components is not a simple one, but an important determinant appears to be the rate at which quartz is deposited in the lung (Heppleston, 1986). Rapid accumulation of larger amounts tends to emphasize lipidosis whilst slower retention of smaller quantities allows silicotic nodules to form. Long-standing accumulations of lipid reveal few, if any, macrophages and quartz particles are isolated from epithelial contact. Localized production of the MFF is thus prevented and epithelial stimulation subsides, so that such fibrosis as occurs is atypical and the condition becomes quiescent. A parallel arose in respect of human pulmonary interstitial fibrosis, where phospholipid in bronchoalveolar lavage was reduced especially in relation to more severe fibrotic changes seen in lung biopsies (Robinson et al., 1988). The suggestion that surface radicals exposed on freshly fractured particles of crystalline silica play a significant role in the genesis of accelerated silicosis (Vallyathan et al., 1988) returns to an old topic, but takes no account of the lipid component or macrophage–fibroblast interaction.

A role for human and animal surfactant lipids may lie in down-regulation of immune reactions within the parenchyma, as suggested by their ability to suppress the proliferative response of peripheral blood lymphocytes to mitogens (Wilsher, Hughes and Haslam, 1988) (see Chapter 4, 'Respiratory bronchioles and alveoli').

Other particles

Carbon dust inhaled by rats led to elevated levels of total phospholipid and lecithin in lung washings (Rhoades, 1972), and alveolar accumulation of phospholipid structures may be seen electron microscopically after *coal-mine dust* exposure.

Long-term exposure of rats to *titanium dioxide* (rutile), which is fibrogenically inert, with excessive pulmonary deposition and consequent impairment of clearance, induced alveolar lipo-proteinosis along with cholesterol granulomas (Lee et al., 1986), and pulmonary phospholipidosis resulted from administration of *diesel particulates* (Eskelson et al., 1987). *Volcanic ash* also proved to be active in animals in this respect (Sanders et al., 1982), as did certain *metals* (Miller et al., 1984; Johansson and Camner, 1986).

Inhalation of *chrysotile* by rats led to a tenfold elevation of lung surfactant (Tetley et al., 1976), whilst lung extract from animals similarly treated showed alterations in surface properties and type II cells became hyperplasic (McDermott et al., 1977).

Alpha-particles emitted by inhaled plutonium dioxide also possess the ability to provoke activity in murine type II cells, their products accumulating in alveolar macrophages (Heppleston and Young, 1985).

The lipid response to mineral particle deposition may therefore be considered a general phenomenon whose intensity varies according to the strength of the irritant. Initially, it may be regarded as a protective mechanism, but one that can lead to deleterious effects.

Diffuse interstitial change in pneumoconiosis

The p and q rounded radiographic opacities seen in coal pneumoconiosis correspond to the usual focal lesions (Figure 5.14), whilst r-type opacities relate to larger fibrotic lesions suggesting silicotic or rheumatoid nodules.

Histologically, pigmented or unpigmented interstitial fibrosis, in contrast to focal dust lesions, has been reported surprisingly often in coal pneumoconiosis, sometimes with no such indication in their gross appearances (Cockcroft et al., 1982). Even in subjects classed as having p-type radiographic opacities, half showed a lattice-work rather than discrete dust foci, although irregular opacities were not considered

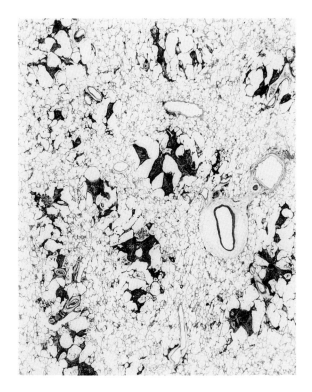

Figure 5.14 Focal dust lesions with proximal acinar emphysema, such as underlie the rounded radiological opacities in coal workers. Magnification × 5; H&E. (Reproduced with permission from Heppleston, 1989b)

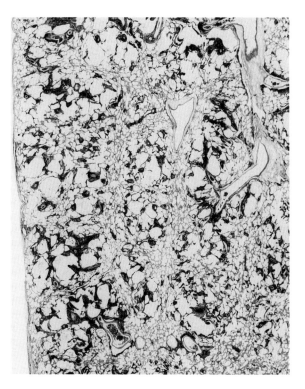

Figure 5.15 Pigmented diffuse interstitial changes with irregular emphysema corresponding to the irregular radiographic appearance in coal workers. Magnification × 5; H&E. (Reproduced with permission from Heppleston, 1989b)

(Ruckley et al., 1981) (Figure 5.15). The irregular radiographic opacities in asbestosis reflect the less circumscribed reaction excited by inhaled fibres. The problem is how to account for diffuse changes when focal features might be expected (see Chapter 13, 'Irregular opacities').

Lipid

By impairing focal aggregation of particles, the lipid component of the pulmonary reaction to inhaled minerals may render fibrosis more diffuse and also diminish the local concentration of the MFF and, hence, the degree of fibrosis. These alterations are particularly evident in silicosis, both human and experimental, but similar effects of a less severe nature occur when animals inhale coal-mine dusts, and different ranks of coal do not necessarily evoke the same degree of lipidosis. Comparison of mine and seam dusts from the same pit revealed the latter to form focal lesions without lipid accumulation and the former more diffuse lesions with the presence of lipid (Civil, Heppleston and Casswell, 1975). Non-

coal minerals such as clays may, therefore, be responsible for the difference, the extent of which could depend on dust composition. If experimental findings may be extrapolated to human beings, variable interference with the macrophage–particle reaction might affect the prevalence of pneumoconiosis in coal workers. Fully developed alveolar lipoproteinosis may occasionally be seen in coal workers, but limited amounts of lipid, although less apparent, will still be able to restrain aggregation and maintain a diffuse distribution of particles.

Particle size

Focal lesions characteristically follow exposure to particles in the micrometre range, up to 5 μm, but 'submicron' particles appear to behave differently. Silica of this size occurs as a fume which is amorphous in physical structure and its effects became evident as Shaver's disease or bauxite fume pneumoconiosis. Later reports confirmed the occurrence of diffuse interstitial fibrosis in exposed workers (Vitums et al., 1977; Brambilla et al., 1980; Robalo-Cordiero et al., 1985), and support also came from experimental evidence (see Chapter 12, 'Fused (vitreous) silica'). Electron microscopic observations in mice which had inhaled droplets of 'submicron' carbon particles provided the probable explanation (Heppleston and Young, 1973). Phagosomes distended with these inert particles lay in the cytoplasm of type I epithelial cells and dust-laden macrophages accumulated interstitially, indicating that carbon had reached its destination by passage through the thin epithelium. Inhaled quartz of 'submicron' size followed the same route and led to interstitial fibrosis in rats (Brody et al., 1982, 1984). Micrometre-sized particles scattered by lipid are associated with disruption of type I epithelium so exposing the interstitium where macrophages and fibroblasts are able to respond to quartz and lead to diffusely oriented collagen deposition; by the transepithelial route the same facility is open to 'submicron' silica. Small chrysotile fibres behaved similarly after inhalation, being taken up by both macrophages and type I cells, to reach the interstitium where contact was established with macrophages and fibroblasts (Brody et al., 1981) and where diffuse fibrosis may ensue.

Because human exposures are generally to particles in the micrometre range, lipid participation may well be a common feature in varying degree. As the stimulus to type II cells increases with lengthening exposure, a diffuse distribution is likely to follow formation of focal lesions and the change from one to the other could be effected by a small amount of lipid, whose subsequent degradation would obscure the relationship.

Diffuse interstitial fibrosis may arise from non-industrial causes and coal workers are not exempt; pigmented honeycombing and focal lesions may coexist (see Chapter 13). Smoking is apparently not a factor (Cockcroft and Andersson, 1987), although viral and bacterial infections could be responsible as well as drugs, hypersensitivity reactions or radiations. Interstitial fibrosis of non-occupational origin may, however, accumulate particles secondarily and be erroneously attributed to them, as happened in an individual exposed to fly ash (Golden et al., 1982) (see Chapter 15). Moreover, the focal lesions of coal workers may in the later stages become so large as to join with neighbouring ones and superimpose a more diffuse pattern.

References

Aalto, M. and Heppleston, A.G. (1984) Fibrogenesis by mineral fibres: an in vitro study of the role of the macrophage and fibre length. *Br. J. Exp. Pathol.* **65**, 91–99

Aalto, M., Kulonen, E. and Pikkarainen, J. (1989) Isolation of a silica-dependent protein from rat lung with special reference to development of fibrosis. *Br. J. Exp. Pathol.* **70**, 167–178

Aalto, M., Potila, M. and Kulonen, E. (1976) The effect of silica-treated macrophages on the synthesis of collagen and other proteins in vitro. *Expl. Cell Res.* **97**, 193–202

Aalto, M., Turakainen, H. and Kulonen, E. (1979) Effect of SiO_2-liberated macrophage factor on protein synthesis in connective tissue in vitro. *Scand. J. Clin. Lab. Invest.* **39**, 205–213

Aalto, M., Kulonen, E., Penttinen, R. and Renvall, S. (1981) Collagen synthesis in cultured mesothelial cells. Response to silica. *Acta Chir. Scand.* **147**, 1–6

Adamson, I.Y.R. and Bowden, D.H. (1987a) Response of mouse lung to crocidolite asbestos. 1. Minimal fibrotic reaction to short fibres. *J. Pathol.* **152**, 99–107

Adamson, I.Y.R. and Bowden, D.H. (1987b) Response of mouse lung to crocidolite asbestos. 2. Pulmonary fibrosis after long fibres. *J. Pathol.* **152**, 109–117

Antoniades, H.V., Bravo, M.A., Avila, R.E., Galanopoulos, T., Neville-Golden, J., Maxwell, M. and Selman, M. (1990) Platelet-derived growth factor in idiopathic pulmonary fibrosis. *J. Clin. Invest.* **86**, 1055–1064

Ashcroft, T. and Heppleston, A.G. (1973) The optical and electron microscopic determination of pulmonary asbestos fibre concentration and its relation to the human pathological reaction. *J. Clin. Pathol.* **26**, 224–234

Baris, Y.I., Bilir, N., Artvinli, M., Sahin, A.A., Kalyoncu, F. and Sebastien, P. (1988) An epidemiological study in an Anatolian village environmentally exposed to tremolite asbestos. *Br. J. Ind. Med.* **45**, 838–840

Barrie, H.J. and Gosselin, L. (1960) Massive pneumoconiosis from a rock dust containing no free silica. Nepheline lung. *Archs Environ. Health* **1**, 109–117

Barry, B.E., Wong, KC., Brody, A.R. and Crapo, J.D. (1983) Reaction of rat lungs to inhaled chrysotile asbestos following acute and subacute exposures. *Expl. Lung. Res.* **5**, 1–21

Bateman, E.D., Emerson, R.J. and Cole, P.J. (1982) A study of macrophage-mediated initiation of fibrosis by asbestos and silica using a diffusion chamber technique. *Br. J. Expl. Pathol.* **63**, 414–425

Bauman, M.D., Jetten, A.M. and Brody, A.R. (1987) Biologic and biochemical characterization of a macrophage-derived growth factor for rat lung fibroblasts. *Chest* **91**, 15S–16S

Bauman, M.D., Jetten, A.M., Bonner, J.C., Kumar, R.K., Bennett, R.A. and Brody, A.R. (1990) Secretion of a platelet-derived growth factor homologue by rat alveolar macrophages exposed to particulates in vitro. *Eur. J. Cell Biol.* **51**, 327–334

Beck, E.G., Holusa, R., Jirakova, D., Kysela, B., Robock, K. and Skoda, V. (1973) On the various effects of two quartzes in animal and cell experiments and their physical semi-conductor properties. *Staub. Reinhalt. Luft* **33**, 3–7

Bégin, R., Massé, P., Sébastien, P., Martel, M., Geoffroy, M. and Labbé, J. (1987) Late aluminum therapy reduces the cellular activities of simple silicosis in the sheep model. *J. Leukocyte Biol.* **41**, 400–406

Behrendt, H. and Seemayer, N.H. (1990) Effect of quartz dust DQ12 on human monocytes/macrophages in vitro. An electron microscopical study. In *Proceedings of the VIIth International Pneumoconioses Conference*, Pittsburgh, US DHSS(NIOSH) Publication no. 90-108, pp. 1459–1465

Behrendt, H., Seemayer, N.H., Braumann, A. and Nissen, M. (1987) Elektronenmikroskopische Untersuchungen zur Wirkung von Quarzstaub DQ12 auf menschliche Monozyten/Makrophagen in vitro. *Silikosebericht Nordrhein-Westfalen* **16**, 213–222

Behrendt, H., Ziesche, R., Stutz, R., Idel, H., Friedrichs, K.H., Hilscher, W. and Magnussen, H. (1990) Role of mast cells in the pathogenesis of silicosis. In *Proceedings of the VIIth International Pneumoconioses Conference*, Pittsburgh, US DHSS (NIOSH) Publication no. 90-108, pp. 1447–1454

Bignon, J., Sebastien, P., Gaudichet, A. and Bonnaud, G. (1978) Measurement of asbestos retention in the human respiratory system related to health effects. In *Proceedings of Workshop on Asbestos: Definitions and Measurement Methods* (eds C.C. Gravatt, P.D. LeFleur and K.F.J. Heinrich), National Bureau of Standards Special Publication 506, Washington, pp. 95–119

Bitterman, P.B., Rennard, S.I., Hunninghake, G.W. and Crystal, R.G. (1982) Human alveolar macrophage growth factor for fibroblasts. Regulation and partial characterization. *J. Clin. Invest.* **70**, 806–822

Böhlen, P. (1989) Fibroblast growth factor. In *Macrophage-derived Cell Regulatory Factors*, vol. 1, *Cytokines* (ed. C. Sorg) Karger, Basel, pp. 204–228

Bonner, J.C. and Brody, A.R. (1991) Asbestos-induced alveolar injury: evidence for macrophage-derived PDGF as a mediator of the fibrogenic response. *Chest* **99**, 54S–55S

Bowden, D.H. and Adamson, I.Y.R. (1982) Alveolar macrophage response to carbon in monocyte-depleted mice. *Am. Rev. Respir. Dis.* **126**, 708–711

Brambilla, C., Brambilla, E., Rigaud, D., Perdrix, A., Paramelle, B. and Fourcy, A. (1980) Pneumoconiose aux fumées de silice amorphe. *Rev. fr. Mal. Resp.* **8**, 383–391

Brightwell, J. and Heppleston, A.G. (1977) A cell kinetic study of the alveolar wall following dust deposition. In *Inhaled Particles IV* (ed. W.H. Walton), Pergamon Press, Oxford, pp. 509–517

Brody, A.R. and Overby, L.H. (1989) Incorporation of tritiated thymidine by epithelial and interstitial cells in broncho-alveolar regions of asbestos-exposed rats. *Am. J. Pathol.* **134**, 133-140

Brody, A.R., George, G. and Hill, L.H. (1983) Interactions of chrysotile and crocidolite asbestos with red blood cell membranes. Chrysotile binds to sialic acid. *Lab. Invest.* **49**, 468–475

Brody, A.R., Hill, L.H., Adkins, B. and O'Connor, R.W. (1981) Chrysotile asbestos inhalation in rats: deposition pattern and reactions of alveolar epithelium and pulmonary macrophages. *Am. Rev. Respir. Dis.* **123**, 670–679

Brody, A.R., Roe, M.W., Evans, J.N. and Davis, G.S. (1982) Deposition and translocation of inhaled silica in rats. *Lab. Invest.* **47**, 533–542

Brody, A.R., Roe, M.W., Evans, J.N. and Davis, G.S. (1984) Deposition and translocation of inhaled silica. In *Occupational Lung Disease* (eds J.B.L. Gee, W.K.C. Morgan and S.M. Brooks), Raven Press, New York, pp. 168–170.

Brown, G.M. and Donaldson, K. (1988) Degradation of connective tissue components by lung derived leucocytes in vitro: role of proteases and oxidants. *Thorax* **43**, 132–139

Brown, G.M., Cowie, H., Davis, J.M.G. and Donaldson, K. (1986) In vitro assays for detecting carcinogenic mineral fibres: a comparison of two assays and the role of fibre size. *Carcinogenesis* **7**, 1971–1974

Brown, R.C., Chamberlain, M., Griffiths, D.M. and Timbrell, V. (1978) The effect of fibre size on the in vitro biological activity of three types of amphibole asbestos. *Int. J. Cancer* **22**, 721–727

Bryant, G., Rao, C.N., Brentani, M., Martins, W., Lopes, J.D., Martin, S.E., Liotta, L.A. and Schiffman, E. (1987) A role for the laminin receptor in leukocyte chemotaxis. *J. Leukocyte Biol.* **41**, 220–227

Bull, T.B., Tetley, T.D., Guz, A., Harris, E. and Fox, B. (1988) Is neutrophil elastase associated with elastic tissue in emphysema? *J. Pathol.* **154**, 64A

Burrell, R. and Anderson, M. (1973) The induction of fibrogenesis by silica-treated alveolar macrophages. *Environ. Res.* **6**, 389–394

Cantin, A.M., Boileau, R. and Bégin, R. (1988) Increased procollagen III amino-terminal peptide-related antigens and fibroblast growth signals in the lungs of patients with idiopathic pulmonary fibrosis. *Am. Rev. Respir. Dis.* **137**, 572–578

Cantin, A., Dubois, F. and Bégin, R. (1988) Lung exposure to mineral dusts enhances the capacity of lung inflammatory cells to release superoxide. *J. Leukocyte Biol.* **43**, 299–303

Caplan, A. (1953) Certain unusual radiological appearances in the chest of coal-miners suffering from rheumatoid arthritis. *Thorax* **8**, 29–37

Chandler, D.B., Kennedy, J.I. and Fulmer, J.D. (1986) Studies of membrane receptors, phagocytosis, and morphology of subpopulations of rat lung interstitial macrophages. *Am. Rev. Respir. Dis.* **134**, 542–547

Chang, L.-Y., Overby, L.H., Brody, A.R. and Crapo, J.D. (1988) Progressive lung cell reactions and extracellular matrix production after a brief exposure to asbestos. *Am. J. Pathol.* **131**, 156–170

Chiappino, G., Friedrichs, K.H., Rivolta, G. and Forni, A. (1988) Alveolar fiber load in asbestos workers and in subjects with no occupational asbestos exposure: an electron microscope study. *Am. J. Ind. Med.* **14**, 37–46

Chiappino, G., Friedrichs, K.H., Forni, A., Rivolta, G. and Todaro, A. (1989) Alveolar and lung fibre levels in non-occupationally exposed subjects. In *Non-occupational Exposure to Mineral Fibres* (eds J. Bignon, J. Peto and R. Saracci). International Agency for Research on Cancer Scientific Publications no. 90, IARC, Lyon, pp. 310–313

Churg, A. (1990) The distribution of amosite asbestos in the periphery of the normal human lung. *Br. J. Ind. Med.* **47**, 677–681

Churg, A. and DePaoli, L. (1988a) Clearance of chrysotile asbestos from human lung. *Expl. Lung Res.* **14**, 567–574

Churg, A. and DePaoli, L. (1988b) Environmental pleural plaques in residents of a Quebec chrysotile mining town. *Chest* **94**, 58–60

Churg, A. and Wiggs, B. (1984) Fiber size and number in amphibole asbestos-induced mesothelioma. *Am. J. Pathol.* **115**, 437–442

Churg. A. and Wiggs, B. (1986) Fiber size and number in workers exposed to processed chrysotile asbestos, chrysotile miners, and the general population. *Am. J. Ind. Med.* **9**, 143–152

Churg, A. and Wiggs, B. (1987) Accumulation of long asbestos fibers in the peripheral upper lobe in cases of malignant mesothelioma. *Am. J. Ind. Med.* **11**, 563–569

Churg, A. and Wiggs, B. (1989) The distribution of amosite asbestos fibers in the lungs of workers with mesothelioma or carcinoma. *Expl. Lung Res.* **15**, 771–783

Churg, A. and Wright, J.L. (1989) Fibre content of lung in amphibole- and chrysotile-induced mesothelioma: implications for environmental exposure. In *Non-occupational Exposure to Mineral Fibres* (eds J. Bignon, J. Peto and R. Saracci), International Agency for Research on Cancer Scientific Publications No. 90. IARC, Lyon, pp. 314–318

Churg, A., Wiggs, B., DePaoli, L., Kampe, B. and Stevens, B. (1984) Lung asbestos content in chrysotile workers with mesothelioma. *Am. Rev. Respir. Dis.* **130**, 1042–1045

Churg, A., Wright, J.L., Gilks, B. and DePaoli, L. (1989a) Rapid short-term clearance of chrysotile compared with amosite asbestos in the guinea-pig. *Am. Rev. Respir. Dis.* **139**, 885–890

Churg, A., Wright, J.L., DePaoli, L. and Wiggs, B. (1989b) Mineralogic correlates of fibrosis in chrysotile miners and millers. *Am. Rev. Respir. Dis.* **139**, 891–896

Churg, A., Wright, J., Wiggs, B. and DePaoli, L. (1990) Mineralogic parameters related to amosite asbestos-induced fibrosis in humans. *Am. Rev. Respir. Dis.* **142**, 1331–1336

Chvapil, M. and Holusa, R. (1965) Zusammenhang der Dosis von Quarzstaub mit der Grösse der Entzündungsreaktion der Lungen. *Int. Archiv. Gewerbepath. Gewerbehyg.* **21**, 369–378

Civil, G.W. and Heppleston, A.G. (1979) Replenishment of alveolar macrophages in silicosis: implication of recruitment by lipid feed-back. *Br. J. Expl. Pathol.* **60**, 537–547

Civil, G.W., Heppleston, A.G. and Casswell, C. (1975) The influence of exposure duration and intermittency upon the pulmonary retention and elimination of dusts from high and low rank coal mines. *Ann. Occup. Hyg.* **17**, 173–185

Cockcroft, A. and Andersson, N. (1987) Radiological irregular opacities and coalwork exposure: a case referent study. *Br. J. Ind. Med.* **44**, 484–487

Cockcroft, A.E.., Wagner, J.C., Seal, R.M.E., Lyons, J.P. and Campbell, M.J. (1982) Irregular opacities in coalworkers' pneumoconiosis – correlation with pulmonary function and pathology. *Ann. Occup. Hyg.* **26**, 767–784

Coffin, D.L., Peters, S.E., Palekar, L.D. and Stahel, E.P. (1989) A study of the biological activity of erionite in relation to its structural characteristics. In *Biological Interactions of Inhaled Mineral Fibers and Cigarette Smoke* (ed. A.P. Wehner), Battelle Memorial Institute, Seattle, pp. 313–323

Conning, D.M. and Heppleston, A.G. (1966) Reticulo-endothelial activity and local particle disposal: a comparison of the influence of modifying agents. *Br. J. Expl. Pathol.* **47**, 388–400

Crapo, J.D., Barry, B.E., Gehr, P., Bachofen, M. and Weibel, E.R. (1982) Cell number and cell characteristics of the normal human lung. *Am. Rev. Respir. Dis.* **125**, 332–337

Davies, P., Allison, A.C. Ackerman, J., Butterfield, A. and Williams, S. (1974) Asbestos induces selective release of lysosomal enzymes from mononuclear phagocytes. *Nature* **251**, 423–425

Davis, J.M.G. and Jones, A.D. (1988) Comparisons of the pathogenicity of long and short fibres of chrysotile asbestos in rats. *Br. J. Expl. Pathol.* **69**, 717–737

Davis, J.M.G., Addison, J., Bolton, R.E., Donaldson, K., Jones A.D. and Miller, B.G. (1985) Inhalation studies on the effects of tremolite and brucite dust in rats. *Carcinogenesis* **6**, 667–674

Davis, J.M.G., Addison, J., Bolton, R.E., Donaldson, K., Jones, A.D. and Smith, T. (1986) The pathogenicity of long versus short fibre samples of amosite asbestos administered to rats by inhalation and intraperitoneal injection. *Br. J. Expl. Pathol.* **67**, 415–430

De Lustro, F., Mackel, A.M., DeLustro, B. and LeRoy, E.C. (1983) Human monocyte regulation of connective tissue growth. *Am. Zoologist* **23**, 213–220

Denny, J.J., Robson, W.D. and Irwin, D.A. (1937) The prevention of silicosis by metallic aluminium I. *Can. Med. Assoc. J.* **37**, 1–11

Denny, J.J., Robson, W.D. and Irwin, D.A. (1939) The prevention of silicosis by metallic aluminium II. *Can. Med. Assoc. J.* **40**, 213–228

Depasse, J. (1980) Mechanism of the haemolysis by colloidal silica. In *The in vitro Effects of Mineral Dusts* (eds R.C. Brown, I.P. Gormley, M. Chamberlain and R. Davies), Academic Press, London, pp. 121–124

Depasse, J. (1982) Influence of the sialic acid content of the membrane on its susceptibility to chrysotile. *Environ. Res.* **27**, 384–388

Dethloff, L.A., Gilmore, L.B., Brody, A.R. and Hook, G.E.R. (1986a) Induction of intra- and extra-cellular phospholipids in the lungs of rats exposed to silica. *Biochem. J.* **233**, 111–118

Dethloff, L.A., Gilmore, L.B., Gladen, B.C., George, G., Chhabra, R.S. and Hook, G.E.R. (1986b) Effects of silica on the composition of the pulmonary extracellular lining. *Toxic. Appl. Pharmacol.* **84**, 66–83

Doll, R. (1987) Symposium on Man-Made Mineral Fibres, Copenhagen, October 1986: Overview and conclusions. *Ann. Occup. Hyg.* **31**, 805–819

Donaldson, K., Slight, J. and Bolton, R.E. (1988) Oxidant production by control and inflammatory bronchoalveolar leucocyte populations treated with mineral dusts in vitro. *Inflammation* **12**, 231–243

Donaldson, K., Slight, J., Brown, G.M. and Bolton, R.E. (1988) The ability of inflammatory bronchoalveolar leucocyte populations elicited with microbes or mineral dust to injure alveolar epithelial cells and degrade extracellular matrix in vitro. *Br. J. Expl. Pathol.* **69**, 327–338

Donaldson, K., Brown, G.M., Brown, D.M., Bolton, R.E. and Davis, J.M.G. (1989) Inflammation generating potential of long and short fibre amosite asbestos samples. *Br. J. Ind. Med.* **46**, 271–276

Dubois, C.M., Bissonnette, E. and Rola-Pleszczynski, M. (1989) Asbestos fibers and silica particles stimulate rat alveolar macrophages to release tumor necrosis factor. *Am. Rev. Respir. Dis.* **139**, 1257–1264

Dubois, F., Bégin, R., Cantin, A., Massé, S. Martel, M., Bilodeau, G., Dufresne, A., Perreault, G. and Sébastien, P. (1988) Aluminum inhalation reduces silicosis in a sheep model. *Am. Rev. Respir. Dis.* **137**, 1172–1179

Elias, J.A., Rossman, M.D. and Phillips, P.D. (1987) Phenotypic variability among density-fractionated human lung fibroblasts. *Am. Rev. Respir. Dis.* **135**, 57–61

Eskelson, C.D., Chvapil, M., Strom, K.A. and Vostal, J.J. (1987) Pulmonary phospholipidosis in rats respiring air containing diesel particulates. *Environ. Res.* **44**, 260–271

Evans, M.J., Shami, S.G. and Martinez, L.A. (1986) Enhanced proliferation of pulmonary alveolar macrophages after carbon instillation in mice depleted of blood monocytes by strontium-89. *Lab. Invest.* **54**, 154–159

Evans, S.M. and Zeit, W. (1949) Tissue responses to physical forces II. The response of connective tissue to piezoelectrically active crystals. *J. Lab. Clin. Med.* **34**, 592–609

Fallon, J.T. (1937) Specific tissue reaction to phospholipids: a suggested explanation for the similarity of the lesions of silicosis and pulmonary tuberculosis. *Can. Med. Assoc. J.* **36**, 223–228

Faulds, J.S. and Nagelschmidt, G. (1962) The dust in the lungs of haematite miners from Cumberland. *Ann. Occup. Hyg.* **4**, 255–263

Gallagher, J.E., George, G. and Brody, A.R. (1987) Sialic acid mediates the initial binding of positively charged inorganic particles to alveolar macrophage membranes. *Am. Rev. Respir. Dis.* **135**, 1345–1352

Gant, V.A. and Hamblin, A.S. (1985) Human bronchoalveolar macrophage heterogeneity demonstrated by histochemistry, surface markers and phagocytosis. *Clin. Exp. Immunol.* **60**, 539–545

Gardner, L.U. (1923) Studies on the relation of mineral dusts to tuberculosis III. The relatively early lesions in experimental pneumokoniosis produced by carborundum inhalation and their influence on pulmonary tuberculosis. *Am. Rev. Tuberc.* **7**, 344–357

Gerwin, B.I., Lechner, J.F., Reddel, R.R., Roberts, A.B., Robbins, K.C., Gabrielson, E.W. and Harris, C.C. (1987) Comparison of production of transforming growth factor-β and platelet-derived growth factor by normal human mesothelial cells and mesothelioma cell lines. *Cancer Res.* **47**, 6180–6184

Godelaine, D. and Beaufay, H. (1989) Comparative study of the effect of chrysotile, quartz and rutile on the release of lympho-cyte-activating factor (interleukin 1) by murine peritoneal macrophages in vitro. In *Non-occupational Exposure to Mineral Fibres* (eds. J. Bignon, J. Peto and R. Saracci), International Agency for Research on Cancer Scientific Publication No. 90, IARC, Lyon, pp. 149–155

Golden, E.B., Warnock, M.L., Hulett, L.D. and Churg, A.M. (1982) Fly ash lung: a new pneumoconiosis? *Am. Rev. Respir. Dis.* **125**, 108–112

Goldstein, B., Rendall, R.E.G. and Webster, I. (1983) A comparison of the effects of exposure of baboons to croci-dolite asbestos and fibrous glass dusts. *Environ. Res.* **32**, 344–359

Goodglick, L.A. and Kane A.B. (1990) Cytotoxicity of long and short crocidolite asbestos fibers in vitro and in vivo. *Cancer Res.* **50**, 5153–5163

Gormely, I.P., Collings, P., Davis, J.M.G. and Ottery, J. (1979) An investigation into the cytotoxicity of respirable dusts from British collieries. *Br. J. Expl. Pathol.* **60**, 526–536

Gough, J. (1940) Pneumoconiosis in coal trimmers. *J. Pathol. Bacteriol.* **51**, 277–285

Gough, J., Rivers, D. and Seal, R.M.E. (1955) Pathological studies of modified pneumoconiosis in coal-miners with rheumatoid arthritis (Caplan's syndrome). *Thorax* **10**, 9–18

Gritter, H.L., Adamson, I.Y.R. and King, G.M. (1986) Modulation of fibroblast activity by normal and silica-exposed alveolar macrophages. *J. Pathol.* **148**, 263–271

Gulumian, M. and Kilroe-Smith, T.A. (1987a) Crocidolite-induced lipid peroxidation in rat lung microsomes I. Role of different ions. *Environ. Res.* **43**, 267–273

Gulumian, M. and Kilroe-Smith, T.A. (1987b) Crocidolite-induced lipid peroxidation II. Role of antioxidants. *Environ. Res.* **44**, 254–259

Gylseth, B., Mowé, G. and Wannag, A. (1983) Fibre type and concentration in the lungs of workers in an asbestos cement factory. *Br. J. Ind. Med.* **40**, 375–379

Gylseth, B., Churg, A., Davis, J.M.G., Johnson, N., Morgan, A., Mowé, G., Rogers, A. and Roggli, V. (1985) Analysis of asbestos fibers and asbestos bodies in tissue samples from human lung. *Scand. J. Work Environ. Health* **11**, 107–110

Hahon, N. (1983) Effect of coal rank on the interferon system. *Environ. Res.* **30**, 72–79

Hahon, N. and Booth, J.A. (1987) Silicate minerals and the inter-feron system. *Environ. Res.* **43**, 395–409

Hahon, N. and Eckert, H.L. (1976) Depression of viral interferon induction in cell monolayers by asbestos fibers. *Environ. Res.* **11**, 52–65

Hansen, K. and Mossman, B.T. (1987) Generation of superoxide (0_2^0) from alveolar macrophages exposed to asbestiform and nonfibrous particles. *Cancer Res.* **47**, 1681–1686

Harington, J.S., Miller, K. and Macnab, G. (1971) Hemolysis by asbestos. *Environ. Res.* **4**, 95–117

Harmsen, A.G., Muggenburg, B.A., Snipes, M.B. and Bice, D.E. (1985) The role of macrophages in particle translocation from lungs to lymph nodes. *Science* **230**, 1277–1280

Heppleston, A.G. (1947) The essential lesion of pneumokoniosis in Welsh coal workers. *J. Pathol. Bacteriol.* **59,** 453–460

Heppleston, A.G. (1958) The disposal of coal and haematite dusts inhaled successively. *J. Pathol. Bacteriolt.* **75**, 113–126

Heppleston, A.G. (1962) The disposal of dust in the lungs of silicotic rats. *Am. J. Pathol.* **40**, 493–506

Heppleston, A.G. (1963) Deposition and disposal of inhaled dust. The influence of pre-existing pneumoconiosis. *Arch Environ. Health* **7**, 548–555

Heppleston, A.G. (1972) The pathological recognition and patho-genesis of emphysema and fibrocystic disease of the lung with special reference to coal workers. *Ann. NY Acad. Sci.* **200**, 347–369

Heppleston, A.G. (1978) Cellular reactions with silica. In *Biochemistry of Silicon and Related Problems* (eds G. Bendz and I. Lindqvist), *Nobel Foundation Symposium 40.* Plenum Press, New York, pp. 357–379

Heppleston, A.G. (1979) Silica and asbestos: contrasts in tissue response. *Ann. NY Acad Sci.* **330,** 725–744

Heppleston, A.G. (1986) Determinants of pulmonary fibrosis and lipidosis in the silica model. *Br. J. Expl. Pathol.* **67**, 879–888

Heppleston, A.G. (1988a) Prevalence and pathogenesis of pneumoconiosis in coal workers. *Environ. Health. Perspect.* **78**, 159–170

Heppleston, A.G. (1988b) Environmental lung disease. In *Pathology of the Lung* (ed. W.M. Thurlbeck), Thième Medical, New York, pp. 591–685

Heppleston, A.G. (1989a) Silicotic fibrogenesis: the contributions of Eino Kulonen. *Br. J. Expl. Pathol.* **70**, 178–182

Heppleston, A.G. (1989b) Relationship of lipid secretion and particle size to diffuse interstitial change in pneumoconiosis: a pathogenetic perspective. *Am. J. Ind. Med.* **15**, 427–439

Heppleston, A.G. (1991) Asbestos fibre content and the pulmonary reaction. In *Asbestos-related Cancer* (ed. Mels Sluyser), Ellis Horwood, Chichester, pp. 61–106

Heppleston, A.G. and Morris, T.G. (1965) The progression of experimental silicosis. The influence of exposure to 'inert' dust. *Am. J. Pathol.* **46**, 945–958

Heppleston, A.G. and Styles, J.A. (1967) Activity of a macrophage factor in collagen formation by silica. *Nature* **214**, 521–522

Heppleston, A.G. and Young, A.E. (1972) Alveolar lipo-proteinosis: an ultrastructural comparison of the experimental and human forms. *J. Pathol.* **107**, 107–117

Heppleston, A.G. and Young, A.E. (1973) Uptake of inert partic-ulate matter by alveolar cells: an ultrastructural study. *J. Pathol.* **111**, 159–164

Heppleston, A.G. and Young, A.E. (1985) Population and ultra-structural changes in murine alveolar cells following $^{239}PuO_2$ inhalation. *J. Pathol.* **146**, 155–166

Heppleston, A.G., Ahlquist, K.A. and Williams, D. (1961) Observations on the pathogenesis of silicosis by means of the diffusion chamber technique. *Br. J. Ind. Med.* **18**, 143–147

Heppleston, A.G., Fletcher, K. and Wyatt, I. (1974) Changes in the composition of lung lipids and the 'turnover' of dipalmitoyl lecithin in experimental lipo-proteinosis induced by inhaled quartz. *Br. J. Expl. Pathol.* **55**, 384–395

Heppleston, A.G., Kulonen, E. and Potila, M. (1984) In vitro assessment of the fibrogenicity of mineral dusts. *Am. J. Ind. Med.* **6**, 373–386

Heppleston, A.G., McDermott, M. and Collins, M.M. (1975) The surface properties of the lung in rats with alveolar lipo-proteinosis. *Br. J. Expl. Pathol.* **56**, 444–453

Heppleston, A.G., Wright, N.A. and Stewart, J.A. (1970) Experimental alveolar lipo-proteinosis following the inhalation of silica. *J. Pathol.* **101**, 293–307

Hoffman, R.M., Claypool, W.D., Katyal, S.L., Singh, G., Rogers, R.M. and Dauber, J.H. (1987) Augmentation of rat alveolar macrophage migration by surfactant protein. *Am. Rev. Respir. Dis.* **135**, 1358–1362

Holborow, E.J., Faulk, W.P., Beard, H.K. and Conochie, L.B. (1977) Antibodies against reticulin and collagen. *Ann. Rheumatol. Dis.* **36** (Suppl.), 51–56

Holt, P.F. and Went, C.W. (1960) Studies on the nature of silicosis. A suggested mechanism of fibrogenesis. *Br. J. Ind. Med.* **17**, 25–30

Holt, P.F., Mills, J. and Young, D.K. (1964) The early effects of chrysotile asbestos dust on the rat lung. *J. Pathol. Bacteriol.* **87**, 15–23

Holt, P.F., Mills, J. and Young, D.K. (1965) Experimental asbestosis with four types of fibers: importance of small particles. *Ann. NY Acad. Sci.* **132**, 87–97

Holt, P.G., Warner, L.A. and Papadimitriou, J.M. (1982) Alveolar macrophages: functional heterogeneity within macrophage populations from rat lung. *Aust. J. Expl. Biol. Med. Sci.* **60**, 607–618

Huybrechts-Godin, G., Peeters-Joris, C, and Vaes, G. (1985) Partial characterization of the macrophage factor that stimulates fibroblasts to produce collagenase and to degrade collagen. *Biochim. Biophys. Acta* **846**, 51–54

Jajte, J., Lao, I. and Wiśniewska-Knypl, J.M. (1987) Enhanced lipid peroxidation and lysosomal enzyme activity in the lungs of rats with prolonged pulmonary deposition of crocidolite asbestos. *Br. J. Ind. Med.* **44**, 180–186

Jajte, J., Lao, I., Wiśniewska-Knypl, J.M. and Wrońska-Nofer, T. (1988) Silica earth provoked lung fibrosis with stimulation of lysosomal enzymes and lipid peroxidation in rats. *Br. J. Ind. Med.* **45**, 239–245

Jaurand, M.C., Renier, A. and Bignon, J. (1980) The adsorption of phospholipids and red blood cell membranes on chrysotile fibres. In *The in vitro Effects of Mineral Dusts* (eds. R.C. Brown, I.P. Gormley, M. Chamberlain and R. Davies), Academic Press, London, pp. 121–124

Jaurand, M.C., Bignon, J., Sebastien, P. and Goni, J. (1977) Leaching of chrysotile asbestos in human lungs. Correlation with in vitro studies using rabbit alveolar macrophages. *Environ. Res.* **14**, 245–254

Johansson, A. and Camner, P. (1986) Adverse effects of metals on the alveolar part of the lung. *Scan. Electron Micros.* **2**, 631–637

Jordana, M., Newhouse, M.T. and Gauldie, J. (1987) Alveolar macrophage/peripheral blood monocyte-derived factors modulate proliferation of primary lines of human lung fibroblasts. *J. Leukocyte Biol.* **42**, 51–60

Jordana. M., Schulman, J., McSharry, C., Irving, L.B., Newhouse, M.T., Jordana, G. and Gauldie, J. (1988) Heterogeneous proliferative characteristics of human adult lung fibroblast lines and clonally derived fibroblasts from control and fibrotic tissue. *Am. Rev. Respir. Dis.* **137**, 579–584

Kagan, E., Oghiso, Y. and Hartmann, D-P. (1983) Enhanced release of a chemoattractant for alveolar macrophages after asbestos inhalation. *Am. Rev. Respir. Dis.* **128**, 680–687

Kalter, V.G. and Brody, A.R. (1991) Receptors for transforming growth factor-β (TGF-β) on rat lung fibroblasts have higher affinity for TGF-β$_1$ than for TGF-β$_2$. *Am. J. Respir. Cell Mol. Biol.* **4**, 397–407

Kampschmidt, R.F., Worthington, M.L. and Mesecher, M.I. (1986) Release of interleukin-1 (IL-1) and IL-1-like factors from rabbit alveolar macrophages with silica. *J. Leukocyte Biol.* **39**, 123–132

Katsnelson, B.A. and Privalova, L.I. (1984) Recruitment of phagocytizing cells into the respiratory tract as a response to the cytotoxic action of deposited particles. *Environ. Health. Perspect.* **55**, 313–325

Keith, I., Day, R., Lemaire, S. and Lemaire, I. (1987) Asbestos-induced fibrosis in rats: increase in lung mast cells and autacoid contents. *Expl. Lung Res.* **13**, 311–327

Kelley, J. (1990) Cytokines of the lung. *Am. Rev. Respir. Dis.* **14**, 765–788

Kilroe-Smith, T.A., Webster, I., van Drimmelen, M. and Marasas, L. (1973) An insoluble fibrogenic factor in macrophages from guinea pigs exposed to silica. *Environ. Res.* **6**, 298–305

King, E.J., Mohanty, G.P., Harrison, C.V. and Nagelschmidt, G. (1953a) The action of flint of variable size injected at constant weight and constant surface into the lungs of rats. *Br. J. Ind. Med.* **10**, 76–92

King, E.J., Mohanty, G.P., Harrison, C.V. and Nagelschmidt, G. (1953b) The action of different forms of pure silica on the lungs of rats. *Br. J. Ind. Med.* **10**, 9–17

Klosterkötter, W. and Robock, K. (1967) Zur Bestimmung der Dehydrogenase – Aktivität als Mass für die cytopathogene Wirkung von Stäuben. *Silikosebericht Nordrhein – Westphalen* **6**, 51–54

Kobzik, L., Goldleski, J.J., Barry, B.E. and Brain, J.D. (1988) Isolation and antigenic identification of hamster lung interstitial macrophages. *Am. Rev. Respir. Dis.* **138**, 908–914

Kovacs, E.J. (1991) Fibrogenic cytokines: the role of immune mediators in the development of scar tissue. *Immunol. Today.* **12,** 17–23

Kriegseis, W. and Scharmann, A. (1982) Specific harmfulness of respirable dusts from West German coal mines V: Influence of mineral surface properties. *Ann. Occup. Hyg.* **26**, 511–524

Kriegseis, W., Scharmann, A. and Serafin, J. (1987) Investigations of surface properties of silica dusts with regard to their cytotoxicity. *Ann. Occup. Hyg.* **31**, 417–427

Kriegseis, W., Biederbick, R., Boese, J., Robock, K. and Scharmann, A. (1977) Investigations into the determination of the cytotoxicity of quartz dust by physical methods. In *Inhaled Particles IV* (ed. W.H. Walton), Pergamon, Oxford, pp. 345–357

Kreiss, K., Danilovs, J.A. and Newman, L.S. (1989) Histocompatibility antigens in a population based silicosis series. *Br. J. Ind. Med.* **46**, 364–369

Kulonen, E., Aalto, M., Aho, S., Lehtinen, P. and Potila, M. (1982) Increase of RNA and appearance of new protein in silicotic lung tissue. *Ann. Occup. Hyg.* **26**, 463–471

Langer, AM., Wolff, M.S., Rohl, A.N. and Selikoff, I.J. (1978) Variation of properties of chrysotile asbestos subjected to milling. *J. Toxicol. Environ. Health* **4**, 173–188

Lassalle, P., Gosset, P., Aerts, C. Fournier, E., Lafitte, J.J., Degreef, J.M., Wallaert, B., Tonnel, A.B. and Voisin, C. (1990) Abnormal secretion of interleukin-1 and tumor necrosis factor α by alveolar macrophages in coal worker's pneumoconiosis: comparison between simple pneumoconiosis and progressive massive fibrosis. *Expl. Lung Res.* **16**, 73–80

Last, J.A. and Reiser, K.M. (1989) Biosynthesis of collagen cross-links III. In vivo labeling and stability of lung collagen in rats with bleomycin-induced pulmonary fibrosis. *Am. J. Respir. Cell Mol. Biol.* **1**, 111–117

Laub, R., Huybrechts-Godin, G., Peeters-Joris, C. and Vaes, G. (1982) Degradation of collagen and proteoglycan by macrophages and fibroblasts. *Biochim. Biophys. Acta* **721**, 425–433

Laurent, GJ. (1986) Lung collagen: more than scaffolding. *Thorax* **41**, 418–428

Le Bouffant, L., Daniel, H. and Martin, J.C. (1977) The therapeutic action of aluminium compounds on the development of experimental lesions produced by pure quartz or mixed dust. In *Inhaled Particles IV* (ed. W.H. Walton), Pergamon Press, Oxford, pp. 389–401

Le Bouffant, L., Daniel, H., Martin, J.C. and Bruyère, S. (1982) Effect of impurities and associated minerals on quartz toxicity. *Ann. Occup. Hyg.* **26**, 625–633

Le Bouffant, L., Daniel, H., Henin, J-P. and Martin, J.C. (1985) Pouvoir carcinogène des fibres de chrysotile de longeur < 5 µm. *Cahiers de notes documentaires* **118**, 83–89

Lee, K.P., Henry, N.W., Trochimowicz, H.J. and Reinhardt, C.F. (1986) Pulmonary response to impaired lung clearance in rats following excessive TiO₂ dust deposition. *Environ. Res.* **41**, 144–167

Lemaire, I., Beaudoin, H. and Dubois, C. (1986) Cytokine regulation of lung fibroblast proliferation. Pulmonary and systemic changes in asbestos-induced pulmonary fibrosis. *Am. Rev. Respir. Dis.* **134**, 653–658

Lemaire, I., Beaudoin, H., Massé, S. and Grondin, C. (1986a) Alveolar macrophage stimulation of lung fibroblast growth in asbestos-induced pulmonary fibrosis. *Am. J. Pathol.* **122**, 205–211

Lemaire, I., Dubois, C., Grondin, C. and Gingars, D. (1986b) Immunoregulation of lung fibroblast growth: alteration in asbestos-induced pulmonary fibrosis. *Clin. Expl. Immunol.* **66**, 201–208

Leslie, C.C., McCormick-Shannon, K., Cook, J.L. and Mason, R.J. (1985) Macrophages stimulate DNA synthesis in rat alveolar type II cells. *Am. Rev. Respir. Dis.* **132**, 1246–1252

Lewis, D.M. and Burrell, R. (1976) Induction of fibrogenesis by lung antibody-treated macrophages. *Br. J. Ind. Med.* **33**, 25–28

Lugano, E.M., Dauber, J.H., Elias, J.A., Bashey, I., Jimenez, S.A. and Daniele, R.P. (1984) The regulation of lung fibroblast proliferation by alveolar macrophages in experimental silicosis. *Am. Rev. Respir. Dis.* **129**, 767–771

McDermott, M., Wagner, J.C., Tetley, T., Harwood, J. and Richards, R.J. (1977) The effects of inhaled silica and chrysotile on the elastic properties of rat lungs: physiological, physical and biochemical studies of lung surfactant. In *Inhaled Particles IV* (ed. W.H. Walton), Pergamon Press, Oxford, pp. 415–425

McDonald, A.D. and McDonald, J.C. (1980) Malignant mesothelioma in North America. *Cancer* **46**, 148–154

McLemore, T.L., Roggli, V., Marshall, M.V., Lawrence, E.C., Greenberg, S.D. and Stevens, P.M. (1981) Comparison of phagocytosis of uncoated versus coated asbestos fibers by cultured human pulmonary alveolar macrophages. *Chest* **80**, 39S–42S

Mancuso, T.F. (1988) Relative risk of mesothelioma among railroad machinists exposed to chrysotile. *Am. J. Ind. Med.* **13**, 639–657

Marks, J. and Nagelschmidt, G. (1959) Study of the toxicity of dust with the use of the in vitro dehydrogenase technique. *Archs. Ind. Health* **20**, 383–389

Maroudas, N.G. (1973) Growth of fibroblasts on linear and planar anchorages of limiting dimensions. *Expl. Cell Res.* **81**, 104–110

Masse, R., Fritsch, P., Nolibe, D., Lafuma, J. and Chretien, J. (1977) Cytokinetic study of alveolar macrophage renewal in rats. In *Pulmonary Macrophage and Epithelial Cells* (eds C.L. Sanders, R.P. Schneider, G.E. Dagle and H.A. Ragan), CONF-760927, Technical Information Center, US Dept. Commerce, Springfield, Virginia, pp. 106–114

Mavrogordato, A. (1926) Contributions to the study of miners' phthisis. *Publications of the South African Institute for Medical Research* No. 19(3), 1–84

Mendez. I. de, Daniel, H., Bignon, J., and Lambré, C.R. (1989) Peroxidase activities in the hamster bronchoalveolar lining fluid: modifications induced by exposure to silica dust. *Expl. Lung. Res.* **15**, 681–694

Miall, W.E., Caplan, A., Cochrane, A.L., Kilpatrick, G.S. and Oldham, P. (1953) An epidemiological study of rheumatoid arthritis associated with characteristic chest X-ray appearances in coal-workers. *Br. Med. J.* **2**, 1231–1236

Miller, A.A. and Ramsden, F. (1961) Carbon pneumoconiosis. *Br. J. Ind. Med.* **18**, 103–113

Miller, B.E. and Hook, G.E.R. (1988) Isolation and characterization of hypertrophic type II cells from the lungs of silica-treated rats. *Lab. Invest.* **58**, 565–575

Miller, B.E., Dethloff, L.A., Gladen, B.C. and Hook, G.E.R. (1987) Progression of type II cell hypertrophy and hyperplasia during silica-induced pulmonary inflammation. *Lab. Invest.* **57**, 546–554

Miller, K., Calverley, A. and Kagan, E. (1980) Evidence of a quartz-induced chemotactic factor for guinea pig alveolar macrophages. *Environ. Res.* **22**, 31–39

Miller, R.R., Churg, A.M., Hutcheon, M. and Lam, S. (1984) Pulmonary alveolar proteinosis and aluminium dust exposure. *Am. Rev. Respir. Dis.* **130**, 312–315

Morgan, A., Davies, P., Wagner, J.C., Berry, G and Holmes, A. (1977) The biological effects of magnesium-leached chrysotile asbestos. *Br. J. Expl. Pathol.* **58**, 465–473

Morinaga, K., Kohyama, N., Yokoyama, K., Yasui, Y., Hara, I., Sasaki, M., Suzuki, Y. and Sera, Y. (1989) Asbestos fibre content of lungs with mesotheliomas in Osaka, Japan: a preliminary report. In *Non-occupational Exposure to Mineral Fibres* (eds J. Bignon, J. Peto and R. Saracci), International Agency for Research on Cancer Scientific Publication No. 90, IARC, Lyon, pp. 438–443

Mossman, B.T., Hansen, K., Marsh, J.P., Brew, M.E., Hill, S., Bergeron, M. and Petruska, J. (1989) Mechanisms of fibre-induced superoxide release from alveolar macrophages and induction of superoxide dismutase in the lungs of rats inhaling crocidolite. In *Non-occupational Exposure to Mineral Fibres* (eds J. Bignon, J. Peto and R. Saracci), International Agency for Research on Cancer Scientific Publications No. 90, IARC, Lyon, pp. 81–92

Nagelschmidt, G. (1960) The relation between lung dust and lung pathology in pneumoconiosis. *Br. J. Ind. Med.* **17**, 247–259

Nash, T., Allison, A.C. and Harington, J.S. (1966) Physico-chemical properties of silica in relation to its toxicity. *Nature* **210**, 259–261

Nolan, R.P., Langer, A.M., Harington, J.S., Oster, G. and Selikoff, I.J. (1981) Quartz hemolysis as related to surface functionalities. *Environ. Res.* **26**, 503–520

Nolan, R.P., Langer, A.M., Weisman, I. and Herson, G.B. (1987) Surface character and membranolytic activity of rutile and anatase: two titanium dioxide polymorphs. *Br. J. Ind. Med.* **44**, 687–698

Norris, D.A., Clark, R.A.F., Swigart, L.M., Huff, J.C., Weston, W.L. and Howell, S.E. (1982) Fibronectin fragment(s) are chemotactic for human peripheral blood monocytes. *J. Immunol.* **129**, 1612–1618

Nourse, L.D., Nourse, P.N., Botes, H. and Schwartz, H.M. (1975) The effects of macrophages isolated from the lungs of guinea pigs dusted with silica on collagen biosynthesis by guinea pig fibroblasts in cell culture. *Environ. Res.* **9**, 115–127

Oghiso, Y. (1987) Heterogeneity in immunological functions of rat alveolar macrophages – their accessory cell function and IL-1 production. *Microbiol. Immunol.* **31**, 247–260

Oghiso, Y. and Kubota, Y. (1986) Interleukin-1-like thymocyte and fibroblast activating factors from rat alveolar macrophages exposed to silica and asbestos particles. *Jap. J. Vet. Sci.* **48**, 461–471

Oghiso, Y. and Kubota, Y. (1987) Interleukin-1 production and accessory cell function of rat alveolar macrophages exposed to mineral dust particles. *Microbiol. Immunol.* **31**, 275–287

Parod, R.J. and Brain, J.D. (1983) Uptake of latex particles by pulmonary macrophages: role of calcium. *Am. J. Phys.* **245**, C227–C234

Piguet, P.F., Collart, M.A., Grau, G.E., Sappino, A-P. and Vassalli, P. (1990) Requirement of tumour necrosis factor for development of silica-induced pulmonary fibrosis. *Nature* **344**, 245–247

Pinkerton, K.E. and Yu, C-P. (1989) Intrapulmonary airway branching and parenchymal deposition of chrysotile asbestos fibers. In *Biological Interaction of Inhaled Mineral Fibers and Cigarette Smoke* (ed. A.P. Wehner), Battelle Memorial Institute, Seattle, pp. 211–222

Pinkerton, K.E., Plopper, C.G., Mercer, R.R., Roggli, V.L., Patra, A.L., Brody, A.R. and Crapo, J.D. (1986) Airway branching patterns influence asbestos fiber location and the extent of tissue injury in the pulmonary parenchyma. *Lab. Invest.* **55**, 688–695

Platek, S.F., Groth, D.H., Ulrich, C.E., Stettler, L.E., Finnell, M.S. and Stoll, M. (1985) Chronic inhalation of short asbestos fibers. *Fund. Appl. Toxicol.* **5**, 327–340

Policard, A., Collet, A. and Martin, J.C. (1963) La mobilité des lésions dans les pneumoconioses. *Beit. Silikose-Forsch.* **Sb5**, 267–272

Policard, A., Letort, M., Charbonnier, J., Daniel-Moussard, H., Martin, J.C. and Le Bouffant, L. (1971) Recherches expéri-mentales concernant l'inhibition de l'action cytotoxique du quartz au moyen de substances minérales, notamment de composés de l'aluminium. *Beitr. Silikose-Forsch.* **23**, 1–58

Pooley, F.D. and Clark, N. (1979) Fiber dimensions and aspect ratio of crocidolite, chrysotile and amosite particles detected in lung tissue specimens. *Ann. NY Acad. Sci.* **330**, 711–716

Postlethwaite, A.E., Seyer, J.M. and Kang, A.H. (1978) Chemotactic attraction of human fibroblasts to type I, II and III collagens and collagen-derived peptides. *Proc. Natl Acad. Sci. USA* **75**, 871–875

Postlethwaite, A.E., Raghow, R., Stricklin, G.P., Poppleton, H., Seyer, J.M. and Kang, A.H. (1988) Modulation of fibroblast functions by interleukin-1: increased steady-state accumulation of type I procollagen messenger RNAs and stimulation of other functions but not chemotaxis by human recombinant interleukin-1α and β. *J. Cell Biol.* **106**, 311–318

Radzun, H.J., Parwaresch, M.R. and Kreipe, H. (1983) Monocytic origin of human alveolar macrophages. *J. Histochem. Cytochem.* **31**, 318–324

Reiser, K.M. and Gerriets, J. (1986) Experimental silicosis: mechanisms of acute and chronic lung changes. In *Silica, Silicosis, and Cancer* (eds D.F. Goldsmith, D.M. Winn and C.M. Shy), Praeger, New York, pp. 93–104

Rennard, S.I., Hunninghake, G.W., Bitterman, P.B. and Crystal, R.G. (1981) Production of fibronectin by the human alveolar macrophage: mechanism for the recruitment of fibroblasts to sites of tissue injury in interstitial lung diseases. *Proc. Natl Acad. Sci. USA* **78**, 7147–7151

Rennard, S.I., Ferrans, V.J., Bradley, K.H and Crystal, R.G. (1982) Lung connective tissue. In *Mechanisms in Respiratory Toxicology*, vol. 2 (ed. H. Witschi), CRC Reviews, Boca Raton, FL, pp. 115–153

Rennard, S.I., Jaurand, M-C., Bignon, J., Kawanami, O., Ferrans, V.J., Davidson, J. and Crystal, R.G. (1984) Role of pleural mesothelial cells in the production of the submesothelial connective matrix of lung. *Am. Rev. Respir. Dis.* **130**, 267–274

Rennard, S.I., Bitterman, P.B., Ozaki, T., Rom, W.N. and Crystal, R.G. (1988) Colchicine suppresses the release of fibroblast growth factors from alveolar macrophages in vitro. The basis of a possible therapeutic approach to the fibrotic disorders. *Am. Rev. Respir. Dis.* **137**, 181–185

Rhoades, R.A. (1972) Effect of inhaled carbon on surface properties of rat lung. *Life Sci.* **11**, 33–42

Robalo-Cordiero, A.J.A., Baganha, M.F., Azevedo-Bernarda, R., Leite, A.C.P. Almieda, U.R.G., Bairos, V.F., Gaspar, E., Garcao, M.F., Lima, M.A.M., Rosa, M.A.S., Pega, A.F. and Bastos, J.M.P. (1985) Biological effects of fume silica (amorphous type). In *In vitro Effects of Mineral Dusts* (eds E.G. Beck and J. Bignon), Springer, Berlin, pp. 489–496

Robinson, P.C., Watters, L.C., King, T.E. and Mason, R.J. (1988) Idiopathic pulmonary fibrosis. Abnormalities in bronchoalveolar lavage fluid phospholipids. *Am. Rev. Respir. Dis.* **137**, 585–591

Robock, K. and Klosterkötter, W. (1973) Investigations on the specific toxicity of different SiO_2 and silicate dusts. *Staub. Reinhalt. Luft* **33**, 60–64

Robock, K and Reisner, M.T.R. (1982) Specific harmfulness of respirable dusts from West German coal mines. I: Results of cell tests. *Ann. Occup. Hyg.* **26**, 473–479

Roggli, V.L. and Brody, A.R. (1984) Changes in numbers and dimensions of chrysotile asbestos fibers in lungs of rats following short-term exposure. *Expl. Lung Res.* **7**, 133–147

Roggli, V.L., George, M.H. and Brody, A.R. (1987) Clearance and dimensional changes of crocidolite asbestos fibers isolated from lungs of rats following short-term exposure. *Environ. Res.* **42**, 94–105

Roggli, V.L., Pratt, P.C. and Brody, A.R. (1986) Asbestos content of lung tissue in asbestos associated diseases: study of 110 cases. *Br. J. Ind. Med.* **43**, 18–28

Rom, W.N., Bitterman, P.B., Rennard, S.I., Cantin, A. and Crystal, R.G. (1987) Characterization of the lower respiratory tract inflammation of nonsmoking individuals with interstitial lung disease associated with chronic inhalation of inorganic dusts. *Am. Rev. Respir. Dis.* **136**, 1429–1434

Ross, H.F., King, E.J., Yoganathan, M. and Nagelschmidt, G. (1962) Inhalation experiments with coal dust containing 5 percent, 10 percent, 20 percent and 40 percent quartz: tissue reactions in the lungs of rats. *Ann. Occup. Hyg.* **5**, 149–161

Rowlands, N., Gibbs, G.W. and McDonald, A.D. (1982) Asbestos fibres in the lungs of chrysotile miners and millers – a preliminary report. *Ann. Occup. Hyg.* **26**, 411–415

Ruckley, V.A., Chapman, J.S., Collings, P.L., Douglas, A.N., Fernie, J.M., Lamb, D. and Davis, J.M.G. (1981) Autopsy studies of coalminers' lungs – phase II. *Technical Memorandum 81/18*. Institute of Occupational Medicine, Edinburgh.

Rüttner, J.R., Bovet, P. and Aufdermaur, M. (1952) Graphit, Carborund, Staublunge. *Dtsche Med. Wochenschr.* **77**, 1413–1415

Sanders, C.L., Conklin, A.W., Gelman, R.A., Adee, R.R. and Rhoads, K. (1982) Pulmonary toxicity of Mount St. Helens volcanic ash. *Environ. Res.* **27**, 118–135

Schmidt, J.A., Oliver, C.N., Lepe-Zuniga, J.L., Green, I. and Gery, I. (1984) Silica-stimulated monocytes release fibroblast proliferation factors identical to interleukin 1. A potential role for interleukin 1 in the pathogenesis of silicosis. *J. Clin. Invest.* **73**, 1462–1472

Schuyler, M.R., Gaumer, H.R., Stankus, R.P., Kaimal, J., Hoffmann, E. and Salvaggio, J.E. (1980) Bronchoalveolar lavage in silicosis. Evidence of type II cell hyperplasia. *Lung* **157**, 95–102

Schwartz, L.W. and Christman, C.A. (1979) Lung lining material as a chemoattractant for alveolar macrophages. *Chest* **75S**, 284S–288S

Schwartz, D.A., Rosenstock, L. and Clark, J.G. (1989) Monocyte-derived growth factors in asbestos-induced interstitial fibrosis. *Environ. Res.* **49**, 283–294

Sebastien, P., Fondimare, A., Bignon, J., Monchaux, G., Desbordes, J. and Bonnaud, G. (1977) Topographic distribution of asbestos fibres in human lung in relation to occupational and non-occupational exposure. In *Inhaled Particles IV* (ed. W.H. Walton), Pergamon Press, Oxford, pp. 435–444

Seemayer, N.H. and Manojlovic, N. (1979) Untersuchungen über die biologische Wirkung von Grubenstäuben II. Vergleichende Prüfung der Zytotoxizität von 16 verschiedenen Grubenstäuben an alveolaren Makrophagen des Meerschweinchens in vitro. *Silikosebericht Nordrhein-Westfalen* **12**, 173–179

Seemayer, N.H, Baumann, A. and Maly, E. (1987) Entwicklung eines "in vitro" Testsystems mit menschlichen Makrophagen und Fibroblasten zur analyse der Wirkung von Quarz-und Grubenstäuben I. Bildung eines Fibroblasten-Proliferationsfaktor. *Silikosebericht Nordrhein-Westfalen* **16**, 191–199

Seppä, H.E.J., Yamada, K.M., Sëppa, S.T., Silver, M.H., Kleinman, H.K. and Schiffmann, E. (1981) The cell binding fragment of fibronectin is chemotactic for fibroblasts. *Cell Biol. Int. Rep.* **5**, 813–819

Shami, S.G., Evans, M.J. and Martinez, L.A. (1986) Type II cell proliferation related to migration of inflammatory cells into the lung. *Expl. Mol. Pathol.* **44**, 344–452

Shaw, R.J., Benedict, S.H., Clark, R.A.F. and King, T.E. (1991) Pathogenesis of pulmonary fibrosis in interstitial lung disease. Alveolar macrophage PDGF(B) gene activation and up-regulation by interferon gamma. *Am. Rev. Respir. Dis.* **143**, 167–173

Shelley, S.A., L'Heureux, M.V. and Balis, J.U. (1975) Characterization of lung surfactant: factors promoting formation of artifactual lipid-protein complexes. *J. Lipid Res.* **16**, 224–234

Shellito, J., Esparza, C. and Armstrong, C. (1987) Maintenance of the normal rat alveolar macrophage cell population. The roles of monocyte influx and alveolar macrophage proliferation in situ. *Am. Rev. Respir. Dis.* **135**, 78–82

Simson, F.W. and Strachan, A.S. (1935) Silicosis and tuberculosis. Observations on the origin and character of silicotic lesions as shown in cases occurring on the Witwatersrand. *Publications of the South African Insititute for Medical Research* **6**, 367–406

Singh, J.P., Adams, L.D. and Bonin, P.D. (1988) Mode of fibroblast growth enhancement by human interleukin-1. *J. Cell Biol.* **106**, 813–819

Sjöstrand, M. and Rylander, R. (1987) Lysosomal enzyme activity and fibroblast stimulation of lavage from guinea pigs exposed to silica dust. *Br. J. Expl. Pathol.* **69**, 309–318

Sluiter, W., Van Hemsbergen-Oomens, L.W.M., Elzenga-Claasen, I., Annema, A. and Van Furth, R. (1988) Effect of lung surfactant on the release of factor increasing monocytopoiesis by macrophages. *Expl. Hematol.* **16**, 93–96

Smither, W.J. (1965) Secular changes in asbestosis in an asbestos factory. *Ann. NY Acad. Sci.* **132**, 166–181

Spurny, K.R., Stöber, W., Opiela, H. and Weiss, G. (1980) On the problem of milling and ultrasonic treatment of asbestos and glass fibers in biological and analytical applications. *Am. Ind. Hyg. Assoc. J.* **41**, 198–203

Spurzem, J.R., Saltini, C., Rom, W., Winchester, R.J. and Crystal, R.G. (1987) Mechanisms of macrophage accumulation in the lungs of asbestos-exposed subjects. *Am. Rev. Respir. Dis.* **136**, 276–280

Summerton, J., Hoenig, S., Butler, C. and Chvapil, M. (1977) The mechanism of hemolysis by silica and its bearing on silicosis. *Expl. Mol. Pathol.* **26**, 113–128

Tainer, J.A., Turner, S.R. and Lynn, W.S. (1975) New aspects of chemotaxis. Specific target-cell attraction by lipid and lipoprotein fractions of *Escherichia coli* chemotactic factor. *Am. J. Pathol.* **81**, 401–410

Tetley, T.D., Hext, P.M., Richards, R.J. and McDermott, M. (1976) Chrysotile-induced asbestosis: changes in the free cell population, pulmonary surfactant and whole lung tissue of rats. *Br. J. Expl. Pathol.* **57**, 505–514

Thomas, E.D., Ramberg, R.E., Sale, G.E., Sparkes, R.S. and Golde, D.W. (1976) Direct evidence for a bone marrow origin of the alveolar macrophage in man. *Science* **192**, 1016–1018

Tilkes, F. and Beck, E.G. (1983) Macrophage functions after exposure to mineral fibers. *Environ. Health. Persp.* **51**, 67–72

Timbrell, V., Ashcroft, T., Goldstein, B., Heyworth, F., Meurman, L.O., Rendall, R.E.G., Reynolds, J.A., Shilkin, K.B. and Whitaker, D. (1988) Relationships between retained amphibole fibres and fibrosis in human lung tissue specimens. *Ann. Occup. Hyg.* **32** (suppl. 1), 323–340

Unsworth, D.J., Scott, D.L., Almond, T.J., Beard, H.K. Holborow, E.J. and Walton, K.W. (1982) Studies on reticulin I: Serological and immunohistological investigation of the occurrence of collagen type III, fibronectin and the non-collagenous glycoprotein of Pras and Glynn in reticulin. *Br. J. Expl. Pathol.* **63**, 154–166

Vallyathan, V., Shi, X., Dalal, N.S., Irr, W. and Castranova, V. (1988) Generation of free radicals from freshly fractured silica dust. A potential role in acute silica-induced lung injury. *Am. Rev. Respir. Dis.* **138**, 1213–1219

Vitums, V.C., Edwards, M.J., Niles, N., Borman, J.O. and Lowry, R.D. (1977) Pulmonary fibrosis from amorphous silica dust, a product of silica vapor. *Archs. Environ. Health.* **32**, 62–68

Voisin, C., Wallaert, B., Aerts, C. and Grosbois, J.M. (1985) Bronchoalveolar lavage in coalworkers' pneumoconiosis: oxidant and antioxidant activities of alveolar macrophages. In *In Vitro Effects of Mineral Dusts* (eds E.G. Beck and J. Bignon), Springer, Berlin, pp. 93–100

Vorwald, A.J., Durkan, T.M. and Pratt, P.C. (1951) Experimental studies of asbestosis *Archs. Ind. Hyg. Occup. Med.* **3**, 1–43

Vuorio, E.I., Makela, J.K., Vuorio, T.K., Poole, A. and Wagner, J.C. (1989) Characterization of excessive collagen production during development of pulmonary fibrosis induced by chronic silica inhalation in rats. *Br. J. Expl. Pathol.* **70**, 305–315

Wagner, J.C. (1990) Biological effects of short fibres. In *Proceedings of the 7th International Pneumoconioses Conference*, US DHHS (NIOSH) Publication, no. 90-108, pp. 835–839

Wagner, J.C., Griffiths, D.M. and Hill, R.J. (1984) The effect of fibre size on the in vivo activity of UICC crocidolite. *Br. J. Cancer* **49**, 453–458

Wagner, J.C, Pooley, F.D., Berry, G., Seal, R.M.E., Munday, D.E., Morgan, J. and Clark, N.J. (1982) A pathological and mineralogical study of asbestos-related deaths in the United Kingdom in 1977. *Ann. Occup. Hyg.* **26**, 423–430

Wagner, M.M.F., Edwards, R.E., Moncrieff, C.B. and Wagner, J.C. (1984) Mast cells and inhalation of asbestos in rats. *Thorax* **39**, 539–544

Wallaert, B., Lassalle, P., Fortin, F., Aerts, C., Bart, F., Fournier, E. and Voisin, C. (1990) Superoxide anion generation by alveolar inflammatory cells in simple pneumoconiosis and in progressive massive fibrosis of nonsmoking coal workers. *Am. Rev. Respir. Dis.* **141**, 129–133

Warheit, D.B., Hill, L.A., George, G. and Brody, A.R. (1986) Time course of chemotactic factor generation and the corresponding macrophage response to asbestos inhalation. *Am. Rev. Respir. Dis.* **134**, 128–133

Warheit, D.B., Overby, L.H., George, G. and Brody, A.R. (1988) Pulmonary macrophages are attracted to inhaled particles through complement activation. *Expl. Lung Res.* **14**, 51–66

Warner, A.E., Barry, B.E. and Brain, J.D. (1986) Pulmonary intravascular macrophages in sheep. Morphology and function of a novel constituent of the mononuclear phagocytic system. *Lab. Invest.* **55**, 276–288

Watson, A.J., Black, J., Doig, A.T. and Nagelschmidt, G. (1959) Pneumoconiosis in carbon electrode makers. *Br. J. Ind. Med.* **16**, 274–285

Webster, I. (1970) Asbestos exposure in South Africa. In *Pneumoconiosis. Proceedings of the International Conference, Johannesburg 1969* (ed. H.A. Shapiro), Oxford University Press, Cape Town, pp. 209–212

Webster, I., Henderson, C.I., Marasas,, L.W. and Keegan, D.J. (1967) Some biologically active substances produced by the action of silica and their possible significance. In *Inhaled Particles II* (ed. C.N. Davies), Pergamon Press, Oxford, pp. 111–119

Welgus, H.G., Campbell, E.J., Bar-Sahvit, Z., Senior, R.M. and Teitelbaum, S.L. (1985) Human alveolar macrophages produce a fibroblast-like collagenase and collagenase inhibitor. *J. Clin. Invest.* **76**, 219–224

Weller, W. (1977) Long-term test on rhesus monkeys for the PVNO therapy of anthracosilicosis. In *Inhaled Particles IV* (ed. W.H. Walton), Pergamon Press, Oxford, pp. 379–386

Whitsett, J.A., Weaver, T.E., Lieberman, M.A., Clark, J.C. and Daugherty, C. (1987) Differential effects of epidermal growth factor and transforming growth factor-β on synthesis of M_r = 35,000 surfactant-associated protein in fetal lung. *J. Biol. Chem.* **262**, 7908–7913

Wiedemann, H.P., Lwebuga-Mukasa, J.S. and Gee, J.B.L. (1985) Asbestos fibers enhance the production of a mesothelial cell-derived soluble factor which stimulates fibroblast DNA synthesis. In *In Vitro Effects of Mineral Dusts* (eds E.G. Beck and J. Bignon), Springer, Berlin, pp. 377–382

Wiessner, J.H., Henderson, J.D., Sohnle, P.G., Mandel, N.S. and Mandel, GS. (1988) The effect of crystal structure on mouse lung inflammation and fibrosis. *Am. Rev. Respir. Dis.* **138**, 445–450

Wiessner, J.H., Mandel, N.S., Sohnle, P.G. and Mandel, G.S. (1989) Effect of particle size on quartz-induced hemolysis and on lung inflammation and fibrosis. *Expl. Lung Res.* **15**, 801–812

Wiessner, J.H., Mandel, N.S., Sohnle, P.G., Hasegawa, A. and Mandel, G.S. (1990) The effect of chemical modification of quartz surfaces on particulate-induced pulmonary inflammation and fibrosis in the mouse. *Am. Rev. Respir. Dis.* **141**, 111–116

Wilsher, M.L., Hughes, D.A. and Haslam, P.L. (1988) Immunoregulatory properties of pulmonary surfactant: effect of lung lining fluid on proliferation of human blood lymphocytes. *Thorax* **43**, 354–359

Yazicioglu, S., Ilcayto, R., Balci, K., Sayli, B.S. and Yorulmaz, B. (1980) Pleural calcification, pleural mesotheliomas, and bronchial cancers caused by tremolite dust. *Thorax* **35**, 564–569

Yeager, H., Russo, D.A., Yañez, M., Gerardi, D., Nolan, R.P., Kagan, E. and Langer, A.M. (1983) Cytotoxicity of a short-fiber chrysotile asbestos for human alveolar macrophages: preliminary observations. *Environ. Res.* **30**, 224–232

Zenker, F.A. (1867) Über Staubinhalationskrankheiten der Lungen. *Dtsches Archiv Klin. Med.* **2**, 116–172

Ziskind, M., Weill, H., Anderson, A.E., Samimi, B., Neilson, A. and Waggenspack, C. (1976) Silcosis in shipyard sandblasters. *Environ. Res.* **11**, 237–243

6

Clinical considerations

W. Raymond Parkes

Medical men . . ., in examining into the symptoms of diseases, sometimes put their questions inaccurately, and not unfrequently mislead patients into a false description, from some opinion about the disease which they have too hastily adopted.

Matthew Baillie (1797)

Systematic and detailed discussion of medical history-taking and clinical examination is to be found in textbooks of respiratory medicine but, in regard to the subject of this book, certain aspects of both topics merit special attention.

First of all, two fundamental points, not always properly considered, should be emphasized:

1. Whether occupational or non-occupational respiratory disease is being considered, the discipline and procedure to be followed for history and examination are, or should be, the same apart from the fact that, in the former, detailed enquiry into conditions of work is required.
2. Pulmonary disease of non-occupational origin may occur in individuals who have been exposed to an occupational risk and, in many instances, its primary cause may lie outside the lungs. This possibility must not be neglected when a worker (or patient) is presented to the clinician as a case of supposed occupational disease if unfortunate errors (which may persist for years) are to be avoided.

Needless to say, it is essential that treatable non-occupational disease should be distinguished from an occupational disease for which there is no treatment as quickly as possible. Misdiagnosis of non-occupational disease as occupational is rarely eradicated from the patient's mind, and leads to resentment and apprehension. The opposite error, though less common, can, nevertheless, subject the patient to unnecessary investigation (including thoracotomy) and treatment, for example, when silicosis is misinterpreted as tuberculosis or sarcoidosis. The situation is well summarized by Turton (1987) echoing Matthew Baillie: 'A general problem in clinical medicine is the inflexible thinking that can follow a confident clinical diagnosis based on initial impressions, even when discordant information becomes available later.'

Occupational history

A detailed history of past and present occupations is the most important means by which the clinician's attention is directed, on the one hand, to the likelihood that the patient's pulmonary disease is caused by exposure to some hazard at work or, on the other hand, to the fact that the disease under investigation is unlikely to be of occupational origin. Yet clinicians are not always well equipped to elicit an occupational history with accuracy due to lack of detailed knowledge of an industry. In such instances they fail to appreciate the nature of a particular process or, if they identify it, are unable to evaluate whether the exposure is, or is not, likely to be significant and the cause of the disease in question. Thus, on the one hand, identification of an occupational cause may be missed or delayed or, on the other, a causal connection between a potential hazard and disease is taken for granted and the correct diagnosis overlooked. Today, the difficulty is all the greater because of the chemical and physical complexities of many industrial processes and an increasing number of sensitizing agents capable of causing asthma or extrinsic allergic alveolitis. In some cases, even the experienced clinician may fail to obtain a history that is adequate to identify a specific risk. This possibility has to be recognized, as does the opposite (all too common) danger of indicting an unfamiliar, but innocent, substance that is not pathogenic. When in doubt, the clinician should seek the assistance of those non-medical experts whose advice will usually help to solve the problem posed: factory inspectors, industrial hygienists, mineralogists, employers and, in the UK, the Health and Safety Executive or Employment Medical Advisory Service, or, in the USA, the Occupational Safety and Health Administration.

The workers, or patients, should be encouraged to explain the details of their jobs freely, with little interruption; they often have detailed knowledge of the process in which they worked, although this is not always so and they may make assumptions that are inaccurate or wrong. Direct questions as to whether there has been exposure to a specific hazard or material should be avoided initially until the overall history has been obtained, when the clinician can decide on which particular processes or jobs to concentrate attention. Inevitably this procedure is time-consuming but a detailed history must never be replaced by a few 'quick-fire' questions if unfortunate errors are to be avoided.

The history must be taken in strictly chronological order starting with details of the first job on leaving school and progressing step by step to the present job or retirement; as far as possible, no gaps or uncertainties should exist when it is complete. It is also necessary to form some idea of the intensity of exposure to a hazard as well as the duration of this exposure.

The description of a job, or the name given to it by the worker, may conceal its true nature and, therefore, an unexpected hazard. For example, a *bricklayer* may have worked with refractory bricks (not house bricks) containing high concentrations of free silica and, furthermore, may have used asbestos fibre or rope for grouting the expansion joints of kilns; a *stoker* may not only have stoked boilers in factory, power station or hospital but may also have been exposed to free silica dust produced when cleaning ('scaling') the tubes, or intermittently to asbestos during the stripping and reapplication of lagging materials around boilers and neighbouring pipes by insulation workers in the immediate vicinity; a *labourer* in a factory producing poultry meal may, until recent times, have operated a flint crushing mill and so have been exposed to the risk of silicosis; a *shot blaster* fettling metal castings may have been well protected during the actual process but not at the end of the shift when used shot and fettled sand may have had to be collected from the trap beneath the cabinet for separation; a *scrap-metal worker* might recall, on further enquiry, that the work included the melting down of beryllium alloys; a *welder* may be exposed to metal fumes such as zinc, iron or cadmium oxides, to gases such as the oxides of nitrogen or ozone, or to asbestos from the

activities of insulation workers in the vicinity; a general *maintenance fitter* may have serviced or repaired asbestos-processing machinery and exhaust ventilation ducts containing dust; and a *clerk* or a *housewife* may have worked in a respiratory hazard many years previously. These few examples emphasize the detail that may be required in occupational histories. Although some of these risks have now been eliminated, this is comparatively recent and so disease resulting from such exposures in the past can be encountered today.

As the popular description of a job may give no clue to the nature of the work involved, it is necessary to establish exactly what the job entails and the materials used. The possibility of multiple risks operating in the one work process, or of an individual having worked in different hazardous industries over the years must always be borne in mind. The worker should also be asked what protective measures were used: in particular, local exhaust and general ventilation, and the wearing and type of respirators and protective clothing. This information enables the physician to form some impression of the concentrations of dust to which that person may have been exposed.

It is important, also, to obtain details of part-time work (other than the habitual occupation) which may, for example, be responsible for asthma or extrinsic allergic alveolitis. Enquiry as to whether fellow workers have, or have had, respiratory disease is important in that it may provide help either in diagnosis or possible identification of a previously unrecognized hazard.

Exposure of workers to a hazardous aerosol from a nearby process and disease which may result from it, and not from their own jobs, is commonly referred to as *paraoccupational*.

Domestic history

Potentially hazardous dusts shaken from a worker's overalls at home during cleaning or preparation for laundering may have been, in the past, a possible risk to the family (see 'Family history', later). Details of hobbies should always be sought. Eliciting a history of bird fancying (chiefly budgerigars and pigeons) is important, especially in those cases where there has been prolonged exposure; under these conditions, chronic extrinsic allergic alveolitis of insidious onset may occur and its relationship with the cause is apt to be unsuspected. The level of exposure to dust is related not to the number of pigeons kept by breeders but to the degree of disturbance of lofts by cleaning and other activities (Anderson et al., 1990). In the UK, pigeon fancying has been a popular hobby among coal miners over many years. The breeding and keeping of a variety of small animals may be a source of asthma.

'Do-it-yourself' enthusiasts, who today are legion, may work with solder fluxes, various woods, epoxy resin hardeners or isocyanate-containing paints, with consequent development of asthma. They may have used asbestos materials and, although exposure has usually been too low to be a hazard to health, it may be responsible for the presence of asbestos bodies in the lungs and sputum (see Chapter 14).

Failure to identify domestic sources of exposure may result in disease being wrongly attributed to occupation.

Smoking habits

Accurate information about past and present smoking habits is most important and must always be obtained and recorded. People fall into one of three groups: smokers, ex-smokers and non-smokers. Cigarette, cigar and pipe smoking must be distinguished and its duration and the question of inhaling established.

As the effects of smoking are related to the duration of the habit and are cumulative and, thus, greater with increasing years, the consumption of cigarettes should be carefully recorded as the number smoked per day from the age at which smoking began. For comparison with other types of smoking, it is helpful to note that one manufactured cigarette is approximately equivalent to 1 g tobacco, and that 1 oz (28 g) tobacco per week equals 4 g daily whether smoked in a pipe or as hand-rolled cigarettes (Higgins, 1959). A useful method of quantifying life-long cigarette consumption is in *'pack-years'* – *the pack-year being defined as one packet of 20 cigarettes per day for one year.*

In the epidemiological studies the importance of obtaining a smoking history that quantifies realistically life-long consumption cannot be too strongly emphasized; relegation simply to 'smoker' (light or heavy), 'ex-smoker' and 'non-smoker' categories at the time of the study is inadequate. 'The simplest and best solution is to make entirely separate analyses' for each of these classes 'which are now not far from equality in numbers' (Oldham, 1987).

The effects that smoking may have on the lungs are discussed in Chapters 3, 9, 10, 13 and 14. It is worth noting here, however, that atopy, as indicated by reactivity to common allergens on skin-prick testing, appears to be associated with an increased susceptibility to bronchoconstriction caused by smoking, and to recurrent chest infections especially in younger subjects (Burrows, Lebowitz and Barbee, 1976).

Medical history

Before considering the medical history in detail, it is as well to recall that disease of the upper respiratory and gastrointestinal tracts, disorders of connective tissue and abnormality of the thoracic skeleton are fairly common causes of bronchopulmonary symptoms and disease – a fact that is often overlooked or forgotten when workers or patients suspected of having an occupational disorder are under investigation. Consequently, both symptoms and disease may be wrongly attributed to a work-related disorder, real or supposed. Brief discussion of these important relationships is, therefore, in order.

Upper respiratory tract

For many years, chronic disease of the nose and paranasal sinuses has been known to be associated with bronchopneumonia (Amberson, 1937), recurrent bronchitis (Hogg and Brock, 1951) and bronchiectasis (Quinn and Meyer, 1929). In 1935 Maurice Davidson (an astute Brompton Hospital physician) wrote that chronic rhinitis with nasal obstruction 'leads in turn to infection of the lower respiratory tract, a vicious circle of infection being constantly maintained'. In recent times, intermittent or chronic infection of the upper respiratory tract has been found in about 42 per cent of patients with proven bronchiectasis, and allergic rhinitis in 56 to 74 per cent of patients with asthma (Mackay and Cole, 1987).

Chronic or recurrent rhinosinusitis is caused by the following:

1. Mechanical obstruction due to congenital or acquired abnormalities of the nose or sinuses, hypertrophy of the adenoids or turbinate bones, and nasal polyposis (see Chapter 1).
2. Allergy, which yields yellow- or green-coloured nasal secretions when their eosinophil count is high.
3. Damage to the ciliated epithelium by recurrent viral infections in childhood or later, with resultant impairment of mucociliary clearance (*secondary ciliary dyskinesia*) of the nose and sinuses, which may be compounded by ciliotoxic sols produced by subsequent, and repeated, bacterial infections (Greenstone and Cole, 1985).
4. Impaired humoral immunity due to selective deficiency of subclasses of IgA, IgM or IgG (Barker and Bardana, 1988).

More than one-third of patients with chronic bronchial sepsis (that is, daily production of purulent sputum) have frank chronic purulent sinusitis, and some 80 per cent have upper respiratory symptoms (Mackay and Cole, 1987). Mucociliary clearance is reduced in patients with mucopurulent sinusitis and, as already noted in Chapter 3, purulent sputum in bronchiectasis appears to be toxic to nasal and bronchial cilia (Smallman, Hill and Stockley, 1984).

Impaired ciliary function may contribute to delayed clearance in all respiratory disorders in which there are purulent secretions (Wilson et al., 1986). Although many humoral deficiencies are congenital, others, which are acquired and of late onset, are being increasingly recognized (Hermans, Diaz-Buxo and Stobo, 1976).

Postnasal discharge (or 'drip') of excessive secretions often occurs and results in persistent cough and clearing of the throat (Irwin, Carrao and Pratter, 1981) and, in many instances, in recurrent pulmonary infection consequent upon aspiration of secretions. With the aid of an inert radioactive tracer, aspiration from the pharynx has been shown to occur in normal subjects during normal sleep – especially if deep (Huxley et al., 1978); in fact, spontaneous coughing is suppressed during deep sleep (Power et al., 1984). Therefore, patients must be questioned specifically about this important symptom – invariably associated with chronic rhinosinusitis – if, as is often the case, they do not volunteer it themselves.

Thus, bronchopulmonary insults from aspiration of infected secretions may result in secondary dyskinesia, impaired mucociliary clearance and recurrent inflammation with destruction and scarring of the epithelium of the airways, and, in vulnerable individuals with acquired humoral deficiency or hyperreactive airways, in diffuse bronchiectasis. In short, there is a 'vicious circle' of bronchial sepsis (Cole, 1986). In less florid form this process is probably more common than is realized in the pathogenesis of chronic disease of the lungs – at least in the UK; it can result in asthmatic airflow obstruction or scarring and shrinkage of the lungs, and should be kept in mind in the differential diagnosis of occupational pulmonary disease.

Upper gastrointestinal tract (gastro-oesophageal reflux)

Aspiration of oesophageal contents has been recognized for years as a cause of pneumonia, bronchiectasis, lung abscess and diffuse (often progressive) pulmonary fibrosis (Belcher, 1949; Belsey, 1960; Hiebert and Belsey, 1961; Pearson and Wilson, 1971). In this connection Barrett, in 1964, wrote that: 'oesophageal and pulmonary diseases are occasionally associated, and quite often neither the patient nor the doctor appreciates that there is a

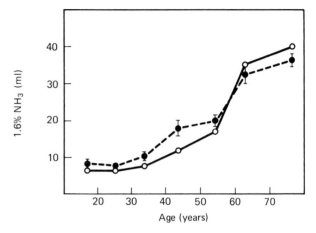

Figure 6.1 Graph showing the decline, in older age groups, of sensitivity of the laryngeal airway to inhalations of 1.6% ammonia gas. The age is the mean for each of the seven age groups and the volume of ammonia is that necessary to check respiration sufficiently to show on spirometer record. ----● Mean curve; —○ median curve; I standard error of the mean. (Reproduced, with permission, from Pontoppidan and Beecher, 1960)

connection.' Gastro-oesophageal reflux is now known to be a common cause of respiratory symptoms and disease, including some cases of intrinsic asthma (Allen and Newhouse, 1984) and of chronic cough without evident pulmonary disease (Irwin and Curley, 1989).

Gastro-oesophageal reflux, whether noticed or not, occurs intermittently in many normal individuals but rarely during recumbency or sleep, and causes no complications (DeMeester et al., 1980). But in patients who have abnormal or inappropriate relaxation of the lower oesophageal sphincter, with or without associated hiatus hernia, 24-hour pH monitoring of the oesophagus shows that reflux occurs more often in the supine position and at night, and may continue for as long as 40 minutes (DeMeester et al., 1976; Jenkinson et al., 1990). Reflux is often, but not always, associated with heartburn. A relationship between chronic bronchopulmonary disease and recurrent gastro-oesophageal reflux is doubted by some clinicians in the belief either that the association is coincidental or that it is improbable that irritant gastric contents can pass the protective laryngeal reflex without provoking obvious symptoms – in particular, paroxysmal coughing. But this reflex is depressed during sleep and is increasingly less active in subjects over 40 years of age (Figure 6.1) when reflux tends to be more prevalent (Pontoppidan and Beecher, 1960), and, as already noted, spontaneous cough is suppressed during deep sleep. Furthermore, the acidity of gastric contents tends to be reduced by saliva, although this is suppressed during sleep.

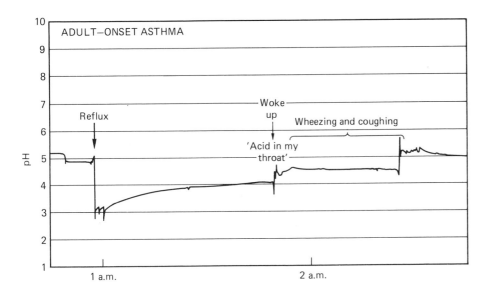

Figure 6.2 Part of a 24-hour oesophageal pH monitoring record in a patient with asthma, showing reflux of gastric juice into the oesophagus during the night, signified by a drop of oesophageal pH from 5 to 3 with a gradual return to pH 5. After this prolonged reflux, during which the patient was supine, she awoke, complained of an acid taste, and started wheezing and coughing. Asthma lasted 35 minutes. (Reproduced, with permission, from DeMeester et al., 1980)

Patients with oesophagopharyngeal regurgitation (the symptoms of which are awareness of spontaneous movement of fluid from the oesophagus to the pharynx, often at night, without associated belching, vomiting, choking or any other warning) have hypotensive lower and upper oesphageal sphincters, diminished response of the upper oesophageal sphincter to intraoesophageal fluid and reduction of peristaltic amplitude. Thus, there is failure of several of the normal barriers against regurgitation (Gerhardt et al., 1980). Relaxation of the lower oesophageal sphincter and reflux occur during transient arousals and longer periods of wakefulness but not during stable sleep (Dent et al., 1980). Yet symptoms of aspiration are often absent. The development of a reliable technique for prolonged (24 hours) recording of intraoesophageal pH has made it possible to identify a potential relationship between abnormal gastro-oesophageal reflux and respiratory symptoms. Symptomless reflux has been found in 21 per cent of patients with chronic cough (Irwin et al., 1988) and in 75 per cent of patients with chronic hoarseness (Castell, 1989). Symptomless ('silent') aspiration was demonstrated with reasonable certainty by radio-isotopic 'tagging' of gastric contents in affected patients before they retired to bed, followed by scanning of their lungs; overnight intraoesophageal pH monitoring confirmed prolonged episodes of reflux (Reich et al., 1977; Chernow et al., 1979). This finding is consistent with the observations of Power et al. (1984) cited earlier.

Because repeated small aspirations tend to escape notice for years, related pulmonary fibrosis occurs insidiously (Iverson, May and Samson, 1973).

Oesophageal reflux is believed to occur in about 50 per cent of asthmatic adults (Allen and Newhouse, 1984). A causal effect is established when – as has been shown – intermittent episodes of asthma are regularly associated with a fall of intraoesophageal pH to less than 4.0 and are directly related to nocturnal wheezing occurring during sleep (Castell, 1989) (Figure 6.2). Even short-lived oesophageal acidification can provoke increased hyperreactivity of the airways in asthmatic and non-asthmatic subjects (Rauscher, Popp and Ritschka, 1989). This relationship is also supported by long-term relief of asthma by treatment with cimetidine or surgical correction of gastro-oesophageal reflux (Larrain et al., 1981; Perrin-Fayolle et al., 1989). Whether asthma is caused by aspiration or by stimulation of vagal afferent arcs in the oesophagus with resultant reflex bronchoconstriction via vagal efferent arcs in the airways (Mansfield and Stein, 1978), or by both, remains to be established. However, although reflux is evidently capable of provoking asthma, this effect appears to be limited to periods of recumbency and sleep and to be absent during waking hours (Orr, Johnson and Robinson, 1984; Ekström and Tibbling, 1989); of course, not all patients with nocturnal asthma have reflux nor do all those with reflux have nocturnal asthma (Ekström and Tibbling, 1988).

Thus, gastro-oesophageal reflux should be suspected as a possible 'aetiological factor in the patient with intrinsic asthma with recurring nocturnal bronchospasm or tracheitis, or both, particularly if symptoms of heartburn and regurgitation have preceded the development of asthma' (Castell, 1989). This applies equally to the differential diagnosis of suspected occupational asthma which is also often nocturnal, that is, of delayed onset at the end of the working day (see Chapter 21).

There is evidence that an important factor in the inappropriate relaxation of the lower oesophageal sphincter – the fundamental cause of gastro-oesophageal reflux – may be vagal dysfunction which tends to increase with age (Ogilvie, James and Atkinson, 1985). It is significant, therefore, that the sphincter is relaxed by anticholinergic drugs, xanthine bronchodilators, such as theophylline, most sedatives and cigarette smoking (Dennish and Castell, 1971). Hence, treatment of airways' obstruction may exacerbate gastro-oesophageal reflux.

Other causes of repeated, frequently occult, aspiration of oesophageal contents include achalasia of the cardia, Zenker's diverticulum and systemic sclerosis. In systemic sclerosis it may contribute to the pulmonary fibrosis that is often associated with the disorder (see Chapter 15).

Conclusion

There is, then, strong evidence that recurrent aspiration of secretions from the upper respiratory tract and gastric contents from the oesophagus can and does occur, is fairly common (especially in older people) and can escape notice, so that related pulmonary fibrosis develops insidiously. Therefore, enquiry into these possibilities should never be omitted or be superficial when taking a history, simply because the patient is suspected of having an occupational respiratory disease; they can, as has been shown, cause chronic cough and sputum, asthmatic syndromes and unilateral or bilateral pulmonary fibrosis. The question of pulmonary fibrosis is discussed in Chapter 15.

Connective tissue (collagen vascular) disorders

Examples of these disorders that frequently involve the lungs or pleura, or both, and may cause dyspnoea on exertion and, to a lesser degree, cough and pain in the chest are: sarcoidosis, rheumatoid disease (with or without arthropathy), Sjögren's disease, systemic lupus erythematosus, polymyositis/dermatomysotitis and systemic sclerosis and its CREST variants – *c*alcinosis, *R*aynaud's phenomenon, *o*esophageal dysfunction, *s*clerodactyly and

*t*elangiectasia, the E representing the American spelling of oesophagus. The association of Raynaud's disease and some of these disorders and diffuse interstitial pulmonary fibrosis (DIPF) is referred to in Chapter 15 ('Associated disorders'). Rheumatoid arthritis has a genetic component and is strongly related to HLA-DR4 (Koenig and Omenn, 1988). It may be associated with diffuse interstitial pulmonary fibrosis (see Chapter 15), bilateral thickening of the pleura, pleural effusion and, as noted in Chapter 10, with chronic obstructive disease of the airways which also appears to be genetically determined.

Although not a connective tissue disorder, inflammatory bowel disease (IBD) – Crohn's disease and ulcerative colitis – is, in a significant number of patients, associated with chronic cough, chronic bronchial suppuration, airways' obstruction (not caused by smoking), reduced gas transfer, and DIPF or bilateral apical pulmonary fibrosis (Hood and Mason, 1970; Meadway, 1974; Higenbottam et al., 1980; Butland et al., 1981; Heatley et al., 1982); there is also an association between ulcerative colitis and pulmonary vasculitis (Forrest and Shearman, 1975). Although sulphasalazine, in the treatment of IBD, can cause inflammatory reactions in the airways and alveoli due to an idiosyncratic response (Tydd and Dyer, 1976), this does not explain the occurrence of these disorders with IBD. That there is such an association should not, perhaps, be unexpected in so far as the non-specific inflammatory changes found below the bronchial epithelium are similar to those under the colonic epithelium in ulcerative colitis (Kirsner, 1970), and lymphocytes sensitized to antigens at one mucosal site tend to circulate and localize at another in the common, mucosal immunological system (Bienenstock et al., 1978) (see Chapter 1). DIPF also occurs in some cases of coeliac disease (Hood and Mason, 1970), a point that is discussed further in Chapter 20 (page 691).

Abnormalities of the thoracic cage

Kyphoscoliosis, ankylosing spondylitis and rheumatoid arthritis cause stiffness of the rib cage with reduction of vital capacity and total lung capacity in advanced disease, and, ultimately, in the case of ankylosing spondylitis, complete rigidity of the cage. As a result, there is apt to be a significant increase in the work of breathing (Bergofsky, 1979). In rheumatoid arthritis in which the costovertebral and costosternal joints are often involved there is, in addition to reduction of total lung capacity, a significant reduction in compliance of the rib cage and impaired expansion of its volume in the absence of disease of the lungs and pleura (Bégin et al., 1988). This situation has to be kept in mind when assessing the significance of dyspnoea or impairment of lung function in cases where one of these abnormalities is accompanied by a work-related respiratory disorder. It must also be remembered that there is an association – undoubtedly underestimated – between ankylosing spondylitis (even when mild) and bilateral fibrosis of the upper lobes of the lungs, sometimes with cavities (Davies, 1972; Hillerdal, 1983).

Past injury to the chest, apart from fractured ribs, may result in unilateral or bilateral thickening of the pleura, the sequela of haemothorax. Injury may affect the conformation and expansion of the chest.

Family history

Ill-health in the family may be of considerable importance. For example: tuberculosis and rheumatoid arthritis, and other connective tissue disorders with a genetic component; familial emphysema and pulmonary fibrosis. Atopy – defined as the propensity to produce IgE in response to common, usually inhaled, allergens and manifested clinically as conjunctivitis, rhinitis or asthma – is transmitted as an autosomal dominant inheritance apparently under the control of a single gene locus, although additional factors (possibly histocompatibility variability or environmental) determine the type and severity of the clinical disease (Hopkin, 1990). Gastro-oesophageal reflux may also be familial due to an autosomal dominant mode of inheritance, often with a long pedigree (Leung, 1988).

Occupations of the family may sometimes be relevant in that one of its members may have habitually returned home in work clothes contaminated, for example, by asbestos, beryllium compounds or allergenic materials such as isocyanate compounds.

Thus, an informed family history may point to the nature of the worker's disease; if, however, it is inadequate or neglected (because an occupational explanation dominates the clinician's mind), temporary or even permanent misdiagnosis may be the consequence.

History of previous illness

A comprehensive history is as important in occupational medical consultations as in those in respiratory medicine in general for, in both, the explanation of much, if not all, of the present disease may be respiratory illness in the past. The chronology of events and the type and duration of treatment must be as accurate as possible; this is assisted by obtaining, whenever possible, past medical records, radiographs and other data.

Careful enquiry into the following details is the minimum required for the identification and evaluation of relevant past disease, on the one hand, or for its exclusion, on the other.

1. Childhood illnesses, including recurrent or chronic rhinosinusitis, chest infections, pulmonary tuberculosis, adenoids and eczema.
2. Illnesses of adolescence and adult life: atopic disorders – urticaria, contact dermatitis, allergic rhinitis, asthma and angioneurotic oedema; upper respiratory tract disease – injury to the nose, chronic infection and postnasal 'drip', and nasal polyposis; pneumonia or pleurisy – whether or not recurrent, and the side or sides affected; recurrent 'bronchitis' or chest infections – whether seasonal, wheezy, productive of purulent or clear sputum, and degree of severity; tuberculosis and type of treatment; gastro-oesophageal reflux; rheumatoid arthritis – which has a significant association with pleural effusion, pleural thickening, DIPF, bronchiolitis obliterans and also bronchiectasis (Solanski and Neville, 1990); and injury to the chest – how sustained, site, severity and whether or not associated with dyspnoea.
3. Drugs used in the treatment of various non-respiratory disorders, and occasionally the cause of pleuropulmonary disease, must always be kept in mind and, when appropriate, carefully enquired about (see Chapter 15).

Current medical history

Symptoms, subjective sensations, differ qualitatively and quantitatively according to whether individuals are being examined as members of a working population or are patients in a hospital or clinic. In the former group, symptoms are likely to be absent or slight but, for various reasons, when present, may not be recounted freely or accurately, whereas in the latter group they are, on the whole, readily volunteered. Thus, answers to questionnaires presented to a workforce may not always be valid. Direct or leading questions can result in invalid deductions which may have important epidemiological as well as clinical implications. In some circumstances, during medical consultations, leading questions are necessary but only after ample opportunity has been given for spontaneous answers to circuitous questions. Furthermore, standardized questionnaires – which are often not appropriate in all parts of the world – should be addressed specifically to the population and work hazard under investigation. Questions, for example, about the occurrence of cough and sputum 'in the winter' as originally posed in the Medical Research Council (1976) questionnaire – but now modified (1986) – are meaningless in many regions (see also Chapter 9). This chapter, however, is concerned with the clinical approach; epidemiological implications are considered in Chapter 8.

Specific symptoms

In many cases of occupational disease there are no respiratory symptoms, but when there are they usually include one or more of the following: cough, sputum, wheeze and dyspnoea on exertion. These symptoms, however, may also be due to non-occupational disease coincident with the occupational disorder, or mistaken for it. An informed history can help to put the clinician on the right track at the outset.

Upper respiratory tract

It is essential to establish the presence or absence of symptoms of rhinosinusitis: namely, mucoid or purulent nasal discharge; awareness of discharge in the back of the throat (postnasal 'drip'), especially when recumbent and on rising in the mornings; nasal obstruction, bilateral or unilateral; and whether persistent throughout the year or intermittent or seasonal. Sneezing, itching and headache may also be complained of. But, equally, the possibility that rhinitis might be due to exposure to some dust, fume or vapour at work rather than being non-occupational must not be overlooked.

Cough

When chronic cough is admitted, details of its type and pattern must be obtained; they often help to identify its cause. The necessary details include: (1) how long it has been present; (2) when it occurs – in the morning on waking, throughout the day, day and night or only at night; (3) if at night, whether or not it is provoked or relieved by recumbency or change in position; (4) its frequency; (5) whether or not it is paroxysmal; (6) whether or not it is provoked by exertion or change in ambient temperature; and (7) the presence or absence of sputum.

Cough is a reflex response to irritation of receptor nerves in a variety of anatomical sites: larynx, trachea and bronchi; pericardium and diaphragm; pharynx; nose and paranasal sinuses; and eustachian (pharyngotympanic) canals and ears (Irwin, Rosen and Braman, 1977). Although usually attributable to a single cause, there are, in many cases, multiple

causes (Irwin, 1989); however, a frequent overriding factor, both in occupational groups and in individuals, is smoking. The most common causes of chronic, non-specific cough are reported to be postnasal 'drip', asthma, chronic bronchitis and gastro-oesophageal reflux (Irwin, Carrao and Pratter, 1981; Ing, Ngu and Breslin, 1991).

The association of cough with disease of the upper respiratory tract has already been referred to.

Patients should be asked, as a matter of routine, about their habitual sleeping posture for this is often relevant to the occurrence of cough, production of sputum or development of wheeze at nights and may suggest that the cause of predominantly unilateral parenchymal disease of the lungs is chronic aspiration.

In general, the earlier stages of occupational disorders are not associated with cough, but the more advanced stages of (for example) silicosis, coal pneumoconiosis and diffuse interstitial pulmonary fibrosis of asbestos, extrinsic allergic alveolitis or chronic beryllium disease may be. Severe, paroxysmal cough may be a feature in some cases of chronic beryllium disease. Intermittent episodes of cough – especially on exertion or at night – may be a variant of asthma (whether occupational or non-occupational) in the absence of other overt symptoms or reduction in ventilatory capacity (Carrao, Braman and Irwin, 1979). This can usually be simply identified if the cough is rapidly relieved by a therapeutic trial with a bronchodilator drug (Lowell, 1979).

A quantitative index of the frequency or severity of cough is important in occupational and other environmental studies, and is referred to in the next section.

The fact that cough is sometimes of psychological origin – an acquired tic or habit – should not be forgotten.

Sputum

Apart from work-related asthma and chronic bronchitis, occupational respiratory diseases, on the whole, produce little or no sputum. Thus, with these exceptions, frequent or persistent sputum usually has some other cause.

Therefore, patients must always be asked whether or not they have sputum and, if so, when it occurs: only with 'colds', seasonally or throughout the year. When, in the 24-hour period, is it most frequent: after getting up in the morning or, if at night, is it influenced by position at rest or a change in position? Is it mucoid or purulent and associated with symptoms of rhinosinusitis or postnasal 'drip'? Thick and tenacious mucoid sputum is produced in some cases of asthma and occasionally in asbestosis and diffuse interstitial fibrosis from other causes, although, in these disorders, it is frequently absent.

In studies of occupational groups an objective index of the production of sputum may be important. This can be achieved by the 'loose cough sign' in which the subject is instructed to take a deep breath and cough hard, the cough being judged to be productive ('loose') or unproductive ('dry') by its sound (Hall and Gandevia, 1971). The test has the advantage of being simple and quick and has been validated by reference to measurements of volume of sputum; it has also been related to the distribution of grades of severity of cough (Field, 1974). However, it is possible that, in some subjects, loose cough, though present early in the day, may be absent later. Thus, it would seem advisable to perform the test at the same time of day in follow-up studies of the same group. The 'loose cough sign' may sometimes occur in the absence of sputum (Forgacs, 1978a).

Haemoptysis rarely occurs in patients with chronic fibrotic occupational diseases unless caused by some other pathological process. It is, however, fairly common (with frothy sputum) in acute pulmonary oedema which can be caused by a variety of irritant gases that may be encountered accidentally in the workplace: ammonia, chlorine, titanium tetrachloride, acrolein and trimellitic anhydride, to name but a few. It can occur in acute pneumonitis due to exposure to beryllium or cadmium fumes, and, on occasion, to extrinsic allergic alveolitis; in infections such as brucellosis and psittacosis; and with physical stresses such as pulmonary barotrauma and high altitude sickness (see relevant chapters).

Wheeze

Often this symptom is not volunteered spontaneously except in severe, episodic asthma. It is, of course, usually a manifestation of obstruction to airflow in the lower respiratory tract and, apart from asthma, may be complained of by some patients with chronic bronchitis. But patients may use the term 'wheeze' for bubbling or rattling sounds caused by excessive secretion in the airways; this difficulty is resolved by clinical examination of the lungs. Apart from asthma and acute exposure to irritant gases, occupational respiratory diseases rarely cause *symptomatic* wheezing.

If wheezing is complained of, it is necessary to establish under what circumstances it occurs. Is it continuous, day and night? If present only during the day, does it happen at work and, if so, at what stage during the shift? If at night, is it affected by recumbency; are there symptoms of oesophageal–pharyngeal regurgitation? Is it associated with dyspnoea and, if so, is breathing normal when there is no wheeze? The fact that wheeze may be complained of in left ventricular heart failure ('cardiac asthma') must not be forgotten.

Not infrequently, when patients do not complain of wheeze, it is evident on auscultation (see page 147).

Pain

Pain in the chest is not a feature of occupational respiratory disease other than that which may be associated with severe acute tracheobronchitis due to accidental exposure to noxious gases or with (usually) unilateral malignancies such as mesothelioma or carcinoma of the lung.

Discomfort or aching in the chest wall, which is commonly bilateral and sometimes referred to as pain by the patient, may be caused by intercostal muscle strain or 'cramps' in individuals with severe dyspnoea, and is often a feature of the 'hyperventilation syndrome'.

Dyspnoea

Breathlessness – the most common symptom of respiratory disease – is a subjective sensation of discomfort caused by a need for increased respiratory effort to a point beyond which it obtrudes unpleasantly into consciousness. It may be acute and episodic, as in asthma, and sometimes nocturnal; or chronic on effort only; or continuous, though worsened by effort. It encompasses various sensations – not merely degree of intensity – which include the feeling of being 'out of breath', inability to take in a full breath, tightness or constriction of the chest, and hunger for more air. It is likely that these sensations are mediated by different physiological mechanisms (Simon et al., 1989).

A variety of disorders other than pleuropulmonary disease may cause dyspnoea and must not be forgotten: obesity and acquired heart disease; metabolic disturbances such as hyperthyroidism and the acidosis of diabetes mellitus or uraemia; anaemia; abnormalities of the thoracic cage, referred to earlier; or it may be psychogenic in origin. Extrathoracic and non-occupational pulmonary causes of dyspnoea, therefore, must be identified and evaluated. Not infrequently one or other of these disorders turns out to be the reason for breathlessness in some individuals with occupational disease.

Impairment (or insufficiency) of any of the components of respiratory function tests is not necessarily associated with respiratory disability – that is, dyspnoea of greater or lesser degree; the two must be clearly distinguished. *Respiratory insufficiency* consists of unsatisfactory performance of one or more tests of respiratory function, whereas *respiratory disability* can be defined as incapacity for competent performance of exercise or effort.

To estimate the degree or severity of shortness of breath the mode of questioning differs according to whether individual patients or members of an occupational population are being examined. In the clinical situation the type and order of questions asked usually have to be varied from patient to patient, according to the way they respond, with the aim of determining the timing and periodicity of dyspnoea, its relationship to effort and comparison with the capacity of other people of the same age and sex under similar conditions. By contrast, in the assessment of breathlessness in an occupational group it is necessary, as far as possible, to eliminate differences in the answers to questions recorded by different observers. To this end some form of standard questionnaire of fixed, graded questions (such as that of the Medical Research Council, 1986) is generally employed. An alternative method with, apparently, good discriminatory capacity, is the simple 'line test' described by Gandevia (1981). One end of a 10-cm line represents extreme breathlessness (0), and the other completely normal breathing (100). Subjects mark their position on the line which is ranked arbitrarily into five grades of dyspnoea. Grading results have been found to correlate well with FEV_1 values in healthy workers and in patients with chronic respiratory disease. The correlation between the symptom of breathlessness and ventilatory function tests, however, is weaker in restrictive than in obstructive pulmonary disease.

When the question of occupational asthma (including byssinosis) is being investigated, a more elaborate form of questioning is required. In this respect it should be noted that, following exposure to a provocative agent, dyspnoea – often with wheeze – may occur within a few minutes (*immediate asthma*) or be delayed for between 1 and 12 hours – usually about 5 hours (*late* or *non-immediate asthma*) – and, therefore, develops mostly at night. Occasionally, late asthma recurs on three or four successive nights without further exposure (see Chapter 21).

Psychological factors

These must also be considered in assessing shortness of breath. Personality and attitude to ill-health – especially when this is attributed, rightly or wrongly, to occupational disease – influence the response of individuals to the subjective experiences of dyspnoea, and the level of their awareness of it. A display of breathlessness, for example, may be suspended during voluble declamation about symptoms, only to return as soon as the recital ends. Mental attitude may affect capacity for exercise, clinical grade of breathlessness and performance of such tests as peak expiratory flow rate (PEFR), forced expiratory volume in 1 second (FEV_1) and forced vital capacity (FVC) (King and Cotes, 1989).

Other tests that rely less on effort and co-operation may be needed to identify impaired function of psychogenic origin, although, on the whole, inappropriate performance of FEV_1 (often with exaggerated reactions) can usually be recognized from the appearance of the spirometry curves. Fear of life-threatening disease – especially among those who have been exposed to asbestos in the past – may be engendered by irresponsible and sensational publicity, by inept medical management or advice, or by involvement in litigation which usually demands multiple medical examinations. The *hyperventilation syndrome* – or 'psychogenic dyspnoea' – is comprised of these features, often with dizziness, paraesthesiae in the hands and feet, painful cramps of the limbs caused by alkalosis resulting from reduced carbon dioxide tension, and pains of muscular origin in the chest (Pincus, 1978). The syndrome is fairly common. Gandevia (1990), for example, has observed it 'in nearly 10 per cent of private patients, 15 per cent of hospital patients and 30 per cent of medico-legal cases'. It may be associated with, or superimposed upon, the dyspnoea of airways' obstruction and, when it occurs during exercise, often results in the patient's dependence upon a bronchodilator aerosol. Urgent and inappropriate resort to such an aerosol during medical interview is diagnostic (Gandevia, 1990). Abnormal hyperventilation may occur not only at rest but also, in some individuals, during exercise (Howell, 1990). Often, however, the complete syndrome does not develop and anxiety may be well disguised; careful clinical appraisal and evaluation of pulmonary function is needed to identify the disorder which, once established, may be difficult to eradicate.

Howell (1990) has given a valuable review of the syndrome under the title 'behavioural breathlessness'.

Tightness of the chest sometimes accompanies shortness of breath, especially when this is acute. The sensation is associated with disease of the lower airways, asthma in particular. It has a vague but more 'internal' localization than the feeling of inability to breathe in 'enough air' as may occur, for example, in cardiac, neurological or restrictive pulmonary disease (Widdicombe, 1979). A sensation of constriction of the lower part of the chest is an early symptom of decompression sickness (see Chapters 24 and 25).

Physical examination

In many cases of occupational disease there are no abnormal physical signs but, when present, they are often due to non-occupational disease. Nevertheless, it is essential, for accurate differential diagnosis, that anyone suspected of, or known to have, an occupational disorder be examined carefully and systemically according to the classic quaternity of inspection, palpation, percussion and auscultation, skills that have been allowed to wane in recent years (Spiteri, Cook and Clarke, 1988).

To begin with, the presence of anaemia, cyanosis (central or peripheral), nasal abnormality, noisy breathing, clubbing of the fingers, rheumatoid arthritis or other connective tissue disorders, and thoracic abnormality should be noted.

Digital clubbing

Apart from some cases of asbestosis and chronic beryllium disease, occupational respiratory disease is infrequently associated with clubbing. Its importance, when present, is that it is more likely to indicate some other disease.

Clubbing (which also affects the toes but is not always recognized as readily as in the fingers) commences simultaneously and progresses uniformly in all digits and, in its early stage, consists of thickening of the nail bed and filling-in of the angle between the nail and nail bed. There is increased longitudinal curvature of the nail and, when advanced, bulbous swelling of the finger tips with pronounced fluctuation and thickening of the nail beds, which may be shiny and red. When clubbing is not advanced, there often is substantial interobserver variation as to its presence or absence, making reports of its prevalence of limited value. Clubbing is said to be present when the hyponychial angle is 195 degrees or more (Regan, Tagg and Thomson, 1967). A simple shadowgraph method for recording its presence and change in severity with the passage of time has been devised (Bentley, Moore and Schwachman, 1976) but, unfortunately, is little used. Even if clubbing is absent at the first examination, it must always be looked for and assessed at all subsequent, routine examinations.

In addition to the well-known causes, clubbing, often severe and progressive, occurs in about 75 per cent of cases of idiopathic diffuse interstitial pulmonary fibrosis (DIPF) – cryptogenic fibrosing alveolitis (CFA) – whether 'lone' or with connective tissue disorders; but, contrary to the widely held belief, clubbing is uncommon in asbestosis and, when it does occur, is usually of mild degree. Indeed, it can be said that clubbing of a moderate-to-severe degree suggests that pulmonary disease is not occupational or that, if it is, there is some coincident complicating disorder – such as carcinoma of the lung. Clubbing may also be familial, being inherited as an autosomal dominant trait with incomplete penetrance, especially in females (Talbot and Montgomery, 1953; Curth, Firschein and Alpert,

1961; Fischer, Singer and Feldman, 1964), and is usually present shortly after birth. It is often found in the absence of accompanying disease, so that, when present, pulmonary disease may be coincidental; in fact, genetic predisposition may explain why clubbing associated with certain acquired diseases occurs only in some patients and not in others (Schneerson, 1981).

Hypertrophic osteoarthropathy, which appears to be a separate entity (Schneerson, 1981), is not associated with occupational pulmonary disease, but may occur coincidently. Thus, it is important to recall that it can closely resemble rheumatoid arthritis especially when the wrists and ankles are affected. Radiology of the joints may be needed for definitive differentiation.

Digital vasculitis

The white fingers of Raynaud's disease, sometimes with the features of digital vasculitis (painful fissures or ulcers of the digits), are seen in some patients with DIPF and systemic lupus erythematosus, rheumatoid arthritis or systemic sclerosis and, occasionally, with 'lone' idiopathic DIPF (Hodson et al., 1984) (see also Chapter 15, page 511).

Upper respiratory tract

To quote Davidson (1935) again: '... *no examination of the chest can be regarded as complete without an examination of the region of the nose and throat*' [his emphasis]. This should be evident from what has been said in Chapters 1 and 3 and earlier in this chapter, and it applies to all individuals with suspected bronchopulmonary disease, be it occupational or non-occupational.

The obvious is often ignored: for example, nasal voice, snuffling, predominance of breathing through the mouth, and the external appearance of the nose; deviation of the septum to right or left (commonly the result of past injury) which is frequently associated with severe, usually unilateral, nasal obstruction and chronic rhinitis. Some other common causes of chronic bilateral or unilateral obstruction have already been referred to. The simple manoeuvre of getting the patient to inhale briskly, with closed mouth, first through one nostril and then the other while the opposite nostril is compressed shut with the examiner's finger, indicates the presence of significant obstruction (in the absence of acute infection) and whether this is bilateral or unilateral, partial or complete.

Both nasal airways should be inspected and the naso- and oropharynx examined for adenoids and enlarged tonsils, and its mucosa for the 'cobble-stone' appearance, caused by inflamed submucosal lymph follicles, that is often associated with postnasal 'drip'.

Such limited, but informative, routine examination is easily within the capability of every clinician. But when significant chronic disease of the nasal airways, accessory sinuses or nasopharynx is suspected, it is imperative that the patient is referred for expert otorhinological examination and assessment.

Peak inspiratory nasal flow rates and a nasal 'patency index' can be measured simply with a standard Vitalograph and have fairly good reproducibility (Eiser, 1990).

Lower respiratory tract

The general principles of inspection, palpation and percussion should be well known and will not be discussed here. It must not be forgotten, however, that persistent breathing through the mouth usually points to chronic nasal obstruction, and expiration through pursed lips (which reduces peak flow at the beginning, and increases flow rate at the end, of expiration), to emphysema. Auscultation, however, demands some attention (regrettably, not accorded to it in the earlier editions of this book) because it is commonly neglected or ill-understood, and is often performed as a perfunctory ritual, an ironic situation in view of its pre-eminence in thoracic medicine from Laënnec's time until the early 1950s – more than 130 years. This lapse is largely attributable to the ascendancy of physiological tests and radiological and other imaging techniques, compounded by a variegated and confused nomenclature of pulmonary sounds over many years, with the consequence that auscultation, despite its simplicity, is often considered to be of little practical value.

Advances in acoustic analysis of normal and abnormal breath sounds and of intrapulmonary adventitious sounds, and the adoption of a simple and valid nomenclature – first suggested by Robertson and Coope (1957) – by the American Thoracic Society (Cugell, 1987), have vindicated and emphasized their clinical importance. In this respect the technique of *time-expanded waveform analysis* has been invaluable. In essence, this consists of recording pulmonary sounds from various sites on the chest wall on magnetic tape and playing this at one-eighth to one-tenth of the speed of the original record, so that the waveforms are spread out and can thus be analysed individually (Murphy, Holford and Knowler, 1977) (Figure 6.3). More recently, computed fast Fourier transformation techniques

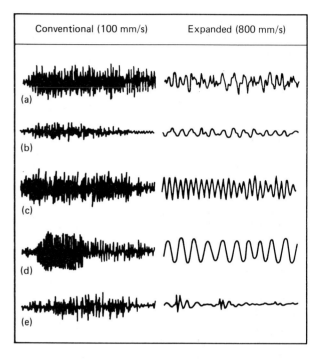

Figure 6.3 Normal and abnormal lung sounds, recorded at conventional trace speed on the left and time-expanded speed on the right. The latter reveals distinct patterns that are not obvious in the former. (a) Normal tracheal inspiration; (b) normal vesicular inspiratory sound; (c) wheeze; (d) rhonchus; (e) inspiratory crackles at posterior lung base. (Modified, with permission, from Murphy, Holford and Knowler, 1977)

(enabling the frequency components to be separated into discrete samples as a histogram spectrum) have been used to analyse the frequencies of the sounds (Stoneman, Parker and Jones, 1989). Although most of the acoustic features revealed by such methods cannot be appreciated by ear, they assist greatly in understanding the sounds heard by clinical auscultation. It is likely, however, that in the very near future, rapid 'on-line' analysis using microcomputers will make these refined techniques readily available clinically and in the field, with the provision of permanent records.

Normal breath sounds

In normal individuals at rest, breath sounds at the mouth are quiet and their frequencies appear to range from about 200 to 2000 Hz. The quality of normal breath sounds in the lungs varies according to the area of the chest where they are heard. Over the trachea, where 'bronchial' or 'tubular' type sounds are heard, their frequencies lie between the threshold of audibility (about 30 Hz) and more than 1000 Hz, and there is a pause between inspiration and expiration.

The mechanism by which normal breath sounds are generated and transmitted in the lungs is complex and incompletely explained. Turbulence of air in larger airways (main, lobar and segmental bronchi) is believed to be their chief source. Sound produced in the trachea is transmitted towards the mouth and, in airways below the trachea, radiates in all directions (Olson and Hammersley, 1985); but, as the lung acts as a low-pass filter and removes the higher frequencies, the normal spectrum of frequencies of the sounds at the chest wall ('vesicular sounds') has been reported to be approximately 100 to 500 Hz with little energy over 500 Hz (Kraman, 1985a). But Ploysongsang, Iyer and Ramamoorthy (1990) have shown that the components of the sound energy of both inspiratory and expiratory breath sounds at the chest wall are similar regardless of the filtering techniques used and, for the most part, are concentrated below 200 Hz, peak power being about 80 to 90 Hz. There is experimental evidence that sound is propagated through the lungs via a longer route (the airways) than a straight transit line between source and receiver but that it changes to parenchymal propagation at airways of approximately 1 to 2 mm diameter (Rice, 1982, 1983). Although airflow in peripheral airways is thought to be laminar and, as such, silent, vesicular sounds may be generated in these airways by some mechanism other than turbulence (Kraman, 1985a). Indeed, the observations of Ploysongsang, Iyer and Ramamoorthy (1990) suggest that both inspiratory and expiratory vesicular sounds are produced in peripheral airways by the same mechanism – whatever that may be.

The important point, however, is that the intensity of vesicular sounds is broadly proportional to regional distribution of ventilation of the underlying lung (Leblanc, Macklem and Ross, 1970; Ploysongsang, 1985); indeed, the amplitude of normal sounds at the chest wall has been found to be directly proportional to the square of overall airflow at the mouth (Shykoff, Ploysongsang and Chang, 1988). Bohadana, Peslin and Uffholtz (1978) showed that, in patients with varying degrees of airflow obstruction, the correlation of intensity of vesicular sounds (assessed clinically) between different examiners and with four indices of airflow velocity was good.

Interestingly, in asthmatic subjects, contrary to current medical understanding, the dominant frequency of breath sounds recorded at the mouth shifts from *lower* to *higher* frequencies before and after treatment with salbutamol, for example, from about 1000 Hz to 2500 Hz, respectively. But this is not detectable using the stethoscope over the lungs owing to the attenuation of the frequencies of the acoustic signal beyond about 2000 Hz during its passage to the chest wall (Stoneman, Parker and Jones, 1989).

In spite of the fact that no more than a weak relationship between intensity of vesicular sounds and regional ventilation has been demonstrated so far by scientific studies, clinical assessment of the intensity of these sounds – which are readily heard through the stethoscope when above about 200 Hz (Kraman, 1985a) – gives valuable information as to whether or not regional ventilation is present and about the severity of airflow obstruction (Ploysongsang, 1985). However, the clinician must constantly be aware that, among healthy subjects of similar bodily habitus, vesicular sounds differ significantly in loudness and, in some individuals, may have an irregular distribution of loudness in different locations on the chest wall (Kraman, 1985a). The reason for this discordancy is uncertain but may be explained, at least in part, by differences in airflow turbulence and sound intensity between the upper and lower reaches of the trachea and the lobar bronchi (Olson and Hammersley, 1985).

Abnormal (adventitious) intrapulmonary sounds

These sounds, superimposed on breath sounds in certain conditions of health and disease, can, as Robertson and Coope (1957) suggested, be distinguished as *continuous* or *interrupted*. They occur in either or both phases of the respiratory cycle. 'Continuous' is taken to mean that the sounds last about 250 ms rather than continuing throughout the respiratory cycle (Loudon and Murphy, 1984), and the term 'interrupted' has now been replaced by *discontinuous*.

Continuous sounds

Wheezes and rhonchi

Continuous sounds having a musical quality, when high-pitched (high frequency), are usually referred to as *wheezes*, and when low-pitched, as *rhonchi* (Figure 6.4). However, in recent years the term 'rhonchus' has been used less in the UK than in North America and replaced by 'low-pitched wheeze'. Wheezes appear to be generated in large airways (main, lobar, segmental bronchi and, possibly, two or three more generations peripherally) narrowed to the point where they are near closure and caused to oscillate by jets of air, the velocity of which at the site of closure largely determines their pitch (Forgacs, 1978a). They are transmitted along the airways to the chest wall, better than through the lung itself, the low-pass filter property of which

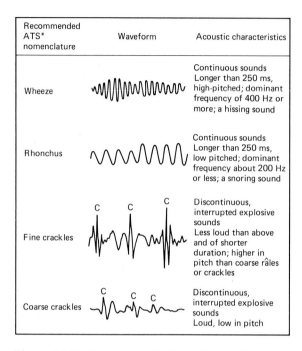

Recommended ATS* nomenclature	Waveform	Acoustic characteristics
Wheeze		Continuous sounds Longer than 250 ms, high-pitched; dominant frequency of 400 Hz or more; a hissing sound
Rhonchus		Continuous sounds Longer than 250 ms, low pitched; dominant frequency about 200 Hz or less; a snoring sound
Fine crackles	C C C	Discontinuous, interrupted explosive sounds Less loud than above and of shorter duration; higher in pitch than coarse râles or crackles
Coarse crackles	C C C	Discontinuous, interrupted explosive sounds Loud, low in pitch

Figure 6.4 Outline of classification of adventitious lung sounds. ATS = American Thoracic Society. (Modified, with permission, from Murphy, 1981)

removes most, if not all, of the higher frequencies before the chest wall is reached (Loudon and Murphy, 1984). *Thus, in suspected cases of asthma, auscultation over the trachea and at the mouth should be standard practice.* Wheezes generated in this way are constant in that they occur repeatedly in the same phase of respiration before and after coughing. Wheezes that are abolished by coughing are wholly or partly related to intraluminal secretions.

Rhonchi, or 'low-pitched wheezes', are usually associated with the production of sputum and may be caused by vibration of flaps of sputum in the air stream; they are cleared or altered by coughing (Murphy and Holford, 1980).

In addition, it should be noted that an uncommon, but important, cause of wheeze is dysfunction of the vocal folds of psychogenic origin, mostly in psychologically unstable women under 40 years of age – 'functional upper airway's obstruction' (Appelblatt and Baker, 1981). Physical signs that help in differentiation from asthma are rapid breathing at low lung volume, wheeze localized to the larynx and heard poorly over the lung fields and absence of hyperinflation. Lung function tests, when possible, show normal airways' resistance. Detection of hypoxia during acute episodes of wheezing distinguishes asthma from vocal fold dysfunction (Goldman and Muers, 1991).

Stridor

This is a loud, continuous sound of similar frequency range to asthmatic wheezing but differs in being more intense, of higher pitch, inspiratory rather than expiratory, and often out of phase with the respiratory cycle. Unlike wheezes, it is loudest at the mouth and inaudible over the lung fields (Forgacs, 1978a; Baughman and Loudon, 1989). Occupational causes of stridor include narrowing of the trachea or large bronchi by lymph nodes enlarged by silicosis or carcinoma of the lung, and sometimes, acutely, by inhalation of an irritant gas, such as ammonia, and by thermal injury from burns.

Discontinuous sounds

Discontinuous sounds, *crackles*, are non-musical, discrete, usually bilateral, explosive sounds, the individual components of which are less than 20 ms in duration, and range in frequency from 200 to 2000 Hz (Forgacs, 1978a). They may be inspiratory and repeated in succeeding inspirations, or expiratory and less often repetitive, or both. The American Thoracic Society nomenclature qualifies crackles as 'fine' (high-pitched) and 'coarse' (low-pitched) (Figure 6.4).

Inspiratory crackles

Time-expanded waveform analysis shows that individual inspiratory crackles – which appear as little more than straight vertical deflections on a conventional phonopneumogram – are transient deflections of some 10 ms which can be characterized by measuring the width of the initial wave deflection and the duration of the first two complete cycles (see Figures 6.3 and 6.4). The auscultatory impression that crackles are 'fine' or 'coarse' may, however, be influenced not only by their waveforms but also by the time interval between successive crackles (Morinari et al., 1980). As crackles span a continuum of sound from high to low pitch, 'medium' crackles with intermediate characteristics can also be expected and are often discernible clinically; they were, in fact, included in the schema proposed by Robertson and Coope (1957). Their acoustic characteristics differ from those of 'fine' and 'coarse' crackles, but their analysis is, as yet, incomplete (Murphy, 1985).

Apart from the bubbling sounds caused by voluminous secretions in larger airways, crackles are believed to be generated by energy released by sudden changes in the calibre of small airways. Individual inspiratory crackles recur at the same volume, or transpulmonary pressure, in each consecutive respiratory cycle (Nath and Capel, 1974a). The

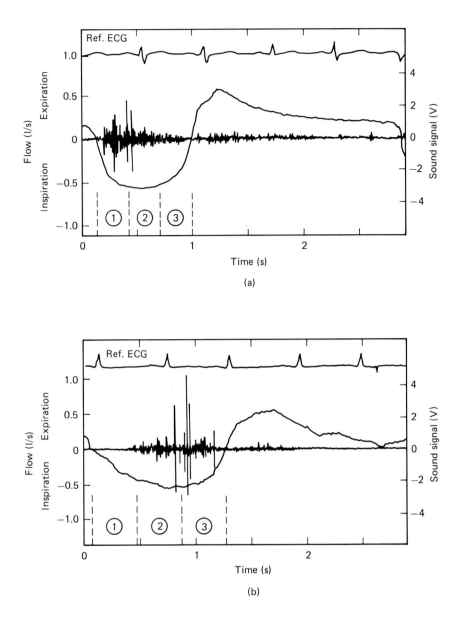

Figure 6.5 (a) Record of patient with chronic obstructive pulmonary disease. Early inspiratory crackles with early end-point of crackling and a short crackling period. In bronchiectasis crackles usually extend further into, and often throughout, mid-inspiration (see Figure 6.7). (b) Record of a patient with idiopathic DIPF (CFA). The peaks of the crackles are seen in the late phase of inspiration, beginning at the end of the mid-phase. There is a fairly long crackling period and late end-point of crackling. In these phonopneumographs inspiration is recorded as a negative, and expiration as a positive, deflection. (1), (2) and (3) indicate early, mid- and late inspiration respectively. (Adapted, with permission, from Piirilä et al., 1991)

most satisfactory explanation to date is that they are sound waves propagated in four directions, or poles (rather than as an expanding sphere), from a point-source in the airways. This so-called *stress–relaxation quadrupole* model is concerned solely with dynamic events that 'occur in or near the airway wall when elastic and surface forces are in transition between static equilibrium states' (Fredberg and Holford, 1983) and not with the dynamics of gas pressure in the airways following abrupt opening, as proposed by Forgacs (1978b). Significantly, the model indicates that the opening time of airways is related to their diameter: it predicts that fine inspiratory crackles originate from small airways (1 to 2 mm in

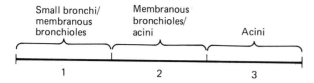

Figure 6.6 Arbitrary division of inspiration into three phases: (1) early, (2) mid and (3) late, and their relationship to the different sites of origin of crackles. (Adapted from Trail, 1948)

diameter) with higher opening pressures and that coarse inspiratory crackles come from larger airways (3 to 5 mm in diameter) at lower opening pressures. Fine crackles are likely to be more numerous than coarse because far more small than larger airways underlie any given site of auscultation on the chest wall (Fredberg and Holford, 1983).

The area of the chest wall covered by a single crackle appears to reflect the area of the lung surface supplied by the airway that generated the crackle. The largest area affected seems to be a very irregular circle with a radius of some 4 to 6 cm. Airways that supply this extent of surface area are in excess of 2 mm in diameter (Kraman, 1980). Experimental evidence that coarse crackles originate in the larger airways has been provided by Kunica et al. (1980). They made simultaneous recordings of fine and coarse crackles at two sites on the chest wall, 6 and 12 cm apart. Coarse crackles were more widely distributed than fine, being present at 6 cm separation in 86 per cent of recordings compared with fine crackles in 22 per cent; at 12 cm they were present, respectively, in 60 per cent and 6 per cent of recordings (see also Loudon and Murphy, 1984). These findings are consistent with the clinical fact that low-pitched, coarse crackles tend to occur earlier, and high-pitched crackles later, in inspiration (Nath and Capel, 1974b; Piirilä et al., 1991) (Figure 6.5).

It seems unlikely that inspiratory crackles are produced by airways more proximal than the peripheral generations of small bronchi. If inspiration is divided arbitrarily into three phases, as Trail (1948) suggested (Figure 6.6), predominance of crackles in the first phase, tailing off into the third, appears to correlate with disease of the smallest bronchi or membranous bronchioles, and predominance of crackles in the third phase, often starting in the second, with disease involving acinar units.

The closure and sudden reopening of small airways in localized areas of deflated (atelectatic) lung resulting in crackles is influenced by the effect of gravity. Thus, they are audible at the pulmonary bases of normal subjects in the upright position during the first few deep inspirations after a period of shallow breathing (that is, from residual volume)

(Workum et al., 1986), and after flight in pilots exposed to sustained positive acceleration in high performance aircraft. In the latter, following exposure, crackles are associated with bilateral, basal subsegmental collapse, both of which tend to clear after several deep inspirations although, in the absence of deep breathing, they can persist for up to 36 hours (Glaister, 1969, 1988) (see also Figure 24.5). Crackles have been shown, experimentally, to be produced by inflation of atelectatic lung (Ploysongsang and Schonfeld, 1980) and, pathologically, their timing appears to be related to the degree of localized atelectasis; the earlier they occur in inspiration, the more severe the atelectasis (Murphy, Del Bono and Davidson, 1989). Low-pitched coarse crackles may occur in the earlier phases of inspiration in chronic bronchitis, bronchiectasis, chronic bronchiolitis and bronchiolectasis (Nath and Capel, 1980) (Figure 6.7 and see Figure 6.5a), and higher-pitched fine crackles, in its mid- to later phases, in the early stage of lobar pneumonia and left ventricular failure. The end-point of crackles is significantly later in patients with idiopathic DIPF (CFA) than in those with bronchiectasis, chronic obstructive pulmonary disease and left ventricular failure (Figure 6.8) (Piirilä et al., 1991) Early inspiratory crackles are often well conducted to the mouth and their character is sometimes modified by cough (Figure 6.9); late crackles are neither heard at the mouth nor altered by cough.

Because of the gravitational effect on the generation of crackles, alteration in the patient's posture (by bending forwards, for example) may, according to the degree of pulmonary deflation, reduce or abolish those which are caused by left ventricular failure and, to a lesser degree, by DIPF in its early, but not in its more advanced, stages in the region of the lung which is uppermost when auscultated (Forgacs, 1974).

There may be some difference in pitch and predominant timing of the crackles of DIPF, depending upon its cause. In both DIPF, whether 'lone' or associated with connective tissue disease, and asbestosis, crackles are generally reported to be similarly fine, numerous and late in inspiration, although often paninspiratory in advanced disease (Forgacs, 1978; Loudon and Murphy, 1984). Reasons for reappraisal of this concept are discussed later. In chronic extrinsic allergic alveolitis, sarcoidosis and chronic beryllium disease, crackles, when they occur, are usually heard in the latter part of inspiration but may, in some cases, be early and of medium-to-coarse quality; in fibrosis associated with aspiration (for example, recurrent gastro-oesophageal reflux), crackles heard over affected areas of the lungs are paninspiratory and range from fine to coarse quality.

An inspiratory musical sound – described as a *squawk*, *squeak* or, by Forgacs (1967), *chirp* – occurs

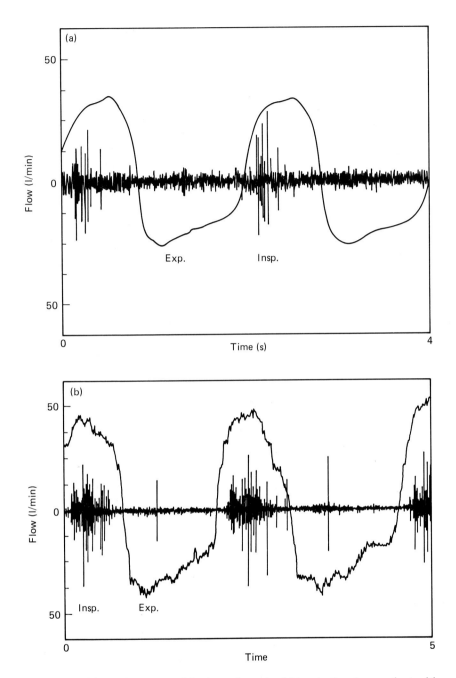

Figure 6.7 (a) Inspiratory crackles in early and mid-inspiration in a patient with chronic bronchitis and bronchiectasis: early end-point of crackling. (b) Shower of inspiratory crackles predominant in mid-expiration with later end-point, and an expiratory crackle in mid-expiration in another patient with bronchiectasis (see Figure 6.8). (Reproduced, with permission, from Dalmasso et al., 1984)

during inspiration (often with varying intensity between breaths) in some patients with fibrosing alveolitis, extrinsic allergic alveolitis or sarcoidosis. It is always associated with inspiratory crackles and tends to occur in middle and late inspiration in extrinsic allergic alveolitis, but in early and mid-

inspiration in chronic bronchiolitis and some cases of DIPF and sarcoidosis (Forgacs, 1967; Earis et al., 1982) and chronic beryllium disease – most probably because larger peripheral airways (1 to 6 mm in diameter) are involved (Geddes et al., 1977). The sound is often audible at the mouth, is only briefly

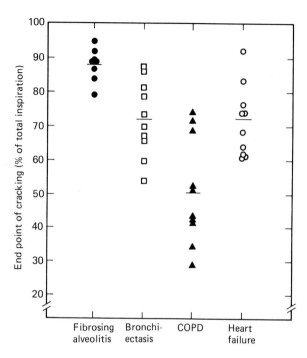

Figure 6.8 End-point of crackling in inspiration in four different disorders. Lines = mean values in the groups. (Reproduced, with permission, from Piirilä et al., 1991)

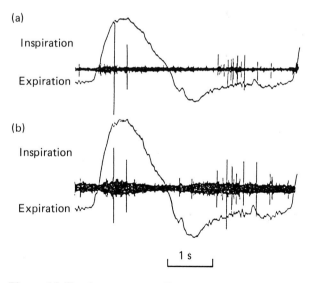

Figure 6.9 Simultaneous recording of early and mid-inspiratory and expiratory crackles heard at the mouth (a) and on the chest wall (b) in the same patient. (Reproduced, with permission, from Nath and Capel, 1974b)

abolished by repeated deep breathing and coughing, and remains constant over years of observation. It may be heard over both the upper and the lower lung fields, sometimes more so in the former.

Expiratory crackles

Although less frequent than inspiratory crackles, expiratory crackles are important. They usually accompany inspiratory crackles and occur at the lower transpulmonary pressures at which small airways close than when they snap open. According to the stress–relaxation quadrupole model, their number and intensity are less than those of inspiratory crackles (as clinical observation confirms), and their initial waveform deflections should be in the opposite direction, as suggested by Fredberg and Holford (1983) and verified by Dalmasso et al. (1984) and Walshaw et al. (1990). They are intermittent and may vary from one respiratory cycle to another. The same criteria of pitch apply as to inspiratory crackles. Their importance lies in the fact that they are often present in bronchiectasis, chronic bronchiolitis, advanced DIPF (fibrosing alveolitis) and in some cases of tuberculosis, and are frequently audible at the mouth (see Figure 6.9). In addition, there appears to be a significant correlation between numbers of expiratory crackles and reduction in gas transfer factor in cryptogenic fibrosing alveolitis, suggesting that they may be an indicator of severity of the disease (Walshaw et al., 1990). Unlike the random, low-pitched, rattling, expiratory crackles, which are caused by air passing through copious secretions, they are not altered by coughing (Nath, 1981).

Figure 6.10 shows the sound pressure and the time variation of the frequency spectrum of inspiratory and expiratory crackles in a respiratory cycle in a patient with idiopathic DIPF (CFA). Note that crackles are predominant in mid-inspiration but continue to the end of inspiration.

To return to the question of adventitious sounds in chronic fibrosing alveolitis (DIPF) and asbestosis, it has been the author's experience over a number of years that, whereas the auscultatory features of crackles may be similar (that is, fine and either late in inspiration or in mid-inspiration with end-inspiratory accentuation) in mild ('early') idiopathic DIPF and asbestosis, they are, by contrast, often coarse in the first and second phases of inspiration as well as at the end, and frequently audible at the mouth in more advanced idiopathic DIPF (and nonspecific, diffuse, pulmonary fibrosis), but not in more advanced asbestosis. In addition, inspiratory 'squawks' and expiratory crackles are heard in some cases of advanced DIPF (Nath, 1981; Walshaw et al., 1990), but not in asbestosis; these sounds, together with coarse inspiratory crackles, often occur in the upper as well as the lower lobe regions but their number and distribution may differ significantly in the two lung fields. By contrast, the inspiratory crackles of asbestosis are invariably confined to the lower halves of the lung fields and are approximately similar in both.

(a)

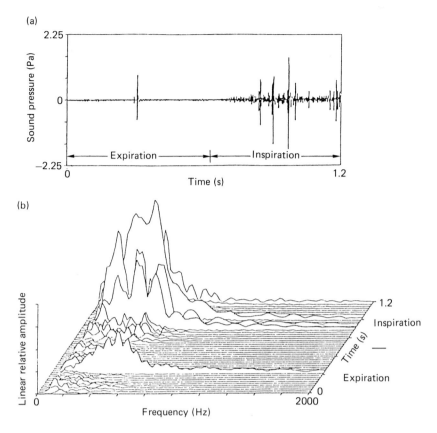

(b)

Figure 6.10 The upper panel shows the time variation of the frequency of crackles in a complete respiratory cycle of a patient with idiopathic DIPF (CFA). One expiratory crackle and a shower of inspiratory crackles are seen. The lower panel shows the frequency spectrum and distribution of these crackles in the same respiratory cycle in three-dimensional display. exp. = expiration; insp. = inspiration. (Reproduced, with permission, from Dalmasso et al., 1984)

The presence of coarse crackles in early inspiration in chronic fibrosing alveolitis and non-specific interstitial fibrosis, but not in asbestosis, is explicable if more of the larger airways (that is, small bronchi and proximal membranous bronchioles) are involved by disease – fibrosis and reversible, local atelectasis – than in asbestosis. Similarly, this would account for the different occurrence of early and mid-inspiratory 'squawks' which have, in fact, been associated with mural scarring of small bronchi (6 mm diameter) and membranous bronchioles (Geddes et al., 1977). Although it is generally held that asbestosis is an 'end-stage' fibrosis that is indistinguishable from other forms of diffuse interstitial fibrosis, apart from the presence of asbestos fibres and bodies (Craighead et al., 1982) there are, nevertheless, significant clinicopathological differences. Indeed, this is supported by the observation that, while cases of asbestosis and idiopathic DIPF may sometimes appear to be similar radiographically, they are quantitatively dissimilar functionally,

function being impaired more in idiopathic fibrosis than in asbestosis at an equivalent degree of parenchymal involvement (Cookson, Musk and Glancy, 1984). (See Chapter 15 for further discussion.)

For some reason, crackles are either absent or scanty, and of limited distribution in some cases of the fibrotic stage of sarcoidosis, beryllium disease and extrinsic allergic alveolitis of radiographic severity comparable to cases of idiopathic DIPF or asbestosis.

The clinical differentiation of idiopathic DIPF, non-specific pulmonary fibrosis and asbestosis is often far from straightforward. It is proposed that careful auscultatory assessment of crackles can, in many cases, assist in this, especially when related to the other clinical features of disease.

The notion that the characteristics of crackles can serve a useful auxiliary role in the differentiation of some forms of diffuse interstitial fibrosis may, perhaps, seem novel, although the author has, over

Table 6.1 Features of crackles in some relevant pulmonary disorders

	Bronchiectasis/ bronchiolectasis	*Chronic bronchitis*	*Chronic fibrosing alveolitis (DIPF)*	*Asbestosis*	*Left ventricular failure*
Inspiratory crackles Typical timing in inspiration	Early and mid	Early	Mid and late in mild disease. Throughout in more advanced disease	Mid and late in mild disease. Throughout in more advanced disease	Latter third or two-thirds
Quality	Medium to coarse	Medium to coarse	Fine in mild disease. Coarse in early and mid-inspiration in more advanced disease	Fine in mild disease. Occasional; medium in mid and late inspiration in more advanced disease	Fine
Numbers	Moderate	Few	Moderate to profuse (except in mild disease)	Few in mild disease. Moderate in more advanced disease	Profuse
Effect of cough	Sometimes reduced, but briefly	May be reduced or discharged	No change	No change	Reduced temporarily
Effect of position	No change	No change	Modified or abolished in mild disease; otherwise unaffected	Modified or abolished in mild disease; otherwise unaffected	Abolished
Intensity	Loud	Faint	Intermediate	Intermediate	Intermediate
Inspiratory 'squawks'	Frequent; early inspiration	Absent	Fairly common; mid or late inspiration	Absent	Absent
Expiratory crackles	Common; throughout; coarse	In some cases	Often in more advanced disease; mid and late; medium to coarse; not numerous; persistent	Absent	In some cases, early; fine
Transmission of crackles to mouth	Both inspiratory and expiratory; inspiratory 'squawks' common	Both, in some cases	Early inspiratory and expiratory, medium to coarse in more advanced disease; often with 'squawks'	Not transmitted	Not transmitted

the years, found good correlation between these characteristics and the morbid anatomy of the lungs. This is considered further in Chapter 15. The earlier observation of Epler, Carrington and Gaensler (1978) that 'coarse' crackles occurred in 18 per cent of cases of chronic fibrosing alveolitis ('usual interstitial pneumonia') compared to 6 per cent of those of asbestosis, and Forgac's (1969) suggestion that they are indicative of advanced fibrosis, had already pointed in this direction, and Murphy and Del Bono (1982) noted that 'patients with interstitial fibrosis and many fine paninspiratory crackles also often

had medium or coarse crackles'. Thus, it is significant that Munakata et al. (1991) have confirmed not only that crackles occur in both inspiration and expiration in some cases of idiopathic DIPF, but that they can be coarse as well as fine in either phase, and that Piirilä et al. (1991) have shown that the waveform characteristics of crackles in such different pulmonary diseases as idiopathic DIPF, bronchiectasis, 'chronic obstructive pulmonary disease' and congestive cardiac failure have clear distinctive features. As Murphy (1985) has said, there is 'reason to believe that lung sounds could reflect abnormalities in some diffuse lung diseases more closely than standard chest roentgenograms do' – and, perhaps, more closely than other imaging techniques. Computer methods of analysing the sound signals and pinpointing their sites of origin (by modifying such techniques as 'triangulation' used in locating submarines, for example) should resolve the matter (Murphy, 1981) (see 'Conclusion').

Table 6.1 summarizes the features of crackles in some pulmonary disorders that are relevant in the present context.

Conclusion

Auscultation is an important aid in the diagnosis and assessment of progression of a variety of occupational disorders of the lungs and in their differentiation from non-occupational disease, and should be carefully cultivated. Two authoritative voices put the matter in a nutshell. First:

> The fact is that the great amount of information gained by listening to the chest is not so easily or cheaply obtained by any other instrument or procedure. The correlation between auscultatory and pathologic conditions is remarkably good.
> (Kraman, 1985b)

Secondly:

> What seems certain is that adventitious sounds can be as rich a source of information as heart sounds *if one pays close attention to their pitch and timing.*
> [Present author's emphasis] (Forgacs, 1967)

Of course, observer variability exists in the auscultation of all pulmonary sounds but, in the case of crackles, this can be substantially reduced when clinicians or medical technicians are trained to auscultate under controlled conditions during tidal, slow, deep breathing in a quiet room, and by listening to play-back of tape-recordings of the sounds. Agreement is good, and screening of industrial workers exposed to asbestos (for example) has proved reliable (Workum et al., 1986). Also, as mentioned earlier, a practical computer-based method for identifying and analysing crackles and of documenting and quantifying them is now feasible. This can be expected to improve the accuracy of diagnosis in both clinical and occupational fields of practice (Murphy, Del Bono and Davidson, 1989; Piirilä et al., 1991).

Auscultation must be performed, without distraction, in a quiet room with the patient sitting or standing upright and the chest completely bare. The patient should be asked to breathe through the open mouth, first quietly at tidal volume and then slowly and deeply from functional residual capacity ('tidal–slow deep breathing'). Inspiratory airflow less than 0.5 to 0.75 l/s causes little or no sound at the chest wall (Kraman, 1985a). Auscultation should proceed in orderly fashion from region to region of the lung fields – anterior, posterior and lateral – comparing like region with like on both sides of the chest wall. Inspiration must first be concentrated upon: the duration and intensity of breath sounds and then the adventitious sounds. The mental device, mentioned earlier (see Figure 6.6), of dividing inspiration into three phases is helpful. Auscultation at the mouth, with the stethoscope bell to one side, and over the trachea must *never* be omitted. Extraneous crackling sounds heard when listening over a hairy chest wall can be abolished by wetting the hair.

It is worth remembering that the sensitivity of the binaural 'stethoscope–ear system' is limited to sound frequencies between, approximately, 50 and 400 Hz; that below 1000 Hz the sensitivity of the ear falls abruptly, so it is relatively insensitive to most normal breath sounds (less than 500 Hz); and that acuity of hearing varies between individuals and declines with age – hence the need for concentration in a quiet environment. The bell of the stethoscope conducts both low- and high-pitched sounds, the diaphragm mainly high-pitched sounds but with the advantage of a larger diameter (Kindig et al., 1982).

Clinical and laboratory tests

The application and relevance of examination of sputum, physiological tests, radiological and other forms of imaging, bronchial provocation tests, bronchoalveolar lavage and immunological and other tests are discussed in appropriate chapters.

Skin-prick tests

These are often necessary in the investigation of occupational asthma and extrinsic allergic alveolitis, and may be helpful in establishing that a known industrial allergen is the likely cause of worker's asthma (see Chapter 20 and 21).

Biopsy

Examinations of a scalene node may help to resolve a difficult diagnosis, especially in the presence of generalized systemic disease. Sarcoid-type granulomas of beryllium disease and silicotic nodules can sometimes be identified.

If clinical and non-invasive investigations fail to establish the diagnosis, biopsy of lung may be indicated:

1. In the hope of providing an accurate diagnosis.
2. To exclude infections or neoplastic disease which may masquerade as an occupational disease.
3. Because of the possibility of identifying, and assessing the activity of, an unsuspected, treatable, disorder.

All available methods have a roughly similar incidence of complications which, though low, can be life-threatening, and to which the patient should not be exposed unnecessarily. In general, thoracotomy (limited or open) is preferable to drill and needle methods (although more unpleasant for the patient) because the most appropriate site for sampling can be selected by inspection and palpation of lung or pleura, and larger and more representative samples of tissue obtained from more than one site. The specimen should, whenever possible, be insufflated with formalin. Sampling of dependent parts of the middle and lower lobes is not advisable because they often contain non-specific fibrosis and arterial vascular changes (Gaensler and Carrington, 1980; Newman, Michel and Wang, 1985). The transbronchial needling technique, although usually the clinician's first choice, should be avoided because it yields such small fragments of lung that either a diseased area is not sampled or differential diagnosis of abnormal tissue may be impossible.

As a rule, it can be said that, if the occupational and medical history, physical examination and appropriate investigations are carefully carried out and their results accurately and logically analysed, sampling of intrathoracic tissues in suspected cases of any type of pneumoconiosis should rarely be necessary. It is axiomatic that inspection of earlier chest radiographs is an integral part of investigation, and this alone may often prevent embarrassing mistakes.

Routine medical examinations

Before entering work in an industry with a known dust, fume, gas or atmospheric pressure hazard, the prospective employee should have a clinical examination, chest radiograph and assessment of FEV_1 and FVC. A basic reference point for future examination is thus established. In general, this examination should exclude persons with chronic chest disease and, where relevant, those with an allergic (or atopic) diathesis. Chronic nasal obstruction should be looked for and, if present and severe, corrective surgery advised; acceptance of individuals with chronic nasal obstruction into work having a potential aerosol hazard is probably undesirable.

Established workers exposed to a potential risk of developing lung disease should be examined regularly; an interval of 2 years is probably most satisfactory for the majority of industries. In some industries, such as those with a 'silica' risk, a chest radiograph is all that is required; but in others, in particular those involving asbestos, clinical, radiological and physiological examinations are mandatory.

Details of examinations must be fully recorded and the records kept readily available. To have maximal prospective value, each·worker's record must include a description of the job and the nature of materials used (that is, their analysis and origin) and, whenever possible, the concentration of the relevant dust or fume in the work environment. Changes in work must also be noted. This demands close co-operation between medical, engineering and production departments and safety personnel. It is clear that such co-operation not only ensures the best information upon the incidence and behaviour of disease in the factory population but also confers the greatest long-term advantage on the worker.

The necessity for these examinations should always be explained to the workers concerned. If this is done, few will fail to understand that they are done for their benefit and will co-operate accordingly.

References

Allen, M.C.J. and Newhouse, M.T. (1984) Gastroesophageal reflux and chronic respiratory disease. *Am. Rev. Respir. Dis.* **129**, 645–647

Amberson, J.B. (1973) Aspiration bronchopneumonia. *Int. Anesthesiol. Clins* **3**, 126–128

Anderson, K., Ewing, R.A.M., Boyd, G. and Morris, G. (1990) Atmospheric air sampling and implication for estimation of antigen exposure in pigeon breeders. *Thorax* **45**, 320P

Appelblatt, N.H. and Baker, S.R. (1981) Functional upper airway obstruction, a new syndrome. *Archs Otolaryngol.* **107**, 305–306

Baillie, Matthew (1797) *The Morbid Anatomy of Some of the Most Important Parts of the Human Body*, 2nd edn, London, p. xv

Barker, A.F. and Bardana, E.J. Jr (1988) Bronchiectasis: update of an orphan disease. *Am. Rev. Respir. Dis.* **137**, 969–978

Barrett, N.R. (1964) Association of esophageal and pulmonary diseases. *Postgrad. Med.* **36**, 470–473

Baughman, R.P. and Loudon, R.G. (1989) Stridor: differentiation from asthma or upper airway noise. *Am. Rev. Respir. Dis.* **139**, 1407–1409

Bégin, R., Radoux, V., Cantin, A. and Ménard, H.A. (1988) Stiffness of the rib cage in a subset of rheumatoid patients. *Lung* **166**, 141–148

Belcher, J.R. (1949) The pulmonary complications of oesophageal disease. *Br. J. Dis. Chest* **54**, 342–348

Belsey, R. (1960) The pulmonary complications of oesophageal disease. *Br. J. Dis. Chest* **54**, 342–348

Bentley, D., Moore, A. and Schwachman, H. (1976) Finger clubbing: a quantitative survey by analysis of the shadowgraph. *Lancet* **2**, 164–167

Bergofsky, E.H. (1979) Respiratory failure of disorders of the thoracic cage. *Am. Rev. Respir. Dis.* **119**, 643–669

Bienenstock, J., McDermott, M., Beyfus, A.D. and O'Neill, M.A. (1978) A common mucosal immunological system involving the bronchus, breast and bowel. In *Secretory Immunity and Infection* (eds J.R. McGhee, J. Mestecky and J.L. Babb), Plenum, New York, pp. 53–59

Bohadana, A.B., Peslin, R. and Uffholtz, H. (1978) Breath sounds in the clinical assessment of airflow obstruction. *Thorax* **33**, 345–351

Burrows, B., Lebowitz, M.D. and Barbee, R. (1976) Respiratory disorders and allergy skin-test reactions. *Ann. Intern. Med.* **84**, 134–139

Butland, R.J.A., Cole, P., Citron, K.M. and Turner-Warwick, M. (1981) Chronic bronchial suppuration and inflammatory bowel disease. *Q. J. Med.* **197**, 63–75

Carrao, W.M., Braman, S.S. and Irwin, R.S. (1979) Chronic cough as the sole presenting manifestation of bronchial asthma. *N. Engl. J. Med.* **300**, 633–637

Castell, D.O. (1989) Asthma and gastroesophageal reflux. *Chest* **96**, 2–3

Chernow, M.D., Johnson, L.F., Janowitz, W.R. and Castell, D.O. (1979) Pulmonary aspiration as a consequence of gastro-esophageal reflux. *Dig. Dis. Sci.* **24**, 839–844

Cole, P.J. (1986) Inflammation: a two-edged sword – the model of bronchiectasis. *Eur. J. Respir. Dis.* **69**, suppl. 147, 6–15

Cookson, W.O.C.M., Musk, A.W. and Glancy, J.J. (1984) Asbestosis and cryptogenic fibrosing alveolitis: a radiological and functional comparison. *Aust. NZ J. Med.* **14**, 626–630

Craighead, J.E., Abraham, J.L., Churg, A., Green, F.H.Y., Kleinerman, J., Pratt, P.C., Seemayer, T.A., Vallyathan, V. and Weill, H. (1982) The pathology of asbestos-associated disease of the lungs and pleural cavities: diagnostic criteria and proposed grading schema. *Archs Pathol. Lab. Med.* **106**, 544–596

Cugell, D.W. (1987) Lung sound nomenclature. *Am. Rev. Respir. Dis.* **136**, 1016

Curth, H.O., Firschein, I.L. and Alpert, M. (1961) Familial clubbed fingers. *Archs Derm.* **83**, 828–836

Dalmasso, F., Guarene, M.M., Spagnolo, R., Benedetto, G. and Righin, G. (1984) A computer system for timing and acoustical analysis of crackles: a study of cryptogenic fibrosing alveolitis. *Bull. Eur. Physiopathol. Respir.* **20**, 139–144

Davidson, M. (1935) *A Practical Manual of Diseases of the Chest.* Oxford University Press, London, New York, Toronto, pp. 58–59

Davies, D. (1972) Ankylosing spondylitis and lung fibrosis. *Q. J. Med.* **41**, 395–417

DeMeester, T.R., Johnson, L.F., Joseph, G.J., Toscano, M.S., Hall, A.W. and Skinner, D.B. (1976) Patterns of gastro-sophageal reflux in health and disease. *Ann. Surg.* **184**, 459–469

DeMeester, T.R., Wang, C-I., Wernly, J.A., Pellegrini, C.A., Little, A.G., Klementschitsch, P., Bermudez, G., Johnson, L.E. and Skinner, D.B. (1980) Technique, indications and clinical use of 24-hour esophageal pH monitoring. *J. Thorac. Cardiovasc. Surg.* **79**, 656–670

Dennish, G.W. and Castell, D.O. (1971) Inhibitory effect of smoking on the lower esophageal sphincter. *N. Engl. J. Med.* **284**, 1136–1137

Dent, J., Dodds, W.J., Friedman, R.H., Seguchi, T., Hogan, W.J., Arndorfer, R.C. and Petrie, D.J. (1980) Mechanism of gastro-esophageal reflux in recumbent asymptomatic subjects. *J. Clin. Invest.* **65**, 256–267

Earis, J.E., Marsh, K., Pearson, M.G. and Ogilvie, C.M. (1982) The inspiratory 'squawk' in extrinsic allergic alveolitis and other pulmonary fibroses. *Thorax* **37**, 923–926

Eiser, N. (1990) The hitch-hikers guide to nasal airway patency. *Respir. Med.* **84**, 179–183

Ekström, T. and Tibbling, L. (1988) Gastro-oesophageal reflux and nocturnal asthma. *Eur. Respir. J.* **1**, 636–638

Ekström, T. and Tibbling, L. (1989) Esophageal acid perfusion, airway function, and symptoms in asthmatic patients with marked bronchial hyperreactivity. *Chest* **96**, 995–998

Epler, G.R., Carrington, C.B. and Gaensler, E.A. (1978) Crackles (rales) in the interstitial pulmonary diseases. *Chest* **73**, 333–339

Field, G.B. (1974) The application of a quantitative estimate of cough frequency to epidemiological surveys. *Int. J. Epidemiol.* **3**, 135–143

Fischer, D.S., Singer, D.H. and Feldman, S.M. (1964) Clubbing: a review with emphasis on hereditary acropachy. *Medicine* **43**, 459–479

Forgacs, P. (1967) Crackles and wheezes. *Lancet* **2**, 203–205

Forgacs, P. (1969) Lung sounds. *Br. J. Dis. Chest* **63**, 1–12

Forgacs, P. (1974) Gravitational stress in lung disease. *Br. J. Dis. Chest* **68**, 1–10

Forgacs, P. (1978a) The functional basis of pulmonary sounds. *Chest* **73**, 399–405

Forgacs, P. (1978b) *Lung Sounds*, Baillière Tindall, London

Forrest, J.A.H. and Shearman, D.J.C. (1975) Pulmonary vasculitis and ulcerative colitis. *Dig. Dis.* **20**, 482–486

Fredberg, J.J. and Holford, S.K. (1983) Discrete lung sounds: crackles (rales) as stress–relaxation quadrupoles. *J. Acoust. Soc. Am.* **73**, 1036–1046

Gaensler, E.A. and Carrington, C.B. (1980) Open biopsy for chronic diffuse infiltrative lung disease: clinical, roentgenographic and physiological correlations in 502 patients. *Ann. thorac. Surg.* **30**, 411–425

Gandevia, B.H. (1981) Clinical techniques. In *Occupational Lung Diseases* (eds H. Weill and M. Turner-Warwick), Marcel Dekker, New York, Basel, pp. 11–33

Gandevia, B. (1990) Behavioural breathlessness. *Thorax* **45**, 716

Geddes, D.M., Corrin, B., Brewerton, D.A., Davies, R.J. and Turner-Warwick, M. (1977) Progressive airway obliteration in adults and its association with rheumatoid disease. *Q. J. Med.* **46**, 427–444

Gerhardt, D.C., Castell, D.O., Winship, D.H. and Shuck, T.J. (1980) Esophageal dysfunction in esophagopharyngeal regurgitation. *Gastroenterology* **78**, 893–897

Glaister, D.H. (1969) Lung collapse in aviation medicine. *Br. J. Hosp. Med.* **2**, 635–642

Glaister, D.H. (1988) The effects of long duration acceleration. In *Aviation Medicine*, 2nd edn (eds J. Ernsting and P. King), Butterworths, London, pp. 150–151

Goldman, J. and Muers, M. (1991) Vocal cord dysfunction and wheezing. *Thorax* **46**, 401–404

Greenstone, M. and Cole, P.J. (1985) Ciliary function in health and disease. *Br. J. Dis. Chest* **79**, 9–26

Hall, G.J.L. and Gandevia, B. (1971) Relationship of the loose cough sign to daily sputum volume. *Br. J. Soc. Prev. Med.* **25**, 109–113

Heatley, R.V., Thomas, P., Propipchuk, E.J., Gauldie, J.,

Sieniewicz, D.J. and Bienenstock, J. (1982) Pulmonary function abnormalities in patients with inflammatory bowel disease. *Q. J. Med.* **203**, 241–250

Hermans, P.E., Diaz-Buxo, J.A. and Stobo, J.D. (1976) Idiopathic late-onset immunoglobulin deficiency. *Am. J. Med.* **61**, 221–237

Hiebert, C.A. and Belsey, R. (1961) Incompetency of the gastric cardia without radiological evidence of hiatus hernia. *J. Thorac. Cardiovasc. Surg.* **42**, 352–359

Higenbottam, T., Cochrane, G.M., Clark, T.J.H., Turner, D., Millis, R. and Seymour, W. (1980) Bronchial disease in ulcerative colitis. *Thorax* **35**, 581–585

Higgins, I.T.T. (1959) Tobacco smoking, respiratory symptoms and ventilatory capacity. *Br. Med. J.* **1**, 325–329

Hillerdal, G. (1983) Ankylosing spondylitis lung disease – an underdiagnosed entity. *Eur. J. Respir. Dis.* **64**, 437–441

Hodson, M.E., Haslam, P.L., Spiro, S.G. and Turner-Warwick, M. (1984) Digital vasculitis in patients with cryptogenic fibrosing alveolitis. *Br. J. Dis. Chest* **78**, 140–148

Hogg, J.C. and Brock, R.C. (1951) Discussion on the role of sinusitis in bronchiectasis. *J. Laryngol. Otolol.* **65**, 442–457

Hood, J. and Mason, A.M.S. (1970) Diffuse pulmonary disease with transfer defect occurring with coeliac disease. *Lancet* **1**, 445–457

Hopkin, J.M. (1990) Atopy and genetics. A review. *J. R. Coll. Physns Lond* **24**, 159–169

Howell, J.B.L. (1990) Behavioural breathlessness. *Thorax* **45**, 287–292 and 716

Huxley, E.J., Viroslav, J., Gray, W.R. and Pierce, A.K. (1978) Pharyngeal aspiration in normal adults and patients with depressed consciousness. *Am. J. Med.* **64**, 564–568

Ing, A.J., Ngu, M-C. and Breslin, A.B.X. (1991) Chronic persistent cough and gastro-oesophageal reflux. *Thorax* **46**, 479–483

Irwin, R.S. (1989) Is the anatomic diagnostic work-up of chronic cough not all that it is hacked up to be? *Chest* **95**, 711-713

Irwin, R.S. and Curley, F.J. (1989) Is the anatomic, diagnostic work-up of chronic cough not all that it is hacked up to be? *Chest* **95**, 711–713

Irwin, R.S., Carrao, W.M. and Pratter, M.R. (1981) Chronic persistent cough in the adult: the spectrum and frequency of causes and successful outcome of specific therapy. *Am. Rev. Respir. Dis.* **123**, 413–417

Irwin, R.S., Rosen, M.J. and Braman, S.S. (1977) Cough. A comprehensive review. *Archs Intern. Med.* **137**, 1186–1191

Irwin, R.S., Zawacki, J.K., Curley, F.J., French, C.L. and Hoffman, P.J. (1988) Twenty-four hour esophageal pH monitoring in evaluating gastroesophageal reflux (GER) as the cause of chronic cough. *Am. Rev. Respir. Dis.* **137**, suppl., 161

Iverson, L.I.G., May, I.A. and Samson, P.C. (1973) Pulmonary complications in benign esophageal disease. *Am. J. Surg.* **126**, 223–228

Jenkinson, L.R., Norris, T.L., Barlow, A.P. and Watson, A. (1990) Acid reflux and oesophagitis – day or night? *Gullet* **1**, 36–44

Kindig, J.R., Beeson, T.P., Campbell, R.W., Andries, A. and Tavel, M.E. (1982) Acoustical performance of the stethoscope: a comparative analysis. *Am. Heart J.* **104**, 269–275

King, B. and Cotes, J.E. (1989) Relation of lung function and exercise capacity to mood and attitudes to health. *Thorax* **44**, 402–409

Kirsner, J.B. (1970) Ulcerative colitis 1970 – recent developments. *Scand. J. Gastroenterol.* **5**, suppl. 6, 63–91

Koenig, J.Q. and Omenn, G.S. (1988) Genetic factors. In *Variations in Susceptibility to Inhaled Pollutants* (eds J.D. Brain, B.D. Beck, A.J. Warren and R.A. Shaikh), Johns Hopkins University Press, Baltimore and London, pp. 59–88

Kraman, S. (1980) Determination of the extent of crackle propagation on the chest wall. In *Fifth International Conference on Lung Sounds*, September 15, 16, Imperial College, London, p. 3

Kraman, S.S. (1985a) Vesicular (normal) lung sounds: how are they made, where do they come from, and what do they mean? *Semin. Respir. Med.* **6**, 183–191

Kraman, S.S. (1985b) New tools in lung sound research. *Semin. Respir. Med.* **6**, 220–228

Kunica, E.S., Holford, S.K., Dewey, C.F. and Murphy, R.L.H. (1980) The distribution of fine and coarse discontinuous adventitious sounds over the chest wall. In *Fifth International Conference on Lung Sounds*, September 15, 16, Imperial College, London, p. 7

Larrain, A., Carrasco, J., Galleguillos, J. and Pope, C.E. (1981) Reflux treatment improves lung function in patients with intrinsic asthma. *Gastroenterology* **80**, 5 (part 2), 1204

Leblanc, P., Macklem, P.T. and Ross, W.R.D. (1970) Breath sounds and distribution of pulmonary ventilation. *Am. Rev. Respir. Dis.* **102**, 10–16

Leung, A.K.C. (1988) Familial gastroesophageal reflux and hiatus hernia. *Proc. R. Coll. Physns Edin.* **18**, 277–280

Loudon, R. and Murphy, L.H. (1984) Lung sounds. *Am. Rev. Respir. Dis.* **130**, 663–673

Lowell, F.C. (1979) 'Asthma', 'rhinitis' and 'atopy' reconsidered. *N. Engl. J. Med.* **300**, 669–670

Mackay, I. and Cole, P. (1987) Rhinitis, sinusitis and associated chest disease. In *Scott Brown's Otolaryngology*, 5th edn, Vol. 3, *Rhinology* (eds I.S. Mackay and T.R. Bull) Butterworths, London, pp. 61–92

Mansfield, L.E. and Stein, M.R. (1978) Gastroesophageal reflux and asthma: a possible reflex mechanism. *Ann. Allergy* **41**, 224–226

Meadway, J. (1974) Ulcerative colitis, colitic spondylitis and associated apical pulmonary fibrosis. *Proc. R. Soc. Med.* **67**, 324–325

Medical Research Council (1976) and (1986) *Questionnaire on Respiratory Symptoms*, MRC, London

Morinari, M., Mori, M., Kinoshita, K. and Honda, N. (1980) Differentiation of fine and coarse crackles by time sequence analysis. In *Fifth International Conference on Lung Sounds*, September 15, 16, Imperial College, London, p. 6

Munakata, M., Ukita, H., Doi, I., Ohtsuka, Y., Masaki, Y., Homma, Y. and Kawakami, Y. (1991) Spectral waveform characteristics of fine and coarse crackles. *Thorax* **46**, 651–657

Murphy, R.L. (1981) Auscultation of the lung: past lessons, future possibilities. *Thorax* **36**, 99–107

Murphy, R.L.H. (1985) Discontinuous adventitious lung sounds. *Semin. Respir. Med.* **6**, 210–219

Murphy, R. and Del Bono, E. (1982) Lung sound mapping. In *Seventh International Conference on Lung Sounds*, October 7, 8, University of California, Davis School of Medicine, Martinez CA; International Lung Sounds Association, p. 21

Murphy, R.L.H., Del Bono, E.A. and Davidson, F. (1989) Validation of an automatic crackle (râle) counter. *Am. Rev. Respir. Dis.* **140**, 1017–1020

Murphy, R.L.H. and Holford, S.K. (1980) Lung sounds. *Basics Resp. Dis.* **8**, 1–6

Murphy, R.H.L., Holford, S.K. and Knowler, W.C. (1977) Lung sound characterization by time-expanded waveform analysis. *N. Engl. J. Med.* **296**, 968–971

Nath, A.R. (1981) Lung sounds. In *Clinical Investigation of Respiratory Disease* (ed. T.J.H. Clark), Chapman and Hall, London, pp. 9–31

Nath, A.R. and Capel, L.H. (1974a) Inspiratory crackles and mechanical events of breathing. *Thorax* **29**, 695–698

Nath, A.R. and Capel, L.H. (1974b) Inspiratory crackles – early and late. *Thorax* **29**, 223–227

Nath, A.R. and Capel, L.H. (1980) Lung capacities in bronchiectasis. *Thorax* **35**, 694–699

Newman, S.L., Michel, R.P. and Wang, N.S. (1985) Lingular lung biopsy: is it representative? *Am. Rev. Respir. Dis.* **132**, 1084–1086

Ogilvie, A.L., James, P.D. and Atkinson, M. (1985) Impairment of vagal function in reflux oesophagitis. *Q. J. Med.* **54**, 61–74

Oldham, P.D. (1987) Decline of FEV$_1$. *Thorax* **42**, 161–164

Olson, D.E. and Hammersley, J.R. (1985) Mechanisms of lung sound generation. *Semin. Respir. Med.* **6**, 171–179

Orr, W.C., Johnson, L.F. and Robinson, M.G. (1984) Effect of sleep on swallowing, esophageal peristalsis and acid clearance. *Gastroenterology* **86**, 814–819

Pearson, J.E.G. and Wilson, R.S.E. (1971) Diffuse pulmonary fibrosis and hiatus hernia. *Thorax* **26**, 300–305

Perrin-Fayolle, M., Gormand, F., Braillon, G., Lombard-Platet, R., Vignal, J., Azzar, D., Forichon, J. and Adeline, P. (1989) Long-term results of surgical treatment for gastroesophageal reflux in asthmatic patients. *Chest* **96**, 40–45

Pincus, J.H. (1978) Hyperventilation syndrome. *Br. J. Hosp. Med.* **19**, 312–313

Piirilä, P., Sovijärvi, A.R.A., Kaisla, T., Rajala, H-M. and Katila, T. (1991) Crackles in patients with fibrosing alveolitis, bronchiectasis, COPD and heart failure. *Chest* **99**, 1076–1083

Ploysongsang, Y. (1985) Lung sounds as indices of ventilation. *Semin. Respir. Med.* **6**, 192–200

Ploysongsang, Y. and Schonfeld, S.A. (1980) Production of rales during low volume breathing. In *Fifth International Conference on Lung Sounds*, September 15, 16, Imperial College, London, p. 21

Ploysongsang, Y., Iyer, V.K. and Ramamoorthy, P.A. (1990) Inspiratory and expiratory vesicular sounds. *Respiration* **57**, 313–317

Pontoppidan, H. and Beecher, H.K. (1960) Progressive loss of protective reflexes in the airway with the advance of age. *J. Am. Med. Assoc.* **174**, 2209–2213

Power, J.T., Stewart, I.C., Connaughton, J.J., Brash, H.M., Shapiro, C.M., Flenley, D.C. and Douglas, N.J. (1984) Nocturnal cough in patients with chronic bronchitis and emphysema. *Am. Rev. Respir. Dis.* **130**, 999–1001

Quinn, L.H. and Meyer, O.O. (1929) Relationship of sinusitis and bronchiectasis. *Archs Otolaryngol.* **10**, 152–165

Rauscher, H., Popp, W. and Ritschka, L. (1989) Effect of short esophageal acidification on airways hyperactivity. *Respiration* **55**, 11–15

Regan, G.M., Tagg, B. and Thomson, M.L. (1967) Subjective assessment and objective measurement of finger clubbing. *Lancet* **1**, 530–532

Reich, S.B., Earley, W.C., Ravin, T.H., Goodman, M., Spector, S. and Stein, M.R. (1977) Evaluation of gastropulmonary aspiration by a radioactive technique: concise communication. *J. Nucl. Med.* **18**, 1079–1081

Rice, D.A. (1982) Airway to pleura sound transmission in excised lung. In *Seventh International Conference on Lung Sounds*, October 7, 8, University of California, Davis School of Medicine, Martinez CA; International Lung Sounds Association, p. 5

Rice, D.A. (1983) Sound speed in pulmonary parenchyma. *J. Appl. Physiol.* **54**, 304–308

Robertson, A.J. and Coope, R. (1957) Rales, rhonchi and Laënnec. *Lancet* **2**, 417–423

Schneerson, J.M. (1981) Digital clubbing and hypertrophic osteoarthropathy: the underlying mechanisms. *Br. J. Dis. Chest* **75**, 113–131

Shykoff, B.E., Ploysongsang, Y. and Chang, H.K. (1988) Airflow and normal lung sounds. *Am. Rev. Respir. Dis.* **137**, 872–876

Simon, P.G., Schwartzstein, R.M., Weiss, J.W., Lahive, K., Fencl, V., Teghtsoonian, M. and Weinberger, S.E. (1989) Distinguishable sensations of breathlessness induced in normal volunteers. *Am. Rev. Respir. Dis.* **140**, 1021–1027

Smallman, L.A., Hill, S.L. and Stockley, R.A. (1984) Reduction of ciliary beat frequency *in vitro* by bronchiectatic secretions. A serine proteinase effect. *Thorax* **39**, 663–667

Solanski, T. and Neville, E. (1990) Bronchiectasis: A forgotten association of rheumatoid disease. *Thorax* **45**, 822

Spiteri, M.A., Cook, D.G. and Clarke, S.W. (1988) Reliability of eliciting physical signs in examination of the chest. *Lancet* **1**, 873–875

Stoneman, S.A.T., Parker, R. and Jones, A. (1989) Correlation of breath sounds with diagnosis of lung dysfunction: experimental observations. *Proc. Instn Mech. Engrs H* **203**, 151–158

Talbot, J.H. and Montgomery, W.R. Jr (1953) Familial clubbing of fingers and toes. *Archs Intern. Med.* **92**, 697–700

Trail, R.R. (1948) *Chest Examination: the Correlation of Physical and X-ray Findings in Disease of the Lung.* Churchill, London, pp. 55–58

Turton, C.W.G. (1987) Troublesome pleural fluid. *Br. J. Dis. Chest* **81**, 217–224

Tydd, T.F. and Dyer, N.H. (1976) Sulphasalazine lung. *Med. J. Aust.* **1**, 570–573

Walshaw, M.J., Nisar, M., Pearson, M.G., Calverley, P.M.A. and Earis, J.E. (1990) Expiratory lung crackles in patients with fibrosing alveolitis. *Chest* **97**, 407–409

Widdicombe, J.G. (1979) Dyspnoea. *Bull. Eur. Physiopathol. Respir.* **15**, 437–440

Wilson, R., Sykes, D.A., Currie, D. and Cole, P.J. (1986) Beat frequency of cilia from sites of purulent infection. *Thorax* **41**, 453–458

Workum, P., Del Bono, E.A., Holford, S.K. and Murphy, R.L.H. (1986) Observer agreement, chest auscultation, and crackles in asbestos-exposed workers. *Chest* **89**, 27–29

7

Imaging in occupational disease of the lung

Peter M. Bretland and W. Raymond Parkes

Introduction

Recent advances in medicine and associated technologies have given physicians a bewildering array of ways of getting pictures of their patients' 'insides', and the term 'imaging' is now in general use. *Conventional radiography* (the transmission image using X-rays) still accounts for about 70 per cent of imaging work overall, and half of this is for chest radiography. *Computed tomography* (CT) uses rotating X-ray tubes and detectors and assigns an attenuation value to each *pixel* (small picture element), producing a similar type of image in shades of grey of a transverse slice of the body. Most radiology departments in developed countries now have access to such apparatus. *Ultrasound* uses the acoustic properties of tissue to measure the timing and magnitude of echoes from the applied pulses and can build up, in almost any plane, anatomical images, although there are limits to its ability to characterize tissue; it cannot traverse gas or bone, which further restricts its application. It is now unusual to find a radiology department not practising ultrasound. *Nuclear medicine* uses radio-isotopes incorporated in radiopharmaceuticals which locate in selected organs by virtue of their physiological properties. It can produce pictures (emission images) from the γ-rays emitted but has the additional, often more important, ability to measure organ function and physiological behaviour. Most large centres now have access to this technique (for example, district general hospitals in the UK). *Magnetic resonance imaging* (MRI), in which the energy changes in spinning hydrogen atoms in response to applied magnetic fields are measured so as to assign a value to each *voxel* (small volume element), is fast developing and can build

up an image of a slice in any plane. The apparatus is expensive and not yet widely available. Although its place in neurology and some parts of orthopaedics is well established, its more general application is not yet fully determined.

It is now the exception rather than the rule, in the UK at least, for departments of chest medicine to run their own X-ray services. Departments of radiology and imaging provide the service required and have other facilities to offer as well as simple chest radiography.

Because, conventionally, the chest radiograph has been for many years the investigation on which most occupational chest disease physicians have relied, it will form the bulk of this chapter, but other imaging techniques do have roles to play which may develop further in the future.

Part I: Chest radiology
Peter M. Bretland

Although the diagnosis of a pneumoconiosis necessarily involves an analysis of occupational history, physical examination and lung function tests, the chest radiograph is without doubt the most informative single investigation available.

The general principles of chest radiography and radiology are admirably discussed, respectively, in *Clark's Positioning in Radiography* (1979) and by Simon (1973), among others. When the pneumoconioses are under consideration, however, it is particularly important that certain principles which determine the appearance of the chest radiograph should be understood if errors of interpretation are to be avoided.

Chest radiography is employed for both clinical and epidemiological purposes: in the former to establish diagnosis, prognosis and guidance of treatment; in the latter to estimate prevalence and behaviour of disease in different communities. Our concern here is mainly with the former. Whichever the purpose, however, the highest possible standard of radiological technique must always be sought.

Relevant X-ray physics

X-rays used for diagnostic purposes are electromagnetic radiations normally within the wavelength range 0.01 to 0.1 nm (0.1 to 1 Å); energy range 12.4 to 24.0 kiloelectron volts (keV). The upper energy level – which determines the quality and penetrating power of the beam – is, in practice, usually denoted by the kilovoltage applied to the X-ray tube, selection of which is an essential part of radiological technique. The X-rays travel in straight lines but, on encountering matter, may be absorbed or scattered in various amounts and directions by its atoms. Whilst such radiation can be considered as having a waveform, its energy can be regarded as travelling in little 'packets' or quanta.

The *atomic number* (that is, the number of electrons around the nucleus in an uncharged atom) of an element decides its character and properties. It is the average atomic number of a body tissue (*not* its atomic weight) that is responsible for the extent to which incident X-rays of given energy will be absorbed or scattered (that is, attenuated) by different tissues. This is the basis of radiographic imaging.

Absorption and scatter

The amount of attenuation is also related to the number of atoms per unit volume and, consequently, to the density or specific gravity of the material. The probability that a quantum of radiant energy will interact with either an atom or molecule is clearly less where the molecules are widely dispersed. Therefore, both absorption and scatter are significantly less in air and other gases than in fluids such as blood or pleural effusion.

Detailed consideration of these processes is inappropriate here. They are well described elsewhere (for example, Selman, 1963; Meredith and Massey, 1977). Two basic facts should, however, be noted:

1. Some radiation is totally or partly absorbed in the material whilst the remainder either has its direction changed or is degraded to lower energy radiation which is scattered in all directions.
2. The amount of scatter is dependent upon the number of electrons per gram of irradiated material. Allowing for density, this is much the same for most elements in biological materials, with the exception of hydrogen which has about twice the number (S.B. Osborn, 1969, personal communication).

Production of the X-ray image

The X-rays emanate from a small source – the focal spot of the X-ray tube. They are produced as a result of the impact on the anode of the evacuated tube by a stream of electrons accelerated from the heated cathode. Of the energy in the electron beam, over 99 per cent is degraded to heat and less than 1 per cent appears as radiant energy. There have been numerous ways of dispersing the heat in the past but for many years now the solution has been a rotating anode made of a material of high specific heat and the tube is immersed in oil also of high specific heat. Collimation produces a beam of the appropriate cross-sectional shape and size which is aimed to pass through the patient on to the film. The effect of X-rays upon the conventional X-ray film is to produce blackening after processing. Conversely, unexposed film is transparent and appears white when viewed against white light. Materials or tissues that absorb X-rays completely and prevent them reaching the film emulsion cast 'shadows' that appear white and are said to be of high radiographic density. Consequently the various tissues of the body, which attenuate X-rays to differing extents, produce a range of effects from black (for example, air) when attenuation is least, through shades of grey (for example, fat and muscle), to white (for example, cortical bone), when attenuation is greatest. It is the *contrast* (a photographic term meaning the relative blackness and whiteness) between various shades of black, grey and white that makes up the image – a *transmission image* that is, in effect, a differential attenuation pattern.

Hence, it is convenient to conceive of four basic radiographic densities: 'air', 'fat', 'water' (equivalent to blood and soft tissues) and 'bone'. With the exception of air the radio-opacity of different tissues is dependent more on their effective atomic number than on their specific gravity (Spiers, 1946) or chemical composition. The *effective atomic number* is an expression of the resultant total absorption of X-rays by atoms of the different elements in a material and is dependent on the percentage by weight, the atomic number and the atomic weight of

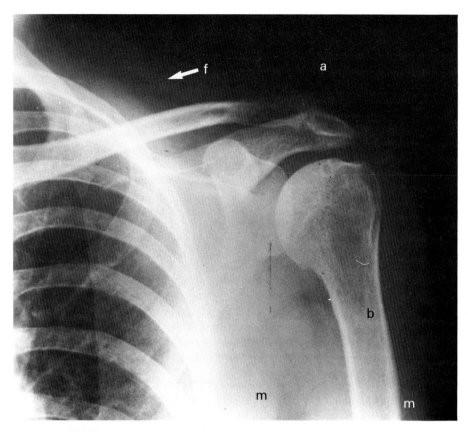

Figure 7.1 Radiographs of a normal shoulder showing the contrast between radio-opacity caused by bone (b), muscle (m), fat (f) and lung compared with air (a)

each element. In the low-voltage region the contribution made by any one element depends on its atomic number raised to about the third power (Johns and Cunningham, 1969). The effective atomic number for fat is given as 5.9, for muscle and water as 7.4, for air as 7.6 and for bone as about 14; the atomic numbers of phosphorus and calcium are 15 and 20, respectively. Air, in spite of its effective atomic number and for reasons given in the next section, is virtually transradiant; fat (which contains less hydrogen than water) produces a grey effect; all body fluids, muscle and solid viscera have a similar radiographic density which is equivalent to that of water, producing a lighter grey effect than fat; and bone gives the most dense, that is, the whitest, 'shadows' of all tissues. A radiograph of a normal shoulder (Figure 7.1) demonstrates these degrees of radio-opacity. The contrast between the various radiodensities makes the total image.

Within the diagnostic range of X-ray energy, the absorption of X-rays is apparently proportional to the second or third power of the effective atomic number (S.B. Osborn, 1969, personal communication), which explains not only why bone stands out so clearly but also why extraneous materials with higher atomic numbers cast denser 'shadows'. It is

on this account that some of these materials, notably iodine and barium, are introduced into the body as contrast media. However, the importance of this principle in the present context is that heavy metals such as iron, tin, antimony and barium, when retained in the lungs, cast particularly dense shadows which contrast sharply with the surrounding lung (see Figure 11.2). Table 7.1 sets out the atomic numbers of the major elements of the body and of some relevant extraneous elements.

In short, the image of the lung fields on the film is caused by the differential attenuation of the X-ray beam by various lung constituents of both endogenous and exogenous origin. Hence, it is the *sum* of superimposed radiodensities of structures and lesions throughout the thickness of the chest. It is essential to appreciate that the X-ray image is a two-dimensional representation of a three-dimensional structure; the body can be considered as if it were flattened against the film.

The effect of air content of the lungs

As the values of the effective atomic numbers given in the last section suggest, air, if compressed to unit

Table 7.1 Atomic numbers of relevant elements

Chief atomic constituents of body tissues and fluids		*Elements of exogenous origin*			
Hydrogen	1	Beryllium	4	Silver	47
Carbon	6	Carbon	6	Cadmium	48
Nitrogen	7	Aluminium	13	Tin	50
Oxygen	8	Silicon	14	Antimony	51
Sodium	11	Titanium	22	Iodine	53
Phosphorus	15	Vanadium	23	Barium	56
Calcium	20	Chromium	24	Rare earth elements	58 to 71
		Manganese	25	Tungsten	74
		Iron	26	Lead	82
		Cobalt	27	Bismuth	83
		Nickel	28	Thorium	90
		Zirconium	47		

density, would in fact absorb more X-rays than unit density muscle or unit density fat. However, air in the lungs is not in this state. Its volume in normal lungs causes their density to be nearer that of ambient air than that of surrounding soft tissues by a factor of about 800. Although air in the lungs contains hydrogen in the water vapour with which it is saturated, it contains only about 0.8 per cent hydrogen by weight compared with 10 per cent in soft tissues. Hence, because the ratio of air density to tissue density is normally 1 : 800, the attenuation of X-rays by air and the lungs as a whole is very substantially less than by other tissues. Furthermore, the lungs cause negligible scatter of radiation because the number of electrons per unit volume in their air is very small in comparison with that of the surrounding tissues. Indeed, it is calculated that the scattering effect (*scatter attenuation coefficient*) of air is almost 1000 times less than that of soft tissues whether these be fat, muscle, blood vessels or fibrous tissue (S.B. Osborn, 1969, personal communication).

Therefore, lung tissue has negligible radiodensity in contrast to that of its pulmonary blood vessels and their blood, mediastinal and other soft tissues, and bone; an increase of soft tissue density within the lungs or the presence of radio-opaque dusts therefore produces additional contrasting opacities on the film. This has a direct and important bearing on an alleged obscuring effect which emphysema is wrongly, but often, supposed to have on the images of pneumoconiotic lesions (see page 175).

Sharpness of the radiographic image on the film

Sharpness on radiographs is limited by three factors:

1. The penumbra around the edges of an image. This is inevitable blurring which is related to the size of the X-ray source (the focal spot) and the distance of the object from the film in relation to the distance of the film from the focal spot (*focus–film distance* or FFD) (Figure 7.2). Penumbra is less with a longer FFD and a smaller focal spot. The effect is known as *geometric blur* or *unsharpness* (Ug).
2. Movement of the object: in the living subject this can be produced by movement of the body, by failure to hold the breath or by pulsation of the

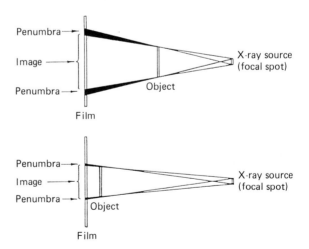

Figure 7.2 Diagram showing the effect of the position of an object on the size of the penumbra around its image on the film. The closer the object to the focal spot from which the X-rays emanate, the larger the image produced. But, because the focal spot has a finite size, the penumbra is also larger, and thus has the effect of blurring the edges of the image. This blurring effect can be decreased by reducing the object–film distance or by reducing the size of the 'focal spot'. It is for this reason that chest films are customarily taken at 6 feet (2 m) using a fine focal spot – preferably under 1 mm diameter

heart and great vessels during X-ray exposure. It is usually called *motional blur* or *unsharpness* (Um).

3. Limitations imposed by the grain size of the film and intensifying screen because all X-ray-sensitive materials are particulate. Large grains are generally more sensitive, needing less X-ray exposure, and vice versa. This determines the speed of the film–screen combination, faster films needing less exposure, so there is a 'trade-off' between image sharpness and radiation dosage. This effect is known as *screen blur* or *unsharpness* (Us).

It follows that there is a lower limit to the size of small lesions that can be shown on a radiograph, although with good apparatus, materials and technique unsharpness can be minimized.

Ug, Um and Us have to be balanced; for example, there is little point in trying to reduce Us by using very fine grain film with its associated high-radiation dosage when Ug cannot be changed on the existing apparatus.

To some extent unsharpness can be compensated for by increased contrast, particularly when the problem is to find the edge of a poorly defined lesion or the lesion differs in attenuation from its surroundings by only a small amount. This is achieved by choice of radiographic factors and by the film–screen combination and film-processing system in use in the department. It is necessary to set up these things to produce an optimum effect: too high a contrast can mask some important appearances in the low density (white) range, and a harsh black and white image can be sufficiently unpleasant to interfere with the mental processes of the observer. Conversely, too low a contrast can mask the edges of lesions in the ranges of grey.

The limitations imposed by the geometric blur may be calculated. Most modern standard X-ray tubes carry two alternative foci: 1.2 mm (broad focus) and 0.6 mm (fine focus). It may readily be calculated from a formula simply derived from the geometry shown in Figure 7.2 that, at the customary FFD of 2 m in a patient whose chest has an antero-posterior (AP) diameter of 20 cm, a fine focal spot of effective diameter 0.6 mm will produce, from the midplane of the chest, a penumbra of 0.03 mm. This means that any nodule less than 0.06 mm in diameter will not be defined by the X-ray beam because the penumbrae on each border of the lesion will touch or even overlap. With a 1.2 mm focus the penumbra will be 0.06 mm and no nodule less than 0.12 mm can be defined. It can be shown that, at a 2 m FFD, the magnification of objects within the chest will not exceed a factor of 1.01, so the difference between the diameter of a lung nodule and that of its image is virtually negligible at these small sizes.

It also follows that widespread nodules, too small to be shown discretely, may still attenuate the X-ray beam to some extent; this is the explanation of the so-called 'ground glass' shadowing described in the early stages of a number of diseases.

The term 'resolution' is often employed to indicate the degree of sharpness in the image but it should be used with caution. In a loose way, it can be said that an imaging system has better or worse resolution to indicate that it shows more or less detail, respectively, of the anatomy or pathology in the patient. Used in this way, no misunderstanding can occur. Unfortunately, resolution is defined and measured differently in the different imaging techniques. In radiology it is measured as the minimum distance apart two lines have to be in the object to be shown separately in the image. *It is usually defined as the visible number of line pairs per millimetre* (LP/mm), as measured on a test film. In CT, nuclear medicine and MRI, in which the mathematical manipulations involve volume averaging, a different concept is needed, and it is different, again, in the USA. So the physician is advised to use the term in a general way only, particularly when comparing imaging techniques.

It may be asked why it would not be possible to have X-ray tubes in routine chest work that have finer foci, so as to achieve better resolution. Although, in theory, this is possible, there are still technical limitations, mostly concerned with heat disposal. Fine focus tubes have to be kept for special purposes and used sparingly.

In any case, the limiting factor in transmission radiography is currently the screen–film blur (Us). Even the best film–screen combinations for general use at the time of writing, commensurate with the accepted levels of radiation dosage, cannot do much better than 10 to 11 LP/mm, so they would not be able to show a nodule smaller than 0.1 mm. There are high-detail systems for bone extremity work which will give up to 15 LP/mm and the special systems for mammography can produce 20 LP/mm, but in both of these the radiographic factors are different and they could not be used satisfactorily in chest work.

X-ray scatter within normal lungs is negligible but may be appreciable from overlying soft tissues and from structures of water density within the thorax, such as pleural effusions or pleural thickening. Scatter does not blur the outlines of the structures on the image but, because the scattered radiations approach the film from all directions, the effect is to produce a generalized greyness of the image. This reduces the contrast between the shadows produced by structures or lesions and the adjacent relatively transradiant lung and can make them difficult or impossible to see. In information theory terms, the signal-to-noise ratio (SNR) is reduced.

It is essential for the physician to appreciate the foregoing principles because, in all forms of occupational lung disease, diagnosis often has to be made on relatively subtle changes in the appearances of the lungs or on the recognition of very small opacities. It will fall to the radiologist and radiographer (or X-ray technician) to produce the best possible images with available equipment, staff and technique. Most radiologists and experienced radiographers or technicians are familiar with the problems – the foregoing paragraphs will have given some evidence of their complexity. For further information, texts such as those by Meredith and Massey (1977) should be consulted. In spite of the advances that have been made in modern equipment, materials and techniques, there are inherent limitations in radiography.

The standard chest radiograph

Conventionally, the routine chest film is a postero-anterior (PA) view and is usually 17 × 14 inches (43 × 35 cm). During X-ray exposure the subject's breath must be held in the deepest possible inspiration. The mid-expiratory position suggested by the International Labour Office (1959) is no longer used; it cannot be accurately controlled and prevents full expansion. In poor inspiration, relative preponderance of vascular markings – especially in the lower zones – can mimic irregular opacities, permitting false positive diagnoses – for example, pulmonary fibrosis (Figure 7.3). The heart shadow is also wider. The technique for taking good quality films is summarized in the International Classification of Radiographs of Pneumoconiosis (International Labour Office, 1970); in the revised edition (1980), objective physical criteria are given by which to judge their quality. Too-white (underexposed) or too-dark (overexposed) films are to be avoided and the quality of serial films should, if possible, be kept comparable. The quality depends on the radiographic factors applied: namely, the voltage across the X-ray tube (kV), the tube current (mA) and the exposure time. Three techniques are available. The well-established 60 to 80 kV technique is still the most common but is now regarded as 'low voltage'. Tube current (mA) and exposure time will vary in different departments depending on the type and power of the apparatus and on the speed of the film–screen combination in use.

Exposure times of less than 0.08 second largely exclude motional blur. Exposure times measured in milliseconds are produced by some powerful apparatus, but the value of this has to be assessed against the other measures of unsharpness. Geometric blur is reduced by using a long FFD, usually 2 m.

Higher voltage techniques (110 to 140 kV), because the higher energy radiation produces more scatter, require the use of a fine stationary lead grid to prevent all except forward scattered radiation reaching the film (Jacobson, Bohlig and Kiviluoto, 1970). Techniques using 150 kV involve an air gap between patient and film for the same reason and a longer FFD, usually 4 m; 350 kV has been used but does not produce satisfactory images (Herman et al., 1982). The subject has been well reviewed by Thomas (1989).

Films must be of an adequate size to include the whole of the thorax from the lung apices to just below the costophrenic angles. This applies equally to routine pneumoconiosis studies as to investigation of the individual so that, unless the patient is obviously small in an individual case, the routine use of 17 × 14 inch (43 × 35 cm) film is advised in occupational lung disease work. In subjects with unduly large chests, the lower parts of the bases may be lost. The radiographer, noticing this on inspection of the film, should then take another film with its long axis horizontal centred lower down to include the costophrenic angles (the so-called 'cross-bases' film). This should be standard practice. A case has been made for a larger film, 16 × 16 inches (40 × 40 cm) (Bohlig and Gilson, 1973) but this size is not readily available from most manufacturers.

The subjects should be unclothed above the waist. Girdles, corsets and lumbar belts should be removed because, in addition to obscuring the lower lung fields, these limit maximal inspiratory descent of the diaphragm. Women should remove brassières because supported breasts can produce remarkably dense soft tissue shadows. Failure to remove clothing, to say nothing of necklaces, beads, charms or other objects worn around the neck or waist, may lead to confusing artefacts. Vigilance is required if these are not to be interpreted as evidence of pathology – especially if obvious clues of pins or buttons are absent and it is taken for granted that the subject was stripped to the waist when the film was taken. This error is more likely to be encountered in periodic radiological examinations of workers in industry than in clinical practice, although the common custom of giving the patient a cotton or disposable paper gown to wear after undressing, particularly with female patients, can conceal the patient's failure to comply fully with instructions.

Consistency of technique is essential at all times in order to detect early radiographic changes and maintain a good comparative standard. This is particularly important in monitoring working industrial populations over a period of years. It is an essential factor to consider when attempting to improve quality, for example, by seeking new apparatus.

Close co-operation is essential between physician and radiologist to ensure that the images convey the required information. The higher voltage techniques tend to reduce contrast but show mediastinal structures better without losing lung detail. Where a

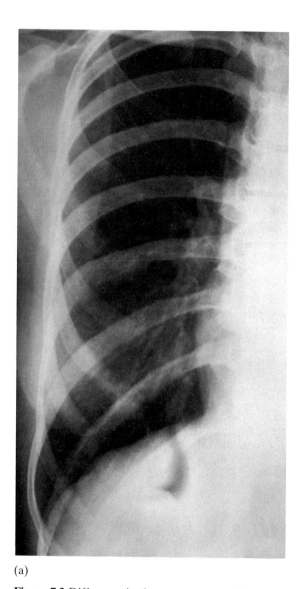
(a)

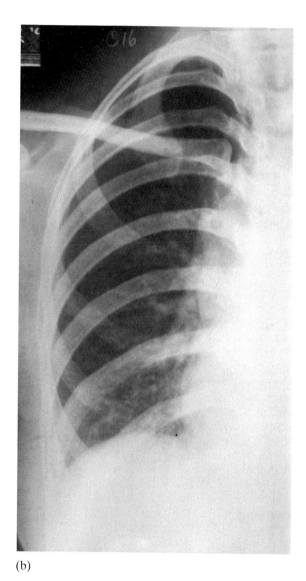
(b)

Figure 7.3 Difference in the appearances of the lower zones of normal lung fields in (a) inspiration compared with (b) expiration. The latter could be interpreted as showing basal, irregular opacities

physician works directly with a radiographer, nothing is lost by periodically consulting a radiologist specializing in chest work to keep pace with the clinical value of technical advances.

Other radiological techniques

Penetrated view

When working with low voltage technique (60 to 80 kV) it sometimes happens that part of the image is not well seen because it is too radiographically dense, that is, there is a 'white-out'. Examples of this are pleural effusion, extensive pleural thickening, collapsed lung tissue and mass lesions in the lung. In these conditions there is always the possibility that within the apparently featureless shadow there may be some useful information concealed. Small increases in voltage will sometimes give a little more information but a really dense shadow will need an 'overpenetrated view'. A substantial increase in voltage is applied (often about 20 kV more) and a grid is needed to minimize the scatter. The exposure is usually also increased. The end result is a film in which the tissues of normal density are blacked out but the region under suspicion may show features not previously visible. Examples are a lung mass

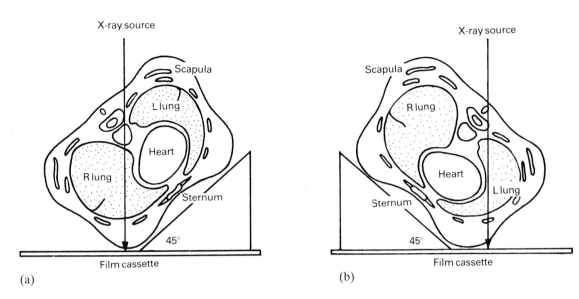

Figure 7.4 Positioning of the thorax for (a) right and (b) left anterior oblique views at 45 degrees showing why these provide invaluable complementary evidence to standard PA and lateral views of disease of the chest wall, pleura and lung. (Adapted, with permission, from *Clark's Positioning in Radiography*, 10th edn, 1979, London, Heinemann Medical)

concealed by a pleural effusion, an obstructed bronchus concealed by other tissue and an air–fluid level in a lung mass. It would be unusual for this technique to be needed in the general run of suspected occupational disease, but it can be a very useful first step in the investigation of a pleural effusion which may be the first evidence of chest disease in, for example, mesothelioma. The adoption of higher voltage techniques (110 or 150 kV) has made the overpenetrated view less necessary but it still has a place.

Lateral view

The value of a lateral view is controversial. In general chest radiology (especially in survey groups), it does not always add enough information to justify the additional radiation dose but there are clear minimum indications: namely, unilateral pathology, mediastinal pathology and suspected hilar abnormalities. In occupational lung disease it is valuable to take a lateral view when the patient is first seen. It will define the spatial relationships of abnormal shadows seen in the PA view and will show the configuration of the chest, the shape and level of the diaphragm, and the dimensions of the retrosternal 'dark' space, which are very valuable in the assessment of hyperinflation. This view also serves as a baseline for comparison with future lateral films.

There is an argument that, where widespread small discrete lesions are suspected on the PA view,

but the appearances are not quite convincing, the superimposition of the two lungs can produce a more diagnostic effect. Although this is true, detail is lost and so the type of lesion is much more difficult to determine. In general, lateral views are confusing and of little value in bilateral disease.

There is never any justification for taking both lateral views.

Anteroposterior (AP) view

An AP view is invaluable for the clarification of uncertain or small and indistinct opacities seen in PA view. It may be that they are situated in the posterior part of the lung and will be better defined because of the lesser penumbra as they will be nearer the film. Some evidence has emerged from CT studies to suggest that this is commonly the case with silicosis (see 'Computed tomography', later). It may therefore be asked why an AP film is not used routinely; the reason is that in an AP film the anterior structures in the thorax, notably the heart and anterior mediastinum, appear larger. Because X-rays emanate from a point source, objects further from the film are more magnified (see Figure 7.2).

Right and left anterior oblique views (RAO and LAO)

These are particularly helpful in demonstrating peripheral disease, such as diffuse pleural thickening or tumour deposition, and hyaline pleural plaques which may be poorly defined or even invisible in a PA view, and also in confirming or refuting the presence of diffuse intrapulmonary fibrosis especially in the lower lung fields (see Chapter 14). As a rule, more informative oblique views are produced if the subject's chest is positioned at 45 degrees to the cassette rather than at the conventional 60 degree angle (MacKenzie and Harries, 1970).

In some cases the RAO is better taken with the subject at 35 or 40 degrees to the cassette to achieve optimal visibility by reducing the obscuring effect of the heart (Figure 7.4). For routine purposes, the LAO is usually the more helpful of the two views but both should be taken when a patient suspected of having asbestos-related pleural or intrapulmonary fibrosis is first examined (see Chapter 14).

Doubt was cast by Reger et al. (1982) on the value of oblique views; interpretation of PA views showed good agreement between observers, but, although adding oblique views increased the detection rate of abnormalities, consistency between observers was appreciably less. They discouraged oblique views except in the hands of those experienced in interpreting them. Nowadays, oblique views are rarely seen in general radiology departments; they are mostly taken in specialized occupational lung disease departments. Many radiologists believe that the same information can be obtained with CT, which has other advantages. Bégin et al. (1984) made a formal comparison, described in 'Computed tomography', later (see page 194).

Macroradiography (magnification technique)

This employs a finer focal spot (0.1 to 0.3 mm) than is used for the routine PA view, and the subject is placed midway between the source and the cassette (Bracken, 1964). It produces larger but less distinct images than the standard film. It is sometimes used in the hope of detecting small discrete lesions of a pneumoconiosis before they give evidence of their presence on standard films.

However, using the geometrical principles on which Figure 7.2 is based, it may be shown that, whereas the magnification of an object in the midplane of the chest would be magnified by a factor of 2 compared with 1.05 in the standard PA radiograph, the penumbra would be the same size as the focal spot. Even with a 0.1-mm focal spot and a consequent 0.1-mm penumbra, it follows that the smallest nodule to be defined would be 0.1 mm in diameter, giving rise to a 0.2-mm image. The image of any nodule smaller than this would be masked by overlapping penumbrae. It will be recalled that in the standard PA radiograph at 2 m FFD with very

little magnification, a 0.12-mm nodule should be demonstrable with a 1.2-mm focal spot and a 0.06-mm nodule with a 0.6-mm focal spot, so there is, on theoretical grounds, virtually no advantage in using macroradiography (see page 163).

It is not surprising therefore that, although macroradiography in readily accessible small parts of the body can be useful (for example, the carpal scaphoid bone and small lesions of the breast), in the chest it has proved misleading. Normal people have been said to have discrete pneumoconiotic lesions and those with proven dust exposure regarded as normal, as the editor of this volume can testify. Careful scrutiny of a standard PA radiograph, followed by inspection with a ×2 or ×4 hand lens, is much more satisfactory. There is good correlation between appearances in standard PA radiographs and postmortem findings.

Apical view

There are occasions when lesions in the lung apical regions (defined as the region above the lower border of the first rib) are poorly defined due to overlying rib shadows, or there are multiple lesions difficult to separate visually. In these cases, the central ray may be made to pass along the lower and posterior surface of the first rib, by tilting the patient backwards and the X-ray tube upwards, and centring on the first anterior interspace, so producing a localized bone-free image at a different angle. It is of great value in distinguishing, for example, tuberculosis or neoplasm from pneumoconiotic apical lesions. In a kyphotic patient it may be easier to do a reversed apical view PA, with the tube angled downwards. The apical view should be distinguished from the *lordotic view* in which the whole thorax is exposed with the patient leaning backwards and a lower centring point; the usual purpose is to see the oblique fissures 'end-on' when there is a possibility of an interlobar effusion. Again, there are those who prefer to use CT to solve these problems but an extra plain radiograph is much easier and cheaper.

Tomography

This technique – in which film and tube move in opposite directions during exposure to 'blur-off' structures other than those in the plane under study, producing an image of a slice or 'cut', from 1 mm to 1 cm thick depending on the angle through which the tube moves – is not used much in occupational disease.

It is sometimes of value in finding cavities, in differentiating a confluent pneumoconiotic mass from other lesions and in identifying such a mass when partly obscured by heart and mediastinal shadows. Both AP and lateral tomography may be needed. Again, many prefer CT for solving these problems but tomography has much to offer, although really thick cuts – zonography – are rarely of use.

Mass miniature radiography (MMR)

In the past, when this was the best case-finding technique for tuberculosis and other readily visible chest pathology, it was very valuable. The disadvantage of most MMR systems using photofluorography (photographing a fluoroscopic screen image) is that they have a short FFD, the mirror optics entail some loss of efficiency (lens cameras are even worse) and the 35 mm or 70 mm films have a slower speed compared with large film–screen combinations. Consequently, there is more geometric blur, preventing the early identification of the early stages of a discrete pneumoconiosis such as silicosis or coal pneumoconiosis, or of the diffuse interstitial fibrosis of asbestosis. The radiation dosage to the patient is higher; it was by a factor of 3 to 4 when the systems were in full use but advances in film–screen speed in conventional large film radiography in recent years have brought this figure up to 8 to 12 or even 20. In most parts of the world, MMR has been generally discontinued and it has very little use now either in general radiology or in screening programmes.

A variation of this technique, using a large screen X-ray image intensifier at 125 kV, is said to produce images of quality comparable with the results of conventional 125 kV technique with four- to sixfold reduction of patient dosage, but the apparatus is expensive and not generally available.

Procedure for inspection of the chest radiograph

The physician must not automatically assume that, because the diagnosis is being considered in an occupational context, any lesions seen are to be regarded as of occupational origin. The film must be approached with an open mind. Failure to do this can lead to an appreciable proportion of diagnostic errors – 11 per cent false positives in one series (Epstein et al., 1984).

Reasonable viewing conditions with reduced ambient light are essential. Complete darkness is unnecessary but the room should not be in bright light such as sun shining through the windows or 100-W bulbs overhead. If a bank of viewing boxes is being used, all should be switched off except those with films on them. Otherwise, the pupillary constriction so produced in the eyes of the observer is enough to prevent much of the weaker light from the image reaching the retina. Strong ambient light may well also interfere with the retinal edge enhancement function due to the Mach band phenomenon (Lane, Proto and Philips, 1976). This results in an impaired appreciation of subtle differences in shades of grey and, hence, of small differences in contrast, particularly in the darker parts of the image. Small lesions against a dark background may just not be perceived. The reduced attenuation of emphysema can produce relative overexposure of the lung fields and lead to a false deduction that the lesions are concealed (see also page 175).

Viewing boxes (illuminators) normally have two 15-W white fluorescent tubes. Various shades are available and are a matter of choice. The author's preference is for a bluer shade (usually designated 'Tropical Daylight') but what really matters is that *all* the illuminators in any given institution should be of the *same* shade and intensity in the clinical and radiological departments, as should the viewing conditions.

A strong light (100 to 150 W) to study darker parts of the film should always be within reach of the observer's hand. The film is best observed at arm's length in the first instance. Gross abnormalities may be well enough seen from distances of 2 to 3 m or more, but the relatively fine abnormalities of occupational lung disease cannot, and sometimes need a hand magnifying lens also within reach. This always presents difficulty in clinical conferences and ward rounds.

Unless a systematic and consistent discipline for examining the film is followed, abnormalities may be overlooked or misinterpreted. The observer should acquire the imaginative ability of 'looking into' the two-dimensional image as if it were three-dimensional, mentally dissecting it in layers. There are several published scrutiny systems, all quite satisfactory (for example, Meschan, 1966; Trapnell, 1967; Simon, 1978; Squire, 1982; Sutton, 1987), and the reader may already be using one. What matters is that there should be no significant omission. Many experienced observers will take in most of the information on the image at first glance, presumably having already gone rapidly through an inspection system, but this process is liable to bias: the eye sees what the mind expects. Some diagnostic image patterns are readily recognizable, but any spot diagnosis thus made should be mentally shelved pending the conscious systematic scrutiny; it may not be confirmed.

The author's preference (Bretland, 1978) is for a scheme that classifies the items to be studied, as shown in Table 7.2, into five anatomical groups of five, which makes it easier to remember them all.

Table 7.2 Scrutiny method

I Soft tissues	II Bony cage	III Central shadow	IV Hila	V Lung fields
Root of neck	Shoulder girdle	Trachea	Shape	Pleura
Axillae	Vertebrae	Superior mediastinum	Size	Horizontal and other fissures
Pectoral muscles	Ribs	Heart shadow – size and shapea	Height	Compare spaces
Breasts	Costal cartilages	Behind heart	Size of vessels	Peripheral lung pattern
Diaphragm and below	Sternum	Heart borders	Distribution of vessels	Abnormal shadows

From Bretland (1978).

An anatomical approach is preferred because, although radiographs and other forms of imaging are very good for locating a lesion in the body, and sometimes describing its physiological behaviour, they are much less effective at saying what it is. Once the location is established, the appearances and behaviour of the lesion noted and the pattern in space and time ascertained, the differential diagnosis can be considered.

If the reader accepts this approach, it may be found useful to have a full-sized, good quality 17 × 14 inch (43 × 35 cm), normal standard PA radiograph available while reading the following paragraphs.

Before starting, there are five routine checks to be made:

1. Name and date (is it the right film?).
2. Side (R or L marker) (remember Kartagener's syndrome of dextrocardia and bronchiectasis).
3. Position (check symmetry of medial ends of clavicles and anterior rib ends for possible rotation).
4. Quality (not over- or underpenetrated or exposed).
5. Respiration (anterior end of right fifth or sixth rib should be visible above the right diaphragm).

The first two groups, the extrathoracic soft tissues and the bones, may be grouped together as the peripheral region.

The soft tissues

The soft tissues of the root of the neck, axillae, chest wall (including the pectoral muscles and breasts) and the diaphragm on both sides are studied and compared. The breast shadows should be noted and checked against the recorded sex, looking for absence, asymmetry or inappropriate presence. The intense radio-opacity of the diaphragm must be 'looked into' carefully to detect abnormal opacities (such as localized pleural thickening) which are only slightly different in density from diaphragmatic muscle. The regions below the diaphragm (liver on the right, gastric air bubble, spleen and splenic flexure on the left) should be noted.

The bones

The shoulder girdle (scapula, clavicle and upper end of humerus on both sides), the vertebrae, the ribs, the costal cartilages and sternum frequently provide clues to disease – pulmonary or otherwise. Much of this is outside the scope of this book, but is discussed elsewhere (for example, Bretland, 1978; Squire, 1982; Sutton, 1987). Mention should be made here of the costal cartilages. The first is almost always calcified in the adult, usually in a bizarre pattern specific for the individual. The others commonly show some calcification, in most people over 30 years of age. Care must be taken not to mistake this for pleural or pulmonary pathology.

Before leaving the peripheral region, the costal margins of the lung fields should be followed from the lung apices to the costophrenic angles and then along the diaphragm to the cardiophrenic angles. One should be familiar with the 'companion shadows' of the lateral chest wall. In the upper zones they are quite fine and of no significance. They may also be seen for a few rib spaces above the costophrenic angles in some normal PA films. These are triangular opacities whose lateral aspects are continuous with the rib shadows and their medial aspects usually well defined and vertical, while their lower parts lack definition. They are bilateral although not necessarily symmetrical, and are caused by the interdigitation of the serratus anterior and external abdominal oblique muscles (Figure 7.5). Slight rotation of the chest makes these shadows more prominent on one side than the other, when they may be misinterpreted as pleural lesions if their true nature is not appreciated. However, they disappear completely on oblique views.

Another important normal anatomical feature is extrapleural costal fat. This is distributed bilaterally beneath the parietal pleura immediately adjacent to the ribs. It tends to be most abundant posteriorly over the fourth to ninth ribs. Although, as a rule, not closely correlated with total body fat, it may be excessive in some subjects in whom there has been a large gain in weight, including those with hyper-corticosteroidism. The deposits cause an undulating opacification along the costal margin of the lung

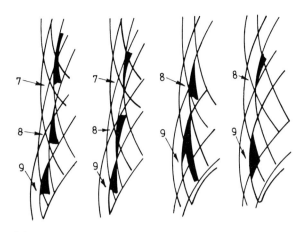

(a)

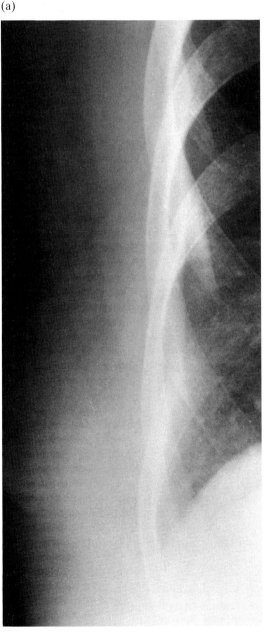

(b)

Figure 7.5 (a) Diagrams of different forms of normal muscle shadows – 'companion shadows' – on the lateral chest wall. (Reproduced, with permission, from Fletcher and Edge, 1970.) (b) Radiograph of type C. (Reproduced by courtesy of L. Preger, *Asbestos-related Disease*, and the Editor, Grune and Stratton.) These shadows are apt to be mistaken for pleural abnormalities, a point which may be important in an asbestos worker

fields (but not in the costophrenic angles) and may be wrongly interpreted as pleural thickening or hyaline plaque formation if the observer is unaware of this normal variant (Gluck et al., 1972; Vix, 1974) (Figure 7.6). They are most clearly demonstrated by anterior oblique views (see page 167).

Fat can also appear beneath the pleura but this is more difficult to distinguish from pleural pathology; CT is usually required (Sargent et al., 1984).

Yet another potential cause of error is the serratus anterior muscle which can cast a shadow over the lateral chest wall on the PA view (Collins, Brown and Batra, 1983). These authors were happy to make the correct diagnosis with oblique views and fluoroscopy but accepted that CT would also solve the problem of a potential false-positive diagnosis of pleural disease (see Chapter 14, page 458).

Scrutiny is now directed to the intrathoracic structures.

The central shadow

The position, size and shape of the trachea should be noted, looking especially for deviation to one side. Above the sternal notch this is usually due to extrinsic pressure, commonly from an enlarged thyroid lobe, even if retrosternal. In the chest it might indicate either loss of volume in the ipsilateral lung due to collapse or fibrosis, or increase in volume on the other side, either by obstructive emphysema or by a pleural effusion. Convex bowing of the trachea to the side of displacement is usually due to upper lobe fibrosis of which the most common cause is old tuberculosis, or to collapse of the upper lobe, whether acute or chronic.

If it is deviated but straight, there is usually loss of volume in the lower lobe on the affected side, which may be the first clue to an obstructing lesion of the lower lobe bronchus. In an adequately penetrated film, particularly in the higher voltage techniques, the bronchial tree can sometimes be followed to the point of obstruction. A central trachea in the presence of a large effusion usually indicates underlying collapse of part or all of the lung on that side. In older people an unfolded atherosclerotic aorta often displaces the trachea to

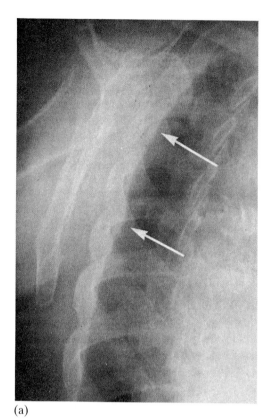

(a)

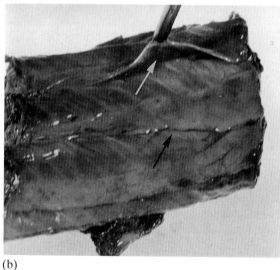

(b)

Figure 7.6 (a) Appearances caused by prominent extrapleural costal fat which may be mistaken for pleural disease. (b) Postmortem appearances of flaps of costal fat (arrowed). (Reproduced, with permission, from Vix, 1974)

the right without indicating lung disease. The bronchi should not normally be seen beyond the origins of the segmental branches. If they are visible further than that, an 'air bronchogram', there must

be increased opacity of the lung tissue. This may be a sign of early widespread pathology, before the lesions are large enough to be shown (see page 164).

The great vessels should be noted together with any change in shape of the superior mediastinum; among other things, the possibility of lymph node enlargement and its differential diagnosis must be considered.

The heart shape and size should be assessed. In many cases chamber enlargement can be identified; although this is controversial, it is commonly possible to distinguish right and left ventricular predominance, and the so-called 'mitral heart' shape can be recognized (Bretland, 1978).

The heart borders are normally sharp due to the contrast between the heart muscle shadow and the relative blackening of the adjacent lung tissue. If they are blurred (the 'outline' or 'silhouette' sign), there is pathology in the adjacent lung, valuable in localizing segmental lesions. Irregular mediastinal pleural thickening can produce the 'shaggy heart' appearance sometimes seen in asbestosis and other types of diffuse interstitial pulmonary fibrosis.

Abnormal appearances of the lungs may have a cardiac origin, and vice versa. It is essential to 'look through' the heart shadow to identify any pathology behind the heart, whether associated with the vertebrae, the lungs or the pleura.

Other texts should be consulted for detailed guidance on the central shadow, such as those quoted earlier.

The hila

The size, shape and height of the hilar shadows should be studied. The left hilum is normally higher than the right by a distance that is somewhere between the width of a rib and that of a rib space. Most of the hilar shadow is due to the pulmonary artery, which normally has a generally concave lateral margin; if it is convex, it is abnormal. At this stage a first look should be taken at the pulmonary artery branches. A convex hilum with large branches indicates big pulmonary arteries, seen in either left to right shunts or pulmonary arterial hypertension. If occupational lung disease has seriously impaired ventilation at an early stage, this may be the first clue. A convex hilum, possibly with a lobulated outline, and normal sized pulmonary arteries, usually indicates the presence of enlarged hilar nodes. Note should be taken here of any calcification, thinking of either an old calcified primary tuberculous complex or the egg-shell calcification sometimes seen in silicosis. Lesser, but appreciable, increase in radiographic density, but not in size, of the hilar nodes may be seen in iron and tin pneumoconioses (see Chapter 11) and, sometimes, in sarcoidosis (Scadding and Mitchell, 1985).

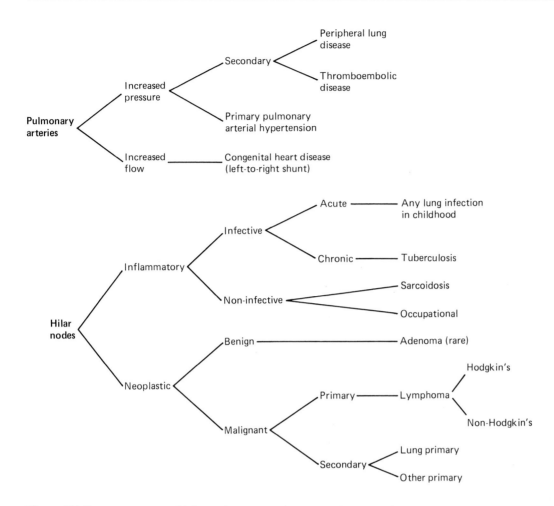

Figure 7.7 Common causes of hilar enlargement. (From Bretland, 1978)

Detailed analysis of hilar shadows and of pulmonary arteries will be found in other texts; assessment can be difficult. A simple classification is given in Figure 7.7 (Bretland, 1978).

Leading on from the hilar scrutiny, the pulmonary arteries should be followed out to the periphery, or at least as far as they go, usually disappearing in the outer third of the lung fields. Their branching, distribution and size should be noted. An abnormal distribution of pulmonary arteries is seen in localized loss of lung tissue, for example, from collapse, lobectomy, localized emphysema or following pulmonary embolus. Vessels lying in a plane roughly parallel to that of the film will show the expected branching pattern, but others seen 'end-on' (remembering the three-dimensional nature of the body) will appear as round or oval opacities. It is important not to mistake such appearances for discrete lesions. In severe pulmonary arterial hypertension the arteries may taper off too soon, the so-called 'peripheral pruning'. This appearance may also be seen in panacinar emphysema. Pulmonary veins are normally not well seen, but if they are enlarged as in moderate pulmonary venous hypertension, they are identifiable in the lower zones by being roughly horizontal. In the upper zones, they are difficult to separate from arteries; however, in more severe pulmonary venous hypertension, the lower lobe veins disappear and only prominent upper lobe vessels are visible.

The lung fields

Before starting to look at the lung fields it is essential to turn attention to the pleura. Concentration on or even a quick look at the peripheral structures can easily cause pleural lesions to be overlooked. Pneumothorax, pleural effusion, pleural thickening (with or without calcification), encysted pleural effusions and even an early mesothelioma can all be missed if specific thought is not given to the possibilities. A shadow within the lung field is not necessarily intrapulmonary, and lateral, oblique or lordotic views or even CT may be necessary to solve such a problem.

Next, the fissures must be considered. The horizontal fissure on the right usually overlies the right fourth rib in front and the sixth rib in the mid-axillary line. The oblique fissures are invisible in the normal PA film unless there is pleural thickening or an encysted effusion. The appearance often described as 'tenting' of the diaphragm is, in fact, pleural thickening at the lower end of the oblique fissure.

The vascular shadows, commonly known as 'normal lung markings', require one further look. Their distribution should be roughly symmetrical and evenly distributed; if they are too sparse generally, especially peripherally, panacinar emphysema may be suspected and, indeed, confirmed by the presence of an expanded rib cage, an increase in the retrosternal transradiant space in the lateral view, a narrow, vertical heart and low, flat diaphragm (Simon, 1964); but it has to be severe to show all these features. It may be mimicked by airways' obstruction; the two may coexist. Localized patches of emphysema produce disturbance of the vascular pattern (see Chapter 9). Bullae contain no lung tissue but some lung pattern will be seen through them. Recent pulmonary embolism also leaves defects in the vascular pattern.

The normal 'lung markings' may now be ignored and the lung tissue, normally invisible on the film, should be studied for evidence of other parenchymal lesions, comparing the two sides by looking at corresponding regions. It is helpful here to use the concept of upper, middle and lower zones, the lung fields being arbitrarily divided by two horizontal lines drawn through the anterior ends of the second and fourth ribs. It is in the study of the abnormal background patterns in the lung fields that clues to the diagnosis are likely to lie. However, it must be emphasized that there is no radiographic appearance unique to any one type of pneumoconiosis. All other relevant information must be considered, radiographic and otherwise; spot diagnosis is particularly dangerous.

Abnormal background patterns

The distribution of the abnormal pattern must first be noted: whether mostly upper, mid or lower zone, and how widespread.

An abnormal pattern largely confined to the lower zones is common in congestive cardiac failure, usually bilateral but not necessarily symmetrical, long-standing mitral valve disease, bronchopneumonia (one or both sides), diffuse interstitial pulmonary fibrosis (fibrosing alveolitis), bronchiectasis and asbestosis. Mid-zone involvement is seen in those types of pulmonary oedema associated with acute left ventricular failure ('bat's wing shadows') and in pulmonary alveolar proteinosis. Mid-zone

and upper zone distribution is usual in silicosis and in coal pneumoconiosis. Apical and upper zone predominance is usual in localized tuberculous and fungal infections. In the absence of a characteristic distribution, other evidence will be required.

The vast majority of such abnormal patterns can be analysed in terms of three types of abnormal shadow, although more than one may be present. These are 'nodular' shadows, linear shadows and ring shadows, illustrated diagrammatically in Figure 7.8.

Nodular shadows

These may be classified as over or under 2 mm in diameter, as 'hard' or 'soft' depending on their radiographic density, as well defined with sharp edges, or poorly defined, even coalescent. Larger nodules of differing sizes are commonly due to successive 'showers' of blood-borne malignant metastases although one major 'shower' may give a uniform nodular pattern. They are usually well defined. Soft, often coalescent, ill-defined nodular shadows of varying sizes up to 4 mm in diameter, mostly basal, are a feature of congestive cardiac failure, due to alveolar oedema. This is often associated with pleural effusions of varying sizes (often quite small) or with short horizontal lines in the costophrenic angles (septal lines, or Kerley 'B' lines, referred to later), enlarged upper lobe pulmonary veins and an enlarged heart. This is an example of a well-known pattern, virtually diagnostic provided it is clinically probable.

If extensive pulmonary oedema is present, coalescence of the soft nodules produces soft fluffy-looking shadows, seen in acute heart failure, drowning and other aspiration situations, including acute heroin, barbiturate and other poisoning.

Generalized nodular shadowing, soft but reasonably well defined and of uniform diameter up to 2 mm, is commonly due to one of four main groups of disease: occupational disorders, sarcoidosis, miliary tuberculosis and miliary carcinomatosis. It is clearly vital to differentiate between these four, although they are sometimes indistinguishable. In miliary tuberculosis the nodules are more uniform in size and density and are evenly distributed (so-called 'snowstorm' appearance) but then a single 'shower' of metastases can look the same. In sarcoidosis the lesions tend not to be so well defined and may present a more reticulated appearance but this disease is a great imitator and may show anything from reticulation through nodular shadows to 2-cm blotches. The presence of hilar glandular enlargement is a help but is not necessary for the diagnosis.

The so-called classic appearance of *Pneumocystis carinii* pneumonia (PCP) is that of a perihilar

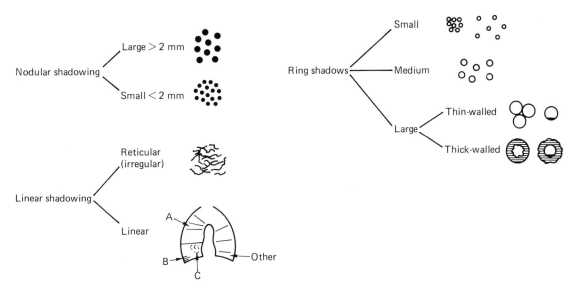

Figure 7.8 Abnormal radiographic patterns in the lung fields

ground-glass appearance which progresses through a reticulonodular appearance to definite nodular shadowing, becoming more extensive (Forrest, 1972). Atypical features are, however, common in this condition, especially when it appears as a complication of the acquired immune deficiency syndrome (AIDS), ranging from no apparent radiographic abnormality to patchy non-specific pneumonic-like shadows (Doppman, Geelhoed and De Vita, 1975; Gedroyc and Reidy, 1985; Heron et al., 1985; Rankin and Pella, 1987).

Well-defined, basal, nodular shadows, which may be calcified or even ossified, are a feature of long-standing mitral stenosis but they may occasionally be more widely distributed. The appearance of the pulmonary veins and the heart shape and size may help to complete the characteristic pattern of mitral disease.

Another nodular pattern is that often seen in old tuberculosis in the lower and mid-zones in the presence of old fibrotic lesions in the shrunken upper zone. These are generally thought to be due to bronchial spread; usually unilateral, they should not cause confusion.

Calcified nodular shadows scattered through the lung, if relatively evenly spaced, are likely to be due to a previous attack of chickenpox in adult life or to old histoplasmosis; if they are in one or two irregular clusters, more in the upper zones, they are likely to be due to old tuberculosis; healed miliary tuberculosis may calcify and leave areas of scattered calcifications.

Occupational lung disease is widely thought to be a common cause of discrete nodular shadowing. This is certainly true for the inert dusts such as those containing tin or iron and for the fibrogenic dusts of silicosis and coal pneumoconiosis; the appearances of beryllium pneumoconiosis are generally believed to be indistinguishable from those of sarcoidosis, which has more of a reticular appearance. Nodular shadowing can also occur in other granulomatous diseases such as those caused by fungi, as in farmers' lung, or avian proteins in bird fanciers' lung, but the nodules are larger, less dense, less well defined and may be 1 to 5 mm in diameter. They tend to be upper and mid-zone lesions and not so uniform (see Chapter 20).

The foregoing has only touched the more common causes of nodular shadows; there are many others listed in Table 7.3.

The presence of emphysema may introduce difficulties. Rarely, in severe, chronic airways' obstruction or severe panacinar emphysema associated with secondary polycythaemia, the pulmonary artery branches in the mid-lung become larger and, where seen 'end-on', can be mistaken for nodular shadows (as may the appearances in pulmonary plethora due to left-to-right shunts). It has been alleged that emphysema may have an obscuring effect so as to conceal small nodules because of increased scatter due to excess air in the lungs (Rappaport, 1936, 1967; Ogilvie, 1970), and thus lead to an underassessment of the category. From the physical principles of differential attenuation already described (page 161), it will be clear that this cannot be so. Furthermore, it has been shown that in the presence of severe emphysema in cases categorized 0/1 there is no excess of pneumoconiotic lesions at postmortem examination (Caplan, 1962) and that so-called 'focal' emphysema, not identifiable radiographically, tends to be associated with overassessment of category (Rossiter et al., 1967).

Table 7.3 Some causes of discrete and irregular opacities

Discrete opacities – round or stellate	*Irregular or linear opacities with or without cystic appearances*
Infections	
Chickenpox (healed calcified lesions) in adults	
Tuberculosis – miliary*	
Blastomycosis*	
Coccidioidomycosis*	
Histoplasmosis*	
Torulosis*	
Schistosomiasis	
Inhalation	
Dusts	
Iron	
Silver	
Barium	
Tin	
Antimony	
Titanium	
Zirconium	
Rare earths	
Coal and carbon	
Free silica	Free silica (occasional)
China clay	
	Asbestos
'Talc' (quartz)	'Talc' (tremolite, anthophyllite)
Beryllium*	Beryllium
	'Hard metal' (cobalt)
Actinomycetes, fungi and other organic materials (extrinsic allergic alveolitis)*	Actinomycetes, fungi and other organic materials (diffuse interstitial fibrosis)
Fumes and gases	
Oxides of nitrogen*	Mercury vapour
Ozone*	Smoking
Phosgene*	
Aspiration	
Pneumonia*	Diffuse interstitial fibrosis
Chronic oronasal sepsis	Chronic oronasal sepsis
Oesophagopharyngeal reflux of gastric contents	Oesophagopharyngeal reflux of gastric contents
Near-drowning	Near-drowning
Liquid paraffin	Liquid paraffin
Diagnostic contrast media*	
Associated with cardiovascular disease	
Alveolar oedema*	Diffuse interstitial oedema*
Mitral stenosis	
Haemosiderosis	
Miliary ossification	
Right-sided infective endocarditis*	
Uncertain cause	
Sarcoidosis*	Sarcoidosis
Associated with erythema nodosum*	Idiopathic diffuse interstitial fibrosis (cryptogenic fibrosing alveolitis)
Idiopathic haemosiderosis	
Alveolar proteinosis*	
Microlithiasis	
Associated with general constitutional diseases	
'Rheumatoid' pneumoconiosis	Developmental
	Diffuse interstitial fibrosis (fibrosing alveolitis) with or without connective tissue disorders (see Table 15.1)
	Xanthomatosis
	Tuberous sclerosis
	Cystic disease of the pancreas
Reticulosis and blood disease	
Leukaemia	
Hodgkin's disease	
Lymphosarcoma	Lymphosarcoma

Table 7.3 *continued*

Discrete opacities – round or stellate	Irregular or linear opacities with or without cystic appearances

Neoplastic
   Primary and secondary carcinoma
   Bronchiolar carcinoma
	Lymphangitis carcinomatosa

Allergic
   Extrinsic allergic alveolitis*
   Eosinophilic infiltration*
   Infiltration during asthma*
   Polyarteritis nodosa*
	Extrinsic allergic alveolitis

Associated with healed inflammatory disease	Fibrosis (organized pneumonia) Bronchiectasis
Familial	Diffuse interstitial fibrosis

*Opacities which may disappear, or regress, spontaneously or with appropriate therapy. Modified from J.G. Scadding (1952) with permission of Emeritus Professor Scadding and the Editor of *Tubercle*.

Displacement of lesions by large emphysematous bullae is a different matter and is usually obvious. Emphysema may, however, cause errors in interpretation if the film is not viewed in reduced ambient light conditions with a strong light readily available, because of the dark appearance of the lung fields caused by their reduced attenuation.

Linear and irregular shadows

These may be classified as normal and abnormal. Almost the only normal linear shadows are the fissures. The main or oblique fissures should be well shown on lateral views and the right horizontal fissure on the PA or AP. Less well known are the very rare left 'horizontal' fissure, sometimes seen sloping obliquely down from the left fourth rib in the mid-axillary line, and the less rare right inferior accessory fissure, which runs downwards and laterally from the right heart border across the cardiophrenic angle to meet the diaphragm about a third of the way from the heart border. In lateral view it seems to run downwards and backwards from the anterior chest wall.

Abnormal linear shadows may again be classified into reticular (irregular) and true linear shadows. 'Reticular' is a descriptive term applied to an appearance that looks like a fine irregular network. There are occasions when it is difficult to be sure whether a fine irregular nodular pattern or a network of lines is being seen. In fact, it has been shown experimentally (Carstairs, 1961) that by passing X-rays through increasing numbers of plastic lattices perpendicular to the beam, eventually an appearance of apparently discrete nodular opacities can be produced. They are a little irreg-

ular with poorly defined areas of relative transradiancy between them but the clear definition of the original lattice is lost (Figure 7.9). It follows that many fibrotic lesions, especially those with finer strands, may produce semi-nodular shadows, which explains some of the appearances that may be observed in extrinsic allergic alveolitis and diffuse interstitial pulmonary fibrosis (DIPF). It also explains the apparent fine nodular appearance seen in cases of uniformly distributed emphysema in dust-pigmented lungs without fibrosis and where there is retention of dusts of low atomic number such as carbon. For these reasons, the term 'reticular pattern' should be used for the radiographic appearance of a fine, somewhat irregular, network which may be very close to a nodular pattern.

Reticular patterns (irregular opacities) are seen in some forms of sarcoidosis, in idiopathic DIPF – 'lone' or associated with connective tissue disorders such as rheumatoid arthritis and systemic sclerosis (see Chapter 15) – and in asbestosis (see Chapter 14).

A term that is capable of misinterpretation is 'mottling', because it has been given different meanings in various places. The British Ministry of Health (1952) defined 'mottling' as multiple discrete or semi-confluent shadows generally less than 5 mm in diameter, and 'miliary mottling' as numerous discrete well-defined shadows not exceeding 2 mm in diameter. Regrettably, all too often these two terms are used to indicate almost any abnormal background pattern by those who have not yet acquired the ability to analyse the pattern properly. Because of potential ambiguity, the term 'mottling' should be avoided, as better terminology is available.

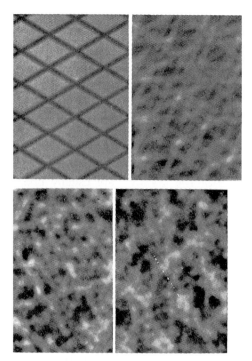

Figure 7.9 The effect produced by superimposing an increasing number of plastic lattices lying at right angles to the X-ray beam. The simple pattern produced by one layer becomes progressively 'nodular' in appearance with ill-defined areas of relative translucency. (Reproduced, with permission, from Carstairs, 1961)

True linear shadows ('A', 'B' and 'C' lines)

These were first described by Kerley – tentatively in 1933, dogmatically in 1950. He described abnormal lines seen in silicosis, pneumoconiosis and other diseases totally different from the normal vascular markings and from the increased streakiness due to oedematous bronchial mucosa. They were quite sharp, 0.5 to 1 mm wide. He classified them as follows:

'A' Lines several inches long, rather ragged and radiating from the hilum. They do not bifurcate and they do not follow the normal branching pattern of bronchi and vessels.
'B' Short sharp lines seen only at the bases, usually less than an inch long and running transversely outwards to touch the pleural margin.
'C' Fine interlacing lines giving the network appearance. It is the fine interlacing lines which have given rise to the term 'reticulation'.

Kerley thought they were due either to strands of fibrous tissue or to choked lymphatics. Trapnell (1963, 1964a) produced evidence to show that 'A' lines could be due to accumulation of dust in deep interlobular septa or in lymphatic anastomotic vessels between the central and peripheral regions, or both, but that 'B' lines could only be due to material in the peripheral interlobular septa because they did not correspond with the anatomy of the lymphatics. The 'C' lines are presumably similar to the 'A' lines but much shorter and run at various angles which foreshorten them on the image.

These lines occur in silicosis and coal pneumoconiosis and in benign pneumoconioses due to inert dusts, such as stannosis and haemosiderosis. They are more common in the higher categories of coal pneumoconiosis (ILO categories 3A, B and C – see Part II), 'B' lines being more common than 'A' (Trapnell, 1964a); and both 'A' and 'B' lines seem to be seen more often in the right lung than in the left (Rivers et al., 1960). They are present in only about half of the cases of coal pneumoconiosis seen by the editor of this volume, a finding confirmed by Trapnell (1964a).

Occupational disease, however, is not the most common cause. These septal lines, particularly the 'B' lines, can also be seen in conditions where there is lymphatic obstruction and those in which there is interstitial oedema, the septa being engorged with fluid. Thus, they appear in cardiac failure, particularly that due to mitral stenosis or left ventricular failure, as a consequence of pulmonary venous hypertension. They can be a transient feature of acute congestive failure and possibly occur in allergic oedema (Prosser and Thurley, 1976). They are occasionally seen locally in some stages of pneumonia. Unilateral 'B' lines may be the first sign of a neoplasm of the bronchus with hilar glandular lymphatic obstruction. Direct invasion by neoplasm of the radiating lymphatics from the hilum can occur, giving rise to the condition known as lymphangitis carcinomatosa. All three types of line may be seen, and superimposition of linear shadows may give rise to an irregular reticular appearance that is difficult to distinguish from a nodular pattern. Enlarged hilar lymph nodes are often present but the heart is usually of normal size.

Trapnell (1964b) found 'A' lines in 10 per cent of 100 cases of proven sarcoidosis and 'B' lines in 5 per cent, but never in the presence of enlarged hilar nodes. He suggested that they were due to perilymphatic sarcoid deposits in the septa. Perilymphatic pathology may also be the explanation for the appearances in some cases of pulmonary fibrosis, neoplasm and haemosiderosis.

True fibrotic linear shadows may be seen in long-standing tuberculosis and also in radiation fibrosis following radiotherapy, usually associated with loss of volume of the affected part of the lung.

Another type of linear shadow is the single horizontal shadow often seen in the lower zone. Although frequently described as 'linear' or 'plate' atelectases or 'Fleischner's lines', many now regard these as fibrous scars of old lung infarcts and of little clinical significance. In the first week of a basal lung infarct, horizontal streaky shadowing at the lung base associated with a raised diaphragm is virtually a diagnostic pattern.

Ring shadows

These may be classified, as in Figure 7.8, into three types: small (up to 3 mm), medium (up to 1 to 2 cm) and large. The term is usually applied to curved lines forming complete circles, usually airspaces bounded by abnormal tissue. In bronchiectasis there are multiple small ring shadows, usually (but not always) basal due to the destruction by infection of alveolar walls and coalescence of the resultant small airspaces – in effect, small abscesses. In other conditions the ring shadows are due to remaining intact air-containing lung tissue in the spaces between pathological tissue, particularly those involving fibrosis. The most common cause is chronic fibrosing alveolitis (DIPF) in which there is a combination of small nodular and small ring shadowing, but they may also be seen in long-standing fibrotic sarcoidosis, 'rheumatoid disease', histiocytosis X and tuberous sclerosis, and can also be a feature of lymphangitis carcinomatosa. When the appearance is more extensive and the ring shadows a little larger, the term 'honeycomb lung' is sometimes used but as many severe generalized lung diseases can end up like this, it is often described as 'end-stage lung'.

Abnormal shadows

These may be roughly classified into five groups: (1) large homogeneous shadows over 1 cm in diameter; (2) irregular shadows of varying density; (3) cavitary shadows; (4) 'fibrotic' shadows; and (5) the 'coin' lesion.

Large homogeneous shadows

The following properties should be noted:

1. Compatibility with lobar or segmental anatomy which might suggest collapse–consolidation or obstructive collapse.
2. Its shape – a well-rounded lesion is likely to be either a cyst (including hydatid disease) or a benign tumour such as adenoma, hamartoma, chondroma or tuberculoma (the last three may contain calcification) whereas lobulation indicates the likelihood of neoplasm.
3. Its borders: if they are well defined, it is rather less likely to be neoplastic, although a single solitary secondary deposit can be well defined

and rounded. Poor definition often indicates neoplasm but it is also seen in encysted pleural effusion seen *en face*. Spiculation is also suggestive of neoplasm but the progressive massive fibrotic shadows of silicosis and coal pneumoconiosis may have irregular borders and, looked at in isolation, may appear to be similar. Progressive massive fibrosis (PMF) commonly arises in relatively advanced occupational disease, and the associated background pattern and distortion of lung anatomy usually allow differentiation. The shadows are usually upper and mid-zone, the latter being the common site for those seen in Caplan's syndrome in rheumatoid arthritis in coal miners. Distinction from neoplasm can be difficult occasionally (Cookson et al., 1985, 1986).

Irregular shadows of varying density

These can be very confusing. Pulmonary oedema, while usually producing basal fluffy shadows, can be perihilar when acute; shifting patches may be seen. Bronchopneumonia and other infections should be considered. They are commonly basal and, if recurrent, may be due to an underlying bronchiectasis. Organisms to bear in mind in distributions other than basal are *Haemophilus* sp., Friedländer's bacillus, fungi and the tubercle bacillus in the upper zones. Perihilar and basal shadowing are common in *Pneumocystis carinii* pneumonia (PCP) complicating AIDS but the shadowing may be anywhere and the nodular appearance may not be seen (Cohen et al., 1984; Gedroyc and Reidy, 1985; Heron et al., 1985). Shifting patches of consolidation are a feature of mycoplasma pneumonia. Legionella infection has, in common with mycoplasma pneumonia and PCP, a tendency to get worse instead of resolving but the shadowing is usually mid-zone and basal. Pneumonias of any kind can complicate any occupational disease, particularly those due to external allergens.

Cavitary shadows (large ring shadows)

These are most commonly due to: necrosis of abnormal parenchyma; tuberculosis with thin walls, lung abscess with thick walls, smooth interior, often irregular outer border but normal surrounding lung; neoplasm, with a thick wall and irregular interior and outer borders. Less common causes of cavitary lesions are hydatid cysts, Hodgkin's lymphoma, rheumatoid nodules, lung infarct and Wegener's granuloma. The lesions of PMF are also occasionally cavitary (see Chapter 13). Any chronic cavity (usually tuberculous) is liable to become secondarily infected with the fungus *Aspergillus* sp. and contains a mycetoma recognizable by the crescents of air separating it from the cavity walls. In the early stages the fungal ball may be seen as an irregularity on the cavity roof.

'Fibrotic' shadows

These are sometimes seen as parallel radiating linear shadows of varying thickness, often coalescing with dense patches and often associated with loss of lung volume. They are a feature of old tuberculosis in the upper zones. Basal fibrosis is a cardinal feature of pulmonary asbestosis, usually bilateral and roughly symmetrical. Fibrosis is also seen as the end-result of many chronic lung diseases, notably sarcoidosis, when it may be widespread.

The coin lesion

This is a colloquial term for a small rounded shadow 0.5 to 2 cm in diameter with well-defined edges and no other distinguishing features; it presents a particular problem. If there are no clues elsewhere (hilar node enlargement, evidence of secondary deposits or of a primary neoplasm), and the lesion is neither cavitary nor containing calcification, it is usual to regard it as neoplastic. It is important to distinguish this appearance from the irregular appearance of PMF lesions because there is an increased liability to neoplasm in long-standing occupational disease.

The foregoing is not intended to be an exhaustive treatise on chest radiology. The intention is to offer a framework on which a scrutiny of the chest radiograph can be based with the hope of omitting no significant consideration and thus contributing to the diagnosis.

Interpretation of the chest radiograph

It must be emphasized that, in general, there is no radiographic appearance unique to any one type of pneumoconiosis. Radiological diagnosis must be deductive in the light of all other relevant data, and spot diagnosis from the image alone must be avoided at all costs.

In the context of suspected occupational lung disease there are three prerequisites:

1. A full clinical and occupational history together with the results of physical examination (see Chapter 6).

2. Previous X-ray films for comparison.
3. A clear understanding of the timescale involved in the disease progression.

The diagnostic problem may take two forms: in the first, the patient has a known or alleged history of exposure to the agent under suspicion and confirmation or refutation is required; in the second, the patient has not hitherto been suspected of having occupational disease. In the former case, the observer must not be biased either way when assessing the radiograph, and must be aware of other causes for the appearances; in the latter, should the observer fail to have the possibility of occupational disease in mind, the diagnosis will be missed and result in inappropriate investigation.

It is important, once the abnormalities have been seen, that their rate of evolution be noted. If the patient is being seen for the first time, there may be clinical evidence from which some deductions can be made, but if previous films are available for comparison the radiographic evolution can be noted. Pneumoconioses are usually slow to evolve and changes in the appearances take many months, usually years, to occur, with the rare exception of 'acute' forms of silicosis, associated with high concentrations of very fine siliceous dust, which can become manifest in a few months (Salyed et al., 1985) (see Chapter 12). Acute infections progress rapidly, appearing in days and resolving in periods measured in weeks, occasionally months. Tuberculosis, whether worsening or resolving, usually does not show appreciable change in less than a month. The same can be said of sarcoidosis and of most neoplasms, though some grow faster than others. Between these two are infections such as PCP and mycoplasma pneumonia whose evolution is measured in weeks and, in common with legionella infection, do not resolve rapidly (may worsen) on the usual antibiotic treatment. These observations alone can be helpful where the radiographic appearances are atypical, as is all too frequently the case.

Descriptions of the radiographic appearances in the various pneumoconioses are given in the respective chapters. In this section some of the more common diagnostic patterns (with possible differential diagnoses) will be discussed as they might arise from systematic scrutiny.

Tracheal deviation should not be overlooked: both tuberculosis and carcinoma can coexist with occupational disease.

Enlarged paratracheal nodes are not a feature of pneumoconioses; they must raise the suspicion of lymphoma or tuberculosis if seen in association with abnormal lung fields. If there is any doubt here, CT will usually resolve it (see pages 193–194).

A cardiac outline that suggests right ventricular preponderance without an increase in heart size usually means pulmonary arterial hypertension and should stimulate search for peripheral lung disease. Pulmonary heart disease may occur in advanced silicosis and other progressive pneumoconioses.

Large main pulmonary arteries, especially with peripheral pruning, could confirm this, provided there is no evidence of a left-to-right shunt.

Hilar lymph node enlargement is seen in silicosis, sometimes with calcification (so-called 'egg-shell' variety), and is associated with nodular and linear shadowing in the lung fields. The differential diagnosis from sarcoidosis may sometimes be difficult because sarcoid nodes do occasionally calcify. Although the peripheral lung pattern of sarcoidosis may look reticular, it does not show the well-defined nodules of silicosis, especially in an upper and mid-zone distribution. The occasional appearance of 'A' and 'B' lines in sarcoidosis may be a source of confusion. Sarcoidosis is the great imitator and can progress to fibrosis, causing just as much respiratory disability as any other fibrotic lung disease (see Chapter 12, page 313).

Dense hilar lymph nodes, which are not enlarged, are a feature of the inert dusts of high atomic number, such as iron, tin and barium (see Chapter 11).

Asymmetrical hilar lymph node enlargement may be seen in primary tuberculosis in susceptible adults; if miliary tuberculosis occurs, the earlier stages of an insidious onset may show a widespread soft nodular pattern, presenting difficulties in diagnosis. In a similar way, a central carcinoma on the right may invade the azygos vein, giving rise to blood-borne metastases, and again produce a similar appearance. In such cases, the further evolution of the disease process will usually make the solution clear.

The pleura deserves particular study in an occupational context. Pleural thickening must be distinguished from the normal 'companion' and fat shadows mentioned earlier. It is important to recognize asbestos-related pleural plaques, calcified or otherwise, commonly bilateral, which usually differ from the bizarre, often extensive, asymmetrical pleural calcifications from previous haemothorax, tuberculous pleurisy or empyema. Differentiation may be difficult and the empyema can coexist with asbestosis. Where pleural thickening is present, careful search must be made for any irregularity or 'lumpiness' which might suggest mesothelioma. If there is any doubt, CT may be of great help (see page 194). The radiology of malignant mesothelioma has been reviewed by Langlois, Glancy and Henderson (1978).

Pleural effusion may have traumatic, inflammatory, immunological, neoplastic and other causes but should prompt study of the occupational history because both benign and malignant effusions may occur in asbestos workers (Cookson et al., 1985) (see Chapter 14). Overpenetrated grid films, ultrasound, CT and MRI all have a place in the investigation (Strankinga et al., 1987).

Summary

Appearances in the lung fields caused by pneumoconioses are of two main types: discrete round opacities of small or large size (nodular shadows) such as occur in siderosis, silicosis and coal pneumoconiosis; and fine-to-coarse linear, curvilinear and irregular opacities such as occur in asbestosis, the fibrotic stage of extrinsic allergic alveolitis, chronic beryllium disease and idiopathic DIPF, accompanied by small ring shadows with central transradiancies in some of these. When discrete round opacities are very small and numerous, they may present an ill-defined ground-glass appearance, but when viewed through a $\times 2$ or $\times 3$ hand lens they are seen never to lose their identity completely. If they are, in fact, too small for this, pathology may sometimes be inferred from an 'air bronchogram' appearance. Indefinite, fine, net-like irregular opacities are sometimes associated with retention of dusts of low atomic number – carbon, for example – and are caused mainly by superimposition of different radiodensities and not by the pathological process. If there is difficulty in differentiating silicosis from sarcoidosis, CT may help to resolve it (see pages 194–195).

Fibrotic conditions may be very difficult to differentiate. Cookson, Musk and Glancy (1984) have shown that the radiographic appearances of cryptogenic asbestosis and fibrosing alveolitis (idiopathic DIPF) may be so similar that they can be distinguished only by clinical and lung function tests, which tend to be worse in fibrosing alveolitis (see Chapter 15).

In considering larger abnormal shadows, such as may occur in silicosis and coal pneumoconiosis (PMF) sometimes with a cavitary appearance, the important decision is to be as sure as possible of their nature. The irregular margins and associated background of nodular and linear pattern together make a well-recognized appearance. Care must be taken to consider the possibility of tuberculous lesions or of neoplasm. Here the complete set of films in chronological order is invaluable. Whilst PMF can appear quite rapidly, its evolution is usually slow and gradual.

It will be clear from the foregoing that any single radiological observation is not of itself enough for a firm diagnosis of a pneumoconiosis, although it may go some way to confirm suspicions based on other evidence. There are, however, a number of characteristic combinations of signs that form patterns which, in the presence of other evidence, are virtually diagnostic. Some of these basic patterns are shown diagrammatically in Figure 7.10 (see also relevant chapters).

It will also be clear that there is nothing easy about radiological interpretation. The existence of observer error (0.5 to 2 per cent would surprise no

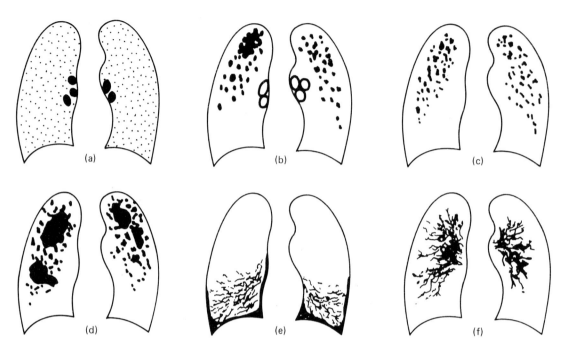

Figure 7.10 Radiographic patterns of some occupational diseases: (a) siderosis, stannosis etc. – dense hilar nodes; (b) nodular silicosis with conglomeration in right upper zone and peripherally calcified hilar nodes; (c) coal pneumoconiosis – early stage; (d) coal pneumoconiosis – PMP; (e) asbestosis; (f) chronic extrinsic allergic alveolitis

one) is well known (see page 190). One way to reduce it is to have the image scrutinized by two observers approaching the problem from different viewpoints. The conventional system of having a radiologist's opinion and that of a chest physician on every image makes such error much less likely.

Part II: Radiographic classification of pneumoconiosis

W. Raymond Parkes

It is important that the technique of interpreting as well as taking films should, as far as possible, be standardized – especially for epidemiological purposes – in order to reduce discrepancies between different observers to a minimum. Hence, over the years various systems of classification have been proposed to standardize the description of radiographs, but that proposed by the International

Labour Office (ILO) in 1930 and subsequently modified in 1950, 1959, 1970 and, most recently, in 1980 has been universally adopted. The present classification, which is accompanied by a set of 22 standard radiographs intended as visual paradigms, is designed to provide 'a means for recording systematically the radiographic abnormalities in the chest provoked by the inhalation of dusts' as seen in standard posteroanterior radiographs (ILO, 1980). In the main it seeks to do two things:

1. To categorize the size and form of opacities.
2. To indicate their profusion or extent in the lung fields.

The Classification is set out in detail in Table 7.4. This is its complete version intended for use in epidemiological studies. The symbols p, q, r, s, t and u refer to small opacities. Irregular opacities s, t and u are defined as having the same widths respectively as the diameters of round opacities p, q and r. Two letters are used to indicate whether small opacities are deemed to be of similar or of different size and shape: for example, q/q if all are round and between 1.5 and 3 mm diameter; and q/t if the q category is predominant but accompanied by 'significant numbers' of irregular t opacities. (Figures 7.11–7.15 – which are *not* ILO films – show examples of the main categories.) There are, in addition, categories

Table 7.4 ILO 1980 International Classification of radiographs of the pneumoconioses: summary of details of classification (complete classification)

Features	*Codes*	*Definitions*
Technical quality	1	Good
	2	Acceptable, with no technical defect likely to impair classification of the radiograph for pneumoconiosis
	3	Poor, with some technical defect but still acceptable for classification purposes
	4	Unacceptable
Parenchymal abnormalities Small opacities Profusion		The category of profusion is based on assessment of the concentration of opacities by comparison with the *standard radiographs*
	0/– 0/0 0/1	Category 0 – small opacities absent or less profuse than the lower limit of category 1
	1/0 1/1 1/2	
	2/0 2/2 2/3	Categories 1, 2 and 3 – represent increasing profusion of small opacities
	3/2 3/3 3/+	as defined by the corresponding standard radiographs
Extent	RU RM RL LU LM LL	The zones in which the opacities are seen are recorded. The right (R) and left (L) thorax are both divided into three zones – upper (U), middle (M) and lower (L) The category of profusion is determined by considering the profusion as a whole over the affected zones of the lung and by comparing this with the standard radiographs
Shape and size Rounded	p/p q/q r/r	The letters p, q and r denote the presence of small rounded opacities. Three sizes are defined by the appearances on *standard radiographs*:
		p = diameter up to about 1.5 mm q = diameter exceeding about 1.5 mm and up to about 3 mm r = diameter exceeding about 3 mm and up to about 10 mm
Irregular	s/s t/t u/u	The letters s, t and u denote the presence of small irregular opacities. Three sizes are defined by the appearances on *standard radiographs*:
		s = width up to about 1.5 mm t = width exceeding about 1.5 mm and up to about 3 mm u = width exceeding 3 mm and up to about 10 mm
Mixed	p/s p/t p/u p/q p/r q/s q/t q/u q/p q/r r/s r/t r/u r/p r/q s/p s/q s/r s/t s/u t/p t/q t/r t/s t/u u/p u/q u/r u/s u/t	For mixed shapes (or sizes) of small opacities the predominant shape and size is recorded first. The presence of a significant number of another shape and size is recorded after the oblique stroke
Large opacities	A B C	The categories are defined in terms of the *dimensions* of the opacities:
		Category A: an opacity having a greatest diameter exceeding about 10 mm and up to and including 50 mm, or several opacities each greater than about 10 mm, the sum of whose greatest diameters does not exceed about 50 mm Category B: one or more opacities larger or more numerous than those in category A whose combined area does not exceed the equivalent of the right upper zone Category C: one or more opacities whose combined area exceeds the equivalent of the right upper zone.
Pleural abnormalities Pleural thickening Chest wall Type		Two types of pleural thickening of the chest wall are recognized: circumscribed (plaques) and diffuse. Both types may occur together
Site	R L	Pleural thickening of the chest wall is recorded separately for the right (R) and left (L) thorax
Width	a b c	For pleural thickening seen along the lateral chest wall the measurement of *maximum width* is made from the inner line of the chest wall to the inner margin of the shadow seen most sharply at the parenchymal–pleural boundary. The maximum width usually occurs at the inner margin of the rib shadow at its outermost point
		a = maximum width up to about 5 mm b = maximum width over about 5 mm and up to about 10 mm c = maximum width over about 10 mm

Table 7.4 *continued*

Features	Codes	Definitions
Pleural abnormalities (contd)		
Face on	Y N	The presence of pleural thickening seen face-on is recorded even if it can be seen also in profile. If pleural thickening is seen face-on only, width can not usually be measured
Extent	1 2 3	Extent of pleural thickening is defined in terms of the *maximum length* of pleural involvement, or as the sum of maximum lengths, whether seen in profile or face-on
		1 = total length equivalent to up to one-quarter of the projection of the lateral chest wall
		2 = total length exceeding one-quarter but not one-half of the projection of the lateral chest wall
		3 = total length exceeding one-half of the projection of the lateral chest wall
Diaphragm		
Presence	Y N	A plaque involving the diaphragmatic pleura is recorded as present (Y) or absent (N), separately for the right (R) and left (L) thorax
Site	R L	
Costophrenic angle obliteration		
Presence	Y N	The presence (Y) or absence (N) of costophrenic angle obliteration is recorded separately from thickening over other areas, for the right (R) and left (L) thorax. The lower limit for this obliteration is defined by a *standard radiograph*
Site	R L	If the thickening extends up the chest wall then both costophrenic angle obliteration and pleural thickening should be recorded
Pleural calcification		The site and extent of pleural calcification are recorded separately for the two lungs, and the extent defined in terms of *dimensions*
Site		
Chest wall	R L	
Diaphragm	R L	
Other	R L	'Other' includes calcification of the mediastinal and pericardial pleura
Extent	1 2 3	1 = an area of calcified pleura with greatest diameter up to about 20 mm, or a number of such areas the sum of whose greatest diameters does not exceed about 20 mm
		2 = an area of calcified pleura with greatest diameter exceeding about 20 mm and up to about 100 mm, or a number of such areas the sum of whose greatest diameters exceeds about 20 mm but does not exceed about 100 mm
		3 = an area of calcified pleura with greatest diameter exceeding about 100 mm, or a number of such areas whose sum of greatest diameters exceeds about 100 mm
Symbols		It is to be taken that the definition of each of the symbols is preceded by an appropriate word or phrase such as 'suspect', 'changes suggestive of', or 'opacities suggestive of' etc.
	ax	– coalescence of small pneumoconiotic opacities
	bu	– bulla(e)
	ca	– cancer of lung or pleura
	cn	– calcification in small pneumoconiotic opacities
	co	– abnormality of cardiac size or shape
	cp	– cor pulmonale
	cv	– cavity
	di	– marked distortion of the intrathoracic organs
	ef	– effusion
	em	– definite emphysema
	es	– eggshell calcification of hilar or mediastinal lymph nodes
	fr	– fractured rib(s)
	hi	– enlargement of hilar or mediastinal lymph nodes
	ho	– honeycomb lung
	id	– ill-defined diaphragm
	ih	– ill-defined heart outline
	kl	– septal (Kerley) lines
	od	– other significant abnormality
	pi	– pleural thickening in the interlobar fissure or mediastinum
	px	– pneumothorax
	rp	– rheumatoid pneumoconiosis
	tb	– tuberculosis

Table 7.4 *continued*

Features	Codes	Definitions
Comments Presence	Y N	Comments should be recorded pertaining to the classification of the radiograph, particularly if some other cause is thought to be responsible for a shadow which could be thought by others to have been due to pneumoconiosis; also to identify radiographs for which the technical quality may have affected the reading materially

© 1980 International Labour Organisation, Geneva. Appendix G, *Guidelines for the use of the ILO International Classification of Radiographs of Pneumoconiosis*, revised edn, 1980, No. 2, pp. 46–48. Occupational Safety and Health Series. Reproduced with permission.

for pleural thickening: whether localized or diffuse, calcified or not.

The specifications of large opacities – categories A, B and C, shown in Table 7.4, which correspond to large masses – are readily defined with a ruler (Figures 7.12 and 7.13). The method of distinguishing between categories B and C is illustrated in Figure 7.14. The terms 'well-defined' and 'ill-defined', which were available for the description of these opacities in the earlier classifications, have, unfortunately, been deleted from the 1980 classification.

It must be emphasized that the allotted category indicates no more than the type and profusion of certain types of opacities in the lung fields. It does not specify a diagnosis or imply respiratory disability or impairment of lung function. The additional symbols, however, do, for the most part, refer to specific pathological states.

A Short Classification, which also employs the standard radiographs, is more appropriate for recording occupational disease in the clinical setting. In this, profusion of small opacities is simply recorded as 0, 1, 2 or 3, and their shape and size, if rounded, as p, q or r and, if irregular, as s, t or u. Large opacities are recorded as A, B or C. However, the list of symbols is the same as in the Complete version.

The 'Guidelines' for the 1980 Classification Systems, Complete and Short (ILO, 1980) include rules for using the system and recommend means for standardizing radiological equipment and technique.

Progression from lower to higher categories of profusion

Because this sort of classification of radiographs is arbitrary, it gives only a semi-quantitative scale of increasing radiographic abnormality. It is conceivable, however, that there is continuum from normality along an abnormality scale, although, of course, a disease process may advance at one time, lag at

another or remain permanently at a standstill at any point. Because a 4-point profusion scale (category 0 to 3) was found to be insufficiently sensitive to assess progression for epidemiological purposes, Liddell (1963) proposed that it be subdivided and converted into a 12-point scale (Figure 7.15). This is employed in the complete Classification.

Use of the classification

Because there are no pathognomonic radiographic features of dust-induced disease, it is recommended that:

1. Films are to be classified only if their appearances are consistent with an occupational disorder.
2. If *all* the appearances are likely to be due to some other cause, they should not be classified.
3. If the appearances are doubtfully those of a pneumoconiosis, they should be classified, but the alternative diagnosis also recorded.

Relegation of a 'case film' to the appropriate category type in the Complete Classification requires comparison with the 'standard' films and the instruction of the ILO guidelines. The radiograph to be categorized has to be compared and matched with the *actual* standard radiograph rather than being classified by the written description of categories. Although, in some circumstances, this may be impractical, the Guidelines state that it is mandatory for the Classification's chief application to epidemiology (where it is most relevant) and the routine surveillance of dust-exposed workers.

Similarly, assessment of profusion in the Complete Classification requires reference to the standard (mid-category) films and the 12-point scale. To do this the observer first classifies the film into one of the four categories, 0 to 3, but if a neighbouring category is considered to be a possible alternative this

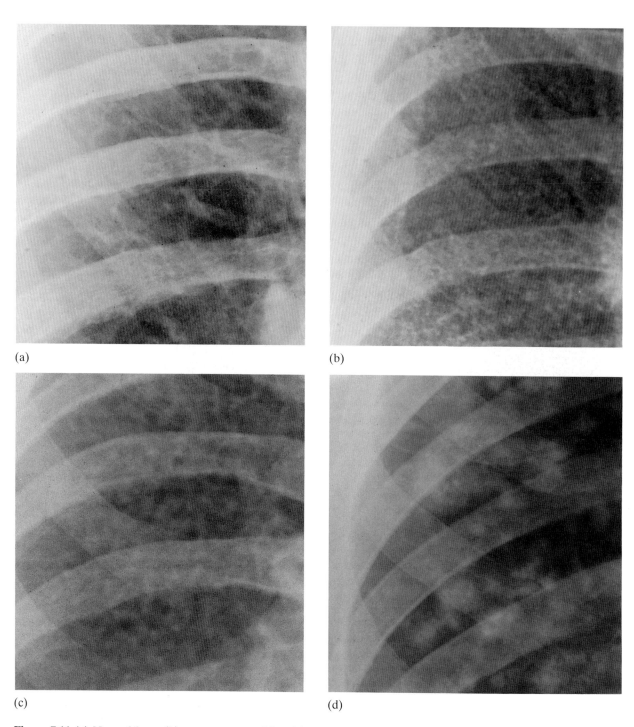

(a)

(b)

(c)

(d)

Figure 7.11 (a) Normal lung; (b) category p opacities; (c) category q opacities; (d) category r opacities. (All of natural size)

must be recorded after the formal category. Thus, if a film is judged to be category 2, although category 1 is given serious consideration, it is expressed as 2/1. A film that is undoubtedly category 2 (that is, mid-category, closely similar to the standard film with neither neighbouring categories considered) is classed as 2/2. Category 0/1 refers to a film that is category 0 though category 1 was seriously considered. This rule has to be followed strictly.

In the Short Classification the features of films are supposed to be recorded in the same way using the

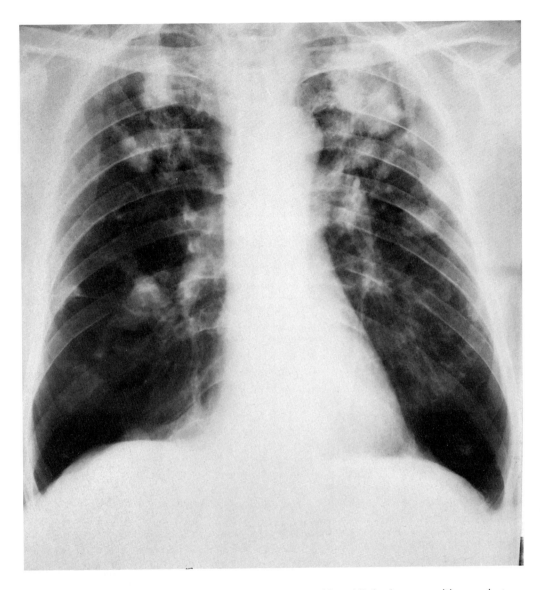

Figure 7.12 Category B with very few small, discrete opacities. All the large opacities can just be aggregated into the right upper zone and, thus, do not exceed one-third of the right lung field, as in Figure 7.14. This is a case of Caplan's syndrome

standard radiographs but the 12-point scale is not employed.

Good examples of the appearances of representative standard films are to be found in an excellent review, 'Classification of radiographs of the pneumoconioses' (1981), in *Medical Radiography and Photography*.

Classification of asbestos-related disease

Because the set of ILO standard films contains only eight that are relevant to description of asbestos-related disease, the Medical Advisory Panel of the Asbestos International Association prepared a supplementary set of 100 films showing the range of appearances of parenchymal and pleural fibrosis attributed to asbestos exposure. All categories of parenchymal lesions between 0/0 and 3/3 are represented with a deliberate bias towards lower categories (where difficulty of interpretation is greatest), together with degrees of pleural change. The set, which is accompanied by a guidebook, is designed for epidemiological and teaching purposes (Browne et al., 1984).

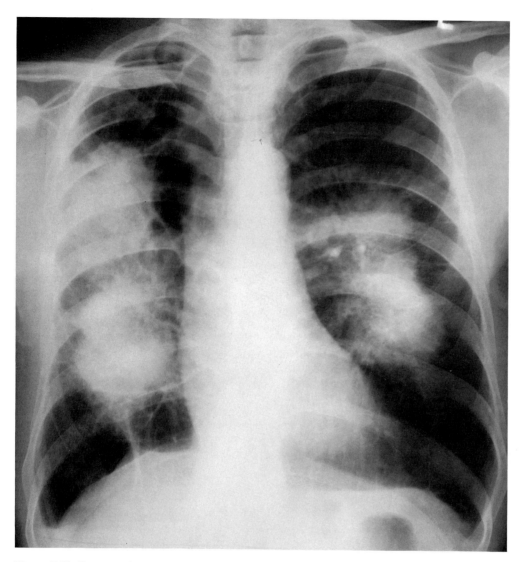

Figure 7.13 Category C: area of large opacities exceeds one-third of the right lung field

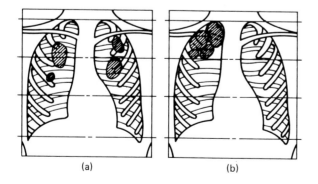

Figure 7.14 Method of categorizing large opacities: (a) represents opacities of massive pneumoconiotic lesions; (b) shows how these are regrouped in the mind's eye or, with the aid of a transparent ruler, into the right lung field. This is category B as the combined area lies within the confines of one-third of the field. An area extending beyond this is classed as category C

The use of radiographs in epidemiology

There are two methods of reading serial films for identification and assessment of progression of disease in individuals: in the first, the films of each are inspected 'side by side' in chronological order; in the second, they are separated and shuffled in with those of all subjects in the group being studied, thus producing a random collection of films. All identifying marks, other than a code, must be masked. The relative accuracy of both techniques has been extensively investigated and evidence produced to indicate that the side-by-side method causes bias in coal pneumoconiosis, tuberculosis and sarcoidosis (Amandus et al., 1973; Reger, Petersen and Morgan, 1974). It is often urged, therefore, that the independent randomized method results in less bias in interpretation of

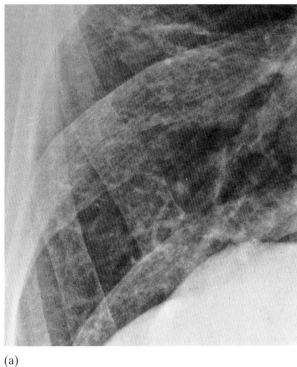

(a)

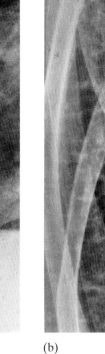

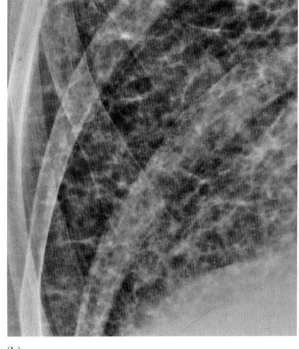

(b)

(c)

Figure 7.15 (a) Category s opacities; (b) category t opacities; (c) category u with some category t opacities. (All of natural size)

progression or regression. But it has been convincingly shown that there is substantially less error when films are viewed together by the side-by-side method and read in known temporal order (Liddell, 1974; Liddell and Morgan, 1978).

Examination of workers' films taken over a specified working period is used to determine the *incidence* (or 'attack rate') of pneumoconiosis and the *rate of progression* of established disease during a particular number of years in defined populations.

Both can be related to cumulative levels of exposure to dust.

It is worth noting that details of categorization in papers published before 1970 may not be comparable with those in later work, in view of the changes in the notation of the system between 1950 and 1980. Valid comparison of incidence or prevalence (especially of small opacities) between studies done at different times, with different observers and in different countries may not be possible if the standard of radiographic technique and method of reading films has varied.

Factors that influence the interpretation of radiographs

Quality of films

Poor quality causes significant variation in the classification of profusion of small opacities (Musch et al., 1984). Of particular importance are thickness of the chest wall (Liddell, 1961) and body weight, which alter both density and contrast of images (Pearson et al., 1965), and penetration of X-rays. Lower categories of discrete opacities tend to be recorded with overpenetrated ('too black') films, and higher categories with underpenetrated ('too white' or 'soft') films. Thus, the quality of films may have a profound effect on prevalence and progression rates (Reger et al., 1972). The lower categories 0/1 to 1/1 are particularly affected by obesity (Musch, Higgins and Landis, 1985).

Films not taken in full inspiration may cause inappropriate recording of irregular opacities or too high a category. In serial films, comparison of degree of inspiration can be made by reference of diaphragmatic levels to rib numbers.

Disagreement on the profusion of small opacities among readers has been found to be greater with increasing age of radiographs (Musch et al., 1984).

Conditions for viewing films

The ILO guidelines indicate a standard optimum illumination (intensity and colour) for viewing screens, but this is by no means always observed. As pointed out earlier in this chapter, intensity of ambient light is also important and should be controlled (see page 169).

Observer error

This is affected not only by the quality of films but also by subjective individual factors. These include the degree and quality of past training and experience of observers. Disagreement between observers is affected by lack of experience of the classification system and of familiarity with the radiographic features of occupational disease; by inadequate knowledge of normal variation in patterns of the lung fields, and by the appearances of unrelated disease. Most important, however, is the fact that perception of contrast in X-ray films by individuals is an inherent ability (and, hence, a variable factor) that is not much affected by practice (Adrian-Harris, 1979). Thus, the performances of individual readers in a group involved in an epidemiological study should be tested and compared at the outset; for this purpose, multiple 'blind' readings are desirable. Readers who differ greatly from their colleagues are then excluded – although it could be that such 'mavericks' are the most accurate. The striking overdiagnosis of asbestos-related disease, for example, that can result from misinterpretation of chest radiographs has been well documented by Reger et al. (1990).

Age and smoking

Increasing age and consumption of cigarettes over the years are significantly associated with an increasing degree of fibrosis of alveolar walls and membranous and respiratory bronchioles, and thickening of pulmonary arterioles and arteries (see Chapters 13 and 14). Irregular opacities of low profusion (categories 0/1 to 1/1), related to these pathological features, are found in low prevalence among smokers (mostly those with a history of 20 pack-years or more) with no known exposure to a hazardous dust (Weiss, 1984, 1988). Thus, it is possible that some smokers with past exposure to asbestos may be wrongly diagnosed as having asbestosis. The prevalence of such opacities is greater in heavy smokers than in non-smokers, both with similar exposure to asbestos (Kilburn et al., 1986; McDonald, Sébastien and Armstrong, 1986). The increased risk of developing small opacities conferred by smoking, compared to non-smoking, is reported to be, on average, one-quarter of that resulting from cumulative exposure to asbestos (Barnhart et al., 1990). A more detailed discussion will be found in Chapter 14. Similar considerations also apply to irregular opacities in radiographs of workers exposed to other dusts; coal miners in particular have received much attention in recent years (see Chapter 13, 'Irregular opacities').

Other non-occupational factors

Of 200 patients with no industrial exposure admitted to an urban hospital, Epstein et al. (1984) found that the radiographs of 22 (11 per cent), classified by the ILO (1980) system, showed unexplained small opacities (mostly 'irregular' and category 1/0 or more) consistent with a pneumoconiosis; another 10 (5 per cent) were explicable by associated disease – such as sarcoidosis, lymphangitis carcinomatosa and congestive cardiac failure. Smoking did not seem to be a significant factor. The authors concluded that small opacities due to some cause other than occupational may be present in the radiographs of about 10 per cent of industrially exposed persons; and they questioned whether non-occupational disorders capable of causing such opacities would be recognized, or considered, when the radiographs of industrial populations were classified. This important potential pitfall should always be borne in mind.

Improvements to the Classification are under discussion internationally for a proposed revision (Kilburn, 1988). However, within the next decade or so, given the potential capacity of computers to process, modify and store detailed images, it seems likely that the standard chest radiograph and its accumulated bulk will become a thing of the past (see pages 203–204). In which case, a completely new approach to a standard classification of 'images' rather than 'opacities' will most probably be needed.

Correlation of radiographic appearances with pneumoconiotic lesions

Correlation between the number and distribution of discrete opacities on chest radiographs and the number and distribution of small pneumoconiotic lesions observed *post mortem* is fairly good, in spite of the fact that, as described in Part I, the appearance of the radiograph is determined not only by the number and composition of the lesions but also by the superimposition of their own radiodensities and those of lung and chest wall structures.

Various factors operate to attenuate X-rays in different types of lesion. The profusion and distribution of silicotic nodules (see Chapter 12) observed *post mortem* show close agreement with radiographic appearances and category; these appearances are due to the combined effect of the concentration of iron within the nodules (Otto and Maron, 1959), to collagen fibrosis, possibly to the

content of free silica and, in some cases, to the deposition of calcium salts. In the case of coal pneumoconiosis, the higher the ILO category of small 'round' opacities, the greater the number of foci of retained dust and the greater the proportion of fibrotic (collagen) nodules found in the lungs (Caplan, 1962). Rossiter (1972) showed that the radiographic appearances in coal miners are correlated most highly with the mineral content of the lungs, although iron also makes a significant contribution. Due to their different X-ray attenuation values, 1.6 g of iron and 5 g of other minerals in the lungs have the same effect as 16 g of coal in increasing the category by one unit (Gilson, 1968). The category of simple coal pneumoconiosis correlates better with the non-haem, endogenous, iron content (which may accumulate during the phagocytosis of dust particles) than with the total iron content of the lungs (Bergman, 1970). It is probable, therefore, that the effect of iron upon category reflects variation in the amount of coal and mineral present (Rossiter, 1972). Coal itself contributes very little to the appearances (see Chapter 13, 'Radiographic appearance').

As might be expected, correlation of radiographic abnormality with large conglomerate or pneumoconiotic masses, of whatever cause, is usually good.

Correlation of radiographic appearances and diffuse pulmonary fibrosis is not, on the whole, as good as that for discrete, round pneumoconiosis lesions, but it improves as the severity of the fibrosis increases from partial loss of alveolar wall architecture to its complete replacement by fibrous tissue, sometimes with the development of multiple cystic spaces ('honeycombing') (Livingstone et al., 1964) (see Figure 7.15c). It is difficult to detect the earlier stages on routine radiographs. These considerations apply not only to diffuse fibrosis of unknown cause but also to asbestosis, chronic beryllium disease and extrinsic allergic alveolitis (see relevant chapters).

Carstairs' (1961) observation (see pages 177–178) that linear networks can be projected as nodular shadows on the radiographic image would explain some of the discrete opacities and relative transradiancies that may be seen in many cases of diffuse fibrosis, and possibly the small p-type opacities sometimes observed on the radiographs of coal workers who are subsequently found to have uniformly distributed emphysema in dust-pigmented lungs without fibrosis (see Figure 13.26). These appearances may be due in some cases to the effective contrast between the increased volume of air in numerous dilated airspaces of panacinar emphysema, on the one hand, and the surrounding lung tissue which possesses greater radiodensity than normal owing to the combined effect of mineral dusts, endogenous iron and coal, on the other (see page 175). In the case of inert dusts of high atomic number the opacities are denser and more clearly demarcated (see Chapter 11).

In general, respiratory symptoms and patterns of impaired lung function correlate very poorly with the radiographic appearances of pneumoconioses and other fibrotic occupational disorders.

Part III: Other imaging techniques
Peter M. Bretland

Computed tomography

There are now few major radiology departments in developed countries that do not have access to computed tomography (CT). Surprisingly, in the last few years, while the cost of general X-ray sets has increased considerably more than the general rate of inflation, that of CT has not; some now cost less than good quality fluoroscopic apparatus. The quality of the image has improved, with shorter scan times and higher definition in most of the models currently available. It cannot replace chest radiology for the first-line investigation of disease of the chest, especially suspected occupational lung disease, but it does have an important place, as will be seen.

It is generally accepted that CT is the best investigation for mediastinal vascular structures and masses (Husband and Fry, 1981) and especially for suspected disease of the lymph nodes (Sagel and Aronberg, 1982). The vascular system of the lung is also well shown. Lung masses are well shown and may be localized much more easily with CT than with routine radiology, especially small solitary nodules and metastatic lung disease (Husband and Fry, 1981). Peripheral lung disease, especially widespread pathology in which the visualization of small lesions in the 1 to 3 mm range is essential to the diagnosis, presents some difficulties, however. In just the same way that the minimum size of nodule demonstrable in a radiograph is limited by the inherent unsharpness in the system, especially geometric blur or unsharpness, U_g (see page 163), there are also limitations with CT. Not only does the X-ray tube and detector system have U_g for the tube depending on the focal spot size plus a further factor for the detector system, but also the pixel size ultimately determines the amount of detail that can

be seen. A brief explanation of how CT works is, therefore, necessary.

A pixel is a small element of the image. Its size is determined by the characteristics of the system in the particular CT set. The patient lies in the centre of a ring gantry having on one side an X-ray tube emitting a narrowly collimated beam, and on the other side one or more detectors. The tube and detectors move and numerous short exposures are made, so that the beam passes through all parts of a narrow transverse 'slice' of the patient at various angles. Data from the detectors are fed into a computer. This conceives the slice as a matrix of small pixels and calculates for each one an attenuation value, usually measured in Hounsfield units (HU) (Sir Godfrey Hounsfield first developed the system). Water is taken as 0 whilst denser tissues have positive and less dense ones negatives values, for example, bone is in the +400 to +1000 range and lung in the –400 to –600 range.

This pattern of numbers in the computer's memory is converted to an image by allocating a shade of grey to each pixel, corresponding to its attenuation value. The number of pixels in the image depends on the matrix size denoted by the product of their horizontal and vertical numbers, and is a measure of the image sharpness. A 160 × 160 matrix produces a pixel size of 1.5 × 1.5 mm, a relatively coarse image, whereas a 320 × 320 matrix has pixels 0.75 × 0.75 mm, a rather sharper image.

Clearly the resolution does not compare at all well with that of the chest radiograph. Whilst there are other ways of expressing resolution in CT (which are not of concern here), one of the current models at the time of writing claims 7 line pairs per cm for routine work and 9 line pairs per cm in high resolution mode. A survey by the Supplies Technology Division of the UK Department of Health (Department of Health, 1989) gives slightly lower figures. Plain radiography can give up to 11 line pairs per mm! (see page 164); this means that nodules really have to be more than 1 mm in size to be shown individually by CT. However, general disturbances in lung pattern, such as may be produced by the fibrosis of asbestosis, may be well seen on account of better contrast resolution.

Because there are many more numbers than there are shades of grey perceptible by the human eye (usually taken as 16), a 'window' is used. In effect, the total range of available shades of grey is set against a selected range of attenuation values so as to produce a grey scale image. The selected range can be extensive or very small; in the first case parts of the body of widely differing attenuation values can be shown on the same image, and in the second case minor differences can be displayed over a limited range of attenuation values. The contrast range can thus be compressed or expanded respectively by altering the window width. It is this facility which to a large extent can compensate for the inherent unsharpness in the image.

Different parts of the body require the grey scale window in different places up and down the number range, for example, the lungs are shown adequately only in the low attenuation range (negative HU value) whereas the abdomen, which mostly contains organs of water density, is demonstrable only by setting the window against the higher attenuation values in the positive HU range. For the abdomen, the window is 'moved up'. In the same way that 'bone windows' in the chest will show the bony structures, windows can be selected to show mediastinal anatomy, details of pleural thickening, intrapulmonary lesions or lung collapse–consolidation. This property of adjusting the image density and contrast range in response to the diagnostic problem gives CT its great advantage over transmission radiography, which relies on X-ray film or other photosensitive material having fixed characteristics. Indeed, it was the capacity to distinguish between brain tissue and cerebrospinal fluid in the ventricles that first demonstrated CT's unprecedented diagnostic value in the study of intracranial pathology.

A further, very important application of this property of the system is in the technique known as *contrast enhancement*. The process by which water-soluble contrast media injected into the vascular system are used to opacify blood vessels or spaces into which these substances are eventually excreted, or to opacify a vascular organ or tumour, is well known in transmission radiology. In CT, small differences in attenuation so produced, not otherwise demonstrable, can be shown by appropriate choice of window; not only can vascular structures in the chest be distinguished from tumour or lymph node but small differences in tissue vascularity may give a clue to the pathology.

To some extent, the ability to show contrast differences so well compensates for the lack of sharpness compared with that of X-ray film. Certainly, in the early days of the technique, when the pixels were clearly visible in the coarser matrices then available, the images were still of great diagnostic value. Modern machines can yield 256 × 256 matrices as standard practice, and 512 × 512 matrices can be achieved. There are so-called 'zooming' techniques which enlarge a small part of the image but do not actually improve the resolution because they are still using the same data. A fresh slice, irradiating only the 'zoomed' region with smaller tube-detector movements, is necessary to produce smaller pixels, a facility offered by some machines. In true *high-resolution computed tomography* (HRCT), sometimes called *high-definition computed tomography* (HDCT), better resolution is achieved with a much thinner slice (as little as 1.0

to 1.5 mm compared with the usual 1 to 1.3 cm thickness). Some models offer a standard choice such as 2, 5 or 10 mm slice thickness.

Application of CT to occupational lung disorders

It will be clear from the foregoing that the technique has both value and limitations. Although it cannot compete with chest radiography in sharpness and detail, it can compensate for this by better contrast resolution and it can show the anatomy and pathology from another angle by producing an image of a transverse slice.

The periphery

In studies of the extrathoracic soft tissues and the bony cage, the visualization in transverse section is useful in distinguishing intrapulmonary shadows from overlying soft tissues. Bony lesions not apparent on the PA radiograph may be shown; Salonen et al. (1986) found that infiltration of the chest wall by mesothelioma was visualized significantly better by CT than by PA radiography. If there is any difficulty in distinguishing the normal extrapleural or subpleural fat pads (Sargent et al., 1984) or the normal shadow of the serratus anterior muscle (Collins, Brown and Batra, 1983) from pleural pathology, CT, particularly HRCT, can usually solve the problem.

The central shadow

In suspected abnormality of the mediastinum, distinction can usually be made between vessels, lymph nodes and other masses, contrast enhancement being particularly useful. Thickened pericardium may be shown (Strankinga et al., 1987), and thickening of the mediastinal pleura not normally visible on the plain radiograph (Salonen et al., 1986).

Hila

The hilar structures are visualized with CT but no authors seem to claim any great advantage over chest radiography, except that, where there are abnormal lymph nodes in both the hila and the mediastinum, CT can show those that are concealed by the shadows of vascular structures in PA radiographs. Pulmonary vessels are well shown.

Pleura

It is in the study of the pleura that most work appears to have been done, particularly in relation to asbestos-related disease. Quite apart from its value (described above) in distinguishing pleural abnormalities from extra- and subpleural fat and the shadows of extrathoracic muscle, Kreel (1976) described its value in showing asbestos-related plaques. Katz and Kreel (1979) found CT more sensitive than plain radiographs in showing small pleural plaques, particularly in the paravertebral region, and, in later stages, circumferential encasement of the lung. They raised the possibility that internal irregularity might be an early sign of mesothelioma. Law et al. (1982) also described the irregular appearance of mesothelioma and found that CT could detect small effusions better than plain radiography but otherwise had no advantage in the group of advanced cases that they studied. They also found that CT did not show diaphragmatic lesions well because the diaphragm would inevitably appear only in part on any one slice. Raithel and Valentin (1983) could show pleural lesions in places such as the retrocardiac space and paravertebral region not visible on plain radiographs and also noted the irregular inner edge of mesotheliomas.

Comparison of CT with four-view plain radiographs (Bégin et al., 1984) showed that CT was better at recognizing lateral pleural sites of plaque formation but worse for diaphragmatic and costophrenic angle sites – again consistent with the differing geometry of the two techniques. CT was better at recognizing calcified pleural plaques. Fourio (1984) found that CT was better than plain X-rays for detecting pleural plaques, including those in the costovertebral grooves, and felt that it had a place in the follow-up of subjects in contact with asbestos showing pleural anomalies. Sluis-Cremer, Thomas and Schmaman (1984) considered that X-rays and CT were about comparable in their detection of pleural plaques, and complementary, each finding a few that the other missed; CT's great advantage lay in clarifying the false appearances due to extra- or subpleural fat or extrathoracic muscle. Salonen et al. (1986) found CT of great value in showing pathology in the mediastinal pleura. High contrast enhancement with a bolus of intravenous contrast medium was observed in mesothelioma tissue although it could not be distinguished from other malignant tissue, and it has also been seen in benign infective lesions of the pleura. If enhancement was slight, the lesion was likely to be benign.

Aberle et al. (1988) found HRCT to be superior to conventional CT in the detection of pleural pathology, as did Gamsu (1989).

Lung parenchyma

In the lung itself, bearing in mind the limitations in resolution, CT has a lot to offer. The horizontal fissure is not well shown because it lies in a plane parallel to those of the slices but the oblique fissures are usually visible and accessory fissures, especially the azygos fissure, are well seen. The so-called 'infolded lung' lesion can be identified. Thickening of fissures is demonstrable.

Where the lung parenchyma is abnormal but the architecture is not visualized on either CT or plain radiography because the individual nodules are too small, the lung may still have an average increase in attenuation which differs to a small, but significant, extent from that of air. It may thus be possible to show an air bronchogram peripherally in the same way that it can be seen in pneumonic consolidation. Depending on the density and extent of the nodular lesions, the effect could be shown by using a narrow window at the appropriate level. It is unlikely to be shown beyond the smallest bronchi (about 2 mm in diameter – see Chapter 1) (Webb et al., 1988). Research is needed to establish whether or not this is so.

It is important to remember, when looking at the lung parenchyma with CT, that there is, in normal lungs, a gravity-dependent perfusion effect. In the supine position, in which the majority of such examinations are carried out, the posterior parts of the lungs show the small vessels to be fuller and more crowded (Kreel, 1976). In the prone position, a similar though lesser effect is shown anteriorly, and in a lateral decubitus position, in the lateral part of the dependent lung; such appearances in the posterior parts of the lung disappear in these other positions (see Figure 14.14).

Katz and Kreel (1979) noted that thickened pleura in the fissures was well shown. In interstitial disease of asbestosis there was a coarse network of linear shadows surrounding spaces of air density, resulting in a 'honeycomb' pattern (Kreel, 1976); in other cases, mixtures of nodular and linear, and sometimes pure nodular, shadows would be seen. These features, when posterior, did not change between the prone and supine positions – a valuable diagnostic clue. They also noted, in four cases of asbestos-related disease, with otherwise normal lungs on both radiograph and CT, loss of the normal gravity-dependent perfusion effect and suggested this as a sign of early interstitial disease. It may well be that a fine interstitial fibrosis is already present but the resolution of the system is not good enough to show it.

Raithel and Valentin (1983) studied with CT, using 4-mm slices with 256×256 or 512×512 matrices, 68 men occupationally exposed to asbestos dust, 36 women with evidence or suspicion of asbestosis, and 24 men with silicosis. In silicosis, the nodular pattern, predominantly posterior and subpleural, was shown, and in asbestosis the dense fibrotic shadowing, also largely posterior and subpleural, was well seen. Pleural thickening was also well shown in asbestos-exposed patients; at least one had mesothelioma. They felt that asbestos-related fibrosis, emphysema, pleural changes and mesothelioma could be identified earlier than on chest radiographs. Their subjects were all examined supine. Whilst this might alter some of the appearances it does not detract from the value of the procedure. They had not, apparently, seen the work of Katz and Kreel (1979) on this aspect.

Bergin and Müller (1985), using standard 1-cm slices in a variety of interstitial lung diseases, could distinguish nodular patterns, seen in sarcoidosis, silicosis and lymphangitic spread of malignancy, from the reticular or irregular linear patterns of idiopathic DIPF and rheumatoid lung (which tended to lie in the lung periphery), hypersensitivity pneumonitis (central predominance) and DIPF of neurofibromatosis (basal with no transverse predominance). Lymphangitic spread of malignancy was distinguished by the accompanying thickened interlobar septa, and silicosis by its predominantly posterior position in the upper and mid-parts of the lungs. In a subsequent study, Bergin and Müller (1987) proposed a three-compartment model, outlined by the three continuous systems of the fibrous skeleton of the lungs (Weibel and Gil, 1977) (see Chapter 1) to describe the distribution of disease. They were able to place lesions due to lymphangitic carcinomatosis, pulmonary lymphoma and sarcoidosis in a compartment, or zone, outlined by the *axial system*, whereas extrinsic allergic alveolitis, pulmonary vasculitis secondary to cryoglobulinaemia, busulphan toxicity, DIPF of neurofibromatosis and silicosis appeared in a middle compartment outlined by the *parenchymatous system*. Silicosis was again distinguished by its uniformly nodular appearance and posterior predominance. The peripheral compartment, delineated by the *peripheral system*, was the site of idiopathic DIPF – 'lone' or associated with connective tissue disorders – with a peripheral rim of irregular (reticular) densities and 'honeycomb' cysts, and with thickened interlobular septa and fine irregularity of the pleura. They felt that these apparently characteristic distributions, if confirmed in larger series, would have considerable diagnostic value.

Bégin et al. (1987) studied established silicosis in 58 subjects and found that, although radiography identified the nodules earlier than conventional CT, the latter could demonstrate coalescence of nodules earlier (see Chapter 12).

Triebel, Jessel and Spielmann (1988) studied fine nodular shadowing in a patient who turned out to have been an arc-welder, and emphasized the difficulty in distinguishing between sarcoidosis and siderosis, even with the aid of HRCT. Their images showed more shadowing posteriorly but they appear to have been done supine so it is not clear whether this is due to the gravity-dependent effect.

Aberle et al. (1988) compared plain radiography, conventional CT and HRCT for parenchymal abnormalities. HRCT proved measurably superior to conventional CT in demonstrating parenchymal lesions, notably curvilinear subpleural lines, thickened interlobular (septal) and interlobular (core) lines, a subpleural-dependent density, parenchymal bands 2 to 5 cm in length extending to the pleural surfaces and subpleural scattered honeycombing, predominantly in the posterior parts of the lower lobes. The posterior lesions were still seen in prone studies, which were considered to be essential to prove the validity of lesions seen in the posterior parts of the lung. Plain radiography proved superior to conventional CT in the detection of lesions assessed 1/0 or 1/1 on the radiograph but HRCT was almost as good.

Lung masses

Putman et al. (1984) reported that CT improved diagnostic accuracy in localized lucent (transradiant) lung lesions. The full extent of cavity formation in the progressive massive fibrotic lesions of silicosis was shown by CT. Bullae were well shown.

Lynch et al. (1988) were able to demonstrate on conventional and HRCT the presence of unsuspected pulmonary masses obscured by parenchymal and pleural abnormalities on the radiographs of asbestos-exposed individuals. These included fissural pleural plaques, round atelectasis, other (presumed) benign masses, (mostly lentiform or wedge-shaped) and carcinomas. The carcinomas were round or lobulated. They emphasized the necessity for HRCT to identify the smaller lesions (under 1 cm) and for routine follow-up to ensure that the lesions were in fact stable.

Diffuse lung disease

The general value of HRCT in chest medicine, including the assessment of asbestosis, has been reviewed by Gamsu and Klein (1989).

General conclusions

The place of CT in the diagnosis and management of occupational disorders of the lung is now becoming clear. Apparatus capable of high-resolution work is highly desirable, and both supine and prone views of the chest should be obtained.

It can never be used as a routine examination and it also does not have a place in screening programmes. It should follow the chest radiograph in the following circumstances:

1. Nodular shadowing is present but of doubtful aetiology. Posterior distribution would favour silicosis. More studies are needed to see if other pneumoconioses behave in a similar fashion.
2. Cases of suspected asbestos-related disease with doubtful X-ray findings, either parenchymal lesions or pleural plaques.
3. Cases of pleural fibrosis, in order to assess extent of involvement, and those of suspected malignant mesothelioma of the pleura.
4. In the course of investigation of a pleural effusion of unknown aetiology if there is a suspicious occupational history.

There is nothing easy in the management and operation of CT apparatus and the interpretation of its images. A wise chest physician will have a close working relationship with a radiologist who is skilled in all aspects of the technique and who has a special interest in chest work.

Other methods involving transmission radiology

A direct quantitative radiological technique

In theory, because each element has a different absorption spectrum (in relation to the range of energies in the X-ray beam) with a particular 'absorption edge' in relation to the electron shell involved (usually the K shell), alteration in penetration due to the differential absorption effect should be demonstrable (McCallum and Day, 1965). Although limited to elements with an atomic number over 40, this has been shown to be true of antimony and tin (McCallum et al., 1971). But it remains an experimental procedure and is not in general use.

Xeroradiography

A xeroradiographic plate, covered with a thin layer of vitreous selenium (a good insulator), if carrying an electrostatic charge, will discharge it if irradiated with X-rays. If it is exposed to the differential absorption pattern in the X-ray beam after passage through the body, the discharges from the plate will also be in accordance with this pattern and so the plate will bear a latent electrostatic image. This is developed by exposing the plate, in a powder chamber, to a cloud of charged fine particles which are electrostatically attracted to the charged areas and so display the image (Meredith and Massey, 1977). The technique has attractive physical properties and has much greater latitude than X-ray film, that is, a wider range of voltage can be used (up to 200 kV) and a wider range of X-ray densities can be shown with less extreme contrast. There is also the edge enhancement effect in which the powder particles appear to pile up like snowdrifts at contrast boundaries.

Linear opacities are shown better than on conventional radiographs but discrete rounded opacities as in silicosis are poorly shown (Thomas and Sluis-Cremer, 1977).

The major disadvantage of the system, apart from the need for special apparatus to produce the high voltage and process the images, is the increased radiation dose involved. Although it has had some success in mammography and bone work, it is not in general use.

Texture analysis

The reading of films with discrete round opacities by computerized techniques is claimed to compare favourably with that of human observers and might be applicable to epidemiological work (Jagoe and Paton, 1975; Ledley, Huang and Rotolo, 1975). There would be, however, numerous variables to be standardized, especially that of film quality. The technique is not in general use.

Ultrasound

Sound is the longitudinal vibration of materials in the direction of propagation, the frequency being measured in hertz (Hz). Sound, transmitted through air and audible to the human ear, is in the frequency range of about 100 to 800 Hz; for example, middle C is 250 Hz. Medical ultrasound uses frequencies from 1.5 to 10 megahertz (MHz), which are inaudible to humans, cannot pass through air or any solid material such as bone, but can pass through fluids and soft tissues. They can be absorbed or scattered to various extents by materials of differing acoustic properties, or reflected or refracted at interfaces between them.

Ultrasound images are produced from the echoes generated from soft tissues and their interfaces. A pulse of ultrasound is emitted by the crystal in the transducer or probe. The time the return echo takes to reach the crystal is measured electronically and the depth of the reflecting surface thus calculated. The underlying physics and electronics and the development of the different kinds of apparatus are complex and have been well described elsewhere (Shirley et al., 1978). For the present purpose, it is enough to know that current apparatus uses hand-held transducers that produce a 'real-time' image which changes as the transducer is moved over the body surface. If the transducer is held still, it can show moving structures such as pulsating vessels or the diaphragm. A coupling medium, such as acoustic gel, is needed between transducer and skin to ensure transmission of the sound waves. Clearly, the process is operator-dependent but ultrasound is now incorporated in the training of nearly all radiologists and of those radiographers, 'ultrasonographers' or technicians specializing in the technique. The major advantage is that no radiation is used and there has been no demonstrable hazard to patient or operator at the power levels used in diagnostic work (about 1 to 5 mW).

The image, an echo pattern based on the acoustic properties of the various tissues, usually shows the echoes in white or shades of grey on a black background (although it can be reversed). It differs from X-ray images in that bony surfaces reflect all the sound, producing strong echoes; interfaces between tissues of differing acoustic properties also produce echoes, and different types of solid tissues are said to be more or less echogenic depending upon whether they produce light or dark grey effects respectively. Fluid is echo-poor and so shows black or dark grey on the image, but flecks of solid matter floating within abscesses will produce echoes. Oedematous tissues are echo-poor, and some solid tissues (for example, lymphoma) cannot be distinguished from fluid. It is therefore not surprising that an echo-poor structure, such as a cyst, transmits more sound than surrounding tissue, producing stronger echoes from, and thus the 'bright-up' effect on, the image of deeper tissues due to through transmission; conversely, echogenic structures cast acoustic shadows, making deeper tissues apparently less echogenic.

The resolution of the image poses physical problems. The depth or axis resolution (that is, in the line of the beam), depending on the electronic analysis of the time of the return echoes, is now very good, usually less than 1 mm (the minimum distance apart of two points that can be shown separately).

The lateral resolution (that is, at right angles to the line of the beam) is dependent on beam width and shape – most beams narrow and then fan out. Hence, a small object anywhere within the beam will be shown on the image at a point corresponding to the centre of the beam; conversely, should there be beam overlap, the same object will be shown more than once. In either case there will be a short streak at right angles to the beam instead of a point on the image. This streak used to be up to 3 mm long, and such effects may still be seen in some of the classic earlier publications. Modern apparatus using focused beams and microprocessors has reduced these figures; one manufacturer claims axial and lateral resolution of 0.4 and 1.7 mm respectively for a 3.5-MHz probe and 0.3 and 1.0 mm for a 7-MHz probe.

The value of the technique in chest medicine can now be seen. In the presence of fluid in the pleural cavity, an intercostal space may be used as a 'window' to obtain access by avoiding the acoustic shadows from the ribs. There will be small echoes from the intercostal and extrapleural tissues, a moderate echo (showing as a line on the image) from the parietal pleural surface, little or none from the pleural fluid and then a moderate echo again from the visceral pleura. Deep to this, the lung produces a strong echo from its superficial layers and then amorphous speckling (Figure 7.16). However, a subpleural mass will transmit some sound and produce echoes from its deep surface, so peripheral tumours or other solid tissues, concealed by the pleural fluid on the radiograph, can become manifest. Thickened pleura is more echogenic than fluid but less so than chest wall and thus can be identified, its thickness measured and irregularities noted.

An approach through a lower space directed downwards can show the diaphragm and its movements. The diaphragm may also be displayed from below through the liver or spleen, and subphrenic fluid collections distinguished from subpulmonary and other pleural fluid.

The literature contains much testimony to the value of ultrasound. Doust et al. (1975), using A-scan and compound B-scan with bi-stable images, showed that pleural fluid over 1 cm in depth could be confidently diagnosed and the diaphragm identified. Curati and Saas (1983) used ultrasound-guided fluid aspiration to obtain cytological or bacteriological diagnosis in 65 cases of pleural effusion, including 26 neoplasms of which 2 were mesotheliomas. Yang et al. (1984) studied 40 patients with radiographic pleural or subpleural opacities and classified the effusions into 'anechoic', 'complex septated' and 'complex non-septated'. Ultrasonically guided percutaneous, transthoracic needle-aspiration of 16 patients with solid subpleural masses yielded 14 positive cytological results, 1 a mesothelioma.

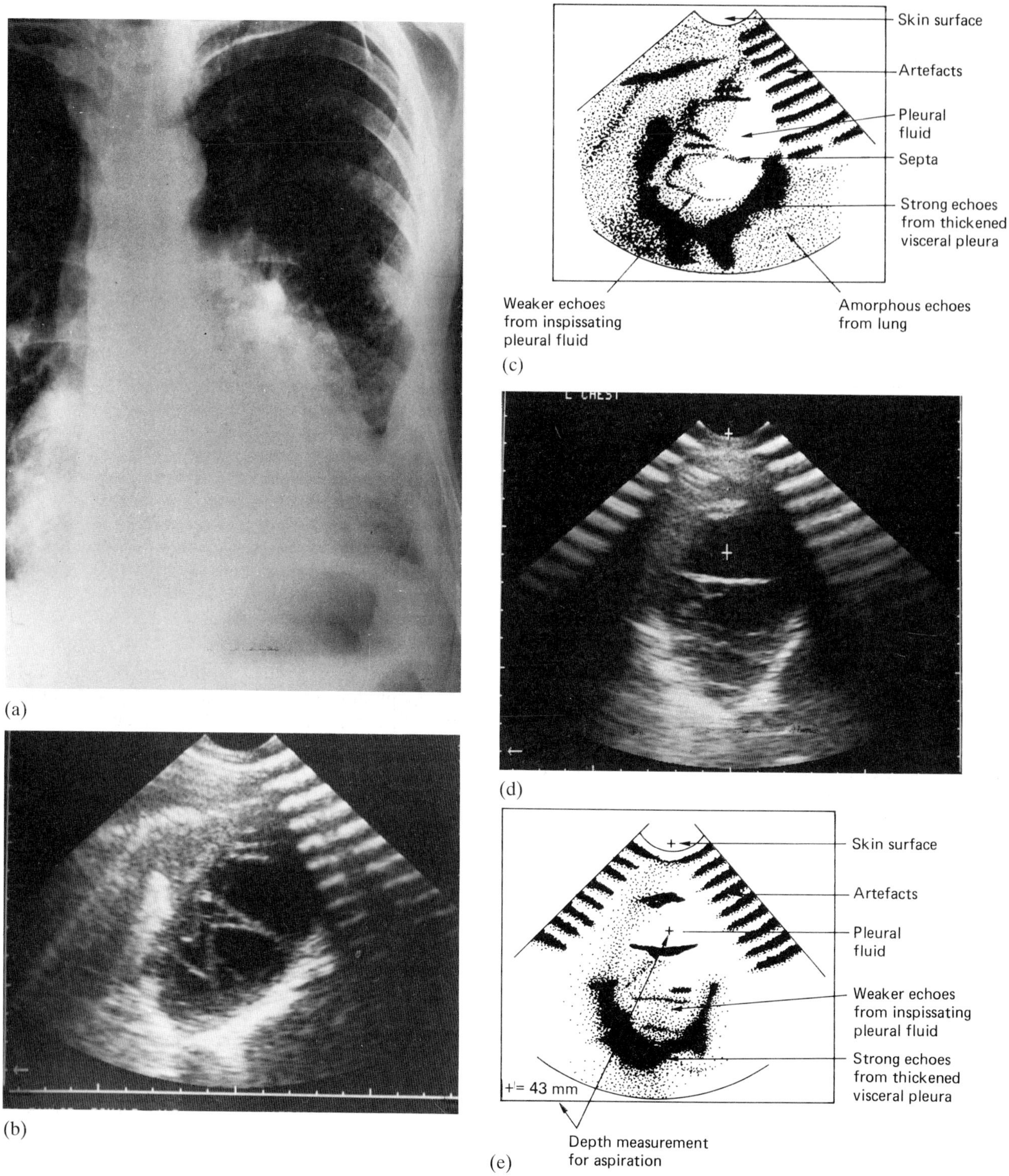

(a)

(b)

(c)

Skin surface

Artefacts

Pleural fluid

Septa

Strong echoes from thickened visceral pleura

Weaker echoes from inspissating pleural fluid

Amorphous echoes from lung

(d)

(e)

Skin surface

Artefacts

Pleural fluid

Weaker echoes from inspissating pleural fluid

Strong echoes from thickened visceral pleura

+ = 43 mm

Depth measurement for aspiration

Figure 7.16 (a) A partly encysted pleural effusion which has not resolved. (b,c) An ultrasound image and line representation of that ultrasound image of the effusion seen to be loculated and septate. Because ultrasound passes readily through fluid it produces no echoes from the effusion which therefore looks black. There is a strong echo from the visceral pleura which is apparently thickened but the effect is potentiated by through transmission, the so-called 'bright-up' effect due to lack of attenuation of the ultrasound beam as it passes through fluid. The inspissating pleural fluid produces rather weaker echoes but is clearly seen. (d,e) Ultrasound image and line representation at the point of access chosen for aspiration. The depth from the skin to the centre of the fluid collection has been measured. (Images by courtesy of Dr B. Gajjar)

Whereas Jay (1985) considered ultrasound to be of little value, Pugatch and Spirn (1985) found it to be an extremely useful, safe and rapid method of defining and localizing pleural fluid and of guiding intervention for diagnostic aspiration, biopsy or drainage. Although CT was superior in providing anatomical representation of pleural and associated thoracic pathology, both methods had much to contribute. Neuhold, Fruhwald and Seidl (1985) emphasized the value of localizing the puncture site for cytology. Kohan et al. (1986) compared decubitus radiography with ultrasound for the detection of small pleural effusions, loculated or otherwise, and found ultrasound superior although there was no advantage in large effusions. Hall (1987), commenting on this, felt that the chief advantage lay in using ultrasound not just to identify the fluid, but also to guide the aspiration which would be performed by the radiologist. Hennighien, Remacle and Bruart (1986) stressed the value and limitations of the technique. O'Moore et al. (1987) reported their results with diagnostic aspiration using 20-gauge needles and catheter placement for drainage or treatment, including the Heimlich valve for pneumothorax, much of the work being done by the radiologist under ultrasound control. Stavaas et al. (1987) reported similar successes, and Halvorsen and Thompson (1986), while describing four CT signs by which ascitic fluid could be differentiated from pleural fluid, also drew attention to the ease with which this could be accomplished by ultrasound. Mueller et al. (1988) described a technique for pleural biopsy in 23 patients using 16- to 20-gauge needles with CT guidance in 1, fluoroscopy in 2 and ultrasound guidance in the remainder, with a high level of diagnostic accuracy.

In general, it is better for the radiologist to undertake ultrasound-guided aspiration or fine-needle biopsy. Merely to locate the abnormality and then leave it to a member of the chest unit to make the puncture subsequently is to invite failure, as the author can testify.

There is widespread reluctance to extract pleural tissue for biopsy where mesothelioma is suspected, for fear of seeding of tumour along the track or surgical scar. Radiologists' abdominal experience shows virtually no hazard to tissue traversed by 20-gauge needles; there do not appear to be any recent reports in the literature of seeding following the fine-needle technique, but this may be because the investigation is often avoided. The question remains open.

Tissue identification by ultrasound is dependent more on anatomical relationships than on the texture in the image, but the latter can be helpful. Agatston et al. (1986) reported unusually strong echoes from the pericardium in a patient thought to have constrictive pericarditis. The pathology *post mortem* was mesothelioma. However, until there is some well-controlled research into the ultrasound appearances of thickened pleura compared with (or progressing to) mesothelioma, the possibility of such a diagnosis by ultrasound must be approached with caution, although the author has seen one case.

The assessment of blood flow and velocity using Doppler shift measurements appears to have little relevance to chest medicine as yet but has a possible application in determining the relative vascularity of tissue. This would be a possible field for research into the differentiation of mesothelioma from thickened pleura.

In summary, the value of ultrasound to the chest physician lies chiefly in the investigation of pleural effusions and of subpleural masses. It depends, critically, on detailed co-operation between the referring physician and a radiologist skilled in the use of the technique. Its place in the investigational algorithm lies after the chest radiograph and before CT.

Nuclear medicine

Diagnostic nuclear medicine is a quantitative technique which counts the numbers of γ-ray high-energy photons emitted by the disintegrating atoms of radioactive substances. An element is said to have isotopes when its atoms exist in different forms having the same atomic number (that is, the same number of electrons in the same electronic shell structure and, therefore, the same chemical properties) but different atomic weights due to differences in their atomic nuclei. They are usually designated briefly by the atomic weight coupled with the chemical symbol. Some isotopes are stable, others are not; they are radioactive because their nuclei disintegrate with the production of radiation characteristic of the isotope. They are known as radio-isotopes or radionuclides.

Although disintegration is random, each radio-isotope has a characteristic half-life ($t_{1/2}$) – that is, the average length of time it takes for the substance to have lost half its atoms and, thus, half its level of radioactivity. The most commonly used diagnostic radio-isotope in medicine is the metastable isotope of the artificial element technetium (^{99m}Tc) which has a half-life of 6.02 hours and a gamma photon energy of 140 keV. Others are used for special purposes.

The rectilinear scanner, in which a small crystal was moved systematically to record the emissions and construct the image, has now been largely replaced by the gamma camera.

A gamma camera head contains a large thin crystal which receives the gamma emissions from the area of the body under study. Each gamma photon produces a flash of light (known as a scintillation) from the crystal. These are counted and located to their point of origin. From the data an emission image is constructed, known as a *planar image* because it receives in the plane of the crystal all the emissions from the corresponding area of the body surface. The procedure is sometimes known as *scintigraphy*. The times of occurrence of the scintillations can be used to generate functional information, usually in the form of time–activity curves.

On some gamma cameras the head can be made to rotate round the patient, and, in a similar way to X-rays, CT can obtain an image of a slice of the patient at right angles to the planar image, using somewhat similar software. This technique is usually known as *single photon emission computed tomography* (SPECT).

The gamma camera image may be on a cathode ray oscilloscope (CRO), when it has a pattern of black dots, each of which represents a scintillation or, on a video screen, as a grey or colour scale, having been digitized by passing through a computer acting as a data processor. Resolution is expressed in a different way in a gamma camera image but in the digitized image is largely governed by the matrix size. Generally it is much less sharp than in CT; a 128×128 matrix is as high as most pieces of equipment go. Both images can be photographed but the digitized or video images can be fed directly into a printer.

In chest medicine, the clinical applications are the assessment of lung perfusion and ventilation and of inflammatory activity.

Lung perfusion studies

If a suspension of fine particles in the size range of 10 to 100 μm is injected intravenously, they will lodge in the pulmonary capillary bed. Current practice in most places is to use *microaggregates of albumin* (MAA) labelled with ^{99m}Tc. A normal lung will produce a homogeneous lung-shaped appearance on the gamma camera image. If the pulmonary arterioles are obstructed by embolus or thrombus, or are narrowed by hypoxic constriction or pressure from pulmonary or interstitial oedema or by fibrosis, or are ablated by the disease process, the particles do not reach the capillary bed in the abnormal area. This shows as a defect in the perfusion image.

Lung ventilation studies

Radioactive gases available for inhalation are krypton (^{81}Kr, $t_{1/2}$ = 13 seconds) and xenon (^{133}Xe, $t_{1/2}$ = 5.3 days; ^{127}Xe, $t_{1/2}$ = 36.4 days). A soluble preparation of ^{99m}Tc can be used as an aerosol provided

the particles are between 0.5 and 2 μm, preferably 1 μm, and there is a dry fine-particle (about 1 μm) preparation of ^{99m}Tc as a carbide (Technegas; Burch, Sullivan and McLaren, 1986). A homogeneous ventilation image of normal lung will be produced by the gamma camera but poorly ventilated regions will show as ventilation defects. Krypton has to be continuously inhaled during image acquisition on account of its short half-life, to give a static equilibrium image. The ^{99m}Tc preparations are inhaled before acquisition. Xenon can be used to assess the rate of uptake by the lung ('wash-in' phase), followed by an equilibrium image and then the rate of disposal of the gas by exhalation ('wash-out' phase), so offering a means of estimating both total and regional lung function. Quantitative studies are possible although not widely used.

Ventilation–perfusion ($\dot{V}/\dot{Q}$) studies, with both types of image simultaneously available for scrutiny, are used chiefly for the diagnosis of suspected thromboembolic disease in which the classic appearance is a perfusion defect in a region with normal ventilation – the so-called *mismatched defect*. If the defect is matched in both images it is presumed that there is lung pathology with both decreased ventilation and perfusion which does not normally occur in simple thromboembolic disease (although it can occur in lung infarct, when the ventilation defect is smaller than the perfusion defect).

In the presence of airways' obstruction, including asthma, mismatched defects also occur. Local hypoxia induces peripheral vascular constriction which will produce a perfusion defect, but enough of the radioactive gas may reach the region involved to produce a normal ventilation image, albeit somewhat patchy. Sometimes there is a reversed mismatch in which poorly ventilated lung retains its blood supply. It follows that radio-isotope lung ventilation–perfusion studies are unreliable as discriminators of thromboembolic disease in the presence of such conditions.

Abnormal appearances are seen in occupational lung disease. Schröder et al. (1969) showed that in silicosis (including coal pneumoconiosis) and silico-tuberculosis there were abnormalities in the perfusion image. Scattered small nodular disease produced widespread patchy defects, and larger nodules had well-marked corresponding defects. Seaton, Lapp and Chang (1971) showed that, in coal pneumoconiosis, conglomerate masses and bullae produced perfusion defects assumed to be due to obliteration of the vessels but similar defects also occurred in lung that looked normal on the radiograph, possibly due to 'compensatory' (irregular) emphysema. However, in simple pneumoconiosis, the perfusion images were normal in the absence of other disease, such as airways' obstruction.

Secker-Walker and Ho (1979), using ^{99m}Tc-labelled MAA and ^{133}Xe, studied lung function in asbestos workers and found defective perfusion in the more fibrotic areas and the bullous areas. Delayed clearance of ^{133}Xe occurred also in fibrotic areas and in the lungs of those with severe airways' obstruction.

Unfortunately, these phenomena are non-specific because they can occur in lung pathology other than that of occupational disease. They have been reviewed by Secker-Walker (1983). They seem to have found little use except in research, although with quantification they might be useful in assessing severity.

The significance of $\dot{V}/\dot{Q}$ studies for the occupational chest physician is that, in investigating a case of dyspnoea without particularly diagnostic signs in the chest radiograph, they may be used to look for thromboembolic disease. In early cases with equivocal radiographic signs, however, abnormal ventilation–perfusion scans not fitting the expected picture will raise suspicion of hitherto unrecognized peripheral lung disease which may turn out to have an occupational origin.

Inflammatory activity studies

The radio-isotope which has found a use here is gallium (^{67}Ga, $t_{\frac{1}{2}}$ = 78 hours) as the citrate. Its mode of action is still not fully understood but it certainly has an affinity for disease processes associated with cellular proliferation and high metabolic activity, and so concentrates in tissues involved in inflammatory disease and tumours. It has an affinity for granulocytes and micro-organisms (Staab and McCartney, 1978). Larson (1978) favoured protein binding involving transferrin taken up by specific receptors on the cell surface. Hoffer (1980) reviewed the chemistry of gallium; it can bind to transferrin, lactoferrin, ferritin and siderophores. At sites of infection, it can enter leucocytes, probably by lactoferrin binding; it may leak through permeable vascular endothelium, either as the ionic form or bound to transferrin, and then bind to apolactoferrin; by binding to siderophores, it may enter bacterial cells. The uptake mechanism in tumours is, apparently, controversial but seems most likely to be via transferrin.

Regions of increased gallium uptake tend to be rather poorly defined on the image, so its manifestations in the pulmonary parenchyma tend to produce somewhat diffuse or patchy appearances. They are best assessed quantitatively. Various types of gallium uptake index have been described, a standard one being that described by Line et al. (1978, 1981), used in the assessment of pulmonary sarcoidosis. McLean, Steele and Murray (1985) reviewed the subject and suggested a simpler method.

Siemsen et al. (1974) demonstrated increased uptake of ^{67}Ga in silicosis (two patterns, one central and located to the mediastinum and hila, the other peripheral and diffuse) and asbestosis (diffuse peripheral pattern only). Peripheral uptake was more extensive than the radiographic signs would suggest, raising the possibility of identifying suspected pathology before the radiographic signs appeared. Reviewing the general application of ^{67}Ga to pulmonary disease, Siemsen, Grebe and Waxman (1978) again suggested that it was more sensitive than radiography in detecting early pneumoconiosis although not specific for any type.

Bégin et al. (1983) studied 58 asbestos workers; 17 of 21 with asbestosis showed increased ^{67}Ga uptake by the lungs, whilst of the other 37, 16 showed an increased gallium index and had abnormal lung function tests. In the experimental sheep model, increased ^{67}Ga uptake was associated with enhanced serum protein leakage and macrophage accumulation as shown by bronchoalveolar lavage (BAL).

Kramer et al. (1987) and Bitran et al. (1987) investigated with ^{67}Ga patients with acquired immune deficiency syndrome, suspected of having *Pneumocystis carinii* pneumonia. In both groups (57 and 32 cases respectively), about half those found positive with ^{67}Ga had normal chest radiographs. This again shows the greater sensitivity of the ^{67}Ga study compared with radiography in an inflammatory condition even if the local reaction is suppressed.

Vanderstappen et al. (1988) investigated 17 patients with idiopathic DIPF and 10 with hypersensitivity pneumonitis (7 with pigeon-fanciers' lung, 2 with farmers' lung and 1 with isocyanate hypersensitivity) and calculated ^{67}Ga indices using the method of Line et al. (1978). The ^{67}Ga indices were lower in those whose condition was unchanged or improved after 1 year, but all those who had higher indices deteriorated. The change in vital capacity correlated closely and inversely with the initial ^{67}Ga index.

Hayes et al. (1988) used an improved method of quantification to assess 24 crocidolite-exposed workers and 8 controls. The gallium index was increased in both the 8 with asbestosis and the 16 with normal or near-normal radiographs, compared with the controls. Delclos et al. (1989) studied 32 asbestos-exposed workers and found increased ^{67}Ga activity in the lung in 56 per cent of those with radiographic evidence of asbestosis and 36 per cent of the others. They also undertook bronchoalveolar lavage.

In summary, the value of nuclear medicine to the occupational chest physician appears to lie in two fields:

1. In the general investigation of dyspnoea, radio-isotope ventilation–perfusion images with unusual defect patterns may raise suspicion of a range of conditions, some of which may be related to occupation.

2. In patients with a history suggesting occupational lung disorder, other than from inert dusts, and no convincing radiographic evidence, a positive gallium study may be a good early sign of lung involvement, although, so far, convincing results have been achieved only with asbestosis; where there are radiographic abnormalities, particularly in asbestosis and hypersensitivity conditions, the gallium index may have prognostic value. Gallium is a relatively expensive radio-isotope and the procedure is somewhat time-consuming, so its use should be reserved for special cases. It must be remembered that the specificity is relatively low but most workers have found it more sensitive than X-rays.

There are also various research studies that are outside the scope of this chapter. Again, the occupational chest physician is urged to keep in touch with a practitioner of nuclear medicine (physician or radiologist) who has an interest in chest disease.

Magnetic resonance imaging (MRI)

This technique (originally called nuclear magnetic resonance (NMR) but now known as MRI) depends upon the fact that the atomic nuclei of some elements (those with an odd number of protons and neutrons) rotate. This spin property is associated with magnetism such that the magnetic moment is in the direction of the axis of rotation. In some ways they resemble minuscule bar magnets. Hydrogen is the most useful of these. Normally the atoms are spinning at random.

In a strong external magnetic field the nuclei tend to align their magnetic moments in the direction of the field, somewhat like an array of spinning tops. If another magnetic field is applied at right angles to the external magnetic field, that alignment will be altered; if the magnetic field is oscillating at the correct frequency, usually in the radio frequency (RF) range, the nuclei will resonate and will rotate round the direction of the external field at an angle to it, somewhat analogous to the movements of a spinning top that is slowing down. They are said to be 'precessing'. When the applied field (RF pulse) is switched off, they will return to their original alignment. The time that the atoms take to realign their magnetic axes (relaxation time, $T1$) is characteristic and depends on the physical and chemical state of the atoms. While precessing, the component

of the magnetic moment at right angles to the main field can induce a current in receiver coils on the surface of the subject. By giving the main magnetic field a gradation, measuring the currents in the surface coils and analysing the data in a somewhat similar way to that used in CT, a pattern of numbers is built up from which an image can be constructed. The difference is that the pattern is in three dimensions, and instead of building the image up in a series of pixels in the planes of the slice, the number pattern relates to small elemental volumes known as voxels. In theory, an image could be constructed in any plane but it is conventional practice to use transverse, coronal or sagittal planes.

There are at least three varieties of image, depending on the lengths and sequences of RF pulses and how the currents in the receiver coils are analysed: a *proton density image* differentiates tissues by the amount of hydrogen they contain; a *T1-weighted image* is dependent on the relaxation time from the precessing angle to the original alignment; the *T2-weighted image* takes account of another aspect of the relaxation time, the time taken for the precessing atoms to lose phase coherence ($T2$) – that is, to cease to rotate 'in step'. Each type of image has a characteristic pattern of differential signal strengths in the various tissues. The mathematics is complex, the terminology has changed over time and there are numerous applied variables, but there is a very readable account in Kean and Smith (1986). The physician is advised to leave the technicalities to radiologists, physicists and others who are familiar with the subject, but it is useful to know the general properties and limitations of the method.

The main magnet is very powerful; strengths from 0.35 to 1.5 teslas (T) may be used (1 tesla (T) = 10 000 gauss (G); the earth's magnetic field is 0.5 gauss). A steel screwdriver would be pulled from one's hand. The equipment usually has to be housed in a separate building, with distance and shielding from other electrical apparatus. Patients with such devices as cardiac pacemakers and implanted items (even surgical clips) which may be ferrimagnetic are liable to considerable hazard and should not go into the machine.

The principal difference from radiographic and CT images is that MRI does not image bones, only soft tissues. It does show bone marrow and pathology therein, but the existence of bone has to be inferred from the shape of the marrow. Many of the images are comparable with CT but the tissue differentiation is not the same and some differences are better shown in MRI, especially in the nervous system. MRI's other great advantage is the capacity to produce coronal and sagittal images which provide information otherwise not readily available. Webb et al. (1988) showed that MRI coronal images of the chest were sometimes better than transaxial CT for evaluating the aorticopulmonary window and masses at the lung apex or base, whereas transaxial images were better for the pretracheal and subcarinal spaces and the hila; coronal images were better at showing lateral hilar masses. Cohen (1984) reviewed the application of MRI to the thorax and noted that pleural fluid tended to give a high signal intensity.

There are several reports to suggest that mesothelioma may give rise to increased signal intensity. Gossinger et al. (1988) described such an appearance in pericardial mesothelioma. Strankinga et al. (1987) reviewed 30 patients with mesothelioma of the pleura. In 6 patients examined by MRI the increased signal intensity on the images demonstrated correctly the site and extension of the tumour. Kanzaki et al. (1988) showed an outer ring of increased signal strength in a localized malignant pleural mesothelioma, whereas Inada et al. (1988) showed only slightly increased signal (midway between muscle and fat) on a $T2$-weighted image in a benign pleural mesothelioma. Lorigan and Libshitz (1989) examined three patients with malignant pleural mesothelioma with circumferential pleural masses. The $T2$-weighted image showed a slight increase of signal intensity, with focal areas of very high signal intensity thought to be due to loculated fluid. Coronal and transaxial images together gave good demonstration of the extent of the tumour, particularly in the mediastinal region. Lymphadenopathy was equally well shown by MRI and CT.

The prospect of finding a mesothelioma at an early stage when surgical removal might be possible is so attractive that it is surprising that more research in this direction has not been done. It is, of course, a relatively rare tumour in general chest medicine.

The application to other types of occupational lung disease does not appear to have been studied, but siderosis seems to be a likely candidate for research into the signal intensity compared with other conditions having similar radiographic appearances.

Clearly, the current place of MRI in occupational lung disease is in the field of research, but its potential clinical value lies in the early diagnosis of mesothelioma and in assessing the prognosis of the established disease.

Magnetopneumography (MPG)

Although not strictly an imaging procedure, this technique makes use of the magnetic properties of dusts containing ferrimagnetic materials. It is based on the observation that a weak magnetic field can be detected with very sensitive apparatus in the chests of individuals with occupational dust exposure (Cohen, 1973) but only significantly with such ferrimagnetic materials (FMM) as magnetite

and hematite. The strength of the field can be augmented by magnetizing the particles with an external magnetic field. This remnant field persists with a half-time of 10–30 minutes. Paramagnetic materials such as asbestos, and endogenous iron in haem and ferritin, do not have this property.

The external field may be uniform over the whole thorax (UFT) or localized (LFT) in which the thorax is studied region by region; it is a much weaker external field than is used in MRI (36 mT) (Cohen, 1975; Kalliomäki et al., 1976; Freedman, Robinson and Green, 1982). With LFT, the results can be plotted as a matrix of numbers somewhat analogous to those produced by a rectilinear scanner in nuclear medicine, so it is possible to work out the distribution of FMM in the lung. This has been shown to correspond to pathological findings.

The content of FMMs (chiefly magnetite) in welding fume and iron and steel foundry dusts may be as much as 30 per cent (Kalliomäki et al., 1979), and has been found to be less than 1 per cent in coal-mine dust and 0.7 per cent in volcanic ash from Mount St Helen's (Freedman, Robinson and Green, 1982). Significant accumulation of ferromagnetic minerals in arc welders, foundry workers and, to a lesser extent in coal miners, has been demonstrated before their presence is detectable radiographically (Kalliomäki et al., 1978a,b; Freedman, Robinson and Johnson, 1980).

The UFT allows differences in thoracic FMMs, both between and within groups of workers, to be detected whilst LFT makes quantitative assessment possible. MPG can be used to monitor accumulation of dusts, in which there is sufficient FMM to act as a tracer, in occupational groups who may be at risk from dust-related disease. However, MPG has no occupational specificity so that comprehensive histories of occupation and hobbies must complement its use (Freedman, Robinson and Green, 1982). It can also measure the translocation and clearance of known trace amounts of inhaled magnetite in the lungs and the extrapulmonary destination of cleared particles (Freedman, Robinson and Street, 1988; Kalliomäki, Kalliomäki and Moilanen, 1988).

At present, however, the technique is largely a research tool of limited availability, but, as it is non-invasive and apparently harmless, its potentialities may well be expanded when further refined.

Storage of images

With few exceptions, occupational lung disorders are chronic conditions even if some manifest in acute phases. Many are slowly progressive, often unnoticed in their early stages. For this reason, as already mentioned, images for comparison over periods of time are essential. It follows that arrangements must be made for the preservation and storage of such images in a retrievable fashion.

The volume of exposed X-ray film in modern health facilities is such that most organizations define a holding policy, a period of years after which the originals are destroyed. In the British National Health Service, the current figure is 8 years (25 years for paediatric images). Even so, sometimes only films from the last 1 or 2 years are readily retrievable. The balance may be held in some other store, not necessarily under the best conditions, or copied onto a small format system to save space, the originals being discarded. Most radiologists can make use of the small format systems, which generally are not accepted into use unless they preserve on the small images all the information present on the originals. Chest physicians working in an organization using one of these systems will need to acquire the art of comparing such images with recent ones and of using the associated equipment.

It is often possible to negotiate with management or imaging departments to set up a system for special preservation of certain classes of image; this could certainly be done for occupational lung disease. This is yet another reason for the chest physician to work in close collaboration with the radiologist.

Computerized systems are under development in which images could be held in digital form, readily retrievable and viewable on digital video monitors at work stations. These are generally known as *picture archive and communication systems* (PACS). Much of ultrasound and nuclear medicine and all of CT and MRI imaging is already digitized and readily susceptible to this form of storage; 128 × 128 or even 256 × 256 matrices can be handled without too much difficulty. However, radiographic images, which constitute over 70 per cent of imaging work over all, half being chest radiographs, present enormous problems on account of the vast amount of data to be stored. Enough has been said about resolution elsewhere in this chapter to make it clear that, if the image sharpness is to be maintained, large matrices will be required; current thinking is that 1024 × 1024 will be needed to reproduce accurately the sort of appearances on which occupational disease diagnosis depends.

Final agreement about the optimum type of system is not, at the time of writing, yet established. The chest physician is advised to maintain close relationships with the radiologists about proposals to introduce PACS locally so as to ensure not only that the image is stored in a large enough matrix but also that the quality of the viewing monitors is adequate.

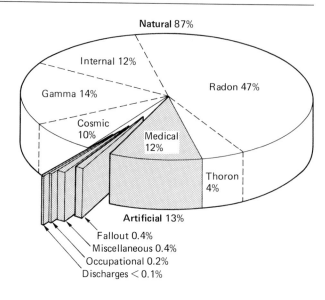

Figure 7.17 Average annual effective dose equivalent to the population of the UK – 2.5 mSv. (Reproduced by permission of the National Radiological Protection Board, 1990)

Radiation hazards

All ionizing radiation can be harmful. In the UK, most of the radiation to which the population is exposed comes from the natural background, but 13 per cent is artificial. X- and γ-rays, used in medical diagnosis and treatment, account for most of this, and amount to 12 per cent of the total to which the population is exposed annually (Figure 7.17). It comprises most (87 per cent) of the artificial radiation, which amounts to 13 per cent of the total overall background radiation (National Radiological Protection Board, 1990). It is therefore essential to keep the radiation dose received *as low as reasonably achievable* (the ALARA principle). It is reasonable to use radiation to make a diagnosis when the benefit is likely to exceed any radiation hazard; this is certainly the case with chest radiographs in which the dose is low. CT and nuclear medicine give rather more than chest radiology. Ultrasound and MRI do not use ionizing radiation at all.

Physicians should bear this in mind and request only those examinations and diagnostic procedures, involving ionizing radiation, that are truly necessary for the proper assessment and management of the patient's condition. Under no circumstances should decisions about such examinations or procedures be delegated to non-medical personnel or to non-medical parts of the organization.

References

Aberle, D.R., Gamsu, G., Ray, C.S. and Feuerstein, I.M. (1988) Asbestos-related pleural and parenchymal fibrosis: detection with high-resolution CT. *Radiology* **166**, 729–734

Adrian-Harris, D. (1979) Aspects of visual perception in radiography. *Radiography* **45**, 237–243

Agatston, A.S., Robinson, M.J., Trigo, L., Machado, R. and Samet, P. (1986) Echocardiographic findings in primary pericardial mesothelioma. *Am. Heart J.* **111**, 986–989

Amandus, H.E., Reger, R.B., Pendergrass, E.P., Dennis, J.M. and Morgan, W.K.C. (1973) The pneumoconioses: methods of measuring progression. *Chest* **63**, 736–743

Barnhart, S., Thornquist, M., Omenn, G.S., Goodman, G., Feigl, P. and Rosenstock, L. (1990) The degree of roentgenographic parenchymal opacities attributable to smoking among asbestos-exposed subjects. *Am. Rev. Respir. Dis.* **141**, 1102–1106

Bégin, R., Cantin, A., Drapeau, G., Lamoureux, G., Boctor, M., Masse, S. and Rola-Pleszczynski, M. (1983) Pulmonary uptake of gallium-67 in asbestosis-exposed humans and sheep. *Am. Rev. Respir. Dis.* **127**, 623–630

Bégin, R., Boctor, M., Bergeron, D., Cantin, A., Bertiaume, Y., Peloquin, S., Bisson, G. and Lamoureux, G. (1984) Radiographic assessment of pleuropulmonary disease in asbestos workers: posteroanterior, four-view films and computed tomograms of the thorax. *Br. J. Ind. Med.* **41**, 373–383

Bégin, R., Bergeron, D., Samson, L., Boctor, M. and Cantin, A. (1987) CT assessment of silicosis in exposed workers. *AJR Am. J. Roentgenol.* **148**, 509–514

Bergin, C.J. and Müller, N.L. (1985) CT in the diagnosis of interstitial lung disease. *AJR Am. J. Roentgenol.* **145**, 505–510

Bergin, C.J. and Müller, N.L. (1987) CT of interstitial lung disease: a diagnostic approach. *Am. J. Roentg.* **148**, 8–15, 9–15

Bergman, I. (1970) The relation of endogenous non-haem iron in formalin-fixed lungs to radiological grade of pneumoconiosis. *Ann. Occup. Hyg.* **13**, 163–169

Bitran, J., Bekerman, C., Weinstein, R., Bennet, C., Ryo, U. and Pinsky, S. (1987) Patterns of gallium-67 scintigraphy in patients with acquired immunodeficiency syndrome and the AIDS-related complex. *J. Nucl. Med.* **28**, 1103–1106

Bohlig, H. and Gilson, J.C. (1973) Radiology. In *Biological Effects of Asbestos* (eds P. Bogovski et al.), IARC, Lyon, pp. 25–30

Bracken, T.J. (1964) The technique of macroradiography in the diagnosis of industrial disease of the chest. *Radiography* **30**, 291–298

Bretland, P.M. (1978) The chest. In *Essentials of Radiology*, Chapter 2, Butterworths, London, pp. 9–62

Browne, K., Lepoutre, J., Mansour, F., Murray, R., Gilson, J.C. and Rossiter, C.E. (1984) Radiology of asbestos-related disease. A supplement to the ILO standard set and a check on its validity. In *Proceedings of the VIth International Conference on Pneumoconiosis*, Bochum 1983. Bergbau-Berufsgenossenschaft, Bochum, pp. 882–888

Buechner, H.A. and Ansari, A. (1969) Acute silicoproteinosis. *Dis. Chest* **55**, 274–284

Burch, W.M., Sullivan, P.J. and McLaren, C.J. (1986) Technegas: a new ventilation agent for lung scanning. *Nuclear Med. Commun.* **7**, 865–871

Caplan, A. (1962) Correlation of radiological category with lung pathology in coal worker's pneumoconiosis. *Br. J. Ind. Med.* **19**, 171–179

Carstairs, L.S. (1961) The interpretation of shadows in a restricted area of lung field in the chest radiograph. *Proc. R. Soc. Med.* **54**, 978–980

Clark's Positioning in Radiography (1979) 10th edn, Vol. 1. (Ilford Publication), Heinemann Medical Books, London

Classification of radiographs of the pneumoconioses (1981) *Med. Radiogr. Photogr.* **57**, 2–17

Cohen, A.M. (1984) Magnetic resonance imaging of the thorax. *Radiol. Clins N. Am.* **22**, 829–846

Cohen, B.A., Pomerans, S., Rabinowitz, J., Train, J.S., Norton, K.I. et al. (1984) Pulmonary complications of AIDS. *AJR Am. J. Roentgenol.* **143**, 115–122

Cohen, D. (1975) Measurement of the magnetic fields produced by the human heart, brain and lungs. *Institute of Electrical and Electronics Engineers Transactions. Mag.* **11**, 694–700

Collins, J.D., Brown, R.K.J. and Batra, P. (1983) Asbestosis and the serratus anterior muscle. *J. Am. Med. Assoc.* **75**, 296–300

Cookson, W.O.C.M., Musk, A.W. and Glancy, J.J. (1984) Asbestosis and cryptogenic fibrosing alveolitis: a radiological and functional comparison. *Aust. NZ J. Med.* **14**, 626–630

Cookson, W.O.M.C., De Klerk, N.H., Musk, A.W., Glancy, J.J., Armstrong, B.K. and Hobbs, M.S.T. (1985) Benign and malignant pleural effusions in former Wittenoom crocidolite millers and miners. *Aust. NZ J. Med.* **15**, 731–737

Cookson, W., De Klerk, N., Musk, A.W., Glancy, J.J., Armstrong, B. and Hobbs, M. (1986) The natural history of asbestosis in former crocidolite workers of Wittenoom Gorge. *Am. Rev. Respir.Dis.* **133**, 994–998

Curati, W.-L. and Saas, E. (1983) Ultrasound of the pleural space with cytological and/or bacteriological correlation: a study of 65 cases. *Ultrasound Med. Biol.* suppl. 2, pp. 245–249

Delclos, G.L., Flitcraft, D.G., Brousseau, K.P., Windsor, N.T., Nelson, D.L., Wilson, R.K. and Lawrence, E.C. (1989) Bronchoalveolar lavage analysis, gallium-67 lung scanning and soluble interleukin-2 receptor levels in asbestos exposure. *Environ. Res.* **48**, 164–178

Department of Health, Supplies Technology Division, NHS Procurement Directorate (1989) *Comparison of the Imaging Performance of CT Scanners*, Issue 6: STD/88/36 (March 1989). Department of Health, 14 Russell Square, London WC1B 5EP

Doppman, J.L., Geelhoed, G.W. and De Vita, V.T. (1975) Atypical radiographic features in pneumocystis carinii pneumonia. *Radiology* **114**, 39–44

Doust, B.D., Baum, J.K., Maldad, N.F. and Doust, V.L. (1975) Ultrasonic evaluation of pleural opacities. *Radiology* **114**, 135–140

Epstein, D.M., Miller, W.T., Bresnitz, E.A., Levine, M.S. and Gefter, W.B. (1984) Application of ILO Classification to a population without industrial exposure: findings to be differentiated from pneumoconiosis. *AJR Am. J. Roentgenol.* **142**, 53–58

Felson, B., Morgan, W.K.C., Bristol, L.J., Pendergrass, E.P., Dessen, E.L., Linton, O.W. and Reger, R.B. (1973) Observations on the results of multiple readings of chest films in coal miners' pneumoconioses. *Radiology* **109**, 19–23

Fletcher, D.E. and Edge, J.R. (1970) The early radiological changes in pulmonary and pleural asbestosis. *Clin. Radiol.* **21**, 355–365

Forrest, J.V. (1972) Radiographic findings in pneumocystis carinii pneumonia. *Radiology* **103**, 539–544

Fourio, M., Dongay, G., Levade, M., Carles, P., Bollinelli, R. and Putois, J. (1984) Apport de la tomodensitometrie dans la pathologie pleuropulmonaire de l'amiante. [Computed tomography investigation of asbestosis.] *J. Radiol.* **65**, 335–339

Freedman, A.P., Robinson, S.E. and Green, F.H.Y. (1982) Magnetopneumography as a tool for the study of dust retention in the lungs. *Ann. Occup. Hyg.* **26**, 319–335

Freedman, A.P., Robinson, S.E. and Johnston, R.F. (1980) Non-invasive magnetopneumographic estimation of lung dust loads and distribution in bituminous coal workers. *J. Occup. Med.* **22**, 613–618

Freedman, A.P., Robinson, S.E. and Street, M.R. (1988) Magnetopneumographic study of human alveolar clearance in health and disease. *Ann. Occup. Hyg.* **32**, 809–820

Gamsu, G. (1989) High resolution CT in the diagnosis of asbestos-related pleuroparenchymal disease. *Am. J. Ind. Med.* **16**, 115–117

Gamsu, G. and Klein, J.S. (1989) High resolution computed tomography of diffuse lung disease. *Clin. Radiol.* **40**, 554–556

Gedroyc, W.M.W. and Reidy, J.F. (1985) The early chest changes of pneumocystis pneumonia. *Clin. Radiol.* **36**, 331–334

Gilson, J.C. (1968) *Classification of Chest Radiographs and its Application to the Epidemiology of Pneumoconiosis.* Report on a Symposium at Katowice, 1967. WHO, Copenhagen

Gluck, M.C., Twigg, H.L., Ball, M.F. and Rhodes, P.G. (1972) Shadows bordering the lung on radiographs of normal and obese persons. *Thorax* **27**, 232–238

Gossinger, H.D., Siostrzonek, P., Zangeneh, M., Neuhold, A., Herold, C., Schmoliner, R., Laczkovics, A., Tscholokoff, D. and Mosslacher, H. (1988) Magnetic resonance imaging findings in a patient with pericardial mesothelioma. *Am. Heart J.* **115**, 1321–1322

Hall, F.M. (1987) Ultrasonography and thoracocentesis (letter). *Am. Rev. Respir. Dis.* **135**, 983

Halvorsen, R.A. and Thompson, W.M. (1986) Ascites or pleural effusion? CT and ultrasound differentiation. *CRC Crit. Rev. Diagn. Imag.* **26**, 201–239

Hayes, A., Cohen, A.T., van der Schaaf, A., Lovegrove, F.T., Thompson, G., Guelfi, G. and Musk, A. (1988) Computer quantitation of gallium-67 uptake in crocidolite-exposed asbestosis workers. *Aust. NZ J. Med.* **18**, 488

Henneghien, Ch., Remacle, P. and Bruart, J. (1986) Interet et limites de l'echographie en pneumologie. *Revue Pneumol. Clin.* **42**, 1–7

Herman, P.G., Drummey, J., Swensson, R.J., Hessel, S.J. and Balikian, J.P. (1982) 350 kV chest radiography has no diagnostic advantage: a comparison with 140 kV technique. *AJR Am. J. Roentgenol.* **138**, 485–489

Heron, C.W., Hine, A.L., Pozniak, A.L., Swinburn, C.R. and Johnson, N.McI. (1985) Radiographic features in patients with pulmonary manifestations of the acquired immune deficiency syndrome. *Clin. Radiol.* **36**, 583–588

Hoffer, P. (1980) Gallium: Mechanism. *J. Nucl. Med.* **21**, 282–285

Husband, J.E. and Fry, I.K. (1981) In *Computed Tomography of the Body.* Chapter 5, Macmillan, London, pp. 40–54

Inada, T., Tada, S., Takahashi, K., Hiraki, S., Nakata, Y., Ohnoshi, T., Kimura, I. and Shimizu, N. (1988) A case of localised pleural mesothelioma examined by magnetic resonance imaging. *Nippon Kyobu Shikkan Gakkai Zasshi* **26**, 893–897

International Labour Office (League of Nations) (1930) *Silicosis.* Records of the International Conference held at Johannesburg 13–27 August 1930. Studies and Reports, Series F (Industrial Hygiene), no. 13. ILO, Geneva, pp. 86–93

International Labour Office (1959) Meetings of Experts on the International Classification of Radiographs of the Pneumoconioses. *Occup. Saf. Health* **9**, No. 2

International Labour Office (1970) *International Classification of Radiographs of Pneumoconioses (1968), Occup. Saf. Health* Series No. 22. ILO, Geneva

International Labour Office (1980) *Guidelines for the Use of ILO International Classification of Radiographs of Pneumoconioses. Occup. Saf. Health* Series No. 22 (Rev. 80). ILO, Geneva

Jacobson, G., Bohlig, H. and Kiviluoto, R. (1970) Essentials of chest radiography. *Radiology* **95**, 445–450

Jagoe, J.R. and Paton, K.A. (1975) Reading chest radiographs for pneumoconiosis by computer. *Br. J. Ind. Med.* **32**, 267–272

Jay, S.J. (1985) Diagnostic procedures for pleural disease. *Clins Chest Med.* **6**, 33–48

Johns, H.E. and Cunningham, J.R. (1969) *The Physics of Radiology*, 3rd edn. Thomas, Springfield, pp. 210–211

Kalliomäki, K., Kalliomäki, P-L. and Moilanen, M. (1988) Magnetopneumography and its application to occupational hygiene. *Ann. Occup. Hyg.* **32**, 821–825

Kalliomäki, P-L., Karp, P.J., Katila, T., Mäkipää, P. and Tos-Savainen, A. (1976) Magnetic measurements of pulmonary contamination. *Scand. J. Work Environ. Health* **4**, 232–239

Kalliomäki, P-L., Korhonen, O., Vaaranen, V., Kalliomäki, K. and Kuponen, M. (1978a) Lung retention and clearance of shipyard arc welders. *Intern. Archs Occup. Environ. Health* **42**, 83–90

Kalliomäki, P-L., Alanko, K., Korhonen, O., Mattson, T., Vaaranen, V. and Koponen, M. (1978b) Amount and distribution of welding fume lung contaminants among arc welders. *Scand. J. Work Environ. Health* **4**, 122–130

Kalliomäki, P-L., Kalliomäki, K., Korhonen, O., Koponen, M., Sortti, V. and Vaaranen, V. (1979) Lung contamination among foundry workers. *Intern. Archs Occup. Environ. Health* **43**, 85–91

Kanzaki, N., Yamamoto, H., Kimoto, S., Inoue, N., Sugita, K., Hiraki, Y. and Aono, K. (1988) A case of malignant localised mesothelioma of the pleura. *Rinsho Hoshasen* **33**, 421–424

Katz, D. and Kreel, L. (1979) Computed tomography in pulmonary asbestosis. *Clin. Radiol.* **30**, 207–213

Kean, D. and Smith, M. (1986) Fundamentals of the NMR experiment. In *Magnetic Resonance Imaging – Principles and Application.* Heinemann Medical, London, pp. 6–20

Kerley, P. (1933) Radiology in heart disease. *Br. Med. J.* **2**, 594–597

Kerley, P. (1950) In *A Textbook of X-ray Diagnosis*, Vol. 2 (eds S.C. Shanks and P. Kerley). Lewis, London, pp. 404–405

Kilburn, K.H. (1988) Does the 1980 ILO Classification of pneumoconiosis need a facelift? *Archs Environ. Health* **43**, 261–262

Kilburn, K.H., Lilis, R., Anderson, H.A., Miller, A. and Warshaw, R.H. (1986) Interaction of asbestos, age and cigarette smoking in producing radiographic evidence of diffuse pulmonary fibrosis. *Am. J. Med.* **80**, 377–381

Kramer, E.L., Stanger, J.J., Garaay, S.M., Greene, J.B., Tiu, S., Banner, H. and McCauley, D.I. (1987) Gallium-67 scans of the chest in patients with acquired immunodeficiency syndrome. *J. Nucl. Med.* **28**, 1107–1114

Kreel, L. (1976) The EMI whole body scanner: an interim clinical evaluation of the prototype. *Br. J. Clin. Equip.* **1**, 220–227

Lane, E.J., Proto, A.V. and Philips, T.W. (1976) Mach bands and density perception. *Radiology* **121**, 9–17

Langlois, S. Le P., Glancy, J.J. and Henderson, D.W. (1978) The radiology of malignant pleural mesothelioma in Western Australia. *Austr. Radiol.* **22**, 305–314

Larson, S.M. (1978) Mechanisms of localization of Ga67 in tumors. *Semin. Nucl. Med.* **8**(3), 193–203

Law, M.R., Gregor, A., Husband, J.E. and Kerr, I.H. (1982) Computed tomography in the assessment of malignant mesothelioma of the pleura. *Clin. Radiol.* **33**, 67–70

Ledley, R.S., Huang, H.K. and Rotolo, L.S. (1975) A texture analysis method in classification of coal workers' pneumoconiosis. *Comp. Biol. Med.* **5**, 53–67

Liddell, F.D.K. (1961) The effect of film quality on reading radiographs of simple pneumoconiosis in a trial of X-ray sets. *Br. J. Ind. Med.* **18**, 165–174

Liddell, F.D.K. (1963) An experiment in film reading. *Br. J. Ind. Med.* **20**, 300-312

Liddell, F.D.K. (1972) Validation of classifications of pneumoconiosis. *Ann. NY Acad. Sci.* **200**, 527–551

Liddell, F.D.K. (1974) Assessment of radiological progression of simple pneumoconioses in individual miners. *Br. J. Ind. Med.* **31**, 185–195

Liddell, F.D.K. and May, J.D. (1966) *Assessing the Radiological Progression of Simple Pneumoconiosis.* Medical Research Memorandum 4. National Coal Board Medical Service

Liddell, F.D.K. and Morgan, W.K.C. (1978) Methods of assessing serial films of the pneumoconioses: a review. *J. Soc. Occup. Med.* **28**, 6–15

Line, B.R., Fulmer, J.D., Reynolds, H.Y., Roberts, W.C., Jones, A.E., Harris, E.K. and Crystal, R.G. (1978) Gallium-67 scanning in the staging of idiopathic pulmonary fibrosis: correlation with physiologic and morphologic features and bronchoalveolar lavage. *Am. Rev. Respir. Dis.* **118**, 355–365

Line, B.R., Hunninghake, G.W., Keogh, B.A., Jones, A.E., Johnston, G.S. and Crystal, R.G. (1981) Gallium-67 scanning to stage the alveolitis of sarcoidosis: correlation with clinical studies, pulmonary function studies and bronchoalveolar lavage. *Am. Rev. Respir. Dis.* **123**, 440–448

Livingstone, J.L., Lewis, J.G., Reid, L. and Jefferson, E.E. (1964) Diffuse interstitial pulmonary fibrosis. *Q. J. Med.* **23**, 71–103

Lynch, D.A., Gamsu, G., Ray, C.S. and Aberle, D.R. (1988) Asbestos-related focal lung masses: manifestations on conventional and high resolution CT scans. *Radiology* **169**, 603–607

McCallum, R.I. and Day, M.J. (1965) *In vivo* method of detecting antimony deposits in the lung by differential absorption of X-radiation. *Lancet* **ii**, 882–883

McCallum, R.I., Day, M.J., Underhill, J. and Aird, E.G.A. (1971) Measurement of antimony oxide dust in human lungs *in vivo* by X-ray spectrophotometry. In *Inhaled Particles 3* (ed. W.H. Walton), Unwin, Woking, pp. 611–618

McDonald, J.C., Sébastien, P. and Armstrong, B. (1986) Radiologic survey of past and present vermiculite miners exposed to tremolite. *Br. J. Ind. Med.* **47**, 445–449

MacKenzie, F.A.F. and Harries, P.G. (1970) Changing attitude to the diagnosis of asbestos disease. *J. R. Nav. Med. Serv.* **56**, 116–123

McLean, R.G., Steele, P. and Murray, I.P.C. (1985) Quantitation of pulmonary gallium-67 uptake: comparison of computer-derived indices. *Nucl. Med. Commun.* **6**, 425–433

Meredith, W.J. and Massey, J.B. (1977) *Fundamental Physics of Radiography*, 3rd edn. Chapters 6–7 and Chapters 18–21. John Wright, Bristol, pp. 57–79, pp. 211–276

Ministry of Health (1952) *Standardization of Terminology of Pulmonary Disease and Standardization of Technique of Chest Radiography.* HMSO, London

Mueller, P.R., Saini, A., Simeone, J.F., Silverman, S.G., Morris, E., Hahn, P.F., Forman, B.H., McLoud, T.C., Shepard, J.O. and Ferrucci, J.T. (1988) Image-guided pleural biopsies: indications, technique and results in 23 patients. *Radiology* **169**, 1–4

Musch, D.C., Higgins, I.T.T. and Landis, J.R. (1985) Some factors influencing interobserver variation in classifying simple pneumoconiosis. *Br. J. Ind. Med.* **42**, 346–349

Musch, D.C., Landis, J.R., Higgins, I.T.T., Gilson, J.C. and Jones, R.N. (1984) An application of Kappa-type analyses to interobserver variation in classifying chest radiographs for pneumoconiosis. *Statist. Med.* **3**, 73–83

National Radiological Protection Board (1990) *Living with Radiation.* Her Majesty's Stationery Office, London

Neuhold, A., Fruhwald, F. and Seidl, G. (1985) Ultraschallgestutzte Punktion wandstandiger intrathorakaler Prozesse. *Ultraschall* **6**, 34–38

O'Moore, P.V., Muelleer, P.R., Simeone, J.F., Saini, S., Butch, R.J., Hahn, P.F., Steiner, E., Stark, D.D. and Ferruci, J.T. (1987) *AJR Am. J. Roentgenol.* **149**, 1–5

Ogilvie, C.M. (1970) Emphysema and coal worker's pneumoconiosis. *Br. Med. J.* **3**, 769

Otto, H. and Maron, R. (1959) Zur Histologie der Eisenablagerungen bei Porzellinersilikosen. *Arch. Gewerbepath. Gewerbehyg.* **17**, 117–126

Pearson, N.G., Ashford, J.R., Morgan, D.C., Pasqual, R.S.H. and Rae, S. (1965) Effect of quality of chest radiographs on the categorization of coal workers' pneumoconiosis. *Br. J. Ind. Med.* **22**, 81–92

Prosser, I.M. and Thurley, P. (1976) Septal lines in a case of asthma with eosinophilia. *Br. J. Radiol.* **49**, 176–177

Pugatch, R.D. and Spirn, P.W. (1985) Radiology of the pleura. *Clins Chest Med.* **6**, 17–32

Putman, C.E., Godwin, J.D., Silverman, P.M. and Foster, W.L. (1984) CT of localized lucent lung lesions. *Semin. Roentgenol.* **19**, 173–188

Raithel, H.J. and Valentin, H. (1983) Computertomographische untersuchungen bei patienten mit Asbestose und Silicose. [Computer-tomographic examination of patients with asbestosis and silicosis.] *Prax. Klin. Pneumol.* **37**, 1119–1129

Rankin, J.A. and Pella, J.A. (1987) Radiographic resolution of pneumocystis carinii pneumonia in response to corticosteroid therapy. *Am. Rev. Respir. Dis.* **136**, 182–183

Rappaport, I. (1936) The phenomena of shadow attenuation and summation in roentgenography of the lungs. *AJR Am. J. Roentgenol.* **35**, 772–776

Rappaport, I. (1967) Overinflation of the lungs of coal miners. *Br. Med. J.* **3**, 493–494

Reger, R.B., Petersen, M.R. and Morgan, W.K.C. (1974) Variation in the interpretation of radiographic change in pulmonary disease. *Lancet* **i**, 111–113

Reger, R.B., Smith, C.A., Kibelstis, J.A. and Morgan, W.K.C. (1972) The effect of film quality and other factors on roentgenographic categorization of coal workers' pneumoconioses. *AJR Am. J. Roentgenol.* **115**, 462–472

Reger, R.B., Ames, R.G., Merchant, J.A., Polakoff, P.P., Sargent, E.N., Silhiger, M. and Whittlesey, P. (1982) The detection of thoracic abnormalities using postero-anterior (PA) vs PA and oblique roentgenograms. *Chest* **81**, 290–295

Reger, R.B., Cole, W.S., Sargent, E.N. and Wheeler, P.S. (1990) Cases of alleged asbestos-related disease: a radiological evaluation. *J. Occup. Med.* **32**, 1088–1090

Rivers, D., Wise, M.E., King, E.J. and Nagelschmidt, G. (1960) Dust content, radiology, and pathology in simple pneumoconiosis of coal workers. *Br. J. Med.* **17**, 87–108

Rossiter, C.E. (1972) Relation between content and composition of coal worker's lungs and radiological appearances. *Br. J. Ind. Med.* **29**, 31–44

Rossiter, C.E., Rivers, D., Bergman, I., Casswell, C. and Nagelschmidt, G. (1967) Dust content, radiology and pathology in simple pneumoconiosis of coal workers (Further Report). In *Inhaled Particles and Vapours*, 2 (ed. C.N. Davies), Pergamon, London, pp. 419–434

Sagel, S.S. (1982) In *Computed Body Tomography* (eds K.J. Lee, S.S. Sagel and K.J.T. Stanley), Raven, New York, pp. 99–129

Sagel, S.S. and Aronberg, D.J. (1982) In *Computed Body Tomography* (eds K.J. Lee, S.S. Sagel and K.J.T. Stanley), Chapter 4, Raven Press, New York, pp. 55–98

Salonen, O., Kivisaari, C.-G., Standerskjold-Anordenstam, K., Somer, K., Mattson, K. and Tammilehto, L. (1986) Computed tomography of pleural lesions with special reference to the mediastinal pleura. *Acta Radiolog. Diagnosis* **27**, 527–531

Salyed, H.N., Parikh, D.J., Ghodasara, N.B., Sharma, Y.K., Patel, G.C., Chatterjee, S.K. and Chatterjee, B.B. (1985) Silicosis in slate pencil workers. 1. An environmental and medical study. *Am. J. Ind. Med.* **8**, 127–133

Sargent, E.M., Boswell, W.D., Ralls, P.W. and Markovitz, A. (1984) Subpleural fat pads in patients exposed to asbestosis: distinction from non-calcified pleural plaques. *Radiology* **152**, 273–277

Schröder, H., Magdeburg, W., Tewes, E. and Rockelsburg, I. (1969) Perfusion scintigraphy of the lungs in patients with silicosis or silicotuberculosis. *Germ. Med. Mth.* **16**, 551–552 [English translation of *Dt. Med. Wschr* (1969) **94**, 1064]

Scadding, J.G. and Mitchell, D.N. (1985) *Sarcoidosis*, 2nd edn, London, Chapman and Hall, pp. 151–159

Seaton, A., Lapp, N.L. and Chang, C.H.J. (1971) Lung perfusion scanning in coalworkers pneumoconiosis. *Am. Rev. Respir. Dis.* **103**, 338–349

Secker-Walker, R.H. (1983) In *Clinical Nuclear Medicine* (eds M.N. Maisey, K.E. Britton and D.L. Gilday), Chapman and Hall, London, pp. 64–65

Secker-Walker, R. and Ho, J.E. (1979) Regional lung function in asbestos workers. *J. Nucl. Med.* **20**, 621

Selman, J. (1963) *Fundamentals of X-ray and Radium Physics*, 3rd edn, Thomas, Springfield, Illinois, pp. 156–161

Shirley, I., Blackwell, R.J., Cusick, G., Farman, D.J. and Vicary, F.R. (1978) *A User's Guide to Diagnostic Ultrasound*, Pitman Medical, London, pp. 16–31

Siemsen, J.K., Sargent, E.N., Griebe, S.F., Windsor, D.W., Wentz, D. and Jacobson, G. (1974) Pulmonary concentration of Ga67 in pneumoconiosis. *Am. J. Roentgenol. Radium Ther. Nucl. Med.* **120**, 815–820

Siemsen, J.K., Grebe, S.F. and Waxman, A.D. (1978) The use of gallium-67 in pulmonary disorders. *Semin. Nucl. Med.* **8**(3), 235–249

Simon, G. (1964) Radiology and emphysema. *Clin. Radiol.* **15**, 293–306

Simon, G. (1973) *Principles of Chest X-ray Diagnosis*, 3rd edn. Butterworths, London

Simon, G. (1978) In *Principles of Chest X-ray Diagnosis*, 4th edn, Anatomical landmarks and variations, Chapter 2. Butterworths, London, p. 8

Sluis-Cremer, G.K., Thomas, R.G. and Schmaman, I.B. (1984) The value of computerized axial tomography in the assessment of workers exposed to asbestos. *Am. J. Ind. Med.* **6**, 27–35

Spiers, F.W. (1946) Effective atomic number and energy absorption in tissues. *Br. J. Radiol.* **19**, 52–63

Squire, L.F. (1982) *Fundamentals of Radiology*, 3rd edn, Harvard University Press, Cambridge MA and London, p. 182

Staab, E.V. and McCartney, W.H. (1978) Role of gallium-67 in inflammatory disease. *Semin. Nucl. Med.* **8**(3), 219–234

Stavas, J., van Sonnenberg, E., Casola, G. and Wittich, G.R. (1987) Percutaneous drainage of infected and noninfected thoracic fluid collections. *J. Thorac. Imag.* **2**, 80–87

Strankinga, W.F.M., Sperber, M., Kainser, M.C. and Stam, J. (1987) Accuracy of diagnostic procedures in the initial evaluation and follow-up of mesothelioma patients. *Respiration* **51**, 179–187

Supplies Technology Division, NHS Procurement Directorate (1989) Comparison of the Imaging Performance of CT Scanners, Issue 6: STD/88/36 (March 1989). Department of Health, 14 Russell Square, London WC1B 5EP

Sutton, D. (1987) *Textbook of Radiology and Imaging*, 4th edn, Churchill Livingstone, London and Edinburgh, p. 328

Thomas, R.G. (1989) In *Radiology of Occupational Chest Disease* (eds A. Solomon and L. Kreel), Springer-Verlag, New York, Berlin, Heidelberg, pp. 1–3

Thomas, R.G. and Sluis-Cremer, G.K. (1977) 200 kV xeroradiography in occupational exposure to silica and asbestos. *Br. J. Ind. Med.* **34**, 281–290

Trapnell, D.H. (1963) The peripheral lymphatics of the lung. *Br. J. Radiol.* **36**, 660–672

Trapnell, D.H. (1964a) Septal lines in pneumoconiosis. *Br. J. Radiol.* **37**, 805–810

Trapnell, D.H. (1964b) Septal lines in sarcoidosis. *Br. J. Radiol.* **37**, 811–813

Trapnell, D.H. (1967) The chest. In *Principles of X-ray Diagnosis*, Chapter 3, Butterworths, London

Triebel, H.-J., Jessel, A. and Spielmann, R.P. (1988) Lungensiderose eines Lichtbogenschweissers. [Pulmonary siderosis (pneumoconiosis) in an arc welder] *Roentgen-Bl.* **41**, 72–74

Vanderstappen, M., Mornex, J.F., Lahneche, B., Chauvot, P., Bouvier, J.F., Wiesendanger, T., Pages, J., Webert, P., Cordier, J.F. and Brune, J. (1988) Gallium-67 scanning in the staging of cryptogenic fibrosing alveolitis. *Eur. Respir. J.* **1**, 517–522

Vix, V.A. (1974) Extrapleural costal fat. *Radiology* **112**, 563–565

Webb, W.R., Stein, M.G., Finkbeiner, W.E., Im, J.-G., Lynch, D. and Gamsu, G. (1988) Normal and diseased isolated lungs: high-resolution CT. *Radiology* **166**, 81–87

Weibel, E.R. and Gil, J. (1977) Structure-function relationships at the alveolar level. In *Lung Biology in Health and Disease* (ed. C. Lenfant), vol. 3: *Bioengineering Aspects of the Lung* (ed. J.B. West), Chapter 1, Section II, Marcel Dekker, New York, pp. 44–47

Weiss, W. (1984) Cigarette smoke, asbestos and small irregular opacities. *Am. Rev. Respir. Dis.* **130**, 293–301

Weiss, W. (1988) Smoking and pulmonary fibrosis. *J. Occup. Med.* **30**, 33–39

Yang, P.-C., Sheu, J.-C., Luh, K.-T., Kuo, S.-H. and Yang, S.-P. (1984) Clinical application of real-time ultrasonography in pleural and subpleural lesions. *J. Formosan Med. Assoc.* **83**, 646–657

8

Epidemiology

Katherine M. Venables

The growth in epidemiological research over the last 30 years has increased our knowledge about occupational lung disease and led to refinements in and standardization of study design and methods of analysis. This chapter describes why and how epidemiological research is done and what questions it can answer. The topics it includes are also relevant to the investigation of epidemics of respiratory disease and to screening programmes to monitor the health of a workforce. Specific occupational lung diseases and the application of particular tests are covered in other chapters. There is a range of textbooks on general epidemiological methodology, and some other reviews with an emphasis on occupational lung disease are by McDonald (1981), Seaton, Seaton and Leitch (1989), and Checkoway, Pearce and Crawford-Brown (1989).

Questions

An understanding of occupational epidemiology depends on knowing what questions it asks and why it asks them. The most important questions are about the relationship between an occupational exposure and disease. Some of these are the following:

1. Does exposure increase the risk of disease?
2. What is the quantitative relationship between exposure and disease?
3. What factors modify the relationship between exposure and disease?
4. Is control of exposure effective in reducing the risk of disease?
5. Is the risk of disease increased at low exposure?

A common question asks simply if exposure increases the risk of disease. More complex questions

ask about the shape and slope of the quantitative relationship between exposure and disease and whether it is influenced by other occupational exposures, age, sex, smoking or other personal factors. The evaluation of the effectiveness of measures to control workplace exposure and the assessment of risk at low exposures, including those experienced by the general population, are special cases of the study of the relationship between exposure and disease.

There are two reasons for posing these questions. The *first* is that answers are clearly essential so that occupational lung disease can be prevented. Quantification of exposure–response relationships is particularly important in providing a rational basis for statutory control limits on exposure in the workplace. The study of low exposures, either directly or by extrapolation from higher exposures, is important for public health in general. McMichael (1989) has discussed the general issues raised by the assessment of risk at low exposure. A topical example is the potential harm to the general public of environmental contamination by asbestos, by radiation or by industrial chemicals.

The *second* reason is that occupational epidemiology can also answer basic aetiological questions. Few lung diseases are caused only by occupational exposure. Even malignant mesothelioma is not confined to asbestos exposure and probably has a low background incidence in the general population. Lung cancer, chronic bronchitis, emphysema and asthma are common conditions with several causes, some of them encountered at work. In aetiological research, occupational exposures are important natural experiments in disease induction. The timing, intensity and duration of exposure are often known more accurately for occupational than for non-occupational causal agents such as dietary factors. It may be possible to extrapolate the general shape of a relationship from an occupational to a non-occupational exposure thought to act by the same mechanism, and vice versa. An interaction between causal factors may suggest that both operate within the same chain of causal events, for example, the effects of asbestos exposure and smoking on the risk of lung cancer.

Epidemiology both tests and generates hypotheses about the causes of lung disease. A hypothesis to test may come from a clinical observation of a cluster of cases of disease within an industry. Of 20 cases of cancer of the paranasal sinuses in High Wycombe, 15 of the patients had worked making wooden chairs; the investigation of this well-known cluster and subsequent studies were reviewed by Acheson (1976). Epidemiology may itself detect disease clusters. Investigations which confirmed the hypothesis of an increased risk of nasal cancer in wood furniture 'workers also found an unexpected excess of nasal cancer among leather workers (Acheson, 1976). Such clusters, whether detected by clinicians or by epidemiologists, may be chance findings; further studies, preferably in a different geographical or time setting, are always necessary to confirm that an increased risk exists and to extend the enquiry to other questions, such as quantification of an exposure–response relationship.

Toxicity testing in animals may also generate hypotheses. Several studies have addressed the carcinogenic potential of formaldehyde to the respiratory tract because it was found to cause nasal tumours in rodents, and the epidemiological evidence suggests that any risk to workers at the usual workplace concentrations, if present, is small (Partanen et al., 1985). Conversely, experimental research on animals can test hypotheses generated by epidemiological research. A study in rats showed that tobacco smoke increased the risk of IgE antibody production against inhaled foreign antigen (Zetterstrom et al., 1985). The stimulus for this experiment was the authors' earlier observation that, in two groups of workers exposed to coffee bean or ispaghula antigen, the prevalence of IgE antibody to these materials was greater in smokers (Zetterstrom et al., 1981) (see Chapter 4, 'Effect of smoking on immune responses').

Important questions about occupational lung disease that are potentially amenable to epidemiological research sometimes cannot be answered, often because the investigator cannot gain access to records or to populations. The Nordic countries make a variety of public records available to researchers but in France and some other countries it is difficult to obtain even the cause of death. Companies differ in their willingness to co-operate with research work and often the most helpful are large organizations that have been successful in controlling occupational exposures. Answers may be imprecise or biased because personnel or exposure records are inadequate. Even apparently good and non-controversial records of employment may be incomplete when checked against external sources

(Enterline and Marsh, 1982). These logistic issues are the major practical constraint to the scope of epidemiology.

Principles of design

Epidemiological research is primarily aetiological and only rarely illuminates disease mechanisms that are more readily investigated by toxicology. In the framework of aetiology, the questions that epidemiology asks are similar to those that are addressed by toxicology but the context of people and their work makes epidemiological findings directly relevant to medicine and industry, whereas the results of a toxicological experiment on animals can only be viewed as supplementary to evidence from man. It is rarely practicable or ethical to apply to human subjects the experimental designs possible in toxicological research. Movement into or out of jobs is not governed by random selection and is outside the control of the investigator. Information on occupational exposure and disease may not be collected 'double-blind' unless it is obtained by the investigator in a special study. The art of epidemiology is in designing a study to prevent or minimize the selection and information bias inherent in normal industrial and medical practice.

Occupational exposure and disease are related in time, and good study design takes account of the temporal dimension. Disease occurs after exposure with a latent interval that varies according to the disease. It may be very short, as in acute lung damage following a gassing accident. Longer intervals are more usual. Figure 8.1 shows results from a

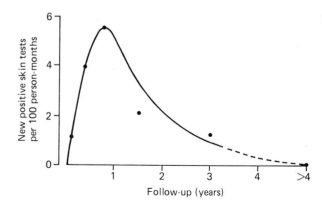

Figure 8.1 Incidence rate of a positive skin test to platinum salts during follow-up of 84 platinum refinery workers from starting work in 1973 or 1974. The study also noted respiratory symptoms that showed a similar pattern. (After Venables et al., 1989, with permission)

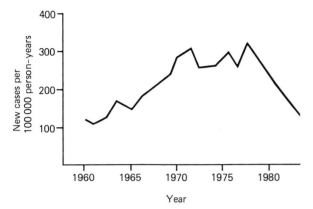

Figure 8.2 Incidence rate, adjusted for age, from 1960 to 1984 of lung cancer in Swedish copper smelter workers. The study also noted a similar pattern for lung cancer mortality. (After Sandstrom, Wall and Taube, 1989, with permission)

study of platinum refinery workers entering the industry in 1973 and 1974 (Venables et al., 1989). The follow-up information that was available included routine records of the results of periodic skin-prick tests with platinum salts during employment. The incidence rate of a positive skin-prick test had a marked peak in the first year of follow-up, reflecting the short latent interval for allergic sensitization. Figure 8.2 shows the age-adjusted incidence rate of lung cancer over time in a cohort of copper smelter workers (Sandstrom, Wall and Taube, 1989), which has been the subject of several studies because the work involves exposure to arsenic and other contaminants. The cohort started work from 1928 onwards, so the peak incidence in the 1970s is clearly some decades after first exposure and reflects the long latent interval for lung cancer.

Studies may be set in a *dynamic population* or in a *cohort*. An administrative grouping, such as the people on a factory's payroll on one day, is a *dynamic population*: there is a constant turnover in the population, so it remains fairly stable in size, age and other characteristics over time. A study of exposure subgroups in a dynamic population cross-section can provide information on the relationship between exposure and disease. Such studies are particularly valuable if repeated so that changes in disease prevalence can be compared to changes in exposure. A difference between exposure subgroups or over time may also be related to a change in turnover. A fall in prevalence of chest radiographic abnormalities in active underground miners might be caused by a reduction in dust exposure but also by removing miners from underground work at the first sign of radiographic changes, with the result that they are not included in subsequent radiographic surveys.

A grouping formed for experimental reasons, such as the patients included in a clinical trial of a

new drug (or the animals studied in a toxicity test), is a *cohort* – that is, a fairly homogeneous group of identified individuals who share a common exposure. A cohort has no turnover but ages with time and becomes smaller as individuals die. Studies of defined cohorts are valuable in examining temporal relationships because exposure and disease information for individuals are linked. There are few administrative reasons for forming occupational cohorts and they are usually constructed by an investigator from records made for other purposes, not necessarily employer records. The practical difficulties in forming a cohort and in following it have led to many ingenious solutions. Union membership (for example, Miller et al., 1989) and local government files (for example, Seniori Costantini, Paci and Miligi, 1989) have been used. McDonald et al. (1978) formed a cohort of miners at the Homestake goldmine in South Dakota from the records of a club which miners joined on achieving 21 years' service. Death from pneumoconiosis (mainly silicosis) and respiratory tuberculosis (including silicotuberculosis) showed a relationship with dust exposure. A common solution is to form a cohort from a previous study of a dynamic population cross-section. This can be done on a national scale by making use of census data (for example, Fraser et al., 1989). A cross-sectional base is not ideal for diseases causing disability that affects continued employment and this is discussed in more detail below in the section on cross-sectional studies.

Epidemiology employs three basic designs: (1) longitudinal observation of a group over time; (2) observation of a population cross-section at one point in time; and (3) comparison of a case series with referents (controls). These approaches are conceptually similar, as the following examples illustrate, but one or other may be more practicable for a particular study.

Longitudinal studies

Longitudinal follow-up of a dynamic population was discussed above and the phrase 'longitudinal study' usually refers to a follow-up of a cohort. It is the only way that changes in lung function or radiographic appearances in individuals can be studied directly. Follow-up can start in the past if adequate historical information is available. A historical cohort study is conceptually identical to one that starts in the present, and both types are prospective in that they follow individuals forward in time.

The simplest variant of the design measures change over a single work shift. A recent example measured forced expiratory volume in 1 second (FEV_1) before and after a shift spent tunnelling, and

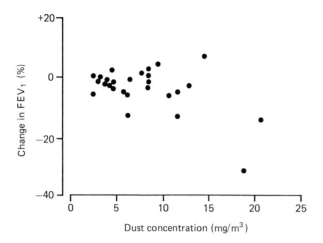

Figure 8.3 Change in FEV₁ across a work shift (percentage of preshift FEV₁) in relation to personal exposure to cement dust in tunnelling. (After Kessel et al., 1989, with permission)

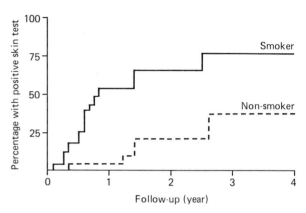

Figure 8.4 Risk of developing a positive skin test to platinum salts by smoking habit at first employment in a platinum refinery. Respiratory symptoms were also related to smoking. (After Venables et al., 1989, with permission)

expressed the difference as a percentage of the preshift value (Kessel et al., 1989). The decrement in FEV₁ increased with increasing cement dust concentration measured by personal sampling (Figure 8.3). The basic design can be extended to follow change in lung function over several years, although logistically this is a far more difficult exercise. Diem et al. (1982) followed almost 300 men from first employment in a new toluene diisocyanate manufacturing plant and measured average annual change in FEV₁ from up to nine tests during follow-up. Exposure to toluene diisocyanate was assessed from the results of over 2000 personal samples. Table 8.1 shows that age-adjusted fall in FEV₁ was related to cumulative exposure to toluene diisocyanate and this was consistent across smoking categories and by level of height-adjusted FEV₁. The differences by exposure were particularly marked in non-smokers.

A longitudinal study measures the *incidence rate* of new cases over time, when the term 'case' is appropriate to the condition under study. Because it

is usual to find that length of follow-up varies, the rate is expressed as *number of new cases divided by 'person-time' of follow-up*. A hundred 'person-years' could represent 100 people followed for 1 year or ten followed for 10 years, so the number of people studied and their average length of follow-up are important pieces of additional information. The incidence rate varies over the period of follow-up, reflecting the latent interval of the disease under study (see Figures 8.1 and 8.2).

The effect of smoking was of interest in a study of platinum refiners (Venables et al., 1989), and an internal comparison was made between those who smoked and those who did not. The risk of developing a positive skin test to platinum salts was increased by four- to fivefold in smokers (Figure 8.4). The study of copper smelters by Sandstrom, Wall and Taube (1989) examined the effect of occupational exposure by both external and internal comparisons. The external comparison was by comparing the observed number of lung cancer cases with the number that would have been

Table 8.1 Average annual change in FEV₁ by smoking and cumulative exposure to toluene diisocyanate, controlling for age, height and FEV₁ level

Cigarette smoking	Average annual change in FEV₁ (ml/year) for FEV₁/height³ of			
	≥550 ml/m³ for exposure of		<550 ml/m³ for exposure of	
	≤68.2 p.p.b. × months	>68.2 p.p.b. × months	≤68.2 p.p.b. × months	>68.2 p.p.b. × months
Never	1	−37	−18	−57
Previous	−12	−15	−32	−35
Current	−26	−37	−46	−57

The annual change in FEV₁ was adjusted to the age 35.6 years – the mean for the study group.
p.p.b. × months = parts per billion × months = exposure units.
After Diem et al. (1982) with permission.

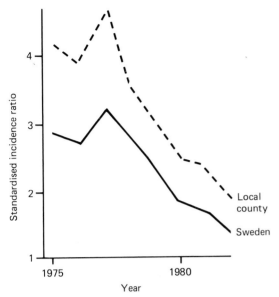

Figure 8.5 Standardized ratio of lung cancer incidence in Swedish copper smelter workers over time with reference to the whole of Sweden and to the local county. A ratio of 1 indicates the same incidence as the comparison population. (After Sandstrom, Wall and Taube, 1989, with permission)

tion that an occupational cohort showed lower mortality than the general population, particularly at the start of follow-up, has been repeatedly confirmed by others and is often termed the 'healthy worker effect'.

Some diseases show wide geographical variation in incidence, and a comparison with local mortality rates may be made to obtain a more comparable reference group than the national population. The earliest example of a local comparison was reported by Doll (1952) in a study of pensioners of a London gas company whose standardized mortality ratio (SMR) for lung cancer fell from 2.40 to 1.81 when a correction was made for London's high mortality from lung cancer. However, using the local lung cancer rates in the study by Sandstrom, Wall and Taube (1989) increased the incidence ratio from lung cancer (see Figure 8.5). A control cohort of other employed persons with similar demographic characteristics to the exposed cohort would be the most appropriate comparison group but this increases logistic difficulties, and by chance or unsuspected bias the control cohort may not be representative of local employed persons as a whole; in particular, it may also be exposed to an agent that causes the disease under study.

expected had the cohort experienced the same incidence as the Swedish population. Figure 8.5 shows that the lung cancer rate in the cohort over time was consistently greater than the overall Swedish rate, as the standardized incidence ratio was always greater than 1. It was even greater using the rates for the rural county in which the smelter was located. Internal comparisons were made using job titles and showed that the lung cancer rate was particularly high in relation to jobs entailing exposure to arsenic, confirming an earlier study (Axelson et al., 1978).

This method of making external comparisons with the general population has become a standard tool in mortality studies. Its advantages and disadvantages have been reviewed extensively by Gardner (1986). It is convenient because national mortality rates are available and based on such a large population that they are very stable. The major disadvantage of using national mortality rates is that people in employment are generally fitter than the general population as a whole. Most employers use health criteria in making appointments and these may be quite stringent for physically demanding occupations such as the fire service. Continuing in employment confers financial and perhaps other material advantages. People who become ill are more likely to leave a job than their healthy peers. Comparing employed persons with the nation as a whole can thus underestimate the effects of occupational exposure. Fox and Collier's (1976) observa-

Cross-sectional studies

A study of a population cross-section measures disease *prevalence*, usually at one point in time (*number of cases at that time as a proportion of all those exposed*). The population may be dynamic or a cohort. The design is often used for studying conditions with a gradual onset in which it is difficult to determine when a non-case becomes a case, such as the symptoms associated with chronic bronchitis or the radiographic changes associated with pneumoconiosis. It is difficult to study the temporal relationship of exposure with a disease of gradual onset, and the cross-sectional design compounds this difficulty by recording both disease and exposure at the same time. Prevalence is dependent on the duration of disease as well as its incidence, so persistent conditions are the most amenable to study by means of prevalence. In contrast, lethal forms of cancer or illnesses in which recovery occurs, such as acute respiratory infections, are not readily detectable by measuring prevalence.

The *cross-sectional design* is common in occupational epidemiology because it is convenient. Descriptive studies are often cross-sectional as are studies of outbreaks such as an outbreak of asthma due to toluene diisocyanate, in a steel coating plant (Venables et al., 1985). They are usually set in dynamic populations of currently employed

Table 8.2 Prevalence of respiratory symptoms and of a positive skin test by degree of animal contact in current job and by quartiles of duration of employment

	Respiratory symptoms* (%)	Positive skin test* (%)
Animal contact		
Regular (animal handlers)	10	12
Intermittent (experimental work)	10	15
Indirect	19	7
Quartiles of duration of employment		
0.24–2.68 years	18	24
2.70–5.92 years	14	16
6.15–11.80 years	3	9
11.86–41.76 years	9	3

*Respiratory symptoms related to work; skin tests with animal antigens; n = 138.
After Venables et al. (1988) with permission.

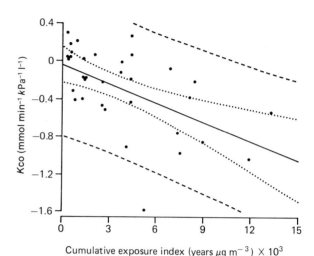

Figure 8.6 Regression line of decrement in gas transfer on cumulative exposure to cadmium with 95% confidence limits for the mean (•••) and for individual values (---) in alloy workers employed for 5 years or more. (Courtesy of Davison et al., 1988)

workers, and this is a disadvantage because such groups may contain a high proportion of 'survivors'. For example, a survey of a group of 138 laboratory workers fulfilled several functions but gave little useful information on the risk of allergy in relation to measures of animal exposure (Venables et al., 1988). The prevalence of respiratory symptoms consistent with occupational asthma and of a positive skin-prick test to one or more animal antigens showed no relationship with a qualitative assessment of the intensity of current animal exposure based on type of work and an inverse relationship to duration of employment (Table 8.2). The most likely explanation was that the risk of allergy was highest soon after first employment (as in Figure 8.1) and that cases – in particular those with the heaviest exposure to animals – left, so differential survival obscured the effect of exposure.

Survivor bias can be minimized by making a cross-sectional study of a complete cohort as in a study of emphysema that included all men who had worked as copper–cadmium alloy workers for at least 1 year from 1926, when the factory opened, to 1983 (Davison et al., 1988). Of 185 men, 103 were alive and resident in the UK; 101 were examined, of whom only 11 were still working in the factory. These figures emphasize that any population cross-section including only currently employed workers is a small fraction of a much larger cohort. Figure 8.6 includes those men who had been employed at the company for at least 5 years. The gas transfer coefficient (*K*CO) was compared with expected values obtained from a group of unexposed men and was less than expected, the decrement increasing with increasing cumulative cadmium exposure. This analysis was carried out to estimate the *K*CO decrement that might occur after working at the current control limit of 50 µg/m³ for a working lifetime. It

was estimated to lie between –0.05 and –0.3 mmol min⁻¹ kPa⁻¹ l⁻¹, which suggested a detrimental effect of such exposure. It illustrates that results from exposures in the past can be applied to current working conditions.

The study also illustrates that there is a relationship between longitudinal and cross-sectional studies when they are set within a cohort. A longitudinal study would have followed the exposed and unexposed groups over time. The study in fact assumed that the two groups had similar lung function in the past and that exposure caused changes over time which resulted in the differences observed in 1983. This assumption is common to most cross-sectional studies and appears to be reasonable.

The departures of lung function from expectation in this study were even greater when published expected values were used. It is more common to find the reverse – that comparisons with published expected values of lung function underestimate the effect of exposure. Firemen, for example, have repeatedly been found to have better lung function than their age and height would predict, but this must be an artefact of selection for work because there is no reason to believe that exposure to smoke improves lung function. Published 'normal' values of lung function should not be used uncritically, as the subjects from whom the values were derived may not be comparable to the workers under investigation.

Case-referent studies

The case-referent study is the logical extension of a description of a case series. Very strong associations between an occupation and a disease may be inferred from a case series, but such descriptions cannot quantify its size. The inclusion of referents who are representatives of the population from which the cases were drawn gives comparative information on the employment histories that might be expected in the base population. In respiratory medicine, the design is used most commonly for lung cancers which are, in general, accurately diagnosed and whose occurrence is noted routinely on death certificates and in cancer registries. It has, on occasion, been used for other conditions: for example, Thoren, Jarvholm and Morgan (1989) reported an almost fourfold increased risk of death from asthma or chronic obstructive pulmonary disease in relation to employment in a soft paper mill.

Case-referent studies are similar to longitudinal studies in conception. This is clearest in the special case of 'nested' case-referent studies set within a cohort study. De Klerk et al. (1989) used a nested case-referent design to model cancer mortality in relation to duration and intensity of exposure to crocidolite at the Wittenoom mine and mill in Australia. This approach allowed tight control of age by matching cases to referents and increased efficiency by including only a proportion of the cohort in the analysis. The authors concluded that both intensity and duration of exposure increased the risk of lung cancer but that intensity was not a major determinant of mesothelioma in the range of exposure at Wittenoom.

Case-referent studies may be efficient in data collection. The cohort study of copper smelter workers by Sandstrom, Wall and Taube (1989), mentioned above, included occupational history information on 3710 workers. The analysis in the full cohort of mortality in relation to arsenic exposure gave similar results to an earlier study by Axelson et al. (1978) which obtained occupational data on only 29 cases of lung cancer and 74 referents. The case-referent study noted lung cancer and referent deaths from one set of parish records, and made use of the fact that the copper smelter was a major employer in the parish.

A case-referent study may be the only feasible design when it is impracticable to enumerate a cohort because an industry is made up of many small firms with poor records. An example is the furniture-making industry which Acheson (1976) described as 'a large number of small firms, most of which had fewer than 50 employees' before the Second World War. One of Acheson's solutions to this difficulty was to carry out a cancer registry-based, case-referent study to compare the occupations recorded in the registry for cases of adenocarcinoma of the nasal sinuses with those of referents with other nasal cancers.

Many case-referent studies take advantage of their small size by collecting detailed information by questionnaire from cases and referents or their relatives. This may be the only practicable way of obtaining exposure information if it is thought that the job title reported on death certificates or in registries will relate poorly to the exposure of interest. It also allows the joint examination of multiple occupational exposures and of personal factors such as smoking. Bourbonnais, Meyer and Theriault (1988) have shown fairly good agreement between occupational histories recorded by individuals and their employment records.

Exposure

Populations with contrasting exposures are needed for assessing whether an exposure causes a disease or for quantifying the relationship between exposure and disease. This will be appreciated by reflecting on what our knowledge would be today of the aetiology of lung cancer if cigarette consumption were not so varied. Occupational groups with an unusually heavy exposure are thus very valuable. Often, only past exposures provide suitable material and this is one major reason why epidemiological studies use historical data. The second is that in diseases with a long latent interval, such as cancer, historical studies allow answers within the lifetime of the investigator.

It will be clear from the examples already cited that there are several different approaches to measuring occupational exposure in epidemiology. The one taken depends on the type of data available. Occupational exposure can be expressed in different ways:

Body burden
Measured air concentration
Ordinal scale of exposure intensity
Cumulative exposure (intensity × duration)
Duration
Exposed/unexposed

The ideal would be a measure of dose at the appropriate target tissue but for many lung diseases we do not know the precise target tissue, nor is dose measurable in practice. Body burden is a potentially measurable surrogate for dose, at least for materials that persist in the body. Sebastien et al. (1989) examined lung tissue from autopsies carried out on members of two cohorts: chrysotile miners from Quebec and chrysotile textile workers from Charleston. The study was prompted by the approximately fiftyfold increased risk of lung cancer in

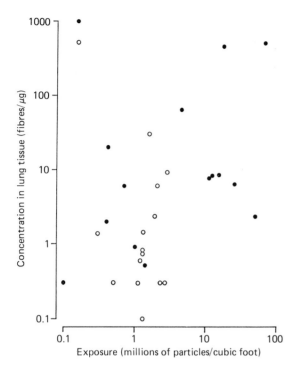

Figure 8.7 Lung fibre burden in relation to chrysotile exposure in chrysotile miners (●) and textile workers (○). (After Sebastien et al., 1989, with permission)

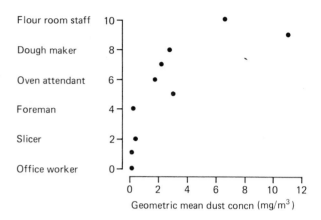

Figure 8.8 An ordinal ranking of job titles by exposure to flour dust in a bakery in relation to measured dust exposure. (After Musk et al., 1989, with permission)

textile workers compared to miners and millers with the same cumulative exposure. The chrysotile and tremolite fibre concentrations in lung tissue from miners were consistently greater than in textile workers and in accord with their greater cumulative exposure (Figure 8.7), suggesting that inaccuracy in exposure measurements in one or both cohorts did not account for their differences in lung cancer mortality and that some other explanation must be sought (see Chapter 14).

In the study of emphysema already mentioned (Davison et al., 1988), comparisons of lung function and other variables were made with liver cadmium concentration measured by neutron activation analysis, and the results confirmed those obtained using cumulative exposure to cadmium, which was closely correlated with liver cadmium (Mason et al., 1988).

It is currently possible to measure body burden for only a fraction of the occupational agents that cause lung disease, and the applicability of the measurements is limited by our uncertain understanding of mechanisms and rates of tissue absorption, metabolism and excretion. The biological response to an exposure is another possible measure of exposure. For example, the antibody response to an antigenic occupational agent can be measured but its value as an exposure index is uncertain

because it is dependent on immunological responsiveness as well as exposure.

The mainstay of most occupational epidemiology is estimation of environmental exposure. Where available, quantitative measures of the air-borne concentration of an occupational agent are often combined with duration of exposure to give *cumulative exposure*. As well as simplifying data analysis, this is done on the assumption that intensity and duration of exposure are equivalent. This may not always be so and it is possible that a high intensity of exposure for a short period may have a different effect from exposure of low intensity over a long period. Duration of exposure is related to tolerance of exposure, and long-term workers may be more resistant to acute adverse effects (as in Table 8.2), and possibly delayed effects also. Nevertheless, the risk of several diseases appears to relate well to cumulative exposure. Decline in lung function over time (Diem et al., 1982; Davison et al., 1988) and lung cancer (De Klerk et al., 1989) are examples from the studies already cited.

Often only job title is available. It is usually possible to rank jobs within one plant on an ordinal scale. Job titles in one bakery were ranked from 0 to 10 for perceived dustiness by experts with experience of the industry (Musk et al., 1989). Figure 8.8 shows that their rankings agreed fairly well with the results of an environmental sampling survey. It also shows that the intervals on the ranking scale are not equidistant. This is often the case with qualitative scales of exposure and underlines the desirability of obtaining at least some quantitative data.

If this degree of detail in ranking is not possible, a classification into 'heavy', 'moderate' or 'light' exposure may be. This is more valuable if some quantification can be provided, as in the classification of arsenic exposure in a copper smelter by

Axelson et al. (1978) into three levels of (1) considerably below current occupational standard, (2) close to but not above it, and (3) above it. The problem of exposure ranking across several industries has been addressed by the development of 'job-exposure matrices' (Medical Research Council, 1983) in which each job title in a particular industry is scored for exposure to agents of interest. A study of lung cancer deaths in England and Wales in men aged from 15 to 64 years during 1970 to 1972 coded the 223 occupational units in the 1971 census data according to five grades of exposure to 14 different agents or activities. There was a significantly raised standard mortality ratio (SMR) with an exposure–response gradient for asbestos, chromates and diesel fumes but these effects disappeared after standardizing for social class (Magnani et al., 1988). The significantly raised SMRs were small, none being greater than 1.5. It is likely that the use of job-exposure matrices within specific industries will be more sensitive than applying them in the general population.

The simplest measure of exposure is that someone has, or has not, worked in an industry that entails exposure to the agent under study. It is usually possible to supplement this by noting duration of employment in the industry. It is important to appreciate that employment in a particular industry, or exposure to what has been or can be measured, may be only a partial measure of the exposure that causes disease. Working in a copper smelter, for example, entails exposure to arsenic, nickel, lead and sulphur dioxide (Axelson et al., 1978; Sandstrom, Wall and Taube, 1989). Exposure to asbestos does not entirely explain the high risk of lung cancer in asbestos textile workers (Sebastien et al., 1989).

No measure of occupational exposure is perfect, and both measurement variability and systematic bias may influence the results of epidemiological research. Random measurement variability always leads to underestimation of the exposure–response relationship. This will be appreciated by imagining what would result if reports of cigarette consumption (which are believed to be accurate) were in fact liable to a random error of plus or minus 20 cigarettes a day. Light smokers would be misclassified as heavy smokers and vice versa, which would obscure disease relationships with smoking. Random variation can be minimized by multiple measurements, as their average will give a more accurate picture of exposure.

The term 'bias' means a systematic underestimation or overestimation. Overestimation of 'usual' exposure may occur when historical occupational hygiene information is used because, until recently, environmental measurements were rarely made in order to describe representative exposures under normal working conditions but to identify processes resulting in high exposure, document the conse-

quences of accidents or monitor compliance with control limits in problem areas. This can lead to overestimation at the upper end of the range of exposure with consequent underestimation of the exposure–response relationship. Bias is also likely when measurement or analytical methods differ between plants or over time as the methods may give different results. The only way to control for this is by calibration of one method against another to achieve standardization.

Disease

The term 'disease' has been used in this chapter to mean any physiological abnormality or pathological state. The lung is very accessible to measurement of a number of parameters, and Table 8.3 lists some indices that have been used in epidemiology. No index in epidemiology is precisely the same as a disease, in the clinical use of the term, but those chosen should be associated with the disease under study. Radiographic opacities in the lungs of workers exposed to asbestos can reasonably be supposed to indicate the presence of asbestosis in the group, even though not necessarily caused by asbestosis in every individual worker. A reduction in gas transfer means little by itself but, taken with other functional and radiographic abnormalities, suggests emphysema in cadmium alloy workers (Davison et al., 1988).

Table 8.3 Some response indices used in epidemiology

Index	Examples
Mortality	Cancer, pneumoconiosis
Cancer registration	Cancer
Radiographic abnormality	Pneumoconiosis, pleural thickening, emphysema
Annual change in FEV_1	Chronic obstructive pulmonary disease
FEV_1	Obstructive pulmonary disease
Change in FEV_1 across a work shift	Acute airways' narrowing
Gas transfer	Emphysema, asbestosis
Bronchial reactivity to histamine, methacholine, exercise	Asthma
Variability in peak expiratory flow	Asthma
Respiratory symptoms	Many conditions
Sputum characteristics	Several conditions
Skin tests, immunological tests on blood	Associated with immunologically mediated lung disease

The choice of index should be informed by knowledge of the pathophysiology and natural history of the disease under study. Mortality is often used as an index of total incidence of cancer because most patients die of their disease in a relatively short time and are accurately certified. It is less useful as a surrogate for the incidence of some other diseases, such as asthma, where the fatality rate is low and certification less reliable. High mortality from asthma in an occupation may have a number of explanations other than that the occupation causes asthma. The study of asthma by methods developed originally for use in surveys concerned primarily with chronic bronchitis and emphysema, such as a single test of FEV_1, also creates difficulty in interpretation. Asthma is characterized by excessive variability in FEV_1 rather than a low mean FEV_1, and requires a different approach, such as measurement of bronchial responsiveness. A rapid method using histamine or methacholine has been described which is suitable for surveys (Yan, Salome and Woolcock, 1983).

Although there is a much greater variety of 'disease' measurements than there are exposure measurements, the same principles apply: a quantitative measurement is more informative, where available and appropriate, than noting the presence or absence of disease, and all measurements are subject to random and systematic variation. Random variation always reduces the strength of an exposure–response relationship. Systematic over- or undermeasurement can increase or reduce its apparent strength.

The random variability in lung function measurements is well documented in textbooks such as that of Cotes (1979), and epidemiological studies usually rely on tests with low variability, such as FEV_1, as a measure of airways' calibre. Observer variation in the reading of chest radiographs is discussed in Chapter 9. Observer variation in the recording of symptoms (Cochrane, Chapman and Oldham, 1951) and physical signs (Fletcher, 1952) is also well documented. As with exposure measurements, it is important to achieve standardization of instruments and observers. Figure 8.9 illustrates that observer C classified 38 per cent of a group of peak expiratory flow records as definitely showing asthma, but observer D so classified only 18 per cent (Venables et al., 1984). Further analysis showed that, when the scale was condensed to asthma and not asthma, the majority of observers agreed on almost all of the graphs. Condensing scales and using the average, or majority, reading is a feature of schemes for dealing with observer variation in a subjective assessment.

Guidelines on the performance of lung function tests have been issued by the American Thoracic Society (1987), and guidance on the interpretation of chest radiographs and a set of standard films are available from the International Labour Office,

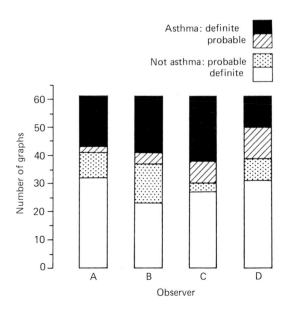

Figure 8.9 Variation between four observers (A to D) in the classification of 61 graphs of peak expiratory flow for the presence of asthma. (After Venables et al., 1984, with permission)

Geneva (see Chapter 7). Bennett and Ritchie (1975) discussed the principles of the design and use of questionnaires, and Samet (1978) reviewed the Medical Research Council questionnaire – the best known respiratory symptoms questionnaire (Medical Research Council, 1960) – whose most recent revision was published in 1986 (MRC, 1986).

Risk

'Risk' is a less emotive term in epidemiology than in everyday English where it implies a probability of an adverse effect that many people would find unacceptable. Some non-occupational factors, such as smoking or abuse of drugs, are a greater threat to individual health than most occupational exposures in the developed world today. Low environmental exposure may, nevertheless, pose a threat to public health. Furthermore, most people are not tolerant of risks over which they have no personal control and about which they have little information. Epidemiology has an important part to play in assessment of risk although decisions on the control of risks are ultimately made by governments.

The simplest way of measuring an occupational risk, in the epidemiological use of the word, is by comparing two groups of exposed and unexposed persons. Conventional summary measures of risk such as the SMR assume a multiplicative effect of exposure and do not provide information directly on absolute differences. A doubling of rate in an exposed group implies a large number of excess cases attributable to exposure if the background rate in unexposed persons is high, but a small number of excess cases if the background rate is low. Expressing lung function as a percentage of predicted values is analogous: an FEV_1 of 80 per cent is 1 litre below predicted if that value is 5 litres, but only 200 ml if the predicted value is 1 litre. A similar multiplicative effect is assumed when change in lung function is expressed as a percentage, as in Figure 8.3. Studies of lung function increasingly use absolute values, as in Figure 8.6 and Table 8.1, and the rate difference is sometimes used in studies of mortality, incidence or prevalence. The presentation of results is always more informative if risk is expressed in different ways.

The interpretation of measures of risk starts with asking if the results could have any other explanation than that exposure increases (or does not increase) the risk of disease. The effect of chance is quantified by statistical tests but factors other than chance are far more likely to give differences (or similarities) between groups in epidemiological studies. Many of the difficulties recognized as occurring in epidemiological studies, such as random measurement error, small sample size or inadequate length of follow-up, mask, rather than enhance, the effects of exposure. Factors leading to underestimation of the effects of occupational exposure include:

1. Small sample size.
2. Study group of 'survivors' in employment.
3. Exposure too low or for too short a time to give an effect.
4. Follow-up time shorter than the latent interval of disease
5. Random variation in measure of exposure.
6. Random variation in index of disease.
7. Overestimation of exposure.
8. Insensitive index of disease.
9. Comparison with the general population.
10. Comparison with a group who are at increased risk of disease because of other exposures.
11. Confounding.

Hernberg (1981) has discussed this in more detail.

However, overestimation of the effects of exposure may occur if disease is more likely to be detected in exposed than in unexposed persons. The autopsy rate may, for example, be higher in workers exposed to a known hazard or they may have examinations such as chest radiographs performed more frequently. This bias is unlikely if no hazard was suspected during the period of the study. Overestimation may occur also if exposure is more likely to be recorded in cases than in non-cases. This is a difficulty only when information on exposure is collected after disease has developed, so is a potential source of bias in case-referent or cross-sectional studies.

'Confounding' may overestimate or underestimate the effects of exposure. A *confounder* is a *risk factor (or protective factor) for the disease under study that is distributed unevenly by exposure category*. Smoking would confound the relationship between an exposure and lung cancer if exposed persons smoked more (or less) than unexposed persons. Confounding by smoking may lead to difficulty in interpreting studies of white-collar workers who smoke less than the general population average. It is often not possible to assess if a disease risk factor is a confounder because information on its distribution by exposure category cannot be obtained. Indirect estimates may be useful: in the study, mentioned earlier, by Thoren, Jarvholm and Morgan (1989) of mortality from asthma and chronic obstructive pulmonary disease in workers in a soft paper mill, a separate survey of smoking habits suggested that local residents who had worked in the mill had smoked more in the past than others, so a confounding effect of smoking was possible. As the risk associated with mill work was fourfold, it was unlikely to be entirely artefactual. Axelson (1989) has estimated that the range of uneven distribution of smokers between exposure groups that is reasonable at current levels of smoking in developed countries is unlikely to elevate the relative risk for lung cancer above 1.5 or depress it below 0.5. As smoking is a potent cause of lung cancer, it is unlikely that factors with weaker effects will exert a stronger confounding influence than this.

Age and sex are always potential confounders and, for lung function, so are height and ethnic background. Confounders need not be factors with a direct biological relationship with disease. Many diseases show a marked social class gradient, for example, which may reflect one or several of the many factors of which social class is an index – including income, education, diet, smoking, alcohol consumption, area of residence, and prenatal and early childhood experience.

Hill's (1984) nine headings for assessing whether an association is causal are valuable when considering all the epidemiological evidence about a relationship between exposure and disease. They include, in particular, the strength of the relationship, its consistency between studies, its temporal pattern, and the presence of a response gradient with exposure. Such a gradient is evidence for a causal relationship regardless of the results of external comparisons which, as discussed above, may not always be appropriate. The effects of any intervention to reduce exposure and the coherence of all the evidence, including that from secular trends in vital statistics and from experimental work, should also be taken into account. Questions to ask in assessing whether the association is causal include:

1. Is it a strong association?
2. What do other epidemiological studies show?
3. Is the epidemiological evidence coherent with other evidence such as secular trends or toxicity testing in animals?
4. Is there a plausible temporal relationship between exposure and disease?
5. Is there a gradient of risk with increasing exposure?
6. Does risk decrease after intervention to reduce exposure?
7. Is there an alternative explanation?
8. Could it be due to chance?

Hill suggested that the specificity of the association should be considered, but current concepts of the causation of disease mean that we readily accept multiple causes and multiple effects. He also listed the plausibility of the causal hypothesis and reasoning by analogy with known causal relationships. Although important, the imagination usually has little difficulty in proposing plausible biological mechanisms and finding supportive analogies for even the most unlikely causal hypotheses. The relationship of crocidolite exposure with mesothelioma is an example of an association that appears to be causal under most of these headings. Others meet only some or none of the criteria and require further investigation (see Appendix VI).

References

Acheson, E.D. (1976) Nasal cancer in the furniture and boot and shoe manufacturing industries. *Prev. Med.* **5**, 295–315

American Thoracic Society (1987). Standardization of spirometry – 1987 update. *Am. Rev. Respir. Dis.* **136**, 1285–1298

Axelson, O. (1989) Confounding from smoking in occupational epidemiology. *Br. J. Ind. Med.* **46**, 505–507

Axelson, O., Dahlgren, E., Jansson, C.-D. and Rehnlund, S.O. (1978) Arsenic exposure and mortality: a case-referent study from a Swedish copper smelter. *Br. J. Ind. Med.* **35**, 8–15

Bennett, A.E. and Ritchie, K. (1975) *Questionnaires in Medicine.* Oxford University Press for the Nuffield Provincial Hospitals Trust, London

Bourbonnais, R., Meyer, F. and Theriault, G. (1988) Validity of self reported work history. *Br. J. Ind. Med.* **45**, 29–32

Checkoway, H., Pearce, N. and Crawford-Brown, D.J. (1989) *Research Methods in Occupational Epidemiology*, Oxford University Press, New York

Cochrane, A.L., Chapman, P.J. and Oldham, P.D. (1951) Observers' errors in taking medical histories. *Lancet* **1**, 1007–1009

Cotes, J.E. (1979) *Lung Function: Assessment and Application in Medicine*, 4th edn, Blackwell Scientific, Oxford

Davison, A.G., Fayers, P.M., Newman Taylor, A.J., Venables, K.M., Darbyshire, J., Pickering, C.A.C., Chettle, D.R., Franklin, D., Guthrie, C.J.G., Scott, M.C., O'Malley, D., Holden, H., Mason, H.J., Wright, A.L. and Gompertz, D. (1988) Cadmium fume inhalation and emphysema. *Lancet* **1**, 663–667

De Klerk, N.H., Armstrong, B.K., Musk, A.W. and Hobbs, M.S.T. (1989) Cancer mortality in relation to measures of occupational exposure to crocidolite at Wittenoom Gorge in Western Australia. *Br. J. Ind. Med.* **46**, 529–536

Diem, J.E., Jones, R.N., Hendrick, D.J., Glindmeyer, H.W., Dharmarajan, V., Butcher, B.T., Salvaggio, J.E. and Weill, H. (1982) Five-year longitudinal study of workers employed in a new toluene diisocyanate manufacturing plant. *Am. Rev. Respir. Dis.* **126**, 420–428

Doll, R. (1952) The causes of death among gas-workers, with special reference to cancer of the lung. *Br. J. Ind. Med.* **9**, 180–185

Enterline, P.E. and Marsh, G.M. (1982) Missing records in occupational disease epidemiology. *J. Occup. Med.* **24**, 677–680

Fletcher, C.M. (1952) The clinical diagnosis of pulmonary emphysema – an experimental study. *Proc. R. Soc. Med.* **45**, 577–586

Fox, A.J. and Collier, P.F. (1976) Low mortality rates in industrial cohort studies due to selection for work and survival in the industry. *Br. J. Prev. Soc. Med.* **30**, 225–230

Fraser, P., Chilvers, C., Day, M. and Goldblatt, P. (1989) Further results from a census-based mortality study of fertiliser manufacturers. *Br. J. Ind. Med.* **46**, 38–42

Gardner, M.J. (1986) Considerations in the choice of expected numbers for appropriate comparisons in occupational cohort studies. *Med. Lav.* **77**, 23–47

Hernberg, S. (1981) 'Negative' results in cohort studies – how to recognise fallacies. *Scand. J. Work Environ. Health* **7**, suppl. 4, 121–126

Hill, A.B. (1984) Statistical evidence and inference. In *A Short Textbook of Medical Statistics*, 11th edn. Hodder and Stoughton, London, pp. 270–279

Kessel, R., Redl, M., Mauermayer, R. and Praml, G.J. (1989) Changes in lung function after working with the shotcrete lining method under compressed air conditions. *Br. J. Ind. Med.* **46**, 128–132

McDonald, J.C. (1981) Epidemiology. In: *Occupational Lung Diseases: Research Approaches and Methods* (eds H. Weill and M. Turner-Warwick), Marcel Dekker, New York, pp. 373–403

McDonald, J.C., Gibbs, G.W., Liddell, F.D.K. and McDonald, A.D. (1978) Mortality after long exposure to cummingtonite–grunerite. *Am. Rev. Respir. Dis.* **118**, 217–277

McMichael, A.J. (1989) Setting environmental exposure standards: the role of the epidemiologist. *Int. J. Epidemiol.* **18**, 10–16

Magnani, C., Pannett, B., Winter, P.D. and Coggon, D. (1988) Application of a job-exposure matrix to national mortality statistics for lung cancer. *Br. J. Ind. Med.* **45**, 70–72

Mason, H.J., Davison, A.G., Wright, A.L., Guthrie, C.J.G., Fayers, P.M., Venables, K.M., Smith, N.J., Chettle, D.R., Franklin, D.M., Scott, M.C., Holden, H., Gompertz, D. and Newman Taylor, A.J. (1988) Relations between liver cadmium, cumulative exposure, and renal function in cadmium alloy workers. *Br. J. Ind. Med.* **45**, 793–802

Medical Research Council: Committee on the Aetiology of

Chronic Bronchitis. (1960) Standardized questionnaires on respiratory symptoms. *Br. Med. J.* **2**, 1665

Medical Research Council: Environmental Epidemiology Unit (1983) *Job-exposure Matrices.* Proceedings of a conference, April 1982, University of Southampton. Medical Research Council, London

Medical Research Council: Committee on Environmental and Occupational Health (1986) *Questionnaire on Respiratory Symptoms.* London, Medical Research Council

Miller, B.A., Blair, A.E., Raynor, H.L., Stewart, P.A., Hoar Zahm, S. and Fraumeni, J.F. Jr (1989) Cancer and other mortality patterns among United States furniture workers. *Br. J. Ind. Med.* **46**, 508–515

Musk, A.W., Venables, K.M., Crook, B., Nunn, A.J., Hawkins, R., Crook, G., Graneek, B.J., Tee, R.D., Farrer, N., Johnson, D., Gordon, D.J., Darbyshire, J.H. and Newman Taylor, A.J. (1989) Respiratory symptoms, lung function, and sensitisation to components of wheat flour in a British bakery. *Br. J. Ind. Med.* **46**, 636–642

Partanen, T., Kauppinen, T., Nurminen, M., Nickels, J., Hernberg, S., Hakulinen, T., Pukkala, E. and Savonen, E. (1985) Formaldehyde exposure and respiratory and related cancers: a case-referent study among Finnish woodworkers. *Scand. J. Work Environ. Health* **11**, 409–415

Samet, J.M. (1978) A historical and epidemiological perspective on respiratory symptoms questionnaires. *Am. J. Epidemiol.* **108**, 435–446

Sandstrom, A., Wall, S.G.I. and Taube, A. (1989) Cancer incidence and mortality among Swedish smelter workers. *Br. J. Ind. Med.* **46**, 82–89

Seaton, A., Seaton, D. and Leitch, A.G. (1989) Epidemiology and respiratory disease. In: *Crofton and Douglas's Respiratory Diseases*, 4th edn. Oxford, Blackwell Scientific, pp. 76–94

Sebastien, P., McDonald, J.C., McDonald, A.D., Case, B. and Harley, R. (1989) Respiratory cancer in chrysotile textile and mining industries: exposure inferences from lung analysis. *Br. J. Ind. Med.* **46**, 180–187

Seniori Costantini, A., Paci, E. and Miligi, L. (1989) Cancer mortality among workers in the Tuscan tanning industry. *Br. J. Ind. Med.* **46**, 384–388

Thoren, K., Jarvholm, B. and Morgan, U. (1989) Mortality from asthma and chronic obstructive pulmonary disease among workers in a soft paper mill: a case-referent study. *Br. J. Ind. Med.* **46**, 192–195

Venables, K.M., Burge, P.S., Davison, A.G. and Newman Taylor, A.J. (1984) Peak flow rate records in surveys: reproducibility of observers' reports. *Thorax* **39**, 828–832

Venables, K.M., Dally, M.B., Burge, P.S., Pickering, C.A.C. and Newman Taylor, A.J. (1985) Occupational asthma in a steel coating plant. *Br. J. Ind. Med.* **42**, 517–524

Venables, K.M., Tee, R.D., Hawkins, E.R., Gordon, D.J., Wale, C.J., Farrer, N.M., Lam, T.H., Baxter, P.J. and Newman Taylor, A.J. (1988) Laboratory animal allergy in a pharmaceutical company. *Br. J. Ind. Med.* **45**, 660–666

Venables, K.M., Dally, M.B., Nunn, A.J., Stevens, J.F., Stephens, R., Farrer, N., Hunter, J.V., Stewart, M., Hughes, E.G. and Newman Taylor, A.J. (1989) Smoking and occupational allergy in workers in a platinum refinery. *Br. Med. J.* **299**, 939–942

Yan, K., Salome, C. and Woolcock, A.J. (1983) Rapid method for measurement of bronchial responsiveness. *Thorax* **38**, 760–765

Zetterstrom, O., Osterman, K., Machado, L. and Johansson, S.G.O. (1981) Another smoking hazard: raised serum IgE concentration and increased risk of occupational allergy. *Br. Med. J.* **283**, 1215–1217

Zetterstrom, O., Nordvall, S.L., Bjorksten, B., Ahlstedt, S. and Stelander, M. (1985) Increased IgE antibody responses in rats exposed to tobacco smoke. *J. Allergy Clin. Immunol.* **75**, 594–598

9

Chronic bronchitis, airflow obstruction and emphysema

W. Raymond Parkes

Chronic bronchitis

In 1959 'chronic bronchitis' was defined by the Ciba Guest Symposium as 'a condition of chronic or recurrent excess of mucus secretion in the bronchial tree'; and in 1965 the Medical Research Council (UK) defined 'chronic' as meaning 'occurring on most days for at least three months in the year for at least two successive years'. This implied persistent production of sputum, expectorated or swallowed, which might or might not be associated with cough. The Council recommended that 'chronic bronchitis' should be classified as follows:

1. *Simple chronic bronchitis* characterized by chronic or recurrent increase in the volume of mucoid bronchial secretion sufficient to cause expectoration.
2. *Chronic or recurrent mucopurulent bronchitis* in which sputum is persistently or intermittently mucopurulent.
3. *Chronic obstructive bronchitis* in which there is persistent widespread narrowing of the intrapulmonary airways causing increased resistance to airflow.

This classification promoted widespread use of the term 'chronic obstructive bronchitis' which implied that associated airflow obstruction was not necessarily related to emphysema. Unfortunately, these three categories fostered the notion of a causally connected sequence of events in which an excess of mucus encourages bronchial infection which, in turn, damages the airways and causes airflow obstruction. Thus, 'chronic bronchitis' was commonly synonymous with 'expiratory airflow obstruction'. Subsequent investigation has altered

these conceptions substantially, and the classification has been revised in 1986 (see 'Revised terminology', page 225).

Hypersecretion of mucus – the hallmark of chronic bronchitis – is produced both by mucous glands and by goblet cells (see Chapter 1, page 7). The mucous glands are enlarged due to hyperplasia of their cells and engorgement with mucus (Douglas, 1980), and goblet cells are increased in number. Enlargement of the glands is conveniently quantified by the ratio of gland-to-wall thickness – the Reid index (see Figure 10.2). The average value of the index in normal lungs is 0.26; in those with chronic bronchitis, it is 0.59 (Reid, 1960, 1967).

Although enlargement of mucous glands and increase in goblet cell numbers are usually contemporaneous and of similar degree, this is not always so. In some cases gland enlargement may predominate with minimal goblet cell activity whereas, in others, there may be an impressive increase in the goblet cells and only minor enlargement of the glands. Such differences in the predominant source of hypersecretion are significant, for although substantially more mucus is produced by mucous glands than by goblet cells, hypersecretion in bronchioles by the latter is considerably more damaging because, due to their small calibre, these airways are readily obstructed (Reid, 1988). Recent investigation has shown that, in cases of established chronic bronchitis, mucus differs from normal, not only in its quantity but also in the presence of epithelial glycolipids which alter the viscoelastic properties of sputum and, thus, the ease with which it can be cleared by the cilia or by cough (Bhaskar et al., 1985).

Cullinan (1991) demonstrated a linear dose–response relationship between the production of sputum and pack-years of smoking; however, using

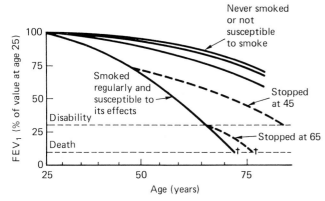

Figure 9.1 Risks for various men if they smoke: differences between these lines illustrate effects that smoking, and stopping smoking, can have on FEV$_1$ of a man who is liable to develop chronic obstructive lung disease if he smokes. † = Death, the underlying cause of which is irreversible chronic obstructive lung disease. Although this curve shows the rate of loss of FEV$_1$ for one particular susceptible smoker, other susceptible smokers will have different rates of loss, thus reaching 'disability' at different ages. (Reproduced, with permission, from Fletcher and Peto, 1977)

matched-pair analysis, he found no significant association with occupational exposure to respirable dusts, fumes and gases, although an exposure–response relationship was apparent.

Fletcher et al. (1976a), in their important prospective study, concluded that neither chronic expectoration nor associated bronchial infection is related causally to the development of airflow obstruction and that production of sputum and obstruction of airflow are, in general, relatively independent responses to cigarette smoke occurring together due to the common factor of smoking.

Forced expiratory volume in 1 second (FEV$_1$), which reflects the average calibre of all the pulmonary airways, has been, and remains, the most commonly used measure of airflow obstruction in such epidemiological studies. It undergoes a slow decline with increasing age (about 20 to 30 ml/year) in most normal adults without the development of dyspnoea (Figure 9.1). But the effects of smoking on FEV$_1$ over the years are complex, as Fletcher and Peto (1977) have shown. The majority of smokers (about 70 to 80 per cent) have either a normal or an increased decline of FEV$_1$, without disabling airflow obstruction. In the remaining 20 to 30 per cent, however, the decline is more rapid (60 to 80 ml/year) and results in disabling airflow obstruction in about the sixth decade (Speizer and Tager, 1979). If smoking is stopped, the progressive fall in FEV$_1$ ceases in most instances, but in many of those with respiratory disability it continues until death from respiratory failure, or until pulmonary heart disease, supervenes (Figure 9.1). The reasons for the

differences in individual responses (or susceptibility), especially in advanced disease, are not understood (Traver, Cline and Burrows, 1979). However, the more susceptible individuals are to the effects of cigarette smoke, the sooner they become disabled if they continue to smoke (Fletcher and Peto, 1977).

It is commonly assumed that the lungs of adults exposed to cigarette smoke or to other respiratory insults – environmental or occupational – have already reached optimal or full physiological development (Speizer and Tager, 1979). But, as shown in Chapters 1 and 3, the morphometry and function of the lungs are apt to vary among individuals. Moreover, there may be subgroups in the population who are vulnerable to a variety of other factors that reduce the likelihood of their lungs ever reaching an optimal state of function (see Chapter 1) and which increase their susceptibility to developing obstructive lung disease. There is some evidence, unrelated to α_1-antitrypsin deficiency (see 'Pathogenesis', page 232), that suggests familial clustering of pulmonary function, chronic bronchitis and chronic obstructive pulmonary disease (Speizer and Tager, 1979), and that implies that chronic bronchitis and chronic obstructive airways' disease may be influenced by polygenic inheritance (Tager et al., 1978). According to Larson et al. (1970), hereditary factors and smoking probably contribute about equally to the likelihood of developing significant airflow obstruction. Indeed, monozygotic twins are more vulnerable to a smoking-related decline in lung function than are dizygotic twins (Zamel et al., 1981), and a family history of allergy appears to be significantly more common among smokers with a rapid decline in FEV$_1$ compared with smokers with a slow annual decline (Taylor et al., 1985).

The lack of close correlation between airflow obstruction and enlargement of mucous glands has been generally confirmed by combined clinicopathological studies, although, in some cases, enlarged mucous glands encroach on the lumina of bronchi (Thurlbeck, 1985). The chief site of irreversible airflow obstruction in smokers is in airways less than about 3 mm diameter in which hyperplasia of goblet cells, hypertrophy of smooth muscle and inflammation in the walls of membranous and respiratory bronchioles are found (Cosio, Hale and Niewoehner, 1980); however, increase in bronchiolar goblet cells and smooth muscle does not, apparently, occur in young smokers. This suggests that these lesions are a later consequence of inflammation (Cosio et al., 1978; Thurlbeck, 1980). In fact, there is a significant association, which increases with age, between inflammatory fibrosis of membranous and respiratory bronchioles and smoking in men who lived in a clean-air environment and were not employed in dusty trades (Adesina et al., 1991). Hyperplasia of goblet cells may, as stated earlier, cause plugging of these airways with mucus and displace the surface layer of surfactant, and so encourage them to close more readily; in addition, they may be blocked by inflammatory exudate, and are thus distorted or even obliterated. The degree to which the bronchioles are involved is the single most important factor in causing respiratory disability. Their structural damage is often demonstrable on bronchograms (Reid, 1988).

In short, there are three separate pathological lesions of the airways that are related to cigarette smoking: large airways' disease, inflammation of membranous bronchioles and inflammation of respiratory bronchioles (Thurlbeck, 1980). These frequently occur together, although with differing severity.

In spite of the fact that the major site of disease responsible for increased resistance to airflow is located chiefly in peripheral airways, tests of function of the larger airways are frequently abnormal, even in young smokers with little disease of their airways (Oxhøj, Bake and Wilhelmsen, 1976; Enjeti et al., 1978). This is consistent with the 'Dutch hypothesis' that smokers with progressive airflow obstruction have increased bronchial reactivity and atopic features similar to, but less marked than, those observed in asthmatic subjects (Orie et al., 1961). Such increased reactivity, even in the absence of airways' obstruction, has been demonstrated in smokers compared with ex-smokers and non-smokers (Burrows, 1981; Cerveri et al., 1989); it develops some years after starting smoking (Taylor et al., 1985). Smoking appears to increase the risk of sensitization to some inhaled antigens encountered in the work environment and, although the increase in the responsiveness of non-specific airways to long-term smoking is small, it may be more pronounced in atopic individuals. However, there is a lack of clear evidence that atopy is a risk factor for irreversible airways' obstruction in individuals without asthma. It is also uncertain whether the risk of airways' hyper-responsiveness precedes and predisposes to the development of chronic airflow obstruction, or is instead a manifestation of inflammation and narrowing of the airways (O'Connor, Sparrow and Weiss, 1989). However, increased bronchial hyper-responsiveness to non-allergic stimuli is common in patients with established chronic airways' obstruction (Yan, Salome and Woolcock, 1985), and seems to be associated with a heightened response of their airways to histamine (De Jongste et al., 1987). There is also evidence that enhanced reactivity of airways usually precedes the development of asthma and may be genetically determined (Hopp et al., 1990).

Thus, the causes of airflow obstruction in smokers, and the reasons for its variability among individuals, are far from straightforward.

Other causes of disease of the airways

A decrease in ventilatory function due to narrowing of larger airways often occurs, and lasts for some weeks, in patients with chronic airways' obstruction following acute viral infections in the upper and lower respiratory tracts, or with acute mucopurulent exacerbations of chronic bronchitis associated with rhinosinusitis. Acute inflammation of the nasal airways and larynx may promote reflex constriction of the intrapulmonary airways through naso- and laryngobronchomotor reflexes (referred to in Chapter 3); indeed, nasal stimulation in patients with asthma or chronic airways' obstruction has been shown to increase bronchoconstriction (Nolte and Berger, 1983).

Lesions of the peripheral airways – in particular, mural fibrosis in membranous bronchioles and respiratory bronchiolitis – are also found among non-smokers (Cosio, Hale and Niewoehner, 1980). It has been known for years that chronic bronchitis with airflow obstruction increases as social class declines, in both men and their wives (Medical Research Council Special Committee, 1966). Fletcher et al. (1976b) pointed out that a large social class difference of mortality from 'bronchitis' in England and Wales 'was present before any social class gradient for cigarette consumption appeared'. In fact, Collis (1923) recorded that in 1916, when widespread cigarette smoking was not yet established, deaths from 'bronchitis and bronchial and nasal catarrh' were 85.3 per 1000, and sickness due to the same causes was 181.3 per 1000. Although he did not define 'bronchitis', he separated it from pneumonia and phthisis (that is, mainly tuberculosis). Indeed, mortality from chronic obstructive pulmonary disease in adults in England has been found to be associated with underweight in the first year of their infancy due, possibly, to adverse environmental effects (Barker, 1991).

Respiratory illness during infancy and childhood, the incidence of which is influenced by a variety of social factors, has been blamed (Holland et al., 1977). However, although there are many reports that such illness predisposes to chronic cough and sputum and impaired lung function in adult life, many have been flawed by the nature of the illness having been decided retrospectively, and often not clearly defined (Glezen, 1989). Nonetheless, two recent prospective investigations have confirmed that there is a strong association (more common in boys) between well-defined acute lower respiratory infection in childhood and impairment of pulmonary function in adolescence and early adult life (Voter et al., 1988; Gold et al., 1989). In some children, infection by influenza A or adenoviruses results in permanent damage in the form of obliterative bronchiolitis or interstitial fibrosis (Becroft, 1971; Lourdes et al., 1974; Laraya-Cuasay et al., 1977); this may also occur in adults.

Airflow obstruction, often without expectoration and independent of smoking, is unusually common in patients with rheumatoid arthritis (with or without the 'sicca' complex), and may also be associated with other connective tissue disorders (Epler et al., 1979; Geddes, Webley and Emmerson, 1979; Segal et al., 1981; Radoux et al., 1987). The underlying cause in the patients with rheumatoid arthritis is an autoimmune, progressive bronchiolitis with lymphocytic infiltration of the mucosa of membranous bronchioles and very small bronchi (Geddes et al., 1977; Herzog, Miller and Hoidal, 1981).

Recent investigations have been interpreted as showing that chronic airways' obstruction itself, independent of age and smoking, may be a risk factor in causation of cancer of the lung (Skillrud, Offord and Miller, 1986; Tockman et al., 1987; Anthonisen, 1989). Evidently, this is a suggestion that needs critical evaluation.

Trends in mortality

Differences in trends in mortality from chronic obstructive airways' disease in the UK over the last 100 years (and currently between countries) have clearly been influenced by differences of terminology and certification practice. Due to changes in respiratory disease coding in the UK between 1983 and 1984, there was a substantial change in the proportion of deaths assigned to different respiratory disease codes. For example, over one-third of the annual increase in deaths classified as 'chronic airways' obstruction' in 1984, would formerly have been assigned to other respiratory categories. This may partly explain an apparent, rather than a real, reversal of a declining mortality trend from this 'cause' in recent years. The trends in mortality in the UK attributed to bronchitis, emphysema and chronic airways' obstruction over the period 1979 to 1986 for people between 45 and 84 years of age show a rise for women over 65 since about 1983, but a slight decline for men in the same age range during this period. Evidently this is not a result of changes in coding practice, which would affect both sexes equally; it is probably due to the fact that (in the UK) the proportion of women who smoke, unlike that of men, has hardly altered between 1979 and 1985 (Backhouse and Holland, 1989). This emphasizes the importance of being aware of alterations in, and the use of, definitions over the years in this as in any other field of medicine.

Revised terminology

The following improvements suggested by Fletcher and Pride (1984) regarding terminology are, therefore, appropriate:

1. The term 'chronic bronchitis' should be used solely to connote chronic or recurrent bronchial hypersecretion, and never to imply the presence of associated obstruction (or limitation) of airflow.
2. The term 'chronic obstructive bronchitis', implying as it does a causal connection between hypersecretion and airflow obstruction, should be abandoned.
3. The term 'chronic obstructive bronchiolitis' seems acceptable for reference to disease of the membranous bronchioles (although it may also involve small bronchi) which, in general, is associated with obstruction to airflow. The term 'small airways' disease', proposed, and much in vogue, a few years ago (Hogg, Macklem and Thurlbeck, 1968), has become an imprecise expression which is used equally for abnormalities of structure and of function and is best avoided.

Objection to the continued use of the term 'chronic bronchitis' has, nevertheless, been made because inflammation of the bronchi is not necessarily a feature of the disorder (Thurlbeck, 1988), but this does not seem realistic in view of the widespread currency of the term and increased awareness of its implications and limitations.

Chronic bronchitis, increased bronchial reactivity, disease of peripheral airways and emphysema do not usually occur as isolated entities but are more often found in varying combinations with differing degrees of severity. Thus, chronic bronchitis as defined (Medical Research Council, 1965), and asthma defined in terms of variable airflow obstruction (Ciba Foundation Study Group, 1971), are not mutually exclusive, and there is no reason why they should be, because their diagnostic criteria are different. Most individuals who satisfy this definition of asthma produce sputum and, of these, about half fulfil the diagnostic criteria for chronic bronchitis (Openshaw and Turner-Warwick, 1989). Not only is bronchial reactivity increased above normal in asthmatic subjects, both with and without associated chronic bronchitis, there is also no difference in its degree between the two. Although all the patients in this investigation were attending an asthma clinic and 75 per cent were atopic, the conclusions emphasize that it is not justifiable to regard individuals with variable airflow obstruction and those who produce sputum as separate, well-defined categories (Openshaw and Turner-Warwick, 1989).

Prevalence

The standard questionnaire for the diagnosis of chronic bronchitis proposed by the British Medical Research Council in 1960, and modified in 1986 to include other respiratory symptoms, has been, and is, widely employed for the assessment of prevalence. But its potential drawbacks (referred to in Chapter 6, page 142) must be kept in mind and, when used, other causes of chronic production of sputum and of cough must be excluded. These include other chronic bronchopulmonary diseases (for example, bronchiectasis and tuberculosis) and disease of the nasal passages and paranasal sinuses which may cause expectoration of 'postnasal drip' secretions. Evidence of such exclusion is not always provided, however, in reported epidemiological and clinical studies of chronic bronchitis. The prevalence of chronic sinusitis, incidentally, is greater in smokers than in non-smokers (Wilson, 1973).

Thus, it is clear that assessment of comparative prevalence in different countries, and even in different parts of the same country, is fraught with difficulty caused by variability of pathogenesis and of the diagnostic criteria that have often been used during life, and for death certification from which mortality rates are calculated. It is certain that 'chronic bronchitis' on some death certificates – especially in countries where the diagnosis is fashionable – may be inaccurate. Furthermore, mortality from so-called 'chronic bronchitis', due primarily to irreversible airways' obstruction, cannot readily be related to past prevalence studies during life, when attention has usually been concentrated on the criterion of production of sputum.

Variation in subjects' answers to questions, differences between observers, inaccuracy in the use of standard questionnaires and failure to exclude other respiratory disease may all cause erroneous or discordant results. It should also be borne in mind that workers in occupations traditionally supposed to be associated with chronic pulmonary disease may, in good faith, give more false-positive answers to a questionnaire than workers in occupations with no such recognized association.

In short, although smoking is the most common factor affecting the prevalence of chronic bronchitis and airflow obstruction that is known to be greatly increased in smokers compared with non-smokers of both sexes in urban and rural populations of the UK, the USA and elsewhere, other factors (referred to earlier) probably affect the susceptibility or resistance of individuals to develop these disorders.

The question of chronic bronchitis, airways' obstruction and occupation is discussed separately in Chapter 10.

Emphysema

Occupational exposures that are believed to cause emphysema are few and not always well authenticated. However, it is appropriate to discuss emphysema briefly because, overall, it is probably the most common pathological disorder of the lungs in the adult population at large; it is thus a frequent incidental finding in individuals with specific occupational diseases whatever their nature.

Because clinical, physiological and radiographic findings are insensitive and imprecise in detecting and quantifying emphysema, the only sure method is inspection of properly prepared lungs (see Appendix III). Therefore, emphysema is best defined and described morphologically.

Some alteration to the definition and categorization of emphysema has been made since that recommended by the Ciba Foundation Guest Symposium in 1959, which was:

Emphysema is a condition of the lung characterized by increase beyond the normal in the size of airspaces distal to the terminal bronchiole either from dilatation or from destruction of their walls.

In this definition, abnormal enlargement of airspaces is not necessarily associated with destruction of their walls although, ultimately, this may be present in the majority of lesions. A revised, and currently recommended, definition embodies a substantial change by separating airspace enlargement into different categories: 'Respiratory airspace enlargement is defined as an increase in airspace size as compared with the airspaces of normal lungs. The term applies to all varieties of airspace enlargement distal to the terminal bronchioles whether occurring with or without fibrosis or destruction' (Snider et al., 1985). According to this system there are three categories of airspace enlargement, of which only one is emphysema: (1) simple enlargement without destruction related to congenital defects or to age; (2) emphysema proper – that is, panacinar, centriacinar and distal acinar types; and (3) enlargement with fibrosis. In this context, then, emphysema is defined as:

a condition of the lung characterized by abnormal, permanent enlargement of the airspaces distal to the terminal bronchiole, accompanied by destruction of their walls, and without obvious fibrosis.

(Snider et al., 1985;
American Thoracic Society, 1987)

As in the earlier (1959) definition, any part or all of the acinus may be involved but destruction of airspace walls is now an *essential* element. Enlargement of airspaces with age, or following lung

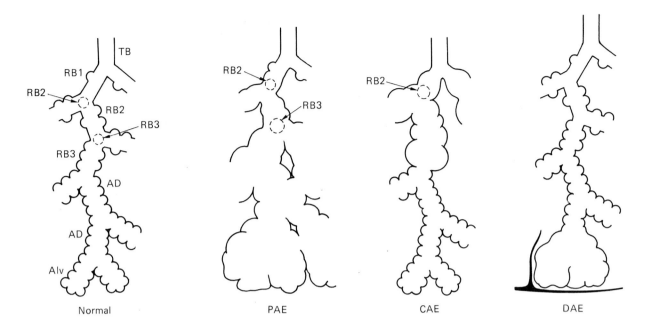

Figure 9.2 Diagram of the anatomical sites of types of emphysema in the acinar architecture. Irregular emphysema is not shown because, in essence, it crosses acinar boundaries. PAE = panacinar emphysema; CAE = centriacinar emphysema; DAE = distal (periacinar) emphysema; TB = terminal bronchioles; RB_1, RB_2, RB_3 = respiratory bronchioles; AD = alveolar ducts: average of nine generations truncated; Alv = alveoli

resection or lobar collapse, is no longer classed as 'emphysema' but as 'ageing lung' and 'compensatory over-inflation', respectively. 'Enlargement', of course, is a relative term and the definition is deemed to depend upon comparison with normal acini but, in practice, airspaces larger than 1 mm have usually been considered as emphysematous. Destruction of airspace walls, however, is not regarded by all authorities as a requisite for the definition of emphysema. Indeed, Reid has emphasized for years, and recently reiterated (1988), that specific reference either to dilatation or to destruction is undesirable, the definition being, in her opinion, most appropriately expressed simply as 'increase beyond the normal in the size of airspaces distal to the terminal bronchiole'.

The recent alterations in definition made, it is said, in the interest of greater precision have, however, caused confusion. So, while having them in mind, it is proposed to discuss emphysema under the four familiar anatomical categories which are characterized by the distribution of enlarged airspaces within the acinus (Figure 9.2).

1. *Panacinar emphysema*, in which all the elements of the acinus – airways and alveoli – are more or less equally involved; when severe, virtually the whole acinus disappears.

2. *Centriacinar emphysema*, in which respiratory bronchioles tend to be enlarged with, in most instances, destruction of related airspaces. As respiratory bronchioles are proximal rather than central in the acinus, it is also referred to as *proximal acinar emphysema* (Heppleston, 1972). It is surprising that the current definition, which is supposedly morphological, subdivides this type according to putative cause: the first being associated with cigarette smoking and airflow obstruction, the second with respiratory bronchiolar dilatation, said to be due to deposition of coal or other mineral dusts and often referred to as 'focal emphysema' (Snider et al., 1985; American Thoracic Society, 1987). As the essence of the latter is said to be dilatation and not destruction – at least as 'a primary event' (Heppleston, 1972) – it might be surmised, according to the terms of the definition, that, like 'ageing lung', it should not be classified as emphysema. The question as to whether or not there are two distinct, recognizable forms of centriacinar emphysema is discussed in Chapter 13. Distribution within the lung, however, is, on the whole, similar.

3. *Periacinar emphysema*, in which the alveolar ducts and sacs at the periphery of the acinus are predominantly affected where it is bordered by

connective tissue (secondary interlobular septa and pleura). Hence, it is also known as *paraseptal* or *distal acinar* emphysema.

4. *Irregular emphysema*, in which there is irregular enlargement and destruction of acini associated with fibrosis but without any uniform or particular anatomical distribution (Thurlbeck, 1976). It is often referred to as *scar emphysema*, its form and extent being determined by the scar. Scarring, however, is sometimes present in panacinar emphysema. Although these features accord with a definition of emphysema in which destruction of airspaces is an essential criterion, it is classified as 'airspace enlargement with fibrosis' and not as emphysema in the updated definition (Snider et al., 1985; American Thoracic Society, 1987). Small, localized lesions of coal, or similar types of pneumoconiosis, in the region of the respiratory bronchioles may cause scar emphysema of central (or proximal) acinar distribution (see Chapter 13).

The term 'bulla' is a general one for an emphysematous space more than 1 cm in diameter in the distended state. Most bullae represent localized accentuation of one of the four types of emphysema (Thurlbeck, 1976) and, thus, are not a specific form of emphysema, although some are independent of associated widespread emphysema. For this reason the terms 'bulla' and 'bullous emphysema' have been eliminated from the recent definition (Snider et al., 1985).

Interstitial emphysema

Interstitial emphysema differs from the other types just considered in the location of the air and in being mainly of traumatic origin. It is the result of the leakage of air into interstitial tissues of the lung from ruptured alveoli. The escaped air tracks along perivascular sheaths to the mediastinum (pneumomediastinum) and pericardium (pneumopericardium), and may reach the subcutaneous tissues of the neck and face; pneumothorax, often bilateral, may develop subsequently.

Important occupational causes include the following:

1. Decompression pulmonary barotrauma, which can result from improperly controlled ascent from depth in diving operations or from sudden failure of cabin pressure in aircraft flying at high altitude, and its consequent equalization with the ambient atmospheric pressure (see Chapters 24 and 25 respectively).

2. Blast injuries in air from explosions, especially in confined spaces, and in water where divers,

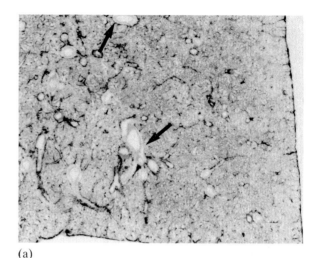

(a)

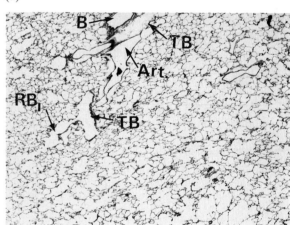

(b)

Figure 9.3 (a) Normal lung: alveolar spaces are less than 1 mm in diameter. Arrows indicate bronchi. (From paper-mounted section, natural size.) (b) Microsection of normal lung: Art = pulmonary artery; B = bronchiole; TB = terminal bronchiole; RB$_1$ = first respiratory bronchiole. Magnification ×10. (By courtesy of Dr David Lamb)

seamen and armed forces' personnel may be affected; pilots who fire their ejection seats to escape from submerged, crashed aircraft may also be affected.

3. Blunt trauma caused by falling into water from great height or by a blow to the chest wall.

The cause of the alveolar rupture in decompression barotrauma is over-inflation but in the other instances it is probably a shearing stress effect.

Alveolar rupture may also occur in medical conditions associated with paroxysmal coughing, vomiting, severe asthmatic episodes and over-enthusiastic positive pressure ventilation.

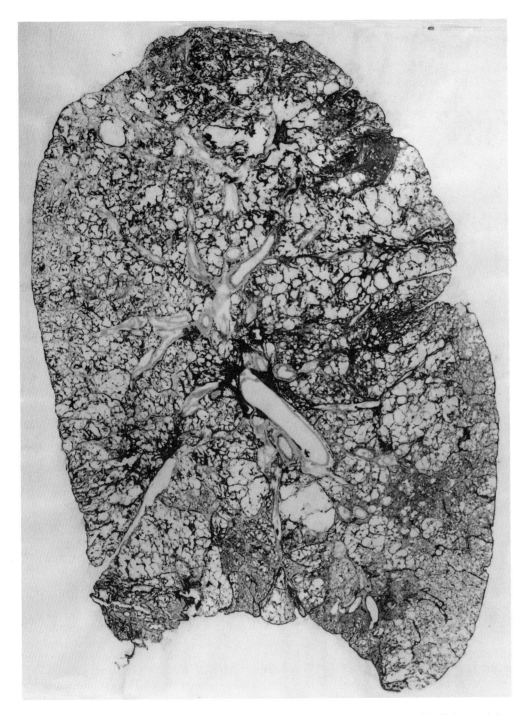

Figure 9.4 Whole lung section of widespread, severe panacinar emphysema with little surviving normal lung

Pathology

Emphysema is common in adult lungs. If irregular emphysema is excluded, about half the lungs examined *post mortem* are emphysematous, centriacinar emphysema being, in general, more common than panacinar, and both increase in frequency with age (Thurlbeck, 1968). Barium-impregnated slices of perfused lung (see Appendix III) are indispensable for proper assessment of emphysema. It is of interest that, internationally, the highest frequency and severity of emphysema appears to be in Cardiff, South Wales, in a diverse, non-mining community (Thurlbeck, Ryder and Sternby, 1974).

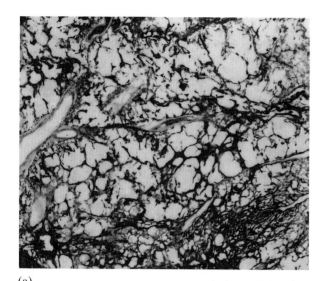

(a)

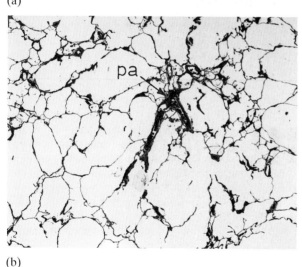

(b)

Figure 9.5 Severe panacinar emphysema: (a) natural size; (b) microsection. pa = pulmonary artery. Magnification ×10. (Courtesy of Dr David Lamb)

Figure 9.3 shows the naked eye and microscopic appearances of normal lung for reference.

Panacinar emphsema

Panacinar emphysema is distributed with equal frequency in both upper and lower parts of the lungs, and may be local or general but with a propensity for their anterior and basal regions. The affected parts do not deflate normally when the thorax is opened at necropsy, and the lung substance may be so attenuated that, when cut, it sags away from the blood vessels and airways.

To the naked eye, the earliest stage consists of isolated enlarged airspaces in any part of the lung,

and the most advanced stage of a total loss of lung architecture with only strands of surviving tissue (Figures 9.4 and 9.5a). Microscopy shows loss of alveolar walls which, consequently, are much reduced in number, and alveolar ducts and respiratory bronchioles are extensively involved (Figure 9.5b). In severe emphysema, the walls of membranous bronchioles are thicker and show substantially more chronic inflammation than those of normal lungs (Linhartová and Anderson, 1983).

Centriacinar (proximal acinar) emphysema

Centriacinar emphysema is characteristically distributed in the upper two-thirds of the lungs, particularly in the apical and posterior segments of the upper lobes and the apical segments of the lower, but it is sometimes scattered throughout the lungs. Typically it consists of localized enlargement of respiratory bronchioles and their alveoli, with subsequent loss – or 'destruction' – of the walls of both in varying degree. These localized lesions coalesce to form sharply outlined emphysematous spaces surrounded by normal lung. The spaces, the walls of which may contain black pigment, vary from 1 mm to 1 cm or more in diameter (Figures 9.6 and 9.7a). Microscopically, alveoli immediately adjacent to the spaces are compressed but the alveolar ducts and sacs are normal (Figure 9.7b). Inflammation is usually present in terminal and proximal respiratory bronchioles with lymphocytes, plasma cells and, occasionally, neutrophils; it may be replaced by fibrosis (Gough, 1968) (see under 'Chronic bronchitis'). There is also a loss of muscle in the inflamed walls of the emphysematous spaces which is indistinguishable from that said to be a feature of 'focal emphysema' (Thurlbeck, 1976) (see Chapter 13).

Centriacinar and panacinar emphysema often coexist in the same lung but, when advanced and widespread, differentiation may not be possible.

Periacinar (distal acinar) emphysema

Periacinar emphysema is uncommon and takes the form of rows of multiple enlarged airspaces from about 0.5 mm to about 2 cm in diameter, distributed typically along the anterior margins of the upper and middle lobes and lingula, at the costophrenic angle of the lower lobes (Figure 9.8). It also occurs along the septa and branches of blood vessels. Some of these airspaces, either on the surface or within the lung, may become bullae, sometimes of great size (Edge, Simon and Reid, 1966; Reid, 1967). Periacinar emphysema is often associated with (usually fine) fibrosis of the pulmonary pleura and interlobular septa but destruction of the

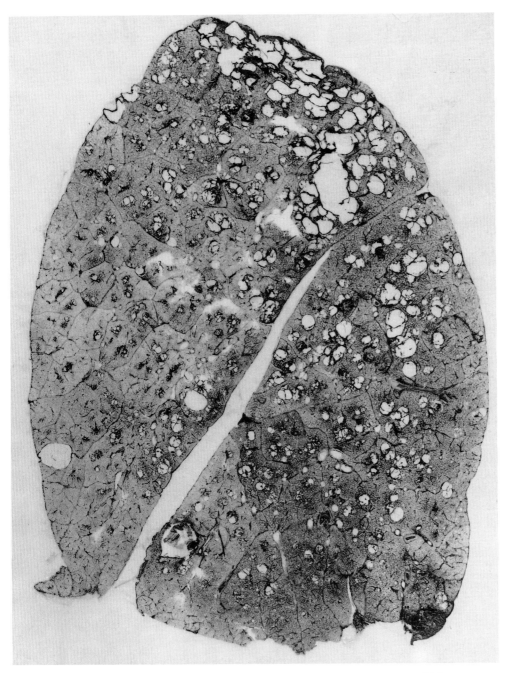

Figure 9.6 Whole lung section of moderate-to-severe centriacinar emphysema which, characteristically, is distributed mainly in the upper regions of the upper and lower lobes. Note that, apart from a few carbon macules, most of the adjacent and intervening lung is normal

parenchyma is dominant. It may simulate the 'honeycombing' of diffuse insterstitial pulmonary fibrosis (DIPF) both subpleurally and within the lung (Gough, 1968). Microscopically, the lesions are characterized by loss of alveolar walls in the distal part of the acinus which contains little or no lung tissue, but adjacent alveoli and lung are normal

(Heard, 1969). Fine fibrosis is also often present in the walls of the bullae (Gough, 1968).

Irregular (scar) emphysema

Irregular emphysema is probably the most common form of emphysema, involving two or more acini

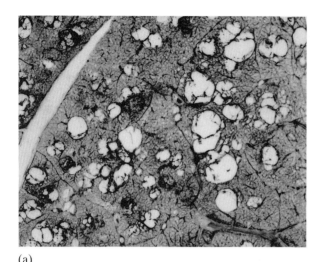

(a)

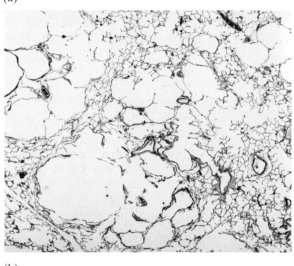

(b)

Figure 9.7 Centriacinar emphysema: (a) natural size –
note sharp demarcation from normal lung; (b)
microsection – normal lung between the lesions.
Magnification ×10. (Courtesy of Dr David Lamb)

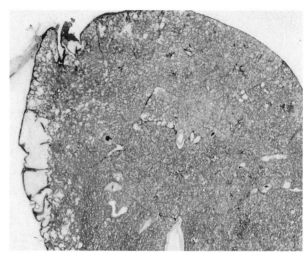

Figure 9.8 Distal acinar (paraseptal) emphysema of
moderate degree in an upper lobe. Most of the
underlying lung is normal. (Naturtal size)

within a lobule and affecting any or all of their
regions in irregular fashion; it is almost always
caused by contracted scar tissue. Scarring, however,
is not necessarily associated with emphysema.
Distension and rupture of alveoli, alveolar ducts and
respiratory bronchioles, to a varying degree, result
from retraction of the scar tissue. Scars may be
minute or large. Fine scarring in small lesions of coal
and similar types of pneumoconiosis in the walls of
respiratory bronchioles may cause emphysema in
the proximal part of the acinus (see Chapter 13).
Irregular emphysema of variable extent is
frequently found in the apices of the upper lobes,
and large areas may occur anywhere in the lungs.
The amount of lung tissue drawn into and lost in
scar tissue is often considerable, and much more

than the size of the scarred area might suggest –
sometimes the greater part of a lobe.

Occasionally, this type of emphysema may be
confused with the 'honeycomb' cysts of DIPF,
especially on paper-mounted whole lung sections,
but gross and microscopic inspection shows thick,
fibrotic lung between these cysts, which is not seen
between the enlarged airspaces of irregular emphysema. Microscopically, a varying degree of infiltration by lymphocyte and plasma cells is commonly
present in DIPF, sometimes with prominent smooth
muscle hyperplasia (see Chapter 15, page 521),
features absent in irregular emphysema in which
fibrous tissue in the distended and destroyed
airspace walls is quantitatively normal.

Pathogenesis

Disruption of the network of elastic fibres in the
lungs is generally held to be a cardinal factor in the
production of emphysema. The now well-known
association of an inherited deficiency of a protease
(elastase)-inhibiting serum protein, α_1-antitrypsin
(α_1-AT), with rapidly advancing emphysema in
some individuals (Laurell and Eriksson, 1963) led,
in combination with the observation that
widespread destructive emphysema developed in
the lungs of experimental animals after installation
of protease (Gross et al., 1965), to the
protease–antiprotease imbalance theory of the
pathogenesis of emphysema in man.

α_1-Antitrypsin, which is synthesized in the liver
and is a powerful inhibitor of elastase produced by

neutrophils, is identified with the protease inhibitor (Pi) chromosome locus; more than 80 phenotypes are known. Individual types are specified, according to their electrophoretic mobility, by the letters F, M, S and Z. The normal phenotype, present in more than 90 per cent of people, is PiM. Low plasma concentrations of α_1-AT and emphysema are associated with a number of α_1-AT phenotypes but the most common is PiZ. Some 80 to 90 per cent of PiZ individuals develop panacinar emphysema – often more severe at the base than elsewhere in the lung – and airflow obstruction that is of earlier onset and increased severity in smokers than in non-smokers with this defect. But this anomaly is rare. However, more significantly, it is now believed that elastase inactivation due to the potent oxidant effects of cigarette combustion (Janoff and Carp, 1977) is the chief cause of non-hereditary emphysema in smokers, although proof that such an event actually occurs in the lungs due to deficient elastase inhibitor (α_1-AT) has been difficult to establish. Nevertheless, three recent observations lend it support:

1. Substantially more neutrophils are present in the alveolar walls of smokers and animals exposed to cigarette smoke than in the alveolar walls of non-smokers (Ludwig et al., 1985).
2. Neutrophil elastase specifically localized in the emphysematous areas of smokers' lungs has been demonstrated immunohistologically (Damiano et al., 1986), although Bull et al. (1988) could not confirm this.
3. The level of plasma neutrophil elastase is significantly increased in healthy cigarette smokers compared with non-smokers (Weitz et al., 1987).

Thus, although some questions remain unanswered, it seems likely that unopposed neutrophil elastase activity makes an important contribution to continuing lung damage in cigarette smokers (Wewers, 1989). But why is it that lobar pneumonia, which is associated with an enormous influx of neutrophils, resolves without any trace of emphysema? The explanation is that pneumococci produce a potent inhibitor of neutrophil elastase and, in addition, α_1-AT concentration is increased in the pneumonic exudate (Janoff, 1985).

Centriacinar emphysema, as just stated, is often associated with chronic inflammation of terminal and respiratory bronchioles which is usually, but not exclusively, linked with smoking; local excess of elastase may well contribute to its development. Both neutrophils and alveolar macrophages accumulate in the lungs as part of the inflammatory response. Smokers' macrophages also produce an elastase which, unlike that from neutrophils, is not inhibited by α_1-AT (Laurent, Janoff and Kagan, 1983; Niederman et al., 1984) and they account for about 9 per cent of the total elastase in lung lavage fluid (McGowan et al., 1983a). Thus, it appears that both cell types cause increased elastolytic activity in the interstitium of the peripheral airspaces of smokers. Alveolar macrophages also ingest neutrophil elastase and, bearing in mind that their lifespan is 80 to 90 days and that of neutrophils is 1 to 2 days, they may act as an elastase reservoir which could have pathogenic significance because they are present in large numbers in the respiratory bronchioles of smokers (McGowan et al., 1983b). The typical distribution of centriacinar emphysema in the upper parts of the main lobes is attributed to the fact that these regions of the lungs are subjected to more gravitational strain than the lower parts (West, 1971; Forgacs, 1974). In addition, alteration in the pattern of ventilation that occurs during smoking tends to shift smoke particles preferentially into the upper lobes (Pearson et al., 1985) and, as perfusion in the lung bases is greater than in the upper parts, the availability of α_1-AT is likely to be greater in the lower zones (Cockcroft and Horne, 1982).

Another neutrophil elastase inhibitor, *antileukoprotease*, which is produced by the mucous glands and, probably, by Clara cells (see Chapter 1, page 8), is also inactivated by oxidants generated by inflammatory cells. However, it is important to note that, in some circumstances, even high concentrations of the protease inhibitors may fail to protect the lung from the proteolytic activity of inflammatory cells. This is because, on the one hand, these cells adhere so tightly to the lung matrix that antiprotease cannot gain access to the interface and, on the other, oxidants from inflammatory cells inactivate the inhibitors in their immediate proximity (Senior and Kuhn, 1988).

If the protease–antiprotease hypothesis is, in fact, correct, it is unlikely to be the only explanation of emphysema in smokers, because smoking not only inhibits the lung's defences against protease activity but it also comprises repair of injured tissue, and the relative importance of these two effects may differ in individuals (Senior and Kuhn, 1988).

At present, however, as Tetley (1992) has concluded, the plain fact is that 'Even after 30 years, we still do not know the exact combination of factors/mechanisms that predispose an individual to the development of emphysema'.

Gough (1947) and Heppleston (1947) attributed centriacinar emphysema of similar distribution in coal-miners' lungs to the action of accumulated coal dust – chiefly in the first and second respiratory bronchioles – and considered it to be a separate and specific form of emphysema – *focal emphysema*, an interpretation still maintained by some pathologists although many do not share this view. The topic is discussed in more detail in Chapter 13.

As stated earlier, irregular emphysema and many cases of periacinar emphysema result from varying degrees of fibrosis. In the case of irregular emphysema it is the sequel, among other causes, of unresolved pneumonia, granulomatous disease (such as tuberculosis and histoplasmosis), sarcoidosis, eosinophilic granuloma or contracted pneumoconiotic masses.

Clinical features

Emphysema of any type, sometimes extensive, may be found – often unexpectedly – in individuals who apparently had few or no respiratory symptoms during life. But the majority of cases of severe emphysema are associated with clinical evidence of chronic airflow obstruction. Physical examination is of limited value and imprecise in the diagnosis and evaluation of severity of emphysema.

As a rule, panacinar emphysema causes gradually increasing breathlessness on exertion and, ultimately, at rest. Abnormal physical signs are absent until it is advanced and widespread, when the chest may be hyperresonant and breath sounds much reduced; in some cases, central cyanosis is present. Centriacinar emphysema alone rarely causes symptoms, and when dyspnoea on exertion is present it is probably due to airflow obstruction resulting from bronchiolar disease. Periacinar emphysema is symptomless unless it gives rise to spontaneous pneumothorax or to large bullae; similarly, irregular emphysema is symptomless unless it is extensive, as is sometimes the case, for example, with healed tuberculosis or large contracted pneumoconiotic lesions. In general, all of the last three types are not detectable clinically, although, when bullous or irregular emphysema is severe, impaired expansion of the chest and intensity of breath sounds may be present on the affected side.

Physiology

Panacinar emphysema is associated with airflow obstruction due to loss of elastic recoil of the lung, and with impaired TLCO and low KCO which is caused by reduction in the area of alveolar capillary interspace available for gas exchange; this, in turn, leads to hypoxaemia and hyperventilation on exertion. Diminution of elastic recoil also results in premature collapse of the airways during expiration and, thus, in air trapping and a consequent increase in residual volume; likewise, the distensibility of the lung is increased and so, therefore, is the total lung capacity. In centriacinar emphysema, airflow obstruction is variable and, in many cases, negligi-

ble; in advanced disease, however, there may be reduction in effective alveolar ventilation with increased ventilation–perfusion inequality and some reduction in TLCO. Bullae may or may not be associated with airflow obstruction, depending upon whether they arise from panacinar or periacinar emphysema; when bullae are large, gas transfer may be impaired – though not in all cases – owing to the presence of a large unventilated space (Davies, Simon and Reid, 1966). When irregular emphysema is extensive, airflow obstruction, alterations of lung volumes and impaired gas transfer are usual.

Ischaemic heart disease

Emphysema and chronic airflow obstruction are known to be associated with a reduced incidence of atherosclerotic heart disease (see also Chapter 13, page 401). This may be due to increased levels of high-density lipoprotein, cholesterol and apolipoprotein AI in chronic airflow obstruction; they are believed to exert a protective effect against the development of ischaemic heart disease (Bolton et al., 1989).

Radiographic diagnosis

On routine chest radiography (posteroanterior (PA) and lateral films), the diagnosis of panacinar emphysema rests on the appearances of over-inflation and reduction in the peripheral branches of the pulmonary artery which are seen in varying degree in moderate-to-severe emphysema. Although Burki (1989) concluded that standard radiographs do not detect emphysema reliably, Lohela et al. (1984) found that, by comparing radiographic appearances of lungs during life and *post mortem*, emphysema of moderate-to-severe degree can be diagnosed with an overall accuracy of 77 per cent on standard PA and lateral films during life using the following well-known criteria: blunting of costophrenic angles, depression of the domes of the diaphragm, widening of the retrosternal translucency and the sternodiaphragmatic angle (lateral films), irregular radiolucencies and reduction in the peripheral vascular pattern in the lung fields (PA films).

Centriacinar (proximal acinar) emphysema, whether or not associated with dust, is not detectable on standard radiographs. Periacinar emphysema, when severe, may be clearly identified on routine PA films as a row of translucent areas at the periphery of the lung field in the upper and midzones; sometimes they are associated with bullae which are easily recognizable and may be very large (Edge, Simon and Reid, 1966). More often, however, this type of emphysema is an unexpected autopsy finding. Irregular emphysema is identifiable, when fairly advanced, as hyperlucent areas of lung around fibrotic lesions.

Irregular linear opacities are sometimes present in the lower lung fields and appear to be the result of an accentuation of the normal differences between absorption of X-rays by air and by lung – approximately 1 : 800); that is, more air and less lung in emphysematous areas increase the radiographic contrast in the image between air and adjacent remaining lung tissue. This contrast effect may be increased by the presence in the lung parenchyma of dusts with atomic numbers greater than carbon (see Chapter 7, page 163). There is also evidence of a significant association between this type of opacity and cigarette smoking (Weiss, 1988). Smoking, in fact, is associated with varying histological degrees of fine DIPF and emphysema, the severity of both being related to the amount smoked. This has relevance to the interpretation of irregular opacities in the radiographs of coal miners, asbestos workers and others, which is discussed in Chapters 7, 13 and 14.

A quantitative, computed tomographic (CT) scanning technique has been reported which appears to be capable of diagnosing, locating and quantifying mild-to-severe emphysema with a high degree of accuracy (Gould et al., 1988), although the conclusion from another investigation in which preoperative scans were compared with the pathology of subsequently resected lungs was that CT images fail to differentiate mild centriacinar and panacinar emphysema from normal parenchyma (Miller et al., 1989). However, high-resolution CT (see Chapter 7) can distinguish both types of emphysema at an early stage (Kuwano et al., 1990).

References

Adesina, A.M., Vallyathan, V., McQuillen, E.N., Weaver, S.O. and Craighead, J.E. (1991). Bronchiolar inflammation and fibrosis associated with smoking: a morphological cross-sectional population analysis. *Am. Rev. Respir. Dis.* **143**, 144–149

American Thoracic Society (1987) Standards for the diagnosis and care of patients with chronic obstructive pulmonary disease (COPD) and asthma. *Am. Rev. Respir. Dis.* **136**, 225–228

Anthonisen, N.R. (1989) Prognosis in chronic obstructive pulmonary disease: results from multicenter clinical trials. *Am. Rev. Respir. Dis.* **140**, 595–599

Backhouse, A. and Holland, W.W. (1989) Trends in mortality from chronic obstructive airways disease in the United Kingdom. *Thorax* **44**, 529–532

Barker, D.J.P. (1991) The intrauterine origins of cardio-vascular and obstructive lung disease in adult life. *J. R. Coll. Physns Lond.* **25**, 129–133

Becroft, D.M.O. (1971) Bronchiolitis obliterans, bronchiectasis and sequelae of adenovirus type 21 infection in young children. *J. Clin. Pathol.* **24**, 72–82

Bhaskar, K.R., O'Sullivan, D.D., Selzer, J., Rossing, T.H., Drazen, J.M. and Reid, L.M. (1985) Density gradient study of bronchial mucus aspirates from healthy volunteers (smokers and non-smokers) and from patients with tracheostomy. *Expl Lung Res.* **9**, 289–308

Bolton, C.H.M., Mulloy, E., Harvey, J., Downs, L.G. and Hartog, M. (1989) Plasma and lipoprotein lipids and apolipoproteins AI, AII and B in patients with chronic airflow limitation. *J. R. Soc. Med.* **82**, 91–92

Bull, T.B., Tetley, T.D., Guz, A., Harris, E. and Fox, B. (1988) Is neutrophil elastase associated with elastic tissue in emphysema? *J. Pathol.* **154**, 64A

Burki, N.K. (1989) Roentgenologic diagnosis of emphysema. *Chest* **95**, 1178–1179

Burrows, B. (1981) An overview of obstructive lung disease. *Med. Clins North Am.* **65**, 455–471

Cerveri, I., Bruschi, C., Zola, M.C., Maccarini, L., Grassi, M., Lebowitz, M.D., Rampulla, C. and Grassi, C. (1989) Smoking habit and bronchial reactivity in normal subjects. *Am. Rev. Respir. Dis.* **140**, 191–196

Ciba Foundation Guest Symposium (1959) Terminology, definitions and classification of chronic pulmonary emphysema and related conditions. *Thorax* **14**, 286–299

Ciba Foundation Study Group No. 38 (1971) In *Identification of Asthma* (eds R. Porter and J. Birch), Churchill Livingstone, Edinburgh

Cockcroft, D.W. and Horne, S.L. (1982) Localization of emphysema within the lung. An hypothesis based upon ventilation/perfusion relationships. *Chest* **82**, 483–487

Collis, E.L. (1923) The general and occupational prevalence of bronchitis and its relation to other respiratory diseases. *J. Ind. Hyg. Toxicol.* **5**, 264–276

Cosio, M.G., Hale, K.A. and Niewoehner, D.E. (1980) Morphologic and morphometric effects of prolonged cigarette smoking on the small airways. *Am. Rev. Respir. Dis.* **122**, 265–271

Cosio, M.G., Ghezo, H., Hogg, J.C., Corbin, R., Loveland, M., Dosman, J. and Macklem, P.T. (1978) The relations between structural changes in small airways and pulmonary function tests. *N. Engl. J. Med.* **298**, 1277–1281

Cullinan, P. (1991) Aetiological factors in chronic sputum production. *Thorax* **46**, 773

Damiano, V.V., Tsang, A., Kucich, U., Abrams, W.R., Rosenbloom, J., Kimbel, P., Fallahnejad, M.K. and Weinbaum, G. (1986) Immunolocalization of elastase in human emphysematous lungs. *J. Clin. Invest.* **78**, 482–493

Davies, G.M., Simon, G. and Reid, L. (1966) Pre- and post-operative assessment of emphysema. *Br. J. Dis. Chest* **60**, 120–128

De Jongste, J.C., Mons, H., Block, R., Bonta, I.L., Frederiksz, A.P. and Kerrebijn, K.F. (1987) Increased *in vitro* histamine responses in human small airways smooth muscle from patients with chronic obstructive pulmonary disease. *Am. Rev. Respir. Dis.* **135**, 549–553

Douglas, A.N. (1980) Quantitative study of bronchial mucous gland enlargement. *Thorax* **35**, 198–201

Edge, J., Simon, G. and Reid, L. (1966) Periacinar (paraseptal) emphysema: its clinical, radiological and physiological features. *Br. J. Dis. Chest* **60**, 10–18

Enjeti, S., Hazelwood, N., Permott, S., Menkes, H. and Terry, P. (1978) Pulmonary function in young smokers; male–female differences. *Am. Rev. Respir. Dis.* **118**, 667–676

Epler, G.R., Snider, G.L., Gaensler, E.A., Cathcart, E.S., Fitzgerald, M.X. and Carrington, C.B. (1979) Bronchiolitis in connective tissue diseases. *J. Am. Med. Assoc.* **242**, 528–532

Fletcher, C.M. and Peto, R. (1977) The natural history of chronic airflow obstruction. *Br. Med. J.* **1**, 1645–1648

Fletcher, C.M. and Pride, N.B. (1984) Definitions of emphysema, chronic bronchitis, asthma, and airflow obstruction: 25 years on from the Ciba symposium. *Thorax* **39**, 81–85

Fletcher, C., Peto, R., Tinker, C. and Speizer, F.E. (1976a) The natural history of chronic airflow obstruction. *Br. Med. J.* **1**, 1645–1648

Fletcher, C., Peto, R., Tinker, C. and Speizer, F.E. (1976b) *The Natural History of Chronic Bronchitis and Emphysema*. Oxford University Press, London

Forgacs, P. (1974) Gravitational stress in lung disease. *Br. J. Dis. Chest* **68**, 1–10

Geddes, D.M., Webley, M. and Emerson, P.A. (1979) Airways obstruction in rheumatoid arthritis. *Ann. rheum. Dis.* **38**, 222–225

Geddes, D.M., Corrin, B., Brewerton, D.A., Davies, R.J. and Turner-Warwick, M. (1977) Progressive airway obliteration in adults and its association with rheumatoid disease. *Q. J. Med.* **184**, 427–444

Glezen, W.P. (1989) Antecedents of chronic and recurrent lung disease. Childhood respiratory trouble. *Am. Rev. Respir. Dis.* **140**, 873–874

Gold, D., Tager, I.B., Weiss, S.T., Tosteson, T.D. and Speizer, F.E. (1989) Acute lower respiratory illness in childhood as a predictor of lung function and chronic respiratory symptoms. *Am. Rev. Respir. Dis.* **140**, 877–884

Gough, J. (1947) Pneumoconiosis in coal workers in Wales. *Occup. Med.* **4**, 86–97

Gough, J. (1968) The pathogenesis of emphysema. In *The Lung* (eds A.A. Liebow and D.E. Smith), Williams & Wilkins, Baltimore, pp. 109–133

Gould, G.A., Macnee, W., McLean, A., Warren, P.M., Redpath, A., Best, J.J.K., Lamb, D. and Flenley, D.C. (1988) CT measurements of lung density in life can quantitate distal airspace enlargement – an essential defining feature of human emphysema. *Am. Rev. Respir. Dis.* **137**, 380–392

Gross, P., Pfitzer, E.A., Tolker, E., Babyak, M.A. and Kaschak, M. (1965) Experimental emphysema. *Archs Envir. Health* **11**, 50–58

Heard, B.E. (1969) *Pathology of Chronic Bronchitis and Emphysema*. Churchill, London

Heppleston, A.G. (1947) The essential lesion of pneumoconiosis in Welsh coal workers. *J. Pathol. Bacteriol.* **59**, 453–460

Heppleston, A.G. (1972) The pathological recognition and pathogenesis of emphysema and fibrocystic disease of the lungs with special reference to coal workers. *Ann. NY Acad. Sci.* **200**, 347–369

Herzog, C.A., Miller, R.R. and Hoidal, J.R. (1981) Bronchiolitis and rheumatoid arthritis. *Am. Rev. Respir. Dis.* **124**, 636–639

Hogg, J.C., Macklem, P.T. and Thurlbeck, W.M. (1968) Site and nature of airways obstruction in chronic obstructive lung disease. *N. Engl. J. Med.* **278**, 1355–1360

Holland, W.W., Colley, J.R.T., Leeder, S.R., Crockhill, R.N. and Halil, T. (1977) Comment absorber en épidémiologie l'étude de la bronchite chronique et de ses signes précurseurs chez l'enfant. *Revue fr. Mal. Respir.* **5**, 87–94

Hopp, J., Townley, R.G., Biven, R.E., Bewtra, A.K. and Nair, N.M. (1990) The presence of airway reactivity before the development of asthma. *Am. Rev. Respir. Dis.* **141**, 2–8

Janoff, A. (1985) Elastase and emphysema. Current assessment of the protease–antiprotease hypothesis. *Am. Rev. Respir. Dis.* **132**, 417–433

Janoff, A. and Carp, H. (1977) Possible mechanisms of emphysema in smokers: cigarette smoke condensate suppresses proteinase inhibition in vitro. *Am. Rev. Respir. Dis.* **116**, 65–72

Kuwano, K., Matsuba, K., Ikeda, T., Murakami, J., Araki, A., Nishitani, H., Ishida, T., Yasumoto, K.K. and Shigematsu, N. (1990) The diagnosis of mild emphysema. Correlation of computed tomography and pathology scores. *Am. Rev. Respir. Dis.* **141**, 169–178

Laraya-Cuasay, L.R., De Forrest, A., Huff, D., Lischner, H. and Huang, N.N. (1977) Chronic pulmonary complications of early influenza virus infection in children. *Am. Rev. Respir. Dis.* **116**, 617–625

Larson, R.K., Barman, M.L., Kueppers, F. and Fudenberg, H.H. (1970) Genetic and environmental determinants of chronic obstructive pulmonary disease. *Ann. Intern. Med.* **72**, 627–632

Laurell, C.-B. and Eriksson, S. (1963) The electrophoretic α_1-globulin pattern of serum in α_1-antitrypsin deficiency. *Scand. J. Clin. Lab. Invest.* **15**, 132–140

Laurent, P., Janoff, A. and Kagan, H.M. (1983) Cigarette smoke blocks cross-linking of elastin in vivo. *Am. Rev. Respir. Dis.* **127**, 189–192

Linhartová, A. and Anderson, A.E. Jr (1983) Small airways in severe panlobular emphysema: mural thickening and premature closure. *Am. Rev. Respir. Dis.* **127**, 42–45

Lohela, P., Sutinen, S., Pääkkö, P., Lahti, R. and Tienari, J. (1984) Diagnosis of emphysema on chest radiographs. *Fortschr. Röntgenstr.* **141**, 395–402

Lourdes, R., Laraya-Cuasay, D.A., Palmer, J., Hugg, D.S., Lischner, H.W. and Huang, N.N. (1974) Chronic pulmonary complications of early influenza virus infection. *Am. Rev. Respir. Dis.* **109**, 703 (abstract)

Ludwig, P.W., Schwartz, B.A., Hoidal, J.R. and Niewoehner, D.E. (1985) Cigarette smoking causes accumulation of polymorphonuclear leukocytes in alveolar septum. *Am. Rev. Respir. Dis.* **131**, 828–830

McGowan, S.E., Arbeit, R.D., Stone, P.J. and Snider, G.L. (1983a) A comparison of the bonding fate of internalized neutrophil elastase in human monocytes and alveolar macrophages. *Am. Rev. Respir. Dis.* **128**, 688–694

McGowan, S.E., Stone, P.J., Calare, J.D., Snider, G.L. and Franzblau, C. (1983b) The fate of neutrophil elastase incorporated by human alveolar macrophages. *Am. Rev. Respir. Dis.* **127**, 449–455

Medical Research Council (1960) Committee on the Aetiology of Chronic Bronchitis. Standardized questionnaires on respiratory symptoms. *Br. Med. J.* **2**, 1665

Medical Research Council (1965) Special Committee on Aetiology of Chronic Bronchitis. Definition and classification of chronic bronchitis of clinical and epidemiological purposes. *Lancet* **1**, 775–779

Medical Research Council (1966) Special Committee. Chronic bronchitis and occupation. *Br. Med. J.* **1**, 101–102

Medical Research Council (1976) *Questionnaire on Respiratory Symptoms*. Medical Research Council, London

Medical Research Council (1986) Committee on Environmental and Occupational Health. *Questionnaire on Respiratory Symptoms*. Medical Research Council, London

Miller, R.R., Müller, N.L., Vedal, S., Morrison, N.J. and Staples, C.A. (1989) Limitations of computed tomography in the assessment of emphysema. *Am. Rev. Respir. Dis.* **139**, 980–983

Niederman, M.S., Fritts, L.L., Merrill, W.W., Fick, R.B., Matthay, R.A., Reynolds, H.Y. and Gee, J.B.L. (1984) Demonstration of free elastolytic metalloenzyme in human lung lavage fluid and its relationship to alpha$_1$-antiprotease. *Am. Rev. Respir. Dis.* **129**, 943–947

Nolte, D. and Berger, D. (1983) On vagal bronchoconstriction in asthmatic patients induced by nasal irritation. *Eur. J. Respir. Dis.* suppl. 128, 110–114

O'Connor, G.T., Sparrow, D. and Weiss, S.T. (1989) The role of allergy and non-specific airway hyperresponsiveness in the pathogenesis of chronic obstructive pulmonary disease. *Am. Rev. Respir. Dis.* **140**, 225–252

Openshaw, P.J.M. and Turner-Warwick, M. (1989) Observations on sputum production in patients with variable airflow obstruction; implications for the diagnosis of asthma and chronic bronchitis. *Respir. Med.* **83**, 25–31

Orie, N.G.M., Sluiter, H.J., de Vries, K., Tammeling, G.J. and Witkop, J. (1961) The host factor in bronchitis. In *Bronchitis, an international symposium*, April 1960, University of Groningen. Royal Van Gorcum, Assen, pp. 43–59

Oxhøj, H., Bake, B. and Wilhelmsen, L. (1976) Spirometry and flow–volume curves in 10-year follow up in men born in 1913. *Scand. J. Respir. Dis.* **57**, 310–311

Pearson, M.G., Chamberlain, M.J., Morgan, W.K.C. and Vinitski, S. (1985) Regional deposition of particles in the lung during cigarette smoking in humans. *J. Appl. Physiol.* **59**, 1828–1833

Radoux, V., Ménard, A., Bégin, R., Décary, F. and Koopman, W.J. (1987) Airways disease in rheumatoid arthritis patients. *Arthr. Rheum.* **30**, 249–256

Reid, L. (1960) Measurement of bronchial mucous gland layer; a diagnostic yardstick in chronic bronchitis. *Thorax* **15**, 132–141

Reid, L. (1967) *The Pathology of Emphysema*, Lloyd Luke, London

Reid, L.M. (1988) Chronic obstructive pulmonary disease. In *Pulmonary Diseases and Disorders*, 2nd edn, vol. 2 (ed. Alfred P. Fishman), McGraw-Hill, New York, pp. 1247–1272

Senior, R.M. and Kuhn, E. III (1988) The pathogenesis of emphysema. In *Pulmonary Diseases and Disorders*, 2nd edn, vol. 2 (ed. Alfred P. Fishman), McGraw-Hill, New York, pp. 1209–1218

Segal, I., Fink, G., Machtey, I., Gura, V. and Spitzer, S.A. (1981) Pulmonary function abnormalities in Sjögren's syndrome and the sicca complex. *Thorax* **36**, 286–289

Skillrud, D.M., Offord, K.P. and Miller, R.D. (1986) Higher risk of lung cancer in chronic obstructive pulmonary disease. *Ann. Intern. Med.* **105**, 503–507

Snider, G.L., Kleinerman, J., Thurlbeck, W.M. and Bengali, Z.H. (1985) The definition of emphysema: report of a National Heart, Lung and Blood Institute Division of Lung Diseases Workshop. *Am. Rev. Respir. Dis.* **132**, 182–185

Speizer, F.E. and Tager, I.B. (1979) Epidemiology of chronic mucus hypersecretion and obstructive airways disease. *Epidemiol. Rev.* **1**, 124–142

Tager, I., Tishler, P.V., Rosner, B., Speizer, F.E. and Litt, M. (1978) Studies of familial aggregation of chronic bronchitis and obstructive airway disease. *Int. J. Epidemiol.* **7**, 55–62

Taylor, R.G., Joyce, H., Gross, E., Holland, F. and Pride, N.B. (1985) Bronchial reactivity to inhaled histamine and annual rate of decline in FEV$_1$ in male smokers and ex-smokers. *Thorax* **40**, 9–16

Tetley, T.D. (1992) Emphysema revisited. *Respir. Med.* **86**, 187–193

Thurlbeck, W.M. (1968) Chronic obstructive lung disease. In *Pathology Annual* (ed. S.C. Sommers), Appleton-Century-Crofts, New York, pp. 367–398

Thurlbeck, W.M. (1976) *Chronic Airflow Obstruction in Lung Disease*, vol. V, *Major Problems in Pathology* (ed. James L. Bennington), W.B. Saunders, Philadelphia, London

Thurlbeck, W.M. (1980) Smoking, airflow limitation and the pulmonary circulation. *Am. Rev. Respir. Dis.* **122**, 183–186

Thurlbeck, W.M. (1985) Chronic airflow obstruction: correlation of structure and function. In *Chronic Obstructive Pulmonary Disease*, 2nd edn (ed. Thomas L. Petty) Marcel Dekker, New York, Basel, pp. 167–168

Thurlbeck, W.M. (1988) Chronic airflow obstruction. In *Pathology of the Lung* (ed. W.M. Thurlbeck), Thième Medical Publishers, New York, p. 529

Thurlbeck, W.M., Ryder, R.C. and Sternby, N. (1974) A comparative study of the severity of emphysema in necropsy populations in three different countries. *Am. Rev. Respir. Dis.* **109**, 239–248

Tockman, A.S., Anthonisen, N.R., Wright, E.C. and Donithan, M.G. (1987) IPPB trial group, Johns Hopkins lung project. Airway obstruction and the risk for lung cancer. *Ann. Intern. Med.* **106**, 512–518

Traver, G.A., Cline, M.G. and Burrows, B. (1979) Predictors of mortality in chronic obstructive pulmonary disease. A 15-year follow-up study. *Am. Rev. Respir. Dis.* **119**, 895–902

Voter, K.Z., Henry, M.M., Stewar, P.W. and Henderson, F.W. (1988) Lower respiratory tract illness in early childhood and lung function and bronchial reactivity in adolescent males. *Am. Rev. Respir. Dis.* **137**, 302–307

Weiss, W. (1988) Smoking and pulmonary fibrosis. *J. Occup. Med.* **30**, 33–39

Weitz, J.I., Crowley, K.A., Landman, S.L., Lipman, B.I. and Yu, J. (1987) Increased neutrophil elastase activity in cigarette smokers. *Ann. Intern. Med.* **107**, 680–682

West, J.B. (1971) Distribution of mechanical stress in the lung; a possible factor in localisation of pulmonary disease. *Lancet* **1**, 839–841

Wewers, M. (1989) Pathogenesis of emphysema. Assessment of basic science concepts through clinical investigation. *Chest* **95**, 190–195

Wilson, R.W. (1973) Increased prevalence of sinusitis among smokers compared with non-smokers. *J. Occup. Med.* **15**, 236–244

Yan, K., Salome, C.M. and Woolcock, A.J. (1985) Prevalence and nature of bronchial hyper-responsiveness in subjects with chronic obstructive pulmonary disease. *Am. Rev. Respir. Dis.* **132**, 25–29

Zamel, N., Webster, P., Lorimer, E., Man, S. and Wolf, C. (1981) Environment versus genetics in determining bronchial susceptibility to cigarette smoke. *Chest* suppl. 80, 57

10

Bronchitis, airways' obstruction and occupation

W.K.C. Morgan

The inhalation and deposition of dust in the lungs have been known for many years to lead to respiratory symptoms and, in particular, shortness of breath, cough and phlegm. Although Thackrah (1832) and Greenhow (1861) assumed these symptoms indicated a diagnosis of bronchitis and inferred that dust was responsible, in retrospect it is apparent that the causes of, and diseases producing, such symptoms in workers in the dusty trades and, indeed, in those who were not exposed to dust were several. With the advent of chest radiography, improvements in bacteriology and, in particular, the isolation of the tubercle bacillus and other respiratory pathogens, as well as the application of epidemiology to the study of respiratory disease, it became possible to distinguish the various diseases that are associated with cough, sputum and shortness of breath.

Early in this century, Haldane (1925) made the observation that coal miners had fewer bronchitic symptoms and a lower mortality than did metal miners. At that time cigarette smoking played a small role in the induction of bronchitis and respiratory impairment. Between 1925 and 1940, British coal mines became mechanized and the dust levels to which coal miners were exposed rose significantly. Concomitant with this was an increase in the incidence and prevalence of respiratory disease. Much of the increased frequency of respiratory disease was subsequently found to be a consequence of coal pneumoconiosis and prompted the government of the day to establish the Pneumoconiosis Research Unit (PRU) of the Medical Research Council (MRC).

In 1961, a 5 per cent sample of the entire population of Great Britain was surveyed by the Ministry of Pensions and National Insurance. The results of this survey indicated that bronchitis was an important cause of absenteeism in the working classes, and that miners and quarrymen were particularly affected. Subsequently, the Ministry of Pensions asked the MRC to set up a committee to study the aetiology of bronchitis with particular emphasis on the role played by occupation.

In 1966, the MRC Committee published a report (Medical Research Council, 1966) that examined the role of bronchitis as a cause of respiratory disability. The Committee also noted that chronic bronchitis had a multifactorial aetiology and that cigarette smoking, air pollution, social class and dust exposure all apparently played a role. The Committee also noted that, because the symptoms of bronchitis were the same whatever the cause, it was not possible to apportion the contribution of a particular exposure or factor, or to know whether any impairment that may be present was a consequence of occupational or other factors. The Committee concluded that, although the dusty occupations had a greater incidence and prevalence of bronchitis, and in this regard it was apparent that coal miners and foundry workers had a greater morbidity and mortality from bronchitis, it was difficult to show a direct cause-and-effect relationship between dust exposure and either morbidity or mortality. Thus, the wives of coal miners and foundry workers were also found to have more cough and sputum and, on occasion, a lower ventilatory capacity than did the wives of non-miners. This suggested that factors other than occupation were important contributory factors to the bronchitis of miners and foundry men. The Committee suggested that dust played only a limited role in the induction of bronchitis and respiratory disability, but they recommended that the situation be kept under review. The MRC Committee's report occasioned several critical responses, but the arguments used to rebut the Committee's conclusions seemed based on clinical impression, sympathy and political ideology rather than objective evidence (Gough, 1966; McLaughlin, 1966; Pemberton, 1966).

Bronchitis, ventilatory impairment and exposure to dust

When compared with a matched reference population, workers in the dusty trades have an increased prevalence of bronchitis as manifested by the presence of cough and sputum (Higgins and Cochrane, 1958; Higgins, 1960). Although many of the initial observations in this regard were made in coal miners (Higgins and Cochrane, 1958; Gilson, 1970), over the years similar findings have been noted in steel workers (Lowe, 1968; Lowe, Campbell and Khosla, 1970), foundry men (Lloyd Davies, 1971), textile workers (Pratt, Vollmer and Miller, 1980; Morgan et al., 1982), gold miners (Irwig and Rocks, 1978), cement workers (Kalačič, 1973a,b) and in those who work with bauxite (Townsend et al., 1985). The increased prevalence of cough and sputum has, in many instances, been accompanied by a slight reduction in ventilatory capacity. This is reflected as a lower forced expiratory volume in 1 second (FEV_1) in the presence of a relatively normal or only slightly reduced forced vital capacity (FVC). Such a reduction in the ventilatory capacity may be seen in coal miners and those exposed to silica in the absence of progressive massive fibrosis or conglomerate silicosis (Higgins, 1972; Irwig and Rocks, 1978).

A number of studies have been carried out in coal miners which make it clear that the ventilatory defect does not appear to be related to the presence of simple coal pneumoconiosis (Cochrane, Higgins and Thomas, 1961; Morgan et al., 1974) (Figure 10.1). (See Chapter 7 for ILO Classification of Radiographs of the Pneumoconioses.) Similar studies have shown an analogous situation in silica-exposed populations, in that a reduced ventilatory capacity may be seen in both those with and without simple silicosis (Irwig and Rocks, 1978). The reduction in ventilatory capacity which occurs in such subjects can be explained in two ways:

1. A condition exists which induces airflow obstruction, this being peculiar to the dusty trades and

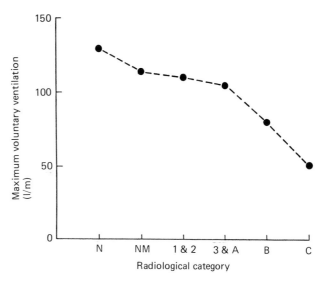

Figure 10.1 The relationship between the ILO radiographic category and ventilatory capacity. N = non-miners, NM = miners with a normal radiograph, 1/2 etc. represent the various categories. Ventilatory capacity was assessed as the $FEV_{0.75}$. This was converted to an indirect MVV by multiplying by 40. (Reproduced, with permission, from Gilson, 1957, derived from the late Professor A.A. Cochrane and I.T.T. Higgins, *Industrial Pulmonary Disease*, with permission from Little, Brown & Co., 1960)

affecting miners with and without simple pneumoconiosis. This condition could be either emphysema or bronchitis, or both.
2. Differential migration is responsible. When new workers are recruited to the industry, and the fitter and younger men subsequently leave within months or a few years of starting work, those who remain in the mines would probably have a lower ventilatory capacity and would not be representative of the total population who started work.

It was noted some years ago that, during hard times and when unemployment was high in the coal industry, those who left the industry and sought employment elsewhere tended to be both fitter and younger (Cochrane, Higgins and Thomas, 1961). Over the last 20 to 30 years, however, this has not been the case and, indeed, a study by McClintock (1971) of new entrants into coal mining in Britain showed that it was the more muscular and, probably, fitter recruits who stayed in the industry. This might, perhaps, also explain why coal miners with categories 2 and 3 simple pneumoconiosis often have a higher ventilatory capacity than those with category 1 and those with normal chest radiographs (see Chapter 7). Thus, the explanation for the increased prevalence of cough and sputum, and of increased airways' obstruction, cannot be explained by selective migration and would seem to be related to the development of either emphysema or chronic bronchitis, or both.

Definition and pathology of bronchitis

Until recently, a diagnosis of bronchitis implied a condition characterized by cough and sputum, and one usually associated with a reduction in ventilatory capacity or likely to lead to such a reduction. The work of Fletcher et al. (1969) provided the stimulus for a definition of bronchitis that depended solely on the symptoms of cough and sputum without reference to lung function. [The currently accepted definition of 'chronic bronchitis' is discussed in Chapter 9.]

The seminal studies of Reid (1960) at the Brompton Hospital characterized the pathological features of bronchitis. She showed that there was an increase in the depth and number of mucus-secreting glands in the airways. The mucous glands of the large airways are mostly responsible for secretion of mucus (see Chapter 9). The ratio of the depth of the mucous glands (gland thickness) to the bronchial wall thickness, measured from the surface of the respiratory epithelium to the cartilage, is known as the *Reid index* and provides a most useful way of quantifying the degree and severity of bronchitis (Figure 10.2).

Bronchitis and mucous gland hyperplasia may occur as a result of long continued exposure to any number of chronic irritants, including cigarette smoke, dust and air pollutants, whether they are particulate or gaseous. Continued exposure to sulphur dioxide, ozone or ammonia may produce chronic bronchitis. When attempting to study the prevalence of bronchitis in a working population, and in trying to determine the cause of the bronchitis, there are two important confounding factors, namely, cigarette smoking and age. In cigarette smokers, the effects of smoking completely overwhelm the effects of air pollution, dust and other factors. In women, the prevalence of bronchitis frequently does not show the same clear-cut relationship to smoking and often appears to be related to social class (Enterline and Lainhart, 1967). This is a consequence of the fact that women in the professional classes tend to be reluctant to admit to coughing up sputum.

Bronchitis, emphysema and cigarette smoking

It is now apparent that cigarette smoking may lead to both bronchitis and emphysema, and that the two are distinct and unrelated responses (Fletcher et al., 1976) (see Chapter 9). Chronic bronchitis, as described by Reid (1960), mainly involves the glands of the larger airways, although the goblet cells of the smaller airways are to some extent affected. Chronic bronchitis tends to be reversible and, after a subject has stopped smoking for 6 to 9 months, his or her cough and sputum usually clear up. As a result of their long-term studies in a cigarette-smoking population, Fletcher et al. (1976) clearly indicated that bronchitis does not invariably lead to emphysema and, moreover, is associated with little in the way of ventilatory impairment. Some degree of bronchial hypersecretion is found in virtually every smoker of more than 10 cigarettes a day who has been smoking for more than 5 years. In contrast, emphysema has been defined as an anatomical alteration of the lungs, characterized by an abnormal enlargement of the airspaces distal to the terminal bronchiole and associated with destruction of the alveolar walls (see Chapter 9). It is associated with irreversible airways' obstruction and cannot be expected to improve when the subject stops smoking. More importantly, as is evident from the studies of Fletcher et al. (1976), Bates (1973), Thurlbeck et al. (1970) and Jamal et al. (1984), chronic bronchitis neither causes significant airways' obstruction nor portends the development of chronic, irreversible airways' obstruction which, in any case, occurs in only 12 to 15 per cent of those who are cigarette smokers. Whilst the presence or absence of airways' obstruction is not an all-or-none

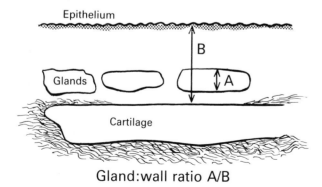

Figure 10.2 Diagrammatic representation of the Reid index. A represents the thickness of the bronchial mucous gland layer whilst B represents the depth from the surface of the respiratory mucosa to the cartilage in the bronchial wall

attribute, and it is clear that a spectrum of suscepti-bility exists, nevertheless, there seem to be two contrasting groups, namely: the susceptible subjects who, in their normal lifespan, may become disabled by obstruction if they happen to be smokers; and the non-susceptibles who will not develop obstruction irrespective of smoking habit.

If a comparison is made of the mean FEV_1 of smokers and non-smokers, in most instances a sizeable disparity is not evident. This results from the fact that the real effect of smoking on the FEV_1 occurs only in the susceptible minority, and is more or less obscured by the virtually normal FEV_1 of the majority. Nevertheless, among the susceptible majority some are severely affected and suffer premature disability and death. It is also abundantly evident that those who are cigarette smokers, and who happen to have airways' obstruction, tend to underestimate their cigarette consumption, or have reduced their cigarette consumption because of their symptoms and imply that their reduced consumption reflects their life-time average cigarette consumption (see also page 223).

Emphysema, airways' obstruction and exposure to coal-mine dust

It is necessary to point out that in the ageing popula-tion emphysema is found frequently *post mortem* without any obvious cause and such subjects may have shown no impairment of ventilatory capacity (see Chapter 9). It is also abundantly clear from the work of Ryder, Dunnill and Anderson (1971) that at least 15 to 20 per cent of the lungs needs to be involved before the subject is likely to complain of shortness of breath or to have a reduced ventilatory capacity. Minor degrees of emphysema, therefore, do not lead to symptoms of breathlessness.

A series of papers from South Wales have put forward the proposition that coal miners have a higher prevalence of emphysema than do non-miners (Ryder et al., 1970; Lyons et al., 1972; Lyons and Campbell, 1976). The authors of these papers have attempted to relate emphysema demonstrated *post mortem* to measurements of lung function *ante mortem* and to radiographic category. The subjects included in these studies had been referred to a pneumoconiosis medical panel. Emphysema was quantified by point counting. All such subjects had claimed compensation and most had serial pulmonary function tests performed as a result of

the compensation they had been awarded. The investigators claimed to have demonstrated a relationship between the presence of simple pneumoconiosis and progressive massive fibrosis (PMF) and pulmonary impairment *ante mortem* as diagnosed by a reduction in the ventilatory capacity, measured by the FEV_1. They suggested that the p type of opacity is associated with emphysema more frequently than the larger q and r types (see 'Radiographic classification of pneumoconiosis', Chapter 7). The statement that 'there is no reason why these deaths should not provide a true sample of experience of men with this disease' (that is, coal pneumoconiosis) appeared in their first paper. This would imply that the sample of subjects was repre-sentative of coal miners not only in Wales, but throughout Britain and, indeed, the rest of the world. The notion that disability claimants can be regarded as a random and unbiased sample was disputed by Gilson and Oldham (1970). By the same token, Ryder et al. (1970) attempted to relate the presence of emphysema to the radiographic category of pneumoconiosis and, in so doing, made no distinction between those subjects who had simple and complicated disease. Since categories B and C of progressive massive fibrosis (PMF) may lead to airways' obstruction in the absence of smoking, such an assumption introduced significant bias. In their second paper (Lyons et al., 1972), the authors still chose not to separate their subjects with simple coal pneumoconiosis from those with PMF, and again they were criticized by Oldham and Berry (1972). Moreover, when an attempt was made to relate the size of the decrements in FEV_1 to radio-graphic category, it was evident that those with categories 2 and 3 simple pneumoconiosis had a lesser decrement (0.8 litre below the predicted value) than those who had a clear chest radiograph (1.25 litres below the predicted value).

Whilst there is no doubt that, *post mortem*, coal miners with coal pneumoconiosis often can be shown to have an increased prevalence of emphy-sema (Heppleston, 1972), the emphysema that occurs in non-smoking pneumoconiotic coal miners is not associated with significant or disabling airways' obstruction (Morgan et al., 1974; Hankinson, Reger and Morgan, 1977). If the emphy-sema were to be associated with airways' obstruc-tion, then increasing category of simple coal pneumoconiosis would be associated with a decre-ment in ventilatory capacity, and this is not the case. Moreover, it is accepted that the higher categories of simple pneumoconiosis are associated with increased dust deposition in the lung (Ruckley et al., 1984). It has likewise been shown that the severity of the category of simple pneumoconiosis increases concomitantly with the extent of 'focal emphysema' (Leigh et al., 1983). Further studies have related the presence of right ventricular hypertrophy in coal miners to the presence of simple pneumoconiosis and PMF and to the miners' smoking habits during life (Fernie et al., 1983). Right ventricular hypertrophy and pulmonary heart disease did not occur in coal miners unless they had been cigarette smokers or had PMF. By the same token, if emphysema had been the cause of this airways' obstruction, then in simple coal pneumoconiosis there should be a reduction of the alveolocapillary surface and this would be associated with a concomitant and significant reduction in the diffusing capacity (gas transfer). This is not the case (Kibelstis, 1973).

Early studies of simple coal pneumoconiosis suggested that the type of emphysema that occurred in this condition was different from that seen in smokers. Gough (1968) and Heppleston (1972) both referred to the condition as 'focal dust emphysema' or 'focal emphysema'. Gough (1968) pointed out that

> ...in the young coal miner with a short exposure to dust, dying of accident or of non-pulmonary disease there is an accumulation of coal dust specifically related to the terminal and respiratory bronchioles. The lungs can evidently withstand this deposition without harm for some years. Emphysema then develops, and, in miners who have been exposed for 20 years, some degree of dilatation of the proximal orders of respiratory bronchioles is usual and may be marked. After 40 years of dust exposure, the majority of miners will show focal dust emphysema, although there is a surprising range in the quantity of dust deposited and the degree of emphysema in miners working under similar conditions.

Heppleston (1954) and Gough (1968) went on to suggest that centriacinar emphysema, although starting in the same site, tended to extend to the alveoli more often and, in addition, was associated with bronchiolitis. Some pathologists, however, now dispute that any distinction can be made between the centriacinar emphysema seen in cigarette smokers and 'focal dust emphysema'; of course, in the cigarette-smoking miner both are likely to coexist. As mentioned earlier, Ruckley et al. (1984) have confirmed a relationship between emphysema and exposure to respirable coal dust, but this can be demonstrated only in those miners showing parenchymal fibrosis (see Chapters 9 and 13). What is clear, however, is that extensive 'focal emphysema' may be present in the absence of any impairment of ventilatory capacity (Cochrane, Higgins and Thomas, 1961; Morgan et al., 1971). This is not true of the subject who has extensive small airways' disease and centriacinar emphysema due to cigarette smoking. Moreover, many other relatively inert dusts may lead to the presence of 'focal emphysema', including hematite, stannic oxide and the common air pollutants (Morgan, 1984). Arguing cogently against the likelihood of emphysema being

responsible for the occurrence of airways' obstruction specifically in coal miners is the fact that similar decrements in lung function have been observed in those exposed both to silica (Irwig and Rocks, 1978) and to asbestos (McDonald et al., 1972), and that such obstruction is independent of radiographic change. In silicosis there is no excess emphysema except in smokers, and in asbestosis the characteristic lesions are of interstitial fibrosis where the lungs become stiffer than normal – the antithesis of emphysema in which the lungs are exceptionally compliant.

It has also been shown that the ventilatory capacity, lung volumes and diffusing capacity of coal miners with the various types of small, rounded opacity differ little except in so far as those miners with simple coal pneumoconiosis and the p type of opacity tend to have a slightly reduced gas transfer (Seaton, Lapp and Morgan, 1972). If significant emphysema leading to obstruction were present in miners with the p type of opacity, the residual volume and total lung capacity would be expected to be significantly increased compared with miners with the q and r type of opacities, but such changes have not been consistently demonstrated (see Chapter 13, 'Lung function: simple pneumoconiosis'). Moreover, a large epidemiological study in a group of working coal miners has shown that miners with and without simple coal pneumoconiosis have a slight increase in total lung capacity and residual volume and that increasing category of simple coal pneumoconiosis is associated with an increase in residual volume (Morgan et al., 1974). These findings suggest either that there is a slight loss of elastic recoil in miners with simple pneumoconiosis or that coal miners often have some small airways' obstruction, that is, dust-induced bronchiolitis. Finally, Waters, Cochrane and Moore (1974) have shown that the p type of opacity is not associated with decreased longevity. If disabling emphysema were present and associated with a lower ventilatory capacity, it could reasonably be expected that miners with the p type of opacity would show a decreased life expectancy. Nevertheless, it is apparent that the p type of opacity is associated with certain physiological abnormalities, indicating that there are anatomical changes present in the lungs that are not present in those who have the q and r type of opacities (Seaton, Lapp and Morgan, 1972). Thus, measurements of airspace size carried out by Hankinson, Palmes and Lapp (1979) have shown that there is a dilatation of the alveoli or the respiratory bronchioles or both. These workers were unable to detect any differences in lung function between those miners with the p, q and r type of opacities.

In conclusion, although coal miners with increasing radiographic category of simple coal pneumoconiosis have an increased prevalence of 'focal emphysema', this is not associated with significant airways' obstruction or with a significant loss of diffusing capacity, unless the miner is a smoker. 'Focal emphysema' is associated with a somewhat abnormal distribution of inspired gas, a slight loss of elastic recoil in the lungs, an increased residual volume and minor ventilation–perfusion inequalities (Morgan and Lapp, 1976), but none of these explains the slight loss of ventilatory capacity that is found in a proportion of coal miners (Morgan and Lapp, 1976; Morgan, 1978).

Effects of dust-induced bronchitis

The majority of studies that have related the prevalence of bronchitis to dust exposure have been carried out in coal miners. As a population, coal miners offer many advantages in that they are usually a well-defined and relatively homogeneous group who, throughout most of their life, tend to work in the same occupation. Although many of the observations and inferences that follow have been derived from studies of coal miners, there is no reason to believe that dust-induced bronchitis of coal miners differs in any way from the bronchitis that is seen in workers exposed to silica, bauxite, or any other mineral or gaseous occupational pollutant.

A number of studies have shown that the prevalence of bronchitis increases with cumulative dust exposure (Ashford et al., 1970; Rae, Walker and Attfield, 1971; Kibelstis et al., 1973). In Britain, it has proved possible to relate cumulative coal-mine dust exposure to the prevalence of bronchitis (Rae, Walker and Attfield, 1971), but long-term dust measurements have been lacking in the USA until recently. In an early study in the USA, Kibelstis et al. (1973) related cough and sputum to surrogate measures of dust exposure and also to cigarette smoking. They were able to show that non-smoking coal miners who worked at the face had a greater prevalence of bronchitis than those in the less dusty jobs. This effect was evident in virtually all age groups. In smoking miners, however, the effects of cigarette smoke completely overwhelmed those of dust. Similar observations have been reported in Belgian coal miners (Vuylsteek and Depoorter, 1978).

Rogan et al. (1973) demonstrated, in British coal miners, that ventilatory capacity was inversely related to lifetime cumulative exposure to coal dust. The presence of pneumoconiosis did not lead to an additional decrement of ventilatory capacity above and beyond those decrements due to cumulative dust exposure, smoking habits and stature. Whilst smokers showed a more rapid decline in the FEV_1 than non-smokers, a cumulative effect of dust exposure was apparent in both smoking and non-smoking miners. Among non-smokers, the FEV_1 was generally lower in those subjects who were the most dust exposed as compared with miners who were less dust exposed. However, the rate of decline of the FEV_1 remained the same in non-smoking miners from age 30 to 60 years, regardless of whether they were exposed to high or low dust levels. At the same time, Kibelstis et al. (1973) were similarly able to show a dust-induced effect on the ventilatory capacity of non-smoking miners. As mentioned earlier, the investigators subdivided their cohort according to their job, namely: face workers; those employed on transportation and in miscellaneous other jobs; and those working on the surface. The length of time worked in each particular job was also known. They were able to show that the FEV_1 of the non-smoking surface workers, when expressed as a percentage of the predicted value, was statistically significantly greater than that of the non-smoking face workers. The difference, however, was relatively small (4.3 per cent). When expressed as a percentage of predicted, a significant difference existed between the FEV_1 of the smoking and the non-smoking face workers (6 per cent), and also between the smoking and the non-smoking surface workers (10.6 per cent). Cigarette consumption, as might be expected, was appreciably higher in the surface workers than it was in the face workers, because the latter are not permitted to smoke while underground. Similarly, airways' obstruction was found to be three times more common in smokers than in non-smokers.

A West German study of some 7000 workers from a variety of dusty trades related respiratory symptoms and lung function to dust exposure, smoking habits and other factors (Deutsche Forschungsgemeinschaft, 1978). Age and smoking habits were the most important factors related to the prevalence of bronchitis and airways' obstruction. There was an additive effect of smoking, age and dust in the younger workers, with the combined decrement of all three variables equalling the sum of their separate effects.

Hankinson et al. (1977) and Hankinson, Reger and Morgan (1977) compared the type of respiratory impairment associated with dust-induced bronchitis and the type of impairment induced by cigarette smoking. They used the same cohort of over 9000 working coal miners who had been studied by Kibelstis et al. (1973). In this study, the ventilatory capacity had been assessed with flow–volume curves and, in addition, dynamic lung volumes had been measured. The total lung capacity (TLC) was calculated using a radiological method (Morgan et al., 1971). The residual volume (RV) was calculated by subtracting the FVC from the TLC. Thus, it was possible to express flow rates as a percentage of vital capacity, of total lung capacity and also at absolute

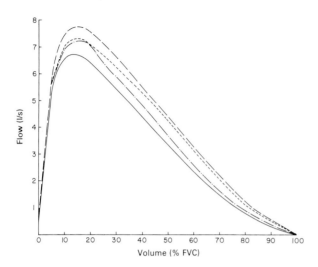

Figure 10.3 Mean flow–volume curve expressed as a percentage of forced vital capacity of four groups of subjects as designated in the figure. There were 428 subjects in each group. In Figures 10.3, 10.4 and 10.5 the following symbols were used: – – – non-smoking, non-bronchitis; ---- non-smoking, bronchitis; – · – · – smoking, non-bronchitis; —— smoking, bronchitis. (Figures 10.3–10.5 were reproduced, with permission, from Hankinson, Reger and Morgan, 1977)

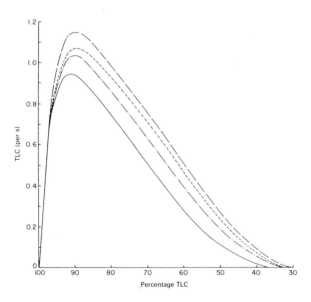

Figure 10.4 Mean flow–volume curve expressed as a percentage of total lung capacity of four groups of subjects as designated in the figure. There were 428 subjects in each group

lung volumes. Hankinson, Reger and Morgan (1977) went on to select four age- and height-matched groups according to whether or not they had bronchitis and to whether or not they were cigarette smokers. Four hundred and twenty-eight subjects

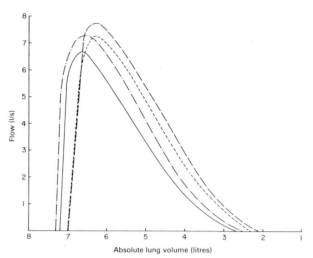

Figure 10.5 Mean flow–volume curve expressed as absolute lung volume of four groups of subjects as designated in the figure. There were 428 subjects in each group

were included in each group. The mean flow–volume curves are shown in Figures 10.3 to 10.5. It is evident from the values that cigarette smoking led to a reduction of flow at all lung volumes. In the subjects who were non-smokers with bronchitis, flows were reduced mainly at high lung volumes, although there was some effect at low lung volumes suggesting that the small airways had not been entirely spared. Flows at absolute lung volumes revealed similar findings, but, more importantly, it was noted that smokers as a whole had an increased RV and an increased TLC. The increase in TLC which occurred in smokers was statistically highly significant and indicates that there is a loss of elastic recoil in the lungs, presumably due to the presence of subclinical emphysema. The TLC of subjects with dust-induced bronchitis was, however, within the normal range. Thus, it would seem that there is little doubt that dust may induce bronchitis and that this is associated with a small reduction in the ventilatory capacity, in particular in the FEV_1, and in flows at high lung volumes (Hankinson, Reger and Morgan, 1977; Hankinson et al., 1977).

Although these data have, in the main, been derived from coal miners, it is noteworthy that, between 1958 and 1972, Brinkman and colleagues (Brinkman and Coates, 1962; Brinkman and Block, 1966; Brinkman, Block and Cress, 1972) carried out a well-planned series of epidemiological investigations in an industrial population who were exposed to various dusts, some of which were inert, but some of which contained a reasonably high percentage of free silica; however few, if any, of the population had silicosis. As in other studies, they came to the conclusion that the main factors affecting the rate of decline of ventilatory capacity were age and cigarette smoking, and that any contribution of dust was relatively small.

A recent study of Kreiss et al. (1989) showed that hard rock mining exposures affected smokers and non-smokers differently. In smokers, flow rates were decreased at all lung volumes and the TLC and RV were increased. In non-smokers, dust exposure was associated with decreased lung volumes and increased flow rates. The authors went on further to state that their results differed from those of Hankinson et al. (1977), who had expressed the opinion that 'industrial bronchitis is limited to the large airways'. In practice, Hankinson and colleagues showed that, although flows in the large airways were predominantly affected, there was also a reduction in flows in the small airways. The apparent disparities in the findings of the two groups of investigators can easily be reconciled. Kreiss et al. (1989) were studying hard rock miners exposed to silica, and exposure to the latter leads to nodular fibrosis and increased stiffness of the lungs, with a decrease in compliance and lung volumes. The opposite situation prevails in coal miners, and the 'focal dust emphysema' that may affect those with pneumoconiosis leads to an increased TLC and an increased RV (Morgan et al., 1971; Nemery, Veriter and Brasseur, 1987).

It is well recognized that maximal expiratory flow rates depend (1) on the elastic recoil of the lung, (2) on the frictional resistance of the small airways and (3) on the cross-sectional area of the large airways. Thus, in a dust-exposed population, flow rates are influenced both by the effects of parenchymal and tracheobronchial dust deposition. Moreover, the lung parenchyma may become either more or less compliant (coal pneumoconiosis vs asbestosis or silicosis). The effects of industrial bronchitis on expiratory flow rates at various lung volumes are, therefore, influenced significantly by the elastic properties of the lung parenchyma. Nevertheless, the predominant effect of industrial bronchitis is on the large airways, just as it is in cigarette smoke-induced bronchitis (Fletcher et al., 1976). Some investigators (Cotes et al., 1989) have claimed that they have been unable to duplicate the findings of Hankinson and colleagues (Hankinson, Reger and Morgan, 1977; Hankinson et al., 1977), and have argued that the effects of industrial bronchitis are not predominantly located in the large airways. However, they expressed their flows as a percentage of vital capacity in the absence of any knowledge of TLC or RV. This, as just indicated, may be misleading and introduces error. This is especially true when the dust to which the subject is exposed is likely to have an effect on the mechanical properties of the lungs, because, under these circumstances, the physiological effects of industrial bronchitis may be dissimulated and it is therefore essential to express the flows at absolute lung volumes.

In those exposed to mineral dusts, ventilatory impairment occurs as frequently in those with radiographic evidence of coal pneumoconiosis or silicosis as it does in those who have a clear chest radiograph. Because the radiographic category of both silicosis and coal pneumoconiosis is related to the weight of dust retained in the lung parenchyma (Nagelschmidt, 1965; Caswell, Bergman and Rossiter, 1971), it is reasonable to infer that the reduction in the FEV_1 seen in dust-exposed workers, and which is independent of radiographic category, originates from dust deposition in the dead space, that is, bronchitis. The apparent lack of association between bronchitis and the presence of silicosis or coal pneumoconiosis suggests that the particles responsible for the two conditions probably differ in size, with those responsible for bronchitis being somewhat larger than those responsible for pneumoconiosis (Morgan, 1978). The particles responsible for bronchitis are mainly deposited as a result of inertial impaction and are removed by the mucociliary escalator, whilst those responsible for pneumoconiosis are more likely to be deposited by sedimentation. There is, moreover, no indication that industrial bronchitis predisposes in any way to the development of the type of small airways' disease and bronchiolitis that may be associated with emphysema (see Chapter 9). Whether the cessation of exposure leads to an improvement in the symptoms of industrial or occupationally induced bronchitis is unknown; however, using the analogy of cigarette smokers' bronchitis, it is likely that this would be the case.

Dust versus cigarette smoke: relative contributions to ventilatory impairment

A few longitudinal studies relating decrements in lung function to cumulative dust exposure have been carried out in coal miners (Love and Miller, 1982; Attfield, 1985) and in those exposed to silica (Glover et al., 1980). Most studies have shown that the mean effects of dust are about equal to one-third to one-fifth of those of cigarette smoke.

Some 1677 miners from five British collieries were studied over a period of 11 years by Love and

Miller (1982). The FEV_1 loss was related to cumulative dust exposure after correction for age, smoking and colliery effect. The cohort was divided according to whether they were non-smokers, ex-smokers or current smokers, and some adjustments were made for the duration and intensity of smoking. Love and Miller showed that cigarette smoking had roughly three times the effect of dust; however, there were a number of flaws in the study, including the fact that smoking was treated as a static unchanging variable – in the same way as, for example, height. Obviously, this is not the case and the effects of cigarette smoking increase with the number of 'pack-years'. Moreover, prospective quantitative data on cigarette smoking habits were not available. Attfield (1985) described his findings subsequently in a 9-year follow-up of US coal miners. Here again, only about one-quarter of the population were available to be included in the final analysis. It was noted that those who left coal mining tended to be older, showed more evidence of bronchitis and ill-health, and were more likely to be smokers. Because much of the difference between those who remained at work and those who left could be accounted for by age, Attfield decided to include only those miners between 29 and 49 years of age. Unfortunately, the older age groups would be comprised of those subjects who were most likely to show the greatest effects of cigarette smoking. He also found that cigarette smoking had three to four times the effects of coal dust exposure. It is interesting to note, however, that dust exposures in US coal miners were significantly less than they were during the comparable period in Britain, despite relatively similar effects on ventilatory capacity.

An additional study of the same cohort of British miners has recently been published and maintains that chronic bronchitis is associated with loss of lung function (Marine, Gurr and Jacobsen, 1988). These authors noted 'that men with bronchitic symptoms have evidence of airway obstruction more often than do men without symptoms', an observation that has been made repeatedly and was to be expected because cigarette smoking is known to be the most common cause not only of bronchitis, but also of irreversible airways' obstruction. Later they maintain that 'dust related increases in symptom prevalence may be regarded as indicators to dust-induced impairment of respiratory function', but then subsequently add 'this association does not necessarily mean that the symptoms are the cause of the obstruction. But it is misleading to state that the conditions are unrelated'. They then go on to say 'that the increased prevalence of potentially lethal obstructive airway disease caused by high exposures to coal-mine dust may be just as great as the smoking-attributable prevalence of the same condition in miners who smoke cigarettes'. If

bronchitis does not lead to the obstruction then the only other possibility would seem to be emphysema; however, in those non-smoking miners who have chronic bronchitis and decrements in airflow, there is no physiological or other indication of emphysema in the absence of coal pneumoconiosis (Hankinson, Reger and Morgan, 1977). Similarly, it is also stated that their interpretation of the results is supported by 'the demonstration of an increase in mortality attributed to bronchitis and emphysema in coal miners who have had relatively high dust exposures' – an observation that several other studies using data collected prospectively have failed to confirm (Ortmeyer et al., 1974; Cochrane et al., 1979; Foxman, Higgins and Oh, 1986). Moreover, with increasing dust exposure there is a concomitant increase in age and also in lifetime cigarette consumption, and the belief that multiple regression analyses will inevitably sort out the relative contributions of each to mortality is now known not to be the case (McGee, Reed and Yano, 1984). Unfortunately, there are a number of anomalies in the three British studies (Rae, Walker and Attfield, 1971; Rogan et al., 1973; Marine, Gurr and Jacobsen, 1988) in that, although the data analysed were derived from exactly the same cohort, the percentage of non-smokers in each varied by almost one-third (Morgan and Lapp, 1988); and there are also discrepancies between the number of subjects in the various dust-exposed groups.

A series of reports from France has claimed that occupational exposure leads to bronchitis that is associated with a sufficiently large reduction in the ventilatory capacity to cause disabling impairment (Kauffman et al., 1982; Annesi and Kauffman, 1986). However, the cohort studied by these investigators comprised workers of multiple occupations with varied exposures, and included metallurgists, chemists, printers and flour millers. Some of those employed in the flour mill would be expected to develop asthma rather than irreversible obstruction, whilst those in the sector described as 'chemistry' would be exposed to paints, varnishes and plastics. Here again, occupational asthma may well have been a factor. More importantly, of the original population of 1002 men, only 71 per cent of the 780 re-examined 11 years later had satisfactory spirometric tracings (Kauffman et al., 1982). With enthusiasm and good quality control, reproducible and acceptable readings of the FVC and FEV_1 should be obtained in 98 per cent of subjects (Morgan et al., 1988).

A number of difficulties exist with regard to comparisons made between the mean decrement in FEV_1 induced by cigarette smoking and that induced by dust. Whilst only 12 to 15 per cent of cigarette smokers develop airways' obstruction (Fletcher et al., 1976), around 40 to 50 per cent of non-smoking miners, who have worked for 20 or more years underground, complain of cough and sputum and are likely to show a minor decrement in FEV_1 (Kibelstis et al., 1973). Thus, to compare the mean decrement in FEV_1 in cigarette smokers with that in non-smokers is misleading in that, of the smokers who develop airways' obstruction, some will have a disabling decrement in ventilatory capacity. In contrast, a far greater percentage of non-smoking coal miners will have bronchitis and a concomitant, but much smaller, dust-induced decrement in FEV_1. Of the 12 to 15 per cent of coal miners who are cigarette smokers, and go on to develop airways' obstruction, the 11-ml decrement noted by Love and Miller (1982) is occurring solely in this susceptible minority. If the whole population were to smoke 20 cigarettes a day, the resultant mean reduction in the FEV_1 would be minor, because, in most subjects, the effects are skewed, with most showing a normal age-related decline in FEV_1, but a few showing clinically significant losses. Thus, the decrement induced by cigarette smoking is likely to lead to severe disability in a minority, whilst the decrement that occurs in a greater percentage of the non-smoking miners who have dust-induced bronchitis is slight and non-disabling. Ryder, Dunnill and Anderson (1971) graphically illustrate this point in their paper relating the prevalence of emphysema found *post mortem* to age and cigarette smoking. The fact that only 19 of the 106 smokers' lungs which they examined showed more than 20 per cent involvement makes it evident that the vast majority of smokers do not go on to develop disabling emphysema.

Other sources of bias – including the healthy worker effect – have also to be taken into account in longitudinal studies. It is frequently assumed that workers leave their occupation prematurely because of exposure to dust or other occupationally related hazards. In reality, the percentage of non-smokers, ex-smokers and smokers in the various age groups change gradually over the working lifetime (Morgan, 1986). Thus, in the older workers, there is a greater percentage of non-smokers and ex-smokers as compared to younger employees. This is particularly true of coal miners (Kibelstis et al., 1973). Moreover, Attfield (1985) showed that it was the smokers who tended to drop out prematurely rather than non-smokers. It would be reasonable, therefore, to infer that the smokers who leave the workforce do so because of premature disability, and those who continue working are likely to be relatively resistant to the effects of cigarette smoking.

Numerous studies have shown that bronchitis is associated with an increased mortality from malignant and non-malignant respiratory disease. However, when an attempt is made to control for the effect of the reduced ventilatory capacity in subjects who have bronchitis, it becomes evident that cough and sputum alone do not lead to decreased longevity from respiratory disease other than that due to lung cancer (Foxman, Higgins and Oh, 1986). Thus, the increased death rate associated with bronchitis is a reflection of cigarette smoking and not an effect of bronchitis. Thurlbeck et al. (1970) and Jamal et al. (1984) have made it clear that, although bronchitis is associated with the development of symptoms, there is only a poor correlation between bronchitis as diagnosed from pathological criteria and a decreased FEV_1.

If it were assumed that a certain proportion of coal miners may develop disabling airways' obstruction in the absence of cigarette smoking, then a similar proportion of miners would be expected to develop right ventricular hypertrophy and pulmonary heart disease. There have been several studies made during life (Thomas, 1948; Lapp et al., 1971), and there has also been a series of postmortem studies that make it clear that neither pulmonary heart disease nor right ventricular hypertrophy occurs in non-smoking miners unless the subject has PMF (Thomas, 1948, 1951; Wells, 1954; James and Thomas, 1956). A more recent postmortem study carried out on a number of British coal miners showed that right ventricular hypertrophy and pulmonary heart disease were absent unless there was a history of cigarette smoking or PMF was present (Fernie et al., 1983).

Recent mortality studies in working coal miners have shown a normal life expectancy (Morgan, 1984; Surgeon-General, US Public Health Service, 1986) and, similarly, Miller and Jacobsen (1985) have shown that British coal miners as a whole have a 13 per cent lower general mortality than other men from the same region. By selecting specific subgroups, these authors concluded that miners with chronic bronchitis have an increased mortality. Cigarette smoking is the most common cause of chronic bronchitis and, because cigarette smoking leads to numerous life-threatening diseases, it is not surprising that those with cough and sputum show an increased standardized mortality ratio (SMR). Because bronchitis has been shown by Fletcher et al. (1976) and by Foxman, Higgins and Oh (1986) to have little or no effect on lung function, it is difficult to see why bronchitic subjects should die prematurely, at least of airways' obstruction. Moreover, Ortmeyer et al. (1974), in a prospective study carried out on a randomly selected population of US coal miners and ex-miners, were unable to show any effect of dust exposure on life expectancy in the absence of PMF. In contrast, the effects of cigarette smoking stood out like a sore thumb. Similar findings were reported by Foxman, Higgins and Oh (1986). Elmes (1981) has comprehensively reviewed the relative effects of cigarette smoking and dust in the induction of irreversible airways' obstruction, and concluded that cigarette smoking is a far more serious hazard.

Bronchitis and airways' obstruction in other occupations

Welders

Over the last few years, a number of studies have shed some light on the chronic effects of welding, especially with regard to the prevalence and effects of bronchitis. In a group of welders from the Newport News shipyard, Hunnicutt, Cracovaner and Miles (1964) found that the prevalence of symptoms such as cough and sputum was significantly higher in welders than in non-welders. There was also an increased prevalence of airways' obstruction, but only smoking welders were affected. Comparable findings resulted from a study of Boston shipyard welders (Peters, Murphy and Ferris, 1973), in which no detectable ventilatory defect was present in welders who did not smoke. In a similar investigation there was no significant difference between 156 Danish welders and controls in the occurrence of chronic bronchitis and ventilatory function after controlling for smoking (Fogh, Frost and George, 1969). Again, Sjögren and Ulfvarson (1985), although able to show an increased prevalence of bronchitis, could detect no effect on lung function in a group of 269 welders of whom 64 were aluminium welders, 56 stainless steel welders and 149 road track welders. Antti-Poika, Hassi and Pyy (1977) found similar results in a group of Finnish arc welders.

In a series of carefully controlled and detailed studies, McMillan and his colleagues investigated the health of welders employed in the Royal Navy dockyards in Britain. In a retrospective study in which he analysed the morbidity and incidence of respiratory disease over a 5-year period, McMillan (1979) included five relatively comparable groups who also worked in the shipyard, as a reference population. He concluded that there was no evidence of a significant excess of chronic respiratory disease in the welders. He noticed, however, that welders suffered more from upper respiratory tract illnesses than other groups, although the absence from work on account of these illnesses was of the same duration.

Furthermore, in a general review of the health of welders in Royal Navy dockyards, McMillan (1983) concluded that there was no evidence of a causal relationship between welding and respiratory diseases or other ill-health, with the exception of injuries. He felt that there may be a small minority of welders who are unusually susceptible to the effects of fumes and gases, and that such people have obstructive airways' disease such as asthma or

emphysema. Neither the asthma nor the emphysema was, however, related to welding exposure.

Owing to the fact that most studies have been carried out in welders with relatively short exposures to welding fumes, that is, less than 15 years, McMillan and Pethybridge (1984) decided to examine 135 welders aged 45 years and over who had had prolonged exposure. The average duration of welding in this group was 33.1 years. Those exposed had detailed clinical, radiological and pulmonary function examinations carried out and were compared with a comparable control group aged 45 years and over. They concluded that prolonged exposure to welding fumes did not cause either significant clinical abnormality or any serious impairment of lung function; however, they expressed the opinion that minimal airways' obstruction may result from exposure to welding fumes. Similar findings have been reported by Hayden et al. (1984) in welders employed in three engineering factories in the British Midlands. These investigators concluded, however, that welders had no increased risk of chronic obstructive lung disease. Analogous conclusions have been reached by Peters, Murphy and Ferris (1973), Fogh, Frost and George (1969) and Antti-Poika, Hassi and Pyy (1977). The subject of airways' obstruction and other hazards that occur in welders has been reviewed by Morgan (1989).

Welding is discussed further in Chapter 18.

Firefighters

The acute effects of smoke inhalation have been well documented, but it has also been suggested that there is an association between firefighting, lung disease and decrements in lung function (Sidor and Peters, 1974a,b). It has been claimed that Boston firefighters showed an increased decline in lung function over a period of a year (Peters et al., 1974). When the lung function measurements were repeated 3 years later, however, no such decline was evident (Musk, Peters and Wegman, 1976). It became apparent that the so-called increased rate of decline was probably a consequence of inadequate quality control during the performance of the spirometry.

Sparrow et al. (1982) described an increased rate of decline in firemen as compared to controls. They maintained that the increased rate could not be explained by smoking habits, age, height or factors other than the firefighters' occupation. Unfortunately, this study relied on current smoking habits rather than lifetime consumption, and the latter correlates far better with ventilatory capacity than do current smoking habits. There seems little doubt that, in the USA, the proportion of cigarette smokers among firemen is higher than among the general population and, moreover, because most of their time is spent waiting in smoke-filled rooms, the prevalence of bronchitis may be increased even among non-smoking firefighters from second-hand smoke effects (passive smoking). A more recent study from Britain has shown that non-smoking firefighters appear to have the same prevalence of symptoms and the same ventilatory capacity as the control subjects selected for this study (Horsfield et al., 1988). The wearing of breathing apparatus during firefighting appeared to be effective in preventing the development of respiratory symptoms. Finally, the SMR of firefighters, at least for respiratory disease, is normal (Mastromatteo, 1959). Thus, there would seem to be no definite evidence that firefighting leads to an increased prevalence of bronchitis or airways' obstruction in non-smoking firefighters.

The effects of 'fire smoke' are also discussed in Chapter 18.

Grain workers

Subjects exposed to grain, particularly those who work in grain elevators, may develop asthma (see Chapter 21). This usually comes on within a short time of the subject being exposed. The symptoms are usually severe and the subject often leaves the job in a relatively short time. Evidently, long continued exposure to grain dust may induce a number of respiratory symptoms including cough, sputum and shortness of breath (Tse et al., 1973; Chan-Yeung, Wong and McLean, 1979; doPico et al., 1984). These symptoms do not appear to be related to any specific allergic response to the dust and the obstruction may be partly reversible. For the most part, those affected seem to be cigarette smokers. Broder et al. (1980) have shown that absence from work because of temporary 'lay-offs' is associated with a decrease in the symptoms of cough and sputum. However, the return to work or continued exposure usually leads to a gradual increase in prevalence and severity of these symptoms. Although, in recent years, there has been much investigation into respiratory disease in grain elevator workers, the evidence so far suggests that it is a non-specific reaction, chronic in nature, similar to industrial bronchitis. Furthermore, there is little to indicate that it ever leads to disabling respiratory impairment. There is some suggestion, however, that the rate of decline in lung function in grain

workers is related to bronchial hyperreactivity (Cookson et al., 1986).

Workers exposed to diesel exhaust emissions

Diesel emissions contain a number of particulates and gases, including carbon monoxide, carbon dioxide, sulphur dioxide, formaldehyde and nitrogen dioxide (Robertson et al., 1984). Nitrogen dioxide is most frequently regarded as responsible for any deleterious effect observed in those exposed to diesel fumes. The acute effects of diesel fumes in coal miners have been studied and no significant decrease found in either the FEV_1 or the forced expiratory flow at 50 per cent of the forced vital capacity (FEF_{50}). Workers in both the control and the exposed groups showed a decline in ventilatory capacity over a workshift, presumably an effect of exposure to coal dust (Ames et al., 1982).

Some studies have suggested that there is a higher prevalence of bronchitis in workers exposed to diesel fumes, although ventilatory capacity is apparently unaffected (Ames, Reger and Hall, 1984). Extensive studies have been carried out in Swedish iron ore workers, all of whom have shown no effect on lung function from continued exposure to diesel fumes (Jorgensen and Svenson, 1970; Jorgensen, Kolmodin-Hedman and Stjernberg, 1988). Although the symptoms of bronchitis were present more frequently in those most exposed, cigarette smoking had a far greater effect on their production. Nevertheless, caution is advisable with regard to those exposed to diesel emissions in that there are occasions when, with poor industrial hygiene, the concentrations of the fumes are greater than usual and can lead to eye and respiratory irritation. Even so, no permanent effects have been noted from acute exposure (see Chapter 18, 'Oxides of nitrogen').

Summary

Long continued exposure to dusts and irritant gases will lead to the development of cough and sputum. This may be associated with a minor reduction of the ventilatory capacity and with increase in residual volume, but not with a loss of elastic recoil or with the development of emphysema. Although the prevalence of bronchitis and the magnitude of the reduction of the FEV_1 are related to cumulative lifetime exposure, dust-induced bronchitis or, as it is often known, industrial bronchitis does not cause disabling respiratory impairment.

References

Ames, R.G., Reger, R.B. and Hall, D.S. (1984) Chronic respiratory effects of exposure to diesel emissions in coal mines. *Archs Environ. Health* **39**, 389–394

Ames, R.G., Attfield, M.D., Hankinson, J.L., Hearl, F.J. and Reger, R.B. (1982) Acute respiratory effects of exposure to diesel emissions in coal miners. *Am. Rev. Respir. Dis.* **125**, 39–42

Annesi, I. and Kauffman, I. (1986) Is respiratory mucus hypersecretion really an innocent disorder? A 22 year mortality study of 1061 working men. *Am. Rev. Respir. Dis.* **134**, 688–693

Antti-Poika, M., Hassi, J. and Pyy, L. (1977) Respiratory diseases in arc welders. *Int. Archs Occup. Environ. Health* **40**, 225–230

Ashford, J.R., Morgan, D.C., Rae, S. and Sowden, R.R. (1970) Respiratory symptoms in British coal miners. *Am. Rev. Respir. Dis.* **102**, 370–381

Attfield, M.D. (1985) Longitudinal decline in FEV$_1$ in United States coalminers. *Thorax* **40**, 132–137

Bates, D.V. (1973) The fate of the chronic bronchitic: A report of the ten year follow up in the Canadian Department of Veterans Affairs coordinated study of chronic bronchitis. *Am. Rev. Respir. Dis.* **108**, 1043–1065

Brinkman, G.L. and Coates, E.L. (1962) The prevalence of chronic bronchitis in an industrial population. *Am. Rev. Respir. Dis.* **86**, 47–54

Brinkman, G.L. and Block, D.L. (1966) The prognosis in chronic bronchitis. *J. Am. Med. Assoc.* **197**, 71–77

Brinkman, G.L., Block, D.L. and Cress, C. (1972) Effects of bronchitis and occupation on pulmonary ventilation over an 11-year period. *J. Occup. Med.* **14**, 615–620

Broder, I., Mintz, S., Hutcheon, M.A., Corey, P.N. and Kuzyk, J. (1980) Effect of layoff and rehire on respiratory variables of grain elevator workers. *Am. Rev. Respir. Dis.* **122**, 601–608

Caswell, C., Bergman, I. and Rossiter, C.E. (1971) The relation of radiological appearance in simple pneumoconiosis of coal workers to the content and composition of the lung. In *Inhaled Particles III*, vol. 2 (ed. W.H. Walton) Unwin Brothers, London, pp. 713–721

Chan-Yeung, M., Wong, R. and McLean, L. (1979) Respiratory abnormalities among grain elevator workers. *Chest* **75**, 461–467

Cochrane, A.L., Higgins, I.T.T. and Thomas, J. (1961) Pulmonary ventilatory function of coal miners in various areas in relation to x-ray category of pneumoconiosis. *Br. J. Prev. Soc. Med.* **15**, 1–11

Cochrane, A.L., Haley, T.J.L., Moore, F. and Hole, D. (1979) The mortality of men in the Rhondda Fach, 1950–1970. *Br. J. Ind. Med.* **36**, 15–22

Cookson, W.O.C.M., Ryan, G., MacDonald, S. and Musk, A.W. (1986) Atopy, non-allergic bronchial reactivity, and past history as determinants of work related symptoms in seasonal grain handlers. *Br. J. Ind. Med.* **43**, 396–400

Cotes, J.D., Feinman, E.L., Male, V.G., Rennie, F.S. and Wickham, C.A. (1989) Respiratory symptoms and impairment in shipyard welders and caulker/burners. *Br. J. Ind. Med.* **46**, 292–301

Deutsche Forschungsgemeinschaft (1978) *Research Report on*

Chronic Bronchitis and Occupational Dust Exposure. Harald Boldt Verlag KG, Boppard, Germany

doPico, G.A., Reddan, W., Tsiatis, A., Peters, M.E. and Rankin, J. (1984) Epidemiologic studies of clinical and physiologic parameters in grain handlers of Northern United States. *Am. Rev. Respir. Dis.* **130**, 759–765

Elmes, P.C. (1981) Relative importance of cigarette smoking in occupational lung disease. *Br. J. Ind. Med.* **38**, 1–13

Enarson, D.A., Vedal, S. and Chan-Yeung, M. (1985) Rapid decline in FEV$_1$ in grain handlers. Relation to level of dust exposure. *Am. Rev. Respir. Dis.* **132**, 814–817

Enterline, P.E. and Lainhart, W.S. (1967) The relationship between coal mining and chronic nonspecific respiratory disease. *Am. J. Public Health* **57**, 484–495

Fernie, J.M., Douglas, A.N., Lamb, D. and Ruckley, V.A. (1983) Right ventricular hypertrophy in a group of coal workers. *Thorax* **38**, 436–442

Fletcher, C.M., Elmes, P.C., Fairbairn, A.S. and Wood, C.M. (1969) The significance of respiratory symptoms and the diagnosis of chronic bronchitis in the working population. *Br. Med. J.* **2**, 257–266

Fletcher, C.M., Peto, R. Tinker, C. and Speizer, F.C. (1976) *The Natural History of Chronic Bronchitis and Emphysema.* Oxford University Press, Oxford

Fogh, A., Frost, J. and George, J. (1969) Respiratory symptoms and pulmonary function in welders. *Ann. Occup. Hyg.* **12**, 213–218

Foxman, B., Higgins, I.T.T. and Oh, M.S. (1986) The effects of occupation and smoking on respiratory disease mortality. *Am. Rev. Respir. Dis.* **134**, 649–652

Gilson, J.C. (1970) Occupational bronchitis. *Proc. R. Soc. Med.* **63**, 857–864

Gilson, J.C. and Oldham, P.D. (1970) Coal workers pneumoconiosis. *Br. Med. J.* **4**, 305

Glover, J.R., Bevan, C., Cotes, J.E., Elwood, P.C., Hodges, N.G., Kell, R.L., Lowe, C.R., McDermott, M., and Oldham, P.D. (1980) Effects of exposure to slate dust in North Wales. *Br. J. Ind. Med.* **37**, 152–162

Gough, J. (1966) Chronic bronchitis and occupation. *Br. Med. J.* **1**, 480

Gough, J. (1968) The pathogenesis of emphysema. In *The Lung* (eds A. Liebow and D.T. Smith), Williams and Wilkins, Baltimore, pp. 109–133

Greenhow, E.H. (1860) *Report of the Medical Officer of the Privy Council* and (1861) Appendix VI. HM Stationery Office, London

Haldane, J.S. (1925) *Historical Review of Coal Mining*, Fleetway Press, London, p. 266

Hankinson, J.L., Palmes, E.D. and Lapp, N.L. (1979) Pulmonary air space size in coal miners. *Am. Rev. Respir. Dis.* **119**, 391–397

Hankinson, J.L., Reger, R.B. and Morgan, W.K.C. (1977) Maximal expiratory flows in coal miners. *Am. Rev. Respir. Dis.* **116**, 175–180

Hankinson, J.L., Reger, R.B., Fairman, R.P., Lapp, N.L. and Morgan, W.K.C. (1977) Factors influencing expiratory flow rates in coal miners. In *Inhaled Particles IV* (ed. W.H. Walton), Pergamon Press, Oxford, pp. 737–652

Hayden, S.P., Pincock, A.C., Hayden, J., Tyler, L.E., Cross, K.W. and Bishop, J.M. (1984) Respiratory symptoms and pulmonary function of welders in the engineering industry. *Thorax* **39**, 442–447

Heppleston, A.G. (1954) The pathogenesis of simple pneumoconiosis in coal workers. *J. Pathol. Bacteriol.* **67**, 51–63

Heppleston, A.G. (1972) The pathological recognition and pathogenesis of emphysema and fibrocystic disease of the lung with special reference to coal workers. *Ann. NY Acad. Sci.* **200**, 347–369

Higgins, I.T.T. (1960) An approach to the problem of bronchitis in industry: Studies in agricultural, mining, and farming communities. In *Industrial Pulmonary Disease* (eds E.J. King and C.M. Fletcher), J and A Churchill Ltd, London, pp. 195–207

Higgins, I.T.T. (1972) Chronic respiratory disease in mining communities. *Ann. NY Acad. Sci.* **200**, 197–210

Higgins, I.T.T. and Cochrane, A.L. (1958) Population studies of miners, foundry workers and others in Staveley, Derbyshire. *Br. J. Ind. Med.* **16**, 255–268

Horsfield, K., Cooper, F.M., Buckman, M.P., Guyatt, A.R. and Cumming, G. (1988) Respiratory symptoms in West Sussex firemen. *Br. J. Ind. Med.* **45**, 251–255

Hunnicutt, T.N., Cracovaner, D.J. and Myles, J.T. (1964) Spirometric measurements in welders. *Archs Environ. Health* **8**, 661

Irwig, L. and Rocks, P. (1978) Lung function and respiratory symptoms in silicotic and nonsilicotic gold miners. *Am. Rev. Respir. Dis.* **117**, 429–435

Jamal, K., Cooney, T.P., Fleetham, J.A. and Thurlbeck, W.M. (1984) Chronic bronchitis: Correlation of morphologic findings to sputum production and flow rates. *Am. Rev. Respir. Dis.* **129**, 719–722

James, W.R.L. and Thomas, A.J. (1956) Cardiac hypertrophy in coalworkers' pneumoconiosis. *Br. J. Ind. Med.* **13**, 24–29

Jorgensen, H. and Svenson, A. (1970) Studies of pulmonary function in respiratory tract syndromes of workers in an iron ore mine where diesel trucks are used underground. *J. Occup. Med.* **12**, 348–354

Jorgenson, H.S., Kolmodin-Hedman, B. and Stjernberg, N. (1988) Follow-up study of pulmonary function and respiratory tract symptoms in workers in a Swedish iron ore mine. *J. Occup. Med.* **30**, 953–957

Kalačič, I. (1973a) Chronic nonspecific lung disease in cement workers. *Archs Environ. Health* **26**, 78–83

Kalačič, I. (1973b) Ventilatory lung function in cement workers. *Archs Environ. Health* **26**, 84–85

Kauffman, F., Drouet, D., Lellouch, J. and Brille, D. (1982) Occupational exposure and 12 year spirometric changes among Paris area workers. *Br. J. Ind. Med.* **39**, 221–232

Kibelstis, J.A. (1973) Diffusing capacity in bituminous coal mine. *Chest* **63**, 501–504

Kibelstis, J.A., Morgan, E.J., Reger, R., Lapp, N.L., Seaton, A. and Morgan, W.K.C. (1973) Prevalence of bronchitis and airway obstruction in American bituminous coal miners. *Am. Rev. Respir. Dis.* **108**, 886–893

Kreiss, K., Greenburg, L.M., Kogut, S.J.H., Lezatte, D.C., Irvin, C.G. and Cherniack, R.M. (1989) Hard-rock mining exposures affect smokers and nonsmokers differently. *Am. Rev. Respir. Dis.* **139**, 1487–1493

Kremer, R. (1982) Pulmonary hemodynamics in coal workers' pneumoconiosis. *Ann. NY Acad. Sci.* **200**, 413–432

Lapp, N.L., Seaton, A., Kaplan, K.C., Hunsaker, M.R. and Morgan, W.K.C. (1971) Pulmonary hemodynamics in symptomatic coal miners. *Am. Rev. Respir. Dis.* **104**, 418–426

Leigh, J., Outhred, K.G., McKenzie, H.I., Glick, M. and Wiles, A.N. (1983) Quantified pathology of emphysema, pneumoconiosis and chronic bronchitis in coal miners. *Br. J. Ind. Med.* **40**, 258–263

Lloyd Davies, T.A. (1971) *Respiratory Disease in Foundrymen. Report of a Survey.* Department of Employment, HM Stationery Office, London

Love, R.G. and Miller, B.G. (1982) Longitudinal study of lung function in coal miners. *Thorax* **37**, 193–197

Lowe, C.R. (1968) Chronic bronchitis and occupation. *Proc. R. Soc. Med.* **61**, 98–102

Lowe, C.R., Campbell, H. and Khosla, T. (1970) Bronchitis in two integrated steel works II. Respiratory symptoms and ventilatory capacity related to atmospheric pollution. *Br. J. Ind. Med.* **27**, 121–129

Lyons, J.P. and Campbell, H. (1976) Evaluation of disability in coal workers' pneumoconiosis. *Thorax* **31**, 527–533

Lyons, J.P., Ryder, R., Campbell, H. and Gough, J. (1972) Pulmonary disability in coal workers' pneumoconiosis. *Br. Med. J.* **1**, 713–716

McClintock, J.S. (1971) The selection of juvenile entrants to mining. *Br. J. Ind. Med.* **28**, 45–51

McDonald, J.C., Becklake, M.R., Fournier-Massey, G. and Rossiter, C.E. (1972) Respiratory symptoms in chrysotile asbestos mine and mill workers of Quebec. *Archs Environ. Health* **24**, 358–363

McGee, D., Reed, D. and Yano, K. (1984) The results of logistic analyses when the variables are highly correlated: An empirical example of using diet and CHD incidence. *J. Chron. Dis.* **37**, 713–719

McLaughlin, A.I.G. (1966) Chronic bronchitis and occupation. *Br. Med. J.* **1**, 354

McMillan, G.H.G. (1979) Studies of the health of welders in naval dockyards, *Ann. Occup. Hyg.* **21**, 377–392

McMillan, G.H.G. (1983) The health of welders in naval dockyards. Final Summary Report. *J. R. Nav. Med. Serv.* **69**, 125–131

McMillan, G.H.G. and Pethybridge, R.J. (1984) A clinical, radiological and pulmonary function case-control study of 135 dockyard welders aged 45 years and over. *J. Soc. Occup. Med.* **34**, 3–23

Marine, W.M., Gurr, D. and Jacobsen, M. (1988) Clinically important respiratory effects of dust exposure in British coal miners. *Am. Rev. Respir. Dis.* **137**, 106–112

Mastromatteo, E. (1959) Mortality in city firemen. II. A study of mortality in firemen of a city health department. *Archs Environ. Health* **20**, 227–233

Medical Research Council (1966) Chronic bronchitis and occupation. *Br. Med. J.* **1**, 101–102

Miller, B.G. and Jacobsen, M. (1985) Dust exposure, pneumoconiosis and mortality of coal miners. *Br. J. Ind. Med.* **42**, 723–733

Morgan, W.K.C. (1978) Industrial bronchitis. *Br. J. Ind. Med.* **35**, 285–291

Morgan, W.K.C. (1984) Coal workers' pneumoconiosis. In: *Occupational Lung Diseases* (eds W.K.C. Morgan and A. Seaton), W.B. Saunders, Philadelphia, chaps 14, 15, 17

Morgan, W.K.C. (1986) On dust, disability, and death. *Am. Rev. Respir. Dis.* **134**, 639–641

Morgan, W.K.C. (1989) On welding, wheezing and whimsy. *Am. Ind. Hyg. Assoc. J.* **50**, 59–69

Morgan, W.K.C. and Lapp, N.L. (1976) Respiratory disease in coal miners: State of the Art. *Am. Rev. Respir. Dis.* **113**, 531–559

Morgan, W.K.C. and Lapp, N.L. (1988) Clinically important respiratory effects of dust, exposure, and smoking in British coal miners. *Am. Rev. Resp. Dis.* **138**, 1643–1644

Morgan, W.K.C., Burgess, D.B., Lapp, N.L., Seaton, A. and Reger, R.B. (1971) Hyperinflation of the lungs in coal miners. *Thorax* **26**, 585–590

Morgan, W.K.C., Handelsman, L., Kibelstis, J., Lapp, N.L. and Reger, R.B. (1974) Ventilatory capacity and lung volumes of U.S. coal miners. *Archs Environ. Health* **28**, 182–189

Morgan, W.K.C., Versterlund, J., Burrell, R. and Gee, J.B.L. (1982) Byssinosis: Some unanswered questions. *Am. Rev. Respir. Dis.* **126**, 354–357

Morgan, W.K.C., Donner, A., Higgins, I.T.T., Pearson, M.G. and Rawlings, W. Jr (1988) The effects of kaolin on the lung. *Am. Rev. Respir. Dis.* **138**, 813–820

Musk, A.W., Peters, J.M. and Wegman, D.H. (1976) Lung function in fire-fighters: A three-year follow-up of active subjects. *Am. J. Public Health* **67**, 626–629

Musk, A.W., Smith, T.J. and McLaughlin, E. (1979) Pulmonary function and fire fighters. Acute changes in ventilatory capacity and their correlates. *Br. J. Ind. Med.* **36**, 29–34

Nagelschmidt, G. (1965) The study of lung dust in pneumoconiosis. *Am. Ind. Hyg. Assoc. J.* **26**, 1–7

Nemery, B., Veriter, C. and Brasseur, L. (1987) Impairment of ventilatory function and pulmonary gas exchange in nonsmoking miners. *Lancet* **2**, 1427–1430

Oldham, P.D. and Berry, G. (1972) Coal miners' pneumoconiosis. *Br. Med. J.* **2**, 292–293

Ortmeyer, C.E., Costello, J., Morgan, W.K.C., Swecker, S. and Peterson, M. (1974) The mortality of Appalachian coal miners, 1963 to 1971. *Archs Environ. Health* **29**, 67–72

Pemberton, J. (1966) Occupational lung disease. *Br. Med. J.* **1**, 609

Peters, J.M., Murphy, R.L.H. and Ferris, B.G. Jr (1973) Pulmonary function in shipyard welders. *Archs Environ. Health* **26**, 28–31

Peters, J.M., Theriault, G.P., Fine, L.J. and Wegman, D.H. (1974) Chronic effect of firefighting on pulmonary function. *New Engl. J. Med.* **291**, 1320–1322

Pratt, P.C., Vollmer, R.T. and Miller, J.A. (1980) Epidemiology of pulmonary lesions in non-textile and cotton textile workers. A retrospective autopsy analysis. *Archs Environ. Health* **35**, 133–138

Rae, S., Walker, D.D. and Attfield, N.D. (1971) Chronic bronchitis in dust exposure in British coal miners. In *Inhaled Particles III* (ed. W.H. Walton), Unwin, Old Woking, Surrey, pp. 883–894

Reid, L. (1960) Measurement of bronchial mucous gland layer: A diagnostic yardstick in chronic bronchitis. *Thorax* **15**, 132–141

Robertson, A., Dodgson, J., Collings, P. and Seaton, A. (1984) Exposure to oxides of nitrogen: respiratory symptoms and lung function in British coal miners. *Br. J. Ind. Med.* **41**, 214–219

Rogan, J.M., Attfield, M.D., Jacobsen, M., Rae, S., Walker, D.D. and Walton, W.H. (1973) Role of dust in the working environment in development of chronic bronchitis in British coal miners. *Br. J. Ind. Med.* **123**, 372–377

Ruckley, V.A., Gould, J., Chapman, J.S., Davis, J.M.G., Douglas, A.N., Fernie, J.M., Jacobsen, M. and Lamb, D. (1984) Emphysema and dust exposure in a group of coal workers. *Am. Rev. Respir. Dis.* **129**, 528–532

Ryder, R.C., Dunnill, M.S. and Anderson, J.S. (1971) A quantitative study of bronchial mucous gland volume, emphysema, and smoking in a necropsy study. *J. Pathol. Bronch.* **106**, 59–71

Ryder, R., Lyons, J.P., Campbell, H. and Gough, J. (1970) Emphysema in coal workers' pneumoconiosis. *Br. Med. J.* **3**, 481–487

Seaton, A., Lapp, N.L. and Morgan, W.K.C. (1972) Relationship of pulmonary impairment in simple coal workers' pneumoconiosis to type of radiographic opacity. *Br. J. Ind. Med.* **29**, 50–55

Sidor, R. and Peters, J.M. (1974a) Fire-fighting and pulmonary function. *Am. Rev. Respir. Dis.* **109**, 249–254

Sidor, R. and Peters, J.M. (1974b) Prevalence of rates of nonspecific respiratory disease in firefighters. *Am. Rev. Respir. Dis.* **109**, 255–261

Sjögren, B. and Ulfvarson, U. (1985) Respiratory symptoms and pulmonary among welders working with aluminium, stainless steel, and railroad tracks. *Scand. J. Work Environ. Health* **11**, 27

Sparrow, D., Bosse, R., Rosner, B. and Weiss, S.T. (1982) The effect of occupational exposure on lung function. A longitudinal evaluation of firefighters and non-firefighters. *Am. Rev. Respir. Dis.* **125**, 319–322

Surgeon General, US Public Health Service (1985) *The Health Consequences of Smoking. Cancer and Chronic Obstructive Lung Disease in the Workplace. A Report of the Surgeon General.* US Office on Smoking and Health, Rockville, MD, pp. 300–304

Thackrah, C.T. (1832) *The Effects of Arts, Trades and Professions and of Civic States and Habits of Living on Health and Longevity*, 2nd edn, Longman, London

Thomas, A.J. (1948) The heart in the pneumoconiosis of coalminers. *Br. Heart J.* **10**, 282–292

Thomas, A.J. (1951) Right ventricular hypertrophy in the pneumoconiosis of coal miners. *Br. Heart J.* **13**, 1–9

Thurlbeck, V.M., Henderson, J.A.M., Fraser, R.G. and Bates, D.V. (1970) Chronic obstructive lung disease. A comparison between the clinical, roentgenologic, functional and morphological criteria in chronic bronchitis, asthma and bronchiectasis. *Medicine* **49**, 81–145

Townsend, M., Enterline, P.E., Sussman, P.E., Bonney, T.B. and Rippey, L.L. (1985) Pulmonary function in relation to total dust exposure at a bauxite refinery and alumina-based chemical products plant. *Am. Rev. Respir. Dis.* **132**, 1174–1180

Tse, K.S., Warren, P., Janusz, M., McCarthy, D.S. and Cherniack, R.M. (1973) Respiratory abnormalities in workers exposed to grain dust. *Archs Environ. Health* **27**, 74–77

Vuylsteek, K. and Depoorter, A.M. (1978) Smoking, occupational dust exposure and chronic non-specific lung disease. *Broncho-pneumologie* **28**, 31–38

Waters, W.E., Cochrane, A.L. and Moore, F. (1974) Mortality in punctiform type of coal workers' pneumoconiosis. *Br. J. Ind. Med.* **31**, 196–200

Wells, A.L. (1954) Pulmonary vascular changes in coal-workers' pneumoconiosis. *J. Pathol. Bacteriol.* **68**, 573–587

11

Non-fibrogenic ('inert') minerals and pneumoconiosis

W. Raymond Parkes

In the strict sense of the word no dust deposited in the lungs is 'inert' – that is, does not produce some reaction no matter how limited, localized and transient. But, in that 'pneumoconiosis' is a broad, generic term used to describe the lodgement of any inhaled *dusts* in the lungs irrespective of the effects (excluding asthma and neoplasia), 'inert' is a useful word to separate, as a class, those dusts that, although they may be a nuisance, are believed to cause no significant structural changes from those that do – usually in the form of granulomas or fibrosis. Thus, pneumoconiosis caused by these dusts has often been called 'benign'. In general they are of mineral (inorganic) origin; if insoluble, they cause no significant proliferation of 'reticulin' fibres and no collagenous fibrosis and, if soluble, are not toxic locally or systemically. Certain fumes (that is, particulate metallic oxides ranging from 0.1 to 0.4 μm in diameter – see Chapter 3) may cause similar 'benign' lesions.

Importance of inert dusts and fumes

Their radiodensity ranges from high to low (see Table 7.1, page 163). They may be inhaled in almost pure form or in association with fibrogenic dusts (usually free silica in the form of quartz) either as an intimate mixture produced simultaneously by one industrial process, or separately and at different times by different occupations. Dusts and fumes of low radiodensity give no evidence of their presence on a chest radiograph whereas those of high radiodensity cast small, round, well-defined and contrasted opacities throughout the lung fields, and often cause pronounced opacity of hilar lymph nodes (due to their concentration in these sites) which may be misinterpreted as calcification.

It is convenient, therefore, to consider inert dusts according to whether they are of high or low radiodensity and whether or not their presence is associated with that of a fibrotic pneumoconiosis (such as silicosis or asbestos), in which case the lesions due to the inert dusts are morphologically distinct from the others. But inert dusts (most notably iron oxides) may modify the fibrogenic effect of quartz, and other forms of free silica, causing 'mixed dust fibrosis' (see Chapter 12) which lacks the characteristic morphology of the silicotic nodule. If dusts of low radiodensity are contaminated by quartz as an accessory mineral of parent rock both may be inhaled when such rocks are mined, quarried, crushed or used in industrial processes. Similarly, cristobalite (see Appendix I) is sometimes associated with an inert dust contaminated by free silica or silicates subjected to high temperature. It is important to be aware of this in order that an inert dust is not, on the one hand, wrongly considered to be fibrogenic or that, on the other, the presence of a free silica risk does not go unsuspected.

Dusts of high radiodensity

The resulting pneumoconiosis is discussed in the approximate order of increasing atomic number of the metal or mineral responsible. Although, apart from that caused by iron (siderosis), it is uncommon, if not rare, it crops up from time to time in young workers as well as in those who were exposed to the relevant agent many years ago, and is often a source of diagnostic puzzlement to clinicians unaware of the occupational sources today and in the past. Thus, it is appropriate to consider the various types of this pneumoconiosis in some detail.

Titanium (atomic number 22)

Titanium occurs in nature as trimorphic titanium dioxide (TiO_2) in *ilmenite*, a mixed oxide of iron titanium found with magnetite or hematite in basic igneous rocks and their high-grade metamorphic derivatives, and in sand deposits. *Rutile* and *anastase* are the polymorphs employed in industry. Rutile occurs in the form of fine acicular particles (or needles) in some slates (*clayslate needles*) and in quartz and feldspar. But, despite its wide dispersal in nature, titanium dioxide has, in recent years, been largely of synthetic origin. Ilmenite ore is converted to synthetic rutile and anastase by a chloride or sulphate process.

Because of its whiteness, high refractive index and light-scattering qualities its most extensive use is in pigments for paints, paper, rubber, plastics, cosmetics, glass and ceramics, and as a mordant in dyeing. It has a relatively minor use in welding-rod coatings.

Elemental titanium, very much a 'space-age' metal, is widely used in the manufacture of high-speed aircraft, missiles, spacecraft and equipment for marine environments because of its high strength–weight ratio, resistance to corrosion and ability to withstand a very wide range of temperature.

Sources of exposure

Exposure to significant amounts of titanium dioxide dust is unlikely to occur in mining of ilmenite rock or collection of ilmenite sands but is possible in processes using the oxide as a pigment and for the manufacture of barium titanate for electronic ceramics, and in the machining of titanium metal, and also from the dust collectors of exhaust ventilation systems employed in such industries. Because titanium is highly reactive with oxygen, nitrogen and carbon and no refractory material is able to resist it when in the molten state, it is fused in an enclosed consumable-arc furnace so that exposure of operatives to fume is improbable, though this could occur in the preparation of alloys in which titanium is used.

Pathology

In individuals previously exposed to titanium dioxide, aggregations of carbon-like particles are present around respiratory bronchioles and in alveolar walls without microscopic evidence of fibrosis (Schmitz-Moorman, Horlein and Hanefield, 1964). Though a mild degree of alveolar fibrosis has been reported on occasions this has almost certainly been attributable to small amounts of associated quartz (Määttä and Arstila, 1975). Titanium particles can be demonstrated by electron microscopy and energy dispersive X-ray analysis in the phagosomes of alveolar macrophages and macrophages in sputum and bronchial aspirations even two or three years after cessation of exposure; the viability of these cells is apparently unimpaired (Määtä and Arstila, 1975). Titanium dioxide particles are extremely birefringent and, therefore, show up brightly under crossed Nicol prisms or polaroid filters.

The lack of fibrogenic potential in human lungs is confirmed in those of experimental animals. Rutile and anastase have been generally reported as being equally non-pathogenic in both animals (Ferin and Oberdöster, 1985; Richard, White and Eik-Nes, 1985) and in vitro studies (Heppleston, 1988). For this reason they have been employed as negative control markers in experiments designed to study the effects of potentially noxious dusts and gases (Ferin and Leach, 1976; Donaldson et al., 1988; Brown et al., 1991). But because some synthetic rutiles apparently possess a similar ability to quartz to lyse erythrocytes in vitro, it has been suggested that the biological activity of natural and synthetic rutiles may differ significantly, and thus explain the anomalous results seen in some animal experiments (Nolan et al., 1987). Clearly, this observation needs to be explored further, especially in view of evidence that haemolysis is not a good measure of the biological activity of minerals (Richards, White and Eik-Nes, 1985).

There is, however, no definitive evidence that titanium dioxide is other than inert in human lungs, and the relevance of putative biological activity of synthetic rutile has yet to be demonstrated. In one epidemiological study of a large number of titanium metal production workers over 30 years, chronic respiratory disease, carcinoma of the lung and radiographic abnormalities were no higher than among control individuals (Chen and Fayerweather, 1988). Workers in whom radiographic evidence consistent with fibrosis was reported had also been exposed to potentially fibrogenic dusts (Elo et al., 1972), so the culpability of titanium was not established. It is possible, however, that an idiosyncratic host response to the metal, genetically determined, might occur. Sarcoid-type granulomatous disease has been described in two cases: in one, concomitant exposure to beryllium was not excluded (Angebault et al., 1979); in the other, a furnace man in an aluminium smelting plant, there was a positive lymphocyte transformation response to titanium chloride – although of lower magnitude than that found in most cases of beryllium disease (see

Chapter 17) – and not to aluminium, beryllium or nickel salts (Redline et al., 1986). Redline and her colleagues also found no evidence of sensitization in three healthy individuals who had had prolonged exposure to titanium. Thus, careful immunological investigation (perhaps using lymphocytes from bronchoalveolar lavage) of workers exposed to titanium is evidently needed. However, the possibility of coincidentally associated disease has, as always, to be kept in mind.

Ferruginous bodies may form on rutile needles and have been reported in the lungs of a miner of igneous rock (Crouch and Churg, 1984). These bodies are readily distinguishable from asbestos bodies because their cores are black and strongly birefringent (see Chapter 14).

Symptoms and physical signs

There are no subjective or objective abnormalities associated with titanium dioxide exposure. Some workers in the sulphuric acid extraction process complain of cough, shortness of breath and chest 'tightness', and wheezes may be heard on auscultation. These symptoms and signs appear to be due mainly, although not entirely, to exacerbation of the effects of smoking by the acid vapour (Daum et al., 1977).

Lung function

There are no abnormalities attributable to chronic exposure to titanium dioxide or titanium tetrachloride. Among workers in the acid extraction process a small proportion of non-smokers with more than 20 years' exposure have been found to have some evidence of airflow obstruction but, as might be expected, this was more widespread among smokers (Daum et al., 1977).

Radiographic appearances

No evidence of pneumoconiosis has been observed in men extracting ilmenite sand (Uragoda and Pinto, 1972) but small discrete opacities similar to mild siderosis (see page 258) have been recorded, especially where titanium dioxide is employed in the manufacture of pigments and 'hard metal' (see page 604) (Schmitz-Moorman, Horlein and Hanefeld, 1964).

Diagnosis

The same principles apply as in the case of other benign pneumoconioses.

The effects of exposure to the sulphuric acid process or acute exposure to titanium tetrachloride should be suspected from the work history (see Chapter 18).

Conclusion

The inhalation of titanium dioxide appears to be harmless whether or not there is radiographic evidence of its presence as a benign pneumoconiosis which is sometimes, but unhappily, referred to as 'titanosis' or 'titanicosis'. The rarity of reports of pneumoconiosis may be due – depending upon the process in question – to absence of titanium dioxide from the air or to dust particles being, in general, too large to reach alveolar level; or to dust concentrations or duration of exposure being too low for sufficient dust (the atomic number of which is only slightly in excess of that of calcium) to accumulate sufficiently in the lungs to cause radio-opacities.

Iron (atomic number 26): siderosis

Sources of exposure

Dust or fume of metallic iron and iron oxide may be encountered in the following processes, although their concentrations in many industries are limited by dust control measures.

1. *Iron and steel rolling mills* in which metal strips are subjected to much agitation with the production of rust and iron scale dust.
2. *Steel grinding.*
3. *Electric arc and oxyacetylene welding.* The high temperature of these types of welding when applied to iron gives rise to iron oxide fume and other fumes and gases. The concentration of fumes in the breathing zone is often high if welders work in confined and ill-ventilated places such as tanks, boilers and the holds of ships.

    Welding methods and their possible hazards are discussed in more detail in Chapter 18.
4. *Polishing of silver and steel with iron oxide powder.* The powder is an especially pure form of ferric oxide in a finely divided state, often referred to as 'rouge' or 'crocus'. Polishing is done by means of power-operated buffing wheels of wool or cotton. Silver polishing is also likely to produce minute particles of metallic silver.

    Ferric oxide is further used to polish glass, stone and cutlery.

5. *Fettling (that is, scouring), chipping and dressing castings in iron foundries.* Until recently this process was a common source of quartz as well as iron dust from attrition of burnt-on moulding sands adhering to the castings (see Chapter 12) and, therefore, liable to cause either 'mixed dust fibrosis' or typical silicosis. Nevertheless, siderosis may occur alone when it may be wrongly diagnosed as silicosis.

   A suvey in a Sheffield steel foundry between 1955 and 1960 revealed that the average prevalence of siderosis among welders and burners in the fettling and grinding shops was 17.6 per cent (Gregory, 1970).

6. *Boiler scaling* involves the cleaning of fireboxes, flues and water-tubes in enclosed spaces in the boilers of ships, factories, power stations and the like. A high concentration of dust is produced which contains iron and carbon, and, in coal-fired – but not oil-fired – boilers, silicates and small quantities of quartz derived from the coal. Although siderosis alone may be produced, mixed dust fibrosis is more likely (see Chapter 12).

7. *Mining and crushing iron ores.* The important ores are magnetite, hematite and limonite.

   Magnetite occurs in several geological environments and ores of the mineral are frequently associated with quartz-bearing rock and contain quartz gangue (as in northern Sweden, where the richest deposits are found). It is also found in beach sands. Therefore, quartz may sometimes be a substantial contaminant of the ore resulting in mixed dust fibrosis or silicosis, in addition to siderosis in miners and crusher operators; but, again, siderosis may be observed alone.

   Hematite (also known as 'specularite' and 'kidney ore') is mined chiefly in Cumberland and, until recently, in the Furness district of Lancashire where it occurs in limestone beds; but some deposits are associated with red ferruginous sandstone and are, therefore, liable to contamination by quartz. One of the largest sources in the world, near Lake Superior in Canada, is also partly contaminated by free silica because it contains interbedded layers of chert, but quartz is virtually absent from deposits at Bilbao and on the Quebec–Labrador border.

   Limonite occurs in 'bog iron ore' and bituminous coals. Contaminating silica is usually absent.

   It will be seen, therefore, that the likelihood of siderosis occurring alone, or accompanied by pure silicosis or 'mixed dust fibrosis', depends to a large extent upon the geographical origin of the ore or the site from which it comes in any one deposit. Dust is produced during mining, loading, crushing and milling of the ores.

   Hematite and limonite are used as pigments in paint manufacture and, together with magnetite, are added in finely divided form to certain fertilizers. It is possible, therefore, for workers in those industries to be exposed to iron oxide dusts.

8. *Mining, milling and mixing emery and its use as an abrasive.* Emery is an intimate mixture of hematite, magnetite and *corundum* (aluminium oxide, Al_2O_3) which, next to diamond, is the hardest natural mineral known. Today Turkey is the largest producer and smaller quantities come from the USA. It is found most commonly in pockets or lenses in crystalline limestone, gneisses and schists, or as a deposit derived from these rocks by weathering. It contains insignificant quantities of quartz, and its abrasive quality is due mainly to the aluminium oxide present.

   Because emery is apt to contain variable amounts of impurities (such as plagioclase feldspar) and a constant composition cannot, therefore, be relied upon, it has been very largely replaced by artificial abrasives – principally Carborundum and synthetic corundum (see pages 276 and 594). However, Turkish emery is still employed in the making of coated abrasives such as emery cloths and papers for hand use, and buffing wheels and mops; it is also used in abrasive pastes and as a non-slip, wear-resisting component of concrete floors and road surfaces, and for polishing rice. High concentrations of emery dust have been, and occasionally still are, produced during the manufacture of most of these materials and the use of the different abrasive preparations for various polishing procedures (Bech, Kipling and Zundel, 1965; Foá, 1967).

   Pneumoconiosis in emery workers, therefore, will almost certainly be siderosis unless there has also been exposure to some other dust hazard (for example, the coal mining, pottery or asbestos industries).

9. *Mining, pulverizing and mixing natural mineral pigments.* Apart from hematite and limonite these include the ferruginous earths – ochre, sienna and umber clays – which consist of iron and aluminium oxides with a variable amount of siliceous impurity. These clays are mined in the USA, the Persian Gulf, Turkey, Cyprus, France, Italy and Andalusia but pulverizing and mixing are usually done by the firm which imports them. Synthetic iron pigments prepared from iron oxides, however, have now largely superseded the natural products.

   Siderosis may occur alone in workers who pulverize and mix natural pigments which, at this stage, have been purified by screening, washing and drying; it also occurs in those engaged in some stages of the manufacture of synthetic pigments and in their use. But disease identical to the 'mixed dust fibrosis' of hematite miners (see page 323) may be found among miners and in operatives involved in crushing and coarse-screening the ore when the quartz content of the clays or other parent rocks is substantial as is the case in Italy where it varies from 2 to 35 per cent (Champeix and Moreau, 1958), and in the Apt area of France where it is as high as 50 per cent (Roche, Picard and Vernhes, 1958).

10. *Magnetic tape industry.* This comparatively small industry began in the mid-1960s. Magnetic iron oxide is produced from non-magnetic α-ferric oxide ($Fe_2O_3·H_2O$) which is converted through non-magnetic ferric oxide to the magnetic oxide in a rotary kiln. Exposure to dry powder can occur during charging and emptying kilns, in bagging the finished oxide and in emptying it into mills in preparation for coating the tape. No evidence of any pulmonary abnormalities has been reported (Stokinger, 1984). It is improbable that the very low magnetic fields of the synthetic oxide which might be retained in the lungs are harmful in any way in so far as magnetic iron (apparently used as a navigational aid) in the heads of dolphins (*Delphinus delphis*), homing pigeons and honey bees has no adverse effect (Zoeger, Dunn and Fuller, 1981; Kuterbach et al., 1982).

Pathology

Some workers, as intimated earlier, exposed to metallic iron dust or iron oxide fume (such as welders, iron foundry men, boiler scalers and miners and millers of iron ores) may also have had significant exposure to other dusts such as quartz, cristobalite or asbestos, so that siderosis may be complicated by the presence of 'mixed dust fibrosis' or by asbestosis.

That iron oxide dust is not fibrogenic in human and animal lungs has been well attested over the years: in the former, for example, by Barrie and Harding (1947), Harding, McLaughlin and Doig (1958), Morgan and Kerr (1963), Kaponen and Gustafsson (1980); and, in the latter, by Harding, Grant and Davies (1947), Vorwald et al. (1950), Gross, Westrick and McNerhey (1960), Holmqvist and Swensen (1963), and Albu and Schuleri (1972). Furthermore, natural emery does not induce collagen formation in the lungs or peritoneum (Mellissonos, Collet and Daniel-Moussard, 1966). In spite of this substantial evidence, interstitial fibrosis in two welders was attributed to iron although 5 per cent of silica was present in the lesions in the one and 2.4 per cent in those of the other (Stettler, Groth and MacKay, 1977). Interstitial fibrosis in another arc welder was associated with silicotic nodules and the presence of

silicon on SEM in addition to iron (Guidotti et al., 1978). It is possible that the silicon in these cases represented cristobalite which is, of course, actively fibrogenic (see Appendix I and Chapters 5 and 12). Volatilization of silicates, and any free silica which might be formed, occurs in consumable electrode coatings at arc temperature. The degree of conversion to cristobalite is uncertain because, owing to the small volume of the high-temperature mass at the welding point, the cooling rate of volatilized silica may be too rapid for substantial amounts to form; however, in some circumstances, welding fume may contain amorphous- coated cristobalite of small particle size (W.A. Bloor, 1980, personal communication). It is difficult to explain a report of 10 welders with 'nodular opacities' in their radiographs, the biopsy sections of whose lungs showed DIPF said to be caused by iron particles because scanning electron microscopy (SEM) and energy-dispersive X-ray analysis (EDXA) revealed, apart from the expected high levels of iron, a silicon content no higher than that of control lungs and 'no other specific foreign element' (Funahashi et al., 1988). Some unidentified cause might, however, be suspected. Pulmonary disease in welders is discussed further in Chapter 18.

Iron hydroxide, similar to aluminium hydroxide, exerts a powerful inhibiting influence on the fibrogenic action of quartz (Reichel, Bauer and Bruckmann, 1977).

Macroscopic appearances

The pulmonary pleura is marbled a rust-brown colour but, in the case of hematite, the colour may be a deep brick-red. This is due to the deposition of iron oxide in the pleural lymphatics similar to the black pigmentation seen in the pleura of coal miners.

The cut surface of the lungs reveals grey to rust-brown coloured macules from 1 to 4 mm in diameter which are impalpable and do not stand up from the surface in contrast to silicotic nodules. They are evenly distributed but may be difficult to distinguish as individual lesions if the lungs are generally dust stained. The appearance of the lungs and lesions where hematite is involved is particularly striking due to the brick-red coloration. Some hematite lungs may also exhibit discrete nodular fibrosis or massive fibrosis when quartz is associated with the iron oxide (see Chapter 12). Typical silicotic lesions are readily distinguishable by the naked eye.

Microscopic appearances

The fundamental lesion consists of a perivascular and peribronchiolar aggregation of dark pigmented iron oxide particles which are present both in macrophages and extracellularly in alveolar spaces

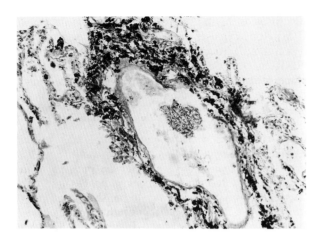

Figure 11.1 Siderosis: there is a perivascular 'cuff' of iron particles and dust-laden macrophages but no fibrosis. The alveolar walls and spaces are normal. Magnification × 225; haematoxylin and eosin

and walls where they are mostly perivascular. Intra- and extracellular collections of these particles are also seen subpleurally and infiltrating interlobular septa. There is no collagenous fibrosis (Figure 11.1). These particles, unlike those of protein-bound endogenous iron, haemosiderin, are not stained, and, therefore, not identified, by Perl's Prussian blue reaction. However, because haemosiderin, together with ferritin, is commonly associated with iron oxide deposition in the lungs a positive reaction may occur. But ferritin – which may be ingested by macrophages containing iron oxide in similar fashion to those containing carbon and quartz – must be separated from the protein apoferritin by a reducing agent, such as hydrosulphite, before it will take the stain.

If fibrotic lesions are seen they are usually caused by tuberculosis or by the additional presence of crystalline silica (Mosinger et al., 1968).

Metallic silver, as well as iron, is present in the lungs of silver polishers. It is taken up as a vital stain by the elastic tissue, and appears grey–black in colour, in the walls of airways and arteries; it is not fibrogenic. This is known as *argyrosiderosis* (Barrie and Harding, 1947). Silver (atomic number 47) contributes significantly to the effective atomic number of the mixture and, therefore, to the density and summation of opacities on the radiograph.

It has been suggested (Sadoul et al., 1979) that the retention of iron dust may cause emphysema in iron miners' lungs, but the evidence for this is unconvincing.

Symptoms and physical signs

Apart from the production of reddish-coloured sputum which sometimes follows exposure to these dusts, there are no symptoms or abnormal physical signs caused by siderosis, and if any are present they are due to some other cause.

Lung function

There is no impairment of any parameter of lung function (Morgan and Kerr, 1963; Fogh, Frost and Georg, 1969; Kleinfeld et al., 1969; Teculescu and Albu, 1973) and, although a greater prevalence of airways' obstruction has been reported among electric arc welders compared with non-welders (Hunnicutt, Cracovaner and Myles, 1964), this was related mainly to cigarette smoking. Impaired lung function in a subject with lone siderosis is due either to the effects of cigarette smoking or to non-industrial lung disease, or a combination of both.

Radiographic appearances

The term 'siderosis' was introduced by Zenker in 1867 when he coined the generic word 'pneumonokoniosis', but the disorder was believed to be fibrosis of the lungs, and cases subsequently reported in the late nineteenth and early twentieth centuries were examples of siderosilicosis. Although it was not until 1936 that Doig and McLaughlin suggested that iron oxide dust itself might be 'opaque to X-rays' and, thus, the reason for the radiographic appearances of the lungs of electric arc welders, it should be acknowledged that, in July 1919, Thurston Holland, a distinguished Liverpool pioneer of radiology, wrote to Collis that hematite dust was 'extremely opaque to X-rays. . . . . Even the finest particles when placed upon the plate leave almost clear glass on development'. Collis replied: 'No one previously appears to have considered the possibility of inhaled dust throwing shadows *per se*, as apart from any fibrosis set up. . . .' (Fawcitt, 1943). This important observation, a valuable clue in the study of the pneumoconioses, seems to have gone unnoticed.

The absorptive capacity of iron for X-rays is considerably higher than that of non-iron lung constituents and of silicate minerals or coal deposits in the lungs; in fact, whereas the mass absorption coefficient for silicate minerals is three to five times greater than carbon, that of iron is 40 times greater (Safety in Mines Research, 1963).

The standard chest radiograph shows a variable, usually large, number of small opacities varying from 0.5 mm to about 2 mm in diameter, of striking density and associated with fewer fine, rather less dense, linear opacities (Figure 11.2). Large, confluent opacities do not occur. In some cases Kerley 'B' lines caused by the accumulation of iron in interlobular septa are prominent. The hilar lymph nodes

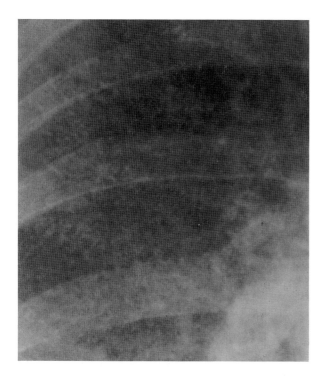

Figure 11.2 Siderosis in an emery worker. Numerous small fairly dense opacities evenly scattered throughout the lung fields – category 3p (natural size)

may appear unusually radio-opaque due to their concentrated iron content, but they are not enlarged.

Prolonged exposure to iron dust or fume is usually required to give these radiographic appearances, but in the event of exposure to high dust concentration they have been observed after as short a period as 3 years (Kleinfeld et al., 1969).

The presence in the lungs of iron-containing dust or fume with a magnetic component can be identified by magnetopneumography with much greater sensitivity than by the standard radiograph (see Chapter 7, page 203). Although this can be of value for serial assessment of the accumulation of dust in the lungs of workers exposed to ferromagnetic mineral particles (lowest in iron and steel workers, higher in foundry workers and highest in arc welders), it is neither practical nor necessary for individual routine examinations.

Diagnosis

This rests upon a history of work in processes known to give rise to iron dust or fume coupled with the radiographic appearances. Siderosis can be easily overlooked if the details of the work are not known as, for example, when it occurs in

woodworkers who have used emery abrasives. Biopsy of lung tissue is rarely justifiable.

The possibility that welders, at some stage in their working lives, may have been in contact with free silica, asbestos or other fibrogenic dusts must not be overlooked.

Differential diagnosis

Other inert dusts of high radiodensity (antimony, tin and barium, for example) may produce almost identical appearances. As a rule the size, density and uniform distribution throughout the lung fields of the opacities of siderosis distinguish them from those of nodular silicosis and coal pneumoconiosis which are larger, less dense, usually less well defined and commonly predominant in the upper and middle zones of the lung fields. Occasionally, tiny 'pinhead' opacities are observed in the radiographs of coal miners (see Chapter 13) but their density is generally less than those of siderosis.

Miliary tuberculosis is readily distinguishable because of the lack of industrial exposure, the illness of the patient and the fact that the opacities tend to be less dense, less well defined and often most profuse in the mid-zones of the lung fields.

Some cases of idiopathic sarcoidosis present a similar appearance but the lack of an industrial history, evidence of enlarged hilar lymph nodes and other clinical and investigatory features of this disorder readily establish the diagnosis. When, however, there is a history of relevant industrial exposure the differentiation may occasionally be sufficiently difficult to indicate lung biopsy, but this should rarely be necessary if the discipline of differential diagnosis is properly followed.

Cryptogenic pulmonary haemosiderosis, which is more common in men than in women and in which opacities similar to those of siderosis follow repeated capillary haemorrhages (Wynn-Williams and Young, 1956; Karlish, 1962), is distinguished by recurrent haemoptysis, hypochromic anaemia and, in some cases, finger clubbing and enlargement of liver and spleen. Haemosiderosis due to mitral stenosis is readily identified in most cases if the presence of the valve disease is recognized and, although differentiation is impossible in the occasional case of a worker with mitral stenosis who has been exposed to iron oxide dusts or fumes, this is of no practical importance.

Prognosis

After the worker leaves exposure, the iron dust is slowly eliminated from the lungs over a period of years. This is reflected in gradual partial or complete disappearance of radiographic opacities

(Doig and McLaughlin, 1948); however, the greater the quantity of dust the longer the period for its elimination.

The benign nature of siderosis has been clearly demonstrated in arc welders (Doig and McLaughlin, 1936; Morgan and Kerr, 1963).

Bronchial carcinoma and iron-dust inhalation

It has been suggested that inhaled iron dust may act as a carcinogen mainly on the grounds that a higher incidence of bronchial carcinoma was calculated to be present in hematite miners in West Cumberland than in the general population (Faulds and Stewart, 1956), but the methods of reaching this conclusion were flawed (Doll, 1959). Other substances (such as tars) with known carcinogenic potential were present in some of the work processes and the smoking habits of the workers were not analysed. An increased mortality (of about 70 per cent) from carcinoma of the lung among miners (Boyd et al., 1970) was subsequently attributed to unusually high concentrations of radon gas in the mine air (Duggan et al., 1970). Similarly, fairly high levels of radon were observed in Swedish iron ore mines before mechanical ventilation was introduced in the 1950s, but an excess of carcinoma of the lung among miners some years later was related to smoking (Edling, 1982).

In a comprehensive review of world literature, Stokinger (1984) found no evidence that iron oxides are carcinogenic in the lungs of man or experimental animals.

Chromite (chrome iron ore)

Chromite is the mineral ore of chromium, and it consists of chromium and iron oxides (Cr_2O_3FeO). The atomic numbers of chromium and iron are 24 and 26 respectively, but the *effective atomic number* of chromite is 22 (see Chapter 7).

The world's largest producers of chromite are Zimbabwe, South Africa, Turkey and the USSR. In the Transvaal it occurs in association with pyroxenite, anorthosite and norite rocks and although there are occasional pegmatite veins which contain some quartz and alkaline feldspar these are few, and the amount of quartz in the mine dust is generally less than 1 per cent (Sluis-Cremer and du Toit, 1968).

Chromite is used in various metallurgical applications, for foundry moulding sands and as a constituent of basic refractories for furnace linings.

The chest radiographs of miners who have been exposed to chromite mine dust for 8 or more years may show small, discrete opacities similar to those of siderosis and increased opacity, but no enlargement, of the hilar shadows. There are no accompanying respiratory symptoms or signs (Sluis-Cremer and du Toit, 1968). No histological studies are available in these cases, but in view of the fact that chromite dust appears to cause only a minor cellular reaction and no fibrosis in the lungs of experimental animals (Worth and Schiller, 1955; Goldstein, 1965), Sluis-Cremer and du Toit (1968) consider that the human lesions are benign and not associated with fibrosis. However, histological examination of the lungs of three men who had worked in a chromate plant in which chromite was one of the three chromium compounds used, revealed large quantities of black pigment (identified as chromite) in the alveolar walls which were thickened, fibrotic and hyalinized (Mancuso and Hueper, 1951). But whether these changes were due to chromium rather than to some past inflammatory process or to other inhaled aerosols was not known.

From the available evidence, therefore, it appears that chromite dust is non-fibrogenic. In contrast to the apparent innocuousness of chromite, however, chromium salts may induce asthma (see Chapter 21), and chromic acid and chromates (hexavalent chromium compounds) are highly irritant to the respiratory tract; furthermore, an increased incidence of carcinoma of the lung is associated with exposure to chromates, but this has not been observed in chromite mine workers (Sluis-Cremer and du Toit, 1968) (see Chapter 19).

Zirconium (atomic number 40) and hafnium (atomic number 72)

Zirconium (Zr) occurs most commonly as *zircon* ($ZrSiO_4$) and *baddeleyite* (ZrO_2). Both zirconium and hafnium (Hf) are closely geochemically associated in zircon, which is the principal ore mineral, in the ratio of 50 to 1. The two are not separated for use other than in nuclear applications (Ampian, 1975). Hafnium oxide is known as *hafnia*. In addition to hafnium, minor amounts of thorium, uranium and rare earth elements are commonly present in the mineral (Klemic, 1975).

Zircon, which is widely distributed in igneous and sedimentary rocks, is recovered commercially from beach sands and river gravels and is concentrated by magnetic and electrostatic separation techniques to remove accessory minerals such as ilmenite, rutile, magnetite and monazite; quartz is removed by gravitation.

Zircon is very heavy, has a very high refractive index and strong birefringence, low solubility and remarkable refractory properties.

Sources of exposure and uses

Zircon dust or fume may be produced when zircon concentrate is dried and calcined to remove organic material; subsequent treatment with magnetic and roll separators to remove quartz and other impurities may also give rise to dust. Dust of zirconium compounds may be produced during many of the processes in which it is used. Quartz dust may be a hazard during the milling of the raw material and in the separation processes, but is otherwise absent.

Probably the largest use of zirconium is in alloy manufacture: with silicon and manganese in steel, and in nickel–cobalt and niobium–tantalum alloys which resist neutron bombardment. This is because zirconium imparts special alloying properties, structural stability at high temperatures, corrosion resistance and low neutron absorption characteristics. For these reasons, it is used inside atomic reactors and to line reaction vessels. It is also employed as an igniter in the manufacture of detonators and munitions.

Zircon is of particular importance in the manufacture of technical refractory ceramics in the form of crucibles, tubes and boats, and for high-temperature work in chemistry and metallurgy. It is increasingly, though not universally, used in foundry work in the form of oil-bonded 'sand', and for mould paints and parting powder in place of quartz sands and 'silica flour' (see Chapter 12). Not only does it eliminate the 'silica' risk – and so may be used for sandblasting – but it possesses the additional advantage of high resistance to thermal shock. In the interest of economy, recovery of zircon sand for re-use in foundries is likely to increase in the future. Zircon and various zirconium compounds are employed as opacifiers in ceramic enamels and in glasses and glazes because of their resistance to acid and to thermal shock, and to impart high dielectric strength to electrical porcelain such as sparking plugs. Zircon is also employed as a polishing agent for glass and television tubes and, in the form of 'pebbles', as a grinding medium in rotary mills. Aluminium oxide and zircon fused in an electric arc furnace produce 'alumina–zirconia' abrasives which are employed in heavy duty grinding wheels.

Zirconium dioxide (*zirconia*), which is produced by reacting zirconium with dolomite at high temperature, plays an important role in turbojet and rocket manufacture because it melts at about 2700°C and, in stabilized form, can withstand temperatures in excess of 1900°C. The powder is also employed in the optical industry for polishing lenses. Some hafnia is invariably present in zirconia but is not a disadvantage to its use as a refractory.

Baddeleyite, which consists chiefly of zirconium dioxide with minor mineral impurities including hafnium up to 1.7 per cent, has similar properties to those of zirconia.

Zirconium is used in the production of photographic flash bulbs, in the surface reflecting material of 'space' satellites and in the chemical and nuclear reactor industries.

Hafnium is used mainly for control rods in naval and, to a lesser extent, in commercial nuclear reactors, and a small amount is employed in optical glass, flash bulbs and as an additive in refractory alloys.

Pathology

The possible biological effect of zircon was investigated in animals by Harding (1948) and Harding and Davies (1952). It was found to be remarkably inert in the lungs. Normal phagocytosis of dust particles and a slight accumulation of small cells occurred but there was no fibrosis or increase of reticulin. Numerous small dense opacities were present throughout the lung fields of radiographs of the animals' lungs due to the atomic number of the retained dust (Harding and Davies, 1952). These observations were confirmed by Reed (1956).

But zirconium-containing compounds can cause non-caseating granulomas in human skin when repeatedly applied in deodorants (Rubin et al., 1956) or injected experimentally especially as sodium zirconium lactate – an observation confirmed in guinea-pigs (Shelley and Hurley, 1958; Epstein, Skahen and Krasnobrod, 1962; Turk and Parker, 1977). Although the granulomas have been referred to as 'allergic type', delayed hypersensitivity has not been successfully demonstrated in animals (Epstein, 1967). This contrasts with the observation that beryllium salts (which cause sarcoid-type granulomas) induce delayed hypersensitivity in both human beings and animals (see Chapter 17). Experimental studies in the rabbit have demonstrated a striking difference between the effects of zirconium compounds and beryllium sulphate. Zirconium aluminium glycate and sodium zirconium lactate when introduced intradermally give rise to small 'foreign body type' (low turnover) granulomas without in vivo and in vitro evidence of delayed hypersensitivity, lymphocyte stimulation or production of macrophage inhibition factor (MIF), whereas beryllium sulphate, as well as inducing local non-caseating granulomas, causes delayed skin reactivity and MIF after repeated injections. Bartter et al. (1991) found that in a worker exposed to zirconium compounds, neither peripheral nor pulmonary (BAL) lymphocytes showed any proliferative response to zirconium. Furthermore, zirconium compounds are much less toxic to alveolar macrophages than beryllium sulphate. Whatever the explanations of the differences between the effects of zirconium and beryllium compounds may be, these observations suggest that the zirconium compounds do not induce delayed hypersensitivity in human beings. It is possible that the insolubility of the zirconium salts limits their dispersal to, and contact with, immunologically competent cells (Kang et al., 1977). There is no cross-sensitivity between beryllium and zirconium (Shelley and Hurley, 1971).

Electron microscopy of epithelioid and multi-nucleate giant cells in granulomas induced by repeated intradermal injection of sodium zirconium lactate shows that they have the same appearances as these cells in granulomas caused by this compound in human skin, but that their ultrastructure differs in a number of respects from similar cells observed in human sarcoidosis (Turk, Badenoch-Jones and Parker, 1978).

There does not appear to be any radiographic or histopathological evidence to indicate that zirconium or its compounds have caused granulomatous or fibrotic disease in human beings (Reed, 1956). Peribronchial granulomas have been induced in rabbits by the inhalation of zirconium lactate (Prior, Cronk and Ziegler, 1960) although, in another inhalation experiment with the same compound in three animal species, no granulomas and only minimal fibrosis were observed (Brown, Mastromatteo and Horwood, 1963). Bartter et al. (1991), however, reported severe DIPF in both lower lung fields in a man who had worked for 39 years, from 1961, as a lens grinder and polisher exposed to zirconia (ZrO_2), talc, asbestos, silica, zinc stearate, iron compounds and traces of other metals. His chief exposure was believed to be a compound containing 90 per cent zirconia and 10 per cent 'respirable quartz'. Quantitative scanning electron microscopy analysis of particles in a biopsy specimen of lungs showed a predominance of zirconia, zirconium silicate and zirconium aluminium silicate with lower concentrations of silica, talc and aluminium silicate which the authors dismissed as being 'well below those associated with pneumoconiosis due to these agents'. Because of these findings and the absence of any non-occupational explanation for DIPF, they suggested that 'zirconium should be considered as a likely cause of pneumoconiosis'. Nonetheless, further critical investigation of the effects of zirconium compounds on human lungs is needed to establish a causal nexus with confidence.

No investigations into the effects of hafnium or hafnia appear to have been done.

Symptoms and physical signs

There is nothing at present to suggest that the inhalation of dust of zirconium or of zirconium compounds causes any clinical effects in human beings.

Lung function

Estimations of ventilatory function (FEV_1 and FVC) and gas transfer in 11 exposed workers with category 1 to 3 radiographic opacities were normal, though low normal gas transfer was observed in two. Repetition of the gas transfer test 2 to 3 years later in five of these men, four of whom were non-smokers, showed a decrease greater than that expected due to age, but there was no clear indication that this change was due to zircon in the lungs. There was no measurable defect in ventilatory capacity. Among 49 other workers with no evidence of pneumoconiosis, employed in the same process, ventilatory function tests were normal, both in smokers and non-smokers (McCallum and Leathart, 1975).

Radiographic appearances

A survey of workers in a factory processing zircon revealed a number with discrete pneumoconiotic opacities though many of the men had also been exposed to antimony, barium and titanium dust. But

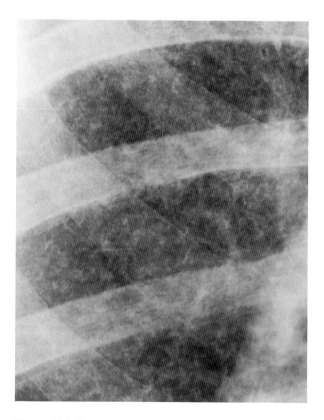

Figure 11.3 Category q opacities in a worker exposed predominantly to zirconium silicate and oxide in a zircon processing plant for about 10 years. (Courtesy of Dr R.I. McCallum)

12 men who had been exposed mainly to zirconium silicate and oxide dusts for periods of 6 to 26 years had small dense opacities ranging from category 1 to 3p. Progression from category 0 to early changes or from one category to a higher category was seen in four men over a period of years although, in general, category did not correlate well with duration of exposure (McCallum and Leathart, 1975) (Figure 11.3). The opacities may gradually regress after exposure ceases. By contrast no radiographic changes 'reasonably attributable to radio-opaque dusts' were found by Reed (1956) in 22 men who worked in a zirconium plant for 1 to 5 years; however, this could well have been due to the short period of exposure. Similarly, a study of 32 men exposed to zirconium-containing dust for an average of 4.9 years showed no radiological abnormality, but concentrations of zirconium were low and time of exposure was relatively short (Hadjimicheal and Brubaker, 1981).

McCallum (R.I., 1977, personal communication) – like Harding and Davies (1952) previously – has produced discrete opacities in the lung fields and dense hilar node shadows in cats (which remained fit and well) following prolonged exposure to pure zirconium silicate dust.

It is likely that the effective atomic number of zirconium compounds – and, hence, their absorptive capacity for X-rays – will exceed that of zirconium according to the amount of hafnium associated with them, though this will usually be small.

Diagnosis

The possibility of a symptomless and benign pneumoconiosis being caused by zirconium dusts should be borne in mind in view of the widespread use of these compounds in industry. It is possible that the small opacities seen in the chest radiographs of some moulders and 'knock-out' men in foundries where moulding sands and parting powders have been replaced by zircon may be caused by zirconium rather than, or in addition to, iron (see 'Siderosis').

Conclusion

Prolonged exposure to zirconium dusts may cause a 'benign' pneumoconiosis similar to siderosis but, at present, there is no consistent evidence that it gives rise to granulomatous or fibrotic lung disease, although evidently, this cannot be dismissed out of hand. The reaction to zirconium compounds in both human beings and animals, appears to be different from that which occurs in the case of beryllium compounds; delayed (type IV) hypersensitivity does not seem to be involved.

Zirconium tetrachloride is referred to in Chapter 18, page 615.

Tin (atomic number 50); stannosis (stannum, tin)

Because the atomic number of tin is almost double that of iron its radiodensity is substantially greater.

Stannosis was first recognized in Germany during the Second World War. Shortly afterwards it was reported in Czechoslovakia (Barták and Tomečka, 1949), in the USA (Pendergrass and Pryde, 1948; Cutter et al., 1949; Dundon and Hughes, 1950) and, in particular detail, in the UK (Robertson and Whittaker, 1955; Robertson et al., 1961). It is much less common than siderosis because the possibilities of industrial exposure are limited. By 1959 over 150 cases were recorded in the world literature (Barnes and Stoner, 1959).

Origins of tin ore

The chief ore is *cassiterite*, tin oxide, from which tin must be recovered by smelting. The main tin fields of the world are in Malaysia, the UK, Thailand, Indonesia, Bolivia, Nigeria and Australia. The metalliferous region of south-west England is the only indigenous source in the UK and production here has increased greatly in recent years after a long period of decline. In spite of this the UK is one of the world's largest importers and consumers of tin in various forms after the USA which possesses no workable tin deposits.

The ore is found only in association with granitic rocks that contain substantial quantities of quartz.

Sources of exposure and uses

Due to the fact that the amount of tin in the crude ore is extremely small, mining procedures (drilling and loading of ore), crushing and screening are unlikely to cause stannosis, but the highly siliceous dust produced is a source of silicosis. Concentrates of cassiterite received by the smelters are largely freed of associated rock and the content of quartz, therefore, almost eliminated.

Processes likely to produce tin dust or fume are as follows: the emptying of bags of crude ore into skips; milling and grinding of ore (Oyanguren et al., 1957); shovelling up of spilt ore; tipping of crushed ore into the calcination furnace; charging smelting furnaces with calcined ore (molten tin issuing from these furnaces gives off tin oxide fume) (Spencer and Wycott, 1954); raking out of refinery furnaces which contain a high percentage of tin oxide and melting down tin scrap to recover tin oxide (Dundon and Hughes, 1950). Solid impurities are removed by heating the impure tin just above melting point. It is then drained off or separated by filtration; little tin oxide fume is likely to be evolved.

Tin dust produced by grinding, briquet making, smelting and casting contains 58 to 65 per cent tin and only 0.2 to 1 per cent quartz (Oyanguren et al., 1957). High concentrations of tin dust and fume are also produced by hearth tinning where the articles to be plated are dipped by hand into molten tin (Cole et al., 1964). Tin plating is now done mainly by electrodeposition methods.

The greatest production of primary refined tin in 1972 was by West Malaysia and then in order, the UK, Thailand, Indonesia, Nigeria, Bolivia, Australia, Spain and the USA (Slater, 1974).

The uses of tin are extensive, the two most important being in tinplating and solders, but also in bronzes, bearing metals, various alloys (such as tin–lead, known as 'Babbitt', and aluminium tin), inorganic tin compounds (employed, for example, in ceramic glazes, vitreous enamels and tooth pastes) and organotins (that is tin-based organic compounds) which are used in the manufacture of certain polyvinyl chloride articles, in fungicides, pesticides, antifouling paints and paper manufacture (Slater, 1974). Wafers of metallic tin are reacted with chlorine to produce stannic chloride (used in electroplating salts) which is further processed into various organotins such as tributyl and dioctyl tin. Opportunity for exposure to metallic tin dust or oxide fume in this process is, however, negligible. Occasional exposure to the irritant vapours of stannic chloride and hydrochloric acid may occur during plant maintenance but simple precautions render this of minor order (D. Fysh, 1977, personal communication). In the float glass process (see Chapter 12), plate glass is floated in molten tin in an enclosed bath, but there is no exposure to tin fume or dust at any stage (J.D. Cameron, 1970, personal communication).

Pathology

Pneumoconiosis in tin miners occurs in the form of nodular silicosis; stannosis is not seen. There is, in some cases, well-marked, grey–black pigmentation of subpleural interlobular septa due to deposition of dust.

Macroscopic appearances

In stannosis, naked-eye inspection of the cut surface of the lungs reveals numerous tiny (1 to 3 mm), grey–black dust macules, soft to the touch and not raised above the cut surface of the lung.

Microscopic appearances

Macrophages containing tin oxide dust particles are present in alveolar walls and spaces, perivascular lymphatics and interlobular septa. The macules, like those of siderosis, consist of dense perivascular and peribronchiolar aggregations of dust-laden macrophages (see Figure 11.1). By light microscopy the intracellular particles are indistinguishable from carbon but they remain after microincineration (Robertson et al., 1961) whereas carbon disappears; X-ray diffraction gives definitive identification. The tetragonal crystals of tin oxide exhibit strong birefringence, unlike crystals of quartz which are poorly birefringent. There is no excess of reticulin or collagen fibres even after 50 years' exposure to tin oxide (Robertson et al., 1961).

The quartz content of the lungs is negligible and has been estimated as substantially less than 0.2 g/lung (Robertson et al., 1961) and in the same cases the amount of tin was estimated as ranging from 0.5 to 3.3 g/lung – the former value related to a man with an 11-year exposure and the latter, one with 50 years. Dust particles, single or aggregated, recovered from the lungs are from 0.1 to 0.5 µm in diameter and closely resemble furnace fume particles in size and appearance (Robertson et al., 1961).

The hilar lymph nodes appear black but are not fibrotic.

Although small quantities of tin oxide have been found in the spleen and liver of a man who had stannosis (Barták and Tomečka, 1949), there is no evidence that it has any systemic toxic effect.

Tin oxide does not cause fibrosis in the lungs (Robertson, 1960; Fischer and Zinnerman, 1969), liver or spleen (Fischer and Zinnerman, 1969) of experimental animals.

Symptoms and physical signs

There are no symptoms or abnormal physical signs due to the inhalation and retention of tin oxide dust.

Lung function

Lung function is unaffected (Robertson, 1960). If there is any associated abnormality it is due to some other cause.

Radiographic appearances

When exposure to tin oxide dust has been heavy or prolonged numerous small, very dense opacities are scattered evenly throughout the lung fields; they may be somewhat larger (2 to 4 mm diameter) and more 'fluffy' or irregular in outline than those of siderosis – possibly due to the combined effect of superimposition and their greater radiodensity (Figure 11.4). Owing to deposition of dust in interlobular septa, Kerley 'B' lines are often clearly

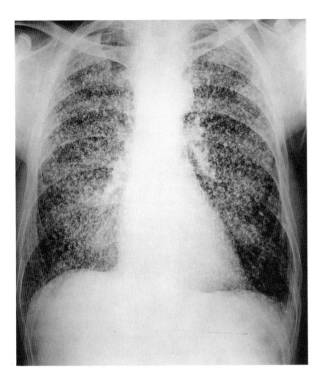

Figure 11.4 Stannosis in a furnace charger in a tin smelting works for 42 years. Note the density of the pulmonary and hilar node opacities. The Kerley 'B' lines in the right costophrenic angle and sharp definition of the lesser fissure are also due to tin deposition

defined and thin dense linear opacities may be seen in the upper lung zones. With lesser degrees of exposure, opacities are fewer, less dense and somewhat larger (Robertson, 1960).

Large confluent opacities do not occur and the hilar shadows, although unduly radio-opaque, are of normal size.

Diagnosis

The occupational history, lack of symptoms and physical signs and the striking density of the opacities on the radiograph are diagnostic. In the absence of a history and when opacities are fairly few they might be mistaken for silicosis, possibly for baritosis or for other causes of discrete bilateral lung lesions.

Prognosis

Stannosis has no known effect upon health or lifespan. It is possible, if sufficient time were to elapse after last exposure to the dust, that the opacities would gradually disappear but this has not been reported.

Antimony (atomic number 51)

Antimony occurs in metamorphic deposits in quartz veins of deep-seated origin which lie in or near intrusive rocks such as the granites and as deposits in limestone and shales. It is mined in South Africa, China, Bolivia, Yugoslavia, Mexico, Canada and Turkey.

It is imported into other countries as *stibnite* (Sb_2S_3) ore or powder. Antimony metal, trioxide, pentoxide, trisulphate and pentasulphide are produced from the ore.

Sources of exposure and uses

Exposure to antimony dust may occur during mining, crushing the ore, and cleaning of extraction chambers which collect the oxide dust from roasting chambers (Renes, 1953). Exposure to fumes has occurred among antimony alloy workers and Linotype setters, but is now likely to be more important among men who smelt and refine the ore in reverberatory furnaces. The mining of antimony can yield dust containing about 25 to 76 per cent of quartz (Potkonjak and Pavlovich, 1983).

In the UK antimony is smelted near Newcastle-upon-Tyne in the largest smelting plant in Europe. The chief centres in the USA are in Pennsylvania and Texas (Cooper et al., 1968). The metal and white antimony trioxide are produced.

Antimony dust apparently remains suspended in the air longer than might be expected of a heavy metal (Fairhall and Hyslop, 1947) which suggests that the particle size is small; the fine white fume of antimony oxide that is produced during smelting consists of particles that, on average, are less than 1 μm diameter (McCallum et al., 1971). Work in the baghouse or at the furnaces is associated with most dust or fume exposure. Pneumoconiosis due to the inhalation of quartz-free powdered antimony trioxide with a particle size of less than 5 μm is recorded (Klučík, Juck and Gruberová, 1962). Quartz is usually absent from the air-borne dust although, in a Yugoslavian smelting plant, it comprised up to 4.7 per cent of the dust, more than 80 per cent of which was antimony oxide (Potkonjak and Pavlovich, 1983).

The metal is used chiefly in semi-conductors and as a component of lead alloys for battery plates, electrodes, pewter, anti-friction metals and printing type. Antimony oxides are employed as pigments for paints, glass and fusable enamels; in the colouring and vulcanizing of rubber, in plastics and the red tips of matches.

Antimony trichloride and pentachloride are referred to briefly in Chapter 18.

Pathology

Histological examination of the lungs of antimony workers has shown an accumulation of dust particles and dust-laden macrophages in alveolar walls and perivascular regions, but no fibrosis or inflammatory reaction (McCallum, 1967); the dust of antimony ore or the trioxide does not cause fibrosis in the lungs of experimental animals (Cooper et al., 1968).

Small amounts of antimony have been detected in the urine of a worker some 4 years after he left the industry, suggesting that antimony is not fixed in the lungs and may be absorbed into the circulation in small quantities and excreted (McCallum, 1963). However, the biological half-life of antimony in the lungs appears to be long (probably more than 20 years), whereas its concentration in the liver and renal cortex of deceased smelters differs little from control subjects; this suggests either that its biological half-life outside the lungs is short or that its systemic absorption is insignificant. Cigarette smoke can contribute to the concentration of antimony in the lungs (Gerhardsson et al., 1982).

Symptoms and physical signs

An orange-coloured staining of the front teeth is characteristic of exposure to antimony oxide in workers with poor oral hygiene but not in those with good hygiene (Potkonjak and Pavlovich, 1983).

There are no symptoms or abnormal physical signs associated with the pneumoconiosis but those of acute chemical pneumonia or pulmonary oedema have occurred rarely in antimony smelters (Renes, 1953).

Some workers may develop rhinitis, perforation of the nasal septum or skin irritation with a papular and pustular rash in the vicinity of sebaceous and sweat glands of the forearms and thighs, especially in the flexures.

Lung function

There is no abnormality of lung function (McCallum, 1963).

Radiographic appearances

These consist of numerous small, dense opacities similar to those of siderosis which vary from ILO categories 1p to 3p. Larger, confluent shadows are not seen but the hilar regions may be denser than normal (Klučík, Juck and Gruberóva, 1962; McCallum, 1963; Cooper et al., 1968) (Figure 11.5). The opacities take 10 or more years of exposure to appear (Potkonjak and Pavlovich, 1983).

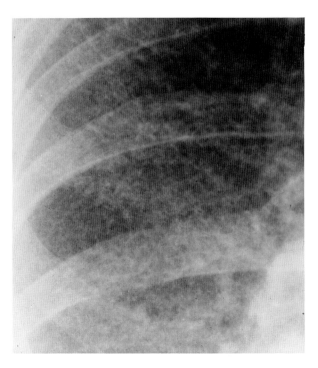

Figure 11.5 Category p opacities (distributed equally throughout the lung fields) in an antimony process worker and weighman for 26 years. Approximately 425 µg antimony/l was present in his urine. (Courtesy of Dr R.I. McCallum)

A radiographic survey of 262 men in an antimony works between 1965 and 1966 revealed the presence of 44 cases (16.8 per cent) of antimony pneumoconiosis (McCallum et al., 1971).

Using in vivo differential X-ray spectrometry in some of these workers, McCallum et al. (1971) observed antimony values ranging from nil to just over 11 mg/cm² , and these tended to rise the longer the period of employment in the industry and the higher the ILO category recorded.

Abnormal chest radiographs have been reported in men mining and smelting antimony ore in Yugoslavia (Karajovic, 1957) but those of the miners appear to have been due to silicosis. The appearances of pulmonary oedema have been reported after heavy exposure to smelting fumes (Renes, 1953), but this does not seem to have been observed by others (Gerhardsson et al., 1982).

Diagnosis

Benign antimony pneumoconiosis is rare but if the clinician is not aware that antimony in the lungs causes radiographic abnormality or, if a history of industrial exposure to antimony is not obtained in the first place, errors in diagnosis (mainly in the direction of non-industrial disease) will probably occur.

The differential diagnosis is generally similar to that of siderosis.

Prognosis

There is no known detrimental effect upon health or life expectancy. An apparent excess of carcinoma of the lung in smelters has not been substantiated as being related to antimony, but the matter is under on-going surveillance (Gerhardsson et al., 1982).

Unlike siderosis and baritosis no evident resolution of radiographic appearances has been recorded.

Barium (atomic number 56): baritosis

The most important compound is *barytes* ($BaSO_4$), known as *barite* in the USA. *Witherite* ($BaCO_3$) is less important.

Although baritosis ('barium lung') was first described by Fiori (1926) in Italy the subject of his report also appears to have had silicosis. One of the first accounts of pure baritosis was given by Arrigoni (1933), and reports from other countries followed over the years. A survey of a barium plant (related to duration of exposure) revealed the presence of baritosis in 48 per cent of 118 workers (Lévi-Vallensi et al., 1966).

Barytes is widely distributed throughout the world together with other minerals and is often associated with igneous, sedimentary and metamorphic rocks. Therefore, such minerals as fluorite, calcite, limestone, witherite, quartz and chert may be intermixed according to the type of deposit in which the barytes is found. In the UK deposits are almost wholly of hydrothermal origin and may thus contain varying amounts of quartz derived from the hydrothermal fluids and not from the surrounding rocks in which they lie. It is evident then that barytes from some areas will contain variable and often significant quantities of free silica.

In 1969 the world's greatest producer of barytes was the USA (mainly from Nevada, Missouri, Arkansas and Georgia), followed in magnitude by Federal Germany, the USSR, Greece, Mexico, the Irish Republic and Canada. It is of particular interest that production by the Irish Republic (County Sligo) has increased almost fortyfold since 1961. The total output by the UK (chiefly as barytes recovered as a byproduct of fluorspar production in Derbyshire) is now very small (Collins, 1972). An underground barytes mine, in limey sandstone, in Ayrshire, Scotland, closed some years ago.

The UK was the sole world supplier of *witherite* which was mined in Northumberland and Durham, but production ceased in 1969.

Sources of exposure and uses

During mining of the crude ore high concentrations of dust may be produced and, as indicated, in some areas this may contain either quartz in hydrothermal deposits or chert from neighbouring rocks. When mining is done by the opencast method the concentration of air-borne dust is greatly reduced.

Barytes is supplied to various industries in crude form, as flotation concentrates from which contaminants have been removed, or in ground and purified form. With the exception of the crude form it is washed, leached out and then crushed or ground in the wet state. The chance of dust inhalation in these circumstances, therefore, is low, but during the drying and bagging of ground barytes, high concentrations of dust may be produced.

Ground barytes is used today chiefly as a weighting agent in muds circulated in the rotary drilling of oil and gas wells, and also as a filler, extender and weighting agent in heavy printing papers, paints, textiles, playing cards, clutch facings, brake linings, soap, linoleum, rubber and plastics. It was used in gramophone records until about 1948 when microgroove records were introduced. A large quantity of the world's barytes is employed in glass manufacture as a flux and to add brilliance, and, because it absorbs γ-radiation efficiently, in aggregates for special concrete ('atomic concrete') and bricks used for radioactivity shields. A hard variety of barytes is used in 'sand blasting' (Collins, 1972).

Barytes is almost the only source of barium used in the manufacture of numerous barium chemicals. Both chemically precipitated barium sulphate, *blanc fixe* (employed as an extender in high opacity white pigments, in 'fining' molten glass and coating photographic papers), and barium sulphate BP have a fine particle size and so may readily become air-borne. Barium carbonate is employed in the UK in the production of glass for television sets (as a barrier to X-rays) and glass of high refractive index, in certain ceramic processes, in some welding rod coatings, and with titanium dioxide to yield barium titanate, the valuable piezoelectric properties of which are exploited in electronic ceramics, digital computers and sonar apparatus. Other barium salts also find a variety of uses, for example, in pyrotechnics, explosives and beet sugar refining.

The likelihood of exposure to barium dust has evidently varied greatly according to the processes involved but, since barium compounds have such a wide application, mild degrees of baritosis may be

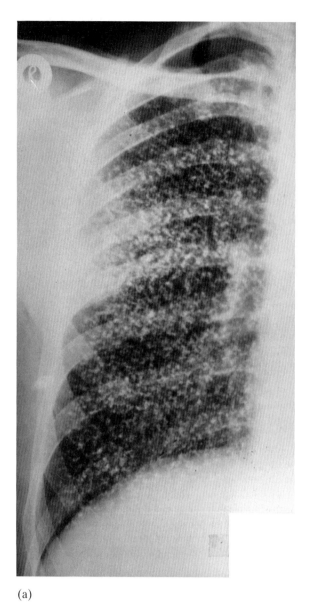
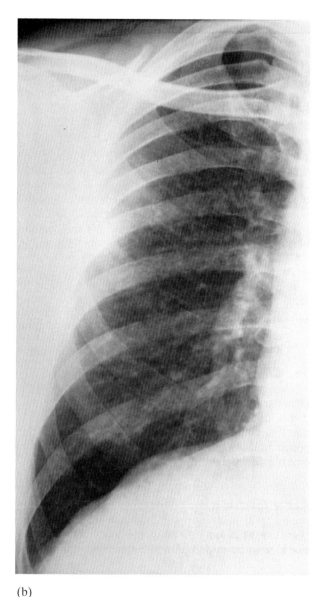

(a)   (b)

Figure 11.6 Very dense, discrete opacities in a miller and grinder of barytes for 15 years. These have steadily regressed in number and density over 18 years from 1961 due to a cessation of exposure and normal pulmonary clearance: (a) 1961; (b) 1979. Ventilatory function tests were normal throughout. (Reproduced, with permission, from Doig, 1976.) In most cases of baritosis, the opacities are less striking than this

more common than is realized. In general, quartz is absent from barytes used in industry but, if present, the amount is minute.

Pathology

Although this section is concerned with baritosis, it should be noted that if exposure has occurred to dust containing both barytes and 'free silica' (as may be the case in some barytes mines) then both barito-

sis and silicosis may be present (Seaton et al., 1986). But there is no evidence that the pathogenesis of the silicotic lesions is modified by barytes.

Macroscopic appearances

Many discrete grey macules are present in the pulmonary pleura and the cut surface of the lungs shows numerous discrete, impalpable macules which resemble those of stannosis. There are no nodules, no confluent massing and no evidence of fibrosis. Hilar lymph nodes are not enlarged.

Microscopic appearances

The appearances of the lesions are similar to those of stannosis and siderosis. The initial reaction is an insignificant mobilization of polymorphonuclear leucocytes but a brisk macrophage response together with a little intra-alveolar exudate. There is no collagenous fibrosis. The lack of fibrotic reaction is confirmed in experimental animals (Huston, Wallach and Cunningham, 1952). Following accidental inhalation of barium meal, barium-containing macrophages fill the alveoli and small airways and some are present in alveolar walls.

If positive identification of the mineral is important, X-ray diffraction or spectrographic methods are advisable. Barytes particles are moderately birefringent.

Symptoms and signs

Baritosis is symptomless and causes no abnormal physical signs. There are no systemic toxic effects due to absorption of barytes and most barium compounds from the lungs as they are poorly soluble and chemically inert.

Lung function

Impairment of lung function has not been recorded nor is it to be expected.

Radiographic appearances

The usual appearances consist of particularly dense, discrete small opacities sometimes of star-like configuration and usually about 2 to 4 mm diameter which are distributed fairly evenly throughout the lung fields, and may develop after only a few months' exposure to the dust (Pancheri, 1950). When the amount of retained barium dust is large (as may be the case after long periods of exposure) the opacities may be bigger and, indeed, large, irregular and densely opaque areas which may give an impression of confluent lesions may be seen. This is due to the superimposition effect of very many highly radiodense deposits. But lack of correlation between duration of exposure and intensity of radiographic abnormality is occasionally encountered and is not readily explicable (Doig, 1976). Kerleys 'B' lines are often prominent and the hilar lymph nodes may be remarkably opaque, though

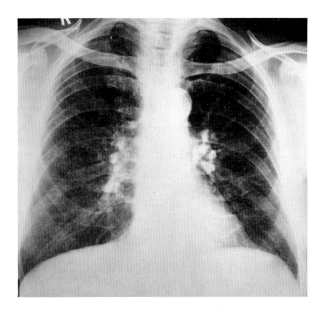

Figure 11.7 Dense opacity of hilar lymph nodes in a man who handled barium carbonate powder for 30 years. Such appearances may be misinterpreted as calcification. The pulmonary opacities are fewer and less dense than those in Figure 11.6a

not enlarged (Figures 11.6a and 11.7). However, in the earlier stages of baritosis the opacities may be indistinguishable from those of nodular silicosis or coal pneumoconiosis (Doig, 1976).

As in the case of siderosis gradual clearing of the opacities occurs after industrial exposure has ceased, due to physiological elimination of the dust (Wende, 1956; Lévi-Valensi et al., 1966; Doig, 1976) (Figure 11.6b).

Diagnosis

A detailed work history presents the necessary clue and the density of the opacities should suggest the possibility of baritosis. But if exposure to the dust has been slight, or if opacities are few, confusion with other causes of discrete opacities may well occur.

It is important to remember that pneumoconiosis in barytes miners is likely to be predominantly silicosis (Seaton et al., 1986). For example, in the case of one such miner (from the now defunct Scottish mine) many characteristic silicotic nodules were found and analysis of the lung ash revealed about 15 per cent SiO_2 by weight but only 4 per cent $BaSO_4$.

Baritosis is rare and many men in whom it is first identified are now elderly and have left the responsible industry years previously. But sporadic new cases can be expected from some among the plethora of processes in which barium compounds are used. This means that consideration of baritosis may occasionally be important in differential diagnosis.

Prognosis

The presence of barytes or witherite in the lungs is not known to have any adverse effect upon health or life expectancy. Gradual clearance of opacities can be expected over years after the worker has left exposure.

The rare earth metal oxides (atomic numbers 57 to 71)

'Rare earths', as a general term, is something of a misnomer in that these elements are widely, though not uniformly, distributed in nature; however, being mixtures of elemental oxides, they are not easily extracted from the minerals with which they are associated – notably fluorospar, calcite and apatite (see Appendix I) whose calcium they replace (Muecke and Möller, 1988). There are 15 rare earth elements whose atomic numbers range from 57 (lanthanum) to 71 (lutetium). Those with lower atomic numbers tend to occur with monazite (cerium phosphate) and those with higher atomic numbers, with *xenotime* (yttrium phosphate). Monazite and bastnaesite are the most important commercially. Monazite also contains up to 30 per cent thorium (atomic number 90), not itself a rare earth element, which is radioactive.

Monazite occurs as a heavy, brown–black sand obtained from alluvial deposits in certain beaches by placer mining methods or by off-shore dredging. Conventional open cast mining is used for bastnaesite deposits. Milling, flotation and electromagnetic techniques are employed to produce pure sands from which the rare earth metals and thorium and yttrium are extracted. Australia, India and Brazil are the chief producers of monazite concentrates and the USA, the chief producer of bastnaesite concentrates.

Sources of exposure and uses

Some exposure to dust may occur during the mining, milling and refining processes but, at most stages, the minerals are either wet or in solution. The use of the cerium subgroup in some industries is more likely to give rise to dust.

Cerium (usually in the form of the dioxide) is employed as a mild abrasive for polishing lenses,

mirrors and prisms; in the manufacture of fireworks, cigarette lighter 'flints'; for high temperature ceramics (such as crucibles); in light metal alloys; and, to increase light brilliance, as the nitrate, fluoride and oxide in the core of carbon arc electrodes. Because many of these processes are dry, substantial amounts of rare earth dust may be generated. The heat of an arc evaporates the salts which accumulate as fine dust on apparatus, on ledges and objects in the work room. Neodymium, dysprosium and holmium (atomic numbers 60 to 67) are employed for certain types of laser crystals; terbium (atomic number 65) and ytterbium (atomic number 70), for magnetic devices in computers; and lanthanums and gadolinium (atomic number 64) in the manufacture of ceramics with superconducting properties at high temperatures. The rare earth elements also catalyse the cracking of petroleum and govern the refractive index of glass lenses and fibreoptics (Muecke and Möller, 1988). Unseparated rare earth elements are also used for various 'misch-metal' alloys some of which, like lighter 'flints', are pyrophoric; the iron alloy, for example, is employed in the manufacture of luminous projectiles and tracer bullets.

Apart from its application in nuclear power reactors thorium is used in the manufacture of incandescent gas mantles and to harden and increase the strength and corrosion resistance of certain alloys. There has been little evidence of radiation injury to the lungs or other organs, although thoron (radon-220) and its decay-products (which are α-emitters with strong ionizing powers) have been related to carcinoma of the lung in some workers processing thorium (Polednak, Stehney and Lucas, 1983) (see also Chapter 19, page 656).

Pathology

In the early 1940s the late Dr L.U. Gardner (then Director of the Saranac Laboratory) suggested that small opacities in the chest radiographs of workmen in Ohio who had been exposed to dusts containing rare earth oxides and fluorides, were caused by the high atomic densities of the rare earth elements. Accordingly, he initiated parallel experiments in guinea-pigs with rare earths in which the ratios of oxides and fluorides were reversed. Intratracheal injection and inhalation techniques were used. The high oxide rare earths produced peribronchiolar and perivascular collections of dust with little or no evidence of fibrosis after 12 months but some small perivascular granulomas developed at the end of about 18 months. Most of the dust was transported to the hilar lymph nodes. The high fluoride rare earths resulted in regional bronchiolar strictures with localized emphysema but no fibrosis or granulomas (Schepers, 1955a,b; Schepers, Delahant and Redlin, 1955). More recently, neither cerium oxide nor cerium fluoride was found to cause fibrosis in lungs in guinea-pigs following intratracheal injections (Hoschek, 1966). In another study the development of peribronchiolar and perivascular, macrophage-rich granulomas has been confirmed in some animals exposed to the inhalation of thorium-free rare earth metals according to intensity and duration of exposure; however, thorium-containing rare earth metals caused fibrosis (Cain, Egner and Ruska, 1977). Inhalation of virtually pure gadolinium oxide with particle diameters of 0.1 to 0.5 μm does not cause fibrosis of the lungs in mice (Ball and Van Gelder, 1966). The level of acid and alkaline phosphatase is not altered in the lungs of rats exposed to monazite, which would seem to imply that this compound is inert in their lungs (Tandon et al., 1977).

Pneumoconiosis attributable to the rare earth elements (to date, chiefly cerium, neodymium and lanthanum) has been reported in workers producing cerium dioxide (Nappée, Bobrie and Lambard, 1972), using carbon arc lamps in the photography, photoengraving and printing industries (Heuck and Hoschek, 1968; Hecht and Wesch, 1980; Sulotto et al., 1986), and polishing lenses (Sinico et al., 1982).

Peribronchiolar inflammatory infiltrates and some adjacent septal fibrosis associated with rare earths (cerium, neodymium, lanthanum and samarium), identified by neutron activation analysis (NAA), has been reported in one case – a photoengraver using carbon arc lamps – with 'reticulonodular' radiographic opacities (Vocaturo et al., 1983). However, severe obstructive airways' disease was also present which would suggest that the peribronchiolar lesions were related to this rather than to retention of rare earths in the lungs. However, thorium – the level of which, in this case, was very low – appears to be capable of inducing fibrosis in human and animal lungs which progresses after exposure has ceased (Heuck and Hoschek, 1968; Cain, Egner and Ruska, 1977; De Vuyst et al., 1990). This possibility, therefore, may have to be considered in cases of rare earth pneumoconiosis in which levels of thorium in the lung or in the expired air are high – other coincident causes having been excluded.

Minute foreign-body granulomas containing cerium dioxide particles have been reported on pulmonary biopsy in one case, a lens polisher, with bilateral 'macro- and micronodular' radiographic opacities which regressed within a year after she had left the work and while under treatment with corticosteroids (Sinico et al., 1982). A causal relationship seems doubtful especially in so far as radiographic appearances have shown little or no regression in the few cases of rare earth pneumoconiosis that have been followed for some years (Sulotto et al., 1986) (Figure 11.8). In this case, and a few others, rare earth elements were identified by NAA, not only in the lungs but also, at lower levels, in lymph nodes,

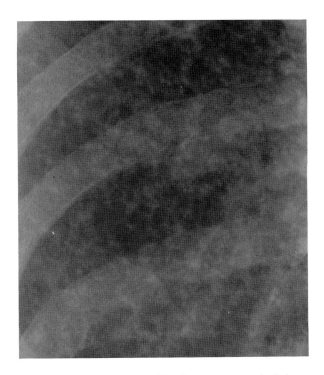

Figure 11.8 Appearances of benign pneumoconiosis in a worker exposed to rare earths, chiefly cerium dioxide, for 16 years. This film was taken 20 years after exposure ceased

blood, urine and nails (Hecht and Wesch, 1980; Sinico et al., 1982); thus, systemic absorption apparently occurs. Similarly, these elements have been identified by NAA in bronchoalveolar lavage fluid of a photoengraver with radiographic appearances consistent with benign pneumoconiosis and concomitant unilateral bronchiectasis (Sulotto et al., 1986).

It can be concluded, therefore, that pulmonary disease in workers with significant exposure to rare earths – although apparently inert – must be critically evaluated, at the same time bearing in mind the risk of wrongly attributing causality of unrelated, coincidental granulomatous or fibrotic pulmonary disease to them, as may occur with other benign pneumoconioses.

Symptoms, signs and lung function

No symptoms, abnormal physical signs or alteration in lung physiology are attributable to these inhaled dusts.

Radiographic appearances

These consist of dense, discrete opacities similar to those of baritosis with increased density of the hilar shadows (Nappée, Bobrie and Lambard, 1972) (Figure 11.8). The ILO/UC categories in the cases described by Heuck and Hoschek (1968) were 2 to 3q. The presence of thoron as [228]Th in their expired air or lungs (measured by the whole body counter) was regarded as confirmation that the opacities were caused by rare earth elements. Indeed, there appears to be a relationship between estimated burdens of thorium in the lungs (calculated from levels of decay products of exhaled thoron gas) and the categories of pneumoconiosis in rare earth miners (Xing-An et al., 1988).

Differential diagnosis

This is similar in all respects to other high-density dusts. Identification of relevant exposure by an informed occupational history is essential. In some cases the demonstration of thorium decay chain elements in exposed air or in the lungs may assist in diagnosis but the availability of this investigation is limited. The diagnosis should be considered in cases in which high density opacities are not readily explicable.

Conclusion

There is no conclusive, consistent evidence to date that the rare earth elements themselves are harmful to the lungs, although the thorium with which they are often associated (especially during extraction from monazite) may, if at high levels, present a long-term hazard. It is important that the clinician should be aware of this pneumoconiosis in view of the increase that has occurred in the use of the rare earths in a wide variety of high- and low-technology industries.

Bismuth (atomic number 83)

Bismuth is obtained by smelting dressed ores of native bismuth or *bismuthinite* (Bi_2O_3) in reverberatory furnaces or crucibles, but some is derived from electrolytic refining of copper and lead with which it is often associated. It is produced mainly in Bolivia, Canada, Mexico and Peru.

Apart from the application of its salts in medicine it is used as a pigment in glass and ceramics, in alloys with low melting points, and alloyed with lead, tin and mercury. Bismuth telluride ($Bi_2(Te·S)_3$) is employed in semi-conductors, and the oxide, hydroxide and oxychloride in cosmetics.

No harmful effects have been reported and, surprisingly, in view of its high atomic number and

the possibility of exposure to dust in some processes, no reports of benign pneumoconiosis caused by bismuth or its compounds appear to be on hand. After inhalation by experimental animals mild granulomas which resolve completely have been described (Rowe, Solomayer and Zenz, 1988).

General conclusions

The importance of inert dusts and fumes of high radiodensity is that they are not responsible for any symptoms, physiological impairment or progressive disease yet they may produce abnormal radiographic appearances which persist either permanently or for many years after the worker has left the relevant industry. It follows that whenever small discrete opacities of emphatic density are observed in the radiographs of a person with no other evidence of pulmonary disease industrial exposure to an inert radiodense dust should always be remembered and investigated.

In some cases the work processes in which these materials were used have been discontinued in recent years or are now carried out only on a small scale. Nevertheless, the chest radiograph may give clear evidence of past exposure years after it has ceased. Failure to recognize present or past exposure to one of these dusts as the cause of an abnormal chest radiograph will inevitably cause misdiagnosis with the possibility of irrelevant investigation and treatment.

Dusts of low radiodensity

Due to their low atomic numbers such dusts cause no evident radiographic abnormality but, when accompanied by free silica in the form of quartz, flint or chert, silicosis may result. In that case the appearances may be interpreted as being caused by the inert dust which is wrongly thought to be fibrogenic or, if the work history is inadequate, to some unconnected disease process.

These dusts are included among the 'nuisance particulates' that are not known to cause lung damage. Five examples are briefly considered so that their negative place in the pathogenesis of pneumoconiosis may be recognized by contrast with the siliceous dusts with which they may be contaminated at some stage or another. They are: limestone, marble, Portland cement and concrete, gypsum and silicon carbide.

Carbon, which in general behaves as an inert dust of low radiodensity, is a special case and is discussed in Chapter 13.

Limestone

Limestones (see Appendix I) generally contain small – usually minute – percentages of quartz and those containing more than about 15 to 20 per cent free silica are rare.

Industrial exposure to 'pure' limestone (that is, of less than 1 per cent quartz content) does not cause a fibrotic pneumoconiosis or abnormality of the chest radiograph even after many years' exposure (Collis, 1931; Davis and Nagelschmidt, 1956), and it has no systemic effect.

Chalk is similarly harmless.

However, when limestone contains flint or chert nodules or significant quantities of quartz grains there is a risk of silicosis. This may occur when siliceous limestone is quarried, crushed, milled, cut or polished (Doig, 1955).

Cement

The terms 'cement' and 'concrete' are frequently confused. Cement is a powder which, when mixed with water, makes a plastic mass that will subsequently harden to a rock-like consistency. The most common varieties (and there are many) are Portland cement in which limestone is the chief ingredient, and Portland–pozzolan cement. A 'pozzolan' is a siliceous or aluminous material, itself possessing no cementing properties, which, in finely divided form and the presence of moisture, reacts at ordinary temperatures with calcium hydroxide to form a material that possesses cementing properties.

Portland cement is manufactured on an enormous scale in large plants throughout the industrialized world, and production has been steadily increasing since the 1960s. The processes involved are often very dusty and, because they are sometimes wrongly regarded as causing fibrotic pneumoconiosis, must be briefly outlined.

There are three main groups of raw materials:

1. *Calcareous:* limestone, marl and chalk.
2. *Argillaceous:* shale, clay, marl, mudstone and, in some countries, volcanic rocks and schists.
3. Gypsum.

The limestone must not contain too high a proportion of quartz but, should this be deficient in the total mix, it is added in the form of quartzite, sand or crushed sandstone.

The process most commonly used involves four stages:

1. Raw materials are crushed in roll, jaw or gyratory crushers and then ground down to optimal size for chemical reaction. Grinding is done either dry in ball or roll mills, or wet in ball mills fed with water.
2. The raw mix is blended to the required composition.
3. It is then calcined at a temperature of about 1430 to 1650°C, usually in rotary kilns, and appears at the far end of the kiln as clinker and is cooled. Calcination drives off moisture, breaks down carbonates to oxides and forms calcium silicates and aluminates so that negligible quantities of quartz remain.
4. Clinker, to which about 5 per cent gypsum has been added, is then ground to a fine powder in ball or race mills. The gypsum controls the setting of the finished product.

Dust collected from grinding mills, crushers and conveyers is returned to the process. Although dust from the kiln stacks may contain some silicon dioxide in addition to other oxides, this is usually collected in electrostatic or mechanical precipitators and likewise returned to the process.

Clearly then, the chance of workers being exposed to significant quantities of free silica is small but, when such exposure does occur, it is in the preparatory stages of the process in those plants where quartz is added or siliceous clays or limestones are used.

The inhalation of cement dust by experimental animals causes neither acute nor chronic pathological changes (Baetjer, 1947). However, Einbrodt and Hentschel (1966) observed an uncommon situation in which dust recovered at the end of the process (in the packaging department) contained 5 per cent quartz and gave rise to atypical collagenous nodules when injected into the peritoneum of rats.

Surveys of large numbers of cement workers in many countries have revealed either no radiographic abnormalities or only an extremely low incidence of discrete opacities (Sayers, Dallavalle and Bloomfield, 1937; Gardner et al., 1939; Sander, 1958; Jenny et al., 1960). In a study of 2557 workers in Argentina, Vaccarezza (1950) did not find a single case of pneumoconiosis. But Hublet (1968) observed discrete opacities – mostly category 1q but also a few 2q – in just over half of 478 men who had worked in a Belgian cement plant from 5 to 20 years. It is not clear what these appearances represented. However, silicotic-type nodules and conglomerate masses have been reported in men who worked at those stages in manufacture where quartz contamination was fairly high (Doerr, 1952; Prosperi and Barsi, 1957).

Asbestos cement – cement reinforced with asbestos fibres – is referred to in Chapter 14.

Concrete

Concrete is a mixture of an inert mineral aggregate with a cementing agent – usually Portland cement – which, on change in temperature or chemical alteration, binds the whole into a solid mass. The purpose of an aggregate is to provide bulk and strength to the mixture. A variety of aggregates, classed as 'coarse' and 'fine' (or light weight), are employed, for example: crushed stone, shale, flint or chert pebbles, blast furnace slag, pumice, breccia, volcanic cinders, vermiculite, perlite, sand and gravel. *Blast furnace slag*, which contains an average of 35 per cent silicon dioxide, is drawn off molten from the furnace at temperatures ranging from 1260 to 1675°C, and, thus, may contain the tridymite and cristobalite phases of silica (see Appendix I). Hence, according to the type of aggregate used, siliceous dust may be produced by the application of powered drills, jack-hammers and the like in construction and demolition work (Figure 11.9) with the possible consequence – often unsuspected – of silicosis or 'mixed dust fibrosis' among the operatives (see Chapter 12).

Conclusion

Cement dust does not cause a pneumoconiosis, but if more than 2 per cent 'free silica' is present as a contaminant, silicosis may occur after some years' exposure. This is most likely to apply to the preparatory stages of cement production. But pneumoconiosis among cement workers is remarkably rare.

The lack of pathogenic effects of cement dust may also be attributed to its actively hygroscopic nature favouring flocculation of its particles so that the resulting aggregates are deposited very largely in the upper respiratory tract and mouth. Certainly rhinolithiasis has been a common annoyance to many workers in the industry.

Dust from concrete with a siliceous aggregate may be a source of silicosis – a situation that, although uncommon, must be kept in mind. It is frequently mistaken for sarcoidosis or inactive tuberculosis.

Gypsum ($CaSO_4 \cdot 2H_2O$)

The geology and mineralogy of gypsum is referred to in Appendix I. As pointed out there, contamination by quartz is variable or absent according to the

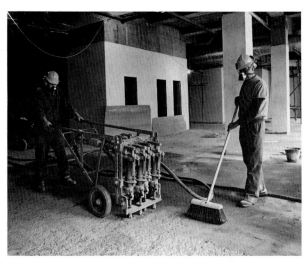

(a)

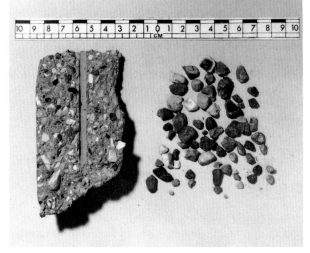

(b)

Figure 11.9 (a) Men lowering level of factory floor of reinforced concrete using compressed air-operated multiple jack-hammers to break up the surface. (b) A fragment of the concrete which contains a coarse aggregate of flint and chert pebbles – shown loose on the right. This type of concrete has been used extensively for numerous construction purposes over many years

geographical location of deposits and whether or not they are associated with shales or mudstones.

It is mined by opencast and underground methods, and is also quarried, the largest of the world's producers being the USA, Canada, France, the former USSR, Spain, Italy and the UK.

First-stage crushing of the rock is done at the main processing plant by ball and hammer mills. Most of the gypsum produced is calcined at low temperature to yield its hemihydrate or anhydrous

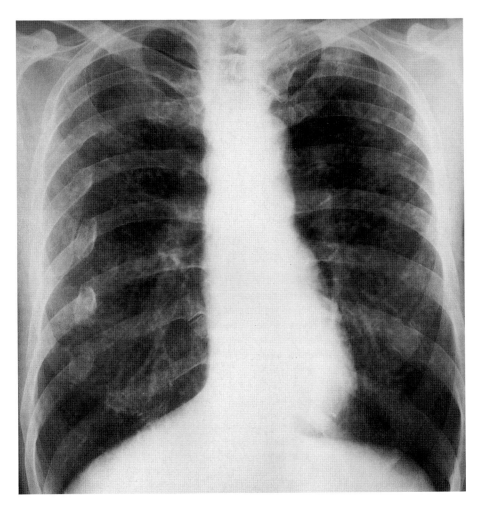

Figure 11.10 Gypsum miner in Sussex (UK) from 1922 to 1956. Category 2qA opacities: gradual increase in their size and density over 25 years. This film was taken 16 years after he had left the industry. (Fractures of ribs due to war injury)

forms. Quartz is usually absent or present only in negligible amounts. Calcined gypsum is widely used in the manufacture of various plasters (such as plaster of Paris and orthopaedic plasters) and wall-boards (often with perlite), for dental moulds, as a soil conditioner, as a 'retarder' in Portland cement manufacture, and for a variety of other purposes.

Gypsum is not cytotoxic to mammalian macrophages and non-macrophage cell lines in tissue culture (Chamberlain et al., 1982), and does not cause fibrosis in experimental animals after prolonged inhalation (Schepers, Durkan and Dellahant, 1955). No evidence of pneumoconiosis or other harmful effect due to gypsum alone has been observed, clinically or pathologically, in human beings, although some peribronchiolar cellular infiltration may occur (Riddell, 1934; Schepers and Durkan, 1955).

In short, gypsum itself does not cause a pneumoconiosis. But small, discrete radiographic opacities, consistent with mild silicosis or 'mixed dust fibrosis' have been observed in British miners who have mined or crushed quartz-contaminated gypsum rock for many years (Figure 11.10). This has occurred more in long-service miners in the Sussex than in the Nottinghamshire mines, owing to a higher content of quartz in the mine dust of the former than in that of the latter (see Chapter 12). It is of interest that these lesions, in cases that the author has followed for some 20 years, have shown little tendency to progress. Subsequent beneficiation of mined ore removes the quartz which, consequently, is not a hazard in manufacturing processes.

Similar cases have not been observed in gypsum miners in the USA.

Silicon carbide

Silicon carbide (SiC) is a synthetic material with a hardness only slightly less than that of diamond; it does not exist in nature. It was first manufactured as an abrasive in 1891, following the invention of the Acheson electric furnace, with the trade name Carborundum by which it is still popularly known. The process consists of heating high-grade quartzite sand (SiO_2) and petroleum coke (as a source of carbon) with sawdust and common salt in an electric furnace according to the reaction:

$$SiO_2 + 3C = SiC + 2CO$$

Furnaces are heated by passing a direct current through powdered graphite which lies as a strip in the charge mixture. This mixture is thermally insulated by the residue ('old-mix') of a charge incompletely converted to SiC in a previous firing; it consists of about 80 per cent sand and 20 per cent SiC (Smith *et al.*, 1984) (Figure 11.11). A number of furnaces operate continuously in staggered fashion which allows periodic dismantling, repair and reconstruction of those that are inactive. This process has changed little over more than 50 years. The temperature at the core of the furnace is about 2200 to 2300°C. If the temperature is too high SiC decomposes, the silica volatilizes and carbon is converted into graphite. The process takes 60 hours: 36 hours heating and 24 hours cooling. When complete the core consists of loosely knit SiC crystals surrounded by a variable amount of unreacted, or partially reacted, raw material. Consequently, the crust of SiC blocks removed from the furnace may contain quartz and cristobalite (Hight, 1975). The quality of the end-product depends not only on the raw materials, but on the accuracy and control of the furnace operations. Carbon monoxide, sulphur dioxide and various hydrocarbons are released during pyrolysis of the petroleum coke.

The blocks, after separation of the crust by men ('carbo-selectors') using pneumatic hand tools, are first ground in jaw crushers and then in hammer or ball mills, and impurities are removed by washing with water or by flotation and sedimentation. At the various stages some of the old-mix is returned to the furnace and re-cycled. The final product is dried and graded on mechanical screens. It is then transported to manufacturers of abrasive products.

It is in the preparation, furnace and crusher areas that 'respirable' dust is most likely to be significant. In the furnace area workers who may be particularly exposed are overhead cranesmen who load old-mix, new-mix and graphite into the furnace, remove contents after firing and transfer SiC to the cleaning floor; loaders, labourers (maintaining and repairing furnaces); payloader operators (cleaning furnaces after SiC has been removed); old-mix operators

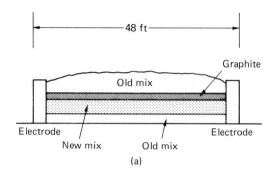

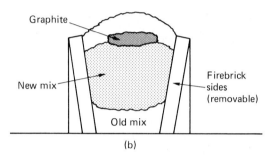

Figure 11.11 Diagrams of the Acheson furnace fired for approximately 36 hours for the production of silicon carbide (see text). (a) Longitudinal section before firing; (b) cross-section before firing. (Reproduced, with permission, from Smith *et al.*, 1984)

(transferring old-mix into the recycling system); and carboselectors. Not unexpectedly, particles of quartz, cristobalite and, of course, SiC have been found in the ambient air (Scansetti, Piolatto and Botta, 1992), although at levels usually below that currently permissible for silica of 100 μg/m (Osterman *et al.*, 1989). However, these levels may well vary during different furnace 'runs'.

In spite of its simple formula, SiC can exist in more than 150 crystal modifications according to differences in the stacking of silicon and carbon layers (Shaffer, 1969). Mostly it occurs in isometric form as grains, but some varieties consist of whiskers or continuous fibres that are generated, possibly, during the sudden escape of gas from forming blocks of SiC in the furnace. Woolly fibrous material containing silicon is sometimes found on the surface of the crusts of blocks. In general, very low levels of air-borne fibres (less than 1 fibre/cm) from 5 to 100 μm in length and less than 0.5 μm in diameter have been recorded in Norwegian plants around furnaces and during separation of the crust. Although, in one plant, significantly higher counts (up to 5 fibres/cm), consistent with the presence of fibres in recycled material, were present in the area in which the raw material was mixed (Figure 11.12a,b). The level of air-borne fibres in the vicinity of the preparation of the final product was negligible (Bye *et al.*, 1985).

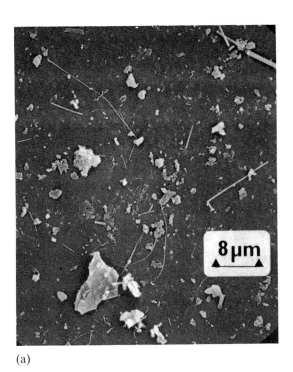
(a)

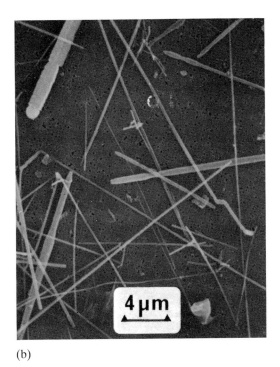
(b)

Figure 11.12 (a) Fibrous and non-fibrous particles of silicon carbide from recycled furnace material (SEM); (b) appearances of isolated fibres of α-silicon carbide by SEM. Range of nominal diameters = 0–1.0 μm; range of length = 0–10 μm. (Reproduced, with permission, from Bye et al., 1985)

Uses

Silicon carbide, chiefly in isometric form, has long been employed for the manufacture of abrasive wheels in place of the previous, hazardous sandstone wheels, but they also find an important use in refractories for boilers and annealing and forging furnaces; in ceramic setter tiles, furnace muffles and electric resistance elements; and, as hot-pressed pieces, for turbine blades.

Silicon carbide fibres are now specifically manufactured as one aspect of a rapidly expanding ceramic-fibre technology (aluminosilicate fibres probably being the most common in this class – see Chapter 18). They are used for the reinforcement of various ceramics and metals and in a variety of engineered products (Griffiths, 1986).

Pathology

Animals exposed to non-fibrous SiC dust do not develop pulmonary fibrosis; it is as inert in the lungs as latex beads (Gardner, 1935; Holt, 1967; Bégin et al., 1989). However, SiC fibres, in cell culture, exhibit comparable cytotoxicity to crocidolite (Birchall et al., 1988), and a recent experiment with sheep has demonstrated that the fibres activate alveolar macrophages to provoke a significant increase in the growth activity of fibroblasts, and cause fibrosis which is nodular rather than diffuse (Bégin et al., 1989). They have also been reported to cause pleural tumours in experimental animals (Stanton et al., 1981).

A post-mortem study of the lungs of three men who had worked in SiC production plants for many years revealed conspicuous silicotic nodules, with heavy black pigmentation, foci of linear interstitial fibrosis of a minor order and occasional ferruginous bodies with black cores believed to be SiC. 'Classic hyalinized silicotic nodules' were also present in hilar and mediastinal lymph nodes, and fragmented or intact ferruginous bodies were seen both within the nodes and lying free in the lymphoid tissue. There was no known exposure to asbestos (Massé, Bégin and Cantin, 1988). To test the possibility that quartz adherent to the SiC particles might explain these lesions, Bégin et al. (1989) investigated the biological activity of raw and ashed SiC particles and found both to be 'completely inert'. However, the quartz or cristobalite responsible would be likely to be found in the partially reacted raw material of block crusts and its fragments, and in old mix. Hayashi and Kajita (1988) reported biopsy of lung from a man who had worked for 10 years up to 1963 in an abrasives plant manufacturing SiC.

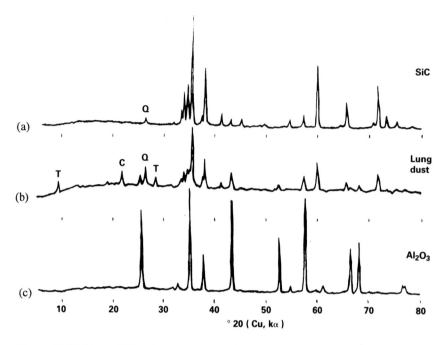

Figure 11.13 X-ray diffraction patterns of (a) commercial silicon carbide, (b) lung dust from a worker in an abrasive manufacturing plant, and (c) aluminium oxide (Cu α-radiation). Q = quartz; C = cristobalite; T = talc. (Reproduced, with permission, from Hayashi and Kajita, 1988)

Conglomerate collagenous lesions and some clusters of ferruginous bodies were observed. Although the authors attributed the lesions to SiC, X-ray diffraction demonstrated the presence of quartz and cristobalite in the dust from the lungs (Figure 11.13): 2.0 and 2.3 per cent, respectively, of the dust content on analytical electron microscopy with 43 per cent SiC and 24 per cent Al_2O_3. Indeed, their illustration of the histology of the periphery of a conglomerate lesion has the appearance of silicosis or 'mixed dust fibrosis' (see Chapter 12). Microprobe analysis showed that the ferruginous bodies contained SiC fibre; asbestos minerals were not identified.

In another report (Funahashi et al., 1984) biopsy analysis of a lung of one of two men (with radiographic evidence of a 'nodular' pneumoconiosis) who, respectively, were exposed for 14 and 20 years to SiC in a factory manufacturing refractory bricks revealed perivascular, nodular fibrosis and abundant ferruginous bodies. On SEM (scanning electron microscopy) most particles in the lung were found to consist of granular (isometric) SiC, although there was a smaller number of fibres 100 μm or more in length. EDXA (electron dispersive X-ray analysis) showed the silicon/sulphur ratio to be similar to that found in a 'fully developed silica nodule', but, as there was a 'lack of strong quartz diffraction', quartz was dismissed as being pathogenically insignificant and SiC suggested as the

likely cause of the fibrosis, although with reservation. Nevertheless, the appearances of the radiographs of both men are wholly consistent with silicosis or 'mixed dust fibrosis'. The cores of the ferruginous bodies were black and, although not specifically identified, were probably SiC.

Associated physiological and radiographic changes

A study of 165 SiC production workers suggests that some restrictive impairment of lung function – seemingly, independent of smoking habit – is associated with length of time spent in the industry and with cumulative exposure to 'respirable' dust (Osterman et al., 1989). The explanation of this finding is uncertain. By contrast, in 141 production workers, a significant decrement of FEV_1 and FVC with radiographic profusion of opacities was found only among smokers (Marcer et al., 1992).

Radiographic evidence of pneumoconiosis (mainly small round opacities) in SiC production workers was reported years ago by Clark (1929), Smith and Perina (1948) and Bruusgaard (1949) and, more recently, especially in older workers, by Peters et al. (1984), Smith et al. (1984) and Gauthier, Ghezzo and Martin (1985). In all these studies men had worked in different stages of the

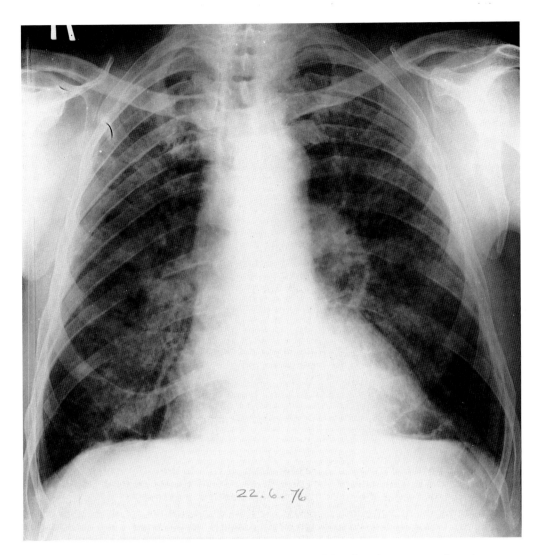

22.6.76

Figure 11.14 Film, taken in 1976, of a mixer and check-weigher in a factory manufacturing silicon carbide (Carborundum) abrasive materials until the mid-1960s. Category 2/3, q/r opacities consistent with silicosis. Exposure to dusts of ceramic bonding materials including ball and china clay, feldspar, flint and frits in addition to silicon carbide and fused aluminium oxide. *Post mortem:* numerous, black-pigmented, silicotic nodules more numerous in the upper than the lower lobes. Some calcifications of hilar lymph nodes. (*Frit:* a calcined mixture of sand and fluxes for melting to form glass)

preparation and production of SiC with the probable consequence of exposure to free silica, but some, in the earlier reports, had, in addition, previously worked in some other dust hazard. Pneumoconiosis has also been attributed to SiC from work in the manufacture of synthetic grindstones. However, materials used to bond SiC grains together contained, until recent years, variable quantities of flint, quartz, feldspar and ball or china clay; so, not surprisingly, silicosis has been recorded in men working in the bonding process (Posner, 1960) (Figure 11.14). Latterly,

bonding material has been largely replaced by a flux (known as 'frit') consisting of silicates or borates, or by rubber, synthetic resins or organic materials.

Irregular radiographic opacities have also been related to work in SiC production for a prolonged period in both smokers and non-smokers (Peters et al., 1984; Gauthier, Ghezzo and Martin, 1985), but a pathological correlation does not seem to have been demonstrated. They may be caused by deposition of dust in interlobular septa (see Chapter 13, 'Irregular opacities').

Mortality

No increase in total mortality or mortality from malignant or non-malignant respiratory disease was observed in a large cohort of men who had worked in an abrasives industry between 1958 and 1983 exposed to SiC and aluminium oxide (Edling et al., 1987).

Conclusion

All the evidence points clearly to granular (isometric) SiC being inert in human lungs and to radiographic, 'nodular'-type pneumoconiosis in workers involved in its production being caused by free silica in one or more of its polymorphs – even at low concentration – resulting either in typical silicosis or 'mixed dust fibrosis'. Indeed, the presence of SiC, as in the case of other non-fibrogenic dusts, may be expected to modify the silicotic process (see Chapter 12). Engelbrecht and Thiart (1972) showed that, in the lungs of rats, SiC and quartz together produced a slight cumulative fibrogenic response over 200 days, less than that caused by quartz alone. Although it has been shown that fibrous SiC can provoke fibrosis in sheeps' lungs the claim that it alone causes characteristic fibrotic lesions in human lungs (Bégin et al., 1989) is by no means substantiated. An association of ferruginous SiC bodies with fibrotic nodules is not proof of cause and effect. Nonetheless, the possibility exists. Thus, careful monitoring of the working environment and medical surveillance of the workforce over a prolonged period are necessary in any process in which SiC fibres might escape into the atmosphere. In evaluating exposure isometric and fibrous particles need to be distinguished. Preferably exposure should be reduced until more information becomes available (Bye et al., 1989).

It should be borne in mind that the use of Carborundum grinding wheels on cast iron or steel may ultimately cause *siderosis* from attrition of the metal (Buckell et al., 1946) and that, when employed for fettling metal castings moulded in siliceous sand, may give rise to silicosis or 'mixed dust fibrosis'.

After this chapter was completed important confirmation that SiC itself has no fibrogenic action in the lungs was provided by Bruch et al. (1993) who, also, believe that accompanying crystalline polymorphs of silica – quartz, cristobalite and tridymite – are the likely cause of instances of fibrosis that have been reported in SiC workers.

Marble

Marble is a metamorphosed carbonate rock consisting predominantly of calcite ($CaCO_3$) and dolomite ($MgCO_3 \cdot CaCO_3$) or both (see Appendix I), but some impurities in the form of talc, chlorite, non-fibrous tremolite, wollastonite (see page 863), diopside (a pyroxene, $CaMgSi_2O_6$) and hematite may sometimes be present in amounts ranging from less than 1 per cent to about 50 per cent. However, it is important to note that commercially the term 'marble' is often used to refer to a variety of other rocks, including serpentines, which have an attractive appearance and will take a polish. Therefore, some stones described as marble may contain significant quantities of quartz so that it is important to know the correct identity of the stones worked by quarrymen, masons and artisans who have supposedly been occupied solely with 'marble'. Conversely, stalagmitic marbles which are calcites with wavy bands similar to onyx are known commercially as 'onyx marbles', which is misleading because true onyx – a banded chalcedony (microcrystalline silicon dioxide) – is, in fact, absent.

Marble proper is quarried by specialized techniques to produce good blocks of uniform quality which are subsequently cut and, for some purposes, polished. It is used for sculpture, various vessels, slabs and dimension stone. White marble is virtually pure (that is, more than 99 per cent) calcium carbonate; coloured marble contains a small percentage of impurities. Hence, true marble offers no risk of silicosis, but some harder varieties, such as those required for decorative flooring and stair treads, may contain a significant amount of quartz. Crushed (or milled) marble is used for the same purposes as crushed limestone.

Both calcite and dolomite are innocuous to the lungs but silicosis or a 'mixed dust fibrosis' (see Chapter 12) may result if the quartz content of the marble or pseudo-marble is significant.

It can be concluded, therefore, that pneumoconiosis does not occur in men working in occupations employing only true marble but may, of course, develop if quartz-containing marbles or pseudo-marbles are worked or quarried.

References

Abrasives (1971) *Ind. Minerals* July, 12–13

Albu, A. and Schuleri, E. (1972) Contribution a l'étude de la ventilation exercise et de la mécanique pulmonaire dans la sidérose professionelles. *Arch. Mal. prof. Méd. Trav.* **33**, 51–58

Ampian, S.G. (1975) Zirconium and hafnium. *Min. Facts and Probl. Bull.* **667**, 1243–1259

Angebault, M., Berland, M., Parent, G. Bonniot, J-P. and Homasson, J.P. (1979) Toxicité pulmonaire du bioxyde de titane, risque lié au ponçage des mastics. *Arch. Mal. prof. Méd. Trav.* **40**, 501–508

Arrigoni, A. (1933) La pneumoconiosi da bario. *Med. Lav.* **24**, 461–467

Baetjer, A.M. (1947) The effect of Portland cement dust on the lungs with special references to lobar pneumonia. *J. Ind. Hyg. Toxicol.* **29**, 250–258

Ball, R.A. and Van Gelder, G. (1966) Chronic toxicity of gadolinium oxide for mice following exposure by inhalation. *Archs Environ. Health* **13**, 601–608

Barnes, J.M. and Stoner, H.B. (1959) The toxicology of tin compounds. *Pharmacol. Rev.* **11**, 211–231

Barrie, H.J. and Harding, H.E. (1947) Argyro-siderosis of lungs in silver finishers. *Br. J. Ind. Med.* **4**, 225–229

Barták, F. and Tomečka, M. (1949) Stannosis (coniosis due to tin). *Proceedings of the Ninth International Congress of Industrial Medicine, London*, Wright, Bristol, pp. 742–754

Bartter, T., Irwin, R.S., Abraham, J.L., Dascal, A., Nash, G., Himmelstein, J.S. and Jederlinic, P.J. (1991) Zirconium compound-induced pulmonary fibrosis. *Archs Intern. Med.* **151**, 1197–1201

Bech, A.O., Kipling, M.D. and Zundel, W.E. (1965) Emery pneumoconiosis. *Trans. Assoc. Ind. Med. Offrs* **15**, 110–115

Bégin, R., Dufresne, A., Cantin, A., Massé, S., Sébastien, P. and Perrault, G. (1989) Carborundum pneumoconiosis. *Chest* **95**, 842–849

Birchall, J.D., Stanley, D.R., Mockford, M.J., Pigott, G.H. and Pinto, P.J. (1988) Toxicity of silicon carbide whiskers. *J. Materials Sci. Lett.* **7**, 350–352

Boyd, J.T., Doll, R., Faulds, J.S. and Leiper, J. (1970) Cancer of the lung in iron ore (hematite) miners. *Br. J. Ind. Med.* **27**, 97–105

Brown, G.M., Brown, D.M., Slight, J. and Donaldson, K. (1991) Persistent biological reactivity of quartz in the lung: raised protease burdon compared with a non-pathologenic mineral dust and microbial particles. *Br. J. Ind. Med.* **48**, 61–69

Brown, J.R., Mastromatteo, E. and Horwood, J. (1963) Zirconium lactate and barium zirconate: Acute toxicity and inhalational effects in experimental animals. *Am. Ind. Hyg. Assoc. J.* **24**, 131–136

Browne, R.C. (1955) Vanadium poisoning from gas turbines. *Br. J. Ind. Med.* **12**, 57–59

Bruch, J., Rehn, B., Song, H., Gono, E. and Malkusch, W. (1993) Toxicological investigations on silicon carbide. 1. Inhalation studies. 2. In vitro cell tests and long term injection tests. *Br. J. Ind. Med.* **50**, 797–806 and 807–813.

Bruusgaard, A. (1949) Pneumoconiosis in silicon carbide workers. *Proceedings of the Ninth International Congress of Industrial Medicine, London*, Wright, Bristol, pp. 676–680

Buckell, M., Garrard, J., Jupe, M.H., McLaughlin, A.I.G. and Perry, K.M.A. (1946) The incidence of siderosis in iron turners and grinders. *Br. J. Ind. Med.* **3**, 78–82

Bye, E., Eduard, W., Gjønnes, J. and Sørbrøden, E. (1985) Occurrence of airborne silicon carbide fibres during industrial production of silicon carbide. *Scand. J. Wk Environ. Health* **11**, 111–115

Cain, H., Egner, E. and Ruska, J. (1977) Deposits of rare earth metals in the lungs of man and in experimental animals. *Virchows Arch [A]* **374**, 249–261

Chamberlain, M., Davies, R., Brown, R.C. and Griffiths, D.M. (1982) *In vitro* tests for pathogenicity of mineral dusts. *Ann. Occup. Hyg.* **26**, 583–592

Champeix, J. and Moreau, H.L. (1958) Observations récentes sur les pneumoconioses par terre d'ocre. *Archs Mal. prof. Méd. Trav.* **19**, 564—573

Chen, J.L. and Fayerweather, W.E. (1988) Epidemiological study of workers exposed to titanium dioxide. *J. Occup. Med.* **30**, 937–942

Clark, W.I. (1929) The dust hazard in the abrasive industry: second study. *J. Ind. Hyg.* **11**, 92–96

Cole, C.W.A., Davies, J.V.S.A., Kipling, M.D. and Ritchie, G.L. (1964) Stannosis in hearth tinners. *Br. J. Ind. Med.* **21**, 235–241

Collins, R.S. (1972) Barium minerals. *Mineral Dossier No. 2*. Mineral Resources Consultative Committee. HMSO, London

Collis, E.L. (1931) Occupational dust disease. *Bull. Hyg.* **6**, 663–670

Cooper, D., Pendergrass, E.P., Vorwald, J.A., Maycok, R.L. and Brieger, M. (1968) Pneumoconiosis among workers in an antimony industry. *AJR Am. J. Roentgenol.* **103**, 495–508

Crouch, E. and Churg, A. (1984) Ferruginous bodies and the histologic evaluation of dust exposure. *Am. J. Surg. Pathol.* **8**, 109–116

Cutter, H.C., Faller, W.W., Stocklen, J.B. and Wilson, W.L. (1949) Benign pneumoconiosis in a tin oxide recovery plant. *J. Ind. Hyg. Toxicol.* **31**, 139–141

Daum, S., Anderson, H.A., Lilis, R., Lorimer, W.V., Fischbein, S.A., Miller, A. and Selikoff, I.J. (1977) Pulmonary changes among titanium workers (abstract). *Proc. R. Soc. Med.* **70**, 31–32

Davis, S.B. and Nagelschmidt, G. (1956) A report on the absence of pneumoconiosis among workers in pure limestone. *Br. J. Ind. Med.* **13**, 6–8

De Vuyst, P., Dumortier, P., Ketelbant, P., Flament-Durand, J., Henderson, J. and Yernault, J.C. (1990) Lung fibrosis induced by Thorotrast. *Thorax* **45**, 899–901

Doerr, W. (1952) Pneumokoniose durch Zementstaub. *Virchows Arch. Pathol. Anat. Physiol.* **322**, 397–427

Doig, A.T. (1955) Disabling pneumoconiosis from limestone dust. *Br. J. Ind. Med.* **12**, 206–216

Doig, A.T. (1976) Baritosis: a benign pneumoconiosis. *Thorax* **31**, 30–39

Doig, A.T. and McLaughlin, A.I.G. (1936) X-ray appearances of lungs of electric arc welders. *Lancet* **1**, 771–775

Doig, A.T. and McLaughlin, A.I.G. (1948) Clearing of X-ray shadows in welder's siderosis. *Lancet* **1**, 789–791

Doll, R. (1959) Occupational lung cancer, a review. *Br. J. Ind. Med.* **16**, 181–190

Donaldson, K., Bolton, R.E., Jones, A., Brown, G.M., Robertson, M.D., Slight, J., Cowie, H. and Davies, J.M.G. (1988) Kinetics of bronch-alveolar leucocyte response in rats during exposure to equal airborne mass concentrations of quartz, chrysotile asbestos, or titanium dioxide. *Thorax* **43**, 525–533

Duggan, M.J., Soilleux, P.J., Strong, J.C. and Howell, D.M. (1970) The exposure of United Kingdom miners to radon. *Br. J. Ind. Med.* **27**, 106–109

Dundon, C.C. and Hughes, J.P. (1950) Stannic oxide pneumoconiosis. *AJR Am. J. Roentgenol.* **63**, 797–812

Edling, C. (1982) Lung cancer and smoking in a group of iron ore miners. *Am. J. Ind. Med.* **3**, 191–199

Edling, C., Jarvolm, B., Andersson, L. and Axelson, O. (1987) Mortality and cancer incidence among workers in an abrasive manufacturing industry. *Br. J. Ind. Med.* **44**, 57–59

Einbrodt, H.J. and Hentschel, D. (1966) Tierexperimentelle Untersuchungen mit Arbeitsplatzstäben ans einem Hüttenzememtwerk. *Int. Arch. Gewerbepath. Gewerbehyg.* **22**, 354–366

Elo, R., Määtä, K. Uksila, E. and Artstila, A.V. (1972) Pulmonary deposits of titanium dioxide in man. *Archs Pathol.* **94**, 417–424

Engelbrecht, F.M. and Thiart, B.F. (1972) The effect of small amounts of aluminium, carbon and carborundum on development of silicosis and asbestosis. *S. Afr. Med. J.* **46**, 462–464

Epstein, W.L. (1967) Granulomatous hypersensitivity. *Progr. Allergy* **11**, 36–88

Epstein, W.L., Skahen, J.R. and Krasnobrod, H. (1962) Granulomatous hypersensitivity to zirconium: Localization of allergen in tissue and its role in formation of epithelioid cells. *J. Invest. Dermatol.* **38**, 223–232

Fairhall, L.T. and Hyslop, F. (1947) *The Toxicology of Antimony*. Suppl. to Publ. Health Rep. No. 195. US Treasury Dept

Faulds, J.S. and Stewart, M.J. (1956) Carcinoma of the lung in hematite miners. *J. Path. Bact.* **72**, 353–366

Fawcitt, R. (1943) Radiological evidence in haematite iron-ore workers. *Br. J. Radiol.* **16**, 323–330

Ferin, J. and Leach, L.J. (1976) The effect of amosite and chrysotile asbestos on the clearance of TiO_2 particles from the lung. *Environ. Res.* **12**, 250–254

Ferin, J. and Oberdöster, G. (1985) Biological effects and toxicity assessment of titanium dioxides: anastase and rutile. *Am. Ind. Hyg. Assoc. J.* **46**, 69–72

Fiori, E. (1926) Contributo alla clinica e alla radiologia delle pneumoconiosi rare. *Osp. magg.* **3**, 78–84

Fischer, H.W. and Zinnerman, G.R. (1969) Lung retention of stannic oxide. *Archs Pathol.* **88**, 259–264

Foá, V. (1967) La pneumoconiosi dei pulitori di oggetti metallici. *Med. Lav.* **58**, 588–602

Fogh, A., Frost, J. and Georg, J. (1969) Respiratory symptoms and pulmonary function in welders. *Ann. occup Hyg.* **12**, 213–218

Funahashi, A., Schlueter, D.P., Pintar, K., Siegesmund, K.A., Mandel, G.S. and Mandel, N.S. (1984) Pneumoconiosis in workers exposed to silicon carbide. *Am. Rev. Respir. Dis.* **129**, 635–640

Funahashi, A., Schlueter, D.P., Pintar, K., Bemis, E.L. and Siegesmund, K.A. (1988) Welders' pneumoconiosis: tissue elemental micro-analysis by energy dispersive X-ray analysis. *Br. J. Ind. Med.* **45**, 14–18

Gardner, L.U. (1935) *Experimental Production of Silicosis*, US Publ. Health Rep. 50, pp. 695–702

Gardner, L.U., Durkan, T.M., Brumfield, D.M. and Sampson, H.L. (1939) Survey in seventeen cement plants of atmosphere dusts and their effects upon the lungs of twenty-two hundred employees. *J. Ind. Hyg. Toxicol.* **21**, 279–318

Gauthier, J.J., Ghezzo, H. and Martin, R.R. (1985) Pneumoconiosis following carborundum (silicon carbide) exposure. *Am. Rev. Respir. Dis.* **134** (Part 2), A191

Gerhardsson, L., Brune, D., Nordberg, G.E. and Wester, P.O. (1982) Antimony in lung, liver and kidney tissue from deceased smelter workers. *Scand. J. Work Environ. Health* **8**, 201–208

Goldstein, B. (1965) Quoted by Sluis-Cremer and du Toit (1968)

Gregory, J. (1970) A survey of pneumoconiosis at a Sheffield steel factory. *Archs Environ. Health* **20**, 385–399

Griffiths, J. (1986) Synthetic mineral fibres. *Ind. Minerals* September, 20–43

Gross, P., Westrick, M.L. and McNerhey, J.M. (1960) Experimental silicosis: the inhibitory effect of iron. *Dis. Chest* **37**, 35–41

Guidotti, T.L., DeNee, P.B., Abraham, J.L. and Smith, J.R. (1978) Arc welders' pneumoconiosis: application of advanced electron microscopy. *Archs Environ. Health* **33**, 117–124

Hadjimichael, M.P.H. and Brubaker, R.E. (1981) Evaluation of an occupational respiratory exposure to a zirconium-containing dust. *J. Occup. Med.* **23**, 543–547

Harding, H.E. (1948) The toxicology of zircon: preliminary report. *Br. J. Ind. Med.* **5**, 75–76

Harding, H.E. and Davies, T.A.L. (1952) The experimental production of radiographic shadows by the inhalation of industrial dusts. Part II. Zircon. *Br. J. Ind. Med.* **9**, 70–73

Harding, H.E., Grant, J.L.A. and Davies, T.A.L. (1947) The experimental production of X-ray shadows in the lungs by inhalation of industrial dusts. I. Iron oxide. *Br. J. Ind. Med.* **4**, 223–224

Harding, H.E., McLaughlin, A.I.G. and Doig, A.T. (1958) Clinical radiographic and pathological studies of the lungs of electric arc and oxyacetylene welders. *Lancet* **2**, 394–398

Hayashi, H. and Kajita, A. (1988) Silicon carbide in lung tissue of a worker in the abrasive industry. *Am. J. Ind. Med.* **14**, 145–155

Hecht, F.M. and Wesch, H. (1980) Beitrag zum röntgenologischen Bild der Cer-Pneumokoniose. *Prax. Pneumol.* **34**, 169–173

Heppleston, A.G. (1979) Cellular reactions with silica. In *Biochemistry of Silicon and Related Problems*, Nobel Foundation Symposium 40 (eds G. Bendz and I. Lindqvist), Plenum Press, New York, pp. 357–359

Heppleston, A.G. (1988) Environmental lung disease. In *Pathology of the Lung* (ed. W.M. Thurlbeck), Thième Medical, New York, p. 660

Heuck, F. and Hoschek, R. (1968) Cer-pneumoconiosis. *AJR Am. J. Roentgenol.* **104**, 777–783

Hight, R.P. (1975) Abrasives. In *Industrial Minerals and Rocks*. (ed.-in-Chief Stanley L. Lefond), American Institute of Mining, Metallurgical and Petroleum Engineers, New York, pp. 28–29

Holmqvist, I. and Swensson, A. (1963) The fibrogenic effect of a granulated iron silicate intended for use in sand blasting. *Arch. Gewerbepath. Gewerbehyg.* **20**, 253–260

Holt, P.F. (1967) *Pneumoconiosis*, Edward Arnold, London, p. 177

Hoschek, R. (1966) Die biologische Wirkung von Seltenen Erden. Tieversuche mit intratrachealer Anwendung. *Zbl. Arb. Med.* **16**, 168–172

Hublet, P. (1968) Enquête relative au risque de pneumoconiose dans la fibrication des ciments de construction. *Arch. belg. Méd. soc.* **26**, 417–430

Hunnicutt, T.N., Cracovaner, D.J. and Myles, J.T. (1964) Spirometric measurements in welders. *Archs Environ. Health* **8**, 661–669

Huston, J., Wallach, D.P. and Cunningham, G.J. (1952) Pulmonary reaction to barium sulphate in rats. *Archs Path.* **54**, 430–438

Jenny, M., Battig, K., Horisberger, B., Havas, L. and Grandjean, E. (1960) Arbeitsmedizinische Intersuchung in Zementfabriken. *Schweiz. med. Wschr.* **90**, 705–709

Kang, K.Y., Bice, D., Hoffmann, E., D'Amato, R. and Salvaggio, J. (1977) Experimental studies of sensitization to beryllium, zirconium and aluminium compounds in the rabbit. *J. Allergy Clin. Immunol.* **59**, 425–436

Kaponen, M. and Gustafsson, T. (1980) Dusts in steel-making plants: lung contamination among iron workers. *Int. Archs Occup. Environ. Health* **47**, 35–45

Karajovic, D. (1957) Pneumoconiosis in workers of an antimony smelting plant. *Proceedings of the Twelfth International Congress on Occupational Health, Helsinki*, Vol. 3, pp. 370–374

Karlish, A.J. (1962) Idiopathic pulmonary haemosiderosis with unusual features. *Proc. R. Soc. Med.* **55**, 223–225

Kleinfeld, M., Messite, J., Keoyman, O. and Shapiro, J. (1969) Welder's siderosis. *Archs Environ. Health* **19**, 70–73

Klemic, H. (1975) Zirconium and hafnium minerals. In *Industrial Minerals and Rocks*, 4th edn (ed. S.J. Lefond et al.) American Institute of Mining, Metallurgical and Petroleum Engineers Inc., New York, pp. 1275–1283

Klučík, I., Juck, A. and Gruberová, J. (1962) Lesions of the respiratory tract and the lungs caused by antimony trioxide dust. *Prac. lek.* **14**, 363–368

Kuterbach, D.A., Walcott, B., Reeder, R.J. and Frankel, R.B. (1982) Iron-containing cells in the honey-bee. *Science* **218**, 695–697

Lévi-Valensi, P., Drif, M., Dat, A. and Hadjadj, G. (1966) A propos de 57 observations de barrytose pulmaire (résultats et une equête systématique dans usine de baryte). *J. fr. Méd. Chir. thorac.* **20**, 443–454

Määtä, K. and Arstila, A.W. (1975) Pulmonary deposits of titanium dioxide in cytologic and lung biopsy specimens. *Lab. Invest.* **33**, 342–346

McCallum, R.I. (1963) The work of an occupational hygiene service in environmental control. *Ann. Occup. Hyg.* **6**, 55–63

McCallum, R.I. (1967) Detection of antimony in process workers' lungs by X-radiation. *Trans. Soc. Occup. Med.* **17**, 134–138

McCallum, R.I. and Leathart, G.L. (1975) Pneumoconiosis in zirconium process workers. September 1975, *XVIII International Congress on Occupational Health*, Brighton, England

McCallum, R.I., Day, M.J., Underhill, J. and Arid, E.G.A. (1971) Measurement of antimony oxide dust in human lungs in vivo by X-ray spectrophotometry. In *Inhaled Particles* (ed. W.H. Walton), Unwin, London and Woking, pp. 611–618

Mancuso, T.F. and Hueper, W.C. (1951) Occupational cancer and other health hazards in a chromatic plant: a medical appraisal. I. Lung cancer in chromatic workers. *Ind. Med. Surg.* **20**, 358–363

Marcer, G., Bernardi, G., Bartolucci, G.B., Mastrangelo, G., Belluco, U., Camposampiero, A. and Saia, B. (1992) Pulmonary impairment in workers exposed to silicon carbide. *Br. J. Ind. Med.* **49**, 489–493

Massé, S., Bégin, R. and Cantin, A. (1988) Pathology of silicon carbide pneumoconiosis. *Mod. Pathol.* **1**, 104–108

Mellissonos, J.C., Collet, A. and Daniel-Moussard, H. (1966) Étude expérimentale d'un émeri naturel des cyclades. *Int. Arch. Gewerbepath. Gewerbehyg.* **22**, 185

Morgan, W.K.C. and Kerr, H.D. (1963) Pathologic and physiologic studies of welder's siderosis. *Ann. Intern. Med.* **58**, 293–304

Mosinger, M., Charpin, J., Rouyer, P., Luccioni, R., Dantin, F. and Dantin, B. (1968) Sur les siderose, sidero-scleroses et siderosilicoses. *Archs Mal. prof.* **29**, 59–66

Muecke, G.K. and Möller, P. (1988) The not-so-rare earths. *Sci. Am.* **258**, 62–67

Nappée, J., Bobrie, J. and Lambard, D. (1972) Pneumoconiose au cérium. *Archs Mal. prof. Méd. Trav.* **33**, 13–18

Nolan, R.R., Langer, A.M., Weisman, I. and Herson, G.B. (1987) Surface character and membranolytic activity of rutile and anastase: two titanium oxide polymorphs. *Br. J. Ind. Med.* **44**, 687–698

Osterman, J.W., Greaves, I.A., Smith, T.J., Hammond, S.K., Robbins, J.M. and Theriault, G. (1989) Work related decrement in pulmonary function in silicon carbide production workers. *Br. J. Ind. Med.* **46**, 708–716

Oyanguren, H., Schüler, P., Cruz, E., Guijon, C., Maturana, V. and Valenzuela, A. (1957) Estanosis: neumoconiosis benigna debida a inhalacion de polvo y humo de estano. *Revta méd. Chile* **85**, 687–695

Pancheri, G. (1950) Su alcune forme di pneumoconiosi particolarmente studiate in Italia. *Med. Lav.* **41**, 73–77

Pendergrass, E.P. and Pryde, A.W. (1958) Benign pneumoconiosis due to tin oxide. A case report with experimental investigation of the radiographic density of tin oxide dust. *J. Ind. Hyg.* **30**, 119–123

Peters, J.M., Smith, T.J., Bernstein, L., Wright, W.E. and Hammond, S.K. (1984) Pulmonary effects of exposures in silicon carbide manufacturing. *Br. J. Ind. Med.* **41**, 109–115

Polednak, A.P., Stehney, A.F. and Lucas, H.F. (1983) Mortality among male workers at a thorium-processing plant. *Health Physics* **44** (Suppl. 1), 239–251

Pontkonjak, V. and Pavlovich, M. (1983) Antimoniosis: a particular form of pneumoconiosis. I. Etiology, Clinical and X-ray findings. *Int. Archs Occup. Environ. Health* **51**, 199–207

Posner, E. (1960) Pneumoconiosis in makers of artificial grinding wheels, including a case of Caplan's syndrome. *Br. J. Ind. Med.* **17**, 109–113

Prior, J.T., Cronk, G.A. and Ziegler, D.D. (1960) Pathological changes with the inhalation of sodium zirconium lactate. *Archs Environ. Health* **1**, 297–300

Prosperi, G. and Barsi, C. (1957) Sulle pneumoconiosi dei lavatori del cemanto. *Rass. Med. Ind.* **26**, 16–24

Redline, S., Barna, B., Tomashefski, J.F. Jr and Abraham, J.L. (1986) Granulomatous disease associated with pulmonary deposition of titanium. *Br. J. Ind. Med.* **43**, 652–656

Reed, C.E. (1956) Effects on the lung of industrial exposure to zirconium dust. *Archs Ind. Health* **13**, 578–580

Reichel, G., Bauer, H-D. and Bruckmann, E. (1977) The action of quartz in the presence of iron hydroxides in the human lung. In *Inhaled Particles IV* (ed. W.H. Walton), Pergamon Press, Oxford, New York, pp. 403–410

Renes, L.E. (1953) Antimony poisoning in industry. *Archs Ind. Hyg.* **7**, 99–108

Richard, R.J., White, L.R. and Eik-Nes, K.B. (1985) Biological reactivity of different crystalline forms of titanium dioxide in vitro and in vivo. *Scand. J. Work. Environ. Health* **11**, 317–320

Riddell, A.R. (1934) Clinical investigation into the effects of gypsum dust. *Can. Publ. Health J.* **25**, 147–150

Robertson, A.J. (1960) Pneumoconiosis due to tin oxide. In *Industrial Pulmonary Diseases* (eds E.J. King and C.M. Fletcher), Churchill, London, pp. 168–184

Robertson, A.J. and Whittaker, P.H. (1955) Radiological changes in pneumoconiosis due to tin oxide. *J. Fac. Radiol.* **6**, 224–233

Robertson, A.J., Rivers, D., Nagelschmidt, G. and Duncomb, P. (1961) Stannosis: Pneumoconiosis due to tin oxide. *Lancet* **1**, 1089–1095

Roche, A.D., Picard, D. and Vernhes, A. (1958) Silicosis in ocher workers: a clinical and anatomo-pathologic study. *Am. Rev. Tuberc.* **77**, 839–849

Rowe, D.M., Solomayer, J.A. and Zenz, C. (1988) Bismuth and compounds. In *Occupational Medicine* (ed. C. Zenz), Year Book Medical, Chicago and London, p. 643

Rubin, L., Slepyan, A.H., Weber, L.F. and Neuheuser, I. (1956) Granulomas of the axillas caused by deodorants. *J. Am. Med. Assoc.* **162**, 953–955

Sadoul, P., Horsky, P., Beigbeider, R., Poncelet, B. and Pham, Q.T. (1979) Siderosis of iron miners in Lorraine. *Arch. Mal. prof.* **40**, 15–23

Safety in Mines Research (1963) *Safety in Miners Research Establishment Report for 1962*, HMSO, London, p. 34

Sander, O.A. (1958) Roentgen re-survey of cement workers. *Archs Ind. Health* **17**, 96–103

Sayers, R.R., Dallavalle, J.M. and Bloomfield, S.G. (1937) *Occupational and Environmental Analysis of the Cement, Clay and Pottery Industries*, Public Health Rep. US No. 238, pp. 1–50

Scansetti, G., Piolatto, G. and Botta, G.C. (1992). Airborne fibrous and non-fibrous particles in a silicon carbide manufacturing plant. *Ann. Occup. Hyg.* **36**, 145–153

Schepers, G.W.H. (1955a) The biological action of rare earths. I. *Archs Ind. Health* **12**, 301–305

Schepers, G.W.H. (1955b) The biological action of rare earths. II. *Archs Ind. Health* **12**, 306–316

Schepers, G.W.H. and Durkan, T.M. (1955) Pathological study of the effects of inhaled gypsum dust on human beings. *Archs Ind. Health* **12**, 209–217

Schepers, G.W.H., Delahant, A.B. and Redlin, A.J. (1955) An experimental study of the effects of inhaled gypsum dust on animal lungs. *Archs Ind. Health* **12**, 297–300

Schepers, G.W.H., Durkan, T.M. and Delahant, A.B. (1955) The biological effect of calcined gypsum dust. An experimental study on animal lungs. *Archs Ind. Health* **12**, 329–347

Schmitz-Moorman, P., Horlein, H. and Hanefeld, E. (1964) Lungenveranderungen bei titandioxyd staub exposition. *Beitr. Silikose forschung* **80**, 1–17

Seaton, A., Ruckley, V.A., Addison, J. and Rhind Brown, W. (1986) Silicosis in barium miners. *Thorax* **41**, 591–595

Shaffer, P.T.B. (1969) A review of the structure of silicon carbide. *Acta Crystallogr.* **B25**, 477–488

Shelley, W.B. and Hurley, H.J. (1958) The allergic origin of zirconium deodorant granulomas. *Br. J. Dermatol* **70**, 75–99

Shelley, W.B. and Hurley, H.J. (1971) The immune granuloma: late delayed hypersensitivity to zirconium and beryllium. In *Immunological Disease*, 2nd edn (ed. M. Samter), Little Brown, Boston, pp. 722–734

Sinico, M., Le Bouffant, L., Paillas, J., Fabre, M. and Trincard, M.D. (1982) Pneumoconiose due au cérium. *Arch. Mal. prof.* **43**, 249–252

Slater, D. (1974) Tin. *Mineral Dossier No. 9*. Mineral Resources Consultative Committee. HMSO, London

Sluis-Cremer, G.K. and du Toit, R.S.F. (1968) Pneumoconiosis in chromite miners in South Africa. *Br. J. Ind. Med.* **25**, 63–67

Smith, A.R. and Perina, A.E. (1948) Pneumoconiosis from synthetic abrasive materials. *Occup. Med.* **5**, 396–402

Smith, T.J., Hammond, S.K., Laidlow, F. and Fine, S. (1984) Respiratory exposures associated with silicon carbide production: estimations of cumulative exposures for an epidemiological study. *Br. J. Ind. Med.* **41**, 100–108

Spencer, G.E. and Wycoff, W.C. (1954) Benign tin oxide pneumoconiosis. *Archs Ind. Hyg.* **10**, 295–297

Stanton, M.F., Layard, M., Tegeris, E., Miller, E., May, M., Morgan, E. and Smith, A. (1981) Relation of particle dimension to carcinogenicity in amphibole asbestos and other fibrous materials. *J. Natl Cancer Inst.* **67**, 965–975

Stettler, L.E., Groth, D.H. and MacKay, G.R. (1977) Identification of stainless steel welding fume particulates in human lungs and environmental samples using electron probe microanalysis. *Am. Ind. Hyg. Assoc. J.* **39**, 76–82

Stokinger, H.E. (1984) A review of world literature finds iron oxides non-carcinogenic. *Am. Ind. Hyg. Assoc. J.* **45**, 127–133

Sulotto, F., Romano, C., Berra, A., Botta, G.C., Rubino, G.F.,

Sabbioni, E. and Pietra, R. (1986) Rare-earth pneumoconiosis: A new case. *Am. J. Ind. Med.* **9**, 567–575

Tandon, S.K., Gaur, J.S., Behari, J., Mathur, A.K. and Singh, G.B. (1977) Effect of monazite on body organs of rats. *Environ. Res.* **13**, 347–357

Teculescu, D. and Albu, A. (1973) Pulmonary function in workers inhaling iron oxide dust. *Int. Arch. Arbeitsmed.* **31**, 163–170

Turk, J.L. and Parker, D. (1977) Sensitization with Cr, Ni and Zr salts and allergic type granuloma formation in the guinea pig. *J. Invest. Dermatol.* **68**, 341–345

Turk, J.L., Badenoch-Jones, P. and Parker, D. (1978) Ultra-structural observations on epithelioid cell granulomas induced by zirconium in the guinea pig. *J. Pathol.* **124**, 45–49

Uragoda, C.G. and Pinto, M.R.M. (1972) An investigation into the health of workers in an ilmenite extracting plant. *Med. J. Aust.* **1**, 167–169

Vaccarezza, R.A. (1950) *Higiene y Salubridad en la Industria del Cemento Portland. Su investigación en las Fábricas Argentinas.* Guillermo, Buenos Aires

Vocatura, G., Colombo, F., Zanoni, M., Rodi, F., Sabbioni, E. and Pietra, R. (1983) Human exposure to heavy metals. Rare earth pneumoconiosis in occupational workers. *Chest* **83**, 780–783

Vorwald, A.J., Pratt, P.C., Durkan, T.M., Delahant, A.B. and Bailey, D.A. (1950) Siderosis – a benign pneumoconiosis due to the inhalation of iron dust. Part II: an experimental study of the pulmonary reaction following inhalation of dust generated by foundry cleaning room operations. *Ind. Med. Surg.* **19**, 170–180

Wende, E. (1956) Pneumokoniose bei Baryt und Lithopocarberten. *Arch. Gewerbepath. Gewerbehyg.* **15**, 171–185

Worth, G. and Schiller, E. (1955). Gesundheitsschädigungen durch Chrom und seine Verbindunge. *Arch. Gewerbepath. Gewerbehyg.* **13**, 673–686

Wynn-Williams, N. and Young, R.D. (1956) Idiopathic pulmonary haemosiderosis in an adult. *Thorax* **11**, 101–104

Xing-An, C., Juan, X.H., Zhihua, D., Min, L.H., Yingjie, Y., Zhong, W.J., Yidien, W., Shou-Hua, L. and Qin, H.Y. (1988) An assessment of the estimated thorium lung burdens of 130 miners in a rare-earth and iron mine in China. *Ann. Occup. Hyg.* **32** (suppl. 1), 871–876

Zenker, F.A. (1867) Über staubinhalations-krankheiten der Lungen. *Dtsch. Arch. Klin. Med.* **2**, 116–172

Zoeger, J., Dunn, J.R. and Fuller, M. (1981) Magnetic material in the head of the Pacific dolphin. *Science* **213**, 892–894

12

Silicosis and related diseases

Hans Weill, Robert N. Jones and W. Raymond Parkes

Silicosis is the lung disease caused by inhaling damaging amounts of respirable free crystalline silica. The first cases must have occurred soon after human labour diversified beyond the simple acquisition of food – when some individuals could devote much of their time to the working of stone. It is thought to be the oldest of the pneumoconioses. Its zenith as a cause of illness and death was doubtless in the early decades of the Industrial Revolution, when powerful machines greatly increased the dustiness of workplaces. In those days, too, tuberculosis was rife, and the interaction between the dust disease and the infection multiplied the baneful effects of dust. The unhealthiness of some dusty trades had been known from antiquity, but more time was required fully to differentiate silicosis from other lung diseases, and to demonstrate its specific cause.

Now, however, there is a respectable body of knowledge concerning silicosis. Although much remains to be learned about its biochemical and cellular mechanisms, the information needed to control silicosis effectively has been available for many decades. This fact has not resulted in its eradication. Outbreaks continue to appear, even in countries with abundant resources for protecting workers' health. As long as human beings must work the earth, silicosis will probably recur: the causative agent is virtually ubiquitous, and ignorance or disregard of health hazards is an all-too-human failing.

Mineralogy

Silicon is, after oxygen, the most abundant element in the earth's crust. The combination of silicon and oxygen as *silica*, or silicon dioxide (SiO_2), is the major constituent of earth's minerals.

Silica may be 'free', that is, not chemically combined with other elements, or may be combined with certain cations to form *silicates*. For more detailed discussion, see Appendix I, 'Silica'.

The three main polymorphic crystalline forms (or phases) of free silica are *quartz*, *tridymite* and *cristobalite*; tridymite and cristobalite are more fibrogenic than quartz. Cryptocrystalline forms (minute grains of quartz cemented together with amorphous silica) include *flint*, *chert* and *chalcedony*. The most important form of amorphous silica, in regard to pulmonary fibrosis, is *diatomite* (or *kieselguhr*), which is non-fibrogenic and consists of the skeletons of diatoms – microscopic marine animals – but, when heated, is converted, depending on the conditions, to tridymite or cristobalite. Another amorphous form is *vitreous silica*, produced by the melting and rapid cooling of crystalline silica.

Sources of exposure

Mining

During the mining of gold, tin, copper, platinum and mica, the operations of drilling, hewing, shovelling, crushing and blasting are all dust producing. Wet rock drilling, introduced in 1897 but not widely used until about 1920 (Holmann, 1947), is only partly successful in suppressing dust even when wetting agents are employed.

The major gold fields are in the Transvaal, the former USSR, Canada, the USA and Australia. The ore usually occurs in quartz veins associated with granite masses.

The chief tin-producing countries of the world have been referred to already in Chapter 11. Tin ore is found in relation to rocks of the granite family.

Copper ores – *chalcopyrite*, *chalcocite* and *bornite*, which may occur in association with igneous rocks, sandstone or shale – are mined in Chile, Zambia (where silicosis among the miners is on record; Paul, 1961), Zaire and the USA.

Mica, which consists of a group of minerals – *muscovite*, *phlogopite*, *biotite*, *lepidolite*, *zinnwaldite*, *roscoelite* and *vermiculite* (see Chapter 16) – is found in rocks of high quartz content (such as pegmatite veins), and these are a source of quartz dust during mining, crushing and milling; hence, silicosis may result from any of these processes (Government of India Ministry of Labour, 1953; Thiruvengadam et al., 1968). India and Brazil are the chief world producers of muscovite sheet mica; the Malagasy Republic has been the major source of phlogopite mica, a lesser producer being Mexico; and the USA is the largest producer of muscovite scrap and flake mica. The question of whether pure mica is capable of causing pulmonary fibrosis is discussed in Chapter 16 (page 558).

Barytes, a cause of inert dust pneumoconiosis after its crushing and milling, may be mined under conditions involving exposure to quartz dust. Fatal silicosis has been diagnosed in Scottish barytes miners (Seaton et al., 1986).

Fluorspar (calcium fluoride, CaF_2), which is worked by underground and opencast mining methods, occurs in vertical veins or flat-lying masses in country rocks so that free silica, as well as other minerals (such as barytes), is often present. In the Derbyshire mine field (the most important in the UK), for example, microcrystalline quartz and chalcedony are widespread in the wall rock, and the fluorspar itself may contain small siliceous nodules. Hence, 15 to 20 per cent SiO_2 may be found in the extracted ore, which may require very fine grinding during beneficiation to remove it. The mineral has many uses: for example, in the manufacture of fluorine chemicals, glass fibre, mineral wool, pottery and microscope lenses; and as a flux in the manufacture of steel ceramics. Its required purity, therefore, varies: acid-grade fluorspar contains a maximum of 1 per cent SiO_2; ceramic-grade, up to 3 per cent; and metallurgical-grade, up to 12 per cent (Notholt and Highley, 1975). Hence, silicosis may occur in fluorspar miners and grinders, but, in the absence of quartz, fluorspar is apparently non-fibrogenic in the lungs of experimental animals (de Villiers and Gross, 1967; South African Medical Research Council, 1974).

Gypsum, hydrated calcium sulphate ($CaSO_4·2H_2O$), is geologically a saline residue and, as such, a non-fibrogenic mineral. It is discussed in more detail in Chapter 11 and Appendix I. But because it was formed in three different ways, according to the local geological conditions, deposits in some regions are associated with intervening shales and mudstones which may contain as much as 30 per cent of fine-grained quartz. These conditions occur in Britain but not in the USA and Germany. Hence, miners and crusher operators in the Sussex and Nottingham gypsum mines – the former more than the latter – may be exposed to dust that contains a variable amount of quartz. This, however, is removed by beneficiation and is not a risk in industrial processes involving gypsum. 'Nodular' silicosis of mild degree has, therefore, occurred after prolonged exposure in British mine workers (Oakes et al., 1982) (see Figure 11.9) but not, as might be expected, in the USA and Germany.

Fireclays – a generic term used to refer to siliceous clays that constitute the seat-earths of some coal seams, and also to a number of differently formed clays suited to various refractory purposes – are today chiefly extracted by opencast methods. Prior to the Second World War, when there were more than 200 mines in the UK, extraction was almost exclusively by underground mining. In 1979, 14 mines were still operating: in Scotland (which has a long history of fireclay mining, as do most coal fields elsewhere), Yorkshire and Cumberland (D.E. Highley, 1980, personal communication). Fireclays are also produced in many other countries, notably the USA, Germany and Japan. Typical coal-measure fireclays have a highly variable composition, consisting predominantly of disordered kaolinite, mica and quartz in varying proportions. The highest quality fireclays contain approximately 1.5 per cent crystalline silica, but those of lower quality may contain as much as 30 per cent. Hence, the mining and bagging of fireclays have caused silicosis in the past, and remain a potential silica hazard. Most of the processing of fireclays in the manufacture of refractory goods, vitrified clay pipes, facing bricks and fireclay sanitary ware is in the wet or semi-wet state, so that a silica risk is usually slight; only small quantities of fireclay are dried or ground.

Ball clays are similar in composition to fireclays, but are less indurated and much more plastic.

Arenaceous (sandy) shales are mined extensively by open-cast methods, for the manufacture of heavy ceramic ware, and for cement and lightweight aggregates. *Oil shales* are also mined almost exclusively by opencast methods (previously, underground mining was not uncommon) for the extraction of crude oil but, as the quartz content of these shales is usually substantial, underground mining and processing has given rise to cases of silicosis in the past, and should still be counted as a potential, although uncommon, silica risk (see page 294).

Tungsten, a metal of fundamental metallurgical importance (see Chapter 18) and application in the electronic, electrical and chemical industries, occurs as *wolframite* [(FeMn)WO$_4$] and *scheelite* (CaWO$_4$) in fissures in association with granite, pegmatite and limestone. In England, it is mined in Cornwall and Cumberland by cross-cutting from main shafts to metal-containing veins (Slater, 1973). Hence, variable amounts of quartz may be present in mine dust, and silicosis has been reported.

Low-grade *iron ores*, known as *taconite* in certain areas, notably the Mesabi Range in Minnesota, have been mined in significant amounts since the 1950s. The material contains substantial quantities of free silica, often in chalcedonic form as chert or as fine-grained quartz (although in some areas the amount of crystalline silica is low), together with silicates. This would appear to be a potential silica risk, but no definite evidence of pneumoconiosis, adverse respiratory symptoms or ventilatory impairment was revealed in a recent survey of 249 men with 20 or more years of mining or processing taconite ore (Clark et al., 1980).

Sandstone or other siliceous sedimentary rocks may be encountered in some coal mines during shaft sinking, and in the development of tunnels and roadways. Surface coal-mine drillers in the USA have been found to have silicosis: 6 per cent had simple silicosis in one survey. A fatal case of (biopsy-proven) silico-lipoproteinosis occurred in one, after 5 years of exposure from rotary drilling using a dry technique (Banks et al., 1983a).

Sand itself is mined, or dredged, for the production of industrial quartz sands. These may be used for fillers, filtration, addition to concrete, production of ceramics, glass and fibrous glass, and blasting abrasives. The silicosis hazard arises from grinding and subsequent operations. Ground silica or 'silica flour', of respirable particle size and approaching 100 per cent quartz, is a highly dangerous material. In eleven cases, radiographic evidence of silicosis (three with large opacities) was found in Illinois silica mining–milling workers with 6 or fewer years' exposure (Banks et al., 1981).

Natural environmental exposure to quartzite sand in dust storms has been reported to cause silicosis in some geographical localities (Policard and Collet, 1952; Hirsch et al., 1974; Norboo et al., 1991).

Quarrying

Granite quarrying

The quartz content of granite varies from 10 to about 30 per cent. Quarrying is carried out with powered drills, wire belt saws fed with an abrasive slurry (usually aluminium oxide) and, in some quarries since the early 1950s, by a flame cutter in which the combustion of oxygen and fuel oil fed through a nozzle produces a flame with a temperature of over 2800°C; a stream of water accompanies the flame and, when it is directed against the rock, the rock disintegrates into fragments. The flame cutter produces a dust consisting of equal numbers of crystalline quartz particles and spheres, both having a geometric mean diameter of 0.3 µm, with the spheres probably composed of amorphous condensed fume. Average dust counts were in the range 5 to 10 ×10^6 particles/ft^3 (Burgess and Reist, 1969). The significance and possible effects of these 'submicron' particles upon the lungs requires further study, but as they undoubtedly consist of 'fused silica' (quartz glass), owing to the high temperature, they may be expected, like Aerosil particles, to have little fibrogenic potential (see 'Fused vitreous silica' later in the chapter).

Small quarries still rely on simple methods with little mechanization, with change to elaborate mechanization in large quarries increasing the concentration of dusts.

Sandstone quarrying

This is carried on in many countries. In the UK, quarries are worked in Cornwall, the Forest of Dean, Lancashire, Cumberland, Yorkshire and Scotland. The quartz content of the stone is always high. It is obtained by drilling and 'channelling' and, if hard, by the use of light blasting charges. It may be cut further and rough hewn in the quarry.

Slate quarrying

Sericite (white mica) is the most abundant constituent of slates, but the quartz content, although it varies widely, is usually in the range 30 to 45 per cent by weight.

The chief slate-producing countries are the USA (Maine, Pennsylvania, Vermont and Virginia), the UK (North Wales – until recently the largest slate-producing area in the world – and Cornwall), Tipperary and Cork in Eire, and France and Germany. Welsh slate has a particularly high quartz content, especially that from Blaenau Ffestiniog.

The fact that the quartz content of slates is variable, and is low in some, probably explains the widely different prevalence of silicosis observed in this industry in different regions.

Exposure to dust occurs during quarrying, in the sawmills where the slate is cut into blocks, and during the splitting of blocks to specified thickness and size by hand or machine. Sawing and splitting are usually done at the quarry site. Slate may still be used for the manufacture of electric panels and switchboards, billiard and other table tops, and fireplaces. It is cut, trimmed and polished in the factory – activities which are also dusty. Production of slate pencils in Mandaur, India has been reported to have caused severe silicosis (Jain et al., 1977).

Production of commercial slate powders for use as fillers leads to some loss of crystalline silica, but their content is seldom less than 25 per cent.

Pumice and pumicite quarrying

This and the subsequent refining processes which may be a source of exposure to crystalline silica are referred to on page 330.

Tunnelling

In civil engineering, cutting tunnels and excavation for a variety of purposes may be unexpectedly hazardous, especially as ventilation is usually poor. Driving sewer tunnels (which may be called 'construction work'), digging graves in sandstone, and excavating deep foundations in sandstone for multistorey buildings (as, for example, in Sydney, NSW, Australia) have all caused silicosis, and are the sort of risks which can be easily overlooked. Perhaps the greatest single-exposure occupational health disaster occurred in 1930 to 1931, as the result of the drilling of the Hawks Nest tunnel through a mountain at Gauley Bridge, West Virginia (Corn, 1980). Approximately 500 workers died of silicosis, and many more were eventually disabled by the disease. Subsequent Congressional hearings documented the appalling dust conditions at the worksite. This tragedy provided early evidence of the rapidly lethal form of silicosis which can result from exposure to enormously high concentrations of crystalline silica (see also 'Acute silicosis', later).

Stoneworking

Structural stone (known as 'dimension stone' in the USA) includes rough building stone, cut stone, ashlar, pavement flags, curbing and monumental stone. The most important materials for these, from the standpoint of silicosis, are sandstone and granite.

Quarried sandstone is cut by hand or machine, dressed, shaped and drilled for building and ornamental purposes, often in closed sheds and, until some 20 years ago (and rarely still), was fashioned into grindstones. Masons and their helpers who work the stone on benches (known as bankers) are likely to be exposed to high concentrations of dust when hygiene measures are inadequate. In some quarries, the stone is crushed and sieved on site for road materials. This is a very dusty process, although in the open air. Many of the

workers who worked Liverpool red sandstone during the building of the Anglican cathedral, or in making graves, developed serious silicosis.

Workers restoring or cleaning sandstone buildings with powered tools may be exposed to high local concentrations of dust.

Quarried granite is cut to specified sizes by wire or gang saws (a gang saw employs steel shot and water), ground to a desired contour or profile, and polished. In large factories, these procedures are highly mechanized and subjected to local and background exhaust ventilation, but in small firms mechanical methods may be limited. Fine cutting and finishing work is carried out with pneumatic hand tools. Designs and inscriptions are cut through stencils by abrasive blasting.

Where standards of local and general exhaust ventilation and enclosure are high – as in the Vermont granite industry (Hosey, Trasko and Ashe, 1957) – the prevalence of silicosis has greatly decreased, but where these are lacking or deficient, it tends to be higher in mechanized than in non-mechanized factories.

Monumental masons and kerbstone dressers were, and occasionally still are, liable to be exposed to dust without protection. Power drilling, chiselling and hammering of floors and walls made of concrete reinforced with chips of flint or quartz-containing rock, if not recognized, remain an important, if limited, hazard.

Manufacture of asbestos cement building products

Manufacturing workers in the USA have contracted silicosis, by itself or in combination with asbestosis, through exposure to raw materials or the dust from machining the finished products. Quartz, as sand or ground silica, may constitute 12 to 15 per cent of the weight of dry ingredients. Users of these products are at little or no risk of silicosis.

Abrasives

Sandstone is now rarely used for the manufacture of grindstones, but such grindstones may still be found in use. Crushed sand, sandstone and quartzite have been used for metal polishes and scouring powders, and flint or quartz are crushed and graded to make sandpaper. Tripoli (see Appendix I) is crushed and made into compositions for finishing and buffing metals, and ground rottenstone is used as a base for polishes.

Crushing and pulverizing these materials, and mixing and sieving them during manufacture, may give rise to a substantial dust hazard, but nowadays the machinery is usually enclosed.

Although it has been known for 30 years or more that high concentrations of the dust of finely powdered quartz, quartzite rock or flint (so-called *silica flour*), used in the manufacture of abrasive soaps and scouring powders, may cause rapidly progressive silicosis, their use in domestic scouring powders has only recently ceased in the UK; however, this may apparently still continue elsewhere (Nelson et al., 1978). Accelerated silicosis developed in jade workers in Hong Kong from the use of silica flour as a polishing agent (Ng et al., 1985).

Carborundum (silicon carbide, SiC) is a synthetic abrasive made by fusing silica and ground carbon at a high temperature. Past silica exposure in its manufacture may have been responsible for cases of pneumoconiosis, but the finished product has been regarded as biologically inert. Exposure of sheep, by instillation, has shown that the particulate form is inert, but a fibrous form is comparable to crocidolite asbestos in its fibrogenicity (Bégin et al., 1989) (see Chapter 11, page 277).

Abrasive blasting

The principle of this technique consists of propelling abrasive grains at high velocity at a target by means of compressed air, water under pressure or a controlled centrifugal force. The grains may be quartzite sands, flint or chert ('sandblasting' proper). Materials with low or absent crystalline silica have been used as substitutes: corundum, iron garnet [usually almandine, $Fe_3Al_2(SiO_4)_3$], coal furnace bottom ash (mainly iron oxides and aluminium silicates), zircon, a hard variety of barytes and silicon carbide. Most are ground to a specified grain size. Steel shot ('shot blasting') has commonly replaced the siliceous grains for some years now, but is more costly, tends to be less hard and deteriorates when stored. Hence, sandblasting has by no means been eliminated from industry, and is still extensively employed in the USA. A severe, accelerated form of silicosis has been observed in the Gulf Coast region, primarily in association with shipbuilding and maintenance of off-shore oil platforms. Both sandblasters and unprotected men working in their neighbourhood have developed silicosis (Ziskind et al., 1976).

Blasting is used to clean metal castings and to remove 'burnt-on' moulding sand in the preparation of metal surfaces for painting or enamelling, for cleaning building stone and concrete, and renovating stone veneer, for making inscriptions on memorial stones, and to etch glass and plastics.

If the size of the article to be blasted is suitable, the process can be enclosed and operated by remote control and, although this does not expose the operator to dust, significant concentrations of dust may be encountered on entering the cabinet or cleaning out spent abrasive from the floor or trap beneath. When enclosure is not possible (for example, sandblasting ships or buildings), the operator must wear a special hood or helmet supplied with uncontaminated compressed air to prevent the entry of dust particles. Enormous concentrations of respirable silica are produced, and some air-supplied respirators and hoods provide flow rates too low to furnish adequate protection (Glindmeyer and Hammad, 1988).

It should be remembered that, even when non-siliceous abrasives are used to clean metal castings, the dust produced from 'burnt-on' moulding sand may contain large amounts of quartz. Until recent times this was a notorious hazard, and dangerous exposure may still be encountered.

Glass manufacture

Pure beach and river sands are employed to produce glass and, until the mid-1960s, sand of graded particle size was used in the form of a slurry to grind and polish plate glass. Subsequently, the 'float glass process' (Pilkington, 1969) has largely replaced the previous techniques for manufacturing plate glass in most major glass industries in the UK and other countries. The earlier grinding and polishing methods, therefore, have now been abandoned by large companies, but may still survive in small firms.

The agate industry

Some 30 000 workers of both sexes are employed in India chipping and grinding agate – banded and variegated chalcedony with a microcrystalline silica content of about 82 per cent – for the manufacture of jewellery and other decorative items. Grinding is particularly hazardous (Rastogi et al., 1991).

Fillers

Finely ground quartz-containing rock is used for some paints and as a filler in the rubber industry: Neuburg chalk (Neuburger Kieselkreide), which contains a high percentage of quartz (Schneider, 1966), is commonly used in Germany. Fillers employed in the manufacture of gramophone records from about 1908 to 1948 (when microgroove records were introduced) included powdered slate and rottenstone of about 10 µm or less particle size. This practice was discontinued in 1948 because of the need to improve the signal-to-noise ratio in the new records (EMI Records (Gramophone Co. Ltd), 1970, personal communication).

Exposure is most likely to occur during the production of fillers, but may exist to a variable degree during their use. An unusual example of this is the development of silicosis in Japanese woodworkers who used tonoko powder (which contains about 78 per cent silicon dioxide) to fill grains in wooden furniture (Kawakami, Sato and Takishima, 1977).

Synthetic mastic asphalt

Synthetic mastic asphalt (in essence a mixture of some type of rock granules and asphalt in proportions that allow it to be worked when heated but to set thereafter into a compact, impervious mass) is employed very widely for roofing, damp courses, skirtings and interior flooring. Asphalt, according to geological origin (see Table AI.2, Appendix I), sometimes contains quartz. Rocks used to make granules are limestones, silica sands, granite, basalt, dolerite (which may contain quartz), and andesite and rhyolite – both lava-forming rocks containing quartz.

Thus, although there is little likelihood of a silica hazard from natural asphalt or from the various uses of synthetic asphalt, this may arise in the quarrying and crushing of the quartz-bearing rocks required, and during the processing of granules and their transfer to silos and trucks. But nowadays, elaborate dust-control systems are normally in place.

In addition, finely ground stabilizers which increase the resistance of asphalt to weathering are also frequently used: for example, those rocks that are used for granules, slate and fly ash. Furthermore, asphalt-coated roof sheeting is dusted with 'backing minerals' to prevent adhesion when rolled; these include finely ground mica, rock dust, slate powder and pyrophyllite, all of which may contain quartz.

Careful enquiry into the nature of materials used and some assessment of dustiness in the past may, therefore, be needed in those who have been involved in the manufacture of asphalt.

Foundry work

Crystalline silica dust is produced in iron and steel foundries in the following ways:

1. Moulding and core making.
2. Application of parting powders.
3. 'Knocking out' or 'shaking out' of castings.
4. Dressing, fettling and abrasive blasting of castings.
5. Contamination of foundry floors.
6. Maintenance and repair of refractory materials.

Moulding and core making

A mould is normally made of highly refractory quartzite sand bonded with a clay (such as china clay or ball clay), and placed in a cast iron or wooden box that splits into two or more parts. The sand is sufficiently plastic to take the 'pattern', or shape, of the casting to be made. If the casting is to be hollow, a core of the desired shape is constructed from oil-bonded sand or plastic, and baked to impart strength. Core strength can also be increased by adding sodium silicate to the sand and passing carbon dioxide gas through it, but there are some technical drawbacks to this method.

Recent core-making processes employ a phenolic resin and catalyst mixed into the sand. When heated by the molten metal, ammonia, formaldehyde, phenol and carbon monoxide are released. A newer technique involves mixing a phenolic resin with an isocyanate in the sand and, when this is in the core box, passing triethylamine through it. These processes have to be subjected to strict hygiene control, to prevent leaking of irritant and toxic gases after metal pouring (see Chapter 18).

When molten metal is poured in, the sand is subjected to a high temperature (about 1600°C in the case of steel), and this is sufficient to convert some of the quartz to cristobalite, which is strongly fibrogenic (see Chapter 5). It may be reused many times over for other moulds.

For a number of years, some foundries have used zircon sands as a substitute for quartzite sands, but these have the disadvantage of being costly. Olivine sands are also used. Olivine consists of magnesium and ferrous orthosilicate, and is non-fibrogenic in animals (see Chapter 16, page 559).

Application of parting powders

Some moulds require dusting with a 'parting powder', which gives increased resistance to thermal shock when the molten metal is run in. Powders of high crystalline silica content have generally been used for this purpose. Inevitably, this is a dusty process and, in the UK, has been controlled since 1950 by the Foundries (Parting Materials) Special Regulations, which forbid the use of materials having more than 3 per cent silicon dioxide by weight of dry material. Replacement with olivine and zircon powders is now common.

'Knocking out' or 'shaking out' of castings

After the metal has cooled, the mould and core are separated, that is, 'knocked out' or 'shaken out', from the casting. This can also be a very dusty job, and a most important potential source of exposure.

If the size of the cast is small enough, it can be enclosed with the vibrating table, which performs the task automatically, but large casts must be done by hand.

Dressing, fettling and abrasive blasting of castings

Sand that is adherent, or burnt on to the casting, must be removed – a process known as 'fettling', 'roughing-off' or 'stripping'. Larger areas are chipped off by hammer and chisel; smaller areas are smoothed down with portable grinding wheels of Carborundum or emery, which is another source of iron oxide dust. Some castings are finished by abrasive blasting (see page 289). Small castings are cleaned in a revolving cylindrical mill, which may contain steel balls (ball mill) as an additional abrasive agent.

All knocking out and fettling operations are potentially very dusty, and various methods of mechanization, enclosure and exhaust ventilation are now applied to eliminate or reduce the dust. In the UK, both the 'knock out' and fettling processes are controlled by the Iron and Steel Foundries Regulations 1953, and abrasive blasting specifically regulated by the Blasting (Casting and other Articles) Special Regulations 1949.

Iron foundry fettling tends to produce a mixed dust consisting of different proportions of iron oxide and quartz, which is an important cause of 'mixed dust fibrosis' described later in this chapter.

Contamination of foundry floors

At one time, all foundries had earth floors; such floors are still occasionally to be found because they have the advantage that they can be dug up to make large moulds. Their disadvantage, however, is that they become highly contaminated with siliceous dust, which it is impossible to eradicate.

Conditions similar to those in iron and steel foundries may be met in some non-ferrous foundries, especially brass foundries and, in the UK, are controlled by the precepts of the Joint Standing Committee in Safety, Health and Welfare Conditions in Non-ferrous Foundries (1957).

Ceramics

Ceramics may be defined as 'man-made articles which have been first shaped or moulded from a wide range of natural earths, minerals and rocks, and then permanently hardened by heat' (Adams, 1961).

Only *pottery* and *whiteware*, that is, bone china, porcelain and earthenware and *refractory ceramics*

are considered here. The manufacture of *structural clay products* (building bricks, floor and roof tiles, piping and chimney pots), the raw materials of which consist of argillaceous clays, does not normally present a 'silica risk', but an exception to this exists in the case of some types of wall and fireplace tiles in which flint and ball clay are used, and have caused, and may still cause, silicosis in men who manufacture, and cut and trim them ('tile-slabbers').

Chinaware, porcelain, stoneware and earthenware

The raw materials for chinaware ('bone china') are china clay, china stone (that is, a granitic rock containing quartz and feldspar, of which a high-quality form called 'Cornish stone' is found in the UK near St Austell), and calcined animal bone; those for stoneware are similar apart from the bone, and some fireclay (a fine-grained equivalent of ganister) may be added. The ingredients for porcelain and vitreous china are china and ball clays, feldspar and quartz or flint; those for earthenware are china and ball clays, feldspar and flint, but fireclay is added for some products, such as sinks. The crystalline silica content of china clay in the refined state, necessary for the ceramic industry, is 2 to 3 per cent; of ball clay, 5 to 25 per cent; and of natural red clay, about 30 per cent (HM Factory Inspectorate, 1959).

Briefly, the manufacturing processes are as follows. Non-plastic raw materials such as china stone, feldspar, fireclay, quartz and calcined flint are crushed and milled, and converted into a 'slip' by the addition of water. The plastic clay materials are also converted into a 'slip'. After the removal of contaminants, the 'slips' are mixed, the mixture pumped through a press where most of the water is extruded and, if required in a plastic state for shaping, the contained air is expelled in a 'pug mill'. The final mixture is known as 'body'.

Crushing and milling calcined flint and quartz is dusty, but the wet process is not. However, spillage and subsequent drying of non-plastic 'slip' and 'body' on benches, equipment, the floor and operatives' clothes can be a source of siliceous dust if the environmental conditions are not rigorously controlled by satisfactory standards of monitoring air-borne dust, local and general exhaust ventilation, and special protective clothing worn by the operatives. Even so, the risk may not be wholly eliminated (see 'Prevention').

Next, 'body' is shaped on a revolving wheel (known as 'jollying' or 'jiggering') or pressed into the desired shapes by machine presses. If the shapes are complex, 'body' is liquefied and poured into a plaster-of-Paris (gypsum) mould ('slip-casting'), and the mould allowed to dry before opening. Obviously, dried 'body' is a source of dust.

As chinaware 'body' contains no flint, it might be thought to offer no silicosis risk. However, silicosis has been observed in exposed workers (Posner, 1961) due, undoubtedly, to the high quartz content (about 30 per cent) of 'Cornish stone'.

The rough surfaces and edges of the ware produced are fettled, usually by women, by applying small knives, abrasive rags and tow to the ware as it stands on a revolving wheel. This operation (known as 'towing') produces much dust and requires strict control.

All shaped ware is then kiln fired between 900 and 1200°C according to the type of ware (Adams, 1961). When removed from the kiln, the ware is known as 'biscuit'. In the British pottery industry before about 1937, ware to be fired was placed in powdered flint for support in fireclay 'saggars'. This exposed kiln workers to high concentrations of crystalline silica dust and, consequently, there was a high prevalence of silicosis. Since that date, flint has been replaced by calcined alumina, with the result that silicosis among these workers has been virtually eradicated (Posner and Kennedy, 1967).

Finally, 'biscuit' ware is glazed with liquid glaze and refired at 1050 to 1400°C. The glaze usually consists of feldspar, quartz, borax, sodium carbonate and zinc oxide. Except for the pulverization of quartz during preparation and the drying of glaze spillage, it does not appear to offer any risk. When ware is decorated, a third 'on glaze' firing at lower temperatures is required. Certain types of ceramics are fired at 1200°C or more in order to produce a large concentration of cristobalite in the ware, because this possesses a very high thermal expansion.

It should be noted that large numbers of women are employed in the pottery industry.

In the UK, pottery manufacture is regulated by the Pottery (Health) Special Regulations 1947, and the Pottery (Health and Welfare) Special Regulations 1950.

In the USA, Finland, Denmark, Mexico and India, wollastonite (see Chapter 16, page 560, and Appendix I) is used as a substitute for flint, quartz sand, feldspar and china clay in 'body' and in 'glazes', with a consequent reduction in the potential silicosis hazard. For economic reasons of import costs and plant design, it is used little in the UK other than for certain glazes and fluxes.

Refractory ceramics

The most important group in the present context is referred to as *acid refractories*. These include lining bricks of various sorts, cements and different types of shaped ware. Bricks and cements are used in kilns, steel furnaces, ovens in gas-making plants, boiler houses and domestic hearths.

The raw materials – ganister or 'silica rock' (that is, quartzite sandstones, sands or grits), which has a very high quartz content – are crushed (usually in dry pans), milled, screened to desired size, and mixed with a controlled quantity of water and, in some cases, with small amounts of paper-mill waste and 'milk of lime'. Power presses shape the resulting material into bricks, or it is made into shapes by hand or by the 'slip casting' method. The bricks and shapes are dried in ovens or on heated floors, and then fired in a tunnel kiln at about 1450°C. Before the bricks are fired, they may be dusted with quartzite sand to prevent adherence, and this is afterwards retrieved, sieved and used again. With recurrent exposure to high temperatures, a significant proportion of the quartz is transformed into cristobalite. In fact, most of the quartz in well-fired bricks is converted gradually to cristobalite and tridymite. The end-product is referred to as 'fireclay brick' when the raw material is ganister, and as 'silica brick' when it is 'silica rock'. Obviously, this process is capable of producing large concentrations of siliceous dust.

Kiln bricklayers and others who maintain and dismantle the refractory bricks of ovens, furnaces, kilns and retorts ('retort setting') are exposed to dust, which may contain up to 10 per cent cristobalite, from disintegrating bricks and, in repair work, there may be an additional hazard in that the interstices of the bricks are often grouted with asbestos fibre mixed with water at the site, or with dry fibre or asbestos rope. This source of asbestos exposure is referred to in Chapter 14.

A coarse-grained quartz sand with natural clay bonding is used to line the dams and runners of blast furnaces. These 'cast house' or 'runner' sands may be a source of dust.

In the presence of small amounts of alkali, quartz is converted to cristobalite at temperatures of about 1200°C instead of about 1400°C (see Appendix I), and as a result cristobalite is the principal constituent of 'silica' refractories; it may also be present in many pottery bodies. Moreover, in the temperature range 1150 to 1250°C, flint is converted to cristobalite more readily than quartz and, in the presence of alkali (for example, chalk), cristobalite may be formed at a temperature as low as 950°C. In view of the fact that cristobalite is apparently more fibrogenic than quartz (see Chapter 5), it may enhance the severity of the resulting lung fibrosis. Calcined flint contains 5 to 10 per cent cristobalite.

Aluminosilicate refractories

Synthetic aluminosilicate ceramic fibre is now used extensively in the lining of high-temperature furnaces, as a substitute for the traditional firebrick. It has superior low thermal capacity and resistance to thermal shock, and is relatively cheap (Griffiths, 1986). It is available in the form of bulk fibre, boards of variously rated insulating capacities and cements. At normal operating temperatures of 1400 to 1700°C, over an extended period, conversion of aluminosilicates with high combined silica content can occur fairly quickly, to give mullite and cristobalite; these transformations commence at temperatures just above 1080°C. Concentrations of cristobalite are higher in the hotter parts of linings closer to the furnace. But cristobalite is not found in high-alumina blankets consisting of virtually 100 per cent Al_2O_3 as there is insufficient silica from which it can be formed (Holroyd et al., 1988). When the alumina content is less than 72 per cent (that of pure mullite) there is insufficient Al_2O_3 available to take up all the SiO_2, and thus free silica, usually in the cristobalite phase, is formed; similarly, where the SiO_2 content of the aluminosilicate is under 28 per cent (that is, the Al_2O_3 content is greater than 72 per cent), cristobalite will not form. Most aluminosilicate refractories (bricks and tiles), however, are not in the form of ceramic fibres (see Chapter 16, 'Kaolin') but, nevertheless, undergo transformation to mullite and cristobalite at similar temperatures (see Appendix I).

Thus, cristobalite-containing dust may be released and inhaled during the stripping of some old aluminosilicate insulating materials exposed to high temperatures for a prolonged period (Holroyd et al., 1988).

Neutral refractories

These are made from chrome ore, aluminium oxides or sillimanite mixed with a small quantity of plastic clay, and fired at temperatures of 1450 to 1650°C. Under these conditions, aluminium oxides do not appear to offer any pneumoconiosis risk. Sillimanite is referred to in Chapter 16 (page 559).

'Basic' refractories

Refractory bricks and other materials are made from magnesium, chert-free dolomite and olivine rock, and they do not present any crystalline silica risk (see Chapter 16, 'Olivine minerals').

Boiler scaling

The tubes, flues and fireboxes of boilers require cleaning and scaling at regular intervals. Coal-fired boilers collect ash and deposits ranging from fireable to lightly sintered or fused deposits. They consist essentially of aluminosilicates derived from decomposed clay particles and, in addition, may contain quartz, iron oxides, unburnt carbon and alkali sulphates. The composition may be very variable depending on that of the coal ash and the temperature at which the deposit is formed. These differences in composition influence the type of lung lesion that may be produced. This is referred to in a later section.

Cleaning is done with brushes, hammer and chisel, and compressed air jets in enclosed and restricted spaces, so that dust concentrations are high. Ash deposited in the gas passages, flues and smoke stacks of oil-fired boilers contains no quartz, but occasionally has a high content of vanadium, which is naturally present in large quantity in some oil – particularly Venezuelan oil (McTurk, Huis and Eckardt, 1956) (see Chapter 18, page 613).

It should be noted that boiler scalers have often worked in close proximity to bricklayers dismantling and replacing refractory brick linings, and may, therefore, have been exposed to quartz dust from this source. Furthermore, in past years, they may have been present during periodic relagging of boiler and neighbouring installations with asbestos-insulating materials, and have even assisted the laggers.

Vitreous enamelling

Enamel consists of quartz, feldspar, metal oxides and carbonates in variable quantities. These ingredients are pulverized, mixed and then fused at temperatures up to 900°C. Although the heat converts much of the quartz into silicates, some remains unchanged. The resulting sinter (referred to as 'frit') is ground with water in a ball-mill, and further quantities of the ingredients may be added. The mix is enamel and the process may be dusty. Enamel spraying, in particular, may present a hazard, especially when the inner surfaces of vessels are sprayed (Friberg and Ohman, 1957). Nowadays, spraying is carried out in booths with special exhaust ventilation, and the sprayer wears a respirator; nevertheless, the potential danger remains.

An additional risk is encountered when some enamelled objects are 'finished off' by sandblasting.

Semi-conductor manufacture

Silica exposures could arise from the production and machining of cultured quartz crystals, but the operations occur on a small scale and are enclosed. Recent concerns have centred on carcinogenesis and other effects or more exotic toxins, for example, gallium arsenide.

Sources of 'mixed dust' exposures

All of the sources listed above are in reality sources of mixed dust exposures, although the effects of crystalline free silica will usually predominate. This section identifies some sources likely to result in 'mixed dust fibrosis' (see later), in which the pathological and clinical effects of silica are conspicuously modified by the presence of another dust.

Occupations in which 'mixed dust fibrosis' have occurred most commonly are casting, fettling, and sand or shot-blasting in iron, steel and non-ferrous foundries; hematite mining, although in the UK this has caused a negligible amount of fibrotic pneumoconiosis since the 1930s, owing to dust suppression measures (Bradshaw, Critchlow and Nagelschmidt, 1962); cleaning and scaling boilers; and electric arc welding and oxyacetylene cutting in foundries where there has also been some exposure to siliceous dusts from neighbouring operations, in addition to iron fumes from welding or cutting.

'Mixed dust fibrosis' has been well documented as occurring in iron and steel foundry workers (Uehlinger, 1946; Rüttner, 1954; McLaughlin and Harding, 1956), non-ferrous foundry workers (Harding and McLaughlin, 1955), boiler scalers (Harding and Massie, 1951), hematite miners (Stewart and Faulds, 1934), and ochre miners (see page 323). It may also occur in potters, in whom there may have been, as stated earlier, an additional exposure to feldspar, kaolinite and other dusts.

Mining of oil shales for extraction of crude oil (see Appendix I, 'Argillaceous rocks') has been associated with pneumoconiosis of mild degree, which consists, microscopically, of small lesions of 'mixed dust' fibrosis, and also, occasionally, of calcification of hilar lymph nodes (Meiklejohn, 1956; Küng, 1979). However, more recently, massive fibrosis has been reported in four main oil shale miners in Scotland (Seaton et al., 1981). Mining has been, or is, carried out chiefly by underground methods in the Scottish Lothians, the USA, Brazil, Sweden and the former USSR. Operations in the Lothians (which commenced in the nineteenth century) and in Sweden ceased in the early 1960s, having become uneconomic (Cameron and McAdam, 1978). In the USA, the rich deposits of the Green River Formation of the Colorado plateau are estimated to be capable of producing 100 000 barrels of shale oil per day (Costello, 1979), but development was abandoned with the fall in crude oil prices of the early 1980s. Although silicates, chiefly kaolinite, are predominant constituents of these shales, their quartz content varies according to site or location of origin, from 3 to 8 per cent to almost 25 per cent in raw Green River shales, and about 40 per cent in Estonian (former USSR) shales. The overall arithmetical mean of quartz in air-borne dust associated with various operations in experimental oil shale mines in the USA in the late 1970s and early 1980s was 3.9 per cent, ranging from 1.8 per cent to 14.0 per cent, some 50 to 60 per cent of which was of respirable size (Hargis and Jackson, 1983). Meiklejohn (1956) warned that increased mechanization (introduced into the Lothian mines in the early 1950s) might increase the pneumoconiosis risk. This is potentially true, although the technology for effective dust control is available (Weaver and Gibson, 1979) if a future 'oil crisis' leads to hasty resumption of mining.

Diatomite

Diatomite, a siliceous sedimentary rock – known also as diatomaceous earth and kieselguhr (see Appendix I) – consists mainly of the fossilized skeletons of a unicellular aquatic plant related to the algae and biologically dependent on silicon. Diatomaceous earth is composed primarily of amorphous silicon dioxide of biogenic origin.

Origins

Commercially, the most important deposits occur in the USA (mainly in California, Nevada, Oregon and Washington), Mexico, South and East Africa, the Massif Central area of France, and Denmark and Germany. Although small quantities are produced in Cumberland and Northern Ireland, the UK relies upon imported diatomite, mainly in the calcined form.

Mining and processing

Mining is carried out almost entirely by the opencast method, and crude diatomite is transferred to the processing plant, where it is crushed, screened, recrushed and put into storage bins for blending into qualities appropriate to various uses. Natural moisture is removed by hot-air heaters at about 260°C, producing *natural dried diatomite*. It is then passed through a series of cyclones and separators to eliminate clays and other contaminants. Further processing may be done in the natural state, but the greater part of the material is calcined. There are two different methods of calcination which were introduced in the 1920s: first, *straight calcination*, in which natural diatomite is heated at approximately 816 to 1100°C in a rotary kiln, thereby removing organic matter, altering its structure and porosity, and converting some of it into cristobalite; secondly, *flux calcination*, in which sodium carbonate or sodium chloride is added as a flux before the diatomite is fired in a kiln at 1100°C or more, resulting in the transformation of a larger portion of the amorphous silica into cristobalite than during straight calcination. These differences in the phases of diatomite silica have important implications in relation to the development of pneumoconiosis (see Chapter 5 'Pathogenesis' and 'Pathology', pages 326 and 327, and Appendix I).

Both natural and calcined forms are next milled, passed again through separators to remove grit and coarse kiln material, and then to a cyclone 'classifier', where they are divided into fine (particles less than 10 μm in size) and coarse products, which are stored in bag-house hoppers, and finally bagged. Straight calcined diatomite is tan or pink in colour due to oxidation of iron, and flux-calcined diatomite is white.

All these processes are potentially dusty, but milling and bagging of calcined diatomite are the chief sources of a pneumoconiosis risk.

Processing diatomite is more advanced in the USA than elsewhere, with annual US production of about 650 000 tonnes, contrasting with world production of 1.7 million tonnes. World industrial demand, mainly of the calcined product, has greatly increased since the Second World War. Rigorous dust controls are now applied in the mines and processing plants.

Diatomite used in the UK is mostly imported in dried and straight or flux calcined forms from the USA and other countries. There is only limited exploitation of UK deposits: in Westmorland where straight calcined powders and granules are produced, and in Northern Ireland, which produces natural grades of dried diatomite; neither produces flux-calcined diatomite.

Uses of diatomite

1. Filtration is the most important use. It is used in the calcined form as a filter aid, and in the manufacture of filters for inorganic and organic liquids, especially in wine, beer and fruit juice production, the manufacture of pharmaceutical liquids and antibiotics (such as penicillin and streptomycin), and in sugar refining. It has to a large extent replaced asbestos filters, which were widely used for this purpose until recently. Berkfeld filters are made from diatomite.
2. Heat and sound insulation: the diatomite is made into refractory bricks, moulded blocks, or used as a binder for pipe covering and insulating cement, for boilers, pipes, stills, furnaces and kilns.
3. Diatomite is used as a filler for plastics, rubber, paper, insecticides, paints, varnishes, linoleums, floor coverings, fertilizers and in special types of paper.
4. Diatomite is used as an adsorbent for industrial floor sweeping powders and chemical disinfectants.
5. Diatomite is used as a mild abrasive in silver, metal and automobile polishes, dental pastes and hand soaps.
6. Other uses are as a carrier for catalysts, a pozzolanic component of certain cements and concrete, for various types of building materials (board, sheets, tiles, blocks and plasters), and in electrode coatings for welding. In the UK, English and Irish diatomite is used especially in cement manufacture, for which purpose it is dried at a low temperature to remove organic matter, such as peat, and hence is unlikely to contain a significant amount of crystalline silica, if any.

Apart from processing, therefore, exposure to diatomite (usually in calcined form) may occur to a varying degree in the manufacture of these products and when mixed by hand for insulation. Maintenance work on processing plants is also a potential source of exposure.

The diseases

Two main types of silicosis may be distinguished: *ordinary silicosis* ('nodular', 'pure' or 'classical' silicosis), whether in a simple or complicated stage, is defined by the formation of characteristic hyaline and collagenous nodules. Accelerated silicosis is a variant developing after more intense exposures, and is characterized by earlier onset and more rapid progression. *Acute silicosis* develops after massive exposures, and the characteristic lesion is similar to alveolar lipoproteinosis.

Mixed dust fibrosis and *diatomite pneumoconiosis* are sufficiently distinctive to warrant separate discussion. It should be remembered that the sources of exposure that produce these conditions will often produce cases of silicosis, depending on the proportion of respirable crystalline silica in mixed dusts or the effects of calcination of diatomite.

Ordinary silicosis

The terms 'simple silicosis' and 'complicated silicosis' are defined radiographically, according to the absence or presence of pneumoconiotic large opacities – irrespective of whether clinical complications, such as tuberculosis, are present.

Incidence and prevalence

Until the Second World War, silicosis was the most important and widespread form of pneumoconiosis. Since then, due mainly to substitution by other materials and hygienic measures, the incidence of new cases appears to have declined dramatically in the majority of industrial countries. Accurate statistics are rarely available, as they are often based on compensation figures and, therefore, on selected cases; diagnostic criteria vary and, in some countries, coal pneumoconiosis is bracketed with 'silicosis'. Furthermore, reliable information about the size of populations at risk is lacking.

The incidence of 'new' cases in the UK is now low. In the USA, although the disease has been virtually eliminated from the Vermont granite (Hosey, Trasko and Ashe, 1957) and metal mining industries (Finn et al., 1963), the evidence of this decline from other industries is not adequate to support a similar conclusion. Some increase (often due to single industrial processes) has been reported in Bulgaria, Spain (World Health Organization, 1968), Sweden (Ahlmark and Bruce, 1967) and Singapore (Khoo and Toh, 1968).

It is of interest that surveys of the granite industry in Cornwall and Devon in 1951 and 1961 (Hale and Sheers, 1963) showed little reduction in the silicosis risk, and that Grundorfer and Raber (1970) found an increase since 1958 among granite workers of lower Austria, due mainly to granite crushing for gravel production. Granite crushing is particularly hazardous when, as in Austria, it is a skilled and continuous occupation, but it is unlikely to be so when workers are casual and unskilled as, for example, they usually are in Sweden (Ahlmark, Bruce and Nyström, 1960) and the UK (Hale and Sheers, 1963). Two surveys of monumental masons in Aberdeen disclosed a 10 per cent prevalence of silicosis in 1951 and 3 per cent in 1970, conglomerate lesions being present in 2 per cent of the former series, but absent in the latter (Lloyd Davies et al., 1973). In 1980, however, an overall prevalence of 10 per cent (ILO categories 2 or 3) was found in slate workers in North Wales between 1971 and 1980 (Glover et al., 1980). Discrete ('simple') pneumoconiosis, but no conglomerate ('massive') disease, was found in 1.6 per cent of 5684 workers in a recent survey of the British pottery industry (Fox et al., 1975).

It should be noted that the use of newly developed, powerful mechanical methods of excavating, tunnelling and quarrying, and for dressing siliceous stones or concrete, or the addition of crushed or powdered quartz or flint to other materials in a variety of industrial processes, may give rise to a serious, often unsuspected silica hazard, even if this only affects a small number of men. For example, silicosis – often in 'semi-acute' form – still appears to occur sporadically as a result of the use of 'silica

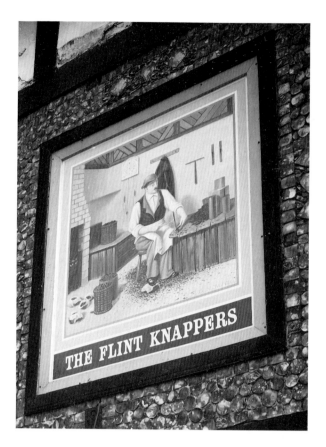

Figure 12.1 Inn sign at Brandon, Suffolk: unworked flint nodules are seen on the floor to the left of the baskets of finished gun-flints. The work place was poorly ventilated. Note the inn wall is constructed of flint nodules. (Reproduced by courtesy of the Managing Director of the Norwich Brewery Ltd)

flour' (see later) in the manufacture of abrasive soaps and cleansers, metal polishing compounds and autoclaved concrete blocks (Salam et al., 1967; Zimmerman and Sinclair, 1977; Nelson et al., 1978).

The ancient occupation of quarrying and fashioning sandstone grindstones in ill-ventilated pits and caves in northern Nigeria has resulted in a 39 per cent prevalence rate of silicosis (Warrell et al., 1975), and the disease is also found in various stages among women in the Transkei District of South Africa who have used similar stones for many years to grind maize and corn (Palmer and Daynes, 1967). A survey of stone cutters in North India revealed a 35.2 per cent prevalence (Gupta et al., 1972), and in agate grinders and chippers in India, 18.4 per cent (Rastogi et al., 1991). These occupations are echoed by the ancient flint knapping industry in Brandon, Suffolk (UK) and the Meusnes district (Loir-et-Cher) in France, in which flint nodules were split and shaped by hand with knapping and flaking hammers to produce bevelled flints about $1 \times \frac{3}{4}$

inches in size for flint-lock guns (still used by 'black powder' enthusiasts) since the late seventeenth century. Although only small numbers of people were involved in the Brandon industry, they suffered 'a terrible mortality from phthisis, induced by flint dust generated in their work' and, at the turn of the century, 77.8 per cent of them died of 'phthisis', compared with 6.5 per cent of the general rural population in the area. Similar depredation occurred among the French knappers (Collis, 1915). Although no pathological details are known, there is little doubt that silicosis was the disease in question. Dust counts of 1313 and 1192 particles (most of which were under 1 μm) per cm³ air were reported by Middleton (1930). Knapping in Brandon is now almost at an end, but the trade is commemorated in the name and sign of a local inn (Figure 12.1).

An up-to-date report on workers in British mechanized iron foundries has shown that 'disabling' pneumoconiosis is now rare, although there is a higher prevalence and rate of progression of pneumoconiosis (which, however, does not exceed category 3 and is normally lower) in some occupations, notably fettlers, than in others (Joint Standing Committee on Health, Safety and Welfare in Foundries, 1977).

In short, although the prevalence of silicosis has, in general, fallen significantly in the last few decades, there is little published information to quantify a continuing reduction during the 1980s. It is still to be reckoned with in differential diagnosis and as a possible cause of respiratory disability.

Pathogenesis

The prevalence and severity of disease are mainly determined by the intensity of exposure to crystalline silica dust; for example, both are greater in sandstone than in granite workers because the quartz content of the former is significantly higher; exposure to high concentrations in confined spaces over a short period – sometimes less than a year – may result in rapidly advancing and often fatal silicosis (Gardner, 1933; Bobear, Hanemann and Beven, 1962; Samimi, Weill and Ziskind, 1974). The authors have cared for several men dying in their thirties and forties of accelerated silicosis, contracted through sandblasting in enclosed spaces.

As pointed out already experimental evidence suggests that cristobalite and tridymite are more fibrogenic than quartz, and observation of isolated cases tends to support this.

Silicosis appears to begin with emigration of macrophages into alveoli. The evolution of the nodules consists of the formation and proliferation of collagenous fibrosis stimulated by the cytological events discussed in Chapter 5, with subsequent

Table 12.1 Prevalence of ANA in relation to radiographic category in silicosis of sandblasters

Total number	Small discrete nodules		Conglomerate lesions					
			A		B		C	
	No.	%	No.	%	No.	%	No.	%
39	5/18	28	2/7	29	6/9	66	4/5	80

χ² P=0.05

Overall prevalence = 44% (17/39).
Adapted with acknowledgement to Turner-Warwick et al. (1977).

hyalinization of the fibrous tissue. The possibility that lung-reactive antibodies (see Chapter 4) might participate – at least in some cases – is suggested by the experimental observations that collagen is the primary antigen that reacts with lung antibodies (Burrell et al., 1966) and that, in vitro, these antibodies stimulate macrophages to release a fibrogenic factor that prompts synthesis of collagen, which, in turn, results in the production of more antigen (Lewis and Burrell, 1976). At present, there is no certainty that such events occur in human subjects. Despite the fact that IgG and IgM have been recorded as occurring among, and bound to, the collagen fibres and fibrohyalin of human silicotic nodules (Pernis, 1968), Wagner and McCormick (1967) failed to identify the presence of rheumatoid factors (RFs).

An unusually high prevalence of circulating antinuclear antibodies (ANAs) related to increasing radiographic severity of disease has been demonstrated in sandblasters with silicosis (Jones et al., 1976; Turner-Warwick et al., 1977) and, although an increased prevalence of RFs was not found among African grindstone cutters with silicosis by Warrell et al. (1975), a slight increase has been observed in ceramic workers (Otto, 1969) and sandblasters with silicosis (Table 12.1 and see Chapter 4, Table 4.4). Certainly RFs may be present, sometimes in high titre, in silicosis that exhibits sudden unexpected progression or enhanced activity in the absence of tuberculosis, and irrespective of whether rheumatoid arthritis is present or not. The significance of these antibodies is uncertain, but they may reflect the severity of macrophage destruction, and release of the nuclear and other contents of these cells caused by crystalline silica (see Chapter 4).

Other observations in workers with silicosis caused by sandblasting have shown no reduction in total numbers of lymphocytes, or the number of T and B cells in the peripheral blood, and no impairment of delayed sensitivity to 'recall' antigens, such as PPD and candida antigen, compared with control individuals. In addition, although there was no evident difference in in vitro responses of T cells to phytohaemagglutinin in the two groups, the responsiveness of these cells to low doses of concanavalin A was depressed in the silicotic group (Schuyler, Ziskind and Salvaggio, 1977). If, as has been suggested, this impairment indicates deficiency of suppressor T cells, it could explain the development of autoantibodies in silicosis and the occasional association of such autoimmune disorders as systemic sclerosis (see page 314), but confirmation of this finding is needed.

The question as to whether a genetic influence may operate has not been much investigated, although a survey of a large number of fluorspar miners and their families in Sardinia suggests that a predisposition for some persons to develop silicosis, and for others to resist it, may be genetically determined (Gedda et al., 1964). One study of Caucasian men found a significant underrepresentation of the antigen HLA-B7 in silicotic individuals (Gualde et al., 1977). Another study found that silicotic individuals were more likely than exposed non-silicotic individuals to have HLA-Aw19 (Koskinen, Tiilikainen and Nordman, 1983), and yet a further study found no differences for HLA-B7 and a significant underrepresentation of HLA-B40, in comparison to normal and to exposed non-silicotic individuals (Sluis-Cremer and Maier, 1984). Excess prevalences of antigens HLA-B44 and HLA-A29 were found in 49 silicotic men, most of whose exposures were in molybdenum mining (Kreiss, Danilovs and Newman, 1989). Clearly, HLA phenotyping has still to disclose a consistent marker of enhanced susceptibility. The red blood cell–plasma anti-oxidant system has also received some scrutiny as a possible susceptibility marker, with encouraging results but a small number of patients (Borm et al., 1986).

Pathology

Macroscopic appearances

The pulmonary (visceral) pleura is usually thickened due to fibrosis, and is often adherent to the parietal pleura, especially over the upper lobes and in the vicinity of underlying conglomerate lesions. Thickening and symphysis may be extensive, but only slight when there are no subpleural nodules.

Nodules are readily felt in the unopened lung, and when it is cut are seen to vary from 2 to 6 mm in diameter, to have a whorled pattern (Figure 12.2), and to be grey–green to dark grey in colour. Similar lesions may be seen in the hilar nodes.

Both discrete nodules and conglomerations of nodules tend to be distributed more in the upper halves of the lungs than in the lower, and more in

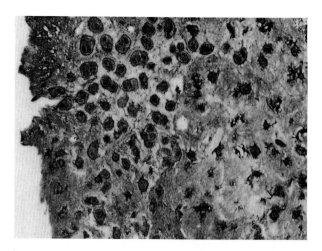

Figure 12.2 Natural size photograph of discrete silicotic nodules. Pigmentation is not uniform and a concentric pattern can be seen. There is no emphysema. Whole lung section

their posterior than their anterior parts; however, exceptions to this are seen. Rarely they are largely confined to a narrow zone adjacent to the pulmonary pleura. When conglomerations of nodules (which may sometimes be large enough to occupy an upper lobe) are examined by reflected light, or in whole lung section against transmitted light, they are clearly seen to consist of closely fused individual nodules (Figure 12.3).

Unlike confluent coal pneumoconiosis (progressive massive fibrosis), conglomerate lesions only rarely develop cavities in the absence of tuberculosis. In some cases, discrete nodules and conglomerations are found subpleurally and, when the conglomerate lesions are calcified and fused to dense pleural fibrosis, the lung is locally encased; this is sometimes referred to as 'cuirass' (armour plate). Occasionally, a large unilateral conglomerate nodular mass occurs with little other evidence of silicosis (Fiumicelli, Fiumicelli and Pagni, 1964), but this should be considered highly atypical.

The gross appearances of nodular silicosis are quite distinct from those of coal pneumoconiosis, but silicotic lesions are sometimes found in the lungs of coal miners who have done a lot of drilling of siliceous rock seams (see Chapter 13).

Enlarged and fixed hilar and paratracheal lymph nodes occasionally cause distortion of the trachea, the main bronchi and branches of the pulmonary arteries near the hilum (Pump, 1968), and similar pulmonary lymph nodes may restrict bronchial movements. In cases with advanced contraction of the upper lobes and elevation of the hila, tracheal deviation is usually the result of redundancy of its length (and most deviate to the right side at the level of the sternal notch).

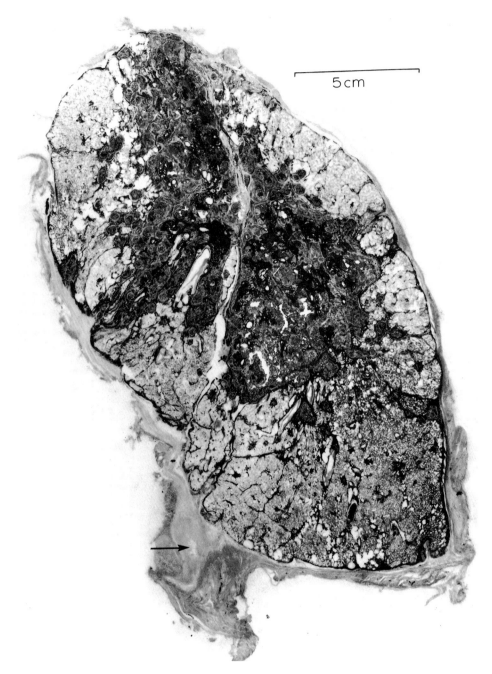

Figure 12.3 Conglomerate or massive silicosis: matting of silicotic nodules many of which, with their whorled pattern, are still individually identifiable. Distribution is predominantly in the upper parts of both lobes. Dense dust pigmentation is limited to a few areas and irregular (scar) emphysema is absent. Note widespread thickening of the pleura which is densely hyalinized in places (lighter areas) and there is a small zone of calcification (arrowed). Whole sagittal section of the left lung

Microscopic appearances

Dust particles are found either in macrophages or in the naked state in the walls of alveoli – chiefly those of respiratory bronchioles – and collected in perivascular areas. They cause cell death, fibroblast proliferation and reticulin formation. The walls of affected alveoli are thereby thickened, in some places sufficiently to obliterate neighbouring alveolar spaces. Collagenous fibrosis follows in a concentric

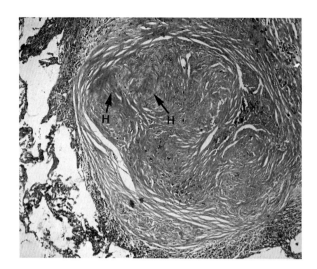

Figure 12.4 Microsection of a typical silicotic nodule showing the concentric ('onion skin') arrangement of collagen fibres, some of which are hyalinized (H), lack of dust pigmentation and the cellularity of the periphery. The lesion is clearly demarcated from adjacent lung tissue which is substantially normal. The appearances are those of a proliferative process. Compare with lesions of coal pneumoconiosis and asbestosis. Magnification × 55; H & E stain

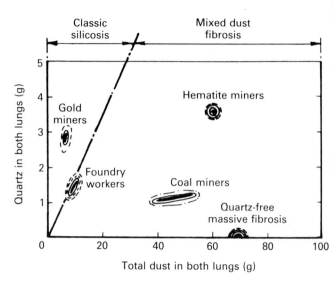

Figure 12.5 Average values of total dust and quartz in lungs with advanced forms of different diseases. (Reproduced, with permission, from Nagelschmidt, 1960)

arrangement. Subsequently, much of the collagen becomes 'hyalinized', and the resulting near-spherical nodules consist of concentrically arranged, or whorled, zones of acellular hyalin, which are enclosed by a moderately cellular collagenous capsule; the cells consist of macrophages (which often contain carbon particles) and plasma cells (Figure 12.4). Giant cells are not seen. Silicotic hyalin resembles amyloid in that it has a higher content of carbohydrate and phospholipids than other forms of hyalin, and is weakly birefringent.

Silicotic nodules, by contrast with the lesions of coal pneumoconiosis (see Chapter 13), are 'proliferative' in that they contain an excess of collagen, but little dust; indeed, the higher the quartz content of a dust, the smaller the amount of dust required to produce a given severity of fibrosis (Figure 12.5) (Nagelschmidt, 1965), and the longer the quartz particles are retained in the lungs, the greater the fibrosis and the smaller the quantity necessary to cause fibrosis (Einbrodt, 1965). Continuous exposure to dust causes existing nodules to increase in size and new ones to form. This progression may occur long after exposure has ceased, and may be due either to a self-perpetuating tendency for quartz-containing macrophages to migrate and die in and around existing lesions (Heppleston, 1962) or to the intervention of a secondary immunological reaction. The distinguishing features between

typical and 'rheumatoid' silicotic nodules are referred to in a later section in this chapter, and between silicotic nodules, 'rheumatoid' coal nodules, and tuberculous lesions in Chapter 13.

Silica content

The silica content of normal lungs with no exposure to industrial dusts has been found to be about 0.1 to 0.2 per cent dried tissue, and that of normal hilar lymph nodes to range from 0.23 to 0.6 per cent dried tissue. The content of silicotic lungs is commonly about 2 to 3 per cent, but may be as high as 20 per cent of the dried weight (Sweany, Porsche and Douglass, 1936; Fowweather, 1939) (Figure 12.5).

Alveoli in proximity to silicotic nodules are usually of normal size; occasionally scar (irregular) emphysema is seen, but is exceptional and of slight order, because the nodules are proliferative and expanding. Associated centrilobular emphysema is not seen.

Nodules tend to occur in clusters, and may subsequently fuse into conglomerations of varying size. These conglomerations are not amorphous masses, because individual nodules do not wholly lose their identity. It is to be noted that calcification (which is sometimes pronounced) may occur in some nodules in the absence of tuberculosis or histoplasmosis, the insoluble calcium salts being deposited mainly in the central hyalin (Moreschi, Farina and Chiappinio, 1968). Central necrosis of conglomerate masses occasionally occurs in the absence of complicating tuberculosis, apparently as a result of ischaemic changes.

Quartz particles can be demonstrated in variable amounts in the central zone of the nodules, and as a halo around their periphery, by accurately oriented polarized light (see Appendix IV) or by dark-ground microscopy after microincineration of the lesions, but they are absent from the collagenous capsule.

The growth of peribronchiolar silicotic nodules may narrow or obliterate these airways, and perivascular nodules may cause obstruction of lymphatics and arteritis, with eventual obliteration of some vessels and destruction of their walls. Larger elastic arteries are rarely obstructed, but may be compressed.

In the rare case in which silicosis develops rapidly from the start – sometimes following work with crystalline silica in a finely divided state – and in which some additional unidentified determining factor (possibly immunological) may play a part, the nodules are very numerous, small and lack the ordered compact pattern of typical nodules (Figure 12.6).

Much of the dust reaching the lymphatics passes to the hilar lymph nodes, but some travels to the internal mammary nodes and to more distant extrathoracic nodes, notably the supraclavicular, cervical and abdominal aortic groups. Particles gaining entry to the blood may give rise to isolated nodules in the spleen (Belt, 1939) and liver (Lynch, 1942), but are too few to cause any functional damage; however, if calcified, they may be radiographically visible.

Affected lymph nodes contain dense fibrosis or typical nodules with quartz particles. The capsular and peripheral regions of these nodes may calcify and resemble the shell of an egg. This change may appear early or late in relation to the evolution of the lung lesions, and may be present when silicotic lung disease is negligible. It has been suggested that this is due to an unusual propensity to deposit calcium salts (Chiesura, Terribile and Bardellini, 1968). There is no evidence that tuberculous infection is involved.

Tuberculosis

It has been established that silicosis predisposes to pulmonary tuberculosis since the beginning of the century, and in those days the majority of silicotic individuals succumbed to it. In 1937, Gardner found evidence of coexistent tuberculosis in 65 to 75 per cent of silicotic individuals from various industries. In recent years, the rate has fallen dramatically in parallel with the general decline of tuberculosis, but, nevertheless, it is still in excess of that in the general population. Bailey et al. (1974) observed 10 cases (12 per cent), 3 of whom died of silicotuberculosis, in 83 sandblasters from New Orleans. Predominant

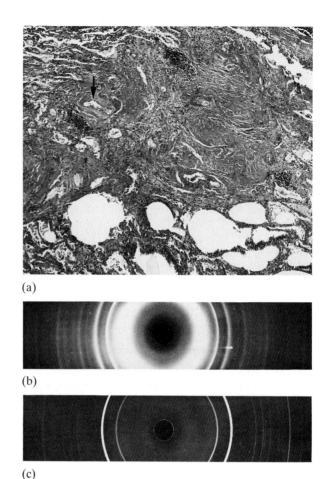

(a)

(b)

(c)

Figure 12.6 (a) Microsection of a representative lesion of rapidly developing atypical silicosis over 3 years in a man exposed to high concentrations of uncalcined quartzite sands. There is only a suggestion of the ordered pattern which characterizes typical silicotic nodules and the fibrosis, which engulfs an artery (arrowed) and is partly hyalinized, extends in places into alveolar walls so that clear demarcation from normal lung is lacking. Numerous plasma cells and lymphocytes were present adjacent to these lesions. Occasional typical silicotic nodules were also present elsewhere in the lungs. (See Figure 12.15 for radiographic features.) Magnification × 55; H & E stain. (b) X-ray diffraction of the lung dust shows a strong quartz pattern. (Analysis by F.D. Pooley, Cardiff.) (c) Standard quartz pattern

involvement of the lower lobes was unusually common. The more advanced the silicosis, the greater the incidence of active tuberculosis is likely to be (Chatgidakis, 1963).

The enhancing effect of crystalline silica on tuberculosis was demonstrated experimentally by Gardner (1929), by the reactivation of previously induced and healing tuberculous lesions in guinea-pig lungs after inhalation of a quartz aerosol, and by the production of tuberculous lesions in guinea-pigs by a normally non-pathogenic strain of tubercle bacillus (R1) in the presence of quartz (Gardner, 1934). More recent experiments have confirmed the potentiating effect of quartz upon tuberculosis in guinea-pigs (Policard et al., 1967), and the demonstration that this occurs at macrophage level has already been referred to in Chapter 5.

Rheumatoid silicotic nodules

Nodules of larger than average size (that is, 3 to 5 mm diameter), frequently with light-grey necrotic centres, may be found in the lungs of silicotic subjects in whom rheumatoid arthritis or circulating rheumatoid factor without arthritis was present in life. The association was noted by Clerens (1953) and Colinet (1953) in women exposed to a crystalline silica hazard, and the pathology has been described in miners of siliceous rocks and in others (Chatgidakis and Theron, 1961; Kurppa et al., 1963). To the naked eye, the lesions look like tuberculous nodules, and are easily misinterpreted as such, but acid-fast bacilli cannot be identified microscopically, nor can *Mycobacterium tuberculosis* be isolated by culture or guinea-pig inoculation. In geographical areas where histoplasmosis is endemic, this may be diagnosed in error, but *Histoplasma* sp. cannot be identified in the nodules (Gough, 1959). Unlike the nodules of rheumatoid coal pneumoconiosis, concentric black rings of deposited coal particles or other pigmented dust are either absent or feeble (Figure 12.7 and see Chapter 13). They are usually scattered discretely, but are occasionally seen in conglomerations.

Microscopically, the lesions consist of an acidophilic, acellular necrotic centre in which there are the remains of collagen fibres and, at the periphery of the necrosis, fibroblasts are arranged in palisade form, although less prominently than in rheumatoid subcutaneous nodules. External to these is a zone of polymorphonuclear leucocytes and macrophages, and there may be clefts containing cholesterol crystals. These are not seen in non-rheumatoid silicotic nodules. Outside this active zone normal reticulin and collagen fibres are arranged in various stages of maturation, also numerous plasma cells, lymphocytes and fibroblasts, but no giant cells. Endarteritis, consisting mainly of plasma cells and lymphocytes, is found in close proximity to the lesions. When activity in the nodules has ceased, they may, as with 'pure' silicotic nodules, become calcified.

Eleven cases (2 per cent) of 'rheumatoid-modified' silicotic nodules were found in 576 autopsies on European gold miners studied at the Johannesburg Pneumoconiosis Research Unit (Chatgidakis and Theron, 1961). In general,

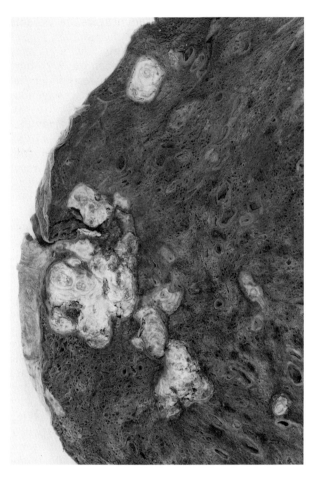

Figure 12.7 Rheumatoid silicotic nodules: note absence of typical silicotic nodules and slightness of dust pigmentation. Microscopy confirmed the presence of necrotic rheumatoid nodules and the absence of tuberculosis. (See Figure 12.17a–d for radiographic features)

however, the prevalence of rheumatoid silicosis may be lower than this.

Clinical features

Symptoms

It is important to emphasize that there may be no symptoms, even though the radiographic appearances may be surprisingly advanced. Early symptoms of airways' inflammation and obstruction are generally associated with smoking. In the absence of smoking, cough may develop as the disease advances, and is of variable severity, mainly in the mornings, but sometimes intermittently throughout the day and night. In the later stages, there may be prolonged and distressing paroxysms due, possibly, to irritation of nerve receptors in the trachea and bronchi by silicotic lymph node masses.

Often there is no sputum, or only a small quantity of mucoid appearance raised from time to time during the day. There is no haemoptysis in the absence of other complicating disease.

Unless there is accompanying chronic obstructive bronchitis or allergic asthma, there is no wheeze, although some patients who have narrowing, distortion and fixity of the trachea and main bronchi, caused by contiguous silicotic nodes, may complain of stridor (see 'Physical signs'), especially during effort, when there is increased velocity of airflow. This is an uncommon symptom.

Breathlessness occurs as the disease advances, first during pronounced effort and later with lesser degrees of effort; it is rarely complained of at rest unless other lung disease is present. The presence and severity of dyspnoea and impairment of lung function correlate poorly with radiographic appearances.

Chest pain is not a feature of silicosis.

General health may become impaired as respiratory failure, with or without congestive heart failure, supervenes, or with the development of tuberculosis. Haemoptysis and loss of weight may signal the presence of tuberculosis.

Physical signs

As indicated previously, the general physical condition is good, but deteriorates with the onset of congestive heart failure and in the presence of tuberculosis. Central cyanosis is absent unless there is complicating heart or lung disease, and dyspnoea at rest suggests disease other than silicosis.

Finger clubbing is not caused by silicosis, and when observed is either of congenital type or evidence of other pathology.

The chest contour is usually normal, but in advanced disease there may be localized flattening of one upper zone, possibly with some degree of dorsal scoliosis. Expansion remains good and equal until a late stage of the disease, when it may be somewhat diminished, often more on one side (where underlying fibrosis is greater) than on the other.

The trachea is sometimes displaced to one side, either by silicotic hilar node masses or a large distorted conglomerate mass in an upper lobe. Occasionally, hard, non-tender, silicotic lymph nodes are palpable in the neck and supraclavicular fossae.

Percussion note is unaffected, unless there are areas of unusually dense pleural fibrosis – mainly in the upper zones.

Breath sounds are normal or reduced by pleural thickening, and inspiratory and expiratory stridor (of greater or lesser intensity) may be heard over the trachea and at the open mouth when there is excessive distortion of the trachea or main bronchi; when this is present, it is persistent. Adventitious sounds are not heard in disease uncomplicated by chronic bronchitis or tuberculosis.

In the advanced stage of silicosis, the signs of pulmonary heart disease may eventually develop, with or without those of congestive heart failure.

Investigations

Lung function

In simple silicosis, impairment of any parameter of lung function is generally absent, but in some cases slight reduction in vital capacity (VC) and of arterial oxygen tension (on effort) may be observed. With more advanced disease, impairment is commonly present, but often of a much lesser degree than the radiographic category might suggest. There is a decrease of total lung capacity (TLC), VC, residual volume (RV), functional residual capacity (FRC) and compliance, with or without evidence of airways' obstruction, and, in some cases, a slight reduction in gas transfer, although this is often remarkably little affected even in the presence of advanced disease. Oxygen desaturation is not present at rest or on moderate effort (300 kg/m per min) in the non-conglomerate stage of disease (Becklake, du Preez and Lutz, 1958), but may be observed on greater effort in some cases. As the disease progresses to massive conglomeration, inequality of gas distribution and of the ventilation–perfusion ratio occurs, resulting in some impairment of gas transfer factor (TL) in addition to the volume changes mentioned. However, in a study of non-smoking men with non-conglomerate (simple) silicosis, TL was not reduced and, even in those with category B and C conglomeration, KCO (carbon monoxide transfer coefficient) was normal in most cases (Tećulescu and Stănescu, 1970). Ventilation–perfusion imbalance, resulting in arterial oxygen desaturation on effort, is determined primarily by the extent and distribution of the silicotic fibrosis.

There is nothing characteristic in the patterns of impaired function in silicosis. Obstruction is likely to be the sole or dominant spirometric abnormality until the disease is radiographically far advanced, usually in association with smoking (Jones, Weill and Ziskind, 1975). Radiographic progression and higher average dust exposures are each associated with more rapid declines in forced expiratory volume in 1 second (FEV_1) and forced vital capacity (FVC) (Ng, Chan and Lam, 1987).

Exercise testing is probably no more useful than tests of resting ventilatory function in assessing

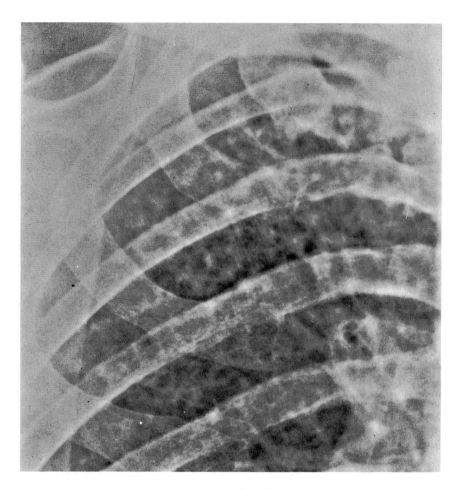

Figure 12.8 Discrete radiographic opacities of typical silicosis at an early stage: category q (natural size)

respiratory impairment in mild simple silicosis (Violante, Brusasco and Buccheri, 1986). The best overall guide to the degree of respiratory disability in conglomerate disease is the ventilatory capacity.

Radiographic appearances

The earliest radiographic evidence of nodular silicosis consists of small discrete opacities of moderate radiodensity, which appear in the upper halves of the lung fields and vary from 1 to 3 mm in diameter (ILO categories p and q) (Figure 12.8). Descriptions and depiction of typical radiographic appearances may be found in the instructions and standard films of the ILO 1980 classification (International Labour Office, 1980). It has been claimed, however, that linear opacities accompanying the normal vascular markings are the earliest evidence of silicosis, but this is not generally accepted (Ashford and Enterline, 1966), and these

appearances (of which it is difficult to be convinced) do not correlate with morbid anatomical evidence of silicosis.

There appears to be a clear relationship between total dust exposure and radiographic evidence of silicosis (Beadle, 1971), and the risk of its progression (Hughes et al., 1982).

As the disease advances, discrete opacities increase in number and may increase in size (ILO category r), and occupy the lower as well as the other zones of the lung fields (Figure 12.9). More often, there is an increase only in profusion and extent, and the background nodules remain the same size as when first detected, even if large opacities develop. In some cases, the development of massive large opacities results in apparent decreasing profusion of the background nodules. In general, the small opacities are roughly symmetrical in the two fields, but are sometimes of disparate size and distribution. Coalescence of rounded small opacities (ILO symbol ax) may be visible; this is probably a

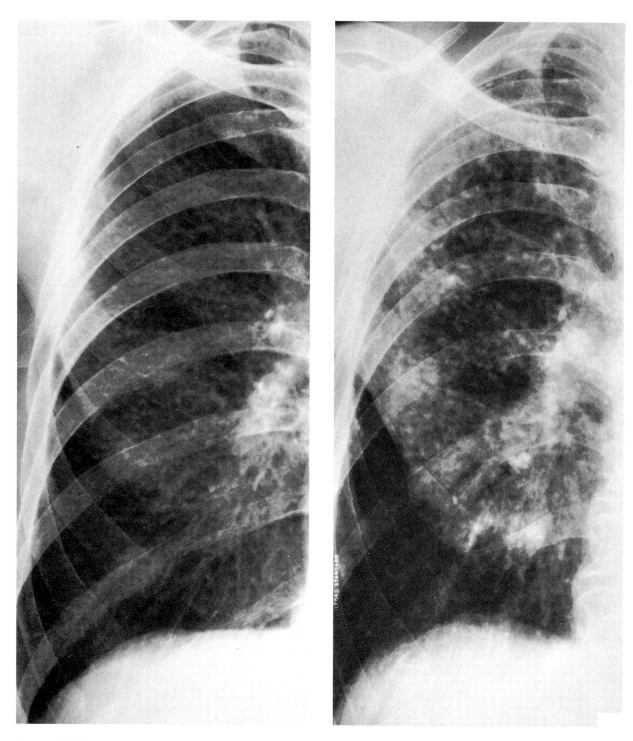

Figure 12.9 (a, b) Progression of discrete 'nodules' of silicosis from low category qq 1/0 to qq 2/2 over 10 years (1958–1968): slate quarry worker

transitional stage between small and large opacities. These conglomerate densities usually occur in the upper zones, and often become ILO category A large opacities, of 10 to 50 mm diameter. Larger (category B) and sometimes massive (category C) opacities may form, and can occupy the greater part of both lung fields (Figures 12.10 and 12.11). Bullae may be seen in the vicinity of conglomerations and at the lung bases, and in some cases there may be significant bowing and distortion of the trachea

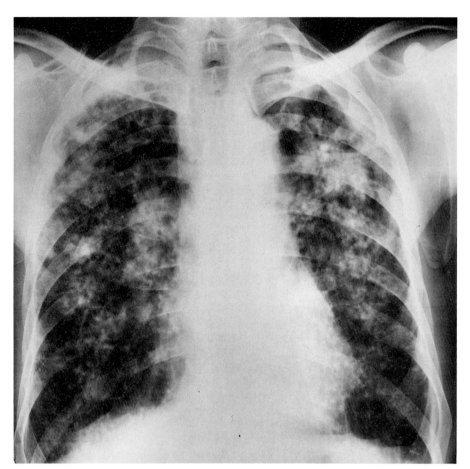

Figure 12.10 Moderately advanced silicosis with bilateral conglomeration. Note bilateral apical thickening of the pleura. Hilar node calcification is not evident. Foundry sandblaster for 16 years and fettler for 5 years

(Figure 12.11). Cavity formation in the absence of complicating tuberculosis is uncommon. Rarely, unilateral conglomeration is present in the absence of other evidence of silicosis; exclusion of cancer in the rare case of solitary pneumoconiotic large opacity usually requires thoracotomy. The curious tendency for the silicotic masses in Lipari pumice workers to occupy the lower lung fields is referred to in Chapter 16 ('Pumice and pumicite').

Occasionally, the discrete opacities are small and very dense, and may closely resemble the appearances of the calcified nodules seen in some cases of rheumatoid coal pneumoconiosis (see Chapter 13, page 389), and in microlithiasis (Figure 12.12). The presence of rheumatoid arthritis is associated with a tendency to present with the coarser (category r) small opacities (Sluis-Cremer et al., 1986).

An important feature of some cases is evidence of lymph node calcification, which is characterized by thin, very dense ring shadows around the nodes – so-called 'eggshell' calcification (Figures 12.13 and 12.14). The nodes most commonly involved are those of the hilar and mediastinal groups, but other intrathoracic nodes (for example, the internal mammary chain) and extrathoracic nodes (notably the supraclavicular, cervical and axillary groups, and occasionally the intra-abdominal and inguinal groups) may also be affected (Polacheck and Pijanowski, 1960). Curiously, there appears to be no correlation between the intensity of the calcification and the amount of silicosis or the presence of pulmonary tuberculosis (Chiesura, Terribile and Bardellini, 1968). Calcification may be prominent when there is little or no obvious

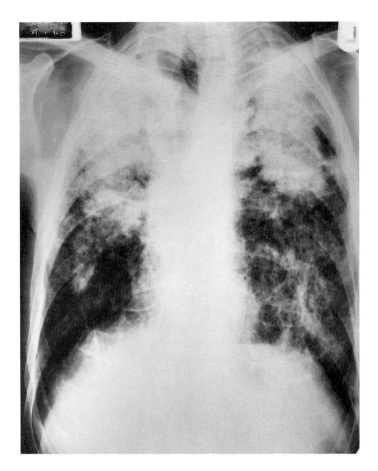

Figure 12.11 Massive silicotic conglomeration with bilateral upper zone pleural thickening and displacement of trachea to the right: crusherman in granite quarry for 26 years

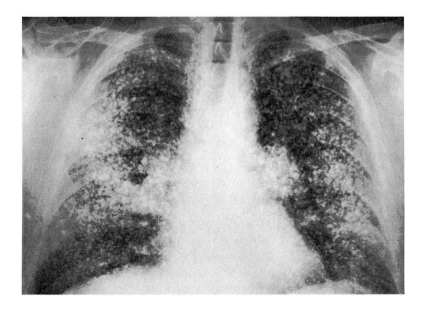

Figure 12.12 Multiple dense small opacities: many of the nodules were calcified. Refractory brick worker for 5 years and granite quarry worker for 3 years

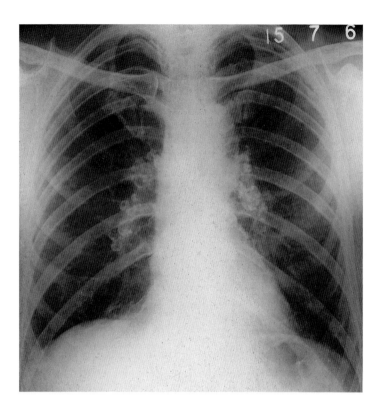

Figure 12.13 Bilateral hilar node: 'egg-shell'-type calcification in a slate worker for 43 years. Note absence of evidence of intrapulmonary disease and pleural thickening

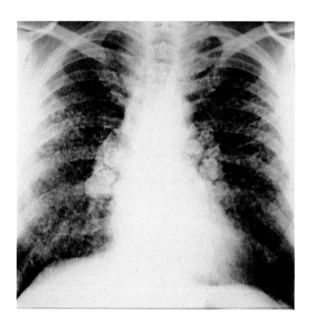

Figure 12.14 Gross egg-shell calcification of hilar nodes with category qq 3/3 discrete silicotic pulmonary lesions: slate rockman for 32 years, North Wales

lung involvement (see Figure 12.13) or absent in the presence of advanced silicosis (see Figure 12.10). Although not a pathognomonic sign – because it is seen rarely in sarcoidosis, tuberculosis, histoplasmosis and following irradiation of mediastinal lymphoma – predominantly peripheral calcification of hilar nodes is highly suggestive of silicosis or of exposure to some form of crystalline silica.

Evidence of diffuse bilateral pleural fibrosis is present in many cases, and in advanced disease may be extensive and partly calcified; occasionally, calcified thickening (see Figure 12.10) occurs with little obvious lung disease.

The radiographic appearances of the rare cases of silicosis which develop exceptionally fast (see 'Microscopic appearances') bear little resemblance to those of typical silicosis. Opacities are numerous, widespread, small and ill-defined, and spontaneous pneumothoraces are apt to occur (Figure 12.15).

It should not be assumed that silicosis progresses at a steady rate in every patient, and there is not necessarily parallel worsening of the radiographic appearance and lung function. Worsening of the radiograph may proceed by fits and starts, and some cases advance steadily to a point, then remain stable for long (perhaps, indefinite) periods. The term

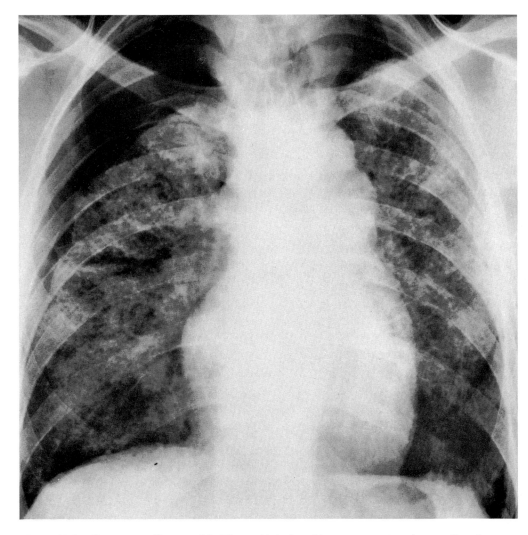

Figure 12.15 Film of case illustrated in Figure 12.6. Opacities are numerous but small and indefinite unlike those caused by nodular silicosis. Bilateral pneumothoraces are present. The patient was in good health 2 years before death. Although there was no arthropathy, latex fixation test was positive, circulating antinuclear antibodies present and serum IgG much increased. Thus, immunological activity may have featured in the development of this disease. (Radiograph by courtesy of Dr K.P. Goldman)

'progressive massive fibrosis', with its connotation of predictable or proven behaviour, should not be automatically applied to all cases with large opacities. Although the different patterns of behaviour of silicosis appear to be determined mainly by the amount of siliceous dust inhaled, idiosyncratic reaction, as stated already under 'Pathogenesis', may also be involved.

In general, sudden changes are most likely to be due to complicating tuberculosis, but occasionally they are associated with rheumatoid disease. Higher odds of progression have been found in silicotic subjects with rheumatoid arthritis (Sluis-Cremer et al., 1986). The typical appearances of Caplan-type

necrobiotic nodules (see Chapter 13) are very uncommon, but have been reported (Chiesura, Bruguone and Mezzanotte, 1961; Kurppa et al., 1963; Gambini, Agnoletto and Magistretti, 1964) (Figure 12.16). Occasionally, large ill-defined opacities develop rapidly, exhibit vacillant behaviour over subsequent years, and are sometimes associated with recurrent, transient pleural effusions in individuals with active rheumatoid arthritis or with high titres of circulating RF without overt arthropathy (Figure 12.17).

In the accelerated form of nodular silicosis, progression is often detectable on radiographs made 2 or 3 years apart. This is in striking contrast to

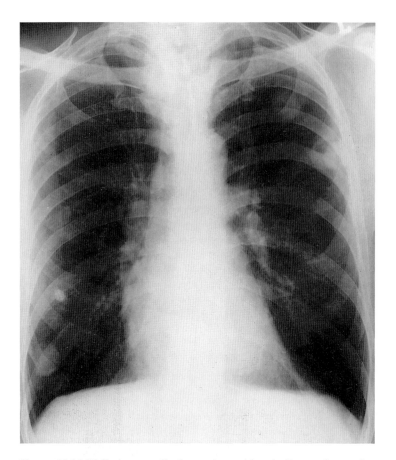

Figure 12.16 Well-circumscribed round opacities similar to those of Caplan's syndrome in coal workers. Patient worked as a dipper in vitreous enamelling for 7 years and as a crusher of reject pottery (containing free silica and china clay) for the manufacture of refractory enamel for 10 years. Note the cavity in lesion in left midzone and the absence of discrete small nodules of silicosis. Rheumatoid arthritis developed 15 years before this film was taken. Circulating rheumatoid factors present. No evidence of tuberculoisis. Lung biopsy confirmed rheumatoid nodules

asbestosis, in which progression is usually difficult to detect on films separated by 5 or more years (Jones et al., 1989). The vagaries of silicosis progression, and the earlier age at which the disease can occur, warrant greater caution in giving a prognosis.

It is rarely necessary to use radiological techniques other than posteroanterior (PA) and lateral views for diagnosis, although tomography may be helpful in demonstrating silicotuberculous cavities. Bronchography may reveal bronchial distortion, filling defects and localized bronchiectasis in cases with conglomerate masses.

Computed tomography (CT) of the chest was compared with plain radiographs in foundry workers. The two modalities were equal in the evaluation of complicated silicosis. CT did not detect more cases of early simple disease, but did detect more cases of early coalescence (Bégin et al., 1987). However, high-resolution CT scan improves identification and gives better definition of silicotic nodules than conventional CT (Bégin et al., 1991). The prognostic significance of early coalescence detected only by CT is a complete unknown. CT is clearly superior to plain radiographs for detecting and grading emphysema. In a study of 17 silicotic subjects, it was grade of emphysema, rather than grade of nodulation, that correlated well with reduced ventilatory and gas transfer function (Bergin et al., 1986) (see Chapter 7).

Bronchial arteriography demonstrates the presence of bronchial artery enlargement and bronchopulmonary shunts in areas of conglomerate masses, but not in discrete nodular disease (Tada et al., 1974).

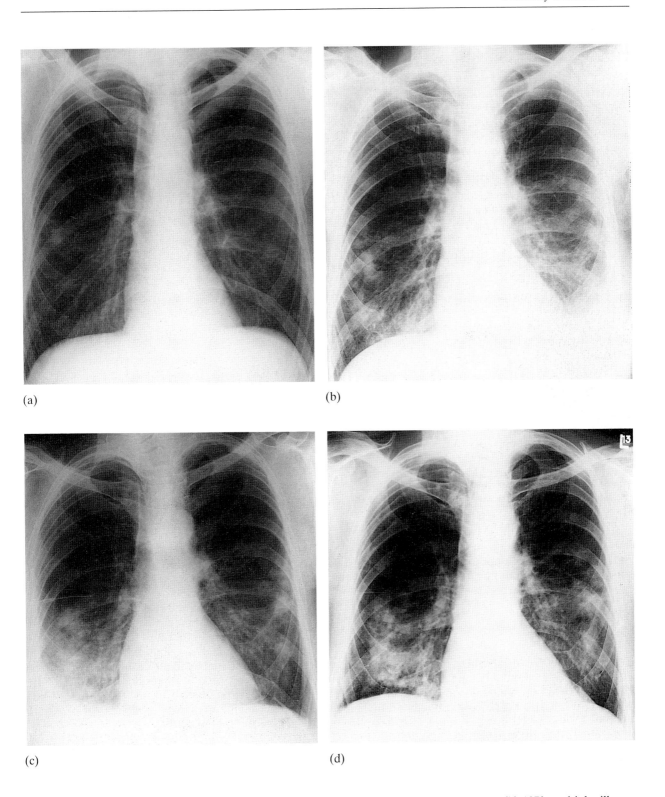

(a)

(b)

(c)

(d)

Figure 12.17 (a) 1967: single small opacity and slight pleural thickening of right lower zone. (b) 1970: multiple, ill-defined, dense opacities of both middle and lower zones with pleural effusion on left. (c) 1972: some increase in size of lower zone opacities; right pleural effusion has now developed. (d) 1976: further slight increase in lung opacities, but complete resolution of effusions. Note that the development, appearance and distribution of the lung opacities are unlike those of typical silicosis. Patient worked as a pottery caster and fettler for 36 years. Rheumatoid arthritis developed about 1962 and was progressive. Circulating rheumatoid factors persistently present in high titre. ANAs negative; no evidence of tuberculosis. *Post mortem*: bilateral diffuse thickening of the pulmonary pleura and well-circumscribed, grey-coloured nodules with a faint concentric pattern in both lower lobes (see Figure 12.7)

Other investigations

Biopsy of lung tissue is seldom required for diagnosis (see below). Sputum culture for mycobacteria is indicated in patients who are tuberculin positive at diagnosis, or who subsequently convert to tuberculin positivity, in cases showing cavitation or progressive contraction, and in patients with unexplained fever.

Tests for circulating rheumatoid and antinuclear antibodies, when positive, suggest the possibility of an underlying immunological cause for suddenly advancing tuberculosis-negative silicosis.

Electrocardiography may be required in advanced cases to establish or refute the presence of pulmonary heart disease.

Investigations for sarcoidosis may be indicated on rare occasions to distinguish the two diseases (see 'Diagnosis').

The erythrocyte sedimentation rate is not raised in the absence of complicating tuberculosis or other disease.

Elevation of serum angiotensin-converting enzyme (ACE) levels has been described in silicotic patients. One study showed association of higher levels with more severe radiographic abnormality (Nordman, Koskinen and Froseth, 1984), whilst another found the opposite (Bucca et al., 1984). A third study found levels elevated and intermediate between control and sarcoidosis values (Inoue et al., 1987). Elevations were produced in experimental silicosis in rats, but serum levels were poorly correlated with histology (Brown et al., 1983). At present, the test is not of accepted value in diagnosis.

Scintigraphic scanning after administration of gallium-67 (^{67}Ga) does not give consistent results in silicosis, nor does it help to differentiate it from other chest diseases (see Chapter 7, page 201).

Diagnosis

Diagnosis may be established by histopathology, although examination of lung tissue is seldom required. As in other pneumoconioses, open biopsy is strongly preferred. The tiny fragments obtained by bronchoscopic biopsy are subject to sampling error and crush artefact, and are usually too small for tissue mineralogy or other specialized examinations. It is reasonable to do bronchoscopic biopsy in those cases in which sarcoidosis or diffuse metastatic cancer is a plausible alternative, but the procedure is then being performed to exclude or establish by tissue diagnosis the alternative disease, not silicosis.

The tissue diagnosis of silicosis should be based upon a finding of silicotic nodules, or silico-lipoproteinosis, supported when necessary by identification and measurement of silica in the tissue. It should be remembered that the finding of silicotic nodules does not mean that silicosis is the only lung disease present; that conclusion should be made in the light of all the relevant clinical and exposure data. The diagnoses 'anthracosis' and 'anthracosilicosis', often reported of tissue obtained by bronchoscopic lung biopsy, mean only 'soot in the lung' – a common finding in adult residents of urban areas – in other words, not even a disease, and certainly neither coal pneumoconiosis nor silicosis.

Diagnosis is usually made by clinical–radiological methods. In general, the criteria are similar to those for other pneumoconioses:

1. An exposure history that connotes a substantial risk of the condition.
2. Radiographic findings consistent with the condition.
3. The absence of any good reason to believe that the radiographic findings are the result of some other condition.

Radiographic findings 'consistent with' ordinary silicosis may range from nodulation that is entirely non-specific in appearance, up to symmetrical large opacities with uniform background nodulation, which look like nothing other than pneumoconiosis. For acute silicosis, the consolidations are entirely non-specific in appearance. For both ordinary and acute silicosis, the abnormality should be bilateral.

When a satisfactory occupational history is combined with good quality radiographs, nodular silicosis should rarely be mistaken for other diseases. The chief cause of misdiagnosis is failure to recognize the 'silica' hazard of a past occupation, and the fact that the prevalence of silicosis is now low increases the possibility of this error.

Silicosis can often be suspected from radiographs that also show tuberculosis, when there is an unusual degree of symmetry of the apical disease, or when a focus of tuberculosis is found against a background of small nodules that are relatively uniform in size and distribution. The latter could represent coexisting miliary tuberculosis, but in clinic patients it usually represents silicosis.

When silicotic lung lesions and hilar and pulmonary lymph nodes are calcified, it is necessary to exclude the following:

1. Tuberculosis.
2. Histoplasmosis: calcified lung nodules (from the so-called 'miliary' form, following a heavy inhalation exposure to the organism) usually show substantial inhomogeneity of both size and distribution. The rare case may mimic simple silicosis, but will lack upper zone predominance. Calcified lymph nodes almost always show a stippled or homogeneous pattern, and larger lung nodules may show a target pattern of concentric calcifications that is not seen in silicosis.

3. Sarcoidosis: confusion occasionally arises here, particularly when silica exposures have occurred in a high-risk group for sarcoidosis. In particular, it should be remembered that pulmonary and hilar node sarcoid lesions may calcify and present a similar radiographic appearance in patients with hilar lymphadenopathy that has been slow to subside (Israel et al., 1961; Scadding and Mitchell, 1985). Non-calcified silicotic lesions, especially in women (from past work in the pottery industry, for example) may be mistaken for sarcoidosis.

4. Pulmonary alveolar microlithiasis: this rare disorder may occasionally be simulated radiographically by silicosis when the lesions are very small and calcified (see Figure 12.12).

5. Calcified lung lesions as a sequel of chickenpox are usually few in number, small (about 2 to 3 mm in diameter), and are not accompanied by the eggshell sign of hilar node calcification.

Silicosis is unlikely to be confused with lung cancer, but it may obscure the early signs of tumour development.

Complications

Tuberculosis and other infections

Silicosis is the only pneumoconiosis that predisposes to the development of tuberculosis. Although the incidence of tuberculosis in silicosis has fallen dramatically since the 1950s, it is still the most common complication. Mortality studies continue to show increased tuberculosis death rates in silicotic patients (Westerholm et al., 1986). Tuberculosis may occur at any stage in the evolution of silicosis, but is most likely in the fifth and later decades in association with a moderate-to-severe degree of silicosis (Chatgidakis, 1963; Jones, Owen and Corrado, 1967).

In the early stage of the tuberculous disease, it is difficult or impossible to recognize any change in the established radiographic appearance of silicosis, and there may be no symptoms; a recently developed cough with scanty greenish sputum may, however, give a warning signal. Subsequently, the characteristic symptoms develop, sometimes with haemoptysis. Rapid radiographic changes consistent with tuberculosis are then seen, possibly with evidence of cavitation. When the disease is of an indolent nature, or after healing, scar emphysema with bullae may be detected radiographically in the areas of fibrosis.

Atypical mycobacteria are sometimes isolated from the sputum of silicotic subjects. These organisms may occasionally be found in association with *Mycobacterium tuberculosis* (Palmhert, Webster and Lens, 1968). Some are not pathogenic, but *M. avium* complex (*Mycobacterium avium-intercellulare* complex) is a serious, if rare, complication, and is poorly sensitive to antituberculous therapy; *M. kansasii* is also pathogenic, but usually responds well to drug treatment, despite nominal isoniazid resistance. Infection by different 'opportunist' mycobacteria has been reported in 37 per cent of foundry workers with silicosis (Rosenzweig, 1967), and by *M. kansasii* in 11 per cent of silicotic sandblasters (Bailey et al., 1974). The pathogenicity of these organisms is probably potentiated by quartz and other forms of crystalline silica, and the importance of distinguishing these organisms from *M. tuberculosis* is evident. Their prevalence is likely to vary according to geographical locality.

A residual tuberculous or ischaemic cavity in a conglomerate silicotic mass may be colonized by *Aspergillus* species. The organism is usually *A. fumigatus*, occasionally *A. niger*, *A. flavus* or *A. nidulans*. As a rule, circulating precipitating antibodies to the relevant organisms are present, but, in a few cases, are absent. The characteristic radiographic appearance of aspergilloma as a cavity containing a central density (due to a fungal ball), partly or wholly surrounded by a 'halo' of air, may be seen, and should alert the physician to the diagnosis. However, a proportion of such aspergillomas are first identified *post mortem*. Slight, recurrent haemoptysis is fairly common, but, occasionally, may be massive and fatal. Therefore, haemoptysis in a silicotic patient may signal the presence of active tuberculosis, bronchial carcinoma or aspergilloma.

Pulmonary heart disease

This may develop in some cases of advanced conglomerate silicosis, but right ventricular failure due to this cause (contrary to popular belief and many textbook descriptions) supervenes in only a small proportion, in whom, however, death is likely to occur in congestive heart failure. At least in past years, the likelihood of pulmonary heart disease causing death has been significantly increased when there is complicating tuberculosis, by contrast with silicosis alone (Becker and Chatgidakis, 1960). The rarity of symptomatic pulmonary heart disease may reflect the tendency of patients with advanced silicosis to die of acute worsenings of respiratory failure, caused by ordinary bacterial or viral respiratory infections.

Bronchitis

Episodes of acute and subacute bronchitis due to infection in deformed and rigid bronchi may occur in advanced stages of silicosis, but there is correlation between chronic obstructive bronchitis, which is very largely associated with cigarette smoking, and silicosis and siliceous dusts. Inhalation of siliceous dust has been viewed as a cause of chronic obstructive bronchitis (Becklake, 1985).

Emphysema

Small areas of scar ('irregular') emphysema are occasionally observed around nodules, and larger bullous areas of the same type of emphysema may be related to conglomerate lesions. Centrilobular and panlobular emphysema may be present, but are pathogenically unrelated to the silicosis (see Chapter 9). Small subpleural emphysematous spaces are commonly seen on the radiograph around the lateral and superior edges of large silicotic masses.

Spontaneous pneumothorax

Spontaneous pneumothorax is an uncommon complication caused by the rupture of a bleb or bulla, and the resulting pneumothorax is often localized due to the limitations imposed by pleural symphysis. Even when localized, however, a pneumothorax may be under tension, and so produce effects on cardiorespiratory function vastly out of proportion to its size. In advanced silicosis, pneumothorax is often difficult to treat: the stiff lung is hard to re-expand, the air leak may be persistent and the poor baseline ventilatory function makes thoracotomy hazardous.

Segmental and middle lobe collapse

Exceptionally, compression or occlusion of small bronchi by enlarged silicotic lymph nodes causes an area of lung collapse.

Rheumatoid syndrome

The progression of silicosis and the appearance of the lesions in the presence of rheumatoid arthritis, or rheumatoid factor without rheumatoid arthritis, has already been alluded to. They are important in that they may be mistaken for active tuberculous disease and, if pleural effusion occurs, carcinoma may be suspected.

Claims of a silica-induced increased risk of rheumatoid arthritis and systemic lupus erythematosus continue to rest mainly upon case reports. An exception is the demonstration of an association between silica exposure and increased incidence and prevalence of rheumatoid arthritis in a cohort of 1026 Finnish granite workers (Klockars et al., 1987). A recent case-control study of gold miners (matched on age) with and without rheumatoid arthritis showed significantly more silicosis in the arthritic subjects; but the arthritic silicotic subjects had developed silicosis after significantly less intense dust exposures (Sluis-Cremer et al., 1986). The latter (with other findings) was interpreted as evidence that rheumatoid arthritis increases the risk of silicosis, and the authors expressed doubt about the existence of a contrary relationship (that is, silicosis increasing the risk of rheumatoid arthritis). This is not conclusive, and the suspicion of such a relationship lingers among both rheumatologists and chest physicians. It is doubtful whether mortality studies would reflect an association, given the low lethality of the rheumatic disorders and the incomplete listing of coincidental diagnoses on death certificates. The most that can be said is that such a causal relationship is possible; if present, it is not very robust.

Systemic sclerosis – SS (scleroderma)

Silicosis appears to be associated with an unusually high prevalence of scleroderma. Byrom Bramwell, in 1914, first drew attention to this association in stonemasons, but, since the late 1950s, there have been many reports of its occurrence in such workers as gold miners, fluorspar miners, sandblasters, and those involved in pottery and foundry processes (Bellini and Ghislandi, 1959; Francia, Monarca and Cavallot, 1959; Erasmus, 1960; Carini and Lo Martire, 1965; Migueres et al., 1966; Rodnan et al., 1967; Gunther and Schuchhardt, 1970; Ziskind et al., 1976). In former East Germany it had been estimated that males exposed to silica were 25 times more likely to develop a systemic sclerosis-type disorder than unexposed males (Zeigler et al., 1982), and SS was regarded as an occupational disease in persons with heavy exposure (Mehlhorn, 1984). But Rowell (1984) is not convinced that the disease described is truly SS, and has pointed out that the reported incidence is much higher than the suspected gene frequency of classic SS.

Interpretation of case reports is often difficult because of authors' failure to distinguish among *acrosclerosis* (distal scleroderma without visceral involvement), *localized scleroderma* (with no visceral involvement or Raynaud's phenomenon) and SS (in which there is always visceral involvement and usually Raynaud's phenomenon). It has been suggested that the skin lesions are, in fact, pseudoscleroderma (localized scleroderma), because in many of the reported cases, Raynaud's phenomenon, microstomia and systemic involvement have been absent, and the skin disease is often localized (Jabłońska, 1975). A 0.6 per cent incidence of scleroderma in silicotic individuals has been reported by Francia, Monarca and Cavallot (1959), who suggest that it adversely affects the course of the silicosis. A high incidence of SS in black South African gold miners has been inferred from diagnosis rates in the clinic: ten men had proximal scleroderma and bilateral basal radiographic abnormality, with only six of them showing radiographic findings consistent with silicosis (Cowie, 1987). Seventy-nine white South African gold miners with SS had no greater prevalence of silicosis than did an age-matched group of miners without SS, but on average they had more intense silica exposures (Sluis-Cremer et al., 1985).

If, in fact, these are not chance associations, it may be that impairment of T-lymphocyte function and consequent autoantibody production, or a common anticollagen antibody against lung and skin, are involved. Certainly, there is an increased prevalence of circulating ANA in silicosis (see 'Pathogenesis') and in scleroderma, in which it may be as high as 90 per cent (Jayson, 1977).

Cancer of the lung

Since the last edition of this book, there has been considerable interest in the issue of whether crystalline silica exposure, or silicosis, increases the risk of lung cancer. This has led to a review by the International Agency for Research on Cancer (IARC, 1987a) which concluded that there was *sufficient* evidence of carcinogenicity of crystalline silica in experimental animals, and *limited* evidence in humans. These findings resulted in a 2A classification for crystalline silica (IARC, 1987b).

The positive evidence for lung cancer in animals comes from inhalation and intratracheal instillation experiments in rats, with negative studies in other species; fibrosis was an associated finding (Holland, 1983, 1986). Intrapleural and intraperitoneal injections of quartz have produced malignant lymphomas in this species (IARC, 1987a).

Epidemiological studies of cancer risk associated with silica exposure in human subjects can be classified by whether the study population is defined by: (1) exposure (studies of workers) or (2) disease (studies of silicotic subjects).

Studies have been reported of workers with silica exposure in three general industrial categories: mining; ceramics, glass and related industries; and the granite and stone industry.

Mining studies have included workers employed in coal, gold and other ore mining. Due to the low levels of silica exposure in coal mining, studies of coal miners cannot, in general, adequately address the question of potential cancer risk. Only one such study assessed risk in relation to estimated silica exposure, finding no relationship.

Studies of gold miners have been generally negative. Of three studies of the Homestake mine in South Dakota, only the first (and smallest) study (Gillam et al., 1976) found an elevated cancer risk. Two much larger studies carried out at a later date (McDonald et al., 1978; Brown et al., 1986), in spite of finding substantial silicosis and tuberculosis risk, and both having a dose–response relationship to estimated total dust exposure, found neither elevated cancer risk nor a relationship to exposure. Three other studies include one from Australia (Armstrong et al., 1979) that found an increased risk of lung cancer which the authors interpreted as more probably related to elevated smoking prevalence than to exposure, and two others from South Africa (Hessel and Sluis-Cremer, 1986; Hnizdo and Sluis-Cremer, 1991), difficult to interpret, both of which included smoking information. In a case-control necropsy study of lung cancer in miners, Hessel, Sluis-Cremer and Hnizdo (1990) found no case-control differences for silica exposure indicators, and no association between lung cancer and the presence or severity of silicosis of any site. The only positive results for gold miners are from a Canadian government study of Ontario miners (Muller et al., 1983) which reported excess respiratory and stomach cancer, but which did not have information on smoking, exposure levels, or radon exposure.

A composite investigation of men with silicosis from metalliferous mines (lead and zinc), granite quarries and coal mines in Sardinia, which took smoking and chronic airways' obstruction into account, did not reveal any clear association between exposure to silica or severity of silicosis and mortality from carcinoma of lung (Carta, Cocco and Casula, 1991).

Of three studies in the ceramics and glass-related industries, a case-control study of lung cancers in Italy (Forastiere et al., 1986) should be ignored because of its strong bias towards a relationship with silica exposure (controls who died of silicosis (10.5 per cent), who probably had extensive silica exposure, were deleted and replaced by other controls). A cohort study was negative (Puntoni et al., 1985), and a proportional mortality study (Thomas, 1982) found inconsistent results: excess lung cancer observed among workers who made plumbing fixtures was not observed in another part of the industry with similar processes and silica exposures (talc was also used in such work).

The most informative data from the granite and stone industries come from a cohort study of 5414 Vermont granite workers (Costello and Graham, 1986), which found a significantly elevated lung cancer risk for shed workers hired before 1930 (a standard mortality ratio, SMR, of 146, based on 51 cases), and a marginally significant ($P = 0.06$) risk for those hired 1930 to 1949 (an SMR of 128 based on 41 cases). Overall, there was a relationship to latency and employment duration, both of which would be correlated with exposure levels, because earlier levels are believed to have been higher than later (dust control measures were instituted around 1940). Employment duration is a reliable surrogate measure for cumulative exposure only when concentration levels have been constant over time, which is known not to be the case for these workers. There was no smoking or quantitative exposure information, and the authors interpreted their findings as positive only for the pre-1930 employees, when exposures were presumably very high.

Two proportional mortality studies did not convincingly demonstrate lung cancer risk to be elevated. In one, a study of 969 deaths among Vermont granite workers (1952 to 1978), lung cancer was slightly elevated (a proportional mortality ratio, PMR, of 1.3), but the rate was lower for those hired before 1940 than for later workers, and there was no trend for any cancer with estimated cumulative dust exposure (Davis et al., 1983). A study of 1905 deaths among members of a granite cutters' union found substantial silicosis and tuberculosis risk, but only slightly elevated lung cancer risk (PMR of 1.2, based on 97 cases), with no trend for employment duration or latency, and no smoking information (Steenland and Beaumont, 1986).

A study of tunnel workers (Selikoff, 1978) reported an elevated lung cancer risk among those employed over 20 years (observed/expected = 12/4.7). There was excess tuberculosis, and 20 cases of pneumoconiosis/silicosis, indicating extensive silica exposure. However, there was no information about smoking, quantitative silica exposure or other exposure.

Finally, there have been a number of studies of silicotic subjects (10 to 15), almost all of them finding an increased risk of lung cancer, generally more than twofold. The IARC working group did not find the results from these studies to be convincing, noting a number of methodological difficulties: potential positive bias from non-comparability of referent subjects, possible differences in disease detection, smoking prevalences and other occupational exposures; and potential negative bias from competing risks among the silicotic subjects (for example, tuberculosis and other infectious diseases; respiratory failure).

In summary, those epidemiological studies that have found excess lung cancer risk in silica-exposed workers are consistent with evidence from animal experiments, which have demonstrated silica to be an animal carcinogen. These supporting human data are primarily from a cohort study of Vermont granite workers and, to a lesser extent, from a study of Canadian miners and one of tunnel workers. In the Vermont study, a statistically significant excess

cancer risk was observed only among those hired prior to 1930, when exposures were substantially higher than in recent decades. Only a few studies included quantitative estimates of exposure concentrations, and these were negative. Consequently, no quantitative dose–response relationship is available for estimating potential cancer risk at current exposure levels. Additionally, an elevated cancer risk among employees exposed to levels comparable to current workplace standards has not been demonstrated. Excess lung cancer risk among silicotic subjects could be directly related to the high silica exposures of this group or to the lung fibrosis. Observations supporting a link between dust-induced lung fibrosis and cancer have recently been reported for asbestos exposure (excess lung cancer risk restricted to workers with radiographic evidence of asbestosis – see Chapter 14). Heppleston (1985) concluded that lung cancer showed no relationship to either the pulmonary accumulation of dust, of high or low silica content, or the presence of silicosis or mixed dust pneumoconiosis. J.C. McDonald, who was Chairman of the IARC Working Group, later wrote that '...it is premature to conclude that exposure to crystalline silica has caused lung cancer in man' (McDonald, 1989). It may be reasonably concluded that the evidence to date that occupational exposure to silica results in excess lung cancer risk is not yet persuasive. This question is also considered briefly in Chapter 19 (page 657).

Neurological

Irreversible abductor paralysis of the left vocal fold is a rare sequel of involvement of the left recurrent laryngeal nerve in a mass of silicotic lymph nodes (Arnstein, 1941). Obviously, all other possible causes of paralysis must be excluded before this diagnosis is accepted.

Oesophageal compression

Oesophageal compression with dysphagia is another rare effect of large masses of silicotic lymph nodes (Longley, 1970).

Nephropathy

Renal lesions, which are claimed to be distinctive, have been attributed to heavy occupational exposure to free silica. They consist of thickening of glomerular capillary loops and basement membranes, increase in the numbers of mesangial and endothelial cells, periglomerular fibrosis and degenerative changes in the proximal convoluted tubules, with deposition of electron-dense particles in cytosomes. Proteinuria and systemic hypertension have been ascribed to these changes (Saldanha, Rosen and Gonick, 1975). The loop of Henle and distal convoluted tubules are apparently normal, as is their function, and mineral particles and silicotic nodules are absent. It has been suggested that autoantibodies may be involved (Kolev, Doitschinov and Todorov, 1970). In a case of acute glomerulonephritis associated with silico-lipoproteinosis, immunofluorescence demonstrated deposits of IgM and C3 component of complement in the mesangium and along the glomerular basement membrane, but no antigen could be identified (Giles et al., 1978). The silicon content of the renal tissue in these cases was much increased. Renal lesions mimicking Fabry's disease (glycosphingolipid lipoidosis), on both light and electron microscopy, were found in a surface coal driller without other evidence of Fabry's disease and with biopsy-proven pulmonary silico-lipoproteinosis (Banks et al., 1983b). That particular patient also had Raynaud's phenomenon, serum ANAs at 1:640 in homogeneous and peripheral distribution, and strong mesangial immunofluorescence for IgM and C3, but no renal silica shown by scanning electron microscopy and back-scatter electron imaging.

An endemic nephropathy with similar lesions in a Yugoslavian population has been attributed to the drinking water, which has a high free silica content derived from rock erosion. Identical lesions consisting of periglomerular, peritubular and perivascular fibrosis have been produced in guinea-pigs by adding 1- to 3-μm quartz particles to their drinking water for several months (Markovic and Arambasic, 1971). The underlying cause of this endemic 'Balkan nephropathy' (which appears to be concentrated in an area around the Danube in Yugoslavia, Bulgaria and Rumania) remains obscure (Leading Article, 1977), although viral infection is considered to be likely in both natural and experimental disease (Apostolov, Spasic and Bojanic, 1975; K. Apostolov, 1977, personal communication).

In 1924, Gye and Purdey observed that glomerular damage and necrosis (primarily of the vascular endothelium) occurred in mice and rabbits after intravenous administration of silicic acid sol. However, a recent review characterized the body of experimental data as inadequately supportive of a causal relationship between silica exposure and human kidney disease (NIOSH: Silicosis and Silicate Diseases Committee, 1988). No pathognomonic lesion of silica-induced nephropathy has been described in human beings.

Interest in an association between silica and renal disease in populations can be traced back to 1933 at least, when excess mortality from chronic nephritis was found in occupations having a silicosis hazard (Collis and Yule, 1933). To date, however, there has been no confirmation of an increased risk of renal disease in large and well-defined groups of silicosis patients or silica-exposed workers. The situation is similar to that described above for various connective tissue diseases: silica may be a cause of kidney disease, but, if so, the effect is not likely to be strong.

Prognosis

In general, it is unusual for normal lifespan to be shortened, or for invalidism to be produced, by uncomplicated silicosis, although respiratory symptoms may be present. However, in a small proportion of cases, the disease becomes complicated and progresses to severe respiratory disability, and death often occurs many years after the person has left the responsible industry. In such cases, the prevalence of which is difficult to determine, the radiographic category may have been as low as 2q at the time of leaving. The likelihood of invalidism and death from pulmonary heart disease is increased by tuberculosis if this is not treated promptly and successfully, which, in the majority of cases, can be achieved (see 'Treatment', below).

The finding of rheumatoid arthritis or rheumatoid factor alone may signal impending progression of the disease. When chronic obstructive bronchitis or emphysema, or both, are present with large conglomerate silicotic masses or silicotuberculosis, serious invalidism and death from respiratory failure are likely.

When silicosis occurs at an early age, the prognosis is poor. There will have been intense exposures, with a correspondingly high risk of progression, and this risk applies over the decades of potential remaining life. Favourable prognostic factors include acquisition through work in a trade associated with lower average exposures, advanced age at diagnosis, early stage at diagnosis and an observed slow rate of progression.

Treatment

Prophylactic

Because it was shown that metallic aluminium dust is capable of preventing silicosis in experimental animals (Denny, Robson and Irwin, 1939), inhalation of aluminium aerosols by men with silicosis, and those exposed to quartz dusts, was advocated and widely employed from the early 1940s to the mid-1950s. Although it was claimed that the development of silicosis and the progression of existing silicosis were prevented, this has not been substantiated, and there appears to have been no difference in the behaviour of the disease in treated and untreated groups (Kennedy, 1956). Aluminium lactate, inhaled 1 month after silica instillation, reduced the histopathology, lavage markers of alveolitis and silica retention in sheep (Dubois et al., 1988).

Therapeutic

There is at present no specific treatment available to halt the progress or to bring about resolution of human silicosis. As described in Chapter 5, polyvinyl pyridine-*N*-oxide (PVPNO) and related substances, and polybetaine, effectively prevent silicosis in experimental animals, but they are not suitable for that use in human subjects; for example, PVPNO is carcinogenic in animals and extremely slowly eliminated. However, it appears to be ineffective in preventing fibrosis due to coal–quartz mixtures (Weller, 1977). Another compound, *N*-oxide-poly-1,2-ethylene piperidine (with the amusing abbreviation 'NO-PEP') is said to alter silica-induced oxidative reactions in an animal model (Ivanova, Puchkova and Nekrasov, 1984). Infusion of PVPNO has been used therapeutically in human disease, and was reported as effective under certain conditions and lacking in 'toxic side effects' (Prugger, Mallner and Schlipkoter, 1984). A related compound, poly-2-vinylpyridine-1-oxide, is apparently neither toxic nor carcinogenic. In theory, agents capable of inhibiting or reversing cross-linking of collagen might be effective in preventing progression of silicosis. The one with most promise is β-aminopropionitrile (BAPN), which has been shown to inhibit its progression in experimental animals (Levene, Bye and Saffiotti, 1968), and has been used successfully in controlling scar tissue in human surgery, but, of course, it does not influence already established fibrosis. It is uncertain, therefore, that such an agent would be of value in clinical practice. All potentially anti-fibrotic agents must at present be regarded as experimental, and proof of their efficacy and safety will require long and carefully controlled trials.

Corticosteroids do not influence or halt the progress of the disease, and are obviously dangerous in the presence of unrecognized tuberculous disease. They may cause resolution of a complicating 'rheumatoid' pleural effusion, but, again, a tuberculous cause must be excluded.

Given the lack of specific treatment of the fibrotic process, the physician should take measures to prevent or promptly treat complications and coexisting disorders. The most important single aspect of care is the patient's continuous access to a knowledgeable physician. At a minimum, there should be an annual visit for interview, examination, radiograph and tuberculin test. If the tuberculin test is found to be positive, isoniazid should be given, and

an argument can be made for use of a second antituberculous drug for prophylaxis (in complicated cases, the authors always use multiple drugs, even in the face of negative sputum cultures). Cultures for mycobacteria (and fungi) should be obtained in patients who develop cavitary lesions, rapid progression or unexplained fever, even if the tuberculin test is negative. The patient with impaired lung function should be given the once-only immunization against the pneumococcus and the annual influenza immunizations. Further occupational exposures to silica or other fibrogenic dusts should be forbidden, and the individual should be warned against taking employment that involves appreciable risk of any other kind of respiratory disease or injury. Finally, the patient should be reminded at every opportunity to seek medical advice without delay in the event of new or worsening respiratory symptoms or intercurrent illness.

Treatment of silicotuberculosis

Treatment of complicating tuberculosis was shown to be effective if a satisfactory combination of antituberculous drugs is administered for a sufficient length of time (Keers, 1969), and this remains true for the more recently introduced drugs. Quiescence of disease is thereby achieved in the great majority of cases. The poor results reported in the 1950s appear to have been due to inadequate regimens. However, a few individuals with advanced cavitary silicotuberculosis may respond poorly (Morgan, 1979), and the development of overall drug resistance greatly increases the likelihood of a fatal outcome.

Acute silicosis

Alveolar silico-lipoproteinosis

Pathology

Macroscopic appearances

The pleura is usually thickened and adherent, but in some cases is free, and the lungs are voluminous, heavy and mostly airless. The hilar lymph nodes are often enlarged, and a tenacious, mucinous material may be present in the large airways.

When the lungs are cut, there is grey–white consolidation interspersed by pink–red areas and diffuse interstitial pulmonary fibrosis (DIPF), which

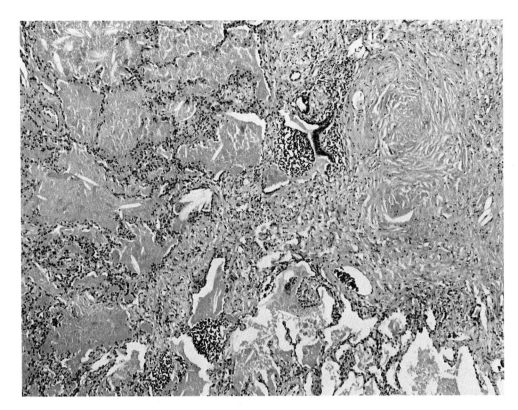

Figure 12.18 Alveolar silico-lipoproteinosis in a man who milled quartz for 7 years. The majority of the alveolar spaces are filled with acellular, finely granular, eosinophilic PAS-positive material with occasional cleft-like spaces. The alveolar walls are mostly normal in appearances but in places are thickened by mild infiltration of mononuclear cells and proliferation of reticulin (centre of field). There are also local aggregations of lymphocytes in the interstitium. On the right there are small, immature, but recognizable, silicotic nodules. Magnification × 40. (Reproduced, with permission, from Xipell et al., 1977)

may be prominent in the upper halves of the lungs. A frothy (often blood-stained) or gelatinous fluid exudes from the cut surfaces. Silicotic nodules are either few and small, or altogether absent.

Microscopic appearances

These are very variable and, as originally described almost 60 years ago (McDonald, Piggott and Gilder, 1930; Chapman, 1932), may consist of areas of acellular fibrosis, sometimes with hyaline centres, around which there is an intense small-cell infiltration; alveolar walls are thickened by fibrous tissue and, in many places, alveolar spaces are filled by an acidophilic, high-protein alveolar fluid containing fine granules and many desquamated cells, to which Mallory drew attention in 1934.

The early stage of the disease exhibits the features of endogenous lipoid pneumonia (Costello et al., 1975). Later, a degree of DIPF is present, accompanied by infiltration of mononuclear and plasma cells and, in alveolar spaces, by desquamated cells and an abundant acidophilic, proteinaceous material that is strongly positive to the periodic acid–Schiff (PAS) stain. The relative amounts and distribution of these entities vary from case to case. Silicotic nodules are usually absent, but, if present, are few in number and smaller and more immature than typical lesions (Hoffman et al., 1973; Roeslin et al., 1980) (Figure 12.18), although exceptions to this, in which there are moderate numbers of fairly mature nodules, are on record (Suratt et al., 1977). Widespread, irregular fibrosis is also seen in cases of prolonged survival. Hyalinized collagenous tissue and birefringent crystals may be found in the hilar lymph nodes (Xipell et al., 1977).

Apart from the presence of occasional silicotic nodules and quartz crystals in the intra-alveolar material, these features are identical with 'idiopathic' alveolar lipoproteinosis (Rosen, Castleman and Liebow, 1958; Heppleston and Young, 1972), in which the alveolar walls are usually, but not always, thickened by cellular infiltration, and the alveolar spaces filled with granular, strongly PAS-positive lipid and proteinaceous material (see Figure 5.11). The proteins are albumin and IgG, apparently derived by transudation from serum proteins; indeed, serum proteins have been identified in bronchopulmonary lavage fluid from human alveolar lipoproteinosis (Hawkins, Savard and Ramirez-Rivera, 1967).

Most of the cells in the alveolar exudate are macrophages that contain numerous osmiophilic lamellar inclusion bodies, which probably originate from disrupted type II cells. These bodies are also free in the phospholipid material, which possesses the hexagonal and parallel lamellated patterns already described in Chapter 5 (see Figure 5.13), and which is probably from an excess of surfactant (Hoffmann et al., 1973). Type I cells are scanty and fragmented. Quartz crystals have been observed in supposedly type II cells (Xipell et al., 1977).

Pathogenesis

Owing to the fact that 'acute silicosis' was first identified in the abrasive soap industry, alkali (sodium carbonate) was considered to be a decisive pathogenic agent, and ingenious chemical theories were advanced suggesting that it exerted an enhancing effect on the fibrogenic potential of quartz; these theories are invalidated by the fact that the same disease process occurs in the absence of exogenous alkali.

At least two conditions are thought to be necessary for the production of the disease:

1. Exposure to high concentrations of quartz, cristobalite or tridymite dust.
2. Small particle size: the disease is usually associated with exposure to finely divided quartz dust, and is reproduced in animals by the inhalation of quartz (or cristobalite) particles of less than 7 or 5 μm diameter (Corrin and King, 1969; Heppleston, Wright and Stewart, 1970) (see Chapter 5, 'Lipidosis').

A third, but speculative, immunological factor may, perhaps, be involved, but remains to be identified (Gough, 1967). Interesting recent work reveals that freshly fractured silica results in silicon-based free radicals, with consequent enhanced potential for lung tissue injury. Because occupations associated with acute silicosis (sandblasting, tunnelling, silica flour mill operations, surface coal-mine drilling) have resulted in inhalation of freshly fractured silica, its role in the pathogenesis of this form of the disease may be relevant (Vallyathan et al., 1988) (see Chapter 5, page 112).

The early changes of the experimental disease consist of a large influx of alveolar macrophages with swollen and vacuolated cytoplasm, followed by production of PAS-positive intra-alveolar material, in which there may be cholesterol crystals. There is some disagreement as to whether pronounced proliferation of type II cells is an early key feature (Corrin and King, 1970; Heppleston and Young, 1972), but these cells appear to be the chief source of the phospholipid (surfactant) accumulation (Heppleston, Fletcher and Wyatt, 1974). The massive production of phospholipid and cell debris appears to isolate the quartz particles from macrophages, thus preventing or reducing the formation of typical silicotic fibrosis (see Chapter 5, page 113). There is some evidence that alveolar clearance may be defective (Kuhn et al., 1966). Macrophages obtained by bronchopulmonary lavage from cases of human idiopathic disease exhibit decreased viability in tissue culture and a reduced capacity to kill candida organisms, although their phagocytic activity is unimpaired, suggesting that they are rendered defective by their abnormal environment. Monocytes from the peripheral blood, however, appear to function normally (Golde et al., 1976).

Alveolar lipoproteinosis seems to be a non-specific, although characteristic, response to a variety of injurious agents in addition to crystalline silica; it has been associated – though often circumstantially – with the inhalation of various dusts, both mineral and organic, and vapours (Davidson and MacLeod, 1969) and, in animals and human beings, with a number of different drugs (Hruban, 1976; Xipell et al., 1977). However, in many cases, there is no identifiable cause.

Clinical features

Symptoms

Symptoms develop quickly over a period of a few weeks, and usually within a year or two of first exposure to the responsible siliceous dust. The subject complains of malaise, fatigue, loss of weight, cough and mucoid sputum, slight or recurrent haemoptysis, and pleuritic type of chest pain; however, the chief symptom is rapidly progressive dyspnoea of sudden onset. In a proportion of cases, however, the onset is insidious and the progression fairly slow.

Physical signs

The patient is usually dyspnoeic at rest and, in the later stages of the illness, orthopnoeic. The reason for this is that a large proportion of the lungs is involved by the disease process, and it is also possible that reflex mechanisms play a part. Central cyanosis may be present, together with fever ranging from 37.2°C (99°F) to 40°C (105°F).

There may be finger clubbing, impaired percussion note and pleural rub. Breath sounds are either diminished or of a bronchial type, depending upon the degree of pleural thickening. Inspiratory crackles are usually heard over the greater part of the lung fields. In some cases, however, there are no abnormal signs.

Investigations

Lung function

Tests reveal a restrictive defect (Buechner and Ansari, 1969) with severe reduction of TLC, compliance and gas transfer, and consequent arterial oxygen desaturation. But these changes have no diagnostic significance.

Radiographic appearances

Early changes often consist of a diffuse haze in the lower zones of both lung fields (Pendergrass, 1958). Thereafter, appearances which may range from those of 'ground glass' type to a mixture of coarse linear and rounded opacities (similar to those of pulmonary oedema) appear rapidly throughout the lung fields. But, in other cases, the pattern of very small round opacities, indicative of alveolar consolidation and resembling miliary tuberculosis, is distributed mainly in the lower lung fields (Figure 12.19). Haziness of both fields, due to diffuse pleural thickening, may also be seen. In cases which take a protracted course, a widespread pattern of irregular fibrosis, sometimes with 'honeycomb cysts', ultimately develops.

Other investigations

Sputum often contains strongly PAS-positive material, and its differentiation from mucinous substances in other diseases by alcian blue, alcian green and mucicarmine stains is quick and simple, and, therefore, a helpful diagnostic aid (Vidone et al., 1966). Electron microscopy of sputum, although a more difficult procedure, may identify lamellar inclusion bodies (Costello et al., 1975). It may be necessary to obtain lung tissue for biopsy to establish the diagnosis beyond doubt, but the discomfort and danger associated with thoracotomy and needle methods in patients with a very severe restrictive functional defect indicate that this should only be done if other methods fail. Sputum must be cultured for *M. tuberculosis* and 'opportunist' mycobacteria as soon as possible.

Diagnosis

If a detailed occupational history is not elicited, the diagnosis will in all probability be missed. Confusion may occur with pulmonary oedema, fibrosing alveolitis, sarcoidosis, tuberculosis and pneumonia of various types. It should also be borne in mind that alveolar silico-lipoproteinosis may occasionally develop in an individual with already established nodular silicosis or 'mixed dust fibrosis' following additional intense silica exposure.

Complications

Tuberculosis and other pathogenic mycobacterial infections are especially apt to occur (Buechner and Ansari, 1969; Bailey et al., 1974) due, no doubt, to the impaired activity of alveolar macrophages already referred to (see page 113); similarly, fungous infection is also common, and may be yet another distraction from the correct diagnosis. Spontaneous pneumothorax sometimes occurs and, in some cases, right heart failure supervenes.

It appears that acute glomerular nephritis, which may be attributable to silicon toxicity, is a rare complication (Giles et al., 1978) (see page 316).

Prognosis

Spontaneously occurring alveolar lipoproteinosis apparently resolves completely in the majority of cases, but 'silica'-induced disease appears to be almost invariably fatal due to cardiorespiratory failure within about 1 year of development of the first symptoms.

Treatment

Bronchopulmonary lavage with isotonic saline has been advocated (Ramirez-R., 1971; Costello et al., 1975), but the authors have no personal knowledge of success with this treatment. The prognosis is so hopeless that it probably should be tried, and electron microscopy of the recovered fluid can confirm the diagnosis. Despite a recent report of partial success in one case, steroids have not, in general, been helpful (Goodman et al., 1992). Inhalation of a trypsin aerosol has been successful in idiopathic alveolar lipoproteinosis (Riker and Wolinsky, 1973), but it may itself produce lung damage and seems to offer little theoretical advantage over lavage. Complicating mycobacterial, fungal or other pulmonary infections should be treated early and vigorously.

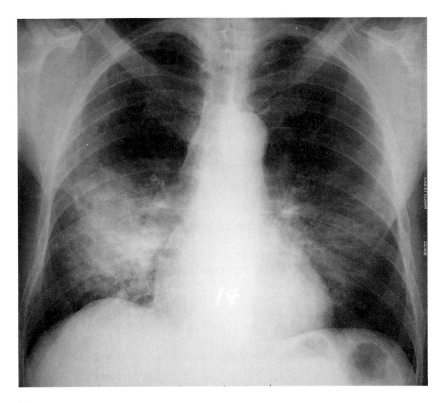

(a)

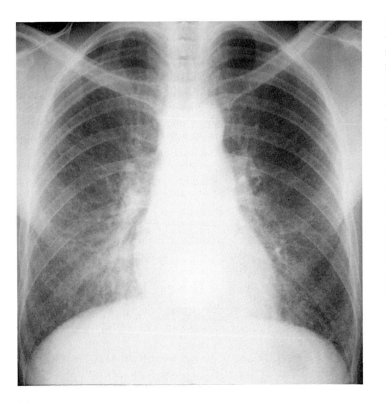

(b)

Figure 12.19 (a) Sandblaster, aged 47 years, who worked at this trade for 7 years in a semi-enclosed 'blasting shed', without an air-supplied respiratory protective device. The lower zone predominance of small opacities, a substantial proportion of which are linear or irregular, and the consolidation are characteristic of acute silicosis (silico-lipoproteinosis). (b) Sandblaster, aged 33 years, with 5 years of indoor work, in 4 of which he wore an air-supplied hood. The uniform distribution of small opacities is not rare in accelerated silicosis. The predominance of the smallest size opacities (p and s) is rare, and the same radiographic pattern has been associated with severe functional impairment in coal pneumoconiosis. This man's diffusing capacity was 32 per cent predicted at the time of this examination, and 6 years later had fallen to 14 per cent predicted

Prevention of ordinary and acute silicosis

This depends upon the recognition of a crystalline silica hazard, and upon a high standard of dust control and disposal, which must be monitored by continual and random analysis of atmospheric dust in the work and 'background' areas. Whenever possible, a harmless material should be substituted.

The principles and methods of dust control are described in 'Occupational exposure to crystalline silica' by the US Department of Health, Education and Welfare (1974), in 'The prevention and suppression of dust in mining, tunnelling, and quarrying' by the ILO (1966) and, as they apply to the pottery industry, in *Health Conditions in the Ceramic Industry* (Davies, 1969).

A 50 µg/m³ time-weighted average permissible exposure limit for respirable crystalline silica was recommended by the US National Institute of Occupational Safety and Health (US Department of Health, Education and Welfare, 1974; Utidjian, 1975). The evidence and assumptions upon which it was based were questioned at the time (Morgan, 1975), and they seem more open to question in light of the subsequent revelations (Graham, O'Grady and Dubuc, 1981) of faulty lung function measurement in the Vermont granite shed studies of 1970 to 1974. The NIOSH recommendation now seems to rest mainly upon the assumption that engineering controls introduced in the granite industry in the late 1930s achieved an almost instantaneous reduction of average dust concentrations, to the 1955 levels reported by Hosey, Trasko and Ashe (1957).

A WHO study group recommended a 40 µg/m³ permissible exposure limit 'almost solely on the basis of what appears to be worst-case situations . . .', citing the (earlier) Vermont granite shed studies of Ashe and Bergstrom (1964) and the gypsum miners study of McDonald and Oakes (1983) as suggesting '. . . a no-effect level below a specific exposure level'. Radiographic data in the gypsum miners came from only 64 men, and the exposure data were not considered very reliable. The study group also issued a plain warning that '. . . there were serious limitations associated with all of the epidemiological exposure–response studies evaluated'.

A recent contribution to defining exposure–response relationships is a retrospective cross-sectional study of Ontario gold and uranium miners (Muir et al., 1989a,b; Verma et al., 1989). Routine surveillance radiographs of 2109 miners were screened: 32 were considered to have nodular opacities of at least ILO category 1/1 by one or more of five readers. Past dust measurements were by konimeter, and extensive simultaneous konimetric and gravimetric sampling was carried out to derive a curve for conversion to gravimetric exposure units.

A curvilinear relationship was found, but the plots furnished do not inspire confidence in conversions at low gravimetric levels (that is, <100 µg/m³). Risks of radiographic silicosis (ILO 1/1), by cumulative silica dose with 5 years' lag time, were computed for each reader. If the exposure levels associated with 1 per cent silicosis risk in a 40-year working lifetime are averaged over the five readers, the mean is 93 µg/m³. If the most sensitive and least sensitive readers are excluded, the mean is 87.5 µg/m³, which is almost identical to the mean of 85 µg/m³ obtained when any three of the five readers agreed in identifying a case. The finding that a 100 µg/m³ exposure level, times 40 years, may result in a silicosis risk greater than 1 per cent seems certain to raise questions about the adequacy of the current US exposure limit. The small number of cases, and the imprecisions in converting particle counts to gravimetric levels, should be kept clearly in mind.

'Mixed dust fibrosis'

Pathogenesis

Lung dust in hematite miners consists of hematite, quartz and mica, with the quartz contributing 4 to 6 per cent of the total dust. This proportion of quartz resembles, but is rather more than that in coal pneumoconiosis (Nagelschmidt, 1965) and, similar to that pneumoconiosis, is not selectively concentrated in the lesions of progressive massive fibrosis (PMF). The more advanced the fibrosis, the higher the quartz content (Faulds and Nagelschmidt, 1962). Hematite does not give a Prussian blue reaction, but intracellular haemosiderin at the periphery of the lesions does (see Chapter 11, page 258).

'Mixed dust fibrosis' appears to be due to modification of the effects of small quantities of crystalline silica (usually quartz) by the accompanying non-fibrogenic dusts. Animal experiments and observations in human subjects have established that iron oxide inhibits or delays quartz-induced fibrosis in the lungs (Kettle, 1932; Gross, Westrick and McNerney, 1960) and that, as hematite, it does not cause fibrosis (Byers and King, 1961). Iron hydroxide encountered by miners in the goethite iron ore mines in the Salzgitter district of Germany appears to be even more effective in preventing fibrotic pneumoconiosis (Reichel, Bauer and Bruckmann, 1977).

According to McLaughlin (1957), the quartz content of the dust responsible for these lesions is under 10 per cent, but later experimental work suggests that it may be appreciably higher than this (Goldstein and Rendall, 1970). If other factors play a part in pathogenesis, they have not been identified. The incidence of complicating tuberculosis approaches that observed in nodular silicosis (Goldstein and Rendall, 1970), but there does not appear to be any evidence that it is involved in pathogenesis of the pneumoconiotic lesions.

The fibrogenic potential of combinations of quartz and kaolinite in animal lungs is referred to in Chapter 16 (page 553).

Coal pneumoconiosis, in some respects, resembles 'mixed dust fibrosis', but there are reasons for treating it as a separate entity (see Chapter 13).

Pathology

Macroscopic appearances

As in the case of nodular silicosis, the pulmonary pleura is often thickened to a variable degree, and may be puckered where it overlies an intrapulmonary fibrotic mass. Distended bullae are sometimes present in these areas.

The cut surfaces of the lungs reveal irregular or stellate fibrous lesions, which may vary in size from about 3 or 4 mm to confluent masses which may occupy the greater part of a lobe or lung. Characteristic whorled silicotic nodules are uncommonly seen either alone or within areas of fibrosis. Confluent massive lesions may be present, irregular in form, and often not limited by the anatomical boundaries of lobes or segments. In some cases of hematite miners, they are identical to the PMF lesions of coal pneumoconiosis (see Chapter 13), although of reddish colour, and do not resemble the conglomerate masses of silicotic nodules. Cavities are rarely seen unless there is complicating tuberculous or opportunist mycobacterial infection, but they can occur from ischaemia, as in coal pneumoconiosis (Gibbs and Wagner, 1988).

Both small and large lesions occur mainly in the upper halves and posterior zones of the lungs (but there are exceptions to this), and are rarely of similar size and distribution in the two lungs. Occasionally, only a few isolated lesions are present.

Grey–black pigment is intimately distributed through the lesions, and in hematite lungs the fibrotic areas are, like the rest of the lungs, brick-red in colour. Coal dust from mould-facing materials is sometimes present in considerable quantity in foundry workers' lungs.

Microscopic appearances

Iron and quartz particles accumulate in alveolar walls adjacent to respiratory bronchioles and small

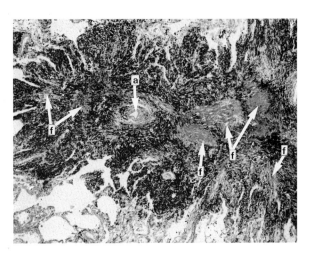

Figure 12.20 'Mixed dust fibrosis' in an iron foundry worker. 'Medusa head' formation with a lot of dust and scattered, collagenous fibrosis some of which is unpigmented (f). The lesion surrounds an artery (a) and extends slightly into some alveolar walls although the adjacent lung is largely normal. Magnification × 55; H & E stain. Compare with Figure 12.4

arteries. In lesions in which there is no quartz, there is no reaction other than a slight increase of reticulin fibres (that is, *siderosis* – see Chapter 11), but when small quantities of quartz are present there is fibroblastic activity leading to peribronchiolar and perivascular collagen fibrosis, which obliterates neighbouring alveoli and spreads, to a greater or lesser degree, further into the lung. Reticulin and collagen fibres are arranged in both linear and radial fashion, so that individual lesions are of irregular or stellate ('Medusa head') form, and not concentrically nodular (Figure 12.20). Separate silicotic nodules may occur, however, in some cases, and occasionally both types of lesions are seen together; the nodular component is usually immature and hyaline changes are absent. Massive lesions consist of much dust, which is mostly extracellular and randomly arranged, often hyalinized, collagenous fibrosis; in other cases, however, the fibrosis has the whorled appearance of nodular silicosis.

Pulmonary arteries in the fibrotic areas may be engulfed by fibrous tissue, and occluded or obliterated. In hematite mixed dust fibrosis, there is an intense accumulation of iron-containing dust in and around pulmonary blood vessels, but muscularized arteries are not evident. This is believed to imply an absence of constriction of the terminal regions of the arterial tree (Heath, Mooi and Smith, 1978).

Scar (irregular) emphysema may be present around some 'mixed' lesions due to their concentration, and bullae with air trapping may be found in relation to larger confluent masses. Scar emphysema is not a constant feature, and in many cases it is absent or of very slight degree. Other types of emphysema which may be present are coincidental and not pathogenically related.

By contrast with nodular silicosis, calcification does not occur in the 'mixed' lesions other than from healing of complicating tuberculosis.

Carbon, iron and other metallic dust particles are present in large quantities and weak doubly refractile particles may suggest the presence of quartz. Siderosis often accompanies mixed dust fibrosis in iron foundry workers.

Clinical features

Symptoms, physical signs and lung function

The same considerations apply as in the case of nodular silicosis.

Radiographic appearances

When lesions in the lungs are small, the opacities they produce on the film may resemble those of discrete 'nodular' silicosis or coal pneumoconiosis; when larger, there are irregular opacities (usually in the upper and middle zones) that may be indistinguishable from those produced by fibrocaseous tuberculosis. As a rule, the well-demarcated opacities of discrete or conglomerate nodular silicosis are not observed. Calcification of lesions is not seen unless caused by quiescent tuberculosis, and 'eggshell' calcification of hilar lymph nodes does not seem to occur (Figure 12.21).

In iron foundry workers, hematite miners and boiler scalers, numerous small radiodense opacities due to siderosis may also be present throughout the lung fields (see Chapter 11). In a survey of 1194 British foundry men, small discrete opacities were observed in 34 per cent of fettlers and 14 per cent of foundry floor men, but larger opacities indicative of conglomerate lesions were not seen (Lloyd Davies, 1971). It is probable that iron, and possibly zircon, dust contributed significantly to these appearances (see Chapter 11).

Diagnosis

The most difficult task is to distinguish radiographically between 'mixed dust fibrosis' and healed or active tuberculosis, but the presence of cavities favours active tuberculosis. However, when there is an appropriate occupational history and a background appearance of radiographic small opacities, and sputum cultures are positive for *M. tuberculosis*, it is virtually impossible to exclude the presence of coexistent 'mixed dust fibrosis'.

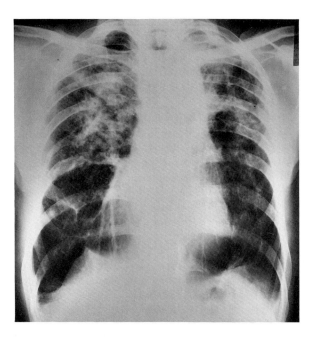

Figure 12.21 Moderately advanced 'mixed dust fibrosis': irregular massive opacities with very few discrete nodules in the rest of the lung fields. Extensive scar emphysema. Investigation for tuberculosis consistently negative

Occasionally, isolated lesions, when seen radiographically for the first time, may suggest collapse consolidation or bronchial carcinoma.

Complications

Complications are similar to those already described for nodular silicosis in regard to tuberculosis and other infections, pulmonary heart disease, chronic bronchitis, emphysema and the 'rheumatoid' changes. Circumscribed 'rheumatoid-modified' nodules, with naked-eye appearances of alternating concentric rings of black pigment and yellow–grey tissue, and the microscopic features described in Chapter 13, have been observed in a boiler scaler (Campbell, 1958) and an iron foundry worker (Caplan, Cowen and Gough, 1958); consistent radiographic characteristics have only been recorded in a roof tile slabber (Hayes and Posner, 1960) and a worker in artificial grinding wheel manufacture (Posner, 1960).

Tuberculosis complicates 'mixed dust fibrosis' less often than it complicates nodular silicosis, but is substantially more frequent than in the general population.

An increased incidence of cancer of the lung among hematite miners is referred to in Chapter 11 (page 260).

Prognosis

This is much the same as in nodular silicosis, but life expectancy is rarely shortened.

Treatment and prevention

The principles are similar to those applying to silicosis.

Diatomite pneumoconiosis

Prevalence

This is an uncommon pneumoconiosis, the severity of which appears to correlate with the cristobalite content of the dust and duration of exposure.

A survey in the diatomite processing industry in 1953 to 1954, which included 869 workers in five facilities, showed that 25 per cent of the 251 workers with more than 5 years' dust exposure, and nearly 50 per cent of 101 workers exposed to high concentrations of calcined dust, had radiographic evidence of pneumoconiosis which, on the whole, indicated nodular and confluent lesions. The majority of these employees had been mill hands handling calcined material. There were no definite cases among the quarry workers (Cooper and Cralley, 1958).

Another radiographic survey of 869 diatomite workers revealed that of those who had been mill hands for more than 5 years, 17 per cent had 'linear–nodular' (simple) pneumoconiosis, and 23.2 per cent had larger confluent opacities (Oechsli, Jacobson and Brodeur, 1961).

Rigorous dust controls in quarrying and processing plants have, however, resulted in the virtual elimination of new cases. For example, by 1974, 14 (3.3 per cent) of a workforce of 428 men, employed since 1953 in an American plant where these measures had been introduced in the mid-1950s, had radiographic evidence of pneumoconiosis, and this did not exceed ILO category 1/1. Of 129 employees exposed before 1953, only 2 mill workers (2.6 per cent) had category A opacities thought to indicate pneumoconiosis (Cooper and Jacobson, 1977). Further follow-up of 473 employees, all with at least 5 years of service at this facility, was subsequently reported (Cooper and Sargent, 1984). Only 11 films were classified as showing definite simple pneumoconiosis, none with large opacities; they all worked

in the mill, and had more than 25 years' employment. The authors commented that these results were in striking contrast to the earlier findings, the result of a smaller proportion of the study population who began work prior to the 1950s, when dust levels were appreciably higher.

There appears to be no information on the prevalence of pneumoconiosis among workers using calcined diatomite in the various manufacturing processes, but the risk is probably low, although it is possible that some cases have passed unrecognized, being interpreted as 'sputum-negative fibrotic tuberculosis'.

Pathogenesis

The structural forms of silicon dioxide that may be found in diatomite have a crucial influence on its fibrogenic potential. Natural diatomite is non-crystalline (amorphous), and is associated with only small quantities of quartz – less than 2 per cent in California, Nevada and Oregon (Cooper and Cralley, 1958) – and trace amounts of tridymite and cristobalite. When it is subjected to high temperature calcination, cristobalite and some tridymite are formed at a rate related to the degree and duration of the applied heat (see Appendix I, page 843); the cristobalite content may be about 21 per cent of the bag-house product (Cooper and Cralley, 1958). Flux calcination greatly facilitates the speed with which cristobalite is produced in the same temperature range as straight calcination (Bailey, 1947), in which case some 60 per cent cristobalite may be present in the bag-house product (Cooper and Cralley, 1958), and tridymite may also be present. Figure 12.22 shows X-ray diffraction patterns of diatomite subjected to the different forms of calcination. The amount of cristobalite evolved is similar whether diatomite is of salt or fresh water origin (Cooper and Cralley, 1958).

Most early reports of animal studies did not indicate the presence or extent of crystalline silica in the test materials, and are therefore of limited value in assessing the lung reaction that results from exposure to natural diatomite. Natural diatomite, without detectable crystalline silica, causes infiltration of alveolar walls by macrophages, many of which contain dust particles, and no proliferation of connective tissue fibres (Tebbens and Beard, 1957). However, experimental fibrosis from natural diatomite contaminated by quartz or cristobalite has been reported (Vorwald et al., 1949; Pratt, 1983).

In human subjects, there is little evidence that it causes lung fibrosis (Vigliani and Mottura, 1948; Luton et al., 1956; Cooper and Cralley, 1958). By contrast, and as noted in Chapter 5, cristobalite and tridymite are more fibrogenic than quartz in experimental animals, and calcined diatomite has been

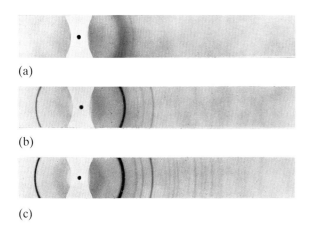

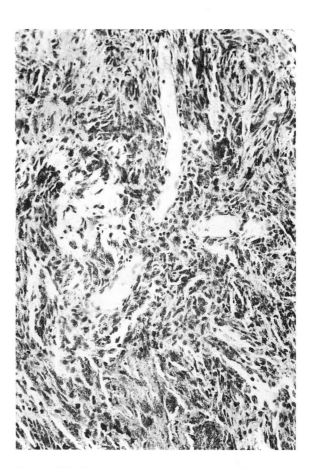

Figure 12.22 X-ray diffraction patterns of diatomite products. (a) Natural diatomite: the presence of the diffuse band and the absence of lines indicate that this is non-crystalline or amorphous. (b) Straight calcined diatomite: the distinct lines are characteristic of cristobalite. (c) Flux-calcined diatomite: lines are further increased in intensity. Disappearance of the diffuse bands indicates conversion of amorphous silicon dioxide to cristobalite. (Reproduced, with permission, from Wagner et al., 1968)

Figure 12.23 Pneumoconiosis due to calcined diatomite. This compact lesion consists of immature collagenous fibrosis which lacks the organized arrangement of typical silicotic nodules and is much more cellular. Magnification × 225; H & E stain. (Section by courtesy of Dr F.R. Dutra)

shown to be fibrogenic in human lungs (Vorwald et al., 1949). The relative rate of lung clearance of diatomite, and, therefore, the relationship between clearance and toxicity, is unclear. Uncalcined amorphous silicon dioxide has been found to be eliminated from the lungs more rapidly than either quartz or cristobalite (Klosterkötter and Einbrodt, 1965), but also less rapidly than cristobalite (Pratt, 1983).

The mean particle size of the final calcined product may be about 0.7 μm (Wagner et al., 1968), which ensures penetration to the alveolar region.

It has been emphasized that any samples of supposedly 'amorphous silica' obtained for workplace analyses or experimental purposes must be shown by X-ray diffraction to be free of any crystalline silica contaminants or products modified by heat treatment if valid interpretations of data are to be made (Bell, Dunnom and Lott, 1978).

Pathology

Macroscopic appearances

The pulmonary pleura is often thickened. Areas of fine and coarse, grey in colour, diffuse interstitial fibrosis of both linear and stellate form are seen in lung slices, usually in the upper halves of the lungs, although the lower halves may be involved, and the subpleural region is a common site of selection. It may be of slight or extensive order. Confluent

masses of fibrosis may also be present, again chiefly in the upper zones, and may contain ischaemic cavities. Characteristic whorled silicotic nodules and conglomerations are absent.

There may be scar emphysema, sometimes with bullae (especially in relation to areas of subpleural fibrosis), but often there is no emphysema.

Microscopic appearances

Early lesions consist of collections of dust-containing macrophages in alveoli, alveolar walls and hilar lymph nodes, either with no connective tissue reaction or with only a delicate reticulin proliferation (Carnes, 1954). As the lesions progress, diffuse collagen fibrosis occurs in the peribronchiolar and perivascular regions with much fibroblast activity, and this extends into surrounding lung tissue as diffuse interstitial fibrosis, producing thickening of

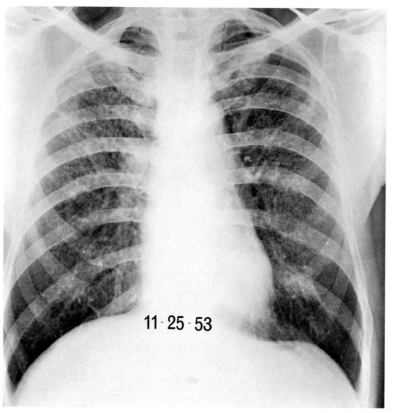

(a)

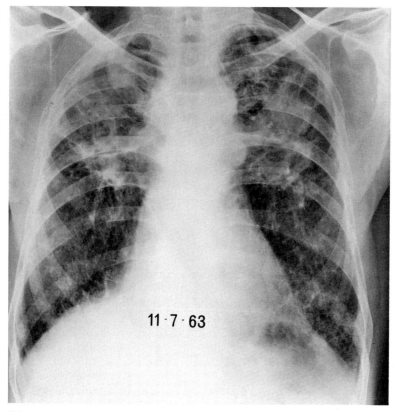

(b)

Figure 12.24 Diatomite pneumoconiosis in a man who spent 25 years in a processing mill with intermittent heavy exposure to flux calcined diatomite. He was removed from risk after the first film (a). The second film (b) was taken 10 years later. Tuberculin tests negative; no bacteriological evidence of tuberculosis. Note the appearances of diffuse interstitial fibrosis in the lower zones. (By courtesy of Dr W. Clark Cooper)

alveolar walls and obliteration of adjacent alveolar spaces (Figure 12.23). The cellular element is often prominent, and the lesions show some predilection for the subpleural zone (Spain, 1965).

Many dust particles which can be identified as fragmented diatoms may be seen in macrophages and fibrous tissue, and rather stubby, pseudoasbestos bodies with rudimentary segmentation are sometimes observed (Nordmann, 1943). The birefringence of cristobalite is low. Characteristic silicotic lesions do not occur, but 'hyalinization' may be seen in some areas of fibrosis (Vorwald et al., 1949; Dutra, 1965). In some cases, both macroscopic and microscopic features are those of 'mixed dust fibrosis' associated, however, with fragments of diatoms.

The confluent masses consist of collagenous fibrosis – often unusually cellular – arranged in random fashion, and showing little or no tendency to whorling. Necrosis may occur in them, sometimes with areas of calcification, due to ischaemic changes and in the absence of tuberculosis. Neighbouring blood vessels may be surrounded, and some obliterated, by fibrosis.

Scar emphysema may be related to the lesions, but this is not a constant finding, and it appears to occur chiefly in the form of small localized bullae in the vicinity of the subpleural fibrosis.

Fibrotic lesions are also seen in the hilar lymph nodes. The quartz content of the lungs is low. In one study, it was less than 2 per cent of the lungs by weight (Vorwald et al., 1949).

Clinical features

Symptoms

In general, respiratory symptoms are uncommon. When they occur, they consist of morning cough, which may be non-productive, and a mild-to-moderate degree of breathlessness on effort; rarely, in advanced cases, there is disabling dyspnoea. Haemoptysis does not seem to occur.

Physical signs

Finger clubbing is not a feature of the disease (Cooper and Cralley, 1958). There may be no abnormal signs, but in some cases breath sounds in the upper halves of the lungs may be of bronchial type accompanied by inspiratory crackles, which may also be heard over the lower lobe regions in some cases. Signs of spontaneous pneumothorax can sometimes be elicited. In advanced cases, the signs of upper zone fibrosis with tracheal displacement may be present.

Evidence of congestive heart failure due to pulmonary heart disease appears to be rare.

Investigations

Lung function

Comprehensive studies have been carried out by Motley, Smart and Valero (1956) and Motley (1960). As in the case of other types of pneumoconiosis, abnormal values correlate poorly with radiographic appearances, and good pulmonary function may be associated with fairly extensive radiographic changes; however, large confluent lesions are usually associated with abnormal function.

Maximum breathing capacity, timed FEV and FVC, may be slightly to moderately impaired, and arterial oxygen saturation often reduced in slight to moderate degree; RV is significantly increased, and there may be some reduction in TLC and gas transfer (TL). Uneven ventilation is present in some cases and, occasionally, there is pronounced airways' obstruction.

Radiographic appearances

The earliest abnormality consists of linear or round ('nodular') opacities, or both ('linear–nodular'), in the upper and mid-zones of the lung fields, and extending to their periphery. These appearances are sometimes fine and 'lace-like'. It is unusual for the discrete round opacities to exceed about 2 mm in diameter, and they have low contrast with the surrounding tissues, rarely possessing the radiodensity of those due to nodular silicosis (Oechsli, Jacobson and Brodeur, 1961).

The opacities become more prominent as they coalesce, and coalescent lesions, which are at first indistinct, later appear as well-circumscribed homogeneous densities (ILO category B or C). These are mainly in the upper zones and usually bilateral, and may exhibit evidence of contraction, distortion or cavities, but rarely calcification. Appearances consistent with DIPF may be seen in the lower zones, but have rarely been reported (Figure 12.24).

Enlargement or eggshell calcification of hilar lymph nodes is not seen.

Other investigations

Apart from obtaining lung tissue for biopsy (which should rarely be necessary), there are no investigations that are likely to give further assistance in establishing the diagnosis.

Diagnosis

This depends upon a history of an exposure of 5 or more years to calcined diatomite in processing or manufacture, and upon radiographic appearances.

Tuberculosis – active or quiescent – is the most important differential diagnosis.

Complications

In common with other forms of advanced silicosis, there is a tendency to spontaneous pneumothorax (Vigliani and Mottura, 1948; Smart and Anderson, 1952), although an increased likelihood of tuberculosis has not been demonstrated. However, when tuberculosis complicates diatomite pneumoconiosis, it tends to pursue an indolent course (Smart and Anderson, 1952). Failure of treatment in cavitary disease has been reported (Spain, 1965).

Prognosis

Progression to the stage of advanced confluent masses may occur years after the worker has left the industry with the disease in an early stage.

Life expectancy appears rarely to be shortened, and pulmonary heart disease is probably exceptional. Occasionally, however, rapidly progressive disease may occur and end in fatal pulmonary heart disease (Luton et al., 1956); this has mainly been associated with disease due to flux-calcined diatomite.

Treatment

There is no treatment to prevent or reverse the course of the disease.

Prevention

A rigid programme of dust control (monitoring of local and atmospheric dust, enclosure systems where possible, exhaust ventilation, good housekeeping and use of respirators) is necessary in diatomite processing and the use of the calcined form in manufacture. These measures, as noted already, have been applied in the major processing plants in the USA since the mid-1950s, with excellent results.

Silicic lavas and volcanic glasses

Volcanic glass is formed when lava is cooled quickly.

Pumice and pumicite

Pumice and pumicite differ only in the size of their particles, those of pumicite being less than 4 mm in diameter. Both, as mentioned briefly in Appendix I (page 864), are lightweight, cellular, glassy rocks consisting of glass-walled, bubble casts formed by rapid frothing of viscous silicic lava (such as rhyolite) due, in turn, to rapid expansion of dissolved gas during sudden cooling and drop in pressure. They occur either as massive blocks in lava flows and vent fillings or they may be more or less fragmented by violent eruption. Although silica is mainly amorphous and glassy, variable amounts of crystalline silica in the form of microcrystals of quartz, tridymite and cristobalite may be present. The silica content has been variously estimated as between 1 to 5 per cent in Messina by Faraone and Majori (1958), and 20 to 25 per cent – about one-quarter of which is crystalline and the rest amorphous – by Pancheri and Zanetti (1963) in pumice on the Island of Lapari. Thus, the amount of crystalline silica present varies from deposit to deposit, but is generally low.

They are usually obtained by opencast mining in the USA, Italy and Greece. Extraneous material is removed by screening through meshes of different sizes and, in general, pumice and pumicite used in industrial processes will contain little, if any, crystalline silica; high-quality powders contain no crystalline silica. The presence of a significant amount of crystalline material, in fact, would adversely affect the products.

Both have been employed increasingly in recent years as aggregate for building block and lightweight concrete, and pozzolan–Portland cement. Pumice concrete is more resistant to heat than ordinary concrete. Due to its low bulk density, pumice has valuable heat- and sound-insulating properties, and is used for loose-fill insulation and in acoustic plasters. High-quality pumice and pumicite are also used as abrasives, especially for fine polishing operations, and in some scouring powders and soaps.

Pneumoconiosis has been described, usually without associated tuberculosis, in men who worked on crushers, pulverizers, drying kilns and screens – the last two processes carrying the greatest risk – at the Lipari Island quarries in the Mediterranean. It has, therefore, sometimes been referred to as 'liparosis', although it has the histological features of silicosis or 'mixed dust fibrosis' (Holt, 1957). Radiographically, it can appear as nodular silicosis (Rizzo et al., 1969) and may progress to large multiple conglomerate opacities (ILO category C), which in some cases have a curious propensity for the lower halves of the lung fields (Pancheri and Zanetti, 1963). However, pneumoconiosis does not seem to have been described in similar workers in the USA. Undoubtedly, therefore, the presence of a crystalline polymorph of silica is required to cause fibrosis.

Perlite

This is a metastable volcanic glass, some ores of which occasionally contain small amounts of quartz ranging, for example, from 1 to 3 per cent (Anderson et al., 1956), and inclusions of feldspar, biotite and horneblende, although high-grade perlite does not contain any crystalline material (Cooper, 1975). It has found increasing use in industry since the Second World War in competition with pumice, owing to its ability to be expanded ('popped') by heating between 760 and 1200°C to a very light material possessing the valuable properties of low density, low thermal conductivity and high sound absorption. It is mined by open-pit methods chiefly in the western USA and, on a smaller scale, in Greece, Hungary, Italy, Sardinia, Turkey and the former USSR. The ore is passed through crushers, grinders and screens until appropriate particle size for introduction into the furnace is achieved. Quartz is usually absent or substantially less than 1 per cent in perlite intended for 'expansion', as its presence in any significant amount impairs the quality of the product.

Expanded perlite is used mainly in plasters and wallboards in combination with gypsum, but also as an aggregate in lightweight concretes, and as a filtration medium and paint filler. Because it possesses excellent insulating and fire-resistant capacities, it is employed for sound-absorbing materials and loose-fill insulations. Like pumice, therefore, it is a good substitute for asbestos in certain insulation products. It is also used in foundry sand mixtures, as an extender and filler in paints, enamels, plastics and rubber, and as a soil conditioner.

Perlite is non-fibrogenic in the lungs of experimental animals (A.J. Vorwald, 1953, quoted by Cooper, 1975), and a preliminary survey of 240 perlite workers with up to 23 years' exposure in different parts of the industry did not reveal radiographic evidence of an associated pneumoconiosis (Cooper, 1975), nor any significant reduction of FEV_1 or FEV_1/FVC (Cooper, 1976). A follow-up study (Cooper and Sargent, 1986) of 152 workers with 5 or more years of mining or milling exposure showed none with radiographic evidence of pneumoconiosis, and no dust effects on cross-sectional or longitudinal (66 workers, 1975 to 1983) lung function.

It may be concluded that perlite itself is unlikely to cause pulmonary fibrosis, but the possibility that occasionally some ores may contain quartz in excess of 2 to 3 per cent has to be borne in mind. There is, in addition, no evidence that fibrous minerals (such as erionite), which were produced in some geological areas by hydrothermal changes of volcanic ash, have been found in perlite production.

Fused (vitreous) silica

Fused, or vitreous, silica is the amorphous (non-crystalline) phase of silica that results when any other phase is melted and cooled. At temperatures well in excess of 1700°C under atmospheric pressure, silica exists in liquid amorphous form and, when cooled at a rate that prevents it from crystallizing, becomes a glass at room temperature (Sosman, 1965) (see Appendix I).

Fused silica is manufactured by fusion of very high quality quartzite sand in various types of electric arc and graphite resistance furnaces. During heating the quartz transforms to different crystal modifications, the exact route depending on the rate of heating. The transformations of α to β quartz, to tridymite and cristobalite and, finally, to liquid silica are typically observed. Any unfused, or partially fused, material – usually cristobalite – must be removed. It is unusual for cristobalite to be present after the ingots are crushed, but this can occur around areas of reduction in the raw material or due to power fluctuations in arc or resistance electrodes (Power, 1985).

Its properties of high purity, low thermal conductivity, low coefficient of thermal expansion and very high refractoriness at temperatures in excess of 1650°C are most valuable in numerous industrial processes, notably a wide range of refractory applications (such as continuous casting processes, mould coatings, coke-oven door liners and crucibles), the manufacture of glass as a refractory roof over the melting tanks (especially the float glass process), for ceramic saggers, and as an inert filler and extender in various resins used in the electronics industry – in particular, semiconductors. A point of importance is that, after prolonged periods of heating above 1150°C (as may occur in refractories), fused silica tends to devitrify (recrystallize) to cristobalite (Power, 1985).

Neither the production nor the use of fused silica in industrial applications appears to have caused any pulmonary disorder.

Microamorphous (submicron) silica is used extensively in industry, as fillers for rubber, paints and paper; in cosmetics, inks, automobile polishes and electric light bulbs; as a diluent for insecticides; and as a carrying agent for catalysts.

Microamorphous silica has, in general, similar properties to those of vitreous silica that has been very finely ground, although the structures are not identical (Sosman, 1965); crystalline and cryptocrystalline phases are absent. It is prepared, at similarly high temperatures, by precipitation from sodium silicate solutions (trade name Hi-Sil), hydrated calcium silicate (trade name Silene) or pure silicon tetrachloride (trade names, Aerosil, Degussa and Dow Corning silica) in the presence of combustible gases, and is, thus, sometimes referred to as synthetic or *precipitated silica*. The particles of these different preparations range in size from 5 to 40 nm and are uniform in each preparation (Volk, 1960). Neosyl, another hydrated silica precipitate, has a particle size range of 100 to 200 nm but these form loose agglomerates of 1 to 10 μm diameter.

Potentially, the most dusty areas in the manufacture of the amorphous silicas have been the furnace room, and the bagging and loading departments, but for some years these have been well controlled by dust suppression measures. In ferrous and non-ferrous metallurgy, the chief sources of amorphous silica are electric-arc furnaces, crucibles and ladles, where it occurs either as silica fume or vapour. The tendency for fume particles to aggregate probably reduces their chances of penetrating to the lower respiratory tract.

Surveys of workers in the Hi-Sil, Silene and Aerosil processes, in which men were observed over periods of 8 to 12 years, revealed no evidence of pneumoconiosis or harmful effects (Volk, 1960; Plunkett and De Witt, 1962). Similarly, pneumoconiosis was not found in men who had worked for some 25 years in the ferroalloy industry, although 'clouds of flocculated particles' of precipitated silica were produced (Roberts, 1965). However, small amounts of quartz have been found in condensed furnace fume in the ferrosilicon industry, but were associated with only minimal evidence of pneumoconiosis (Swensson et al., 1971). A report that 'amorphous silica dust' of 0.05 to 0.75 μm particle size originating from an electric-arc furnace in a metallurgical process, in which quartz was 'vaporized' at high temperature, caused 'nodular' fibrotic pneumoconiosis can hardly be correct, in view of the fact that the dust from this plant, which was shown to provoke pulmonary fibrosis of similar severity to that of quartz in animals, was, as the authors themselves state, identified by the American National Institute of Occupational Safety and Health (NIOSH) as cristobalite with a layer of amorphous silica (Johnson, Lewis and Groth, 1973; Vitums et al., 1977). Brambilla et al. (1980) also suggested that microamorphous silica was the cause of micronodular fibrosis in six workers exposed to 'amorphous silica smoke', although they were also exposed to quartz dust – in 'limited' amount – during the initial milling of sand.

Experimental work in rats exposed to microamorphous silica particles, which are completely lacking in cytotoxicity to macrophages (Kessel, Monaco and Marchisio, 1963), has demonstrated that they are eliminated from the lungs more rapidly than quartz, although they are still detectable after a period of 12 months. The resulting lesions, which consist mainly of macrophage accumulations and reticulin proliferation akin to the effect of an inert dust, regress as the silica disappears from the lungs (Byers

and Gage, 1961). A similar lack of significant collagen formation has also been observed in guinea-pigs and rabbits (Schepers et al., 1957a,b). However, it should be noted that, although some authors have claimed that microamorphous silica does cause fibrosis in animals (for example, Swensson, 1967; Zaidi, 1969), satisfactory evidence that the material administered was unadulterated has not been provided. More recently, in a general review of the question, Ferch (1985) concluded that synthetic amorphous silica is innocuous in both human beings and animals.

It should be noted, however, that some cristobalite (which, as stated earlier, is likely to be more fibrogenic than quartz) can survive temperatures above its melting point of 1723°C, so that its crystals may be present in the silica which results on cooling (see Appendix I); indeed, the white powder deposited when silica condenses out of its gas phase may contain finely divided (microcrystalline) cristobalite in addition to microamorphous silica (Sosman, 1965). In short, any experimental or epidemiological study which purports to show that fused amorphous silica is, itself, fibrogenic must demonstrate beyond doubt that the material studied is, in fact, truly amorphous and free of contaminating crystalline or cryptocrystalline silica.

Thus, fused silica in general does not cause pneumoconiosis in human beings, although cristobalite, which in some circumstances may be associated with it, can.

References

Adams, P.J. (1961) *Geology and Ceramics*, Department of Scientific and Industrial Research, Geological Survey and Museum. HMSO, London

Ahlmark, A. and Bruce, T. (1967) The current pneumoconiosis situation in Sweden. *Scand. J. Respir. Dis.* **48**, 181–188

Ahlmark, A., Bruce, T. and Nyström, A. (1960) *Silicosis and Other Pneumoconioses in Sweden*, Svenska Bokforlaget, Stockholm and Heinemann, London

Apostolov, K., Spasic, P. and Bonjanic, N. (1975) Evidence of a viral etiology in endemic (Balkan) nephropathy. *Lancet* **2**, 1271–1273

Armstrong, B.K. McNulty, J.C., Levitt, L.J., Williams, K.A. and Hobbs, M.S.T. (1979) Mortality in gold and coal miners in Western Australia with special reference to lung cancer. *Br. J. Ind. Med.* **36**, 199–205

Arnstein, A. (1941) Non-industrial pneumoconiosis, pneumonio-tuberculosis and tuberculosis of the mediastinal and bronchial lymph glands in old people. *Tubercle (London)* **22**, 281–295

Ashe, H.B. and Bergstrom, D.E. (1964) Twenty-six years' experience with dust control in the Vermont granite industry. *Ind. Med. Surg.* **33**, 73–78

Ashford, J.R. and Enterline, P.E. (1966) Radiological classification of pneumoconiosis. *Archs Environ. Health* **12**, 314–330

Bailey, D.A. (1947) Conversion of silica during ignition. *J. Ind. Hyg. Toxic.* **29**, 242–249

Bailey, W.C., Brown, M., Buechner, H.A., Weill, H., Ichinose, H. and Ziskind, M. (1974) Silico-mycobacterial disease in sandblasters. *Am. Rev. Respir. Dis.* **110**, 115–125

Banks, D.E., Morring, K.L., Boehlecke, B.A., Althouse, R.B. and Merchant, J.A. (1981) Silicosis in silica flour workers. *Am. Rev. Respir. Dis.* **124**, 445–450

Banks, D.E., Bauer, M.A., Castellan, R.M. and Lapp, N.L. (1983a) Silicosis in surface coal mine drillers. *Thorax* **38**, 275–278

Banks, D.E., Milutinovic, J., Desnick, R.J., Grabowski, G.A., Lapp, N.L. and Boehlecke, B.A. (1983b) Silicon nephropathy mimicking Fabry's disease. *Am. J. Nephrol.* **3**, 279–284

Beadle, D.G. (1971) The relationship between the amount of dust breathed and the development of radiological signs of silicosis: and epidemiological study in South African gold miners. In: *Inhaled Particles III* (ed. W.H. Walton) Unwin Brothers, Old Woking, Surrey, pp. 953–964

Becker, R.J.P. and Chatgidakis, D.B. (1960) The heart in silicosis. *Proceedings of Pneumoconiosis Conference, Johannesburg, 1959* (ed. A.J. Orsenstein), Churchill, London, pp. 205–216

Becklake, M.R. (1985) Chronic airflow limitation: its relationship to work in dusty occupations. *Chest* **88**, 608–617

Becklake, M.R., du Preez, L. and Lutz, W. (1958) Lung function in the silicotics of the Witwatersrand gold mines. *Am. Rev. Tuberc. Pulm. Dis.* **77**, 400–412

Bégin, R., Bergeron, D., Samson, L., Boctor, M. and Cantin, A. (1987) CT assessment of silicosis in exposed workers. *AJR Am. J. Roentgenol.* **148**, 509–514

Bégin, R., Dufresne, A., Cantin, A., Masse, S., Sebastien, P. and Perrault, G. (1989) Carborundum pneumoconiosis. Fibers in the mineral activate macrophages to produce fibroblast growth factors and sustain the chronic inflammatory disease. *Chest* **95**, 842–849

Bégin, R., Ostinguy, G., Fillion, R. and Colman, N. (1991) Computed tomography scan in the early detection of silicosis. *Am. Rev. Respir. Dis.* **144**, 697–705

Bell, Z.G. Jr., Dunnom, D.D. and Lott, H. (1978) Basis for exposure standards for amorphous silica dusts. *Am. Ind. Hyg. Assoc. J.* **39**, 418–421

Bellini, F. and Ghislandi, E. (1959) Su due casi di silicosi e sclerodermia. *Med. Lav.* **50**, 63–70

Belt, T.H. (1939) Silicosis of the spleen: a study of the silicotic nodule. *J. Pathol. Bacteriol.* **49**, 39–44

Bergin, C.J., Muller, N.L., Vedal, S. and Chan-Yeung, M. (1986) CT in silicosis: correlation with plain films and pulmonary function tests. *AJR Am. J. Roentgenol.* **146**, 477–483

Bobear, J.B., Hanemann, S.J. and Beven, T. (1962) Silicosis in Louisiana: new or unrecognized hazard. *J. Louisiana State Med. Soc.* **114**, 391–397

Borm, P.J., Bast, A., Wouters, E.F., Slangen, J.J., Swaen, G.M. and de Boorder, T. (1986) Red blood cell and anti-oxidant parameters in silicosis. *Int. Archs Occup. Environ. Health* **58**, 235–244

Bradshaw, F., Critchlow, A. and Nagelschmidt, G. (1962) A study of airborne dust in hematite mines in Cumberland. *Ann. Occup. Hyg.* **4**, 265–273

Brambilla, C., Brambilla, E., Rigaud, D., Perdrix, A., Paramelle, B. and Fourcy, A. (1980) Pneumoconiose aux fumées de silice amorphe. *Rev. fr. Mal. Resp.* **8**, 383–391

Bramwell, B. (1914) Diffuse scleroderma: its frequency; its occurrence in stonemasons; its treatment by fibrinolysin-elevations of temperature due to fibrinolysin injection. *Edinburgh Med. J.* **12**, 387–401

Brown, D.P., Kalplan, S.D., Zumwalde, R.D., Kaplowitz, M. and Archer, V.E. (1986) Retrospective cohort mortality study of underground gold mine workers. In: *Silica, Silicosis, and Cancer. Controversy in Occupational Medicine* (eds D.F. Goldsmith, D.M. Winn and C.M. Shy), Praeger, New York, pp. 335–350

Brown, R.C., Munday, D.E., Sawicka, V.M. and Wagner, J.C. (1983) Angiotensin converting enzyme in the serum of rats with experimental silicosis. *Br. J. Exp. Pathol.* **64**, 286–292

Bucca, C., Veglio, F., Rolla, G., Cacciabue, M., Cicconi, C., Ossola, M., Nuzzi, A., Avolio, G. and Angeli, A. (1984) Serum angiotensin converting enzyme (ACE) in silicosis. *Eur. J. Respir. Dis.* **65**, 477–480

Buechner, H.A. and Ansari, A. (1969) Acute silico-proteinosis. *Dis. Chest* **55**, 174–284

Burgess, W.A. and Reist, P.C. (1969) An industrial hygiene study of flame cutting in a granite quarry. *Am. Ind. Hyg. Assoc. J.* **30**, 107–112

Burrell, R., Esber, H.J., Hagadorn, J.E. and Andrews, C.E. (1966) Specificity of lung reactive antibodies in human serum. *Am. Rev. Respir. Dis.* **94**, 743–750

Byers, P.D. and Gage, J.C. (1961) The toxicity of precipitated silica. *Br. J. Ind. Med.* **18**, 295–302

Byers, P.D. and King, E.J. (1961) Experimental infective pneumoconiosis with *Mycobacterium tuberculosis* (var. *muris*) and hematite by inhalation and by injection. *J. Pathol. Bacteriol.* **81**, 123–134

Cameron, I.B. and McAdam, A.D. (1978) *The Oil-Shales of the Lothians, Scotland: Present Resources and Former Workings*, Report 78/28, Institute of Geological Sciences, HMSO, London

Campbell, J. A. (1958) A case of Caplan's syndrome in a boiler scaler. *Thorax* **13**, 177–180

Caplan, A., Cowen, E.D.H. and Gough, J. (1958) Rheumatoid pneumoconiosis in a foundry worker. *Thorax* **13**, 181–184

Carini, R. and Lo Martire, N. (1965) Sclerosi sistematica progressiva e silicosi pulmonare. *Med. Lav.* **56**, 708–715

Carnes, W.H. (1954) Quoted by Oechsli, Jacobson and Brodeur (1961)

Carta, P., Cocco, P.L. and Casula, D. (1991) Mortality from lung cancer among Sardinian patients with silicosis. *Br. J. Ind. Med.* **48**, 122–129

Chapman, E.M. (1932) Acute silicosis. *J. Am. Med. Assoc.* **98**, 1439–1441

Chatgidakis, C.F. (1963) Silicosis in South African white gold miners. *Med. Proc.* **9**, 383–392

Chatgidakis, C.F. and Theron, C.P. (1961) Rheumatoid pneumoconiosis (Caplan's syndrome). *Archs Environ. Health* **2**, 397–408

Chiesura, P., Bruguone, F. and Mezzanotte, S. (1961) Due osservazioni di sindrome di Caplan in minatori di galleria. *Lav. Umano* **13**, 203–213

Chiesura, P., Terribile, P.M. and Bardellini, G. (1968) Le calcificazioni à guscio d'uovo nella silicosi: elementi tratti dall' osservazioni di 52 casi. *Minerva Med. Roma* **59**, 5960–5968

Clark, T.C., Harrington, V.A., Asta, J., Morgan, W.K.C. and Sargent, E.N. (1980) Respiratory effects of exposure to dust in taconite mining and processing. *Am. Rev. Respir. Dis.* **121**, 959–966

Clerens, J. (1953) Silicose pulmonaire et rheumatisme ou syndrome de Colinet-Caplan. *Arch. Belg. Med. Soc.* **11**, 336–342

Colinet, E. (1953) Polyarthritis chronique evolutive et silicose pulmonarie. *Acta Physiother. Rheum. Belg.* **8**, 37–41

Collis, E.L. (1915) Industrial pneumoconioses with special reference to dust-phthisis. *Public Health* **28**, 252–264

Collis, E.L. and Yule, G.U. (1933) The mortality experience of an occupational group exposed to silica dust, compared with that of the general population and an occupational group exposed to dust not containing silica. *J. Ind. Hyg.* **15**, 395–417

Cooper, W.C. (1975) Radiographic survey of perlite workers. *J. Occup. Med.* **17**, 304–307

Cooper, W.C. (1976) Pulmonary function in perlite workers. *J. Occup. Med.* **18**, 723–729

Cooper, W.C. and Cralley, L.J. (1958) *Pneumoconiosis in Diatomite Mining and Processing*, Public Health Service Publication No. 601, US Department of Health, Education and Welfare, Washington DC

Cooper, W.C. and Jacobson, G. (1977) A 21-year radiographic follow-up of workers in the diatomite industry. *J. Occup. Med.* **19**, 563–566

Cooper, W.C. and Sargent, E.N. (1984) A 26-year radiographic follow-up of workers in a diatomite mine and mill. *J. Occup. Med.* **26**, 456–460

Cooper, W.C. and Sargent, E.N. (1986) Study of chest radiographs and pulmonary ventilatory function in perlite workers. *J. Occup. Med.* **28**, 199–206

Corn, J.K. (1980) Historical aspects of industrial hygiene. II. Silicosis. *Am. Ind. Hyg. Assoc. J.* **41**, 125–133

Corrin, B. and King, E. (1969) Experimental endogenous lipid pneumonia and silicosis. *J. Pathol.* **97**, 325–330

Corrin, B. and King, E. (1970) Pathogenesis of experimental pulmonary alveolar proteinosis. *Thorax* **25**, 230–236

Costello, J. (1979) Morbidity and mortality study of shale oil workers in the United States. *Environ. Health Perspect.* **30**, 205–208

Costello, J. and Graham, W.G.B. (1986) Vermont granite workers' mortality study. In *Silica, Silicosis, and Cancer. Controversy in Occupational Medicine* (eds D.F. Goldsmith, D.M. Winn and C.M. Shy) Praeger, New York, pp. 437–440

Costello, J.F., Moriarty, D.C., Branthwaite, M.A., Turner-Warwick, M. and Corrin, B. (1975) Diagnosis and management of alveolar proteinosis; the role of electron microscopy. *Thorax* **30**, 121–132

Cowie, R.L. (1987) Silica-dust-exposed mine workers with scleroderma (systemic sclerosis). *Chest* **92**, 260–262

Davidson, J.M. and MacLeod, W.M. (1969) Pulmonary alveolar proteinosis. *Br. J. Dis. Chest* **63**, 13–28

Davies, C.N. (Ed.) (1969) *Health Conditions in the Ceramics Industry*, Pergamon, Oxford, pp. 101–170

Davis, L.K., Wegman, D.H., Monson, R.R. and Froines, J. (1983) Mortality experience of Vermont granite miners. *Am. J. Ind. Med.* **4**, 705–723

de Villiers, A.J. and Gross, P. (1967) The pulmonary response of rats to fluorspar and radiation. In: *Inhaled Particles and Vapours II* (ed. G.N. Davies). Pergamon Press, Oxford, pp. 135–140

Denny, J.J., Robson, W.D. and Irwin, D.A. (1939) Prevention of silicosis by metallic aluminum. *Can. Med. Assoc. J.* **40**, 213–228

Dubois, F., Begin, R., Cantin, A., Masse, S., Martel, M., Bilodeau, G., Dufresne, A., Perreault, G. and Sebastien, P. (1988) Aluminum inhalation reduces silicosis in a sheep model. *Am. Rev. Respir. Dis.* **137**, 1172–1179

Dutra, F.R. (1965) Diatomaceous earth pneumoconiosis. *Archs Environ. Health* **11**, 613–619

Einbrodt, H.J. (1965) Quantitative and qualitative Untersuchungen uber die Staubretention in der menschlichen Lungen. *Beitr. Silkosforsch.* **87**, 1–105

Erasmus, L.D. (1960) Scleroderma in gold miners. *Proceedings of Pneumoconiosis Conference, Johannesburg* (ed. A.J. Orenstein), Churchill, London, pp. 426–435

Faraone, G. and Majori, L. (1958) Determiazoni conimetriche e granulometriche nelle varie fasi lavorative della industria della pomice in Canneto-Lapori (Messina). *Acta Med. Leg. Soc.* **11**, 83–94

Faulds, T.S. and Nagelschmidt, G.S. (1962) The dust in the lungs of hematite miners from Cumberland. *Ann. Occup. Hyg.* **4**, 255–263

Ferch, H. (1985) Zur Gewerbehygienischen unbedenklichkeit: Pulverförmige Amorphe Synthetische Kieselsäuren. *Staub. Reinhalt. Luft.* **45**, 236–239

Finn, R.H., Brinton, H.P., Doyle, H.N., Cralley, L.J., Harris, R.L., Westfield, J., Bird, J.H. and Berger, L.B. (1963) *Silicosis in the Metal Mining Industry. A Revaluation. 1958–1961*, Public Health Service Publication No. 1076, US Government Printing Office, Washington DC

Fiumicelli, A., Fiumicelli, C. and Pagni, M. (1964) Contributo allo studio della silicosi massiva unilarale isolata. *Med. Lav.* **5**, 516–530

Forastiere, F., Lagorio, S., Michelozzi, P., Cavariani, F., Arca, M., Borgia, P., Perucci, C. and Axelson, O. (1986) Silica, silicosis and lung cancer among ceramic workers: case-referent study. *Am. J. Ind. Med.* **10**, 363–370

Fowweather, F.S. (1939) Silicosis and the analyst. *Analyst* **64**, 779–787

Fox, A.J., Greenberg, M., Ritchie, G.L. and Barraclough, R.N.J. (1975) *A Survey of Respiratory Disease in the Pottery Industry*, Health and Safety Executive, HMSO, London

Francia, A., Monarca, G. and Cavallot, A. (1959) Osservazioni clinico-roentzenologische sull' assazione silicosi-sclerodermia. *Med. Lav.* **50**, 523–540

Friberg, L. and Ohman, H. (1957) Silicosis hazards in enameling. A medical, technical and experimental study. *Br. J. Ind. Med.* **14**, 85–91

Gambini, G., Agnoletto, A. and Magistretti, M. (1964) Tre casei di sindrome di Caplan. *Med. Lav.* **55**, 261–271

Gardner, L.U. (1929) Studies on experimental pneumoconiosis. *Am. Rev. Tuberc.* **20**, 833–875

Gardner, L.U. (1933) Pathology of the so-called acute silicosis. *Am. J. Public Health* **23**, 1240–1249

Gardner, L.U. (1934) *Pathology, Human and Experimental* (ed. B.E. Kuechle) First Saranac Symposium on Silicosis, Trudeau School of Tuberculosis, Saranac Lake, New York

Gardner, L.U. (1937) *The Significance of the Silicotic Problem* (ed. B.E. Kuechle) Third Saranac Symposium on Silicosis, Trudeau School of Tuberculosis, Saranac Lake, New York

Gedda, L., Bolognesi, M., Bandino, R. and Brenci, G. (1964) Ricerche di genetica sulla silicosi die minatori delia Sardegna. *Lav. Umano* **16**, 555–562

Gibbs, A.R. and Wagner, J.C. (1988) Diseases due to silica. In: *Pathology of Occupational Lung Disease* (eds A. Churg and F.H.Y. Green), Igaku-Shoin, New York, pp. 155–175

Giles, R.D., Sturgill, B.C., Suratt, P.M. and Bolton, W.K. (1978) Massive proteinuria and acute renal failure in a patient with acute silicoproteinosis. *Am. J. Med.* **64**, 336–342

Gillam, J.D., Dement, J.M., Lemen, R.A., Wagoner, J.K., Archer, V.E. and Blejer, H.P. (1976) Mortality patterns among hard rock gold mines exposed to an asbestiform mineral. *Ann. NY Acad. Sci.* **271**, 336–344

Glindmeyer, H.W. and Hammad, Y.Y. (1988) Contributing factors to sandblasters' silicosis: inadequate respiratory protection equipment and standards. *J. Occup. Med.* **30**, 917–921

Glover, J.R., Bevan, C., Cotes, J.E., Elwood, P.C., Hodges, N.G., Kell, R.L., Lowe, C.R., McDermott, M. and Oldham, P.D. (1980) Effects of exposure to slate dust in North Wales. *Br. J. Ind. Med.* **37**, 152–162

Golde, D.W., Territo, M., Finley, T.N. and Cline, M.J. (1976) Defective lung macrophages in pulmonary alveolar proteinosis. *Ann. Intern. Med.* **85**, 304–309

Goldstein, B. and Rendall, R.E.G. (1970) The relative toxicities of the main classes of minerals. *Pneumoconiosis. Proceedings of the International Conference, Johannesburg, 1969* (ed. H.A. Shapiro), Oxford University Press, Capetown, pp. 429–434

Goodman, G.B., Kaplan, Stachura, I., Castranova, V., Pailes, W.H. and Lapp, N.L. (1992) Acute silicosis responding to corticosteroid therapy. *Chest* **101**, 366–370

Gough, J. (1959) Rheumatoid pneumoconiosis. *Bulletin of Postgraduate Community Medicine, University of Sydney* **15**, 280–284

Gough, J. (1967) Silicosis and alveolar proteinosis. *Br. Med. J.* **1**, 629

Government of India Ministry of Labour (1953) *Silicosis in Mica Mining in Bihar*, Report No. 3, Office of the Chief Advisor Factories

Graham, W.G.B., O'Grady, R.V. and Dubuc, B. (1981) Pulmonary function loss in Vermont granite workers. A long-term follow-up and critical reappraisal. *Am. Rev. Respir. Dis.* **123**, 25–28

Griffiths, J. (1986) Synthetic mineral fibres. *Industr. Minerals (London)* September, 20–43

Gross, P., Westrick, M.L. and McNerney, J.M. (1960) Experimental silicosis: the inhibitory effect of iron. *Dis. Chest* **37**, 35–41

Grundorfer, W. and Raber, A. (1970) Progressive silicosis in granite workers. *Br. J. Ind. Med.* **27**, 110–120

Gualde, N., de Leobardy, J., Serizay, B. and Malinvand, G. (1977) HL-A and silicosis. *Am. Rev. Respir. Dis.* **116**, 334–336

Gunther, G. and Schuchardt, E. (1970) Silikose und progressive sklerodermie. *Deutsch. Med. Wschr.* **95**, 467–468

Gupta, S.P., Baja, A., Jain, A.L. and Vasudeva, Y.L. (1972) Clinical and radiological studies in silicosis: based on a study of the disease amongst stone cutters. *Indian J. Med. Res.* **60**, 1309–1315

Gye, W.E. and Purdey, W.J. (1924) The poisonous properties of colloidal silica. III. *Br. J. Exp. Pathol.* **5**, 238–250

Hale, L.W. and Sheers, G. (1963) Silicosis in West Country granite workers. *Br. J. Ind. Med.* **20**, 218–225

Harding, H.E. and McLaughlin, A.I.G. (1955) Pulmonary fibrosis in non-ferrous foundry workers. *Br. J. Ind. Med.* **12**, 92–99

Harding, H.E. and Massie, A.P. (1951) Pneumoconiosis in boiler scalers. *Br. J. Ind. Med.* **8**, 256–264

Hargis, K.M. and Jackson, J.O. (1983) Industrial hygiene aspects of underground oil shale mining. In *Health Issues Related to Metal and Non-metallic Mining* (eds W.L. Wagner, W.M. Rom and J.A. Merchant), Boston, London, Sydney, Butterworths, pp. 463–484

Hawkins, J.E., Savard, E.V. and Ramirez-Rivera, J. (1967) Pulmonary alveolar proteinosis. Origins of proteins in pulmonary washings. *Am. J. Clin. Pathol.* **48**, 14–17

Hayes, D.S. and Posner, E. (1960) A case of Caplan's syndrome in a roof tile maker. *Tubercle (London)* **41**, 143–145

Heath, D., Mooi, W. and Smith, P. (1978) The pulmonary vasculature in hematite lung. *Br. J. Dis. Chest* **72**, 88–94

Heppleston, A.G. (1962) The disposal of dust in the lungs of silicotic rats. *Am. J. Pathol.* **40**, 493–506

Heppleston, A.G. (1985) Silica, pneumoconiosis, and carcinoma of the lung. *Am. J. Ind. Med.* **7**, 285–294

Heppleston, A.G. and Young, A.E. (1972) Alveolar lipo-proteinosis: an ultrastructural comparison of the experimental and human forms. *J. Pathol.* **107**, 107–117

Heppleston, A.G., Fletcher, K. and Wyatt, I. (1974) Change in the composition of lung lipids and the 'turnover' of dipalmitoyl lecithin in experimental alveolar lipo-proteinosis induced by inhaled quartz. *Br. J. Exp. Pathol.* **55**, 384–395

Heppleston, A.G., Wright, N.A. and Stewart, J.A. (1970) Experimental alveolar lipo-proteinosis following the inhalation of silica. *J. Pathol.* **101**, 293–307

Hessel, P.A. and Sluis-Cremer, G.K. (1986) Case-control study of lung cancer and silicosis. In: *Silica, Silicosis and Cancer. Controversy in Occupational Medicine* (eds D.F. Goldsmith, D.M. Winn and C.M. Shy), Praeger, New York, pp. 351–355

Hessel, P.A., Sluis-Cremer, G.K. and Hnizdo, E. (1990) Silica exposure, silicosis, and lung cancer: a necropsy study. *Br. J. Ind. Med.* **47**, 4–9

Hirsch, M., Bar-Ziv, J., Lehmann, E. and Goldberg, G.M. (1974) Simple siliceous pneumoconiosis in Bedouin females in the Negev desert. *Clin. Radiol.* **25**, 507–510

HM Factory Inspectorate (1959) *Industrial Health. A Survey of the Pottery Industry in Stoke-on-Trent*, HMSO, London

Hnizdo, E. and Sluis-Cremer, G.K. (1991) Silica exposure, silicosis, and lung cancer: a mortality study of South African gold miners. *Br. J. Ind. Med.* **48**, 53–60

Hoffman, E.O., Lamberty, J., Pizzolato, P. and Coover, J. (1973) The ultrastructure of acute silicosis. *Archs Pathol.* **96**, 104–107

Holland, L.M., Gonzales, M., Wilson, J.S. and Tillery, M.L. (1983) Pulmonary effects of shale dusts in experimental animals. In: *Health Issues Related to Metal and Nonmetallic Mining* (eds W.L. Wagner, W.N. Rom and J.A. Merchant), Butterworths, Boston, pp. 485–496

Holland, L.M., Wilson, J.S., Tillery, M.I. and Smith, D.M. (1986) Lung cancer in rats exposed to fibrogenic dusts. In: *Silica, Silicosis and Cancer. Controversy in Occupational Medicine* (eds D.F. Goldsmith, D.J. Winn and C.M. Shy), Praeger, New York, pp. 267–279

Holmann, A.T. (1947) Historical relationship of mining silicosis and rock removal. *Br. J. Ind. Med.* **4**, 1–29

Holroyd, D., Rea, M.S., Young, J. and Briggs, G. (1988) Health-related aspects of the devitrification of aluminosilicate refractory fibres during use as a high-temperature furnace insulant. *Ann. Occup. Hyg.* **32**, 171–178

Holt, P.F. (1957) *Pneumoconiosis.* Edward Arnold, London, p. 174

Hosey, A.D., Trasko, V.M. and Ashe, H.B. (1957) *Control of Silicosis in the Vermont Granite Industry*, PHS Publication No. 557, US Department of Health, Education and Welfare, Washington DC

Hruban, Z. (1976) Pulmonary changes induced by ammophilic drugs. *Env. Health Perspect.* **16**, 111–118

Hughes, J.M., Jones, R.N., Gilson, J.C., Hammad, Y.Y., Samimi, B., Hendrick, D.J., Turner-Warwick, M., Doll, N.J. and Weill, H. (1982) Determinants of progression in sandblasters' silicosis. *Ann. Occup. Hyg.* **26**, 701–712

IARC (International Agency for Research on Cancer) (1987a) *Silica and Some Silicates*, IARC Monographs on the Evaluation of the Carcinogenic Risk of Chemicals to Humans, Volume 42, IARC, Lyon, pp. 39–144

IARC (International Agency for Research on Cancer) (1987b) *Overall Evaluations of Carcinogenicity: An Updating of IARC Monographs*, IARC Monographs on the Evaluation of the Carcinogenic Risk of Chemicals to Humans, Volumes 1–42, Supplement 7, IARC, Lyon, pp. 341–343

Inoue, Y., Hashimoto, A., Takada, Y., Nishimura, K., Hiwada, K. and Kokubu, T. (1987) Angiotensin converting enzyme in sarcoidosis and in silicosis. *Clin. Exp. Hypertens.* **9**, 481–485

International Labour Office (1966) *The Prevention and Suppression of Dust in Mining, Tunnelling and Quarrying.*

Third International Report 1958–1962, ILO, Geneva

International Labour Office (1980) *Guidelines for the Use of ILO International Classification of Radiographs of Pneumoconiosis*, revised edn, ILO, Geneva

Israel, H.L., Sones, M., Roy, R.L. and Stein, G.N. (1961) The occurrence of intrathoracic calcification in sarcoidosis. *Am. Rev. Respir. Dis.* **84**, 1–11

Ivanova, A.S., Puchkova, N.G. and Nekrasov, A.V. (1984) Effect of synthetic regulators of radical reactions on the course of experimental silicosis. *Vopr. Med. Khim.* **30**, 22–25

Jablońska, E. (1975) *Scleroderma and Pseudoscleroderma*, Polish Medical Publishers, Warsaw; Dowden, Hutchinson and Ross, Pennsylvania

Jain, S.M., Sepaha, G.C., Khare, K.C. and Dubey, V.S. (1977) Silicosis in slate pencil workers. *Chest* **71**, 423–426

Jayson, M.I.V. (1977) Collagen changes in the pathogenesis of systemic sclerosis. *Ann. Rheumatol. Dis.* **36** (suppl.), 26–28

Johnson, G.T., Lewis, T.R. and Groth, D.H. (1973) *Evaluation of Health Hazard of Amorphous Silica-coated Cristobalite following Intratracheal Injection in Rats*, Publication No. SR-35, US Department of Health, Education and Welfare, National Institute for Occupational Safety and Health, Cincinnati

Joint Standing Committee on Health, Safety and Welfare in Foundries (1977) *Some Aspects of Pneumoconiosis in a Group of Mechanised Iron Foundries*, Health and Safety Executive, HMSO, London

Joint Standing Committee on Safety, Health and Welfare Conditions in Non-ferrous Foundries (1957) *Ministry of Labour and National Service. First Report*, HMSO, London

Jones, J.G., Owen, T.E. and Corrado, H.A. (1967) Respiratory tuberculosis and pneumoconiosis in slate workers. *Br. J. Dis. Chest* **61**, 138–143

Jones, R.N., Weill, H. and Ziskind, M. (1975) Pulmonary function in sandblasters' silicosis. *Bull. Physiopathol.* **11**, 589–595

Jones,R.N., Turner-Warwick, M., Ziskind, M. and Weill, H. (1976) High prevalence of antinuclear antibodies in sandblasters silicosis. *Am. Rev. Respir. Dis.* **113**, 393–395

Jones, R.N., Diem, J.E., Hughes, J.E., Hammad, Y.Y., Glindmeyer, H.W. and Weill, H. (1989) Progression of asbestos effects: a prospective longitudinal study of chest radiographs and lung function. *Br. J. Ind. Med.* **46**, 97–105

Kawakami, M., Sato, S. and Takishima, T. (1977) Silicosis in workers dealing with tonoko. *Chest* **75**, 635–639

Keers, R.Y. (1969) The treatment of silicotuberculosis. In: *Health Conditions in the Ceramic Industry* (ed. C.N. Davies), Pergamon, Oxford, pp. 63–69

Kennedy, M.C.S. (1956) Aluminium powder inhalations in the treatment of silicosis of pottery workers and pneumoconiosis of coal miners. *Br. J. Ind. Med.* **13**, 85–99

Kessel, R.W.I., Monaco, L. and Marchisio, M.A. (1963) The specificity of the cytotoxic action of silica: a study *in vitro. Br. J. Exp. Pathol.* **44**, 351–364

Kettle, E.H. (1932) The interstitial reactions caused by various dusts and their influence on tuberculous injections. *J. Pathol. Bacteriol.* **35**, 395–405

Khoo, O.T. and Toh, K.K. (1968) Morbidity of silicosis in Singapore. *Singapore Med. J.* **9**, 186–191

Klockars, M., Koskela, R-S., Jarvinen, E., Kolari, P.J. and Rossi, A. (1987) Silica exposure and rheumatoid arthritis: a follow-up study of granite workers, 1940–1981. *Br. Med. J. [Clin. Res].* **294**, 997–1000

Kolsterkötter, W. and Einbrodt, H.J. (1965) Quantitati tiexperimentelle Untersuchungen uber den Abtransport von Staub aus den Lugen in die regionalen Lymphknoten. *Archs Hyg.* **149**, 367–384

Kolev, K., Doitschinov, D. and Todorov, D. (1970) Morphologic alterations in the kidneys by silicosis. *Med. Lav.* **61**, 205–210

Koskinen, H., Tiilikainen, A. and Nordman, H. (1983) Increased prevalence of HLA-Aw19 and of the phenogroup Aw19, B18 in advanced silicosis. *Chest* **83**, 848–852

Kreiss, K., Danilovs, J.A. and Newman, L.S. (1989) Histocompatibility antigens in a population-based silicosis series. *Br. J. Ind. Med.* **46**, 364–369

Kuhn, C., Gyorkey, F., Levine, B.E. and Ramirez-Rivera, J. (1966) Pulmonary alveolar proteinosis: a study using enzyme histochemistry, electron microscopy and surface tension measurements. *Lab. Invest.* **15**, 492–509

Kung, V.A. (1979) Morphological investigations of fibrogenic action of Estonian oil shale dust. *Environ. Health Perspect.* **30**, 153–156

Kurppa, K., Gudbergsson, H., Hannunkari, I., Koskinen, H., Hernberg, S. and Lamvik, J. (1963) Rheumatoid pneumoconiosis. *Acta Pathol. Microbiol. Scand.* **57**, 169–174

Leading Article (1977) Balkan nephropathy. *Lancet* **1**, 683–684

Levene, C.I., Bye, I. and Saffiotti, U. (1968) The effect of beta-aminopropionitrile on silicotic pulmonary fibrosis. *Br. J. Exp. Pathol.* **49**, 152–158

Lewis, D.M. and Burrell, R. (1976) Induction of fibrogenesis by lung antibody-treated macrophages. *Br. J. Ind. Med.* **33**, 25–28

Lloyd Davies, T.A. (1971) *Respiratory Disease in Foundry Men. Report of a Survey*, HMSO, London

Lloyd Davies, T.A., Doig, A.T., Fox, A.J. and Greenberg, M. (1973) A radiographic survey of monumental masonry workers in Aberdeen. *Br. J. Ind. Med.* **30**, 227–231

Longley, E.O. (1970) Oesophageal compression due to silicotic mediastinal lymph glands. *Trans. Soc. Occup. Med.* **20**, 69

Luton, P., Champeix, J., Ravet, M. and Vallaud, A. (1956) Observations recentes sur la pneumoconiose parterre a diatomees. *Archs Mal. Prof. Med. Trav.* **17**, 125–148

Lynch, K.M. (1942) Silicosis of systemic distribution. *Am. J. Path.* **18**, 313–321

McDonald, G., Piggott, A.P. and Gilder, F.W. (1930) Two cases of acute silicosis with a suggested theory of causation. *Lancet* **2**, 846–848

McDonald, J.C. (1989) Silica, silicosis, and lung cancer. *Br. J. Ind. Med.* **46**, 289–291

McDonald, J.C. and Oakes, D. (1983) Exposure-response in miners exposed to silica. *VIth International Pneumoconiosis Conference, 1983*, Volume 1, ILO, Geneva

McDonald, J.C., Gibbs, G.W., Liddell, F.D.K. and McDonald, A.D. (1978) Mortality after long exposure to cummingtonite–grunerite. *Am. Rev. Respir. Dis.* **118**, 271–277

McLaughlin, A.I.G. (1957) Pneumoconiosis in foundry workers. *Br. J. Tuberc.* **51**, 297–309

McLaughlin, A.I.G. and Harding, H.E. (1956) Pneumoconiosis and other causes of death in iron and steel foundry workers. *Archs Ind. Health* **14**, 350–378

McTurk, L.C., Huis, C.H.W. and Eckardt, R.E. (1956) Health hazards of vanadium containing residual oil ash. *Ind. Med. Surg.* **25**, 29–36

Mallory, T.B. (1934) Case records of the Massachusetts General Hospital, Case 20102. *N. Engl. J. Med.* **210**, 551–554

Markovic, B.L. and Arambasic, M.D. (1971) Experimental chronic interstitial nephritis compared with endemic human nephropathy. *J. Pathol.* **103**, 35–40

Mehlhorn, J. (1984) Is scleroderma without silicosis also an occupational disease? *Z. Erkr. Atmungsorgane* **163**, 65–69

Meiklejohn, A. (1956) Silicosis and other fibrotic pneumonioses. In: *Industrial Medicine and Hygiene*, Volume 3 (ed. E.R.A. Merewether), Butterworths, London, p. 120

Middleton, D.L. (1930) Flint knapping. In: *Silicosis. Records of International Conference, Johannesburg, August, 1930*, International Labour Office, Geneva, pp. 478–479

Migueres, J., Layssol, M., Moreau, G., Jover, A. and Tricoire, J. (1966) Sclerodermie pulmonaire et silicose du spath fluor associee rapports entre sclerodermie et silicose. *J. fr. Med. Chir. Thorac.* **20**, 603–618

Moreschi, N., Farina, G. and Chiappinio, G. (1968) La silicosi pulmonaire calcificata. *Med. Lav.* **59**, 111–124

Morgan, E.J. (1979) Silicosis and tuberculosis. *Chest* **75**, 202–203

Morgan, W.K.C. (1975) The walrus and the carpenter, or the silica criteria standard. Commentary. *J. Occup. Med.* **17**, 782–783

Motley, H.L. (1960) Pulmonary function studies in diatomaceous earth workers. 2. A cross-section survey of 98 workers on the job. *Ind. Med. Surg.* **24**, 370–378

Motley, H.L., Smart, R.H. and Valero, A. (1956) Pulmonary function studies in diatomaceous earth workers. 1. Ventilatory and blood gas exchange disturbance. *Archs Ind. Health* **13**, 165–174

Muir, D.C.F., Julian, J.A., Shannon, H.S., Verma, D.K., Sebestyen, A. and Bernholz, C.D. (1989a) Silica exposure and silicosis among Ontario hardrock miners: III. Analysis and risk assessment. *Am. J. Ind. Med.* **16**, 29–43

Muir, D.C.F., Shannon, H.S., Julian, J.A., Verma, D.K., Sebestyen, A. and Bernholz, C.D. (1989b) Silica exposure and silicosis among Ontario hardrock miners: I. Methodology. *Am. J. Ind. Med.* **16**, 5–11

Muller, J., Wheeler, W.C. Gentleman, J.F., Suranyi, G. and Kusiak, R.A. (1983) *Study of Mortality of Ontario Miners, 1955–1977. Part I*, Toronto: Ontario Ministry of Labour/Ontario Workers' Compensation Board/Atomic Energy Control Board of Canada

Nagelschmidt, G. (1960) The relationship between lung dust and lung pathology in pneumoconiosis. *Br. J. Ind. Med.* **17**, 247–259

Nagelschmidt, G. (1965) A study of lung dust in pneumoconiosis. *Am. Ind. Hyg. Assoc. J.* **26**, 1–7

Nelson, H.M., Rajhans, G.S., Morton, S. and Brown, J.R. (1978) Silica flour exposures in Ontario. *Am. Ind. Hyg. Assoc. J.* **39**, 261–269

Ng, T.P., Allan, W.G.L., Tsin, T.W. and O'Kelly, F.J. (1985) Silicosis in jade workers. *Br. J. Ind. Med.* **42**, 761–764

Ng, T.P., Chan, S.L. and Lam, K.P. (1987) Radiological progression and lung function in silicosis: a ten-year follow-up study. *Br. Med. J.* **295**, 164–168

NIOSH: Silicosis and Silicate Diseases Committee (1988) Diseases associated with exposure to silica and non-fibrous silicate minerals. *Archs Pathol. Lab. Med.* **112**, 673–720

Norboo, T., Angchuk, P.T., Yahya, M., Kamat, S.R., Pooley, F.D., Corrin, B., Kerr, I.H., Bruce, N. and Ball, K.P. (1991) Silicosis in a Himalayan village population: role of environmental dust. *Thorax* **46**, 341–343

Nordman, H., Koskinen, H. and Froseth, B. (1984) Increased activity of serum angiotensin-converting enzyme in progressive silicosis. *Chest* **86**, 203–207

Nordmann, M. (1943) Die Staublunge der Kieselgurarbelter. *Virchows Arch. Pathol. Anat. Physiol.* **311**, 116–148

Notholt, A.J.G. and Highley, D.E. (1975) *Fluorspar, Mineral Dossier No. 1*, Mineral Resources Consultative Committee, HMSO, London

Oakes, D., Douglas, R., Knight, K., Wusteman, M. and McDonald, J.C. (1982) Respiratory effects of prolonged exposure to gypsum dust. *Ann. Occup. Hyg.* **26**, 833–840

Oechsli, W.R., Jacobson, G. and Brodeur, A.E. (1961) Diatomite pneumoconiosis: roentgen characteristics and classification.

AJR Am. J. Roentgenol. **85**, 263–270

Otto, H. (1969) Results of latex tests in 6,000 porcelain workers. In: *Health Conditions in the Ceramic Industry* (ed. C.N. Davies) Pergamon, Oxford, pp. 91–98

Palmer, P.E.S. and Daynes, G. (1967) Transkei silicosis. *S. Afr. Med. J.* **41**, 1182–1188

Palmhert, H., Webster, I. and Lens, C. (1968) Atypical mycobacteria and infections of the lung in the South Africa mining industry. *S. Afr. Pneumocon. Rev.* **3**, 6

Pancheri, G. and Zanetti, E. (1963) L'aspetto radiologico della silicosi da pomice (Liparosi). *Rass. Med. Ind.* **32**, 432–445

Paul, R. (1961) Silicosis in Northern Rhodesian copper mines. *Arch. Environ. Health* **2**, 96–109

Pendergrass, E.P. (1958) *The Pneumoconiosis Problem.* Thomas, Springfield, pp. 95–97

Pernis, B. (1968) Silicosis. In: *Textbook of Immunopathology*, Volume 1 (eds P.A. Meischer and H.J. Muller-Eberhardt) Grune and Stratton, New York, London, pp. 293–301

Pilkington, L.A.B. (1969) The float glass process. *Proc. R. Soc. Med.* **314**, 1–25

Plunkett, E.R. and De Witt, B.J. (1962) Occupational exposure to Hi-Sil and Silene. *Archs Environ. Health* **5**, 469–472

Polacheck, A.A. and Pijanowski, W.J. (1960) Extrathoracic egg-shell calcifications in silicosis. *Am. Rev. Respir. Dis.* **82**, 714–720

Policard, A. and Collet, A. (1952) Deposition of silicosis dust in the lungs of inhabitants of the Sahara regions. *Arch. Ind. Hyg. Occup. Med.* **5**, 527–534

Policard, A., Gernez-Rieux, C., Tacquet, A., Martin, J.C., Devulder, B. and Le Bouffant, L. (1967) Influence of pulmonary dust load on the development of experimental infection by *Mycobacteria kansasii. Nature, London* **216**, 177–178

Posner, E. (1960) Pneumoconiosis in makers of artificial grinding wheels, including a case of Caplan's Syndrome. *Br. J. Ind. Med.* **17**, 109–113

Posner, E. (1961) Pneumoconiosis and tuberculosis in the North Staffordshire pottery industry. *Symposium on Dust Control in the Pottery Industry*, Publication No. 27, British Ceramic Research Association, Stoke, pp. 5–18

Posner, E. and Kennedy, M.C.S. (1967) A further study of china biscuit placers in Stoke-on-Trent. *Br. J. Ind. Med.* **24**, 133–142

Power, T. (1985) Fused minerals – the high purity, high performance oxides. *Ind. Minerals* **214**, 37–57

Pratt, P. (1983) Lung dust content and response in guinea pigs inhaling three forms of silica. *Archs Environ. Health* **38**, 197–204

Prugger, F., Mallner, B. and Schlipkoter, H.W. (1984) Polyvinylpyridine N-oxide (Bay 3504, P-204, PVNO) in the treatment of human silicosis. *Wien. Klin. Wochenschr.* **96**, 848–853

Pump, K.K. (1968) Studies in silicosis of the human lung. *Dis. Chest* **53**, 237–246

Puntoni, R., Vercelli, M., Bonassi, S., Valerio, F., DiGiorgio, F., Ceppi, M., Stagnaro, E., Filiberti, R. and Santi, L. (1985) Prospective study of the mortality in workers exposed to silica [in Italian]. In *Silice, silicosi e cancro* (eds E.I. Deutsch and A. Marcato) University of Padua, Padua, pp. 79–92

Ramirez-R., J. (1971) Alveolar proteinosis: importance of pulmonary lavage. *Am. J. Respir. Dis.* **103**, 666–678

Rastogi, S.K., Gupta, B.N., Chandra, H., Marthur, N., Mahendra, P.N. and Husain, T. (1991) A study of the prevalence of respiratory morbidity among agate workers. *Occup. Environ. Health* **63**, 21–26

Reichel, G., Bauer, H-D. and Bruckmann, E. (1977) The action of quartz in the presence of iron hydroxides in the human lung. In: *Inhaled Particles and Vapours IV* (ed. W.H. Walton), Pergamon Press, Oxford, pp. 403–410

Riker, J.B. and Wolinsky, H. (1973) Trypsin aerosol treatment of pulmonary alveolar proteinosis. *Am. Rev. Respir. Dis.* **108**, 108–113

Rizzo, A., Agati, G., LoCoco, A. and Candela, L. (1968) Sulla pneumoconiosi da pomice aspetti di fuzionalita respiratoria. *Med. Lav.* **59**, 641–648

Roberts, W.C. (1965) The ferro-alloy industry: hazards of the alloys and semi-metallics. Part II. *J. Occup. Med.* **7**, 71–77

Rodnan, G.P., Benedek, T.G., Medsger, T.A. and Cammarata, R.J. (1967) The association of progressive systemic sclerosis (scleroderma) with coal miners pneumoconiosis and other forms of silicosis. *Ann. Intern. Med.* **66**, 323–334

Roeslin, N., Lassabe-Roth, C., Morand, G. and Batzenschlager, A. (1980) La silico-proteinose aigue. *Archs Mal. Prof.* **41**, 15–18

Rosen, S.H., Castleman, B. and Liebow, A.A. (1958) Pulmonary alveolar proteinosis. *N. Engl. J. Med.* **258**, 1123–1142

Rosenzweig, D.Y. (1967) Silicosis complicated by a typical mycobacterial infection. *Transactions of 26th VA–Armed Forces Pulmonary Disease Research Conference*, United States Government Printing Office, Washington, p. 47

Rowell, N.R. (1984) Systemic sclerosis. *J. R. Coll. Phys. London* **19**, 23–30

Rüttner, J.R. (1954) Foundry worker's pneumoconiosis in Switzerland (anthra-silicosis). *Archs Ind. Hyg.* **9**, 297–305

Salam, M.S.A., El-Samra, G.H., El-Alamy, M.A. and Gomaa, T. (1967) Pulmonary manifestations in workers exposed to dusts of synthetic detergents and abrasive soaps. *Ann. Occup. Hyg.* **10**, 105–112

Saldanha, L.F., Rosen, V.J. and Gonick, H.C. (1975) Silicon nephropathy. *Am. J. Med.* **59**, 95–103

Samimi, B., Weill, H. and Ziskind, M. (1974) Respirable silica dust exposure of sandblasters and associated workers in steel fabrication yards. *Archs Environ. Health* **29**, 61–66

Scadding, J.G. and Mitchell, D.N. (1985) *Sarcoidosis*, 2nd edn. Chapman and Hall, London, pp. 151–159

Schepers, G.W.H., Delahant, A.B., Schmidt, J.G., von Wecheln, J.C., Creedon, F.T. and Clark, R.W. (1957a) The biological action of Degussa submicron silica dust (Dow Corning silica), 3. *Archs Ind. Health* **16**, 280–301

Schepers, G.W.H. Durkan, T.M., Delahant, A.B., Creedon, F.T. and Redlin, A.J. (1957b) The biological action of Degussa submicron silica dust (Dow Corning silica), 1. *Archs Ind. Health* **16**, 125–146

Schneider, H. (1966) Silikosegefahrrdung durch Neuburger Kieselkreide. *Int. Arch. Gewerbepath. Gewerbehyg.* **22**, 323–341

Schuyler, M., Ziskind, M. and Salvaggio, J. (1977) Cell-mediated immunity in silicosis. *Am. Rev. Respir. Dis.* **116**, 147–151

Seaton, A., Lamb, D., Browne, W.R., Sclare, G. and Middleton, W.G. (1981) Pneumoconiosis in shale miners. *Thorax* **36**, 412–418

Seaton, A., Ruckley, V.A., Addison, J. and Brown, W.R. (1986) Silicosis in barium miners. *Thorax* **41**, 591–595

Selikoff, I.J. (1978) Carcinogenic potential of silica compounds. In: *Biochemistry of Silicon and Related Problems* (eds G. Bendz and I. Lindquist), Plenum, New York, pp. 311–336

Slater, D. (1973) *Tungsten*, Mineral Dossier No. 5, Mineral Resources Consultative Committee, HMSO, London

Sluis-Cremer, G.K. and Maier, G. (1984) HLA antigens of the A and B locus in relation to the development of silicosis. *Br. J. Ind. Med.* **41**, 417–418

Sluis-Cremer, G.K., Hessel, P.A., Hnizdo, E., Churchill, A.R. and

Zeiss, E.A. (1985) Silica, silicosis, and progressive systemic sclerosis. *Br. J. Ind. Med.* **42**, 838–843

Sluis-Cremer, G.K., Hessel, P.A., Hnizdo, E. and Churchill, A.R. (1986) Relationship between silicosis and rheumatoid arthritis. *Thorax* **41**, 596–601

Smart, R.H. and Anderson, W.H. (1952) Pneumoconiosis due to diatomaceous earth. Clinical and x-ray aspects. *Ind. Med. Surg.* **21**, 509–518

Sosman, R.B. (1965) *The Phases of Silica*, Rutgers University Press, New Jersey

South African Medical Research Council (1974) *Biological Effects of South African Minerals, Fourth Annual Report*, National Research Institute for Occupational Disease, Johannesburg, p. 19

Spain, D.M. (1965) Editorial to diatomaceous earth pneumoconiosis by F.R. Dutra (1965). *Archs Environ. Health* **11**, 619

Steenland, K. and Beaumont, J. (1986) A proportionate mortality study of granite cutters. *Am. J. Ind. Med.* **9**, 189–201

Stewart, M.J. and Faulds, J.S. (1934) Pulmonary fibrosis in hematite miners. *J. Pathol. Bacteriol.* **39**, 233–253

Suratt, P.J., Winn, W.C. Jr, Brody, A.R., Bolton, W.K. and Giles, R.D. (1977) Acute silicosis in tombstone sandblasters. *Am. Rev.Respir. Dis.* **115**, 521–529

Sweany, H.C., Porsche, J.D. and Douglass, J.R. (1936) Chemical and pathological study of pneumoconiosis with special emphasis on silicosis and silico-tuberculosis. *Archs Pathol.* **22**, 593–633

Swensson, A. (1967) Tissue reaction to different types of amorphous silica. In: *Inhaled Particles and Vapours II* (ed. C.N. Davies), Pergamon Press, Oxford, pp. 95–102

Swensson, A., Kvarnstrom, K., Bruce, T., Edling, N.P.G. and Glomme, J. (1971) Pneumoconiosis in ferrosilicon workers – a follow-up study. *J. Occup. Med.* **13**, 427–432

Tada, S., Yasukochi, H., Shida, H., Chiyotani, K., Saito, K., Mishina, M. and Kozuka, Y. (1974) Bronchial arteriography in silicosis. *AJR Am. J. Roentgenol.* **120**, 810–814

Tebbens, B.D. and Beard, R.R. (1957) Experiments on diatomaceous earth pneumoconiosis. 1. Natural diatomaceous earth in guinea pigs. *Archs Ind. Health* **16**, 55–63

Teculescu, D.B. and Stanescu, D.C. (1970) Carbon monoxide transfer factor for the lung in silicosis. *Scand. J. Respir. Dis.* **51**, 150–159

Thiruvengadam, K.V., Anguli, V.C., Shetty, P., Sanibandam, S. and Kosairam, R. (1968) Silicosis in a mica-mine worker. *J. Indian Med. Assoc.* **51**, 248–250

Thomas, T.L. (1982) A preliminary investigation of mortality among workers in the pottery industry. *Int. J. Epidemiol.* **11**, 175–180

Turner-Warwick, M., Cole, P., Weill, H., Jones, R.N. and Ziskind, M. (1977) Chemical fibrosis: the model of silica. *Ann. Rheumat. Dis.* **36** (supplement), 47–50

Uehlinger, E. (1946) Ubermischstaubpneumo-Koniosen. *Schweiz. Z. Path. Bakt.* **9**, 692–700

Department of Health, Education and Welfare (1974) *Criteria for a Recommended Standard. Occupational Exposure to Crystalline Silica.* National Institute for Occupational Safety and Health (NIOSH), pp. 75–120

Utidjian, H.M.D. (1975) Recommendations for a crystalline silica standard. Criteria documents. *J. Occup. Med.* **17**, 775–781

Vallyathan, V., Shi, X., Dalal, N.S., Irr, W. and Castranova, V. (1988) Generation of free radicals from freshly fractured silica dust. *Am. Rev. Respir. Dis.* **138**, 1213–1219

Verma, D.K., Sebestyen, A., Julian, J.A., Muir, D.C.F., Schmidt, H., Bernholz, C.D. and Shannon, H.S. (1989) Silica exposure and silicosis among Ontario hardrock miners: II. Exposure estimates. *Am. J. Ind. Med.* **16**, 13–28

Vidone, R.A., Hoffmann, L., Hukill, P.B., Nesbitt, K.A. and McMahon, F.J. (1966) The diagnosis of pulmonary alveolar proteinosis by sputum examination. *Dis. Chest* **49**, 326–332

Vigliani, E.C. and Mottura, G. (1948) Diatomaceous earth silicosis. *Br. J. Ind. Med.* **5**, 148–160

Violante, B., Brusasco, V. and Buccheri, G. (1986) Exercise testing in radiologically-limited, simple pulmonary silicosis. *Chest* **90**, 411–415

Vitums, V.C., Edwards, M.J., Niles, N.R., Borman, J.O. and Lowry, R.D. (1977) Pulmonary fibrosis from amorphous silica dust, a product of silica vapour. *Archs Environ. Health* **32**, 62–68

Volk, H. (1960) The health of workers in a plant making highly dispersed silica. *Archs Environ. Health* **1**, 125–128

Vorwald, A.J., Durkan, T.M., Pratt, P.C. and Delahant, A.B. (1949) Diatomaceous earth pneumoconiosis. In: *Proceedings of the Ninth International Congress on Industrial Medicine, Bristol*, Wright, Bristol, pp. 726–741

Wagner, J.C. and McCormick, J.N. (1967) Immunological investigations of coal workers' disease. *J. R. Coll. Physns Lond.* **2**, 49–56

Wagner, W.D., Fraser, D.A., Wright, P.G., Dobrogorski, O.J. and Stokinger, H.E. (1968) Experimental evaluation of the threshold limit of cristobalite-calcined diatomaceous earth. *Am. Ind. Hyg. Assoc. J.* **19**, 211–221

Warrell, D.A., Harrison, B.D.W., Fawcett, I.W., Mohammed, Y., Mohammed, W.S., Pope, H.M. and Watkins, B.J. (1975) Silicosis among grindstone cutters in North Nigeria. *Thorax* **30**, 389–398

Weaver, N.K. and Gibson, R.L. (1979) The U.S. oil shale industry: a health perspective. *Am. Ind. Hyg. Assoc. J.* **40**, 460–467

Weller, W. (1977) Long-term test on rhesus monkeys for the PVNO-therapy of anthraco-silicosis. In: *Inhaled Particles and Vapours IV* (ed. W.H. Walton), Pergamon Press, Oxford, pp. 379–386

Westerholm, P., Ahlmark, A., Maasing, R. and Segelberg, I. (1986) Silicosis and risk of lung cancer or lung tuberculosis: a cohort study. *Environ. Res.* **41**, 339–350

World Health Organization (1968) *Pneumoconiosis. Report on the Katowice Symposium, 1967*. Copenhagen: WHO Regional Office for Europe

Xipell, J.M., Ham, K.N., Price, C.G. and Thomas, D.P. (1977) Acute silicoproteinosis. *Thorax* **32**, 104–111

Zaidi, S.H. (1969) *Experimental Pneumoconiosis*, The Johns Hopkins Press, Baltimore, pp. 113–117

Zeigler, V., Pampel, W., Zschunke, E., Munzberger, H., Mahrlein, W. and Kopping, H. (1982) Kristalliner Quarz-(eine) Ursache der progressiven Sklerodermie? *Dermatol. Monatsschr.* **168**, 398–401

Zimmerman, P.V. and Sinclair, R.A. (1977) Rapidly progressive fatal silicosis in a young man. *Med. J. Aust.* **2**, 704–706

Ziskind, M.M., Jones, R.N. and Weill, H. (1976) Silicosis: state of the art. *Am. Rev. Respir. Dis.* **113**, 643–665

Ziskind, M.M., Weill, H., Anderson, A.E., Samimi, B., Neilson, A. and Waggenspack, C. (1976) Silicosis in shipyard sandblasters. *Environ. Res.* **11**, 237–243

13

Pneumoconiosis associated with coal and other carbonaceous materials

W. Raymond Parkes

Although this chapter does not follow the usual systematic order of carbon science it is convenient, in the present context, to discuss coal and its combustion products before other forms of solid carbon that are important to industry. The order in which the materials are presented is as follows:

Coal and its derivatives:
  Pulverized fuel and its ash
  Pitches and cokes
  Furnace slag
Graphite: natural and synthetic
  Composite graphites
Other carbon materials:
  Carbon blacks
  Carbon electrodes
  Activated carbon
  Mesocarbon microbeads
  Carbon fibres

For the interested reader a useful introductory text to carbon science is given by Marsh (1989).

Solid carbons are derived from organic precursors by *carbonization*, that is, 'formation of material with increasing carbon content from organic material, usually by pyrolysis, ending with an almost pure carbon residue at temperatures up to 1600 K [about 1330°C]' (Edwards, 1989). By contrast coal, which is mainly of vegetable origin, is part of a gradually formed sedimentary series ranging from peat, through lignites, sub-bituminous and bituminous coals to anthracite with time and rising temperature, and with increasing depth and tectonic pressure.

Coal

The degree of coalification that occurs with time is defined, among other things, by the carbon : hydrogen ratio and by reflectance (the amount of light reflected from coal macerals). The carbon content increases progressively from peat through various stages to anthracites. Increased maturity is expressed in terms of *rank:* the *higher the rank* the greater the maturity of the coal and its content of carbon (anthracite); the *lower the rank*, the more this relationship is inverted and the greater the content of non-coal minerals including volatile substances (bituminous, sub-bituminous coals and lignite). More details are provided in Appendix I (page 852), but it should be noted here that, although there are different methods of measuring rank, for medical research purposes it is usually expressed in terms of relative amounts of coal (carbon) and non-coal minerals in coal samples or seams.

Thus, amounts of quartz are relatively low in coals of high rank (about 2.2 to 3.8 per cent), but are substantially higher (up to 30 per cent or more) in coals of lower rank (lignite and sub-bituminous), although this varies according to geographical location (Raask, 1985). Chalcedony and cristobalite are also present in some coals (Swaine, 1990) but not in the UK. In addition, adjacent strata between coal seams (sandstone, shales and the like) may contribute significant quantities of quartz to dust in the mines, but this, too, is a very variable factor. The

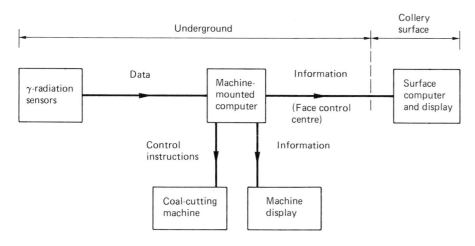

Figure 13.1 Diagram showing the relationship of radiation sensors and computer equipment mounted on coal-cutting machines, and the distribution of data received. Separate information of underground conditions (for example, levels of oxides of nitrogen and methane) are also relayed to the surface computer by the MINOS system (see text for details). (Courtesy of the Director of Research and Scientific Services, British Coal Corporation)

mineral (non-coal) content of coal-mine dust – that is, quartz, muscovite-illites, kaolinite and other silicates – has, in fact, been shown to vary markedly, not only between samples in different collieries, but also in the same colliery and the same coal seams. Furthermore, pronounced differences occur in samples taken in the same sites at different times some months apart: for example, at one coal face the level of quartz increased from 2.1 to 15.7 per cent; at another, kaolin and mica fell from 39.3 to 10.8 per cent (Gormley et al., 1980). Such variations are almost certainly relevant to the manner in which non-coal minerals affect the pathogenesis of coal pneumoconiosis (see 'Pathogenesis' later).

A wide range of trace elements which differ greatly in different geological regions may also be present – although in very small amounts – in all except some low-rank coals; there are also variations within the seams of different stratigraphic sequence as well as lateral and vertical differences in one particular seam (Swaine, 1990). However, they probably have no biological significance to the lungs (see page 374).

Coal mining

Coal is obtained underground by driving tunnels to the face of the coal seam. In Britain and continental Europe it is extracted from long, narrow ('longwall') coal faces which are advanced between parallel entry and exit tunnels on either side of the face. In the USA this method is replacing less

efficient 'room and pillar' mining in which solid pillars of uncut coal are left between communicating tunnels to support the roof as the face is advanced. Dust conditions produced by these two methods differ. Mechanical shearing and cutting machines, introduced in Britain in the 1960s, replaced the old 'pick and shovel' and hand-powered drills by the end of that decade.

However, a disadvantage of mechanical methods has, until recently, been that machines, unlike coal miners, do not distinguish between rock intrusions and coal so that, in some mines, more quartz was contributed to the atmosphere than by hand-derived methods. This potential hazard is now much reduced by important technological advances such as the introduction of the 'Integrated Face' to British coal mines. In this system, coal-cutting machines, which 'sit over' and travel along open armoured conveyor belts, are equipped with sensors that detect differences in the levels of natural γ-radiation that emanate from coal seams and from intervening non-coal strata. The information, passed to a computer mounted on the machine, displays some data on the machine itself and gives it control instructions by calculating the position of its cutting elements relative to the roof of the seam, thus preventing non-coal rock from being cut by directing these elements to a predetermined horizon. It relays all the data to a single computer system – the Face Control Centre – on the mine surface for further display and analysis (Figure 13.1) (D. J. Buchanan, 1991, personal communication). The coal face is extended ('developed') by the machine driving a roadway at a height usually greater than the thickness of the coal seam. In addition, the quality of coal, both underground and on the surface in coal preparation plants, is similarly monitored by evaluation of differences in γ-radiation, thereby quantifying and controlling non-coal minerals.

Although, theoretically, a pulse laser can cut coal, this is not practical in that its energy is focused on a very small area, and the power needed for cutting would not meet the safety requirements of coal mining (D. J. Buchanan, 1991, personal communication).

Cut coal is collected on the conveyor belts and transported to trucks drawn on a railway by diesel or electrical locomotives. Continuous integrity of, and access to, the coal face was, until recent years, maintained by workers who made new underground roadways ('developers'), increased the height of the 'roof' and erected supports ('rippers'), increased the dimensions of other roadways and airways ('dinters') or kept roadways in good repair ('repairers'). Variable amounts of 'stone' dust were produced, the composition of which differed according to the type of rock intrusion: shale being usual and sandstone common. However, many of these operations are now mechanized. In general, concentrations of dust are very low in haulage roadways and in the vicinity of the pit-shaft bottom.

Until recently the development of longwall seams involved placing and firing explosive charges (Hydrox shells) in bore holes ('shot-firing') which give rise to a local, transitory presence of oxides of nitrogen. All personnel withdrew from the environment during, and for a period after, firing. However, this practice has now been largely replaced by methods that do not involve explosives. The possibility that nitrogen dioxide from this source and in exhaust emissions from diesel engines underground might cause chronic airways' obstruction was suggested by Kennedy (1972), but has not been substantiated (see Chapter 18, 'Oxides of nitrogen: mining', page 621).

In the last 25 years exposure to dust in British coal mines has been greatly reduced by increasingly efficient bulk circulation of air along tunnels and faces, improved water infusion and the use of efficient, disposable, personal respirators.

Nowadays, in British collieries, an automatic monitoring system – known as environmental MINOS (Mine Information Operating System) – distinct from that described earlier, detects the presence of gases and assesses other important underground conditions (such as the state of conveyor belts) by a variety of sensors linked to a communications unit which transmits their data to the MINOS computer on the surface for analysis and display (Figure 13.1). Measurement of dust levels is carried out separately, throughout work shifts, at strategic points in the mine.

Opencast mining

Coal from seams close to the surface is obtained by large capacity shovels and excavators. Although the operations are often dusty, individual exposure is usually relatively low. However, the uncovering of coal seams requires removal of overlying strata, first by the drilling of holes with large, mobile drill-rigs (the drill operators being seated in cabs close to the drills), and then by explosive charges placed in the holes to break up the overburden. This is removed by heavy, earth-moving equipment. If the overlying rock is siliceous (as, for example, in West Virginia, USA), drill-crew members are at risk of developing silicosis, whereas the coal miners who follow on these operations are at little risk (Banks et al., 1983).

Colliery surface work

Miners who work as sorters on the 'screens' (that is, conveyors carrying coal) remove shale and rock, and break and grade the coal by hand. Dust concentrations are low and ventilation is good.

Coal trimming

This involved loading, stowing and levelling of coal, previously washed with water, in the holds and bunkers of ships and in large stores where concentrations of dust were high. In latter years this practice has been replaced by mechanical methods. Pneumoconiosis among trimmers was first described by Collis and Gilchrist (1928) and its pathology by Gough (1940). It has often been supposed, but wrongly, that washing coal frees it of non-coal minerals; in fact, much of the mineral matter is so intimately mixed with coal material that, unless the coal is very finely ground, this matter is inaccessible to water. Thus, in practice, washing coal with water does not remove finely disseminated mineral matter (quartz and clay silicates) from within the coal itself or extraneous matter attached to it, although, of course, it does free it of run-of-mine dirt and, to that extent, it is cleaned (J. W. Patrick, 1991, personal communication; see 'Pathogenesis', page 368 and Appendix I, page 854).

Uses of coals

Raw coal for domestic heating now has a greatly limited use because of the undesirable products of combustion, and has been replaced by several commercial types of smokeless fuels produced by its carbonization at low temperatures. The industrial combustion of coal generates much ash, and its industrial carbonization produces coal-tar, coal-tar pitch and metallurgical cokes.

Pulverized fuel ash

Pulverized bituminous (high ash) coals have been burned in coal-fired power stations in place of lump coal for about 50 years. Coal is conveyed from dumps to ball mills which grind the coal to fine size to give particles ranging from 1 to 200 μm, 70 per cent being less than 80 μm. This fine powder is blown into boilers to be burnt as jets of air-borne particles at temperatures around 1600°C. About 80 per cent of the original inorganic matter present in the coal is collected as pulverized fuel ash (PFA) in electrostatic precipitators. The remainder of the ash leaves the boiler as a fused slag via the ash hopper. Most of the PFA is removed before it reaches the smoke stack – some 99.8 per cent in modern power stations in the UK and North America (Bonnell, Schilling and Massey, 1980). Ash that escapes into the stack is commonly called *fly ash*, that is, 'the solid material extracted by electrical or mechanical means from flue gases of a boiler fired with pulverized coal' (Swaine, 1990).

As a result of the high temperature of combustion, most of the constituents of the ash are fused forming spherical particles of aluminosilicate which make up 60 to 80 per cent of its weight. These 'microspheres', approximately 8 to 10 μm in diameter, are composed of quartz, mullite and magnetite particles in a vitreous matrix. A small percentage of unburnt carbon char is usually present (Figure 13.2). Thus, free particles of quartz are very rarely present. The enveloping glass can be dissolved, or etched, by hydrochloric or hydrofluoric acids (Hulett et al., 1980). A water-soluble fraction of PFA particles (2 to 4 per cent of its weight) consists of calcium, sodium and potassium sulphates in a soluble glassy phase with a rough-appearing surface (Raask and Schilling, 1980). The mean particle size of gas-borne ash which reaches electrostatic precipitators is smaller than that of the bulk PFA and ranges from 0.5 to 5 μm (Raask, 1985). Although temperatures are well in excess of 1470°C they are too short-lived ('flash' temperatures) to convert quartz – the content of which ranges from 1 to 9 per cent (Schilling et al., 1988) – to tridymite or cristobalite (see Appendix I, page 842). Indeed, little if any, is melted, but its enclosure in a glassy envelope renders it non-fibrogenic. The high combustion temperatures also destroy the polycyclic aromatic hydrocarbons evolved during devolatilization of the coal, so that they do not present a hazard.

The handling of PFA is chiefly mechanical and plants are enclosed. Nevertheless, some of the ash

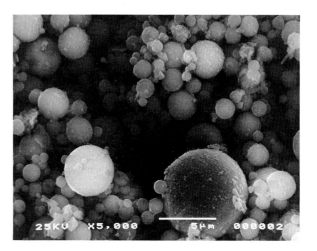

Figure 13.2 Typical scanning electron micrograph appearances of particles of PFA produced by burning coal in a UK power station. White scale bar: 5 μm. (Courtesy of Drs F. Wigley and F. Williamson, Imperial College, London)

may escape to be deposited, sometimes in fairly large quantity, on near-by surfaces. Electrical and mechanical maintenance fitters (especially of precipitators) are, thus, most likely to be exposed. In general, boilers are cleaned by remote control methods, although some of this work is still done manually (Bonnell, Schilling and Massey, 1980). However, it must be borne in mind that many power station workers have been exposed to the dust of silica bricks (containing varying quantities of quartz, tridymite and cristobalite) used, until recently, for the refractory lining of boilers, and to the dust of asbestos from periodic stripping and repairing of lagging by insulation workers in their vicinity (see Chapter 14).

PFA is used in Portland–pozzolanic cements, for lightweight aggregates, abrasives and ceramics, in the manufacture of breeze blocks and cements for road surfaces and, since the mid-1970s, as a filler in asbestos–cement products where it constitutes 10 to 13 per cent of the ingredients. However, it is most extensively employed for land-fill material.

The amount of mullite in the ash may be substantial and undoubtedly explains its presence, often in considerable quantity, in the lungs of boiler men and other workers at coal-fired power stations, and is probably the chief reason for it being found in the lungs of some insulation and other asbestos workers. Mullite, which has valuable refractory properties itself, is normally manufactured by heating aluminium silicates to high temperatures in electric-arc furnaces (see Chapter 16, 'Mullite', page 554).

Pitches

These consist of carbonaceous materials derived from mixtures of organic precursors produced, usually by heating, from coal-tar and petroleum residues. Asphalt, a carbonaceous rock, is discussed briefly in Chapter 12 and Appendix I.

Coal-tar pitches

Coal-tar pitches are a product of heating bituminous coals to yield cokes (see next section). They form the residue of distillation or pyrolysis of coal-tar (after creosote and anthracene oil fractions have been removed), and are mixtures of several hundred organic compounds (including aromatic hydrocarbons such as benzopyrenes and benz[α]anthracene); their exact composition and properties vary according to the original tar and the method of extraction of the low-molecular-weight species (Rand, Hosty and West, 1989). Because they are formed by volatilization, followed by condensation of coal organic matter, the pitches are unlikely to contain quartz. However, in some working practices, fine particulate matter may be 'carried over' into the by-product plant during the charging of coke ovens, but the amount of quartz will be extremely small – probably no more than trace amounts (J. W. Patrick, 1991, personal communication).

Coal-tar pitch and coal-tar are widely used in industry because of their binding properties, for example, in the manufacture of electrodes and of briquettes for industrial heating; in products for road surfaces and flat-topped roofs, and waterproofing pipes and tanks; and for impregnation of bricks for blast and other types of furnace (Moulin et al., 1989).

Petroleum pitches

As a rule, these are produced from the residues of cracking naphtha and gas oils, or of the distillation and refining of crude oil by a variety of methods including thermal and vacuum treatments. Their chemical and physical properties, as for those of coal-tar pitch, depend, in particular, upon the degree and duration of heating. In general, they contain much smaller amounts of aromatic hydrocarbons than coal-tar pitches (Rand, Hosty and West, 1989).

In one form or another, petroleum pitches are essential precursors to the fabrication of a whole variety of carbon and graphite artefacts which are referred to subsequently under the appropriate headings. The process usually involves combining a coke filler material (derived from the carbonization of petroleum pitches or coal-tar pitches by the delayed coking process) with coal-tar pitch as a binder.

Cokes

A variety of cokes is produced for different specialized purposes by heating coals and petroleum pitch. Blends of bituminous coals heated to about 1100°C in an 18- to 24-hour cycle in byproduct coke ovens form 'hard' *metallurgical coke* for blast furnaces and foundries. The properties of coke are standardized by the composition of the average rank of the blend of coals employed and by carbonization temperatures, rate of heating and the design of ovens (Patrick and Clarke, 1989). Despite modern methods of cleaning coal, coke oven charges still contain non-coal mineral matter associated with coal, that is, quartz and the silicon-rich clay minerals kaolinite, illite (hydrous mica), montmorillonite and chlorite, sometimes sericite or biotite micas, and feldspar (J. W. Patrick, 1991, personal communication) (see Appendix I, 'Beneficiation of coal'). Because the highest temperatures involved are around 1100°C (the maximum temperature attained in the production of oven coke), resultant cokes contain much of the quartz of the original coal with little, if any, alteration to tridymite because the time required for it to form is longer than that of the normal coke oven operation; in fact, tridymite has not been detected in metallurgical coke at room temperature (J. W. Patrick, 1991, personal communication). However, tridymite is formed in refractory silica bricks lining the ovens because they are subjected to these temperatures for prolonged periods and held within its stability range of 867 to 1470°C (see Appendix I). Thus, it is present in the oven dust; in fact, coke ovens have been a good source of tridymite (Sosman, 1965).

The slag of iron-making blast furnaces, which is drawn off at higher temperatures of 1400 to 1675°C, is likely to contain some cristobalite and mullite. It is used in Portland cement concrete, as well as in bituminous mixtures of all types and as a component in the production of fibreglass (see Chapters 11, page 274 and 16, page 561).

During the coke process vapours containing various polycyclic aromatic hydrocarbons (PAHs), such as benzo[α]pyrene and 2-naphthylamine, with carcinogenic potential may be evolved. Workers on coke ovens and in tar distillation plants have been found to have an increased mortality from carcinoma of the lung and non-malignant respiratory disease (Swaen et al., 1991). This relationship, which is far from simple, is discussed in more detail in Chapter 19. Measurement of a urinary metabolite of PAHs, 1-hydroxypyrene, has, incidently, been found to be a reliable indicator of total exposure to PAHs (British Coal Medical Service, 1992).

Lignite

This term denotes a number of different substances which, with regard to carbonization, fall midway between peat and bituminous coal. The rock is widely distributed in the western USA and Europe, and is mined by opencast methods. It is normally compact and dull black, and contains variable, often considerable, quantities of detrital quartz (see Appendix I, 'Carboniferous rocks: coal'). Lignite is used for the production of activated carbons. It is of interest to recall that *jet*, a particularly hard, compact and black form of lignite which is not laminated, has little tendency to split and takes a brilliant polish, and was worked in Britain from prehistoric times until some 50 years ago for jewellery, ornaments and buttons. It was a very prosperous industry in Whitby, Yorkshire, until the fashion for jet declined and it was replaced by coloured plastic. It is possible that silicosis or 'mixed dust fibrosis' may have occurred in workers cutting, lathing and polishing the rock.

Graphite

Graphite is an allotropic form of elemental carbon, either natural or synthetic, with a high crystallographic order that differentiates it from non-graphitic carbons. Non-graphitic, but graphitizable, carbons can be converted into graphitic carbons by pyrolysis at temperatures in excess of 2200°C. This transformation ('graphitization') involves a progressive increase in its molecular order, the degree of which is dominantly determined by temperature. Synthetic graphite is also produced by chemical vapour deposition of hydrocarbons at temperatures in excess of 1800°C (Edwards, 1989).

Natural graphite

Known also as *plumbago*, this is elemental crystalline carbon mixed with a variety of mineral impurities. When the crystals are visible to the naked eye it is called 'flake' graphite; when they are small, or cryptocrystalline, it is known as 'amorphous' graphite. Most commercial natural graphites are flake graphites that contain other minerals. Graphite is widely distributed geographically in igneous, sedimentary and metamorphic rocks; the most important commercial flake graphite occurs in metamorphic siliceous sediments (as in Sri Lanka, Madagascar, Madras and Brazil). Its principal impurities are the other minerals of the enclosing schistose rocks: quartz, mica, feldspar and clay. When mined, therefore, it contains variable quantities of quartz: 3.6 to 10 per cent 'free silica' has been reported in samples from Sri Lanka, Korea and south-west Africa (Harding and Oliver, 1949), about 11 to 13 per cent in samples of Italian graphite (Parmeggiani, 1950; Casalone and Rasetti, 1963), and 5.24 per cent in samples from Pennsylvania (Ladoo and Myers, 1951). But the quartz content of graphite ash can be as high as 30 to 52 per cent (Casalone and Rasetti, 1963; Holt, 1987). Iron oxides and other minerals (including tremolite in Sri Lanka) may also be present although these vary considerably in different deposits.

Uses

Refractory ceramics and crucibles

Graphite is very resistant to thermal shock.

Natural flake graphite mixed with various proportions of bond clay and sand is used to make blast furnace hearths and linings, and, with the addition of china clay, to make crucibles and ladles for the chemical and non-ferrous metallurgical industries. The preparation of these materials and subsequent trimming of the products before firing were, until recently (and in some instances may still be), very dusty processes. It is evident that there was a possibility of exposure to quartz dust as well as to graphite (see under 'Pathology'). These ingredients have been replaced to a large extent by artificial graphite, bitumen and certain metals.

Natural graphite has many applications in rockets, missiles, furnaces and moulds.

Foundry facings

Pulverized natural graphite is mixed with sand, clay or talc to give a smooth surface to the mould sand before molten metal is added. It is important in the casting of bells.

Steel and cast iron manufacture

Flake graphite is used to increase the hardness and strength of the metal.

Pencils

Natural graphite of high purity is mixed in varying proportions with clays to produce 'leads' of different hardness. The wet mix is extruded through dies and fired. The famous mines in Borrowdale, Cumberland, which produced graphite solely for this purpose and started in the sixteenth century, were exhausted early in this. Graphite from Texas and Sri Lanka is now commonly used.

Lubricants

Natural graphite of high purity is used after being ground to a fine powder and either mixed with oil or employed untreated.

Brake linings

Natural graphite is used for heavy duty vehicles.

Synthetic graphite

Graphitization is defined as 'solid-state transformation of thermodynamically unstable, non-graphitic carbon into graphite by thermal activation' (Edwards, 1989). Cokes produced from petroleum pitch (a residue from heat treatment and distillation of petroleum fractions) are more anisotropic and, hence, more 'graphitizable' than coal-derived cokes, and relatively free from mineral matter impurities. A highly anisotropic 'needle coke' (with long unidirectional needles) is used to manufacture graphite electrodes, nuclear-grade graphite and aerospace components.

Green (that is, raw) petroleum coke is first calcined in kilns and ground in crushers and sized in mesh screens. Sized coke is mixed with solid pitch binder and heated at 150 to 160°C, cooled and shaped into rods and more massive electrodes or blocks (Figure 13.3). These shapes are then packed in waste coke powder or silica sand (as insulation) in sagger or bulk-bake furnaces, and heated at about 1400°C for 90 to 120 days. On carbonization the pitch generates a second carbon phase bonding together what, in essence, becomes a particulate composite material. This is then impregnated with liquid pitch at high pressure and higher temperature than previously (that is, autoclaved) to increase its strength and electrical conductivity, and the carbonization–graphitization process is consolidated by heating at about 3000°C, thus yielding composite graphite (Rand, Hosty and West, 1989). Finally, the graphite shapes are lathed and planed.

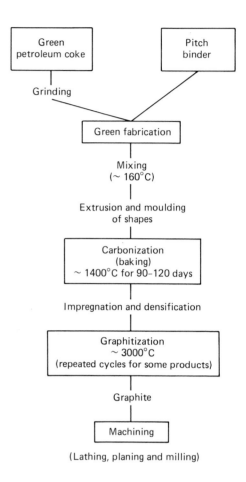

Figure 13.3 Flow diagram of production of granular carbons/graphites. (Modified from Rand, Hosty and West, 1989, with permission)

The grinding and mixing stages, graphitization and machining of the finished products have, over the years, been dirty and dusty and, despite advances in dust control measures, have remained so until recent years (Petsonk et al., 1988). In particular, dust-containing coke, mullite, quartz and, possibly, cristobalite or tridymite may be produced from the insulation materials during the packing and unpacking of shapes at the baking stage. After being heated to high temperatures silica sand recrystallizes (see Appendix I, 'The principal phases of silica'). However, mineral inclusions in the resulting graphite products are very low – at the milligram per kilogram (mg/kg) level – but not absent (H. Marsh, 1991, personal communication).

Coal-tar pitch vapour and polycyclic aromatic hydrocarbons (PAHs) as dust or vapour, or both, may be evolved at different stages of the process, although amounts vary in different plants (Moulin et al., 1989).

Asbestos may be present in insulation cloths and refractory materials in the kiln and furnace areas.

Uses

The advantage of manufactured graphite is that abrasive mineral inclusions can be carefully controlled.

Graphite electrodes

These, often of massive size, are capable of carrying heavy electric currents under great thermal stress. They are important in the production of steel, in the fused mineral industry where they are deployed in two- or three-phase electrode systems (in particular for electrofused alumina, silica, magnesia, zirconia and mullite) (Power, 1985), and in the chemical industry.

Neutron moderators

Large blocks of graphite of high chemical purity are used as neutron moderators in atomic reactors to impede low energy neutrons.

Milled graphite

This is employed either alone, or as a component, for lubricants of high purity.

Graphite miners (notably in Sri Lanka) may develop pneumoconiosis after some 15 to 20 years in the industry (Dassanayake, 1948; Ranasinha and Uragoda, 1972). Grinding, mixing and bagging graphite is a potential source of high concentrations of dust often containing significant quantities of quartz; as much as 52 per cent silica was recorded in the dust of the workplace air of a factory using natural graphite as a lubricant in the manufacture of steel pipes (Casalone and Rasetti, 1963). Today, dust control measures are applied and, in most large industries, are very efficient. Pneumoconiosis both in discrete and progressive massive fibrosis forms is well documented among natural graphite workers (Faulkner, 1940; Dunner and Bagnall, 1949; Gloyne, Marshall and Hoyle, 1949; Parmeggiani, 1950; Jaffé, 1951; Haferland, 1957; Gaensler et al., 1966), and it has also been described in workers in synthetic graphite (Watson et al., 1959; Zahorski, 1961).

Other carbon materials
Carbon blacks

Carbon blacks are manufactured carbon materials of spherical shape ranging from 10 to 1000 nm in size, according to the method of preparation. Thus, a variable proportion of air-borne particles is 'respirable'. Deposited carbons (similar to the 'lamp black' of old) are produced by 'chemical vapour deposition' of carbon from volatile compounds on carbonaceous, metallic or ceramic substrates thereby ensuring a homogeneous microstructure of the material (Edwards, 1989). Carbon blacks exist as individual spheres, as aggregates of spheres or as compact pellets to facilitate handling, packing and transportation.

As refractory chambers are employed in the manufacture of carbon blacks (other than deposited carbon), quartz, or other polymorphs of crystalline silica, are likely to be present and, possibly, survive in small amounts in the final products. However, specific data about such impurities are, apparently, lacking (H. Marsh, 1991, personal communication), although the products from five British factories were reported to be 99 per cent carbon with traces of polycyclic aromatic hydrocarbons (Hodgson and Jones, 1985).

Uses

Carbon black is most extensively employed as a filler and colouring agent in rubber, plastics, gramophone records (in which it constitutes some 2 per cent of the ingredients) and printing inks; it is also used in paints and enamels, in the manufacture of carbon arc rods and carbon paper, and as a filter aid, decolouring agent and clarifier.

Significant exposure to the dust has occurred mainly in the production of carbon black, while being emptied from bags, and weighed and mixed with other materials.

Carbon electrodes

In general, these are smaller than graphite electrodes and, because they are not usually required to withstand the high electrical and thermal pressures for which those electrodes are intended, the production process may not be continued to the stage of graphitization but is otherwise similar, as are the conditions encountered in the workplace (see Figure 13.3). Any mineral inclusions are also low.

Other electrical uses include carbon brushes, carbon arcs and sliding contacts.

Polycyclic aromatic hydrocarbons, evolved from pitch binder in the electrodes during their operation in aluminium smelters, are believed to underlie an excess of cancer of the lung in the workers (see Chapter 19, 'Polycyclic hydrocarbons').

Activated carbons

These are produced from *chars* (charcoals) made by carbonization of peat, lignite, coal, wood, bagasse or coconut shells; they are also manufactured from synthetic materials such as resins. Either steam or air is then introduced as an 'activating' agent to increase and control their porosity and capacity for adsorption (Edwards, 1989; Uragoda, 1989). The presence of quartz in the process will depend upon the source of the parent char. Quartz, pyrites and clay materials are present in variable and often substantial amounts in peat, lignite and bituminous coals (Milner, 1962); they are negligible in woods and absent in coconut shells and synthetic materials. Mineral matter in the final product is usually finely and evenly dispersed with ferrosilicates often being prominent (H. Marsh, 1991, personal communication).

Production involves crushing the char (whatever its origin) into small fragments by rollers, firing at low temperatures (about 510 to 540°C) in rotary kilns during which gas or steam is introduced. The resultant activated carbon is milled and sifted into desired graded sizes and transferred for packing. Most of these operations were very dusty in the past and, in some circumstances, may still be. Thus, it is during manufacture using natural materials, and not from the final product, that quartz-contaminated dust may be encountered; for example, in one instance when lignite was used, the content of quartz was found to be reduced from 3.0 to 0.12 per cent (Gross and Nau, 1967). The ash made from coconut shells is reported to contain 92 per cent carbon but no free silica. Most of the air-borne dust particles in this process were between 12.5 μm and 3.5 μm in diameter but a small proportion was from 3.5 μm to less than 1.2 μm (Uragoda, 1989).

Uses

Activated carbon is used in filters for the purification of water, foods, chemicals, perfumes and air; for removal of offensive tastes and smells; and for clarification of alcoholic drinks and treatment of sewage. None of its uses presents a respiratory hazard.

Mesocarbon microbeads

These consist of microspheres produced by heating pitches to specific temperatures above 390°C to form a liquid crystal system (*mesophase pitch*) in the form of spheres or beads about 25 μm in diameter which are separated from the parent stock by extraction with solvents or by centrifuge. They are materials of increasing interest, with many possible uses as filters and adsorbents, and for mechanical applications (Edwards, 1989). Their manufacture or use does not appear to offer any potential hazard from dust but polycyclic aromatic hydrocarbons are produced during the heating of pitch, and the use of solvents (such as carbon tetrachloride) and the handling of various solutions are potential sources of different types of hazard.

Carbon fibres

These are fibres (filaments, yarns and rowings) which consist of at least 92 per cent carbon, usually in non-graphitic form, first successfully produced in the Royal Aircraft Establishment at Farnborough in England.

One or other of two precursor materials is used in their manufacture: *polyacrylonitrile* or *mesophase pitch*.

Polyacrylonitrile (a probable carcinogen – see Chapter 19) is first heated in air at temperatures of about 220°C to form a ladder polymer under tension, after which it is subjected to a continuously rising temperature gradient up to about 2500°C in an inert atmosphere such as nitrogen. In the earlier stages of the process volatile products – in particular, hydrogen cyanide, ammonia, acrylonitrile and propionitrile – are evolved.

In the mesophase pitch process fibres are drawn from pitch (of which there are many types protected by patent) at 450°C, subjected to an oxidative thermosetting stage and then heated to about 2500°C. Details of the production methods using this precursor and their chemistry is fully described by Donnet and Bansal (1984). The most extensive uses to which carbon fibres are put is in the manufacture of *carbon fibre-reinforced plastics* (CFRP) which often involves epoxy resins.

The production of carbon fibres is an advancing and expanding technology, and considerable improvements in their tensile strength have been made in recent years.

A dust hazard is unlikely in these processes. In the production and winding areas air-borne fibres are reported to be 8 to 10 μm in diameter, fractured laterally but not longitudinally (Jones, Jones and Lyle, 1982). In the polyacrylonitrile process there is a theoretical possibility of exposure to hydrogen cyanide, ammonia, acrylonitrile and polycyclic hydrocarbons and, during heat treatment in CFRP processes, to vapour of the curing agents of epoxy compounds (for example, phthalic acid anhydride and trimellitic acid anhydride) (see Chapter 21).

Uses

One of the most important applications of carbon fibres is in CFRPs. In the aerospace industry, for example: in the manufacture of jet turbine blades, tail fins and tail planes and wings of military aircraft; in the wings and secondary structures of civil aircraft and the composite rotor blades of helicopters; and in satellites and other space-craft.

Non-aerospace uses are numerous. The high tensile strength and low weight of CFRPs is exploited widely in all manner of sports goods such as tennis, squash and badminton rackets, golf clubs, fishing rods, skis, surf boards, racing craft, bicycle frames and the bodies of racing cars. Because of their physical characteristics CFRPs are employed in absorptive cloths for respirators, for 'audio' equipment and in high-speed machinery; its biological inertness is valuable in the making of artificial limbs and other protheses.

Carbon fibre-reinforced carbon has proved to be a significant advance in the manufacture of brakes for aircraft and other vehicles because of its light weight and ability to absorb energy at high temperatures.

The full potential of carbon fibres has yet to be realized (Johnson, 1989).

Terminology

The pathological appearances and behaviour of this pneumoconiosis are similar whether it is the result of exposure to coal or other carbonaceous material, and so is its pathogenesis. The terms 'simple pneumoconiosis' and 'progressive massive fibrosis' have been used to describe the lesions. Simple pneumoconiosis refers to small, discrete dust macules (macula: a stain or spot) or nodules not larger than about 5 mm in diameter. Progressive massive fibrosis (PMF) describes confluent masses of dust and collagen fibrosis more than 1 cm in diameter, although these lesions are not always continuously progressive and do not consist of solid collagenous masses.

As in the previous editions of this book, the term 'coal pneumoconiosis' rather than 'coal workers' pneumoconiosis' is used. However, some authorities prefer the latter on the grounds that 'coal pneumoconiosis' implies disease caused by the response to coal and its inherent mineral matter alone and ignores the effect of the accompanying extraneous minerals, that is, the total 'respirable dust' (A.G. Heppleston and W.K.C. Morgan, personal communication). The addition of 'workers' is meant to imply this. To the point, as explained in Appendix I, some of the accompanying extraneous non-coal minerals attached to the coaly matter are not removed by routine washing.

The term 'black lung' is uninformative and capable of including any of the 'pulmonary conditions which may be present in a coal-miner's chest' (Gross and de Treville, 1970); it should have no place in medical terminology.

Epidemiology

Coal pneumoconiosis

Incidence and prevalence

The incidence, or *attack rate*, of simple pneumoconiosis – that is, the number of men who develop pneumoconiosis per 1000 workers per year or over some other specified period – is related chiefly to the overall mass of 'respirable' dust to which miners are exposed during that period (Walton et al., 1977). It is not affected by smoking habits (Jacobsen, Burns and Atfield, 1977). A clear association between dust retained in the lungs and profusion of small opacities was demonstrated some years ago by Rivers et al. (1960), Casswell, Bergman and Rossiter (1971) and by Rossiter (1972a) who showed that the higher the proportion of coal in the dust the more dust that is needed to produce a given radiological category. At the time, epidemiological evidence as to whether non-coal minerals affected attack rate was controversial. More recently, Hurley et al. (1982) found that, among workers with similar cumulative exposures to coal-mine dust over a 10-year period, those with a longer time of exposure had a higher *prevalence* of simple pneumoconiosis (Figure 13.4). Although these authors did not unmask any clear evidence of an overall effect of quartz (average level in the dust of 5 per cent) on the likelihood of developing pneumoconiosis, they did observe that some miners exposed to dust with a relatively high content of quartz had a more rapid increase in category on the 12-point scale (see Chapter 7) than others during the same period. They pointed out that a slight overall effect of quartz may have been obscured by the estimated lifetime exposures of miners to quartz being less accurate than corresponding estimates of exposures to mixed dust. Variations – and, thus, transient peaks – in the amounts of quartz in 'respirable' coal-mine dust may be significant in this respect.

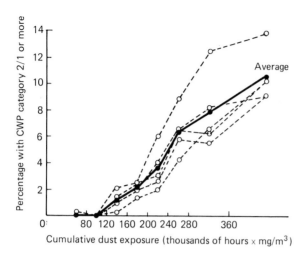

Figure 13.4 Separate (independent-randomized) classification and average classification of radiographs of 2600 coal miners by five readers related to mean cumulative exposures to mixed respirable coal-mine dust from entry into coal mining to time of radiological survey: grouped data. (Reproduced, with permission, from Hurley et al., 1982)

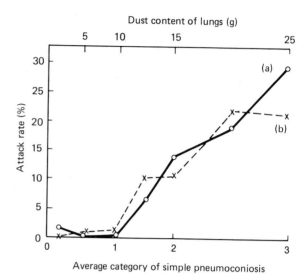

Figure 13.5 (a) Attack rate of PMF among miners and ex-miners aged 25 to 64 in South Wales over 8 years by average category of simple pneumoconiosis and related to average quantity of coal-mine dust in right lungs (Cochrane, 1962). (b) National Coal Board (UK) data over a 5-year period, adjusted linearly to 8 years for comparison. These data were 10 years later than Cochrane's and covered miners in most British collieries (McLintock, Rae and Jacobsen, 1971). Apart from the substantially lower attack rate for category 3 in the latter, the similarity is striking. (The scale is based on average quantity of dust in the lung)

Some of the earlier contradictions between epidemiological and pathological conclusions regarding the effect of the quartz content of mine dust and radiological category have been resolved to a large extent by Jacobsen and Maclaren (1982) who confirmed that an unusual rate of development of simple pneumoconiosis in some workers is associated with exposure to mixed coal-mine dust containing a relatively high percentage of quartz, and by Ruckley et al. (1984a) who showed that both the amount and composition of dust retained in the lungs contribute to the type and profusion of small opacities, and that the rank of coal plays an important role (see 'Radiographic appearances').

Lange et al. (1980) stated that, although quartz is only a minor part of the total dust deposit, it affects the tissue reactions critically. Walton et al. (1977), in fact, anticipated these observations by showing that, of the non-coal minerals the level of quartz increased the attack rate of simple pneumoconiosis but that this affect was offset when exposures to kaolin and mica were relatively high (see 'The role of quartz'). Bennett et al. (1979) reported that the prevalence of profusion category 0/1 or more simple pneumoconiosis increases progressively in the range of low- to high-rank coals from about 4 to 21 per cent respectively, and that this was not explained by higher mass concentrations of dust in high-rank collieries, although they suggested that this might have had an effect before the period of their investigations (1969–1973). However, it is clear that factors other than rank operate as they found a three- to fivefold difference in prevalence in workers from collieries of equal rank (see 'Pathogenesis').

Epidemiological studies have also shown clearly that individual differences in the attack rate of pneumoconiosis occur even in miners with comparable exposures to the same coal-mine dust. The reason for this remains illusive. One explanation is that there are individual differences in retention of quartz within the lungs (see 'The role of quartz'). General discussion of other possibilities is to be found in Chapters 1 and 3.

The attack rate of PMF increases with rising initial profusion of small opacities (simple pneumoconiosis – category 2 or more) and with the rate of their progression during the period of study (McLintock, Rae and Jacobsen, 1971; Jacobsen and Maclaren, 1982) (Figure 13.5). A three- to fourfold increase in the risk of developing PMF has been reported in miners with category 2 or 3 simple pneumoconiosis compared to those with category 1, and cumulative exposure to 'respirable' dust is the major factor in its development (Figure 13.6) (Hurley et al., 1987). In recent years, however, more than half the new cases of PMF, although few, have been reported to occur in men with a radiological category of 1 or less (Shennan et al., 1981); this may be due, at least in

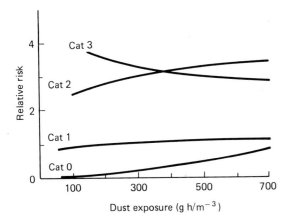

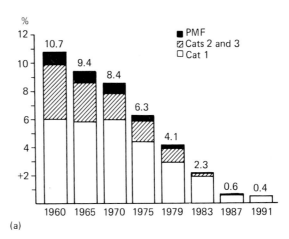

(a)

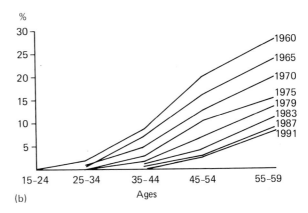

(b)

Figure 13.6 Risks of PMF incidence over a 5-year period at various levels of cumulative exposure and attained category of simple pneumoconiosis relative to the risks for a miner with category 1 pneumoconiosis and of 200 g h/m³ exposure. There is a three- to fourfold increase in the risk of developing PMF with categories 2 and 3 compared with category 1. (Reproduced, with permission, from Hurley et al., 1987)

Figure 13.7 (a) Prevalence of pneumoconiosis in British coal miners 1960–1991. It should be noted that these figures, from all regional coalfields, do not relate to an identified and exclusive cohort of miners followed over time. This is because populations of men who had radiographs taken in the corresponding year of each survey have changed over the years owing to retirement, recruitment, closure of pits and movement of workers between collieries. Nevertheless the data give a valuable indication of the trend of pneumoconiosis over these years. (b) Prevalence of pneumoconiosis according to age at collieries surveyed in the same years (percentage of men who had radiographs taken). This shows that the onset of radiographic changes has been progressively delayed over the years. (Reproduced from the British Coal Medical Service Annual Report 1991–1992 by courtesy of the Director of Medical Services)

part, to temporal variations in radiological techniques and reading of films over the years. Nevertheless, the incidence is not negligible in men with category 0 films in all age groups (Hurley et al., 1987). It varies in different coal fields and is higher in ex-miners – whether of retirement or of working age – than in working miners; this is a finding that does not appear to be explained by differences in dust exposure, although age is an important factor and the risk of attack increases more steeply with age among working miners (Hurley and Maclaren, 1988). In miners in the former Federal Republic of Germany, Lange et al. (1980) found an almost linear correlation between prevalence of PMF and age which, they suggested, implied that the 'activity of the fibrotic process does not diminish with age'. The attack rate is not influenced by expenditure of energy at work, smoking habits or tuberculous infection (Cochrane, 1962), but is by physique as it tends to favour workers who are lighter in weight for their height than others (Maclaren, 1985).

It has been recognized for years that PMF may develop after miners have left the coal mines (Cochrane, 1962) – a fact not often reflected in most incidence and prevalence studies. However, Maclaren and Soutar (1985) reported an attack rate of 94 per 1000 (usually with a simple pneumoconiosis) among 4526 miners who had left the industry up to about 26 years earlier. If the clinician is unaware of this, and especially if the patient has long been resident far from a mining area, PMF observed for the first time in later years is apt to be unrecognized and misdiagnosed.

However, as Figure 13.7a shows, there has been a striking decline in prevalence of PMF in British miners between 1960 and 1991, due to progressive improvements in dust control. Similar trends over the same period appear to have occurred in the USA, Australia, Germany, France and Belgium. However, it is not possible to make valid comparisons of prevalence between different countries because of differences in composition of coal-mine dust, working conditions and the technique and standards of radiological surveys, and other criteria. There is good evidence that rank of coal influences pathogenesis and, therefore, prevalence, and, in this respect, the role of non-coal minerals that show profound regional variations is clearly important (Walton et al., 1977) (see 'Pathogenesis').

Rate of progression

Over a specified time, this appears to be related to the radiological category when the worker is first seen (Jacobsen et al., 1971) and tends to be more rapid where there have been relatively high levels of quartz in the coal-mine dust (Hurley and Maclaren, 1982).

The rate of progression of PMF is influenced chiefly by age: the younger the worker with a category A radiograph, the more likely is progression to occur; this is true, although not inevitable, when he leaves the mining industry. Rheumatoid pneumoconiosis, however, undoubtedly contributes to rapid radiographic progression of both simple pneumoconiosis (usually category r) and PMF – at least in the UK (see page 387).

Mortality

A detailed 20-year follow-up study of miners and ex-miners in South Wales (Rhondda Fach) showed that those with simple pneumoconiosis (categories 1, 2 and 3) and category A opacities survive as well as those with no evidence of pneumoconiosis (category 0) (Cochrane et al., 1979). This confirmed the findings of earlier surveys in Britain (Higgins et al., 1968a; Cochrane, 1973; Cochrane and Moore, 1978) and in the USA where the life expectancy of miners as a whole is the same as that of the general population (Ortmeyer et al., 1974). Interestingly, among Pennsylvanian miners with category B pneumoconiosis mortality was higher in those who worked in anthracite mines than in those in bituminous mines (Ortmeyer, Baier and Crawford, 1973). The fact that only miners with category B and C pneumoconioses had a raised mortality (although low relative to other causes) in the Rhondda valley in South Wales was confirmed by Atuhaire et al. (1985), although this excess was not observed in the Lancashire and Derbyshire coal fields. Rooke et al. (1979) found that the mean age of death among Lancashire miners with PMF was 72 years. Miller and Jacobson (1985) reported an absence of any tendency for mortality to increase with increasing category of simple pneumoconiosis but concluded that 'miners exposed to excessive amounts of respirable coalmine dust are at increased risk of premature death, either from progressive massive fibrosis or from chronic bronchitis or emphysema'. But, Morgan (1986) pointed out that adjustment for smoking habits does not seem to have been made in this study. It also has to be borne in mind that the accuracy of death certificates is often uncertain and can lead to flawed conclusions (Cochrane and Moore, 1981).

In general, it can be concluded that simple pneumoconiosis does not curtail life expectancy and that advanced PMF – the prevalence of which is now low (see Figure 13.7a) – affects mortality in only a minority of subjects most of whom have chronic airflow obstruction related to smoking.

Pneumoconiosis associated with other carbonaceous materials

Pneumoconiosis in the carbon industries in general has not received comprehensive study comparable to that given over the years to pneumoconiosis in coal miners and coal workers in the silica-associated industries. This has probably contributed to some unjustified conclusions in respect of pathogenesis (see 'Pathogenesis', under 'The role of quartz'). As the preceding pages show, the technology of, and the conditions within, the various carbon processes differ considerably.

Globally, a substantial number of workers have been, and still are, employed in these industries but, overall, reliable figures are not available. When pneumoconiosis has been reported its radiological features have been identical to those that characterize coal pneumoconiosis.

Prevalence

Details are limited and often unreliable in almost all of these industries. Before 1982, for example, there were 18 reported epidemiological studies of natural and synthetic graphite workers internationally between 1928 and 1981 which showed prevalence rates of pneumoconiosis ranging from 1 to 73 per cent. Apart from changes in production conditions which have occurred over the years, this wide, if not wild, variation has been attributed to significant differences in: (1) definition of populations at risk; (2) methods of sampling; (3) methods and standards of examination of workers; and (4) classification of pneumoconiosis – the ILO classification, in most instances, was not used and radiological techniques were not uniform. Thus, it is impossible to relate these prevalence rates to varying silica contents of graphite dust in the different processes (Hanoa, 1983).

Epidemiological data in the other carbon industries (to which similar criticism applies) have been more limited and often less detailed though, latterly, a few comprehensive and important reports have appeared. Among 356 workers in the activated carbon industry, 9.6 per cent were reported to have 'definite' low category p simple pneumoconiosis (Wehr et al., 1975); in a survey of 35 men from 11 carbon black plants in western Europe, 6 with more than 10 years' exposure had simple pneumoconiosis of ILO category 2 or less (Crosbie, 1986). No definite relationship between exposure to pulverized fuel ash in English power stations for up to 20 years and radiographic changes has been established (Bonnell, Schilling and Massey, 1980; Schilling et al., 1988). Also no radiographic abnormality, attributable to dust, was found in 98 carbon fibre process workers with 8 years' exposure (Jones, Jones and Lyle, 1982).

There have, of course, been occasional reports over the years of isolated cases of pneumoconiosis in the different industries. Some of these are referred to under 'The role of quartz' (page 371).

Mortality

A survey of 2219, male, long-term employees in the carbon production division (electrodes, carbon arcs and brushes) of the Union Carbide Company (USA) between 1974 and 1983 revealed no increased mortality from non-malignant respiratory disease or from carcinoma of the lung (Teta, Ott and Schatter, 1987). Similarly, with polycyclic aromatic hydrocarbons in mind, no significant excess from carcinoma of the lung was found among workers employed for many years in the carbon black industry (Robertson and Ingalis, 1980; Hodgson and Jones, 1985).

Conclusion

As the foregoing account indicates, quartz and, at times, other polymorphs of silica are often present at some stages of the manufacture of carbon products, although they are usually absent, or of very small quantity, in the end-products. Furthermore, there have often been, and may still be, extraneous sources of free silica dust, such as furnace bricks and waste coke or silica sand used for the packing of furnaces. Workers confined to handling or machining carbon materials of high purity were, until recent times, likely to have had some exposure to silica-containing dust of similar origin. In addition, asbestos cement, rope and blankets were often used, until about the mid-1970s, for thermal insulation of calcination, autoclave and furnace areas, although they probably offered little

or no hazard to the process operatives themselves. That exposure has occurred solely to unadulterated carbon dust over a working life in any of these industries must, therefore, have been highly exceptional. A common assumption that silica (in any of its phases) was absent in some of the processes has not been adequately validated (see 'Pathogenesis', under 'The role of quartz').

The question of a possible relationship between the evolution of polycyclic aromatic hydrocarbons at different stages and carcinomas of the lung is discussed in Chapter 19.

Although control of dust in these industries has been much improved over the years, many processes, by their very nature, are still potentially dusty and dirty, and require the use of efficient hygienic measures.

Pathology

The pathology of pneumoconiosis associated with coal and other carbonaceous materials is similar.

Extrapulmonary appearances

The intercostal parietal pleura is often tattooed with black lines running parallel to the ribs caused by coal dust in and around extrapleural perivascular lymphatic vessels. The pulmonary pleura is marbled blue–black by subpleural deposits of dust and is not thickened unless it overlies a confluent mass of pneumoconiosis (PMF), in which case it may be fibrotic and puckered, occasionally in the form of a hyalinized plaque. Apart from this, pleural fibrosis should lead to suspicion of the presence of some other disease process.

Hilar and mediastinal lymph nodes are densely black and may be slightly enlarged.

Discrete, round lesions – simple pneumoconiosis

Macroscopic appearances

When the lungs are cut through with a knife, a variable number of black dust macules (ranging from few to numerous) are seen and are commonly predominant in the upper halves of the lungs, but may be distributed symmetrically throughout (Figure 13.8). Between these lesions the lung tissue

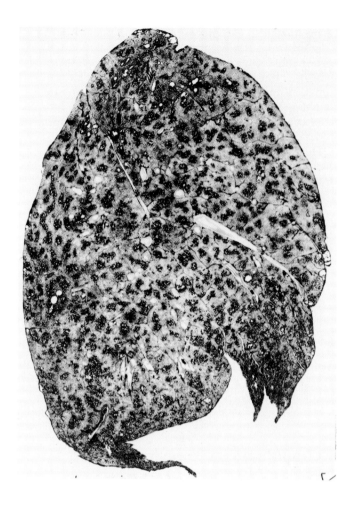

(a)

Figure 13.8 (a) Multiple coal macules (dust pigmentation) distributed fairly evenly in the lung. Only very slight centriacinar emphysema limited to the upper quarter. (Paper-mounted section.)

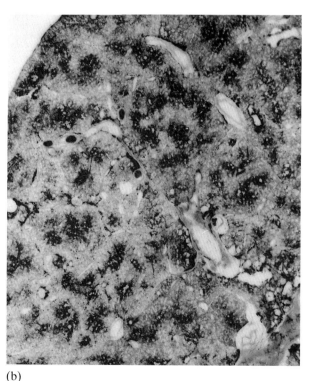

(b)

Figure 13.8 (b) Coal dust macules, without associated emphysema. (Paper-mounted section; slightly enlarged)

is frequently free of dust pigment. Some lungs are uniformly black so that individual macules are not discernible, but much of the coal dust can usually be washed away by a stream of water to reveal the macules. The fact that diffuse and dense black staining is found in some cases, but not in others, although in both instances pneumoconiotic lesions of similar severity may be present, is not readily explicable, and seems at odds with the total dust hypothesis of pathogenesis (see page 368). Macules are not raised above or depressed below the cut surface and they yield no sense of induration to the touch. Interlobular septa and the subpleural region are often dust pigmented – in some cases, deeply.

Black, indurated nodules, some 2 to 5 mm in diameter, which stand out from the cut surface and are readily palpable, may also be present – again in variable numbers – and are usually distributed in the upper parts of the upper and lower lobes but, in some cases, nearly all the lesions are nodular (that is, almost spherical) and may be evenly scattered throughout the lungs, dust macules being virtually absent. Some nodules may exhibit slight scar emphysema (Figure 13.9b). They may also occur in satellite

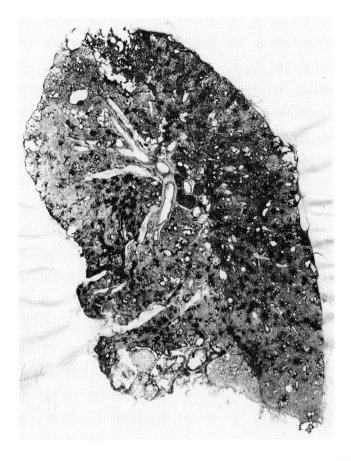

(a)

Figure 13.9 (a) Multiple coal (fibrotic) nodules: intervening lung appears normal (compare Figure 12.2).

groups around areas of PMF. More often, however, the lesions are of stellate or irregular linear shape (Figure 13.10; see also Figures 5.3 and 5.14).

In some lungs the nodules are almost uniformly black, in which case they are readily distinguished from silicotic nodules (Figure 13.9b) but, in others, they are less pigmented towards the centre and bear a superficial resemblance to silicotic nodules. Rheumatoid coal nodules (see page 362), which are usually larger, can also be mistaken for silicotic nodules (see Figure 13.19). Accumulations of dust are also found in the lymphoreticular aggregates at the bifurcations of respiratory bronchioles, and in the adventitia of accompanying arterioles which otherwise remain intact. Capillaries may be obliterated (Wells, 1954a).

The association of emphysema with simple pneumoconiosis is discussed on pages 357 to 360.

Microscopic appearances

Accumulation of free and intracellular particles of coal-mine dust occurs mainly in the walls of respiratory bronchioles (predominantly their first and

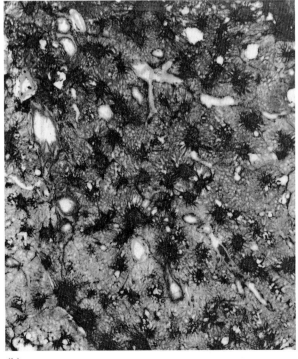

(b)

Figure 13.9 (b) Part of the same lung, slightly magnified, shows mild, scar emphysema around some nodules

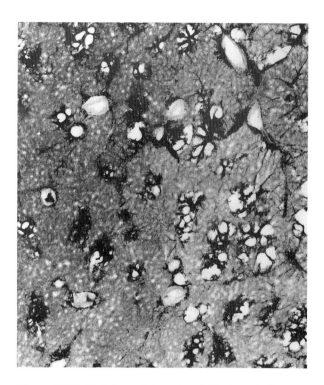

Figure 13.10 Stellate nodules of coal-blackened, fibrous tissue with surrounding centriacinar scar (irregular) emphysema to the right of the field (see also Figure 5.14). To the left of the field there are a few emphysema-free macules and nodules. (Paper-mounted section; slightly enlarged)

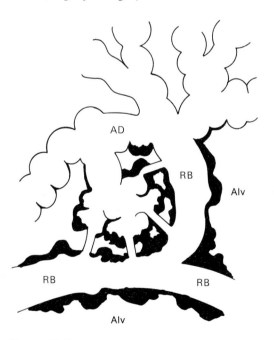

Figure 13.11 Composite reconstruction from serial sections showing four tubules (canals of Lambert) connecting one alveolar system with its neighbouring respiratory bronchioles. AD = alveolar duct; RB = respiratory bronchiole; Alv = alveolus. (Modified, with permission, from Duguid and Lambert, 1964)

second generations), the adventitia of accompanying blood vessels, and in the bronchioloalveolar canals of Lambert (Figure 13.11) and intersegmental respiratory bronchioles (see Chapter 1, page 5). These interconnecting airways most probably influence the distribution of dust within the acinus. Small collections of dust-laden macrophages accumulate on the walls of the airways, especially at their bifurcations, and silt up alveoli which open into or are adjacent to them. Many of these cells are incorporated into the interstitium and covered over by a new lining of type I cells. Deposition of reticulin fibres (type III collagen) and, later, type I fibres gradually occurs in varying degrees. Dust also accumulates in alveoli which border fibrous structures such as the pleura and interlobular septa (Duguid and Lambert, 1964). The fact that consolidations of dust associated with respiratory bronchioles are proximal to their outlets was attributed by Duguid and Lambert (1964) to the presence, in particular, of Lambert's canals. These communications are fairly numerous, although not easily recognized without serial sections, and connect parabronchiolar dust consolidations with dust-laden cells in terminal and respiratory bronchioles. They tend to persist and may sometimes be seen passing through thick layers of solid blackened tissue, maintaining connections between the bronchioles and more outlying alveoli.

The amount of 'packing' of dust within the lesions varies considerably: in some it is very dense with only a small number of intervening cells of any type and few reticulin and collagen fibres; in others, the density is low, the dust particles being interspersed by macrophages and fibroblasts, and the quantity of reticulin and collagen fibres is increased (Figure 13.12). Duguid and Lambert (1964) observed that the 'importance of the parabronchiolar consolidations [of dust] lies in the fact that they undergo organisation and form permanent fibrous scars which in course of time shrink and lead to distortion of the lung structures', although this process does not occur either in all cases or in all lesions. Many of these lesions (which are evenly pigmented and seldom exceed 3 mm in diameter) have a rosette or stellate pattern that becomes more striking the more fibrotic they are (see Figure 13.10). The distinction between macules and these micronodules – which, at times, may be fine – rests on there being a more organized and dense, central, dust-pigmented area in micronodules (Davis et al., 1983). Round nodules tend to be larger and the degree of coal pigmentation in them variable. Although it is evenly dense in some lesions, more often it is uneven, being most prominent towards their periphery. The lower the quantity of coal dust they contain the more collagen is present, and the more rounded and harder they are, that is, the more they resemble silicotic nodules.

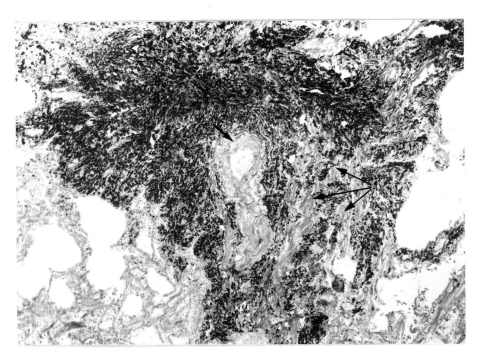

Figure 13.12 Coal nodule showing collagen fibres (arrowed) of irregular distribution with a large quantity of coal dust which is both intra- and extracellular. The appearances are in striking contrast to those of typical silicotic nodules (compare Figures 5.2 and 12.4). 'a' = artery; H & E stain; Magnification × 55

The variability in the appearances of these lesions is related to the composition of the dust retained in the lungs. In fact, macules and black, stellate micronodules are associated with coals of high rank in which the content of carbon is high and that of non-coal minerals, including quartz, is low, but not absent; rounded nodules are associated with lower-rank coal in which the content of carbon is low and that of non-coal minerals – in particular, quartz – is relatively high (Davis et al., 1983). The opinion commonly held until recent years (at least in the UK) that quartz was not involved in the pathogenesis of these lesions (Nagelschmidt et al., 1963) no longer appears to be tenable. Further, there appears to be some form of differential retention of non-coal minerals that is progressively more pronounced in men with more advanced degrees of pneumoconiosis (Davis et al., 1983) (see 'Differential retention of coal and non-coal minerals', page 370).

Foci of plasma cells and lymphocytes may be present around some nodules, and rheumatoid factor (IgM) has been found in coal nodules with no histological evidence of rheumatoid changes (Wagner and McCormick, 1967).

'Curious' bodies, known also as pseudo-asbestos bodies or *coal bodies*, may be found in areas of dust concentration in both coal and graphite pneumoconiosis (Tylecote and Dunn, 1931; Williams, 1934; Town, 1968). They vary from 30 to 70 μm in length,

are clubbed at both ends and their cores consist of black splinters of coal or carbon. As with asbestos bodies (see Chapter 14) their coating is golden yellow, giving a positive reaction to Perl's Prussian blue reagent, and their refractive index is similar (Gloyne, 1932–33). However, they are distinguished from asbestos bodies in being coarser and in having a continuous, non-segmented coat and a black core (Figure 13.13). They are found only in a minority of cases and may be numerous or scanty. Their presence is unrelated to the severity of pneumoconiosis. They have no known pathogenic significance and their mode of formation is not understood.

Emphysema

The relative frequency of both centriacinar and panacinar emphysema in coal miners increases with age and both occur more frequently in smokers than in non-smokers (Ruckley et al., 1984b).

Centriacinar emphysema (CAE) with dust

Emphysema in the centriacinar or proximal acinar location may appear either as dilated spaces with

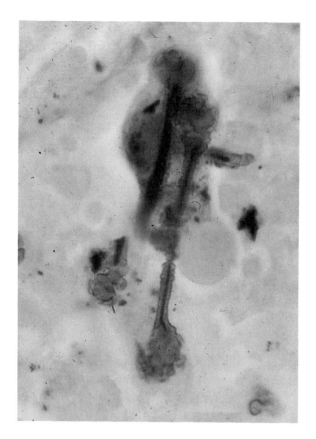

Figure 13.13 Coal bodies: these bear a superficial resemblance to asbestos bodies. Although their coating is golden coloured it lacks definition and clear segmentation, and the core is densely black, often splinter-like. Fragments of bodies may be seen. Graphite bodies are similar. Magnification × 500

pigmented walls without significant fibrosis ('focal emphysema') or as black, stellate, fibrous nodules with surrounding emphysematous spaces – that is, diminutive lesions of scar emphysema. As mentioned in Chapter 9, 'focal emphysema' is regarded by some as a distinct type of emphysema specifically attributable to the effect of accumulated coal or similar dust. However, this appears unlikely for the following reasons.

1. The distribution in the lungs of CAE with dust and no fibrosis is similar to that of CAE without dust (see Chapter 9) and many pathologists have found it difficult, if not impossible, to make any morphological distinction apart from the presence of dust (Wyatt, 1959; Mitchell, 1962; Duguid and Lambert, 1964; Reid, 1967; Heath, 1968). Nonetheless, Heppleston (1972) maintains that 'focal emphysema' is essentially a non-disruptive dilatation of respiratory bronchioles distinct from CAE proper which is only distinguishable by a painstaking, three-dimensional,

microanatomical technique which does not seem to have been repeated by others.
2. Heavy deposition of coal dust is often seen without attendant emphysema, even in elderly coal miners.
3. Macules with and without emphysema, rounded nodules without emphysema, and CAE without dust may all be found, at times, in the same lung.
4. In cases with apparently similar exposure to dust CAE is associated with most of the macules in some but with only a minority in others; in others still, it is absent.

Three features which are said to distinguish 'focal emphysema' should be considered.

1. 'Inflammatory changes in bronchiolar walls are inconstant' (Heppleston, 1972). Thus, these changes, although variable, may be associated with 'focal emphysema' as they are with CAE without dust (see Chapter 9). Duguid and Lambert (1964) found bronchiolar inflammation to be common in coal pneumoconiosis, and Churg and Wright (1983) reported fibrosis – not, apparently, attributable to smoking – in membranous and respiratory bronchioles and alveolar ducts of workers exposed to non-asbestos mineral dusts.
2. 'Disruption of bronchiolar and alveolar walls is not a primary event although it may be seen in advanced lesions . . .' (Heppleston, 1972). This would imply that disruption of airways' walls, of greater or lesser degree, is common to both 'focal emphysema' and CAE without dust.
3. Atrophy of smooth muscle in the walls of affected bronchioles (Heppleston, 1953, 1972). This is also found in CAE without dust (Thurlbeck, 1976) and, thus, cannot be a characteristic feature.

It appears, therefore, that 'focal emphysema' – that is, dilatation or disruption of respiratory bronchiolar walls without scarring – is, except for the presence of dust, morphologically indistinguishable from CAE without dust, commonly associated with smoking. Moreover, as Heppleston (1984) says, it is found 'in many, though not all cases' of coal pneumoconiosis, its absence or lack of universality being due to the 'requisite conditions' not always being achieved by the time the lesions are seen (A.G. Heppleston, 1988, personal communication). However, what these conditions are is unclear. Thus, it may reasonably be concluded that this form of emphysema is not a pathognomonic (that is, an integral or specifically characteristic) feature of simple coal pneumoconiosis.

Accordingly, statements such as the following are misleading in being either incorrect or semantically inconsistent. 'Focal emphysema is sufficiently common to be considered an integral part of the lesion of simple coal workers' pneumoconiosis and is a necessary criterion for its diagnosis' (Green, 1988). Again: '... dilatation of respiratory bronchioles with accumulation of dust laden macrophages in and around respiratory bronchioles ... has been referred to as focal emphysema. However, in those exposed to coal dust, the term coal pneumoconiosis is preferable' (American Thoracic Society, 1987). As has been suggested, emphysema is not an 'integral part' (that is, necessary for the existence of the whole) of the simple pneumoconiosis lesion, and 'emphysema' and 'pneumoconiosis' can hardly be treated as synonymous or interchangeable terms.

Nonetheless, in spite of the fact that dust-associated CAE is a variable and inconstant finding in cases of coal pneumoconiosis, CAE is more common in coal-miners' lungs than in those of the general population, even after smoking is taken into account (Lamb, 1976; Cockcroft et al., 1982a). The explanation appears to be as follows. The probability of dust-associated emphysema being present in the centriacinar location increases with increasing cumulative exposure to coal-mine dust, but the decisive factor in its development is the composition of the dust. This, as stated earlier, is determined by the rank of coal in the lungs, so that the *higher* the rank (and, thus, the lower the quantity of non-carbon minerals, including quartz), the greater the likelihood of stellate nodules with surrounding scar emphysema developing, whereas, the *lower* the rank (and, thus, the greater the quantity of quartz and other non-coal minerals), the less likely this becomes and the more individual pneumoconiosis lesions resemble 'proliferative' silicotic nodules without emphysema (see Chapter 12, page 300).

In short, the emphysema tends to be found in lungs with dust-related fibrosis of milder rather than of more severe degree – that is, central, dust-pigmented, stellate scars (see Figure 13.10) – which appears to be decisive for its development (Davis et al., 1983; Ruckley et al., 1984b). The number and size of such lesions, therefore, are very variable. Individual differences in the levels of retention of quartz in the lungs and apparent differences in its cytotoxic activity, according to petrogenic origin and to other minerals with which it is associated, most probably contribute to this variability (see pages 370 to 372).

To summarize, dust-associated CAE in coal miners consists of: (1) CAE with black pigmented walls but no fibrosis ('focal emphysema') which, apart from the dust pigmentation, is indistinguishable from CAE in the general population; or (2) minute stellate, fibrotic nodules with surrounding emphysematous spaces in the proximal or centriacinar location; or (3) both. The stellate pattern of scar emphysema (which accounts for an excess of CAE in non-smoking coal miners) is the histological pattern most often illustrated in medical tests (Duguid and Lambert, 1964; Heppleston, 1972; Lyons et al., 1981; Ruckley et al.,

1981; Davis et al., 1983). However, both forms – which, incidentally, were distinguished by Gough in 1947 – may be absent, of minor degree or widespread in the lungs of coal miners with simple pneumoconiosis. Davis et al. (1983) have aptly summarized the situation thus: the lesions of coal pneumoconiosis 'should be considered as a variable entity, the exact pattern of which depends on the composition of the dust in the lungs'.

All things considered, misunderstanding or ambiguity of meaning would be avoided if the term 'focal emphysema' were discarded.

Panacinar emphysema

Contrary to the conclusions of Ryder et al. (1970) and Lyons et al. (1972), there is no significant association between the prevalence or the extent of panacinar emphysema and the amount or composition of dust (ash or coal fractions) in coal-miners' lungs (Ruckley et al., 1981, 1984b), although airspace walls are often blackened.

Irregular emphysema

This can occur as the result of contraction of PMF lesions and is present in widely varying degrees in the lungs of some coal miners. In some cases shrinkage of PMF results in bullous-type emphysema which can be severe (see next section).

Conclusions

1. The relative frequency of emphysema in general in coal miners increases with age at death, and both CAE and panacinar emphysema are more prevalent among the smokers than the non-smokers (Ruckley et al., 1984b).
2. The association between exposure to 'respirable coal-mine dust' and emphysema is such as to suggest a causal relationship.
3. This association, however, is only demonstrable for CAE, and is positively and significantly related to an increasing amount of dust in the lungs, although not to its percentage composition. It is confined to lungs with dust-related fibrosis. The 'extent and nature of such fibrosis may be a crucial factor in determining the presence of CAE' (Ruckley et al., 1984b).
4. The degree of CAE in miners' lungs varies substantially. The absence of a quantitative relationship between coal dust and the extent of CAE suggests that its initiation and progression are caused by different factors (Ruckley et al., 1984b).

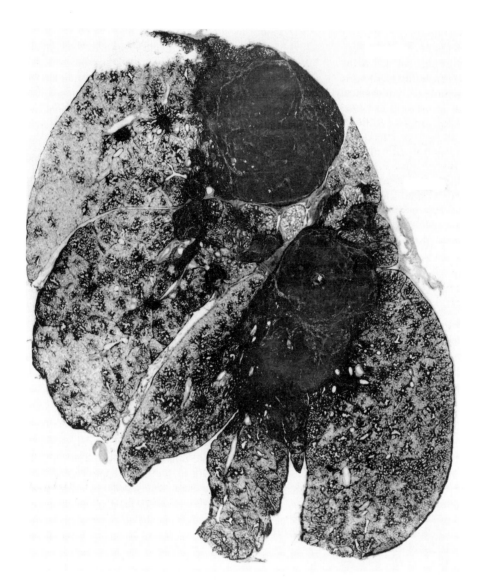

Figure 13.14 Advanced PMF in upper and lower lobes of right lung. Both masses are well circumscribed and demarcated from the rest of the lung – in essence, space-occupying lesion. In this specimen roughly circular and irregular grey areas are evident – a not uncommon appearance. In many cases masses are homogeneously black. Multiple large nodules are also present. Note: emphysema is minimal and irregular (scar) emphysema is absent. (Paper-mounted section)

5. There is no evidence of a causal nexus between exposure to coal-mine dust and panacinar emphysema.
6. There is no convinving evidence to support the view that emphysema, *other than irregular or scar emphysema associated with minute scars and with some cases of PMF*, is more common in coal miners (or carbon workers) than in the population at large.

For further discussion of emphysema in coal miners, see Chapter 10, 'Emphysema, airways' obstruction and exposure to coal-mine dust'.

Progressive massive fibrosis

Macroscopic appearances

These masses (more than 1 cm diameter) usually favour the upper halves and posterior parts of the lungs but there are many exceptions to this. They may be found in the centre of the lung, in the base of a lower lobe, or in the lingula or middle lobe (Figure 13.14). They may be bilateral and roughly symmetrical in size and outline but, more commonly, are of disparate shape, size and distribution in the two lungs. Sometimes only a single mass occurs. When a mass is near the periphery the overlying pulmonary pleura is often puckered and fibrotic, and may be adherent to the parietal layer. A remarkable feature of these lesions is their variable conformation and the fact that they are frequently not confined by the anatomical boundaries of lobes, segments or septa. Therefore, when cut across they may be round, elliptical or linear in shape and so well circumscribed that they appear almost encapsulated and as though they have been dropped into the lung when it is neither distorted nor evidently compressed adjacently; in other cases, they are of irregular shape with poorly defined margins which extend in stellate fashion into the surrounding lung. Scar emphysema, sometimes with bullae, may surround some irregular masses, but is exceptional and does not occur in relation to circumscribed masses (Figure 13.15). Bullae may remain distended due to air trapping after the lung has been removed from the thorax. The cut surface of the lesion may be homogeneously black, although grey, sometimes round areas are often seen, and it is uniformly hard or rubbery. Some masses, however, contain black, pultaceous, necrotic material or fluid which may scintillate due to the presence of cholesterol crystals; others are black, shaggy-walled cavities caused by the previous evacuation of the necrotic contents into a connecting airway. This necrosis is primarily of ischaemic origin (see next section). After evacuation such cavities often refill with fluid of similar composition to blood plasma (Gernez-Rieux et al., 1958). Exceptionally, small caseous or calcified areas which might suggest tuberculosis are seen within a mass. A well-demarcated PMF may appear encapsulated but, in fact, there is no true capsule.

PMF of coal or other carbonaceous pneumoconiosis is readily distinguished from a silicotic conglomeration by the excess of black dust, and by the absence of individually identifiable silicotic nodules with their distinctive whorled pattern in the aggregate. Simple dust macules or nodules, or both, are usually present to a greater or lesser degree in the rest of the lung, but in some cases they are virtually absent. In graphite and other forms of carbon pneumoconiosis, the lungs may be intensely and uniformly black.

If there has been past exposure to relatively high concentrations of quartz as well as to coal or carbon dust, typical – but, more often, immature – silicotic nodules or areas of 'mixed dust fibrosis' (see Chapter 12) may be present in addition to the coal or carbon lesions; there may be egg-shell calcification of the hilar lymph nodes. This is seen particularly in coal miners who have done a lot of rock drilling in shaft sinking or road developing or repairing, or who worked in collieries with heavily faulted ground. Indeed, in some mining areas, silicotic

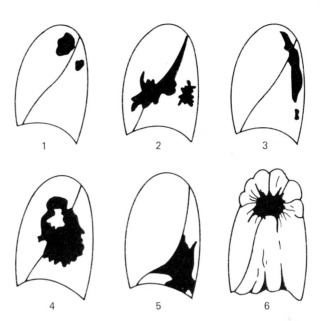

Figure 13.15 Diagram of some of the variable conformations of PMF seen on cutting lungs in the sagittal plane. (1) Solid, well-circumscribed masses without scar emphysema. (2,3) Roughly linear or irregular masses without attendant emphysema. (4) Large, well-circumscribed, cavitary mass and no scar emphysema. When bilateral, such masses can cause obliteration of many pulmonary artery branches and, ultimately, pulmonary heart disease. (5) Irregular contracted mass in the uncommon location of the lower lobe. (6) Contracted irregular mass in upper part of lung with severe scar and bullous emphysema. It will be noted that masses may cross lobar, septal boundaries which are obliterated – (2), (3), (4) and (6)

nodules – both discrete and conglomerate – may predominate, there being only very little characteristic coal pneumoconiosis, for example, in the UK, in the Wigan area of Lancashire (Spink and Nagelschmidt, 1963) and in the West Cumberland area (Faulds, King and Nagelschmidt, 1959). Silicotic nodules have also been observed with carbon pneumoconiosis in men who worked with natural graphite in the manufacture of carbon refractories (Gloyne, Marshall and Hoyle, 1949).

Hilar lymph nodes are usually black, firm and slightly enlarged.

Microscopic appearances

The structure of PMF is identical to that of coal nodules and consists of a large quantity of coal (or carbon) dust, lymphocytes, dust-laden macrophages and dense bundles of reticulin and collagen fibres, some of which are hyalinized. Bronchioles are usually annihilated but remnants of small pulmonary arteries and arterioles may be found in which there is progressive invasion by dust-bearing fibrous tissue, from adventitia to intima, to the point of obliteration; at this stage fragments of elastic lamina (revealed by elastic tissue stains) are the only evidence that these vessels existed (Wells, 1954a). At the periphery of PMF, arteries are partly or completely obstructed by endarteritis and the bigger the mass, the larger and more proximal the arteries involved. Thrombosis may occur in these arteries and spread in retrograde fashion, sometimes as far as the main pulmonary artery branches (Wells, 1954b). Arterial obstruction may cause ischaemic, colliquative necrosis within the mass and, if a bronchus is eroded, the necrotic material expelled in the sputum resulting in the formation of a cavity. Similar changes may be found in the small arteries around coal nodules and in pneumoconiosis due to graphite (Pendergrass et al., 1968).

In some cases plasma cells are very prominent in endarteritis adjacent to PMF and immunofluorescent techniques have demonstrated that rheumatoid factor (IgM) is present in these cells even though the masses show none of the features of rheumatoid coal nodules (see 'Pathogenesis', page 373).

Typical or immature silicotic lesions may be found in some masses, but the amount of collagen in PMF is substantially less than in silicotic conglomerations. Analysis of PMF indicates that, although collagen is present in the peripheral zone, it is replaced near and at the centre by fibrinogen and fibronectin, a protein of the glycosaminoglycan series of acid mucopolysaccharides. One-third of the weight of the masses is attributed to the protein complex and the remaining two-thirds to approximately equal amounts of mineral dusts and calcium phosphate (Wagner et al., 1975, 1982). IgG and IgA may also be present and, in association with fibrinogen, suggest exudation rather than immunological activity.

Rheumatoid coal pneumoconiosis

The *clinical syndrome*, first enunciated by Caplan (1953), is strictly defined as *multiple, large (0.5 to 5 cm diameter), round, radiographic opacities frequently associated with evidence of cavity formation or calcification, usually unaccompanied by the small opacities of simple pneumoconiosis, in coal miners with rheumatoid arthritis.* The lesions causing the opacities have gross and microscopic features unlike those of coal pneumoconiosis (Gough, Rivers and Seal, 1955). Its existence as a distinct entity has been widely confirmed, and the

concept extended beyond the original syndromal confines to include the occurrence of similar, as well as less distinctive and pleomorphic, opacities in the absence of rheumatoid arthritis but associated wth circulating rheumatoid factor (Caplan, Payne and Withey, 1962). The typical radiographic appearances are completely unlike those of non-rheumatoid pneumoconiosis in character and behaviour in time, and the variant form of rheumatoid pneumoconiosis is usually different (see 'Radiographic appearances'). Rheumatoid arthritis may precede or succeed the appearance of lung lesions by a number of years and, in some cases, never develops. There is no evident relationship between severity of rheumatoid arthritis when present and that of rheumatoid pneumoconiosis.

It is difficult to assess prevalence (which rests chiefly on clinical and not on pathological observations) with any accuracy because, owing to its diverse radiographic appearances (see page 387), 'rheumatoid' coal pneumoconiosis has been, and is often, unrecognized; because many individuals have been followed for too short a time for its development to be observed; and because of differing test standards for rheumatoid factor. Most commonly it has been expressed in terms of the number of cases occurring in coal-mining populations. Lindars and Davies (1967) found that the prevalence among 21 557 miners with and without pneumoconiosis from the east Midlands' collieries of Britain was 0.26 per cent, but among those with pneumoconiosis it lay between 2.3 and 6.2 per cent – a similar range, in fact, to that of the prevalence of circulating rheumatoid factor in European populations (Ball and Lawrence, 1961) (see page 376). Among 896 Welsh miners with pneumoconiosis, there were 20 (2.2 per cent) with rheumatoid pneumoconiosis (Miall et al., 1953). Whether the apparent rarity of rheumatoid coal pneumoconiosis in the USA is due to cases going unrecognized or unreported, or to some other reason, has not been established, although, recently, in a personal review of 4000 cases examined for the US National Coal Workers Autopsy Study, Green (1988) found only 3 cases. It is possible that, pathologically, some cases have been misdiagnosed as 'silicosis'.

Conversely, when rheumatoid pneumoconiosis was sought radiologically in coal miners with rheumatoid arthritis, no cases were identified among 100 Pennsylvanian miners and there was no increase in pneumoconiosis prevalence (Benedek, Zawadski and Medsger, 1976). It is, of course, true that in some miners and ex-miners with rheumatoid arthritis pneumoconiosis has no rheumatoid features, and in others no radiological evidence of pneumoconiosis ever develops. The reason for these discrepancies is not clear.

Incidence among workers in the non-coal carbon industries is unknown.

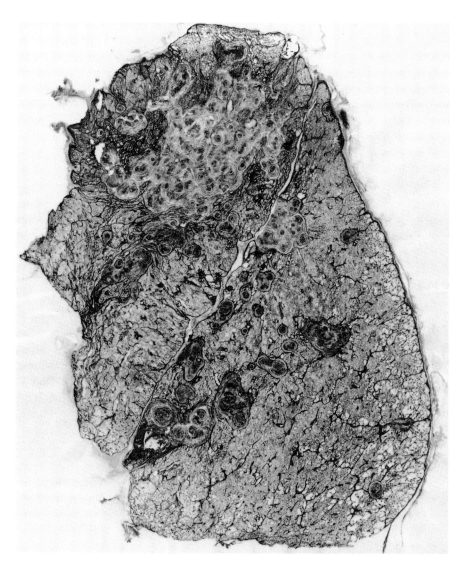

Figure 13.16 Left lung of coal miner who had severe rheumatoid arthritis. Multiple necrobiotic (Caplan) nodules, many of which are matted together, though they retain their identity. Their concentric pattern is clearly visible especially in the lower lobe. Note the virtual absence of non-rheumatoid pneumoconiosis and emphysema. The left lung contained similar, but fewer, lesions. (Paper-mounted section)

Macroscopic appearances

The pulmonary pleura is thickened in a proportion of cases, often more on one side than on the other. Individual nodules vary from about 0.3 to 3.0 cm diameter but may be grouped into aggregates of up to 5 cm overall diameter (Figure 13.16), and are scattered irregularly in any part of the lungs although with some propensity for the periphery and upper zones. Rarely, only a single large nodule may be present. The cut surface of the nodules has a distinctive concentric arrangement of alternating black and grey–white to yellow rings due respectively to laminated collections of dust and necrotic collagen (Figure 13.17a). Liquefaction in the lighter areas may appear as clefts and may contain collections of cholesterol crystals (Figure 13.17b). Indeed, whole nodules may become necrotic and, if connected with airways, discharge their contents into them leaving small cavities which subsequently close in most cases (Figure 13.18); however, if their contents are not discharged they may calcify. These typical features are not, however, always seen and, in some cases, the nodules are uniformly small (that

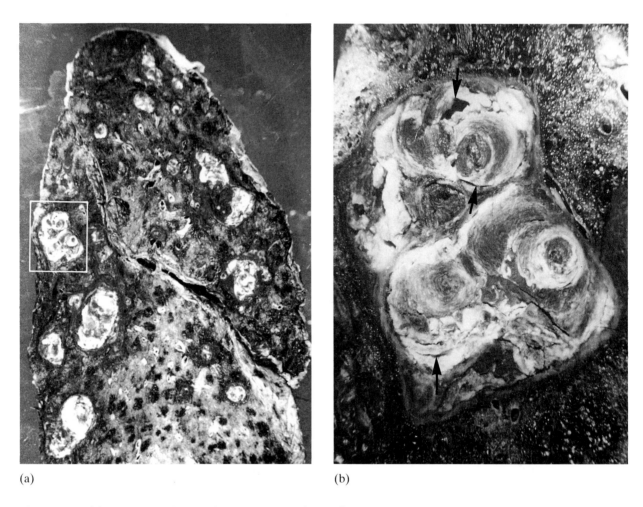

(a)   (b)

Figure 13.17 (a) Large, well-circumscribed necrobiotic (Caplan) nodules in a coal-miner's lung. Non-rheumatoid pneumoconiotic nodules are also present in unusual numbers (compare with Figure 13.16). (Lung slice, three-quarters natural size.) (b) Detail of cluster of nodules enclosed by rectangle in (a). Note circular zones of dust and peripheral clefts (arrowed). Magnification × 275. (Lung slice, courtesy of Dr R.M.E. Seal)

is, less than about 1 cm), perhaps with an occasional larger nodule, either scattered or clustered into composite groups, and may be calcified. In these circumstances they may bear a close resemblance to silicotic nodules (Figure 13.19). Inspection of a rheumatoid coal nodule with a hand lens helps to distinguish its features from those of a silicotic nodule, but microscopy may be necessary for confirmation.

General dust pigmentation is slight and ordinary coal macules and nodules are often absent or fairly few in number in most of these cases; occasionally, isolated Caplan nodules are seen in lungs with otherwise typical non-rheumatoid, simple pneumoconiosis and PMF, indicating that the rheumatoid process is not necessarily present in all lesions.

Microscopic appearances (Figure 13.20)

The centres of most of the nodules consist of necrotic tissue in which there are no surviving cells; this tissue stains pink with haematoxylin and eosin, its collagen content being variable. A blue-staining area of cellular infiltration surrounds this zone; in some instances it forms a complete circle and in others a segment only, depending upon the plane of section. The cells are macrophages, polymorphonuclear leucocytes, fibroblasts and, occasionally, multinucleated giant cells. More peripherally there are circumferentially arranged collagen fibres, fibroblasts and numerous plasma cells. Fibroblasts adjacent to the necrotic area are often grouped in palisade formation although not so strikingly as in distributed in concentric rings that alternate with the other zonal changes. Necrosis in these active zones causes the segmental clefts. Numerous plasma cells and lymphocytes are an important feature in the collagenous zones.

Arteries around the nodules exhibit endarteritis in which plasma cells are significantly more prominent than in non-rheumatoid pneumoconiosis; IgM is present in the arterial walls and in the cells (Wagner and McCormick, 1967; Wagner, 1971).

When activity in the nodule has ceased the necrotic areas tend to calcify, in which case the multiple concentric rings of dust are the only remaining evidence suggestive of their rheumatoid origin. In those cases where the nodules are small (4 to 5 mm diameter) and numerous, their microscopic features are similar to those of larger nodules.

Unlike Caplan nodules, rheumatoid necrobiotic nodules not associated with occupational exposure do not have an annular pattern of dust.

Bacteriology

Tubercle bacilli cannot be isolated by culture or guinea-pig inoculation from the lesions.

Distinguishing features of the nodules

Clearly, rheumatoid coal nodules are distinct from the typical nodules of coal pneumoconiosis or silicosis, and they show evidence of immunological reactivity. The features that differentiate Caplan-type necrobiotic nodules, typical silicosis and tuberculosis may be summarized as follows.

Gross appearances

Caplan nodules   These are generally discrete, up to 3 cm in diamter although they may be larger, and they are sometimes formed into composite groups. They are distributed at random in the lungs. There is a clear-cut concentric ring pattern of dust in nodules sectioned through or near their centres, and cavitary necrosis is fairly common in one or more lesions.

Typical silicotic nodules   These may also be discrete but, as a rule, are smaller than Caplan nodules and tend to occupy the upper halves of the lungs. Conglomerations of nodules are usually more closely matted than composite Caplan nodules. Concentric rings of dust are either absent or very poorly defined but occasionally the gross appearances may be identical. Central necrosis is rare (see Chapter 12). The occupational history should point to silicosis.

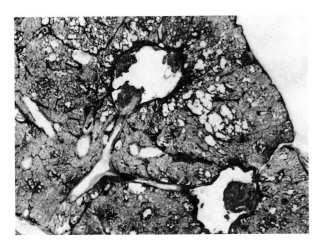

Figure 13.18 Cavitary Caplan nodules communicating with small, adjacent bronchi into which some of the contents have been expelled: dust macules, very scanty. This is from a collier with active rheumatoid arthritis; DAT 1:128. (Paper-mounted section, natural size)

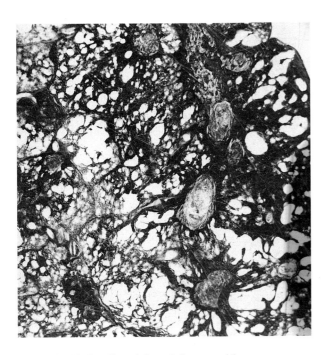

Figure 13.19 Small nodules of rheumatoid pneumoconiosis resembling silicotic nodules. Histological confirmation. (Paper-mounted section, natural size)

subcutaneous rheumatoid nodules. Special stains for 'fibrinoid' material are not helpful (Gough, Rivers and Seal, 1955). By contrast with silicotic nodules, clefts containing cholesterol crystals are often present. During periods of activity, dust-containing macrophages migrate into the lesions, later disrupting and discharging their dust load which remains

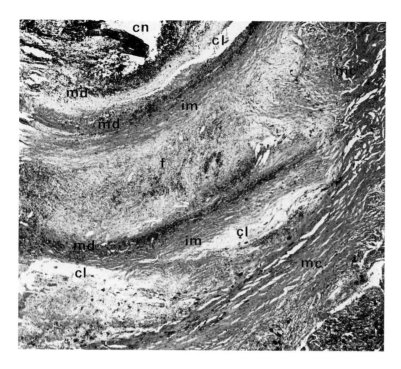

Figure 13.20 Microsection of a rheumatoid pneumoconiotic (Caplan) nodule showing characteristic concentric, alternating, tidal-like zones. Central area of necrosis (cn); macrophage infiltration and coal dust (md); fibroblasts and other cells (f); immature collagen (im); clefts containing cholesterol crystals (cl); mature collagen with cellular infiltration, including many plasma cells, at the periphery (mc). Martius scarlet blue stain; magnification × 45. From a coal-face worker for 18 years, with rheumatoid arthritis; DAT 1:1024. (See also Figure 5.9)

Tuberculous lesions These are not defined or circumscribed as the Caplan nodules are and they tend to agglomerate in irregular form, occupying the upper parts of the lungs. Dust rings are rarely present and caseation is often evident.

Microscopic appearances

These features and the bacteriological findings are shown in Table 13.1.

Differentiation on histological grounds alone may present some difficulty at times, but the correct diagnosis of rheumatoid pneumoconiosis can be made in almost all cases by gross inspection of the lesions – possibly with the aid of a hand lens – by an experienced observer.

Occasionally multiple, well-circumscribed, pulmonary nodules, with central necrosis (sometimes calcified) and dense fibrosis surrounded by an inflammatory reaction of lymphocytes, some plasma cells and a few giant cells follow chickenpox (varicella-zoster virus) in adults (Tulippe-Hecq et al., 1989),

and, in coal miners, may be dust pigmented. Differentiation from Caplan nodules rests on careful comparison of the histological details, and a history of chickenpox in recent years will help. With time, calcification of these nodules increases.

Diffuse interstitial pulmonary fibrosis with coal and other carbonaceous pneumoconioses

Pathologically, diffuse interstitial pulmonary fibrosis (DIPF) of varying severity is sometimes found in the lungs of workers with coal pneumoconiosis. Its appearances and distribution are often similar to those of idiopathic DIPF except that, in most cases, it is heavily pigmented by coal although, in some, it is unpigmented. This is not a new phenomenon. It was observed by Gough and Heppleston and by Caplan and the author, as well as by others, on

Table 13.1

	Nodules of coal pneumoconiosis	Caplan nodules	Typical silicotic nodules	Tuberculosis and dust
Dust lamination	−	+++	−	+
Palisading of fibroblasts	−	+	−	+
Cholesterol crystal spaces	−	++	−	+
Central necrosis	−	++	+ (rare)	++
Calcification	+ (rare)	++	+	++
Excess of peripheral lymphocytes and plasma cells	+ (occ.)*	+++	+	+
M. tuberculosis (culture or guinea-pig inoculation)	−	−	−	++

*Occasional.

routine post-mortem examination of miners' lungs some 30 or more years ago (and often referred to as 'fibrocystic disease') but, as with idiopathic DIPF in general, it appears to have become more common with the passing years (Heppleston, 1972) (see Chapter 15). It has also been reported in workers exposed to natural graphite (with varying amounts of 'free silica') by Gaensler et al. (1966) and Pendergrass et al. (1968). Occasionally, Caplan-type nodules, with or without clinically evident rheumatoid arthritis, are associated with DIPF (Figure 13.21).

A combined study of the lungs of coal miners from South Wales and West Virginia (USA) suggested that the overall incidence of DIPF of moderate or severe degree is approximately 5 per cent (milder forms accounting for a further 10 to 12 per cent), and pigmented fibrosis appeared to be associated with continuing exposure to coal-mine dust after it had been recognized radiologically (McConnochie et al., 1988). In a study of 46 cases in South Wales, Cockcroft et al. (1982b) reported that, although some cases were typical of idiopathic DIPF or had features consistent with extrinsic allergic alveolitis, others showed 'appearances not explained by other diseases'. Many British miners are, or have been, devoted to breeding and racing pigeons or breeding budgerigars, and those who, until collieries were fully mechanized, looked after haulage ponies underground handled potentially mouldy hay and straw. A probable case of the DIPF of extrinsic allergic alveolitis in an underground stable hand is on record (National Coal Board, 1977). It is relevant, in this respect, to note that it is improbable that organic allergens with the potential to cause alveolitis are present in coal (see Appendix I, page 853). Some cases examined personally over the years have had the clinical and immunological stigmata of rheumatoid arthritis or other connective tissue disease and, on occasion, in others the fibrosis appeared to be dust-pigmented organized pneumonia (see Chapter 15, 'Extrapulmonary disorders associated with DIPF').

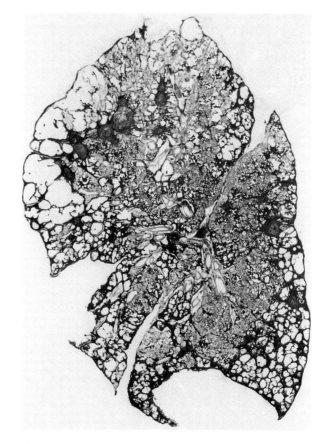

Figure 13.21 Moderately extensive DIPF of right lung with coarse cyst ('honeycomb') formation in all lobes. Typical Caplan-type nodules in upper and lower lobes. Areas of DIPF are sharply demarcated from adjacent lung and deeply pigmented with coal dust. Pigmentation elsewhere is negligible and lesions of non-rheumatoid pneumoconiosis very few. This is from a coal miner with advanced rheumatoid arthritis. (Paper-mounted section)

An interesting point to emerge from the study of McConnochie et al. (1988) is that survival after diagnosis was significantly longer in miners with

DIPF than that reported in some of the earlier series of cases of idiopathic DIPF in the general population.

The significance of irregular radiographic opacities – which do not necessarily signify DIPF – in coal miners is discussed later on page 383.

Pathogenesis of coal and carbon pneumoconiosis

Some aspects of the aetiology of coal pneumoconiosis are discussed in Chapter 5. In this section it is given further consideration, in particular the question of participation of quartz in pathogenesis.

First of all it must be emphasized that 'there is no such thing as "pure" coal' (Wender et al., 1981) – that is, coal completely free of non-coal minerals – and that coal miners inhale a variable mixture of coal and non-coal dust as a result of frequent working of adjacent non-coal strata. As stated at the beginning of this chapter (page 340), the quartz content of coal-mine dusts ranges from low to high depending upon the geological horizons of mines and types of mining operations involved. The average range of 2.02 per cent in South Wales anthracite mines to 12.78 per cent in the East Midlands bituminous collieries reported by Bergman and Casswell (1972) is similar to that in German, French and Belgian collieries despite discrepancies apparently caused by different calibration standards (Davis et al., 1982).

Levels of quartz occurring in natural graphite, and the variability of the associated sources of silica and of its polymorphs in synthetic graphites, carbon blacks, carbon electrodes and activated carbon have also been referred to earlier.

The effect of quantity and rank of coal

Simple pneumoconiosis and PMF considered together

In the UK during the 1930s, there was much confusion regarding the nature of pneumoconiosis in coal miners and the terminology used among the leading authorities of the day. A good measure of this confusion is provided by the participants (among whom were E. L. Collis, Lyle Cummins, J. S. Haldane, E. H. Kettle and E. J. King) in a protracted, but highly instructive, discussion which followed a medical paper read before The Institution of Mining Engineers in 1935 (Fisher, 1935). Until the 1940s coal-miners' pneumoconiosis was generally believed to be silicosis. However, early observations in South Wales, where the histological pattern of disease bears little resemblance to that of typical silicosis, seemed to indicate that the pathological severity of pneumoconiosis was directly proportional to the mass of coal dust recovered from the lungs *post mortem* (King, McGuire and Nagelschmidt, 1956), and that the composition of pulmonary dust was similar to that of the colliery dust inhaled (King and Nagelschmidt, 1945). In other words, the aetiological emphasis was placed more on the accumulated mass of dust than on its composition – an opinion still held by some authorities. PMF was considered to be the result of a 'complicating factor' believed, almost exclusively, to be tuberculosis – hence, the old term 'complicated pneumoconiosis'.

Subsequently, it was found that there were differences in the prevalence of pneumoconiosis, especially PMF, elsewhere in the UK. The quantity of dust in the lungs of men from coalfields in north-west England (Cumberland and Lancashire), for example, was lower than that in South Wales, and the ash content (non-coal minerals) was much higher (Faulds, King and Nagelschmidt, 1959; Spink and Nagelschmidt, 1963). Bergman and Casswell (1972) then showed that the composition of dust in the lungs of men from all the major coalfields in Britain was related to the rank of coal which, of course, varies in different regions: the higher the rank, the higher the percentage of coal and the lower that of quartz in the lung dust. They also demonstrated that the *rate* of accumulation of dust was related to rank (Figure 13.22), being faster for both simple pneumoconiosis and PMF in men mining high-rank coal than in those from low-rank collieries, and also in men with PMF than in those without. But the fact that high-rank coals are associated with a higher prevalence of pneumoconiosis than low-rank coals may, it has been suggested, be due to high-rank collieries having produced a greater mass of 'respirable' dust in the past (Bennett et al., 1979).

Accurate analyses of 'respirable' underground dust carried out by British Coal's Pneumoconiosis Field Research Study – initiated in 1957 (Fay and Rae, 1959) – in various collieries over at least 20 years has enabled valid comparison of the composition of pulmonary dust to be made with that of inhaled colliery dust – an important advantage that was lacking in earlier pathological studies. Using this information, Douglas et al. (1986) were able to show that the lungs of men with PMF contain, on

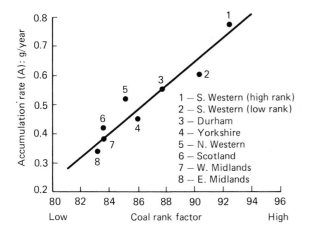

Figure 13.22 Relation between accumulation rate of total dust and rank of coal mined. Each point represents an average value for a particular coalfield. (Reproduced, with permission, from Bergman and Casswell, 1972)

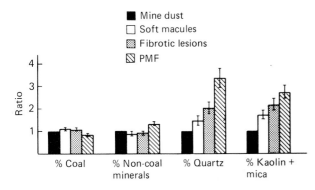

Figure 13.23 This shows degrees of 'enrichment' of particular minerals in lung dust compared with the composition of coal-mine dust to which the individual was exposed in relation to type of pneumoconiosis, expressed as a ratio. A notable increase in quartz, kaolin and mica is present in all cases, but especially those with PMF. The ratio for quartz in PMF lungs is significantly higher than for lungs with soft macules (*P*<0.01) or fibrotic lesions (*P*<0.05). (Reproduced, with permission, from Davis, Ottery and Le Roux, 1977)

average, more dust than the lungs of men without PMF and that they accumulate more dust per unit exposure than those without. This implies that the burden of dust in the lungs is not related simply to the quantity of dust inhaled but to differences in its deposition or clearance, or both, in men who develop PMF and those who do not. Furthermore, dust from lungs of miners with fibrotic nodules or PMF who mined low-rank coals contains a higher proportion of non-coal minerals – including quartz – than was in fact present in the mine dust to which

they had been exposed (Figure 13.23) (see next section).

However, whereas quartz has consistently been regarded as an important factor in the development of coal pneumoconiosis in Germany (Di Biasi, 1949; Reisner et al., 1982), in the UK it has, until recently, been widely believed to play little or no part (Nagelschmidt et al., 1963; Walton et al., 1977). This belief seems to have been spurred by Gough's (1940) observation that the pathology of pneumoconiosis in coal trimmers was similar to that in South Wales' coal miners, and, because water-washed coal, to which the trimmers were exposed, was mistakenly thought to be virtually free of non-coal minerals (see page 342 and Appendix I, 'Beneficiation of coal'), it was subsequently concluded that quartz played little or no part in the pathogenesis of coal pneumoconiosis. An apparent absence of free silica in some cases of similar pneumoconiosis in carbon workers has generally been taken as substantial support for this hypothesis – including this discussion in the previous editions of this book. (This point is discussed later in more detail.) Thus, the total amount of 'respirable' coal dust in the lungs has been regarded as the decisive factor, and levels of quartz averaging 5 per cent of mixed dust, for example, have been considered to have no influence on the probability of developing simple pneumoconiosis (Hurley et al., 1982). Hence, silicotic-type lesions found in some coal-miners' lungs were deemed to be a coincidentally separate silicosis resulting, say, from drilling siliceous rock strata.

It is of interest, therefore, to recall exactly what Gough wrote in 1940:

> . . . the coal trimmer acquires a similar lesion [to that in the coal miner], presumably due to some substance in the coal dust, which may be silica. Although analyses of the lungs show comparatively small amounts of silica in trimmers as compared with miners [no analytical data provided] this does not necessarily mean that the silica content of the dust is proportionately less. It may only indicate a difference in the degree of retention of silica in the lungs.

The last sentence is notable in its anticipation of later evidence of 'enrichment' of quartz in the lungs.

It has been demonstrated by Davis et al. (1983) that, in the UK, coal pneumoconiosis can in fact be regarded as a 'variable entity the exact pattern of which depends on the composition of the dust retained in the lung' – in effect a spectrum of tissue response: they also demonstrated that relatively high percentages of quartz in mixed coal-mine dust are an important factor in its development. Unusually rapid progression of coal pneumoconiosis has been shown by Seaton et al. (1981) and Jacobsen and Maclaren (1982) – thus confirming the earlier findings in the Cumbrian and Lancashire coalfields. However, the possibility that factors other than quartz may be involved is indicated by Seemayer's (1985) observation that the cytotoxicity of coal-mine dusts, although correlating with their quartz content, increases as the overall size of their particles decreases. The question of the influence of quartz in pathogenesis is discussed further in the next section.

Differential retention of coal and non-coal minerals

The concept of differential retention of coal and non-coal minerals in the lungs is in harmony with the results of inhalation experiments in animals exposed to dust at constant respirable concentration over prolonged periods, which showed that the pulmonary burden of deposited dust increases progressively with exposure time and eventually becomes linear (Weller, 1971; Vincent et al., 1985), rather than reaching a constant equilibrium of deposition and clearance as earlier kinetic models had envisaged. Thus, it is concluded that a proportion of inhaled dust, instead of being cleared, is entrapped – or 'sequestered' – in various locations in the lung (Vincent et al., 1987; Strom, Chan and Johnson, 1988) (see Chapter 3, page 45), although substantial accumulation in the lymph nodes does not appear to occur until the burden of dust in the lungs has reached a certain threshold which is lower for toxic (quartz) than for non-toxic dusts (Vincent et al., 1987). Histological confirmation of this concept was provided by Robertson et al. (1988a) in the lungs of rats exposed to coal-mine dust with either 'high' or 'low' content of quartz; they also verified that the proportion of quartz in the lung dust can be greater than that in the 'respirable' dust. Such preferential retention, or 'enrichment', of quartz in coal-miners' lungs, which tends to increase as pneumoconiosis advances, was also observed by Leiteritz, Einbrodt and Kosterkötter (1967), Davis, Ottery and Le Roux (1977), Davis et al. (1983) and Douglas et al. (1986) (Figure 13.24), and in gold-miners' lungs by Verma et al. (1982). This is well summarized by Pooley and Wagner (1988):

> . . . dusts retained in the lungs following [total life] exposures are never pure and frequently there is selective retention of certain particles, which may only have been a minor fraction of the total exposure as measured by environmental sampling, but will be the predominant mineral recovered from the lung tissue.

In addition to selective retention and sequestration of quartz, Brown et al. (1991) showed that it continues to exert a harmful inflammatory effect for up to 48 days in rats after intratracheal injection; they believe that this is due to the particle : macrophage ratio changing with increasing recruitment of macrophages replacing those killed (see Chapter 5,

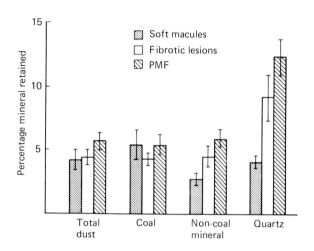

Figure 13.24 The amount of dust retained in the lungs is expressed as a percentage of coal-mine dust inhaled. The percentage of quartz and other non-coal minerals in lungs with soft macules is significantly lower than in those with fibrotic nodules ($P<0.05$) or PMF ($P<0.001$). (Reproduced, with permission, from Davis, Ottery and Le Roux, 1977)

'Macrophage mobilization'), so that the number of quartz particles per cell gradually becomes too low to kill the cells although continuing to activate them to produce proteases – an effect that may be greater in human than in animal macrophages in that they have a substantially higher resistance to the cytotoxic effects of quartz (Seemayer and Braumann, 1988). Enhanced production of proteases associated with a higher percentage of macrophages has been demonstrated in bronchoalveolar lavage fluid from men with coal pneumoconiosis compared with control subjects (Sablonniere et al., 1983). That retention, or sequestration, of dust particles as such is not, however, the major factor causing chronic inflammation is indicated by the fact that only a transient inflammatory response is provoked by the durable, but non-toxic, dust of titanium dioxide. Thus, it appears that the difference between harmful – in this case, quartz – and non-harmful particles (such as carbon) in the lungs is related to their ability to exercise an on-going inflammatory stimulus on pulmonary tissue (Brown et al., 1991). Similar preferential accumulation of quartz no doubt occurs with other dust–quartz mixtures, such as carbon/graphite and china clay, as long as exposure to dust continues.

Differences in susceptibility

As only a minority of coal miners with comparable exposure to coal-mine dust develop simple pneumoconiosis, and even fewer develop PMF, individual susceptibility has been proposed as a possible determining factor. However, because an immunological explanation has now been largely discounted (see page 373) – except in the case of rheumatoid pneumoconiosis – it seems likely that individual differences in deposition and clearance of dust may play an important role (see Chapter 3), in particular, selective clearance of coal dust but retention of quartz, especially in areas of fibrosis, and its preferential transference to lymph nodes (Reisner et al., 1982). With overloading of clearance mechanisms by dust, differing degrees of selective retention and persistence (or sequestration) of quartz and other non-coal minerals govern the type of lesions that develop (Davis et al., 1983). Thus, low levels of quartz in coal-mine and other carbonaceous dusts may be gradually concentrated in the lungs to levels that are decisive in the pathogenesis of pneumoconiosis.

A genetic influence, as reflected by histocompatibility antigens, plays no part in the development of either simple pneumoconiosis or PMF (see page 373).

The role of quartz

Carbon and almost 'pure' coal dusts are not cytotoxic. Pure carbon and natural graphite of high purity, administered by inhalation or intratracheal injection to various species of animals over prolonged periods, do not show any pathological changes in the lungs other than accumulation of dust in macrophages and in alveolar walls and hilar lymph nodes (Ray, King and Harrison, 1951). As the burden of inhaled 'submicron' particles of carbon black increases in the lungs of rats their clearance decreases and transport to lymph nodes increases (Nau et al., 1962; Holt, 1982; Strom, Johnston and Chan, 1987). Pulverized lignite, and bituminous and anthracite coal dusts, alone are not fibrogenic in various experimental animals (Zaidi et al., 1955a; Gross and Nau, 1967; Gross, Braun and de Treville, 1972; Martin, Daniel and Le Bouffant, 1977). The 'coal dust alone' employed by Martin, Daniel and Le Bouffant (1977) in their long-term experiments contained 0.4 per cent quartz and produced a slight increase in reticulin formation. Ray, King and Harrison (1951) showed that, although 'clean' coal (that is, pulverized anthracite containing 0.9 per cent ash with 0.2 per cent silica) and 'pure' pulverized graphite (containing 0.72 per cent ash with 0.24 per cent silica), administered similarly to rats, were deposited in the alveolar interstitium and did not cause fibrosis, the addition of a small quantity of quartz (2 mg) to either resulted in fibrotic lesions in the lungs. In addition,

Martin et al. (1972) found that, when rats were exposed by inhalation to samples of crushed, *uncleaned*, coal with differing contents of non-coal minerals for 21 months, there was a three- to fivefold increase in the development of fibrosis with samples containing, respectively, 5 and 10 per cent quartz compared with animals exposed to coal dust only; fibrosis occurred earlier and was more severe in the sample having the higher content of quartz. This, and similar observations, strongly suggest that coal dust inhibits, in varying degrees, the fibrogenic action of quartz – an affect that has been attributed mainly to aluminium in the non-coal minerals, kaolinite and muscovite–illite, and not to coal itself (Le Bouffant et al., 1982; Reisner et al., 1982; Davis et al., 1983). The inhibitory action of aluminium silicates on the fibrogenic effect of quartz in rats is greater the higher the content of silica in the dust, and is absent with 'pure' coal with less than 0.5 per cent quartz (Le Bouffant, Daniel and Martin, 1977). Indeed, the surface of quartz particles in dust from lower-rank coal seams has been found to be more contaminated with non-coal minerals, and, thus, less biologically active, than that from higher-rank seams (Kriegseis and Scharmann, 1985). The ability of aluminium clay compounds to release aluminium also varies considerably according to their type and structure, illite being the most active (Le Bouffant et al., 1982). It is possible, too, that other substances, such as organic matter, may exert an inhibiting effect, but evidence for this is lacking. However, the protective action of aluminium appears to be transient so that the toxicity of quartz with its fibrogenic potential gradually reasserts itself (Le Bouffant et al., 1982). Preferential clearance from the lungs of non-coal minerals, other than quartz, and consequent alterations in their relative concentrations could account for this. Differing ratios of quartz to other non-coal minerals in various coal-mine dusts may, in fact, explain the apparent contradiction of a higher prevalence of coal pneumoconiosis in high-rank mines with lower contents of non-coal minerals than in low-rank mines in which there is greater non-coal content, including quartz. In the former, although quartz levels are lower, the accompanying aluminium minerals which are also low may have less of an inhibitory effect on its fibrogenicity whereas, in the latter, although the level of quartz is higher, there is substantially more micaceous mineral to suppress its fibrogenic activity (Le Bouffant et al., 1988).

It is of interest that on the basis of their experimental observations of various German coal-mine dusts, Bruch and Hilscher (1988) stated that '. . . the widely fluctuating range of fibrogenicity can only be explained by a corresponding wide variation of inhibiting factors' and that 'the inhibiting effects increase proportionally more than the mineral content'. They concluded: 'a relatively strong inhibition is inherent with dusts of high non-coal mineral content, whereas the specific activity of quartz in dust containing much carbon is higher. Thus, some equalizing function may be deduced which increases the fibrogenic effects of dusts low in non-coal minerals.' These conclusions are consonant with those of Davis et al. (1983) discussed earlier.

However, the contrary hypothesis that concentration of dust in itself is more important than its composition and that minor quantities of quartz can be discounted still receives support (Heppleston, Kulonen and Potila, 1984; Heppleston, 1991a) (see Chapter 5, 'Fibrogenesis: coalmine dust'). The work of Gosset et al. (1991) has lent some support to the hypothesis that either compounds other than quartz or a complex interaction between different particles may play a part in pathogenesis, and has also shown that, in vitro, coal-mine dust (containing 3.2 per cent quartz) induced the release of the cytokines tumour necrosis factor α and interleukin-6 (IL6) (see Chapter 4) from human alveolar macrophages – a phenomenon that is not exclusively related to the effects of crystalline silica.

Heppleston (1991b) has suggested that differing compositions of coal-mine dust in miners' lungs during a working life may result in varying participation of lipid with corresponding variable separation of mineral particles from macrophages and, thus, of the degree of resultant fibrotic response; this could, perhaps, account for discrepancies of prevalence of pneumoconiosis between collieries. Removal of lipid by normal degradation would, of course, leave no trace that this interesting, but conjectural, process had in fact occurred (see Chapter 5, under 'Lipidosis').

Specific aspects of the pathogenesis of PMF

There are five possible factors that may be involved: (1) total burden of dust; (2) quartz; (3) infection; (4) immunological; and (5) central lymph node changes.

Total burden of dust

For some years the most favoured hypothesis in the UK has been that cumulative exposure to respirable dust is decisive because the probability of developing PMF increases with rising radiological category of simple pneumoconiosis (Cochrane, 1962). However, recent studies – already referred to under 'Incidence and prevalence' – showed that about half the cases of PMF, although clearly related to exposure, occurred in men with radiographs of category 0 or 1 (Shennan et al., 1981; Hurley et al., 1987). This suggests that some factor other than, or in addition to, total dust is operating; indeed, Hurley et al. (1987) concluded that 'the carbon content of coal was not obviously related to PMF risks among men with categories 2 or 3 simple pneumoconiosis' and 'that the association between the carbon content of the coal and incidence of simple pneumoconiosis is not strong'. Moreover, there are the further difficulties that similar amounts of dust have been found in the lungs of miners with simple pneumoconiosis to those found in miners with PMF (King, Maguire and Nagelschmidt, 1956), and that PMF lesions occur as either single or bilaterally asymmetrical masses, whereas simple pneumoconiosis has a more or less symmetrical distribution. Further, there is the seeming paradox that, on the one hand, PMF may never develop in category 3 simple pneumoconiosis whereas, on the other, PMF can occur in category 0 or 1, that is, in lungs that have a significant difference in their total burden of dust. The possibility that differences in deposition or clearance of dust, or both, influence events is referred to earlier (page 371), and factors that affect the rate of progression of PMF are mentioned on page 352.

Quartz

The tendency for accumulation and enrichment of quartz in lungs with PMF is seen in Figure 13.23, although this was not found in all cases (Davis, Ottery and Le Roux, 1977). However, higher mean total dust and lower ash content (quartz, kaolinite and mica) were present in lungs with homogeneous, black, PMF lesions that had no particular association with fibrotic nodules, in contrast to PMF with an ill-defined nodular structure where the content of ash components was higher. Nevertheless, quartz was present in the lungs with all types of PMF (Davis et al., 1983). Furthermore, as noted earlier, the case for quartz-free carbon dust as a cause of PMF appears weak, to say the least, on the evidence as it now stands.

Infection

The theory that tuberculosis modified by coal-mine dust is an important determinant held a dominant place for some years, based mainly on the postmortem bacteriological evidence of James (1954) and Rivers et al. (1957) in miners in South Wales, where endemic tuberculosis had recently been prevalent. However, it failed to explain all cases even during that period when tuberculosis was far more prevalent than it is today.

Concentration of soot and pigment in areas of tuberculous disease in the lungs of city dwellers was often observed until recent times owing to migration of carbon-laden macrophages to those sites; it is likely that a similar process occurs when tuberculosis develops in lungs containing coal dust. However, in spite of persuasive experimental evidence such as that of Zaidi et al. (1955b), in which the combined administration of coal dust and tubercle bacilli of low virulence to guinea-pigs produced lesions akin to PMF, although neither did alone, it is difficult to sustain the tuberculosis hypothesis as the chief or sole explanation of PMF in human subjects.

No difference in tuberculin reactivity was found in miners and ex-miners with different categories of pneumoconiosis, or no pneumoconiosis, in South Wales and the Netherlands (Hart, Cochrane and Higgins, 1963; Hendriks and Bleiker, 1964), although Fritze et al. (1969) and Fritze (1975) observed an above-average prevalence of positive reactors in coalminers in the Ruhr. No decline in attack rate of PMF occurred, as might have been expected, in parallel with the fall in incidence of tuberculosis (Cochrane, 1962); PMF progresses in the absence of any evidence of active tuberculosis. Prolonged treatment with antituberculous drugs in 'sputum-negative' miners does not prevent progression of PMF (McCallum, 1961; Ball et al., 1969), and it is most exceptional to find any microscopic evidence of tuberculosis in these lesions today. Finally, it appears that, although the collagen content is significantly increased in lungs with fibrocaseous and inactive fibrotic tuberculous lesions, it is only slightly increased in PMF compared with the rest of the lung (Wagner, 1970).

Other infective agents, notably atypical (type IV) mycobacteria which may occur as secondary invaders, have also been indicted. However, although Gernez-Rieux et al. (1972) showed that experimental infection with *Mycobacterium kansasii* in guinea-pigs exposed to inhalation of quartz-free coal dust for a prolonged period can result in lesions similar to PMF, proof that similar events occur in human disease has not been forthcoming. There is also no evidence that other types of bacterial infection, acute or chronic, are involved in pathogenesis.

Nevertheless, Heppleston (1988) maintains that the 'evidence pointing to an infective factor in the genesis of PMF is too strong to be discounted . . '.

Immunological

Reference has already been made to immunological events in this context in Chapter 5 (under 'The immunological component').

Immunologically competent cells and rheumatoid factor (IgM) were demonstrated by Wagner and McCormick (1967) at the periphery of many PMF lesions with obliterative vasculitis in which plasma cells featured, and also in hilar lymph nodes, but rheumatoid factor was found infrequently in PMF without vasculitis. Thus, it was proposed that PMF with vasculitis may be of rheumatoid origin – a variant of Caplan-type nodules in fact (Wagner, 1971). Subsequent evidence, however, suggests that neither humoral nor cellular components of immune activity have a primary role in pathogenesis of coal pneumoconiosis, and that the inconstancy of circulating antinuclear or rheumatoid factors in cases of PMF indicates that they are most probably provoked by the disease process itself. The development of PMF is not related to levels of circulating antibodies, and the competence of humoral immunity is not affected (Boyd, Robertson and Davis, 1982; Robertson et al., 1984). In addition, there appears to be no relationship between radiological category of pneumoconiosis and levels of circulating T and B lymphocytes (Robertson et al., 1983). Even so it may, perhaps, be premature to dismiss an immunological component completely. Immunological factors do, however, intervene decisively but exceptionally in the genesis of so-called rheumatoid pneumoconiosis (see page 376).

There is no evidence to date that a *genetic influence* operates, in that none of the histocompatibility locus antigens (HLA) tested is associated with a significantly altered risk – positive or negative – of developing pneumoconiosis (Heise et al., 1979; Wagner and Darke, 1979; Souter et al., 1983).

Central lymph node changes

Seal et al. (1986) have suggested that hilar lymph nodes, enlarged by dust-induced necrotic collagenous fibrosis, ulcerate into adjacent bronchi (locally replacing ciliated epithelium by cuboidal epithelium) or pulmonary arteries with the release of dust-laden material into the associated area of lung, thereby initiating the development of PMF. The mechanism of this putative process is far from clear, although local impairment of mucociliary or lymphatic clearance may be envisaged, and the hypothesis accords with preferential migration of quartz to hilar lymph nodes mentioned earlier.

Summary

The stimulus for the formation of PMF, which occurs in some men but not in others, is not known; it is likely that more than one factor is involved. Tuberculous infection probably accounted for some cases in areas of endemic tuberculosis in the past, and whereas the influence of quartz may have been underestimated that of immunological factors (apart from rheumatoid pneumoconiosis), though now difficult to sustain, should not be too hastily rejected. Differences in deposition and clearance of coal-mine dust between individuals (see Chapter 3) may, perhaps, explain susceptibility and, hence, prevalence of PMF in the same coalfield, in particular, differences of enrichment of quartz in the lungs and central lymph nodes. The 'central lymph node hypothesis' requires further investigation.

Trace metals and organic constituents in coal

The lungs of miners of bituminous coal in West Virginia have been found to contain higher concentrations of trace metals than those of the general population but there was no correlation between severity of pneumoconiosis and chromium, copper, iron, manganese, nickel, titanium or zinc (Sweet, Crouse and Crable, 1974). Sorenson, Köber and Petering (1974) reported a higher content of copper, iron, nickel, lead and zinc in the lungs of bituminous miners in Pennsylvania with a high prevalence of pneumoconiosis compared with miners of similar coal with a low incidence of pneumoconiosis in Utah. They suggested that certain trace metals in coal might play a role in the pathogenesis of coal pneumoconiosis. But there is no evidence to support this contention. Exceptionally, coals with high concentrations of one or other trace elements do occur, for example, high selenium-containing coals in Enshoi province in China (Yang et al., 1983). In his authoritative study of this question, Swaine (1990) has stated: 'In general, it seems that trace elements cannot be regarded as a hazard during coal mining and usage, assuming that due care is taken to ensure proper operational conditions.'

The aliphatic and aromatic hydrocarbons which may be present in coal can be leached out by biological fluids and, according to Harrington (1972), should be considered as possible factors in pathogenesis. Small amounts of organic humic and fulvic acids, which have the capacity to bind trace metals, are, apparently, more prevalent in some coals than in others, and it has been postulated that they may be slowly leached out in the lungs and exert a harmful effect by interfering, for example, with metal-dependent enzymes (Kober et al., 1976). However, a pathogenic relationship between these factors and coal pneumoconiosis is unlikely.

Pulverized fuel ash

Cytological studies indicate that the dust is not fibrogenic and no pulmonary disease has been observed in animals or in human beings exposed to PFA or fly ash alone or mixed with sulphur dioxide (McFarland et al., 1971; Alarie et al., 1975; Bonnell, Schilling and Massey, 1980; Raask and Schilling, 1980; Raabe et al., 1982). In rats pre-exposed to fly ash, the fibrotic reaction in their lungs after subsequent exposure to quartz dust was significantly more retarded and less extensive than when they were exposed to quartz dust only (Kaw and Khana, 1988).

A case of diffuse interstitial fibrosis which was conjectured to be caused by fly ash was unconvincing, particularly as asbestos bodies were present in the lungs (Golden et al., 1982).

Non-coal carbonaceous minerals

Justification for the contention that silica, even in small amounts, plays no part in the genesis of coal pneumoconiosis has relied heavily on cases of radiologically and pathologically indistinguishable pneumoconiosis in coal trimmers and workers in carbon manufacturing processes – notably, synthetic graphite and carbon black – in which quartz was supposed to be absent or present in only trace amounts. But, as mentioned earlier (page 342), washed coal (to which coal trimmers were exposed) retains its non-coal minerals and, in his valuable review of the aetiology of graphite pneumoconiosis, Hanoa (1983) showed that valid evidence for this hypothesis is both exiguous and uncertain.

Between 1924 and 1983 approximately 540 cases of graphite pneumoconiosis had been reported. In 167 of these there is no indication as to whether exposure had been to natural or synthetic graphite, and, of the remainder, the majority had worked with natural graphite and the rest with synthetic graphite. Most were diagnosed solely on clinical grounds, and only 39 on biopsy or autopsy findings. In 25 of these cases no information about the type of graphite or its content of silica was provided. Thus, only 14 fairly well-documented cases remained. Ten of these were exposed to natural graphite containing at least 2.7 per cent free silica, three to natural graphite with a silica content of 4 to 10 per cent and one case of exposure to synthetic graphite supposedly containing less than 0.02 per cent silica (Hanoa, 1983). This last case (Lister and Wimborne, 1972) comes from one of some five reports of carbon-related pneumoconiosis which have usually been taken to provide telling evidence against the 'quartz hypothesis', and should, therefore, be looked at in some detail. The man had worked from 1942 to 1959 turning and grinding bars of synthetic graphite but no details of the process or surrounding workshop conditions were given. Chemical analysis of dust taken from the work bench about the time of diagnosis (some 17 years after exposure commenced) yielded a quartz content of 0.02 per cent (Lister, 1961). The lungs contained numerous fibrous nodules some of which consisted of 'whorls of fibrous tissue' thought to be caused by 'nearly pure carbon' because ashed lung 'showed little or no birefringent particles, indicating the *absence of siliceous material*' (original emphasis): an invalid conclusion (see Appendix IV).

Other reports include one of a carbon black worker, and another of carbon electrode workers. The carbon black worker, who had PMF, was employed in a rubber factory for 31 years until 1958. From 1927 to 1948 he weighed and dispensed carbon black powder in the stores, but, for the remaining 11 years, he operated a rubber-extruding machine in which 'french chalk' ('talcum' powder) was used – a possible source of quartz (see Chapter 16). Post-mortem examination of his lungs showed nodules of 5 to 10 mm diameter which 'consisted of densely pigmented, whorled hyaline fibres showing some resemblance to silicotic nodules', and X-ray diffraction revealed the presence of 'a little mullite, talc and doubtful traces of quartz and cristobalite' (Miller and Ramsden, 1961). In two men, both with PMF, who had worked 'in the manufacture of carbon electrodes' (but at which stage of the process is not stated) during the 1930s and 1940s, the amount of quartz in their lungs was estimated by X-ray diffraction to be less than 0.03 and 0.07 g respectively (Watson et al., 1959). In addition, small quantities of mica and mullite (formed by high-temperature transformation of aluminium silicates in coke) were found in both so that some cristobalite may well have been present (see Appendix IV, under 'Routine optical microscopy'), but, if so, the amount would have been small.

Three additional cases include one of PMF in a grinder of graphite (whether natural or synthetic is not clear) whose lungs were reported to contain no quartz (Rüttner, Bovet and Aufdermaur, 1952), and two of PMF in Japanese carbon electrode workers in whose factory samples of dust deposited on work benches contained less than 0.1 per cent free silica by X-ray diffraction, although the amount in their lungs was not reported (Okutani, Shima and Sano, 1964).

Another, sometimes quoted, case of a severe degree of pneumoconiosis thought to be caused solely by carbon in an electrode moulder exposed to graphite is unreliable because X-ray diffraction analysis revealed 'undetermined crystalline impurities' in the dust, and the author himself concluded that 'the question whether graphite can cause pneumoconiosis was not solved' (MacMahon, 1952).

Epidemiological studies of graphite pneumoconiosis – of which there are 18 – have differed so much in definition of populations at risk, in methods of examination and of sampling of workplace dust (usually single random tests, if done at all), and in the radiological techniques and classifications used that they do not conform to the basic requirements for such studies; thus, the reported incidence rates of pneumoconiosis (which vary from 4 to 73 per cent) cannot be validly related to different contents of silica in graphite dust (Hanoa, 1983). It is probable that the incidence of pneumoconiosis associated with the production of any type of non-coal carbon materials is now very low but, as Hanoa (1983) pointed out, there 'is still a need for well-designed epidemiologic studies which could help to establish the dose–response relationship between graphite dust with different quartz contents and pneumoconiosis'.

Conclusion

1. Pure carbon and 'cleaned' or almost quartz-free coal do not cause fibrosis in the lungs of animals. In human beings they may, as in the case of other non-fibrogenic dusts, form non-fibrotic macular lesions of simple pneumoconiosis. However, the hypothesis that the quantity of carbon (or coal) dust alone may cause nodular or PMF lesions when its rate of deposition exceeds that of its clearance from the lungs – whereas other 'inert' dusts under similar circumstances do not – may appear incongruous.

2. Overall, the evidence is in favour of quartz playing a significant, specific or catalytic role in the genesis of the nodular and PMF lesions of coal pneumoconiosis. Reciprocal differential clearance or 'enrichment' of coal or carbon and non-coal (non-carbon) minerals and of quartz, respectively, migration of quartz to the lymphatic system, and the variable influence of non-coal minerals on the cytotoxicity of quartz are each clearly important in their own way, although the details of these complex relationships still have to be properly defined.

3. Evidently there are incompatibilities in some of the reports that claim that similar pneumoconiotic lesions may be caused by almost silica-free carbon, although, if the analytical techniques in the remaining cases were accurate, the possibility would not be excluded. However, this small handful of cases (of which only that of Watson et al. (1959) carries a degree of conviction) hardly seems adequate evidence to override or reject the 'silica hypothesis' outright in favour of one that relies soley on the burden of carbonaceous dust in the lungs – especially when differential 'enrichment' and clearance of the different mineral components are considered.

4. Thus, composition of the dust and, possibly, the size of particles, and not simply its accumulation or total load in the lungs, appear to be key

factors (in which crystalline silica is prominent) in pathogenesis; because of the various permutations in composition, a spectrum of pathological response ensues.

5. These conclusions have a bearing on the standards of exposure limits for quartz in 'respirable' dust, not only in coal mining, but also in other dusty industries (Seaton et al., 1981). They also indicate the protean nature of coal pneumoconiosis in general and the complexity of the interrelationships between the many factors that appear to be involved in its pathogenesis.

Associated DIPF

There is no evidence of a specific causal relationship between coal or carbon dust and DIPF. However, Heppleston (1991a) has suggested that DIPF, rather than nodular or circumscribed lesions, may be caused by a limited degree of lipidosis formed by carbonaceous or siliceous dust prompting type II alveolar cells to secrete excessive surfactant lipid (see page 124). The lipidosis is envisaged as modifying and dispersing the usually localized pneumoconiotic process within the interstitium. Proof that such events occur and give rise to DIPF in coal-miners' lungs is lacking.

Whatever its cause, DIPF that develops in lungs containing coal or carbon dust is likely to become heavily pigmented. The dose-related association of cigarette smoking with minor degrees of DIPF is discussed elsewhere in this chapter (page 383) and in Chapters 7 and 14.

Rheumatoid coal nodules

A significant association of circulating rheumatoid factor and radiographic evidence of rheumatoid coal pneumoconiosis, with and without arthritis, by comparison with simple coal pneumoconiosis and PMF without arthritis, was demonstrated by Caplan, Payne and Withey (1962) (Figure 13.25). Thus, the rheumatoid diathesis was taken as intervening in the determination of an exceptional reaction to the inhaled dust.

The pathogenesis of the lesions is uncertain but, as the presence of immunologically competent cells and rheumatoid factor (IgM) in and around the nodules suggests, it is most probably determined by an immunological reaction (Robertson et al., 1984). However, the respective roles of cellular and humoral immunity have yet to be clearly defined. It is not known, for example, whether the lymphocytes

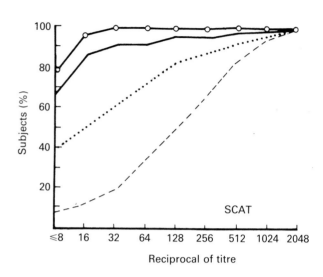

Figure 13.25 Cumulative distribution of sensitized sheep cell agglutination (SCAT) titres expressed as reciprocals in 269 Welsh coal miners. (o-o-o) No pneumoconiosis or simple pneumoconiosis and no arthritis; (——) PMF without arthritis; (. . . . .) rheumatoid pneumoconiosis suspected radiographically without arthritis; (- - - -) rheumatoid pneumoconiosis suspected radiographically with rheumatoid arthritis. (Reproduced, with permission, from Caplan, Payne and Withey, 1962)

are B or T cells and, if the latter, whether helper or suppressor cells; nor is it known whether cytokines are involved. This is a matter of interest because a relationship between prostaglandin E_2 (PGE_2) and interleukin-1 (IL1) (see Table 4.5), which are known to influence formation and necrosis of collagen, has been observed in rheumatoid nodules of the skin – lesions that are histologically similar to Caplan nodules without dust (Myasaka et al., 1989). Although the association of antinuclear antibodies is generally regarded as a non-specific finding, they are now known to consist of about 12 separate entities (Bernstein, 1990); thus, a possible special role of one or more of these in pathogenesis cannot, at present, be confidently excluded.

As described earlier, lungs with typical Caplan nodules usually contain substantially less dust than those with non-rheumatoid PMF as is evident from the post-mortem appearances and the fact that, as a rule, there is little or no radiographic 'background' of simple pneumoconiosis. But, in the variant cases in which nodules are of mixed type (that is, large and small) or are all small and widely scattered, a category 2 (rarely category 3) 'background' may be present (Davies and Linders, 1968) (see under 'Radiographic appearances'). This paucity of dust in so many of these cases is difficult to explain. The presence of immunological reactivity is supported by the observation, referred to already on page 362, that the prevalence of typical rheumatoid pneumoconiosis may be similar to that of circulating rheumatoid factor in the general population. The prevalence of immunological reactivity, however, may vary significantly in different geographical areas.

Just as rheumatoid arthritis presents a variable picture, ranging from a fulminant onset with high titres of rheumatoid factor at one extreme, through mild, sometimes transient, arthritis with fluctuating levels of rheumatoid factor to the presence of rheumatoid factor without arthritis at the other extreme, there is a corresponding scale of pulmonary lesions. At the one end, there are necrobiotic nodules in individuals with rheumatoid arthritis but no known dust exposure (Locke, 1963; Noonan, Taylor and Engleman, 1963) and typical Caplan nodules with past dust exposure; in between, mixed nodules with or without rheumatoid arthritis, or scattered small nodules often without arthritis and, in some cases, rheumatoid factor; and, at the other end, non-rheumatoid PMF with simple pneumoconiosis and no arthritis. Thus, Caplan nodules appear to be associated with (1) high immunological activity and low dust content; (2) the variant type of rheumatoid pneumoconiosis, with transient or lower immunological activity and larger quantities of dust; and (3) non-rheumatoid PMF, with low or absent immunological activity and high dust content (see Figure 13.45). Whether or not this notional scale has pathogenic validity remains to be established but it correlates reasonably well with clinical and autopsy observations in Britain.

Miall (1955) showed that there was no increased prevalence of rheumatoid arthritis among miners and ex-miners with PMF compared with an agricultural population, indicating that the pathogenesis of the arthritis is not related either to dust exposure or to the PMF process in the lungs.

The status of the *tuberculin test* in rheumatoid pneumoconiosis does not appear to be known, but proven coexistent tuberculosis has been extremely rare.

The question of circulating rheumatoid factor and antinuclear antibody in non-rheumatoid coal pneumoconiosis is discussed on pages 394 to 397.

disease – most frequently, in the UK, chronic bronchitis with airflow obstruction. Among British coal miners, smoking has been found to be the chief factor contributing to respiratory symptoms (Ashford et al., 1970).

There is little correlation between respiratory symptoms and radiological category of PMF. Category A lesions cause no symptoms and larger masses may be associated with either no symptoms or those of respiratory disability ranging from trivial to very severe. The reasons for this variability are referred to in the section lung function. Dyspnoea in coal miners with no radiographic evidence of pneumoconiosis is due to unrelated non-occupational disease. The question of chronic bronchitis is discussed in Chapters 9 and 10.

There is usually no sputum associated with PMF if the subject is a non-smoker; when there is, it is generally small in volume but may be large if there is infection in distorted and dilated bronchi in proximity to a mass of PMF. In the absence of active tuberculosis (or other causes), haemoptysis is rare in cases of PMF but is not uncommon – although consisting of little more than staining of the sputum with blood – in cases of rheumatoid pneumoconiosis; in association with the radiographic appearance of cavities (see 'Radiographic appearances'), this may compound a mistaken diagnosis of 'sputum-negative' tuberculosis. Large haemoptysis is very rare. Jet-black sputum is produced by the occasional rupture of PMF with ischaemic necrosis into a bronchus; it may be large in amount, suddenly raised by distressing paroxysmal coughing and may continue in smaller amounts for some days. It consists of mucus containing large quantities of coal (or carbon) dust with cholesterol crystals and, occasionally, small amounts of blood.

Cough is, in general, related to cigarette smoking and the quantity or viscidity of the sputum. But, in some cases of large PMF lesions, cough may be frequent, severe and paroxysmal and often provoked by effort. The reason for this is uncertain; it may be related to 'irritation' of the trachea and main bronchi by large adjacent masses.

Men with PMF uncomplicated by severe scar emphysema or chronic airways' obstruction rarely complain of breathlessness at rest but may do during or after effort.

Clinical features

Symptoms

Simple pneumoconiosis is symptomless. When cough, sputum, wheeze and breathlessness are complained of they are due to coincidental lung

Physical signs

There are no characteristic abnormal physical signs. Finger clubbing is not a feature of either simple pneumoconiosis or PMF. Central cyanosis is not seen in the absence of airways' obstruction of 'blue bloater'-type or unrelated heart disease.

Simple pneumoconiosis and most cases of PMF (even category C) cause no abnormal signs. The trachea is occasionally drawn to one side by contractile PMF, and inspiratory and expiratory stridor caused by distortion of large airways may be heard at the mouth in such cases. Impaired breath sounds and expiratory wheezes are found when massive lesions are associated with severe scar emphysema. Wheezes and rhonchi are most commonly due to coincidental chronic obstruction bronchitis. In some men with 'irregular' radiographic opacities persistent inspiratory crackles may be heard at the bases of the lungs.

Rheumatoid arthritis and subcutaneous rheumatoid nodules should be looked for. The signs of pleural effusion may occasionally be present and mark the onset or exacerbation of rheumatoid disease.

Large, bilateral PMF lesions may be accompanied by signs of pulmonary heart disease and, ultimately, congestive failure, but this is rarely seen today.

Lung function

There are no abnormal physiological changes that are characteristic of coal or other types of carbonaceous pneumoconiosis. Thus, pulmonary function tests have no value in establishing diagnosis.

Simple pneumoconiosis

Most studies of coal miners have shown little or no decrement of ventilatory capacity (measured as FEV_1) with increasing category of simple pneumoconiosis when age has been taken into account (Cochrane and Higgins, 1961; Higgins and Oldham, 1962; Ashford et al., 1968; Morgan et al., 1974), but significant reduction is often associated with smoking (Rogan et al., 1973; Morgan and Lapp, 1976). In 36 life-long, non-smoking Welsh miners with simple pneumoconiosis, mean values of FEV_1 and FVC were found to be similar to those predicted for healthy non-miners of similar age and height, although significantly lower than those of the non-smoking control group; however, this group consisted of only 10 subjects with exceptionally high normal levels of FEV_1 and FVC (Legg, Cotes and Bevan, 1983). Nemery et al. (1987) described a slight, significant fall in FEV_1, although with similar FVC, in 32 non-smoking, symptomless Belgian coal miners with and without simple pneumoconiosis (10 mostly less than category 3 and 22 with no evidence of pneumoconiosis) compared with non-smoking steelworkers of similar age; they attributed the difference to exposure to coal dust. It has been

suggested that slight decline of FEV_1 in some cases of simple pneumoconiosis in French miners (smokers and non-smokers) is accounted for by reduction in FVC (Bates et al., 1985). From a study of 7139 US coal miners, Attfield and Hodous (1992) concluded that exposure to dusty conditions (6 mg/m³) had an adverse effect on their ventilatory capacity (FEV_1, FVC and FEV_1/FVC) not unlike that of smoking cigarettes even in the absence of radiographic evidence of pneumoconiosis. However, because standard deviation of the important variables in the study are very large, and estimates of the coefficients may be far from their true values due to multicollinearity of the variables, the conclusions should be treated with some reserve.

Whether or not there is a relationship between impairment of ventilatory capacity and cumulative exposure to coal-mine dust is discussed in Chapter 10.

Some loss of elastic recoil has been demonstrated in all categories of simple pneumoconiosis in life-long, non-smoking and non-bronchitic Welsh coal miners. This was associated with significantly increased RV and RV/TLC ratio in categories 2 and 3 (Legg, Cotes and Bevan, 1983). However, no relationship between increased RV with increasing category of simple pneumoconiosis and cigarette smoking on airflow obstruction of larger airways (normal FEV_1/FVC) was found in an earlier study of American bituminous coal miners (Morgan et al., 1971). By measuring the response of forced expiratory flow (FEF) at 50 per cent FVC (FEF_{50}) during breathing of helium dioxide, Legg, Cotes and Bevan (1983) also observed changes that may be consistent with slight intrinsic narrowing of small airways with increasing category of simple pneumoconiosis.

Static compliance is reported to be unaffected (Seaton, Lapp and Morgan, 1972a; Murphy et al., 1982), although a tendency towards slightly increased compliance in some men with p-type opacities compared with those with q-type opacities was noted by Musk et al. (1981).

Earlier studies indicated that gas transfer (T_L) is normal in men with category q and r pneumoconiosis but may be reduced to a minor degree in those with p-type opacities (Englert and de Coster, 1965; Cotes et al., 1971; Cotes and Field, 1972; Seaton, Lapp and Morgan, 1972a; Frans, Veriter and Brasseur, 1975). Not all investigators have detected any reduction in T_L (Pivoteau and Dechoux, 1972); Nemery et al. (1987) found no difference in T_L in non-smoking Belgian coal miners with simple or no pneumoconiosis and non-smoking steelworkers of similar age. But in subjects with predominantly p-type opacities, Musk et al. (1981) observed slight reduction of T_L and K_{CO}, increase of static compliance and some physiological features of emphysema. These findings are consistent with some

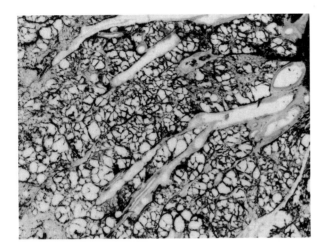

Figure 13.26 Coal-dust pigmented panacinar emphysema which was uniformly spread throughout both lungs: radiographic category 3p. (Paper-mounted section, natural size)

increase in airspace size – confirmed by Ruckley et al. (1984a) – and with a longer residence time of inhaled 0.5-μm particles in the lungs of subjects with category p, compared with those with categories q and r, and with normal miners (Hankinson, Palmes and Lapp, 1979) (Figure 13.26) (see under 'Irregular opacities').

Although slight hypoxia – reduction of partial pressure of arterial oxygen (PaO_2) – has been reported at rest and during exercise in some, especially older, miners both with and without simple pneumoconiosis (Frans et al., 1975; Smidt, Worth and Bielert, 1977), many were smokers and had respiratory symptoms. Nemery et al. (1987) found that PaO_2 'values were abnormal although not pathological' at rest and on exercise in a small group of non-smoking Belgian coal miners (20 of 32) with or without simple pneumoconiosis. However, Lapp and Seaton (1971) had earlier observed that mean PaO_2 lies within normal range during exercise in all categories of simple pneumoconiosis.

The alveolar–arterial oxygen gradient (A–aPO_2) is reported to be increased at rest in men with simple pneumoconiosis (Frans et al., 1975) and in miners without pneumoconiosis or large airways' obstruction (Lapp and Seaton, 1971). More recently, however, Roy et al. (1989) found no significant reduction in resting A–aPO_2 compared with age-predicted normal values in a large cohort (2297) of non-smoking, bituminous, American coal miners with all categories of simple pneumoconiosis, and no significant difference between categories 0 to 3. Thus, they concluded that smoking is the decisive factor in increasing the A–aPO_2 gradient at rest.

Progressive massive fibrosis

There is wide variation in the severity of functional impairment associated with PMF which correlates poorly with radiographic appearances. Responsible factors include, in varying degree, the size and anatomical site of the masses, the amount of associated vasculitis and the presence or absence of scar (irregular) or panacinar emphysema and chronic airways' obstruction.

Ventilatory capacity (FEV_1 and FVC) is usually reduced in greater or lesser degree in subjects with PMF categories B and C. This deficiency, which is often associated with irreversible airflow obstruction, appears to be caused either by distortion and narrowing of airways (as by any large space-occupying lesion) or by irregular emphysema associated with contracting PMF lesions (see Figure 13.15).

In some cases RV is increased but, in others, decreased, possibly due to the space-occupying effect. TLC is usually reduced, as is static compliance in most, but not all, instances.

Gas transfer (TL), in general, is impaired to a varying degree but remains normal in some individuals; although hypoxaemia (reduced PaO_2) is often present during exertion, it is absent at rest in most cases. The A–aPO_2 gradient increases on exertion in most subjects and, in some, is raised at rest (Morgan and Lapp, 1976). These changes are related to significant reduction in the vascular bed caused by the associated arteritis and, in particular, by centrally located masses; they may result in pulmonary hypertension and pulmonary heart disease (Navrátil, Widmisky and Kasalicky, 1968).

Typical, Caplan-type rheumatoid coal pneumoconiosis is usually accompanied by remarkably little, if any, impairment of function, probably because only a small amount of lung tissue is involved, and scar emphysema is absent. For example, the volumes occupied by five separate Caplan nodules of 1 cm diameter and by one non-rheumatoid PMF lesion of 5 cm diameter are, respectively, 2.6 ml and 65.4 ml. Abnormalities of FEV_1, FVC, FEV_1/FVC, VC and TLC have been shown to be significantly less in men with Caplan's syndrome than in those with non-rheumatoid PMF of similar radiological category, age, years worked underground and smoking habits having been taken into account (Constantinidis et al., 1978). However, atypical rheumatoid cases with confluent lesions may exhibit the range of functional changes associated with non-rheumatoid PMF in varying degree and, rarely, can be seriously disabling (see Figure 13.42).

Summary

Impairment of pulmonary function attributable to simple and category A pneumoconiosis is of minor

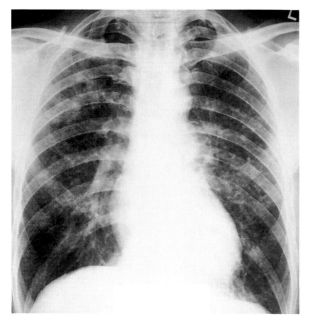

(a) 1959

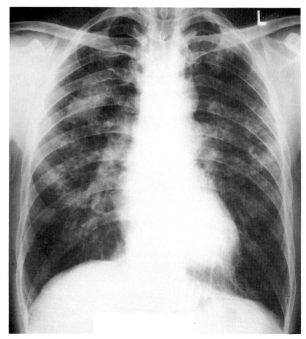

(b) 1965

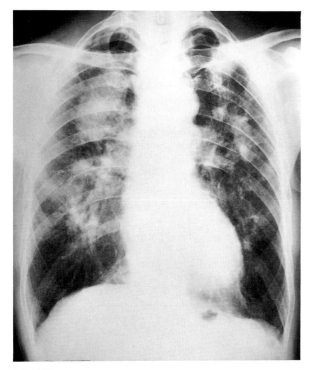

(c) 1976

Figure 13.27 Radiographs showing progression of coal pneumoconiosis in a miner who worked 16 years at the coal face and left the mines in 1960. The 1959 film (a) shows early confluence in the right upper zone (category 2qA). Both the 1965 (b) and 1976 (c) films show category 2qB. In 1976 the PMF opacity is well circumscribed: note the presence of linear opacities radiating from the PMF opacities. It is of interest that circulating rheumatoid factor (DAT 1:128) and antinuclear antibodies were present in 1976 but there were no rheumatic symptoms and no clinical arthropathy

degree and is related mostly to category p cases. Such changes are laboratory observations which, in the main, are not associated with any respiratory disability.

In the case of PMF categories B and C functional abnormalities are usually present, although of varying severity: reduction of ventilatory capacity and T_L, increased $A-aP_{O_2}$ at rest and with exercise, and hypoxaemia on exertion are the most significant. Consequent respiratory disability, which ranges from slight to severely incapacitating, correlates poorly with the radiographic appearances. The older the age at which PMF develops, the less likely it is that severe respiratory dysfunction will occur.

Coke oven workers

No adverse effect on ventilatory function was observed in a study of 354 retired French coke oven plant operators (Chau et al., 1992).

Carbon black and activated carbon workers

No association between total dust exposure and impairment of a range of ventilatory function tests – other than the effects of age and smoking – has been detected in a large number of workers in either industry in western Europe and the USA (Wehr et al., 1975; Crosbie, 1986; Robertson et al., 1988b).

Radiographic appearances

Ordinary (non-rheumatoid) pneumoconiosis

As stated earlier (under 'Incidence and prevalence') the profusion category of simple pneumoconiosis increases with the quantity of dust in the lungs (Rossiter, 1972a; Davis et al., 1979) (see Figure 13.5).

The earliest abnormal appearances consist of a few small, ill-defined, round opacities (distinguishable from vascular shadows) in the outer third of the lung fields and mainly in the upper and middle zones. Subsequently, they are more clearly defined and more widely distributed.

The size of simple pneumoconiosis opacities most commonly seen is category q; category r is less common and category p (the interpretation of which is often difficult) least common. Opacities of different category may be present in the one film but one category is usually predominant, and this is the category quoted. There is good correlation between the profusion of opacities (categories 1 to 3) and the lesions found in the lungs *post mortem*, and a clear relationship to the total content of dust in the lungs (see Figure 13.5) (Davis et al., 1979; Ruckley et al., 1981). It has been computed that the relative contributions of coal and other minerals to the radiological score of simple pneumoconiosis is 1 : 3.8 which is similar to the X-ray mass absorption coefficients of these two fractions (Rossiter, 1972b); in particular, the iron content of the lungs is especially well correlated with category (Bergman and Casswell, 1972; Rossiter, 1972b). Cases of p opacities are associated with the highest mean content of dust in the lungs regardless of rank of the coal mined (Ruckley et al., 1981), and sometimes with widespread emphysema (Figure 13.26).

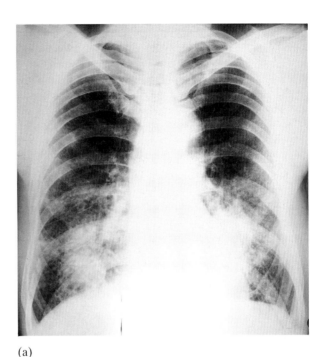

(a)

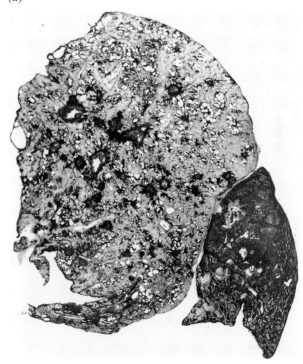

(b)

Figure 13.28 (a) Bilateral lower PMF in a coal miner for 46 years: category 2qB. PMF confirmed *post mortem* when distribution was similar to that seen in (b) (from another subject) which shows PMF occupying a shrunken lower lobe and a few large nodules, some containing ischaemic cavities, in the upper lobe. Note that the slight, but widely scattered, emphysema is not associated with dust, although four or five small stellate nodules with scar emphysema may be discerned posteriorly. (Paper-mounted section)

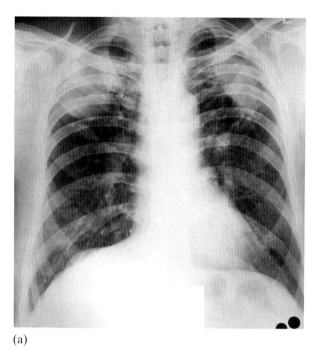
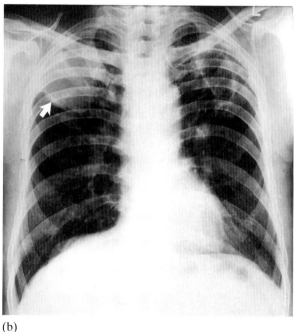

(a)   (b)

Figure 13.29 (a,b) Development of ischaemic cavity in left upper lobe PMF within 12 months associated with episodes of paroxysmal cough and jet-black sputum. A rim of calcification (arrowed) is also seen at the periphery of the lower pole of the PMF in the right lung. This appearance is a feature in some PMF lesions

The opacities of simple pneumoconiosis tend to be distributed in the upper halves of the lung fields until the category 3 stage is reached when the whole of the lung fields are more or less equally involved. PMF opacities – which, arbitrarily, are those larger than 1 cm in diameter (see Table 7.4) – are also more commonly seen in the upper than in the lower halves of the lung fields. They may be unilateral or bilateral and, if the latter, may be distributed roughly symmetrically or asymmetrically (Figure 13.27). In a minority of cases they are confined to the lower lung fields (Figure 13.28). An opacity caused by a single lesion may be obscured by the heart shadow on the standard posteroanterior (PA) film and is only clearly seen in lateral or oblique radiographs. Normally there is a 'background' of category 2 or 3 simple pneumoconiosis with PMF but in a few cases this is absent.

PMF opacities vary greatly in shape as well as in size. They may be round, ovoid, sausage-like or linear in outline, and, as a rule, are well demarcated from the adjacent lung (compare Figure 13.15). Occasionally linear markings radiate from the PMF into the lung field and may reach the chest wall. The development of a cavity within a PMF lesion is indicated by a well-defined, circumscribed translucency (Figure 13.29) in

which there may be evidence of fluid. In most cases the cavity vanishes sooner or later and appearances return wholly or partly to normal. An occasional feature of PMF is a dense peripheral arc or rim at its lower pole which represents calcification. This may be a sequel to accumulation of fluid in a previous cavity and, although probably not pathognomonic, the appearance is rarely seen in other diseases (Figure 13.29b). Evidence of dense calcification within the lesion is also sometimes seen (Figure 13.30). PMF of irregular or stellate outline is often associated with the signs of bullous emphysema, distortion of the lung, and shift of the trachea and mediastinum to the affected side caused by fibrotic scarring. Sometimes a mass alters position over a period of years due mainly to hyperinflation of adjacent emphysematous lungs when its appearance can be mistaken for that of a tumour (Figure 13.31a,b).

The opacities of PMF can be ill or well defined, often the former, in the early stages of disease – a feature more common in the carbonaceous pneumoconioses and 'mixed dust fibrosis' than in silicosis. It is, therefore, unfortunate that the terms 'ill defined' and 'well defined' (and their appropriate symbols) have been omitted in the 1980 ILO Classification (see Table 7.3).

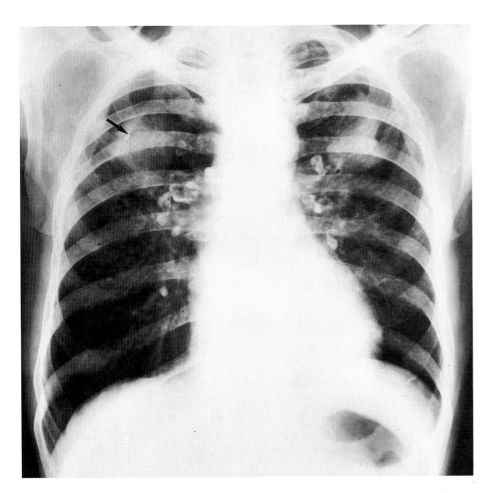

Figure 13.30 'Eggshell' calcification of the hilar lymph nodes and bilateral PMF. Note calcification (arrowed) within the mass in the right lung; standard tomography on CT scan may demonstrate this with greater clarity. Coal miner who worked 30 years underground, part of the time drilling rock for roadway development

The signs of 'eggshell' calcification of hilar lymph nodes, similar to those which may occur in silicosis (see Chapter 12), are present in a small proportion of cases of coal and natural graphite pneumoconiosis. They are more often found with PMF than with simple pneumoconiosis (Jacobsen et al., 1967) (see Figure 13.30). These appearances are related to past exposure to dust from siliceous rocks in shaft sinking or maintaining colliery roads and airways, or to the quartz of natural graphite.

Irregular opacities

Irregular, mainly basal, opacities may also be seen on standard PA radiographs in a minority of coal miners especially in later life; although much attention has been paid to these appearances in recent years, they do not have the significance of small round opacities. A number of different factors, in various permutations, are responsible for their production.

The quality of the chest radiograph is often decisive. As pointed out in Chapter 7 the two important factors that influence radiographic quality are density and contrast, both of which are affected by the thickness of the tissue and the length of the pathway through which X-rays pass. Thus, there is a greater likelihood of increased summation effects contributing to the appearance of irregular opacities in the lower, compared with the upper, lung fields. A spurious appearance of basal irregular opacities in the standard PA film is often caused by poor film quality in subjects who are obese or have significant dorsal kyphosis – abnormalities, incidently, that can impair expansion of the lungs with resultant restriction of ventilatory capacity.

Basal irregular opacities of low profusion (categories 0/1 to 1/2) seen in the radiographs of some cigarette smokers with no known occupational

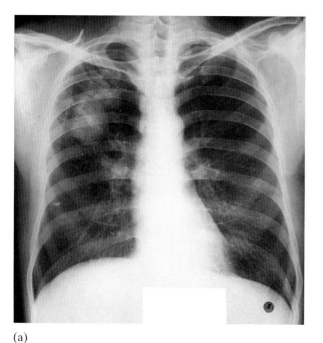

(a)

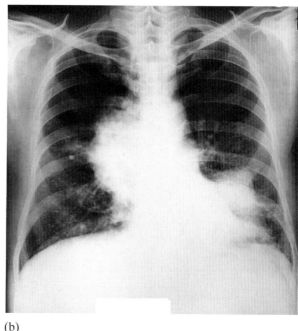

(b)

Figure 13.31 (a) Right upper zone PMF with very few accompanying discrete opacities of simple pneumoconiosis. (b) Twenty years later PMF is larger, well circumscribed and has shifted to the right hilar region. Another PMF is now present in the lower left lung field. There is severe hyperinflation – lung markings absent in upper halves of lung fields. Seen in isolation the appearances of either lung field might be mistaken for other pathology. Note linear opacities radiating from PMF in (a). Post-mortem confirmation

exposure to dusts have been correlated with smoking (Carilli, Kotzen and Fischer, 1973; Weiss, 1988), a relationship that has also been observed in workers exposed to non-hazardous dusts (Weiss, 1991). By contrast, from a study of the radiographs of 1422 subjects, also without known dust exposure, Castellan, Sanderson and Petersen (1985) concluded that, although there was an infrequent association between smoking and small irregular opacities, this was insignificant. But, as most (82 per cent) of their population – in what has been regarded as a 'most convincing study' (Blanc and Gamsu, 1989) – were under 45 years of age (mean age 33 years) (Weiss, 1991), a quantitative association with smoking would have been missed. From their analysis of this and four other studies, Blanc and Gamsu (1989) concluded that cigarette smoking alone is not associated with radiographic opacities consistent with pneumoconiosis, but this, as Weiss (1991) has shown, is most questionable.

Auerbach et al. (1963) and Auerbach, Garfinkel and Hammond (1974) showed a clear correlation between increasing cigarette consumption and DIPF and fibrosis of bronchiolar walls and arterioles (Figure 13.32). More recently, Adesina et al. (1991)

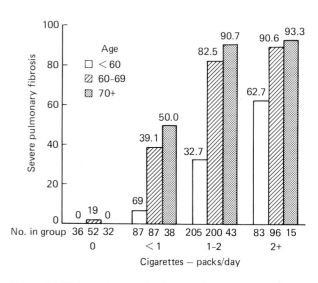

Figure 13.32 Prevalence of microscopic, severe, interstitial pulmonary fibrosis at autopsy in men in relation to age and cigarette-smoking habit. (Reproduced, with permission, from Weiss, 1988; source of data was Auerbach et al., 1963)

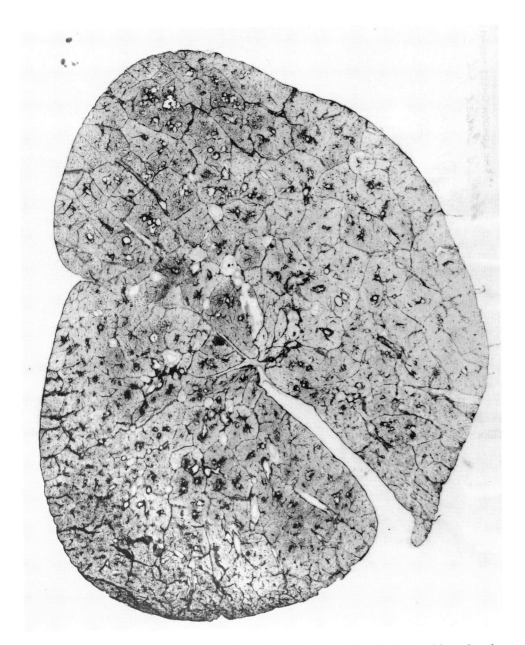

Figure 13.33 Sagittal section of a coal-miner's lung showing well-marked deposition of coal dust in interlobular septa, especially in the peripheral posterior and diaphragmatic zones of the lower lobe; a variable, but fairly common, finding in such lungs. Considered three-dimensionally, these deposits contribute significantly to the total radiographic image. A few nodular lesions of coal pneumoconiosis are also seen. Note sparsity of emphysema. (Paper-mounted section)

also found a significant association between smoking and fibrosis of membranous and respiratory bronchioles in the absence of any occupational exposure. This matter is discussed further in Chapter 7 and, in greater detail, in Chapter 14.

Smoking-related bronchiolar fibrosis and DIPF would be expected to have an additive effect on any other diffuse abnormal source of X-ray attenuation, with a consequent summation effect in the radiographic image. Deposition of substantial amounts of mineral dusts of various types – in this case coal – in interlobular fissures (Figure 13.33) may result in irregular, or Kerley 'B' linear, opacities in the lower lung fields (Trapnell, 1964) (see Chapter 7, 'Production of radiographic image'). The prevalence of 'B' lines increases with increasing category of

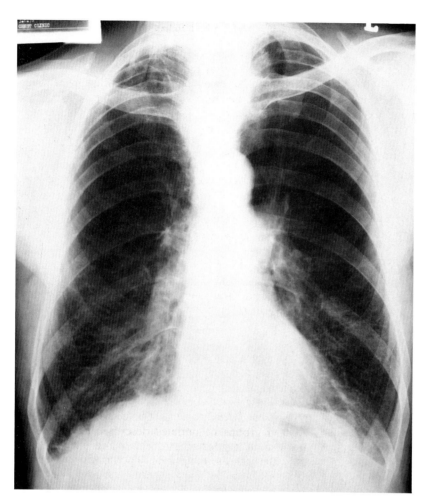

Figure 13.34 Severe hyperinflation of both upper lobes causing, by compression of the lower lobes, appearances that simulate slight DIPF. These could be interpreted as category s opacities. No occupational hazard

pneumoconiosis. Should panacinar emphysema be present in heavily dusted lungs the air–dust contrast effect on the image is likely to be enhanced, resulting in either irregular or p-type opacities, or both, according to the degree and distribution of pathological change (see Figure 13.26) (Hankinson, Palmes and Lapp, 1979) (see Chapter 7, page 177).

Basal irregular opacities are also caused if radiographs are inadvertently taken in full expiration or in inadequate inspiration (see Figure 7.3), by bilateral, severe hyperinflation of the upper lobes (Figure 13.34) especially when air–dust contrast is increased by the mass of coal dust in the lungs, and, of course, by asbestosis and other known causes of DIPF (see Table 7.3 and Chapter 15). The pathological features of DIPF seen in coal miners are described on pages 366 to 368.

In 1974 Lyons et al. found that irregular opacities in coal miners correlated positively with the extent of emphysema of unspecified type (their illustrated 'typical case' being one of mixed centriacinar and panacinar emphysema) and impairment of FEV_1, whereas rounded opacities did not. Later, Cockcroft et al. (1983) reported that these opacities were related to duration of exposure to coal-mine dust underground, and concluded that they were associated, pathologically, with emphysema and, to a lesser degree, with diffuse interstitial fibrosis, often in combination (Cockcroft et al., 1982a). However, apparently inconsistent lung function findings have been described in several similar investigations. In an unselected group of coal miners, Amandus et al. (1976) found that irregular opacities were predominantly associated with smoking, and, to a lesser degree, with age and years worked underground and that FEV_1, FVC and FEV_1/FVC were reduced, whereas no such functional decrements were present in non-smokers with irregular opacities.

After taking the effects of age, height and smoking into account, Cockcroft et al. (1982b) found a significant reduction in ventilatory capacity and T_L, but normal TLC, in coal miners with irregular opacities; they suggested that the lack of increased TLC pointed to the presence of diffuse fibrosis as well as to emphysema. However, their results also showed increased values of RV in those men with a greater number of irregular opacities compared with those with round opacities – a finding that reflects the presence of emphysema more faithfully than does an increase in TLC because TLC is often normal, or only slightly increased, in emphysematous subjects. Musk et al. (1981) also suggested that the functional abnormalities they found in coal miners with irregular opacities can be explained by the coexistence of emphysema and diffuse fibrosis, although their values of FEV_1 and FVC were almost identical in workers with and without irregular opacities; however, T_L and K_{CO} were reduced in those with irregular opacities. Again, Collins et al. (1988) reported that the impairment of FEV_1 and FVC they found in workers with irregular opacities, but not in those with round opacities, was not explicable in terms of age, bodily size or smoking habits, but was 'attributable to the miners' dust exposure as such'.

However, these and several similar studies of this topic do not quantify smoking in terms of life-long consumption, but simply categorize men as 'non-smokers', 'ex-smokers' and 'smokers' (subdivided, in some instances, into 'light' and 'heavy'). This is plainly wrong in that the effect of smoking is not an unchanging state, like sex and height (in adult life), but is cumulative with age in the same way as exposure to dust; both should be considered as continuously changing variables in multiple regression analyses (see Chapter 6, page 137).

The reality of the matter seems to be that irregular opacities – the recognition of which, incidently, is subject to considerable interobserver error (Amandus et al., 1974) – in coal miners can be caused by any of the factors just discussed, alone or in combination according to the circumstances. In other words, by the summation effect of accumulated coal-mine dust on the radiographic image, especially if associated with widespread emphysema (which, of course, is more common in smokers), and by the additional effect of smoking-induced changes in the lungs on the total image especially when these are associated with DIPF of whatever cause. Given these circumstances some apparent inconsistency in patterns of impairment of lung function in different subjects might be expected.

Altogether, the evidence gives little support to the suggestion of Cockcroft et al. (1983) that 'irregular opacities . . . should probably be considered to be part of simple coalworkers' pneumoconiosis'.

Rheumatoid pneumoconiosis

It has already been noted (page 362) that the radiographic, as well as the pathological, features of this variant of the disease differ from those of ordinary coal pneumoconiosis both in appearance and behaviour. The radiographic changes that may occur vary widely and can be enumerated as follows:

1. Typical Caplan-type opacities.
2. Scanty, large round opacities.
3. Mixed, small and large, round and irregular opacities.
4. Scanty, small, round opacities.
5. Multiple, small, round opacities.
6. One or other of these in association with pneumoconiosis of non-rheumatoid, or usual, appearance.
7. Sudden development of widespread, ill-defined opacities.

Caplan-type opacities (Caplan, 1953)

Typically these are round, fairly dense, vary from about 0.5 to 3.0 cm in diameter (occasionally up to 5 cm) and correspond to the discrete nodules or matted groups of nodules described earlier. They are usually moderate in number and are scattered irregularly in the lung fields. The density of individual opacities is variable and rarely completely homogeneous. Evidence of calcification within the lesions is fairly common. Ring shadows caused by excavation of nodules are common and, in some, there are signs of fluid.

Subsequently these ring shadows either disappear leaving little or no trace or resume their original appearance (Figure 13.35). Disappearance of pre-existing opacities and development of new ones in different locations are usual. Appearances may change in a period of months or remain unaltered for years, after which erratic behaviour may resume, sometimes during an exacerbation or first evidence of arthropathy. The superimposition effect of a number of nodules in the X-ray beam may, exceptionally, give the appearances of large lobulated masses (Figure 13.36).

Unlike most cases of ordinary PMF there is, as a rule, no 'background' of simple pneumoconiosis, but exceptions to this occur (Figure 13.37).

Scanty, large, round opacities

These are identical in appearance and behaviour to typical Caplan opacities but are rarely more than about three or four in number. Occasionally only one opacity is evident.

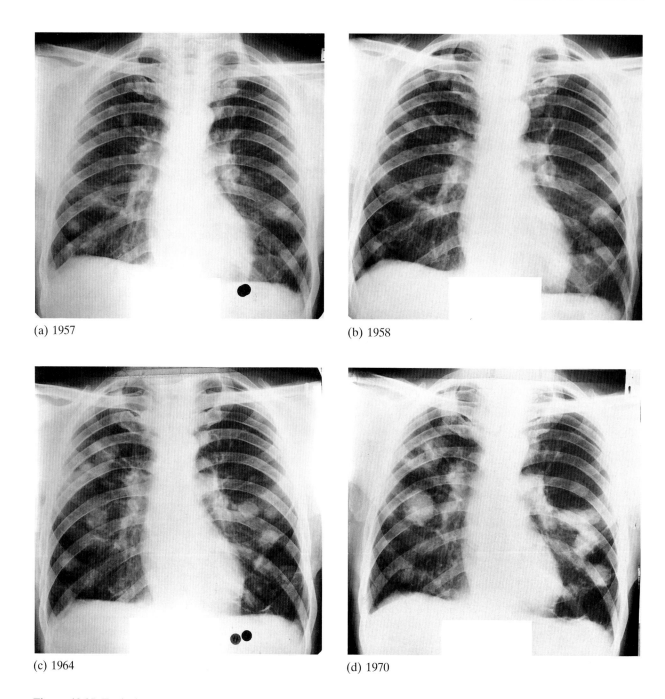

(a) 1957

(b) 1958

(c) 1964

(d) 1970

Figure 13.35 Typical appearances and development of Caplan-type necrobiotic nodules (confirmed histologically) in a coal miner with 20 years at the coal face: mild, active rheumatoid arthritis. A background of simple, non-rheumatoid pneumoconiosis is absent throughout. (a) 1957. In 1958 (b), some lesions seen in the right lung field in 1957 have disappeared. In 1964 (c), new nodules have appeared and, by 1970 (d), have enlarged, with some confluence on the left. Note the clear demarcation of most opacities. The disease was heralded by small haemoptyses when the differential diagnosis was multiple metastatic carcinomas or tuberculomas. Cultures for *Mycobacterium tuberculosis* were consistently negative

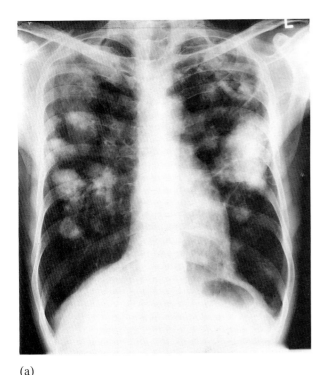

(a)

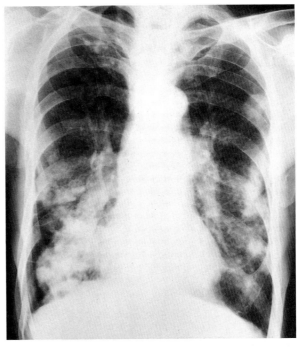

(c)

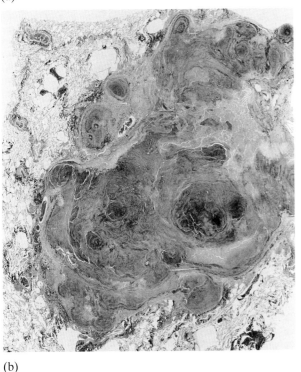

(b)

Figure 13.36 Two cases of multiple large opacities caused by aggregation of nodules of rheumatoid coal pneumoconiosis. In both cases pulmonary metastasis was mistakenly diagnosed many years after the men had left the coal mines. (a) Note the cavitary lesion in the left upper zone. Severe rheumatoid arthritis, sputum consistently negative for *Mycobacterium tuberculosis*. *Post mortem*: discrete masses of matted nodules present in both lungs. (b) This section (from left mid-zone lesion) shows typical agglomeration of nodules – a common feature of rheumatoid pneumoconiosis – and, although the amount of coal dust accumulation is slight, a number of thin, 'tidal' circles, crescents and arcs of dust are clearly visible. Microscopic appearances characteristic and acid-fast bacilli absent. Magnification, approximately × 2; H & E stain. (c) The appearances in the right lower zone are unusual but *post mortem* the lesions were grossly and microscopically characteristic

Mixed, small and large, round and irregular opacities

These are of widely disparate size but the majority range from less than 0.5 cm to about 1 cm in diameter and only a few are larger. Often they exhibit a

less well-defined appearance than those of typical Caplan type. In other respects their development and behaviour are similar though they are especially prone to calcification (Figure 13.38). In some cases their distribution is chiefly peripheral, sometimes with signs of related diffuse pleural thickening

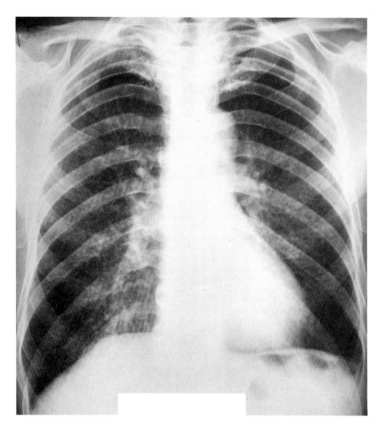

(a) 1967

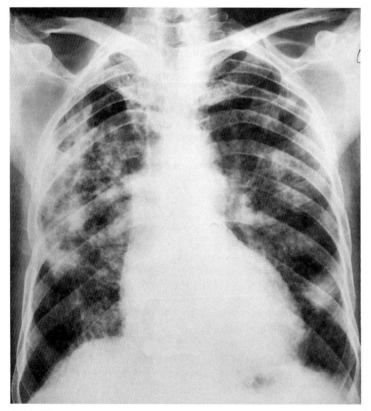

(b) 1972

Figure 13.37 (a) 1967: category 2q simple pneumoconiosis present for about 12 years in a natural graphite worker of 24 years; (b) 1972: the subsequent fairly rapid development of multiple, rounded opacities with ill-defined boundaries bore some resemblance to the appearance of typical Caplan-type nodules (compare Figure 13.35). Note the absence of right sixth rib due to thoracotomy for exclusion of carcinoma. *Biopsy*: necrobiotic nodules with prominent palisading; no tumour. Recurrent joint pains but no clinical arthropathy. *Post mortem*, 2 years later: multiple black nodules of non-rheumatoid pneumoconiosis (up to 4 mm diameter) with several typical Caplan-type nodules up to 2 cm diameter (some cavitary) in both lungs.

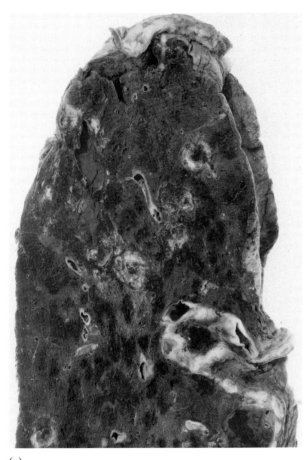

(c)

Figure 13.37 (contd) (c) Slice of unperfused lung showing these nodules (main bronchus and pulmonary artery on the right); no emphysema (compare Figure 13.17). *Microscopy*: typical appearances of rheumatoid pneumoconiosis and numerous graphite bodies; no evidence of tuberculosis or growth

(Figure 13.39). In others, they are clustered into one or two zones of the lung fields.

Scanty, small, round opacities

Opacities of this type, which are few in number, do not, on the whole, vary greatly in size. They may be grouped together in one lung field or scattered in both fields (Figure 13.40).

Multiple, small, round opacities

As a rule these are more or less similar in size and usually widely scattered although some clustering may be seen.

One or other of the foregoing with non-rheumatoid pneumoconiosis

In these cases, which seem to be rare, the appearance of ordinary simple pneumoconiosis or PMF has usually been present for years when additional changes consistent with rheumatoid pneumoconiosis develop within a short period of time, sometimes in relation to the onset or exacerbation of rheumatoid arthritis (see Figures 13.37 and 13.41).

Widespread, ill-defined opacities of sudden onset

This is another rare phenomenon in which bilateral opacities appear and progress with extraordinary rapidity and become widespread. The disease may be fatal within 2 to 3 years and can reasonably be described as acute rheumatoid coal pneumoconiosis (Figure 13.42).

Of the first five of these variants, the mixed and small nodular types are probably the most common, with the typical Caplan type next and the scanty large type least common. Occasionally, however, one type changes into another. Important additional features which may develop in any of the first six variants include the following:

1. Calcification of some or all of the lesions (see Figures 13.38 and 13.40).
2. Signs of pleural effusion – a recognized complication of rheumatoid disease (Ward, 1961; Walker and Wright, 1967) – first remarked upon by Fuller in 1860. Effusion may be single or recurrent on the same or opposite sides. Its development does not correlate with the amount of intrapulmonary disease (Figure 13.43).
3. Diffuse interstitial pulmonary fibrosis (Figure 13.44).

Although a coal miner with rheumatoid arthritis, even of severe degree, may show no evidence of rheumatoid pneumoconiosis, continued observation is essential as the possibility of its subsequent development is always present even in old age. Likewise, the appearances of non-rheumatoid pneumoconiosis may remain unchanged for many years in a person with active rheumatoid arthritis, and rheumatoid pneumoconiosis may never develop.

Thus, there appears to be some overlap of rheumatoid and non-rheumatoid pneumoconiosis both radiologically and immunologically. The range of radiographic appearances of rheumatoid pneumoconiosis, compared with ordinary PMF, and their possible relationship to the levels of dust exposure and immunological activity are summarized diagrammatically in Figure 13.45.

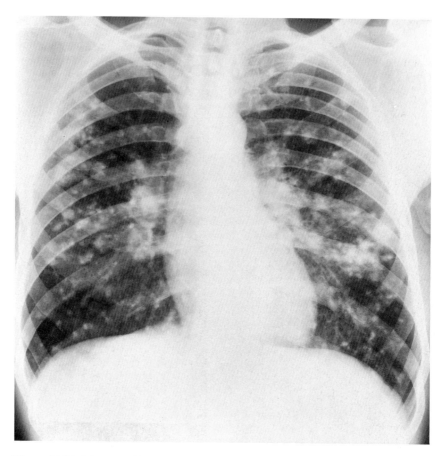

Figure 13.38 Rheumatoid coal pneumoconiosis with small and large ('mixed') opacities resembling silicosis. Calcification of some lesions apparent 5 years after development of rheumatoid arthritis. DAT titres consistently high (1:256 or more). Coal miner for 45 years. Family history of rheumatoid arthritis

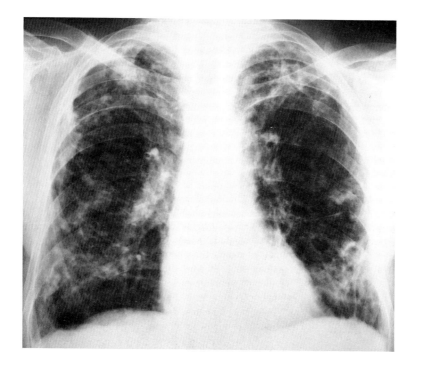

Figure 13.39 Peripheral 'mixed' type of rheumatoid pneumoconiosis in a man exposed to coal and graphite dust. Cavities are seen in some lesions and there is some pleural thickening. Severe rheumatoid arthritis with numerous subcutaneous nodules. DAT titres 1:64 or higher. *Post mortem*: moderate diffuse thickening of pulmonary pleura and many typical Caplan necrobiotic nodules, some containing cavities, within 2 to 3 cm of the pleura; rheumatoid vasculitis widespread in the lungs and elsewhere. No evidence of tuberculosis

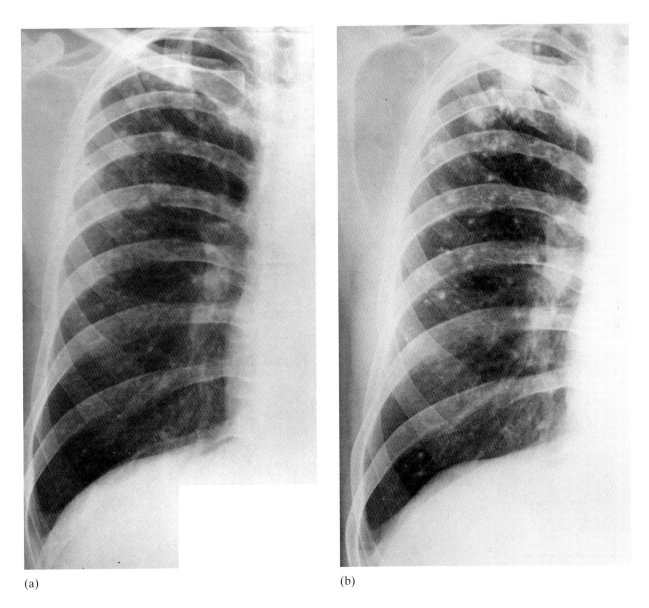

(a)   (b)

Figure 13.40 Small round lesions of rheumatoid coal pneumoconiosis (verified histologically) many of which have subsequently calcified. Time between films (a) and (b) is 15 years. The subject had been a coal miner for 15 years, and had moderately severe rheumatoid arthritis; DAT 1:256. Sputum cultures for *M. tuberculosis* negative

Computed tomography

Standard and high-resolution CT (see Chapter 7) are reported to give better assessment of 'overall disease' and its distribution than standard radiographs because CT, in focusing on transverse sections of lung, reduces the effect of superimposition of lesions seen in PA films. For this reason, it is suggested that over-diagnosis may occur on PA films. CT appears to detect simple pneumoconiosis in its early stages better than the standard radio-

graph but, apart from showing cavitary changes in PMF lesions more clearly, has no superiority in the more advanced stages of pneumoconiosis (Remy-Jardin et al., 1990). High resolution on CT is needed to visualize minute discrete lesions (p opacities) (Akira et al., 1989). However, for all practical purposes, CT has little advantage over technically good PA films.

It is worth remembering too that, in some cases in which the presence of simple pneumoconiosis is uncertain, the combination of anteroposterior (AP)

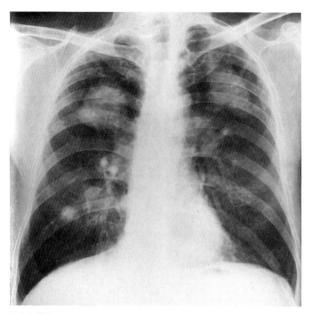

(a) 1971

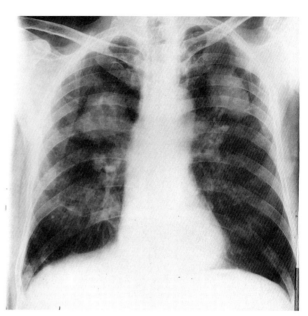

(b) March 1977

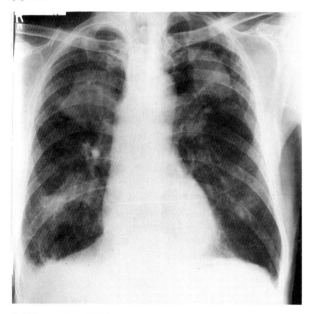

(c) November 1977

Figure 13.41 (a) Bilateral, non-rheumatoid PMF present for years when small, right middle and lower zone opacities appeared in 1968; neoplasm suspected (1971). (b) Appearances unchanged for about 6 years after which the lesions virtually disappeared (March 1977). (c) Reappearance of lower zone lesion, now increased in size, and right basal pleural effusion (November 1977). Rheumatoid arthritis developed suddenly in 1973. Latex test, positive; DAT 1:1024. *Post mortem*: rheumatoid necrobiotic nodules confined to right lower lobe; no evidence of neoplasm or tuberculosis. Histological confirmation. Coal miner for 29 years

and standard PA views may increase the definition of small opacities without having to resort to CT (see Chapter 7, page 167).

in rheumatoid pneumoconiosis whether or not the lesions are excavated.

Bacteriology

When the radiograph shows a cavitary PMF or opacities of recent development, sputum should be cultured for tubercle bacilli and opportunist mycobacteria. Tubercle bacilli are very rarely found

Immunology

Rheumatoid factor

The differential agglutination test (DAT) is positive in almost all cases of rheumatoid pneumoconiosis, often in high titre whether or not there is

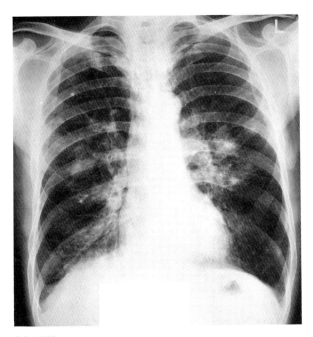

(a) 1958

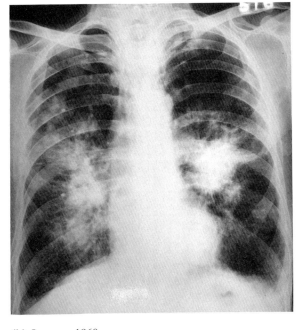

(b) January 1960

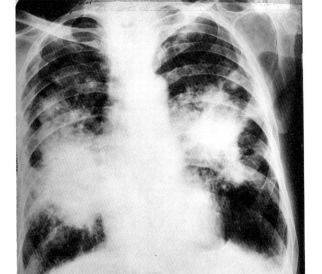

(c) November 1960

Figure 13.42 Dramatically fast development of rheumatoid coal pneumoconiosis with atypical radiographic appearances; from a coal miner aged 60, who had spent 40 years underground. (a) 1958: opacities are consistent with necrobiotic nodules but a few are ill defined. Abrupt onset of severe polyarthropathy at this time; DAT 1:1024. (b) January 1960: crippling, extensive rheumatoid arthritis at this time. (c) November 1960: bilateral changes now far advanced within 10 months with a few Caplan-type nodules discernible in both upper lung fields; severe impairment of respiratory function. *Post mortem* (1961): large, grey–black masses with necrotic cavities in the centre of both lungs. *Microscopy*: multiple, typical, rheumatoid coal nodules in these lesions

accompanying arthritis, but variations in titre may be observed over a period of time. The later fixation test is less consistently positive. The occasional seronegative case usually proves to be positive subsequently if tests are repeated over a period of months.

Circulating rheumatoid factor, detected by DAT, was found in 6 per cent of a small group of British coal miners with simple pneumoconiosis and in 18 per cent of those with category C non-rheumatoid PMF (Soutar, Turner-Warwick and Parkes, 1974). However, Lippman et al. (1973), using a latex test in American miners, found no increase. In a later study of a large number of miners throughout Britain, Boyd, Robertson and Davis (1982) reported the presence of rheumatoid factor detected by DAT in 5.3 per cent that correlated significantly with all categories of pneumoconiosis, particularly in the

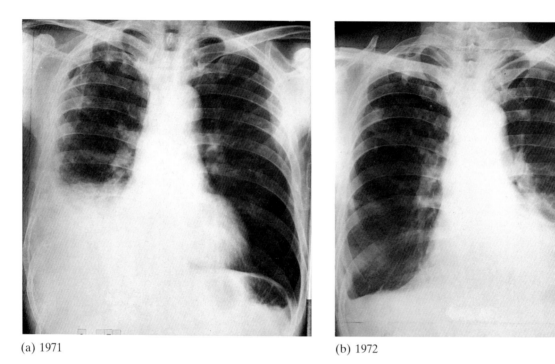

(a) 1971   (b) 1972

Figure 13.43 Scanty, small opacities of rheumatoid coal pneumoconiosis in upper zones of both lungs and recurrent transient pleural effusions on opposite sides: (a) 1971; (b) 1972. Moderately severe rheumatoid arthritis of rapid development in 1970 at age 59 years; DAT consistently positive (range 1:16 to 1:1024); antinuclear antibody positive. No evidence of tuberculosis or cause of pleural effusion other than rheumatoid disease. *Post mortem*: moderate thickening of pulmonary pleura; a few dust macules and small coal pneumoconiosis nodules (2 mm diameter) and several subpleural, Caplan necrobiotic nodules up to 1 cm diameter in both lungs (confirmed microscopically). The subject had been a coal miner for 26 years

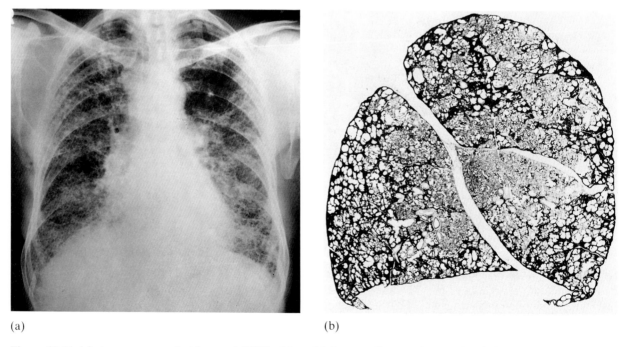

(a)   (b)

Figure 13.44 (a) Appearances of widespread DIPF with multiple cysts diagnosed, wrongly, during life as coal pneumoconiosis; a collier of 20 years who suffered from rheumatoid arthritis in later years. (b) Section of right lung with deeply black-pigmented DIPF and numerous cysts in all lobes. Clear demarcation from unaffected lung. No lesions of coal pneumoconiosis

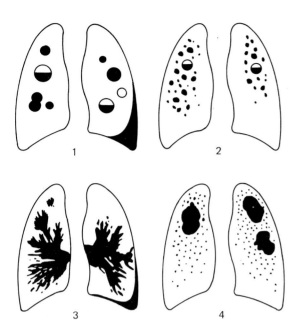

Figure 13.45 Possible relationships of the relative intensities of dust exposure and immunological activity to the range of radiographic appearances in coal pneumoconiosis. (1) Low dust, high immunoactivity. 'Classic' Caplan-type necrobiotic nodules. (2) Intermediate dust, intermediate immunoactivity. Mixed small and large round lesions of rheumatoid pneumoconiosis, and uniform, small round opacities. (3) High dust, high immunoactivity. 'Acute' rheumatoid pneumoconiosis (rare). (4) High dust, absent or low immune activity. PMF and simple pneumoconiosis

few men with PMF and rheumatoid disease, but not with age. However, they concluded that the evidence overall did not suggest a particular association of rheumatoid factor with the development of PMF except for Caplan-type nodules with rheumatoid disease.

Antinuclear antibody

Circulating antinuclear antibody appears to be provoked as a secondary phenomenon by a variety of pathological processes and, thus, is not an indication of specific disease. Antinuclear antibody has been found more often in coal miners with pneumoconiosis – especially those with PMF – than in the general population (Kang et al., 1973; Lippman et al., 1973; Soutar, Turner-Warwick and Parkes, 1974). It is of interest that in American miners their prevalence was reported to be signif-

icantly greater in anthracite than bituminous coal miners with PMF (Lippman et al., 1973). Boyd, Robertson and Davis (1982), in their study referred to in the preceding paragraph, found antinuclear antibody in 23.1 per cent of coalminers with all categories of pneumoconiosis compared with 21.5 per cent of control subjects. These investigations, however, did not identify different types of antinuclear antibody. Although Soutar, Turner-Warwick and Parkes (1974) reported that an increased prevalence of autoantibodies in higher categories of pneumoconiosis was greatest when rheumatoid factor and antinuclear antibody were present together, this was not confirmed by Boyd, Robertson and Davis (1982) who concluded that there was probably no significant relationship between rheumatoid factor and antinuclear antibody in coal pneumoconiosis.

The presence of these antibodies in the serum therefore appears, on present evidence, to have no value in detecting predisposition to the development of PMF apart from men with rheumatoid disease. Both antibodies are often found when DIPF and coal pneumoconiosis coexist.

Serum immunoglobulins

Compared with non-miners British miners with radiographic evidence of coal pneumoconiosis have significantly raised levels of serum IgA and IgG with increasing category of pneumoconiosis. Even miners with no radiographic evidence of pneumoconiosis have a significantly higher mean level of IgA than non-miners. Whether these changes signify an important immunological process in the development of pneumoconiosis or are merely a passive response to dust in the lungs is uncertain (Robertson et al., 1984).

Peripheral blood lymphocytes

Cell-mediated immune responses to pulmonary tissue in chronic disease of the lungs are discussed in Chapter 4. A study of miners from British coalfields in different areas gave no indication that systemic anti-lung antibodies are produced in response to exposure to coal-mine dust, and little to suggest that levels of peripheral T and B lymphocytes alter as radiological category of pneumoconiosis increases. However, a consistent increase in absolute numbers of lymphocytes was evident in smoking compared with non-smoking coal miners (Robertson et al., 1983).

Diagnosis

Occupational and medical histories, and the radiographic appearances, together usually provide the diagnosis. The presence of blue–black, coal tattoo marks in the skin of the hands, forearms, face and torso is additional evidence of past coal mining, and is a valuable sign in men who have been away from the industry for years and in whom the relevant history has been missed or is unobtainable. Lung biopsy is never indicated except to exclude other pathology.

Occasionally the radiographic appearances of miliary tuberculosis, sarcoidosis or systemic connective tissue diseases (such as polyarteritis nodosa and systemic lupus erythematosus) resemble simple pneumoconiosis but, in most cases, the patient is ill. The causes of small discrete opacities are summarized in Table 7.3. Opacities caused by the 'benign' pneumoconioses are denser and, as a rule, more widely scattered in the lung fields than those of simple pneumoconiosis (see Chapter 11).

It should be remembered that, as a result of change in occupation, coal pneumoconiosis and some other type of pneumoconiosis – for example, asbestosis – occasionally coexist (see Chapter 14).

Widespread DIPF in coal miners is sometimes misinterpreted as pneumoconiosis. However, the irregularity of the opacities and the frequent presence of a 'cystic' or 'honeycomb' pattern should prevent this mistake. In some of these cases the fibrosis is deeply pigmented with coal dust (see Figure 13.44); in others it is dust-free.

A close resemblance between PMF opacities and those caused by other disease may sometimes give rise to difficulty or errors in diagnosis in either direction.

Tuberculosis

Large fibrocaseous tuberculous lesions and PMF may be mistaken for each other especially in the presence of category 2 or 3 simple pneumoconiosis. In the former case the patient is unwell, his sputum usually yields tubercle bacilli, and antituberculous treatment causes complete or partial resolution of the radiographic appearances. In the latter, the man is in good health even if complaining of some respiratory disability. PMF with ischaemic cavity formation is frequently mistaken for active tuberculous disease, but there is a history of coughing up jet-black sputum from which tubercle bacilli cannot be isolated. When active tuberculosis and coal pneumoconiosis with PMF coexist, the extent of the pneumoconiosis can only be judged when antituberculous treatment has achieved maximal resolution of the tuberculosis.

Tuberculous bronchial 'abscesses' (Clegg, 1953) – now rare – cause fairly dense, round, radiographic opacities 1 to 2 cm in diameter which are identical in appearance to typical Caplan lesions but are usually few in number, and tubercle bacilli may be cultured from the sputum. Rheumatoid arthritis and circulating rheumatoid factor are absent.

Rheumatoid pneumoconiosis

A diagnostic feature of many of these cases, if serial radiographs are available, is the appearance of lesions within a few months and the equally rapid disappearance of some of them with or without evidence of cavity formation. In the absence of earlier radiographs, a history of past coal mining and the presence of rheumatoid arthritis or circulating rheumatoid factor should suggest the diagnosis. When, however, the lesions are few and contain cavities, or are small and clustered, they are particularly likely to be diagnosed as tuberculosis even when no tubercle bacilli are cultured from the sputum; when they are small, scattered and apparently calcified they may be interpreted as calcified silicotic nodules or healed lesions of tuberculosis, histoplasmosis or pulmonary chickenpox. Lesions which are neither cavitary nor calcified may be mistaken for secondary tumour deposits (from carcinoma of the prostate and kidney especially), although tumour opacities usually have a more homogeneous appearance. Rare disorders which may simulate rheumatoid pneumoconiosis of mixed type in appearance and speed of development are nodular sarcoidosis, Wegener's granuloma, chickenpox nodules and multiple nodular pulmonary amyloidosis (Lee and Johnson, 1975; Holmes, Desai and Sapsford, 1988). The appearance of acute blastomycosis may imitate typical Caplan-type lesions fairly closely (see Figure 22.6).

The usual absence of a 'background' of simple pneumoconiosis is of limited value as an additional pointer to rheumatoid pneumoconiosis, and the latter is sometimes associated with non-rheumatoid PMF (see Figure 13.41).

Sputum cultures are consistently negative for *Mycobacterium tuberculosis*, and large haemoptysis is strongly against rheumatoid pneumoconiosis. In many cases there is a family history of rheumatoid disease.

The pathological diagnosis is discussed on pages 363 to 366.

Carcinoma of the lung

It is obviously important to distinguish between PMF and bronchial carcinoma radiologically and

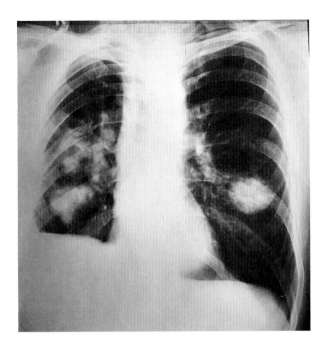

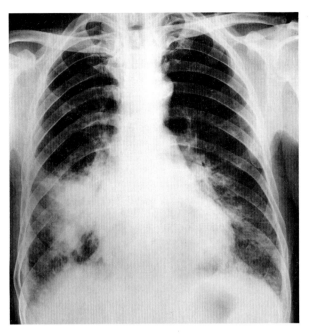

Figure 13.46 Secondary pulmonary tumour deposits resembling PMF and initially diagnosed as such in a coal miner. *Post mortem*: adenocarcinoma in both lungs; very occasional small coal nodules but no PMF. He had been a miner for 8 years

Figure 13.47 Lipoid pneumonia (paraffinoma) resembling, and diagnosed as, lower zone PMF in an aged ex-coal miner addicted to medicinal paraffin oil. Radiographic appearances unchanged for a few years before death. *Post mortem:* moderate numbers of dust macules and occasional small coal pneumoconiosis nodules but no PMF; mass in right lower lobe thought, naked eye, to be a carcinoma but frozen and H & E microsections demonstrated lipoid pneumonia (compare Figure 13.28a)

this is possible in most cases. But difficulty may arise when a patient is seen for the first time or after the lapse of a number of years when the evolution of the opacities in question is not known. Features, referred to earlier, which may be helpful in distinguishing PMF are variable radiodensity of the opacities, linear markings at its periphery and evidence of calcification within the lesions. However, spiculation or scalloping of the periphery of a mass may be seen both in PMF and peripheral carcinoma, although the latter lacks the other features of PMF. Calcification is rare in carcinomas and almost never demonstrable during life, and, although it may be seen in benign adenomas and hamartomas, it does not display the patterns illustrated in Figures 13.29b and 13.30. Tomography may clarify these features. A cavitary lesion may be difficult or impossible to differentiate but, in the case of PMF, there may be a recent history of expectoration of jet-black sputum, often over a number of consecutive days.

Earlier radiographs should be obtained for comparison whenever there is uncertainty about the nature of the lesion. An opacity that is seen to appear and enlarge rapidly in a series of films is most likely to represent carcinoma, whereas one that results from the aggregation of earlier small opacities is probably due to PMF.

When a rheumatoid pneumoconiosis lesion increases in size over a short period of time in a man with rheumatoid arthritis, it may be mistaken for carcinoma with hypertrophic pulmonary osteoarthropathy especially if the two arthropathies are not distinguished. In the case of a single nodule of 'rheumatoid' pneumoconiosis, it may be possible to reach the diagnosis without thoracotomy and biopsy, otherwise this method of investigation should rarely be necessary. Multiple large opacities of rheumatoid pneumoconiosis – especially if they develop quickly – can be misinterpreted as metastatic tumours.

Bronchoscopy is not always helpful in differential diagnosis but bronchography, in cases of PMF, shows that bronchi adjacent to the mass, although distorted and displaced, are not occluded whereas in peripheral carcinoma of the lung they are often abruptly occluded or gradually narrowed to the point of disappearance ('rat-tail' sign) (Goldman, 1965a). CT may be of value in such cases.

Occasionally metastatic tumours in the lungs may simulate PMF very closely but the opacities are usually sharply circumscribed and of uniform density (Figure 13.46).

Sarcoidosis

Apart from small, discrete opacities referred to already large, rounded opacities resembling PMF occur exceptionally in sarcoidosis (Scadding and Mitchell, 1985). Differentiation rests primarily on having this possibility in mind and then excluding sarcoidosis; biopsy may be necessary.

Exogenous lipoid pneumonia

An uncommon simulator of both simple pneumoconiosis and PMF is discussed in more detail in Chapter 23 (pages 778 to 782). An example, probably the result of medicinal liquid paraffin and misinterpreted as PMF, is shown in Figure 13.47.

Prognosis and complications

The influence of the radiological category of simple pneumoconiosis on the development of PMF, and the effect of PMF on life expectancy, are discussed under 'Epidemiology' (page 349). On occasion PMF may, after many years of apparent inactivity, progress to considerable size in the elderly (see 'Incidence and prevalence'). Prognosis is not worsened by the presence of ischaemic cavities unless they are infected by pathogenic atypical mycobacteria (see later). In view of the apparent association of a mild reduction of TL or of the presence of emphysema in some category p cases, in comparison with category q and r cases (see page 378), it is interesting to note that the mortality rate in Welsh miners and ex-miners with punctiform opacities is, if anything, lower than those with other categories of pneumoconiosis (Waters, Cochrane and Moore, 1974).

Pulmonary heart disease

Pulmonary heart disease is not caused by simple pneumoconiosis and is now rare in PMF cases in the absence of concomitant, severe, chronic airflow obstruction.

Tuberculosis and other infections

If tuberculosis develops in the presence of PMF, permanent decline in ventilatory capacity may occur in some cases, in spite of effective antituberculous treatment. Antituberculous treatment was earlier reported to be less effective in men with coal pneumoconiosis than in men with tuberculosis alone (Medical Research Council/Miner's Chest Diseases Treatment Centre, 1963), but there is reason to believe that this was due to irregularity of treatment (Annotation, 1967); at least one other study has shown satisfactory results (Ramsey and Fines, 1963), and more recent experience has confirmed this.

Opportunist mycobacteria are apt to establish themselves in lungs with PMF especially if there is an ischaemic cavity (Marks, 1970).

Infestation of ischaemic cavities by *Aspergillus* sp. sometimes occurs, the circumstances and clinical features of which are identical to those described in Chapter 12 (see under 'Complications', page 313).

Rheumatoid pneumoconiosis

As described already this behaves erratically and may progress suddenly in a short time, but it rarely threatens life and only occasionally causes significant respiratory disability. However, the highly exceptional case in which the course of the disease is acute and the patient seriously ill may end fatally within 2 to 3 years. The occasional development of pleural effusion (which may be recurrent) is generally due to the rheumatoid process although other causes, especially neoplasia, must be excluded. Rheumatoid effusions often have an unusually low glucose content. Rupture of a peripheral nodule through the pulmonary pleura may result in spontaneous pneumothorax, hydro-pneumothorax, pyo-pneumothorax or, occasionally, bronchopleural fistula.

Chronic bronchitis

This is discussed in Chapters 9 and 10.

Carcinoma of the lung

There is no evidence of a causal relationship between coal pneumoconiosis and carcinoma of the lung (Rooke et al., 1979). The death rate due to this tumour is lower in British and American coal miners than in non-miners of a comparable age (Kennaway and Kennaway, 1947; Goldman, 1965b; Liddell, 1973; Costello, Ortmeyer and Morgan, 1974). A lower post-mortem incidence of the growth in Welsh miners with pneumoconiosis than in age-matched non-miners from the same area was reported by James (1955). Furthermore, the survival time of men with this tumour is longer in those with category 2 or 3 simple pneumoconiosis than in those with category 0 (Goldman, 1965c). This lower rate of lung cancer, which is not adequately explained by differences in smoking habits as miners – in Britain at any rate – do not appear to smoke less than non-miners (Jacobsen, 1977; Rooke et al., 1979), seems to be a specific effect of occupation. In France, Dechoux and Wantz (1985) were also unable to detect any correlation between work underground, the presence of pneumoconiosis and lung cancer. However, an apparent excess of lung cancer has been reported in coal miners with pneumoconiosis compared with non-miners in the Wyoming Valley of Pennsylvania. This may be explained by a higher than normal background of ionizing radiation from black shales associated with the coal measures in this region (Myers, 1967; Scarano, Fadali and Lemole, 1972). It should be noted, however, that in Myers' report miners and non-miners were not matched for age or smoking habits and, in that of Scarano et al., only the ages of the cancer patients were recorded and not those of all the miners and non-miners in the survey. The question of ionizing radiation in other mines is discussed in Chapter 19 (under 'Radon and radon daughters', page 656).

Ischaemic heart disease

Higgins et al. (1969) found no difference in prevalence of chest pain and electrocardiographic abnormalities between miners, ex-miners and non-miners in an American mining community. The standard mortality ratio of working miners for ischaemic heart disease in Britain and the USA is lower than that of the general population except for maintenance workers in whom it is slightly increased; in non-working miners it is similar to that of the general population (Higgins et al., 1969; Liddell, 1973; Costello, Ortmeyer and Morgan, 1975).

It has been postulated that chronic hypoxaemia associated with some cases of advanced PMF, as in many other types of advanced lung disease, predisposes to myocardial infarction. But all the evidence is against this. The incidence of myocardial infarction and the death rate from ischaemic heart disease are, in fact, lower than average in PMF and chronic respiratory insufficiency (Nonkin et al., 1964; Samad

and Noehren, 1965; Mitchell, Walker and Maisel, 1968; Sanders, 1970; Lindars et al., 1972; Cochrane, Moore and Montcrieff, 1982; Atuhaire et al., 1985). Chronic hypoxaemia appears to exert a protective rather than a precipitating effect. It causes dilatation and increased interarterial anastomoses of the coronary arteries (Zoll, Wessler and Schesingler, 1951; Keele and Neil, 1971) and coronary artery blood flow is not reduced in patients with emphysema and pulmonary heart disease (Rose and Hoffman, 1956). On the contrary, vascularization of the myocardium down to capillary level is greatly increased in people living in chronic hypoxia at high altitudes compared with those at sea level (Heath and Williams, 1989), and a significant serial decline in mortality from ischaemic heart disease, which is not associated with racial differences, has been observed in people residing at increasingly high altitudes (Mortimer, Monson and MacMahon, 1977; Heath and Williams, 1989). Furthermore, the risk of cardiac arrhythmia does not appear to be increased by chronic hypoxia (Parkes, Phillips and Williamson, 1976).

Systemic sclerosis

Although systemic sclerosis (scleroderma) is reported to occur with unusual frequency in coal miners as well as in men with silicosis (Rodnan et al., 1967) (see Chapter 12, page 314), there is no obvious association with radiographic evidence of pneumoconiosis. No cases appear to have been identified in British coal miners.

Miscellaneous

PMF is not a cause of fatal haemoptysis but intermittent blood streaking of sputum may occur from time to time. Copious jet-black sputum due to rupture of the contents of a cavitary PMF into an airway, although alarming, is usually harmless, and aspiration sequelae do not appear to have been reported.

Proximal retrograde spread of a pulmonary artery thrombus adjacent to a PMF lesion may occasionally lead to embolism and consequent pulmonary infarction, but this is rarely fatal.

Other complications, remarkable for their rarity, are spontaneous pneumothorax (which is often partial) and permanent dysphonia due to paralysis of the left recurrent laryngeal nerve from involvement by PMF in the upper part of the left lung near the hilum.

The question as to whether oxides of nitrogen from shot firing and diesel locomotives in coal mines have any permanent effect on miners' lungs is discussed in Chapter 10, page 249 and Chapter 18, pages 621–622. However, at this point, it is relevant to state that the levels detected underground in British coal mines over the decade before 1982 had no adverse effect on the health of the miners, there being no relationship between exposure and respiratory symptoms or decline in FEV_1 (Robertson et al., 1984).

Treatment

No treatment affects the pneumoconiosis. However, early effective treatment is indicated for chronic airflow obstruction, pulmonary heart disease, tuberculosis and infection by opportunist mycobacteria which need to be carefully typed. In cases where sudden expectoration of large amounts of black sputum has occurred from excavated PMF, reassurance and mild sedation may be indicated, and similarly in the uncommon event of minor haemoptysis associated with rheumatoid pneumoconiosis or non-rheumatoid PMF.

There is no evidence that 'rheumatoid' pneumoconiosis is influenced in any way by corticosteroids but they should be tried in the rare case of fulminant progressive disease. Neither, apparently, does penicillamine have any effect.

Prevention

This rests on three principles:

1. 'Permitted' dust levels.
2. Control of dust production, and regular dust measurements and monitoring of the underground environment.
3. Regular medical supervision.

'Permitted' dust levels

These were introduced by the National Coal Board (now British Coal) as 'approved dust conditions' in 1949 and were originally based on concentrations of 'respirable dust' measured in terms of the *number*

of compact particles being 1 to 5 μm/ml. Since 1969, however, dust levels have been determined in terms of *mass concentration* of particles 1 to 7 μm in diameter expressed as milligrams per cubic metre (mg/m^3) which is a better index of the risk of developing pneumoconiosis (Jacobsen et al., 1971; Hurley et al., 1982). It is derived by gravimetric analysis using a standard, size-selective elutriator (Dunmore, Hamilton and Smith, 1964).

The present standards in the UK are as follows:

1. A maximum of 7 mg/m^3 air (equivalent to a mean concentration of 4 mg/m^3) for operations at longwall coal faces.
2. A maximum of 3 mg/m^3 for operations in drivages and headings where the average quartz content exceeds 0.45 mg/m^3.
3. A maximum of 5 mg/m^3 for operations in other localities.

Control of dust production

This is achieved by special attention to mining techniques, suppression of dust to a minimum, and the wearing of respirators at times when exposure is heaviest.

Medical supervision

In the UK this consists of medical examination and a standard chest radiograph when a worker first enters the industry, and, thereafter, a radiograph every 4 years with ventilatory function tests – both offered on a voluntary basis.

Coal-mine dust standards in the USA

This is 2 mg/m^3 for an 8-hour working shift. It corresponds to 3.2 mg/m^3 using the UK method of gravimetric sampling. Dust is collected by personally carried Atomic Energy Commission cyclone samplers.

References

Adesina, A.M., Vallyathan, V., McQuillen, E.N., Weaver, S.O. and Craighead, J.E. (1991) Brochiolar inflammation and fibrosis associated with smoking; a morphological cross-sectional population analysis. *Am. Rev. Respir. Dis.* **143**, 144–149

Akira, M., Higashitiara, T., Yokouama, K., Yamamoto, S., Kita, N., Morimoto, S., Ikezoe, J. and Kozuka, T. (1989) Radiographic type p pneumoconiosis: high-resolution CT. *Radiology* **171**, 117–123

Alarie, Y.C., Krumm, A.A., Busey, W.M., Ulrich, C.E. and Kantz, R.J. II (1975) Long-term exposure to sulfur dioxide, sulfuric acid mist, fly ash and their mixtures. *Archs Environ. Health* **30**, 254–262

Amandus, H.E., Pendergrass, E.P., Dennis, J.M. and Morgan, W.K.C. (1974) Pneumoconiosis: inter-reader variability in the classification of the type of small opacities in the chest roentgenogram. *Am. J. Roentgenol. Rad. Ther. Nucl. Med.* **122**, 740–743

Amandus, H.E., Lapp, N.K., Jacobsen, G. and Reger, R.B. (1976) Significance of irregular small opacities in radiographs of coal miners in the USA. *Br. J. Ind. Med.* **33**, 13–17

American Thoracic Society (1987) Standards for the diagnosis and care of patients with chronic obstructive pulmonary disease (COPD) and asthma (Chapter 1). *Am. Rev. Respir. Dis.* **136**, 225–228

Annotation (1967) Tuberculosis and pneumoconiosis. *Lancet* **2**, 410

Ashford, J.R., Brown, S., Morgan, D.C. and Rae, S. (1968) The pulmonary ventilatory function of coal miners in the United Kingdom. *Am. Rev. Respir. Dis.* **97**, 810–826

Ashford, J.R., Morgan, D.D., Rae, S. and Sowden, R.R. (1970) Respiratory symptoms in British coal miners. *Am. Rev. Respir. Dis.* **102**, 370–381

Attfield, M.D. and Hodous, T.K. (1992) Pulmonary function of US coal miners related to dust exposure estimates. *Am. Rev. Respir. Dis.* **145**, 605–609

Atuhaire, L.K., Campbell, M.J., Cochrane, A.L., Jones, M. and Moore, F. (1985) Mortality of men in the Rhondda Fach 1950–1980. *Br. J. Ind. Med.* **42**, 741–745

Auerbach, O., Garfinkel, L. and Hammond, E.C. (1974) Relation of smoking and age to findings in the lung parenchyma. *Chest* **65**, 19–35

Auerbach, O., Stout, A.P., Hammond, E.C. and Garfinkel, L. (1963) Smoking habits and age relation to pulmonary changes. *N. Engl. J. Med.* **269**, 1045–1054

Ball, J.D., Berry, G., Clarke, W.G., Gilson, J.C. and Thomas, J. (1969) A controlled trial of anti-tuberculosis chemotherapy in early complicated pneumoconiosis of coal workers. *Thorax* **24**, 399–406

Ball, J. and Lawrence, J.S. (1961) Epidemiology of the sheep cell agglutination test. *Ann. Rheum. Dis.* **20**, 235–245

Banks, D.E., Bauer, M.A., Castellan, R.M. and Lapp, N.L. (1983) Silicosis in surface coalmine drillers. *Thorax* **38**, 275–278

Bates, D.V., Pham, Q.T., Chau, N., Pivotea, C., Dechoux, J. and Sadou, P. (1985) A longitudinal study of pulmonary function in coal miners in Lorraine, France. *Am. J. Ind. Med.* **8**, 21–32

Benedek, T.G., Zawadzki, Z.A. and Medsger, Jr T.A. (1976) Serum immunoglobulins, rheumatoid factor, and pneumoconiosis in miners with rheumatoid arthritis. *Arth. Rheum.* **19**, 731–736

Bennett, J.G., Dick, J.A., Kaplan, Y.S., Shand, P.A., Shennan, D.H., Thomas, D.J. and Washington, J.S. (1979) The relationship between coal rank and the prevalence of pneumoconiosis. *Br. J. Ind. Med.* **36**, 206–210

Bergman, I. and Casswell, C. (1972) Lung dust and lung iron contents of coal workers in different coalfields in Great Britain. *Br. J. Ind. Med.* **29**, 160–168

Bernstein, R.M. (1990) Humoral autoimmunity in systemic rheumatoid disease. *J. R. Coll. Physns (Lond.)* **24**, 18–25

Blanc, P.D. and Gamsu, G. (1988) The effect of cigarette smoking on the detection of small radiographic opacities in inorganic dust disease. *J. Thorac. Imaging* **3**, 51–56

Blanc, P.D. and Gamsu, G. (1989) Editorial. Cigarette smoking and pneumoconiosis: structuring and debate. *Am. J. Ind. Med.* **16**, 1–4

Bonnell, J.A., Schilling, C.J. and Massey, P.M.O. (1980) Clinical and experimental studies of the effects of pulverized fuel ash – a review. *Ann. Occup. Hyg.* **23**, 159–164

Boyd, J.E., Robertson, M.D. and Davis, J.M.G. (1982) Auto-antibodies in coal miners: their relationship to the development of progressive massive fibrosis. *Am. J. Ind. Med.* **3**, 201–208

British Coal Medical Services (1992) *Annual Report 1991–1992*, pp. 23–24, British Coal

Brown, G.M., Brown, D.M., Slight, J. and Donaldson, K. (1991) Persistent biological reactivity of quartz in the lung: raised protease burden compared with non-pathogenic mineral dust and microbial particles. *Br. J. Ind. Med.* **48**, 61–69

Bruch, J. and Hilscher, W. (1988) Effects of particle size of coal mine dusts in experimental anthracosilicosis. III. Tissue reactions in lymph nodes. *Ann. Occup. Hyg.* **32** (suppl. 1), 603–610

Caplan, A. (1953) Certain unusual radiological appearances in the chest of coal miners suffering rheumatoid arthritis. *Thorax* **8**, 29–37

Caplan, A., Payne, R.B. and Withey, J.L. (1962) A broader concept of Caplan's syndrome related to rheumatoid factors. *Thorax* **17**, 205–212

Carilli, A.D., Kotzen, L.M. and Fischer, M.J. (1973) The chest roentgenogram in smoking females. *Am. Rev. Respir. Dis.* **107**, 133–136

Casalone, E. and Rasetti, L. (1963) Rischio silicotigeno in operati esposti ad inalazioni di polvere di grafite. *Med. Lav.* **54**, 597–600

Casswell, C., Bergman, I. and Rossiter, C.E. (1971) The relation of radiological appearance in simple pneumoconiosis of coal workers to the content and composition of the lung. In *Inhaled Particles III* (ed. W.H. Walton), Unwin Brothers, London, vol. II, pp. 713–724

Castellan, R.M., Sanderson, W.T. and Petersen, M.R. (1985) Prevalence of radiographic appearance of pneumoconiosis in an unexposed blue collar population. *Am. Rev. Respir. Dis.* **132**, 684–686

Chau, N., Bertrand, J.P., Guenzi, M., Mayer, L., Téculescu, D., Mur, J.M., Patris, A., Moulin, J.J. and Pham, Q.T. (1992) Lung function in retired coke oven plant workers. *Br. J. Ind. Med.* **49**, 316–325

Churg, A. and Wright, J.L. (1983) Small airways lesions in patients exposed to non-asbestos mineral dust. *Hum. Pathol.* **14**, 688–693

Clegg, J.W. (1953) Ulcero-caseous tuberculous bronchitis. *Thorax* **8**, 167–179

Cochrane, A.L. (1962) The attack rate of progressive massive fibrosis. *Br. J. Ind. Med.* **19**, 52–64

Cochrane, A.L. (1973) Relation between radiographic categories of coalworkers' pneumoconiosis and expectation of life. *Br. Med. J.* **1**, 532–534

Cochrane, A.L. and Higgins, I.T.T. (1961) Pulmonary ventilatory functions of coal miners in various areas in relation to the X-ray category of pneumoconiosis. *Br. J. Prev. Soc. Med.* **15**, 1–11

Cochrane, A.L. and Moore, F. (1978) Preliminary results of a twenty-four hour follow-up of a random sample of an industrial town. *Br. Med. J.* **1**, 411–412

Cochrane, A.L. and Moore, F. (1981) Death certification from the epidemiological point of view. *Lancet* **1**, 742–743

Cochrane, A.L., Moore, F. and Montcrieff, C.B. (1982) Are coal miners with low risk factors for ischaemic heart disease at greater risk of developing progressive massive fibrosis? *Br. J. Ind. Med.* **39**, 265–268

Cochrane, A.L., Haley, T.J.L., Moore, F. and Hole, D. (1979) The mortality of men in the Rhondda Fach, 1950–1970. *Br. J. Ind. Med.* **36**, 15–22

Cockcroft, A., Wagner, J.C., Ryder, R., Seal, R.M.E., Lyons, J.P. and Anderson, N. (1982a) Post-mortem study of emphysema in coal workers and non-coal workers. *Lancet* **2**, 600–603

Cockcroft, A., Barry, G., Cotes, J.E. and Lyons, J.P. (1982b) Shape of small opacities and lung function in coal workers. *Thorax* **37**, 765–769

Cockcroft, A.E., Wagner, J.C., Seal, R.M.E., Lyons, J.P. and Campbell, M.J. (1982c) Irregular opacities in coalworkers' pneumoconiosis – correlation with pulmonary function and pathology. *Ann. Occup. Hyg.* **26**, 767–787

Cockcroft, A., Lyons, J.P., Anderson, N. and Saunders, M.J. (1983) Prevalence and relation to underground exposure of radiological irregular opacities in South Wales coal workers with pneumoconiosis. *Br. J. Ind. Med.* **40**, 169–172

Collins, H.P.R., Dick, J.A., Bennett, J.G., Pern, P.O., Rickards, M.A., Thomas, D.J., Washington, J.S. and Jacobsen, M. (1988) Irregularly shaped small shadows on chest radiographs, dust exposure, and lung function in coal workers' pneumoconiosis. *Br. J. Ind. Med.* **45**, 43–55

Collis, E.L. and Gilchrist, J.C. (1928) Effects of dust on coal trimmers. *J. Ind. Hyg. Toxic.* **10**, 101–109

Constantinidis, K., Musk, A.W., Jenkins, J.P.R. and Berry, G. (1978) Pulmonary function in coal workers with Caplan's syndrome and non-rheumatoid complicated pneumoconiosis. *Thorax* **33**, 764–768

Costello, J., Ortmeyer, C.E. and Morgan, W.K.C. (1974) Mortality from lung cancer in US coal miners. *Am. J. Public Health* **64**, 222–224

Costello, J., Ortmeyer, C.E. and Morgan, W.K.C. (1975) Mortality from heart disease in coal mines. *Chest* **67**, 417–421

Cotes, J.E. (1979) *Lung Function*, 4th ed. Blackwell, Oxford

Cotes, J.E. and Field, G.B. (1972) Lung gas exchange in simple pneumoconiosis of coal workers. *Br. J. Ind. Med.* **29**, 268–273

Cotes, J.E., Deivanayagam, C.N., Field, G.B. and Billiet, L. (1971) Relation between types of simple pneumoconiosis (p or m) and lung function. In *Inhaled Particles III* (ed. W.H. Walton), Unwin, Woking, pp. 633–641

Crosbie, W.A. (1986) The respiratory health of carbon black workers. *Archs Environ. Health* **41**, 346–358

Dassanayake, W.L.P. (1948) The health of plumbago workers in Ceylon. *Br. J. Ind. Med.* **5**, 141–147

Davies, D. and Lindars, D.C. (1968) Rheumatoid pneumoconiosis. *Am. Rev. Respir. Dis.* **97**, 617–629

Davis, J.M.G., Ottery, J. and Le Roux, A. (1977) The effect of quartz and other non-coal dusts in coal workers' pneumoconiosis. Part II Lung autopsy study. In: *Inhaled Particles IV* (ed. W.H. Walton), Pergamon Press, Oxford, pp. 691–700

Davis, J.M.G., Chapman, J., Collings, P., Douglas, A.N., Fernie, J., Lamb, D., Ottery, J. and Ruckley, A. (1979) Autopsy study of coal miners' lungs. Edinburgh, Institute of Occupational Medicine. Report No. RM/789/9 (Eur. P27)

Davis, J.M.G., Chapman, J., Collings, P., Douglas, A.N., Fernie, J., Lamb, D. and Ruckley, V.A. (1983) Variation histological patterns of the lesions of coal workers' pneumoconiosis in Britain and their relationship to lung dust content. *Am. Rev. Respir. Dis.* **128**, 118–124

Davis, J.M.G., Addison, J., Bruch, J., Bruyere, S., Daniel, H., Degueldre, G., Dodgson, J., Gade, M., Gormley, I.P., Le

Bouffant, L., Martin, J.C., Reisner, M. et al. (1982) Variations in cytotoxicity and mineral content between respirable mine dusts from the Belgian, British, French and German coalfields. *Ann. Occup. Hyg.* **26**, 541–549

Dechoux, J. and Wantz, J.M. (1985) Le cancer bronchique chez les mineurs des Houllières du Bassin de Lorrain. *Rev. mal. Resp.* **2**, 69–74

Di Biasi, W. (1949) Pathologische Anatomie der Silkose. *Beiträge zur Silikose-Forschung Heft* **3**, 1–95

Donnet, J.B. and Bansal, R.P. (1984) *Carbon Fibres*. Marcel Dekker, New York

Douglas, A.N., Robertson, A., Chapman, J.S. and Ruckley, V.A. (1986) Dust exposure, dust recovered from the lung, and associated pathology in a group of British coal miners. *Br. J. Ind. Med.* **43**, 795–801

Duguid, J.B. and Lambert, M.W. (1964) The pathogenesis of coal miners' pneumoconiosis. *J. Pathol. Bacteriol.* **88**, 389–403

Dunner, L. and Bagnall, D.J.T. (1949) Pneumoconiosis in graphite workers. *Br. J. Radiol.* **22**, 573–579

Dunmore, J.H., Hamilton, R.J. and Smith, D.S.G. (1964) An instrument for the sampling of respirable dust for subsequent gravimetric assessment. *J. Sci. Instrum.* **41**, 669–672

Edwards, I.A.S. (1989). Structure in carbons and carbon forms. In *Introduction to Carbon Science* (ed. H. Marsh), Butterworths, London, pp. 1–36

Englert, M. and De Coster, A. (1965) La capacité de diffusion pulmonaire dans l'anthrasilicose micronodulaire. *J. fr. Med. Chir. thorac.* **19**, 159–173

Faulds, J.S., King, E.J. and Nagelschmidt, G. (1959) The dust content of the lungs of coal workers from Cumberland. *Br. J. Ind. Med.* **16**, 43–50

Faulkner, W.B. (1940) Bilateral pulmonary abscess secondary to pneumoconiosis. *Dis. Chest* **6**, 306–307

Fay, J.W.J. and Rae, S. (1959) The Pneumoconiosis Field Research of the National Coal Board. *Ann. Occup. Hyg.* **1**, 149–161

Fisher, S.W. (1935). Silicosis in British coal mines. *Transactions of Institute of Mining Engineers (London)*, Vol. 88, Part 5, 377–409; Part 6, 409–414

Frans, A., Veriter, C. and Brasseur, L. (1975) Pulmonary diffusing capacity for carbon monoxide in simple coal workers' pneumoconiosis. *Bull. Physiopathol. Respir.* **11**, 479–502

Frans, A., Veriter, C., Gerin-Portier, N. and Brasseur, L. (1975) Blood gases in simple coal workers' pneumoconiosis. *Bull. Physiopathol. Respir.* **11**, 503–526

Fritze, E. (1975) Zur Tuberkulinsensitivität von staubbelstaten Kohlenbergarbeitern und von niemals staubexponierten Bevolkerungsgruppen des Ruhrgebiets. *Int. Archs Occup. Environ. Health* **35**, 201–215

Fritze, E., Gundel, E., Ludwig, E., Muller, G., Muller, H.O. and Petersen, B. (1969). Die gesundheitliche Situation van Bergar beiten einer Kohlenzeche. *Dtsche Med. Wsche* **94**, 362–367

Fuller, H.W. (1860) *On Rheumatism, Rheumatic Gout and Sciatica, their Pathology, Symptoms and Treatment*, 3rd ed, Churchill, London, pp. 305–326

Gaensler, E.A., Cadigan, J.B., Sasahara, A.A., Fox, E.O. and MacMahon, H.E. (1966) Graphite pneumoconiosis of electrotypers. *Am. J. Med.* **41**, 864–882

Gernez-Rieux, C., Balgaires, E., Fournier, P. and Voisin, C. (1958) Une manifestation souvent méconus de la pneumoco- niose des mineurs: La liquéfaction aseptique des formations pseudotumorales. *Sem. Hôp. Paris* **34**, 1081–1089

Gernez-Rieux, C., Tacquet, A., Devulder, B., Voisin, C., Tonnel, A. and Aerts, C. (1972) Experimental study of interactions between pneumoconiosis and mycobacterial infections. *Ann. NY Acad. Sci.* **200**, 106–126

Gloyne, S.R. (1932–33) The morbid anatomy and histology of asbestos. *Tubercle (Edin.)* **14**, 445–451; 493–497; 550–558

Gloyne, S.R., Marshall, G. and Hoyle, C. (1949) Pneumoconiosis due to graphite dust. *Thorax* **4**, 32–38

Golden, E.B., Warnock, M.L., Hulett, L.D. and Churg, A.M. (1982) Fly ash lung: a new pneumoconiosis? *Am. Rev. Respir. Dis.* **125**, 108–112

Goldman, K.P. (1965a) The diagnosis of lung cancer in coal miners with pneumoconiosis. *Br. J. Dis. Chest* **59**, 141–147

Goldman, K.P. (1965b) Mortality of coal miners from carcinoma of the lung. *Br. J. Ind. Med.* **22**, 72–77

Goldman, K.P. (1965c) Prognosis of coal miners with cancer of the lung. *Thorax* **20**, 170–174

Gormley, I.P., Brown, G.M., Collings, P.L., Davis, J.M.G. and Ottery, J. (1980) The cytotoxicity of respirable dust from collieries. In *The In Vitro Effects of Mineral Dusts* (eds R.C. Brown, M. Chamberlain, R. Davies and I.P. Gormley, Academic Press, London, New York, Toronto, pp. 19–24

Gosset, P., Lassalle, P., Vanhee, D., Wallaert, B., Aerts, C., Voisin, C. and Tonnel, A-B. (1991) Production of tumour necrosis factor-α and interleukin-6 in human alveolar macrophages exposed *in vitro* to coal mine dust. *Am. J. Respir. Cell. Mol. Biol.* **5**, 431–436

Gough, J. (1940) Pneumoconiosis in coal trimmers. *J. Pathol. Bacteriol.* **51**, 277–285

Gough, J. (1947) Pneumoconiosis in coal workers in Wales. *Occup. Med.* **4**, 86–97

Gough, J. (1968) The pathogenesis of emphysema. In *The Lung*, (eds A.A. Liebow and D.E. Smith), Williams & Wilkins, Baltimore, pp. 109–133

Gough, J., Rivers, D. and Seal, R.M.E. (1985) Pathological studies of modified pneumoconiosis in coal miners with rheumatoid arthritis (Caplan's syndrome). *Thorax* **10**, 9–18

Green, F.H.Y. (1988) Coal workers' pneumoconiosis and pneumoconiosis due to other carbonaceous dusts. In *Pathology of Occupational Lung Disease* (eds A. Churg and F.H.Y. Green), Igaku-Shoin, New York, Tokyo, pp. 89–154

Gross, P., Braun, D.C. and de Treville, R.T.P. (1972) The pulmonary response to coal dust. *Ann. NY Acad. Sci.* **200**, 155–165

Gross, P. and de Treville, R.T.P. (1970) Black lungs. *Archs Environ. Health* **20**, 450–451

Gross, P. and Nau, C.A. (1967) Lignite and the derived steam-activated carbon. *Archs Environ. Health* **14**, 450–460

Haferland, W. (1957) Graphitstaublunge und Silikose. *Arch. Gewerbepath. Gewerbehyg.* **16**, 53–62

Hankinson, J.L., Palmes, E.D. and Lapp, N.L. (1979) Pulmonary air space size in coal miners. *Am. Rev. Respir. Dis.* **119**, 381–387

Hanoa, R. (1983) Graphite pneumoconiosis. *Scand. J. Work Environ. Health* **9**, 303–314

Harding, H.E. and Oliver, G.B. (1949) Changes in the lungs produced by natural graphite. *Br. J. Ind. Med.* **6**, 91–99

Harrington, J.S. (1972) Investigative techniques in the laboratory study of coal workers' pneumoconiosis: recent advances at the cellular level. *Ann. NY Acad. Sci.* **200**, 816–834

Hart, J.T., Cochrane, A.L. and Higgins, I.T.T. (1963) Tuberculin sensitivity in coal worker's pneumoconiosis. *Tubercle, Lond.* **44**, 141–152

Heath, D. (1968) Discussion. In *Form and Function in the Human Lung* (eds G. Cumming and L.B. Hunt), Livingstone, Edinburgh, London, p. 35

Heath, D. and Williams, D.R. (1989) *High-altitude Medicine and Pathology*, Butterworths, London, Boston, Singapore, pp. 188–189

Heise, E.R., Mentnech, M.S., Olenchock, S.A., Kutz, S.A., Morgan, W.K.C., Merchant, J.A. and Major, P.C. (1979) HLA-A1 and coal workers' pneumoconiosis. *Am. Rev. Respir. Dis.* **119**, 903–908

Hendriks, C.A.M. and Bleiker, M.A. (1964) Tuberculin sensitivity in coal miners with pneumoconiosis. *Tubercle, Lond.* **45**, 379–383

Heppleston, A.G. (1953) The pathological anatomy of simple pneumoconiosis in coal workers. *J. Pathol. Bacteriol.* **66**, 235–246

Heppleston, A.G. (1972) The pathological recognition and pathogenesis of emphysema and fibrocystic disease of the lung with special reference to coal workers. *Ann. NY Acad. Sci.* **200**, 347–369

Heppleston, A.G. (1984) Pulmonary toxicology of silica, coal and asbestos. *Environ. Health Perspect.* **55**, 111–127

Heppleston, A.G. (1988) Prevalence and pathogenesis of pneumoconiosis in coal workers. *Environ. Health Perspect.* **78**, 159–170

Heppleston, A.G. (1991a) Minerals, fibrosis and the lung. *Envir. Health Perspect.* **94**, 149–168

Heppleston, A.G. (1991b) Current status review. The role of surfactant in the pulmonary reaction to mineral particles. *Int. J. Exp. Pathol.* **72**, 599–616

Heppleston, A.G., Kulonen, E. and Potila, M. (1984) In vitro assessment of the fibrogenicity of mineral dusts. *Am. J. Ind. Med.* **6**, 373–386

Higgins, I.T.T. and Oldham, P.D. (1962) Ventilatory capacity in miners. *Br. J. Ind. Med.* **19**, 65–76

Higgins, I.T.T., Gilson, J.C., Ferris, B.G., Waters, W.E., Campbell, H. and Higgins, M.W. (1968a) IV Chronic respiratory disease in an industrial town; a nine-year follow-up study. Preliminary report. *Am. J. Publ. Health* **58**, 1667–1676

Higgins, I.T.T., Higgins, M.W., Lockshin, M.D. and Canale, N. (1968b) Chronic respiratory disease in mining communities in Marion County, West Virginia. *Br. J. Ind. Med.* **25**, 165–175

Higgins, I.T.T., Higgins, M.W., Lockshin, M.D. and Canale, N. (1969) Coronary disease in mining communities in Marion County, West Virginia. *J. Chron. Dis.* **22**, 165–179

Hodgson, J.T. and Jones, R.D. (1985) A mortality study of carbon black workers employed at five United Kingdom factories between 1947 and 1980. *Archs Environ. Health* **40**, 261–268

Holmes, S., Desai, J.B. and Sapsford, R.N. (1988) Nodular pulmonary amyloidosis: a case report and review of literature. *Br. J. Dis. Chest* **82**, 414–417

Holt, P.F. (1982) Submicron carbon dust in the guinea pig lung. *Envir. Res.* **28**, 434–442

Holt, P.F. (1987) *Inhaled Dust and Disease*, John Wiley & Sons, Chichester, New York, Brisbane, pp. 241–242

Hulett, L.D.Jr, Weinberger, A.J., Northcutt, K.J. and Ferguson, M. (1980) Chemical species in fly ash from coal-burning power plants. *Science* **210**, 1356–1358

Hurley, J.F. and Maclaren, W.M. (1988). Factors influencing the occurrence of progressive massive fibrosis (PMF) in miners and ex-miners. *Ann. Occup. Hyg.* **32** (suppl. 1), 575–583.

Hurley, J.F., Burns, J., Copland, L., Dodgson, J. and Jacobsen, M. (1982) Coal workers' simple pneumoconiosis and exposure to dust at 10 British coal mines. *Br. J. Ind. Med.* **39**, 120–127

Hurley, J.F., Alexander, W.P., Hazledine, D.J., Jacobsen, M. and Maclaren, W.M. (1987) Exposure to respirable coalmine dust and incidence of progressive massive fibrosis. *Br. J. Ind. Med.* **44**, 661–672

Jacobsen, M. (1977) Discussion. In *Inhaled Particles IV*, Vol. 2 (ed. W.H. Walton), Pergamon Press, Oxford, p. 772

Jacobsen, M. and Maclaren, W.M. (1982) Unusual pulmonary observations and exposure to coal mine dust: a case-control study. *Ann. Occup. Hyg.* **26**, 753–765

Jacobsen, M., Burns, J. and Attfield, M.D. (1977) Smoking and coal workers' simple pneumoconiosis. In *Inhaled Particles IV*. Vol. 2 (ed. W.H. Walton), Pergamon Press, Oxford, pp. 759–771

Jacobsen, M., Rae, S., Walton, W.H. and Rogan, J.M. (1971) The relation between pneumoconiosis and dust-exposure in British coal mines. In *Inhaled Particles III* (ed. W.H. Walton), Unwin, Woking, pp. 903–917

Jacobson, G., Felson, B., Pendergrass, E.P., Flinn, R.H. and Lainhart, W.S. (1967) Eggshell calcification in coal and metal miners. *Semin. Roentgenol.* **2**, 276–281

Jaffé, F.A. (1951) Graphite pneumoconiosis. *Am. J. Pathol.* **17**, 909–923

James, W.R.L. (1954) The relationship of tuberculosis to the development of massive pneumoconiosis in coal workers. *Br. J. Tuberc.* **48**, 89–101

James, W.R.L. (1955) Primary lung cancer in South Wales coal miners with pneumoconiosis. *Br. J. Ind. Med.* **12**, 87–91

Johnson, D.J. (1989) Carbon fibres: manufacture, properties, structure and applications. In *Introduction to Carbon Science* (ed. N. Marsh), Butterworths, London, pp. 197–228

Jones, H.D., Jones, T.R. and Lyle, W.H. (1982) Carbon fibre: results of a survey of process workers and their environment in a factory producing continuous filament. *Ann. Occup. Hyg.* 26 (1–4), 861–868

Kang, K.Y., Yagura, T., Sara, Y., Yokoyama, K. and Yamamura, Y. (1973) Antinuclear factor in pneumoconiosis and idiopathic pulmonary fibrosis. *Med. J. Osaka Univ.* **23**, 249–256

Kaw, J.L. and Khanna, A.K. (1988) Development of silicotic lesions in the lungs of rats pre-exposed to coal fly ash. *Br. J. Ind. Med.* **45**, 312–319

Keele, C.A. and Neil, E. (1971) *Samson Wright's Applied Physiology*, 12th ed, Oxford University Press, London, p. 141

Kennaway, E.L. and Kennaway, N.M. (1947) A further study of the incidence of cancer of the lung and larynx. *Br. J. Cancer* **1**, 260–298

King, E.J. and Nagelschmidt, G. (1945) The mineral of the lungs of workers from the South Wales coalfield. In: *Medical Research Council. Chronic Pulmonary Disease in South Wales Coalmines III. Experimental Studies*. HMSO, London, MRC Special Reports Series No. 250

King, E.J., Maguire, B.A. and Nagelschmidt, G. (1956) Further studies of the dust in lungs of coal miners. *Br. J. Ind. Med.* **13**, 9–23

King, E.J., Zaidi, S.H., Harrison, C.V. and Nagelschmidt, G. (1958) The tissue reaction of the lungs of rats after the inhalation of coal dust containing 2% of quartz. *Br. J. Ind. Med.* **15**, 172–177

Kober, T.W., Sorenson, J.R.L., Menden, E.E. and Petering, H.G. (1976) Some natural products from two soft coals. Their removal, metal-binding and enzyme inhibitory activity. *Archs Environ. Health* **31**, 182–188

Kriegseis, W. and Scharmann, A. (1985) Determination of free quartz surfaces in coal mine dust. *Ann. Occup. Hyg.* **29**, 91–99

Ladoo, R.B. and Myers, W.M. (1951) *Non-metallic Minerals* McGraw-Hill, New York, London, p. 250

Lamb, D. (1976) A survey of emphysema in coal workers and the general population (abstract). *Proc. R. Soc. Med.* **69**, 14

Lange, R., Worth, G., Smidt, W. and Stahlmann, W. (1980) Longitudinal study of the radiology of coal workers' pneumoconiosis. 1. Small and large opacities. *Int. Archs Occup. Environ. Health* **45**, 1–13

Lapp, N.L.R. and Seaton, A. (1971) Pulmonary function. In *Pulmonary Reactions to Coal Dust* (eds M.M. Key, L.E. Kerr, and M. Bundy), Academic Press, New York, London, pp. 153–177

Le Bouffant, L., Daniel, H. and Martin, J.C. (1977) The therapeutic action of aluminium compounds on the development of experimental lesions produced by pure quartz or mixed dust. In *Inhaled Particles IV* (ed. W.H. Walton), Pergamon Press, Oxford, New York, pp. 389–400

Le Bouffant, L., Daniel, H., Martin, J.C. and Bruyere, S. (1982) Effect of impurities and associated minerals on quartz toxicity. *Ann. Occup. Hyg.* **26**, 625–634

Le Bouffant, L., Addison, J., Bolton, R.E., Bruch, J., Bruyet, B., Daniel, H., Davis, J.M.G., Degueldre, G., Demarez, J., Dodgson, J., Gormley, I.P., Hadden, G.G., Kovacs, M.P., Martin, J.C., Reisner, M.T.R., Robertson, A. and Rosmanith, J. (1988) Compared *in vitro* and *in vivo* toxicity of coal mine dusts. Relationship with mineralogical composition. *Ann. Occup. Hyg.* **32** (suppl. 1), 611–620

Lee, S.C. and Johnson, H.A. (1975) Multiple nodular amyloidosis. *Thorax* **30**, 178–185

Legg, S.J., Cotes, J.E. and Bevan, C. (1983) Lung mechanics in relation to radiographic category of coal workers' simple pneumoconiosis. *Br. J. Ind. Med.* **40**, 28–33

Leiteritz, H., Einbrodt, H.J. and Klosterkötter, W. (1967) Grain size and mineral content of lung dust of coal miners compared with mine dust. In *Inhaled Particles and Vapours II* (ed. C.N. Davies), Pergamon Press, Oxford, London, pp. 381–390

Liddell, F.D.K. (1973) Mortality of British coal miners in 1961. *Br. J. Ind. Med.* **30**, 15–24

Lindars, D.C. and Davies, D. (1967) Rheumatoid pneumoconiosis. A study in colliery populations in the East Midlands coalfield. *Thorax* **22**, 525–532

Lindars, D.C., Rooke, G.B., Dempsey, A.N. and Ward, F.G. (1972) Pneumoconiosis and death from coronary heart disease. *J. Pathol.* **108**, 249–259

Lippmann, M., Eckery, H.L., Hahon, N. and Morgan, W.K.C. (1973) Circulating antinuclear and rheumatoid factors in coal miners. *Ann. Intern. Med.* **79**, 807–811

Lister, W.B. (1961) Carbon pneumoconiosis in a synthetic graphite worker. *Br. J. Ind. Med.* **18**, 114–116

Lister, W.B. and Wimborne, D. (1972) Carbon pneumoconiosis in a synthetic graphite worker. *Br. J. Ind. Med.* **29**, 108–110

Locke, G.B. (1963) Rheumatoid lung. *Clin. Radiol.* **14**, 43–54

Lyons, J.P., Ryder, R., Campbell, H. and Gough, J. (1972) Pulmonary disability in coal workers' pneumoconiosis. *Br. Med. J.* **1**, 713–716

Lyons, J.P., Ryder, R.C., Campbell, H., Clarke, W.G. and Gough, J. (1974) Significance of irregular opacities in the radiology of coal workers' pneumoconiosis. *Br. J. Ind. Med.* **31**, 36–44

Lyons, J.P., Ryder, R.C., Seal, R.M.E. and Wagner, J.C. (1981) Emphysema in smoking and non-smoking coal workers with pneumoconiosis. *Clin. Respir. Physiol.* **17**, 75–85

McCallum, R.I. (1961) Treatment of progressive massive fibrosis in coal miners. *Proceedings XIIIth International Congress on Occupational Health*, New York, pp. 741–745

McConnochie, K., Green, P.H.Y., Vallyathan, V., Wagner, J.C., Seal, R.M.E. and Lyons, J.P. (1988) Interstitial fibrosis in coal workers – experience in Wales and West Virginia. *Ann. Occup. Hyg.* **32** (suppl. 1), 553–560

McFarland, H.N., Ulrich, C.E., Martin, A., Krumm, A., Busey, W.M. and Alarie, Y. (1971) Chronic exposure of cynamolgus monkeys to fly ash. In *Inhaled Particles and Vapours III* (ed. W.H. Walton), Unwin, Woking, pp. 313–326

Maclaren, W.M. (1985) Using discriminant analysis to predict attacks of complicated pneumoconiosis in coal workers. *The Statistician* **34**, 197–208

Maclaren, W.M. and Soutar, C.A. (1985) Progressive massive fibrosis and simple pneumoconiosis in ex-miners. *Br. J. Ind. Med.* **42**, 734–740

McLintock, J.S., Rae, S. and Jacobsen, M. (1971) The attack rate of progressive massive fibrosis in British coal miners. In *Inhaled Particles III* (ed. W.H. Walton), Unwin, Woking, pp. 933–950

MacMahon, H.E. (1952) The application of X-ray diffraction in pathology (with particular reference to pulmonary graphitosis). *Am. J. Pathol.* **28**, 531–532

Marks, J. (1970) New mycobacteria. *Health Trends* **3**, 68–69

Marsh, H. (1989) *Introduction to Carbon Science*, Butterworths, London, Boston, Sydney

Martin, J.C., Daniel, H. and Le Bouffant, L. (1977) Short and long-term experimental study of toxicity of coal mine dust and some of its constituents. In *Inhaled Particles IV* (ed. W.H. Walton), Pergamon Press, Oxford, New York, pp. 361–370

Martin, J.C., Daniel-Moussard, H., Le Bouffant, L. and Policard, A. (1972) The role of quartz in the development of coal workers' pneumoconiosis. *Ann. NY Acad. Sci.* **200**, 127–141

Medical Research Council/Miners Treatment Centre (1963) Chemotherapy of pulmonary tuberculosis with pneumoconiosis. *Tubercle, Lond.* **44**, 47–70

Miall, W.E. (1955) Rheumatoid arthritis in Wales. An epidemiological study of a Welsh mining community. *Am. Rheum. Dis.* **14**, 150–158

Miall, W.E., Caplan, A., Cochrane, A.L., Kilpatrick, G.S. and Oldham, P.D. (1953) An epidemiological study of rheumatoid arthritis associated with characteristic chest X-ray appearances in coal miners. *Br. Med. J.* **2**, 1231–1236

Miller, A.A. and Ramsden, F. (1961) Carbon pneumoconiosis. *Br. J. Ind. Med.* **18**, 103–113

Miller, B.G. and Jacobsen, M. (1985) Dust exposure, pneumoconiosis and mortality of coal miners. *Br. J. Ind. Med.* **42**, 723–733

Milner, H.B. (1962) *Sedimentary Petrography. II Principles and Applications*, Allen and Unwin, London, pp. 262–264

Mitchell, R.S. (1962) Diffuse pulmonary emphysema and occupation. *J. Am. Med. Assoc.* **181**, 71–77

Mitchell, R.S., Walker, S.H. and Maisel, J.C. (1968) The causes of death in chronic airway obstruction. II. Myocardial infarction. *Am. Rev. Respir. Dis.* **98**, 611–612

Morgan, W.K.C. (1986) On dust, disability and death. *Am. Rev. Respir. Dis.* **134**, 639–641

Morgan, W.K.C., Burgess, D.B., Lapp, N.L. and Seaton, A. (1971) Hyperinflation of the lungs in coal miners. *Thorax* **26**, 585–590

Morgan, W.K.C. and Lapp, N.L. (1976) Respiratory disease in coal miners. *Am. Rev. Respir. Dis.* **113**, 531–559

Morgan, W.K.C., Handelsman, L., Kibelstis, J., Lapp, N.L. and Reger, R.B. (1974) Ventilatory capacity and lung volumes of US coal miners. *Archs Environ. Health* **28**, 182–189

Mortimer, E.A., Monson, R.R. and MacMahon, B. (1977) Reduction in mortality from coronary heart disease in men residing at high altitude. *N. Engl. J. Med.* **296**, 581–585

Moulin, J.J., Wild, P., Mur, J.M., Lafontaine, M., Lefer, M., Mercier-Gallay, M., Villemot, P., Whebi, V. and Coulon, J.P. (1989) Risk of lung, larynx, pharynx and buccal cavity cancers among carbon electrode manufacturing workers. *Scand. J. Work Environ. Health* **15**, 30–37

Murphy, D.M.F., Metger, L.F., Silage, D.A. and Fogarty, M.C. (1982) Effect of simple anthracite pneumoconiosis on lung mechanics. *Chest* **82**, 744–750

Musk, A.W., Cotes, J.E., Bevan, C. and Campbell, M.J. (1981) Relationship between type of simple coal workers' pneumoconiosis and lung function. A nine-year follow-up study of subjects with small rounded opacities. *Br. J. Ind. Med.* **38**, 313–320

Myasaka, N., Sato, K., Yamamoto, K., Goto, M. and Nishioka, K. (1989) Immunological and immunohistochemical analysis of rheumatoid nodules. *Ann. Rheum. Dis.* **48**, 220–226

Myers, C.F. (1967) Anthracosilicosis and bronchogenic carcinoma. *Dis. Chest* **52**, 800–805

Nagelschmidt, G., Rivers, D., King, E.J. and Trevella, W. (1963) Dust and collagen content of lungs of coal workers and progressive massive fibrosis. *Br. J. Ind. Med.* **20**, 181–191

National Coal Board (1977) *Medical Service Annual Report* 1978–1979, NCB, London

Nau, C.A., Neal, J., Stembridge, V.A. and Cooley, R.N. (1962) Physiological effects of carbon black. *Archs Environ. Health* **62**, 415–431

Navrátil, M., Widmisky, J. and Kasalicky, J. (1968) Relationships of pulmonary haemodynamics and ventilation and distribution in silicosis. *Bull Physiopathol. Respir. (Nancy)* **4**, 349–359

Nemery, B., Brasseur, L., Veriter, C. and Frans, A. (1987) Impairment of ventilatory function and pulmonary gas exchange in non-smoking coal miners. *Lancet* **2**, 1427–1430

Nonkin, P.M., Dick, M.M., Baum, G.L. and Gables, C. (1964) Myocardial infarction in respiratory insufficiency. *Archs Intern. Med.* **113**, 42–45

Noonan, C.D., Taylor, F.B.Jr and Engleman, E.P. (1963) Nodular rheumatoid disease of the lung with cavitation. *Arth. Rheum.* **6**, 232–240

Okutani, H., Shima, S. and Sano, T. (1964) Graphite pneumoconiosis in carbon electrode makers. In *XIVth International Congress of Occupational Health*, 1963, Vol. 2 (International Congress Series No. 62), Excerpta Medica, Amsterdam, pp. 626–632

Ortmeyer, C.E., Baier, E.J. and Crawford, G.M.Jr (1973) Life expectancy of Pennsylvania coal miners compensated for disability. *Archs Environ. Health* **27**, 227–230

Ortmeyer, C.E., Costello, J., Morgan, W.K.C., Swecker, S. and Petersen, M. (1974) The mortality of Appalachian coal miners 1963–71. *Archs Environ. Health* **29**, 67–72

Parkes, W.R., Phillips, T. and Williamson, R.G.B. (1976) Coronary artery disease and coal workers' pneumoconiosis. *Br. Med. J.* **2**, 1319–1320

Parmeggiani, L. (1950) Graphite pneumoconiosis. *Br. J. Ind. Med.* **7**, 42–45

Patrick, J.W. and Clarke, D.E. (1989) Mechanical properties of cokes and carbon composition. In *Introduction to Carbon Science* (ed. N. Marsh), Butterworths, London, Boston, Singapore, pp. 230–258

Pendergrass, E.P., Vorwald, A.J., Mishkin, M.M., Whildin, J.G. and Werley, C.W. (1968) Observations on workers in the graphite industry. Part 2. *Med. Radiogr. Photogr.* **44**, 1–17

Petsonk, E.L., Storey, E., Becker, P.E., Davidson, C.A., Kennedy, K. and Vallyathan, V. (1988) Pneumoconiosis in carbon electrode workers. *J. Occup. Med.* **30**, 887–891

Pivoteau, C. and Dechoux, J. (1972) Le retentissement des pneumoconioses à opacités fines de mineurs de charbon sans tombes ventilatoires. *Respiration* **29**, 161–172

Pooley, F.D. and Wagner, J.C. (1988) The significance of the selective retention of mineral dusts. *Ann. Occup. Hyg.* **32** (supp. 1), 187–194

Power, T. (1985) Fused materials – the high purity, high performance oxides. *Ind. Minerals* **214**, 37–57

Raabe, O.G., Tyler, W.S., Last, J.A., Schwartz, L.W., Lollini, L.O., Fisher, G.L., Wilson, F.D. and Dungworth, D.L. (1982) Studies of the chronic inhalation of coal fly ash by rats. *Ann. Occup. Hyg.* **26**, 189–211

Raask, E. (1985) *Mineral Impurities in Coal Combustion – Behaviour, Problems and Remedial Measures*, Springer-Verlag, London

Raask, E. and Schilling, C.J. (1980) Research findings on the toxicity of quartz particles relevant to pulverized fuel ash. *Ann. Occup. Hyg.* **23**, 147–157

Ramsey, J.H.R. and Pines, A. (1963) The late results of chemotherapy in pneumoconiosis complicated by tuberculosis. *Tubercle, Lond.* **44**, 476–479

Ranasinha, K.W. and Uragoda, C.G. (1972) Graphite pneumoconiosis. *Br. J. Ind. Med.* **29**, 178–183

Rand, B., Hosty, A.J. and West, S. (1989) Physical properties of pitch relevant to the fabrication of carbon materials. In *Introduction to Carbon Science* (ed. H. Marsh), Butterworths, London, Boston, pp. 75–106

Ray, S.C., King, E.J. and Harrison, C.V. (1951) The action of small amounts of quartz and larger amounts of coal and graphite on the lungs of rats. *Br. J. Ind. Med.* **8**, 68–73

Reid, L. (1967) *The Pathology of Emphysema*. Lloyd-Luke London

Reisner, M.T.R. and Robock, K. (1977) Results of epidemiological, mineralogical and cytological studies on the pathogenicity of coal mine dusts. In *Inhaled Particles IV* (ed. W.H. Walton), Pergamon Press, Oxford, pp. 703–715

Reisner, M.T.R., Bruch, J.R., Hilscher, W., Kriegseis, W., Prajsnar, D., Robock, K., Rosmanith, J., Scharmann, A., Schlipkötter, H.W., Strubel, G. and Weller, W. (1982) Specific harmfulness of respirable dusts from West German coal mines. VI: Comparison of experimental and epidemiological results. *Ann. Occup. Hyg.* **26**, 527–539

Remy-Jardin, M., Degreef, J.M., Beuscart, R., Voisin, C. and Remy, J. (1990) Coal workers' pneumoconiosis: CT assessment in exposed workers and correlation with radiographic findings. *Radiology* **177**, 363–371

Report of the Pneumoconiosis Committee of the College of American Pathologists to the National Institute for Occupational Safety and Health (1979) Pathology Standards for Coal Workers' Pneumoconiosis. Kleinerman, J. (Chairman). *Archs Pathol. Lab. Med.* **103**, 375–432

Rivers, D., James, W.R.L., Davies, D.G. and Thomson, S. (1957) The prevalence of tuberculosis at necropsy in massive fibrosis of coal workers. *Br. J. Ind. Med.* **14**, 39–42

Rivers, D., Wise, M.E., King, E.J. and Nagelschmidt, G. (1960) Dust content, radiology and pathology in simple pneumoconiosis of coal workers. *Br. J. Ind. Med.* **17**, 87–108

Robertson, A., Dodgson, J., Collings, P. and Seaton, A. (1984) Exposure to oxides of nitrogen: respiratory symptoms and lung function in British coal miners. *Br. J. Ind. Med.* **41**, 214–219

Robertson, A., Bolton, R.E., Miler, B.G., Chapman, J.S., Dodgson, J., Jones, A.D., Niven, J. and Davis, J.M.G. (1988a) The effect of quartz content on the pathogenicity of coal mine dusts. *Ann. Occup. Hyg.* **32** (suppl. 1), 621–633

Robertson, J. McD. and Ingalls, T.H. (1980) A mortality study of carbon black workers in the United States from 1935 to 1974. *Environ. Health* **35**, 181–186

Robertson, J. McD., Diaz, J.F., Fyfe, I.M. and Ingalls, T.H. (1988b) A cross-sectional study of pulmonary function in carbon black workers in the United States. *Am. Ind. Hyg. Assoc. J.* **49**, 161–166

Robertson, M.D., Boyd, J.E., Fernie, J.M. and Davies, J.M.G. (1983) Some immunological studies on coal workers with and without pneumoconiosis. *Am. J. Ind. Med.* **4**, 467–476

Robertson, M.D., Boyd, J.E., Collins, H.P.R. and Davis, J.M.G. (1984) Serum immunoglobulin levels and humoral immune competence in coal workers. *Am. J. Ind. Med.* **6**, 387–393

Rodnan, G.P., Benedek, T.G., Medsger, T.A. and Cammarata, R.J. (1967) The association of progressive systemic sclerosis (scleroderma) with coal miners' pneumoconiosis and other forms of silicosis. *Ann. Intern. Med.* **66**, 323–334

Rogan, J.M., Attfield, M.D., Jacobsen, M., Rae, S., Walker, D.D. and Walton, W.H. (1973) Role of dust in the working environment in development of chronic bronchitis in British coal miners. *Br. J. Ind. Med.* **30**, 217–226

Rooke, G.B., Ward, F.G., Dempsey, A.N., Dowler, J.B and Whitaker, C.J. (1979) Carcinoma of the lung in Lancashire coal miners. *Thorax* **34**, 229–233

Rose, L.B. and Hoffman, D.L. (1956) The coronary blood flow in pulmonary emphysema and cor pulmonale. *Circ. Res.* **4**, 130–132

Rossiter, C.E. (1972a) Relation between content and composition of coal workers' lungs and radiological appearances. *Br. J. Ind. Med.* **29**, 31–44

Rossiter, C.E. (1972b) Relation of lung dust content to radiological changes in coal workers. *Ann. NY Acad. Sci.* **200**, 465–477

Roy, T.M., Walker, J.F., Snider, H.L. and Anderson, W.H. (1989) Resting gas exchange in non-smoking bituminous coal miners with simple pneumoconiosis. *Respiration* **55**, 28–32

Ruckley, V.A., Chapman, J.S., Collings, P.L., Douglas, A.N., Fernie, J.M., Lamb, D. and Davis, J.M.G. (1981) *Autopsy studies of coal miners' lungs* – Phase II Edinburgh: Institute of Occupational Medicine (Report No. TM/81/18)

Ruckley, V.A., Fernie, J.M., Chapman, J.S., Collings, P., Davis, J.M.G., Douglas, A.N., Lamb, D. and Seaton, A. (1984a) Comparison of radiographic appearances with associated pathology and lung dust content in a group of coal workers. *Br. J. Ind. Med.* **41**, 459–467

Ruckley, V.A., Gauld, S.J., Chapman, J.S., Davis, J.M., Douglas, A.N., Fernie, J.M., Jacobsen, M. and Lamb, D. (1984b) Emphysema and dust exposure in a group of coal workers. *Am. Rev. Respir. Dis.* **129**, 528–532

Rüttner, J.R., Bovet, P. and Aufdermaur, M. (1952) Graphit, Caborund, Staublunge. *Dtsche Med. Wschr.* **77**, 1413–1415

Ryder, R., Lyons, J.P., Campbell, H. and Gough, J. (1970) Emphysema in coal workers' pneumoconiosis. *Br. Med. J.* **3**, 481–487

Sablonniere, B., Scharfman, A., Lafitte, J.J., Laine, A., Aerts, C. and Hayem, A. (1983) Enzymatic activities of broncho-alveolar lavage in coal workers pneumoconiosis. *Lung* **161**, 219–228

Samad, I.A. and Noehren, T.H. (1965) Myocardial infarction in pulmonary emphysema. *Dis. Chest* **47**, 26–29

Sanders, W.L. (1970) Heart disease and pneumoconiosis. *Thorax* **25**, 223–225

Scadding, J.G. and Mitchell, D.N. (1985) Lung changes. In *Sarcoidosis*, 2nd ed. Chapman and Hall, London, pp. 101–180

Scarano, D., Fadali, A.M.A. and Lemole, G.M. (1972) Carcinoma of the lung and anthracosilicosis. *Chest* **62**, 251–254

Schilling, C.J., Tams, I.P., Schilling, R.S.F., Nevitt, A., Rossiter, C.E. and Wilkinson, B. (1988) A survey into the respiratory effects of prolonged exposure to pulverised fuel ash. *Br. J. Ind. Med.* **45**, 810–817

Seal, R.M.E., Cockcroft, A., King, I. and Wagner, J.C. (1986) Central lymph node changes and progressive massive fibrosis in coal workers. *Thorax* **41**, 531–537

Seaton, A., Lapp, N.L. and Morgan, W.K.C. (1972a) Lung mechanics and frequency dependence compliance in coal miners. *J. Clin. Invest.* **51**, 1203–1211

Seaton, A., Lapp, N.L. and Morgan, W.K.C. (1972b) The relationship of pulmonary impairment in simple coal pneumoconiosis to type of radiographic opacity. *Br. J. Ind. Med.* **29**, 50–55.

Seaton, A., Dick, J.A., Dodgson, J. and Jacobsen, M. (1981) Quartz and pneumoconiosis in coal miners. *Lancet* **2**, 1272–1275

Seemayer, N.H. (1985) Importance of grain size and mineral content of coalmine dusts for cytotoxicity on macrophages *in vitro*. In *In Vitro Effects of Mineral Dusts: Third International Workshop* (eds E.G. Beck and J. Bignon), Springer-Verlag, Berlin, Heidelberg, New York, pp. 497–503

Seemayer, N.H. and Braumann, A. (1988) Effects of particle size of coal mine dusts in experimental anthrasilicosis. *In vitro* studies on human macrophages. *Ann. Occup. Hyg.* **32** (suppl. 1), 1178–1179

Shennan, D.H., Washington, J.S., Thomas, D.J., Dick, J.A., Kaplan, Y.S. and Bennett, J.G. (1981) Factors predisposing to the development of progressive massive fibrosis in coal miners. *Br. J. Ind. Med.* **38**, 321–326

Smidt, U., Worth, G. and Bielert, D. (1977) Lung function and clinical findings in cross sectional and longitudinal studies in coal workers from the Ruhr area. *Int. Archs Occup. Environ. Health* **40**, 45–70

Sorenson, J.R.J., Köber, T.E. and Petering, H.G. (1974) The concentration of Cd, Cu, Fe, Ni, Pb and Zn in bituminous coals from mines with differing incidences of coal workers' pneumoconiosis. *Am. Ind. Hyg. Assoc. J.* **25**, 93–98

Sosman, R.B. (1965) *The Phases of Silica*, 2nd ed, Rutgers University Press, New Brunswick, New Jersey

Soutar, C.A., Turner–Warwick, M. and Parkes, W.R. (1974) Circulating antinuclear antibody and rheumatoid factor in coal pneumoconiosis. *Br. Med. J.* **3**, 145–147

Soutar, C.A., Coutts, I., Parkes, W.R., Dodi, I.A., Gauld, S., Castro, J.E. and Turner-Warwick, M. (1983) Histocompatibility antigens in coal miners with pneumoconiosis. *Br. J. Ind. Med.* **40**, 34–38

Spink, R. and Nagelschmidt, G. (1963) Dust and fibrosis in the lungs of coal workers from the Wigan area of Lancashire. *Br. J. Ind. Med.* **20**, 118–123

Strom, K.A., Chan, T.L. and Johnson, J.T. (1988) Pulmonary retention of inhaled submicron particles in rats: diesel exhaust exposures and lung retention model. *Ann. Occup. Hyg.* **32** (suppl. 1), 645–657

Strom, K.A., Johnston, J.T. and Chan, T.L. (1987) Retention and clearance of inhaled submicron carbon black particles. *Toxicologist* **7**(29) (Abstract 114)

Swaen, G.M.K., Slangen, J.J.M., Volovies, A., Hayes, R.B., Scheffers, T. and Sturmans, F. (1991) Mortality of coke plant workers in the Netherlands. *Br. J. Ind. Med.* **48**, 130–135

Swaine, D.J. (1990) *Trace Elements in Coal*, Butterworths, London, Boston, Sydney

Sweet, D.V., Crouse, W.E. and Crable, J.V. (1974) The relationship of total dust, free silica, and trace metal concentrations to the occupational respiratory disease of bituminous coal miners. *Am. Ind. Hyg. Assoc. J.* **35**, 479–488

Teta, M.J., Ott, M.G. and Schatter, A.R. (1987) Population based mortality surveillance in carbon products manufacturing plants. *Br. J. Ind. Med.* **44**, 344–350

Thurlbeck, W.M. (1976) Chronic airflow obstruction in lung disease. In: *Major Problems in Pathology*, Vol. 5 (ed. J.L. Bennington), W.B. Saunders, Philadelphia

Town, J.D. (1968) Pseudoasbestos bodies and asteroid giant cells in a patient with graphite pneumoconiosis. *Can. Med. Assoc. J.* **98**, 100–104

Trapnell, D.H. (1964) Septal lines in pneumoconiosis. *Br. J. Radiol.* **37**, 805–810

Tulippe-Hecq, C., Zgheib, A., Borlée-Hermans, G. and Radermecker, M. (1989) Multiple pulmonary nodules. *Eur. Respir. J.* **2**, 119–120

Tylecote, F.E. and Dunn, J.S. (1931) Case of asbestos-like bodies in the lungs of a coal miner who had never worked in asbestos. *Lancet* **2**, 632–633

Uragoda, C.G. (1989) Clinical and radiographic study of activated carbon workers. *Thorax* **44**, 303–304

Verma, D.K., Muir, D.C.F., Stewart, M.L., Julian, J.A. and Ritchie, A.C. (1982) The dust content of the lungs of hard-rock miners and its relationship to occupational exposure, pathological and radiological findings. *Ann. Occup. Hyg.* **26**, 401–409

Vincent, J.H., Johnston, A.M., Jones, A.D., Bolton, R.E. and Addison, J. (1985) Kinetics of deposition and clearance of inhaled mineral dusts during chronic exposure. *Br. J. Ind. Med.* **42**, 707–715

Vincent, J.H., Jones, A.D., Johnston, A.M., McMillan, C., Bolton, R.E. and Cowie, H. (1987) Accumulation of inhaled mineral dust in the lung and associated lymph nodes: implications for exposure and dose in occupational lung disease. *Ann. Occup. Hyg.* **31**, 375–393

Wagner, J.C. (1970) Complicated coal workers' pneumoconiosis. In *Pneumoconiosis. Proceedings of International Conference, Johannesburg 1969* (ed. H.A. Shapiro), Oxford University Press, Cape Town, pp. 306–308

Wagner, J.C. (1971) Immunological factors in coal workers' pneumoconiosis. In *Inhaled Particles III* (ed. W.H. Walton), Unwin, Woking, pp. 573–576

Wagner, J.C. and McCormick, J.M. (1967) Immunological investigations in coal workers' disease. *J. R. Coll. Physns London* **2**, 49–56

Wagner, J.C., Wusteman, F.S., Edwards, J.H. and Hill, R.J. (1975) The composition of massive lesions in coal miners. *Thorax* **30**, 382–388

Wagner, J.C., Burns, J., Munday, D.E. and McGee, J.O'D. (1982) Presence of fibronectin in pneumoconiosis lesions. *Thorax* **37**, 54–56

Wagner, M.M.F. and Darke, C. (1979) HLA-A and B antigen frequencies in Welsh coal workers with pneumoconiosis and Caplan's syndrome. *Tissue Antigens* **14**, 165–168

Walker, W.C. and Wright, V. (1967) Rheumatoid pleuritis. *Ann. Rheum. Dis.* **26**, 467–474

Walton, W.H., Dodgson, J., Haddon, G.G. and Jacobsen, M. (1977) The effect of quartz and other non-coal dusts in coal workers' pneumoconiosis. Part I: Epidemiological studies. In *Inhaled Particles IV* (ed. W.H. Walton), Pergamon Press, Oxford, pp. 669–700

Ward, R. (1961) Pleural effusion and rheumatoid disease. *Lancet* **2**, 1336–1338

Waters, W.E., Cochrane, A.L. and Moore, F. (1974) Mortality in punctiform type of coal workers' pneumoconiosis. *Br. J. Ind. Med.* **31**, 196–200

Watson, A.J., Black, J., Doig, A.T. and Nagelschmidt, G. (1959) Pneumoconiosis in carbon electrode makers. *Br. J. Ind. Med.* **16**, 274–285

Wehr, K.L., Johanson, W.G., Chapman, J.S. and Pierce, A.L. (1975) Pneumoconiosis among activated carbon workers. *Archs Environ. Health* **30**, 578–582

Weiss, W. (1988) Smoking and pulmonary fibrosis. *J. Occup. Med.* **30**, 33–39

Weiss, W. (1991) Cigarette smoking and irregular opacities. *Br. J. Ind. Med.* **48**, 841–844

Weller, W. (1971) The relationship between duration of dust inhalation of a coal quartz mixture and dust retention, lung function and pathology on rats. In: *Inhaled Particles III*, Vol. 1 (ed. W.H. Walton), Unwin, Woking, pp. 337–344

Wells, A.L. (1954a) Pulmonary vascular changes in coal workers' pneumoconiosis. *J. Pathol. Bacteriol.* **68**, 573–587

Wells, A.L. (1954b) Cor pulmonale in coal workers' pneumoconiosis. *Br. Heart J.* **16**, 74–78

Wender, I., Heredy, L.A., Neuworth, M.B. and Dryden, I.G.C. (1981) Chemical reactions and the constitution of coal. In *Chemistry of Coal Utilization: Second Supplementary Volume.* (ed. M.A. Elliot), New York, Wiley, pp. 425–521

Williams, E. (1934) 'Curious bodies' found in the lungs of coal workers. *Lancet* **2**, 541–542

Wyatt, J.P. (1959) Macrosection and injection studies of emphysema. *Am. Rev. Respir. Dis.* **80** (suppl. 1), 94–103

Yang, G., Wang, S., Zhou, R. and Sun, S. (1983) Endemic selenium intoxication of humans in China. *Am. J. Clin. Nutr.* **37**, 872–881

Zahorski, W. (1961) Pneumoconiosis dans l'industrie du graphite artificiel. *Proceedings of the XIIIth International Congress on Occupational Health*, New York, pp. 828–832

Zaidi, S.H., Harrison, C.V., King, E.J. and Mitchison, D.A. (1955a) Experimental pneumoconiosis II. Coal mine dust with attenuated tubercle bacilli (BCG) in the lungs of immunised guinea pigs. *Br. J. Exp. Pathol.* **36**, 543–544

Zaidi, S.H., Harrison, C.V., King, E.J. and Mitchison, D.A. (1955b) Experimental pneumoconiosis IV. Massive pulmonary fibrosis produced by coal mine dust and isoniazid-resistant tubercle bacilli of low virulence. *Br. J. Exp. Pathol§* . **36**, 553–559

Zoll, P.M., Wessler, S. and Schlesinger, M.J. (1951) Interarterial coronary anastomoses in the human heart with particular reference to anaemia and relative cardiac anoxia. *Circulation* **4**, 797–815

14

Asbestos-related disorders

Kevin Browne

Introduction

Asbestos-related disorders can be divided into non-malignant and malignant. The non-malignant ones consist of:

1. Asbestosis (diffuse interstitial pulmonary fibrosis).
2. Hyaline plaques of the parietal pleura.
3. Diffuse thickening of the pulmonary pleura.
4. Benign pleural effusion.
5. Skin corns.

The malignant disorders consist of:

1. Lung cancer.
2. Malignant mesothelioma of the pleura and peritoneum.

The terminology employed for such widely disparate disorders should be free of any ambiguity. Cooke (1924) named the diffuse intrapulmonary fibrosis asbestosis by analogy with 'silicosis', and the term was restricted to this sense until recent times. Lately there has been a tendency to use it for other asbestos-related disorders. To safeguard against avoidable confusion, it seems preferable to confine this term to its original sense of a fibrotic pneumoconiosis.

The estimated number of asbestos workers 'at risk' in the UK in 1958 was 18 700, in 1967 20 000 and in 1970 30 000. By 1988 the number had declined to 9500. However, the figures do not include the unknown number of people working regularly or intermittently in the vicinity of asbestos operations. In the USA, the estimated number of 'exposed workers' was 1600 000 in 1975. Changes in world output of asbestos are shown in Table 14.1.

Classification and characteristics of asbestos minerals

Asbestos (ἄσβεστος, unquenchable) is a collective term for some of the metamorphic, fibrous, mineral silicates of the serpentine and amphibole groups (see Appendix I). They have different physical and chemical properties, but share a fibrous form or habit. Mineralogists have generally taken a particle with a length-to-breadth ratio (aspect ratio) of 10 : 1 or more to be a fibre. In milled asbestos most of the particles have aspect ratios that range from 5 : 1 to 20 : 1 or more and, in the case of chrysotile, mostly greater than 50 : 1. However, for milled non-asbestos amphiboles the ratio of the majority of particles (most of which are cleavage fragments) is less than 3 : 1. Unfortunately, with the introduction

Table 14.1 World production of asbestos

Year	Annual average ($\times 10^3$ tonnes) of			
	Amosite	Crocidolite	Chrysotile*	Total*
1920	<1	3	184	187
1950	38	29	930	1000
1960–64	66	87	2500	2700
1965–69	84	117	2900	3100
1970–74	100	154	3550	3800
1975–79	63	160	4800	5000
1980–84	45	103	4200	4350
1985	38	65	4200	4300
1986	36	63	4000	4100
1987	26	21	4050	4100

*Approximate quantity.
After British Geological Survey.

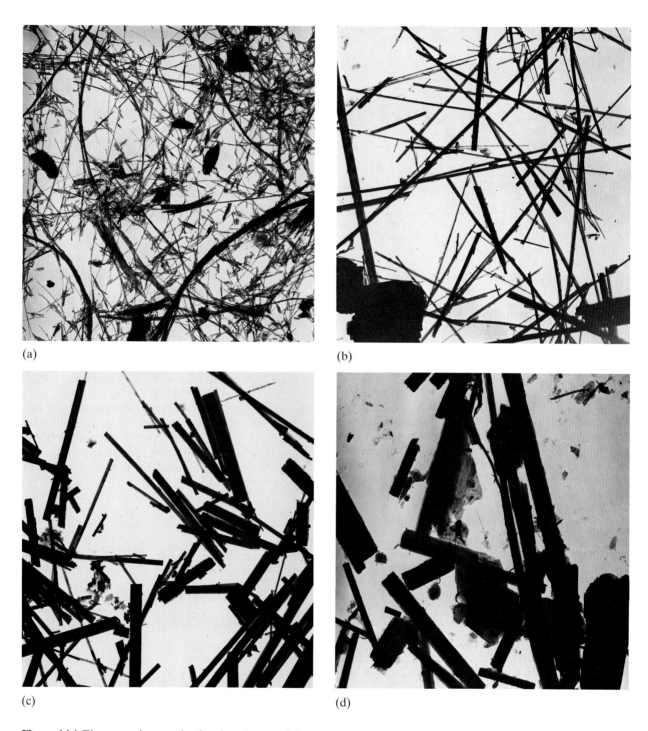

(a)

(b)

(c)

(d)

Figure 14.1 Electron micrographs showing characteristics of the four important asbestos fibre types: (a) chrysotile; (b) crocidolite; (c) amosite; (d) anthophyllite. Magnification × 4500. (By courtesy of Dr F.D. Pooley)

of the membrane filter method of counting, a fibre was arbitrarily defined in the medical and environmental literature as a mineral particle the length of which is at least three times greater than its diameter (Holmes, 1965). This definition has been the basis of all fibre counting for dose–response studies

since that time, and for this reason has been retained despite general agreement that it is inappropriate (see Appendix I, 'The amphiboles').

Economically and technically the most important forms of asbestos are chrysotile, crocidolite and amosite (grunerite). Anthophyllite, actinolite and tremolite have much less commercial value owing to their limited availability and low tensile strength.

Chrysotile is mined extensively in Canada and Russia. It is also mined in Brazil, in South Africa and Zimbabwe, in China, in Greece, Italy and Cyprus, and in the USA, India and small amounts elsewhere. The production of amphiboles is almost entirely confined to South Africa. Crocidolite occurs in isolation in North Cape Province (Cape Blue asbestos) and amosite in the Eastern Transvaal. However, smaller deposits of crocidolite, which are noteworthy for their close association with amosite, are exploited in the Eastern Transvaal (Transvaal Blue asbestos) and veins of both amphiboles are often found in the same reef (Hodgson, 1977). Crocidolite was also mined in Wittenoom in Western Australia on a small scale in the 1930s and on a larger scale from 1943 to 1966. Anthophyllite mines operated in Finland until 1977.

Tremolite has been mined on a small scale in China, Turkey and elsewhere. From the standpoint of human disease, however, tremolite owes its importance to its presence, first, in the soil in certain regions and, secondly, as a contaminant in many chrysotile mines and in the possibility that it is responsible for the cases of mesothelioma that occur in chrysotile miners (see page 468).

Since the introduction of asbestos minerals into modern industry, their production and consumption have grown to enormous proportions (Table 14.1). Because crocidolite has been particularly associated with malignant mesothelioma its use in the UK came under a voluntary ban in 1969, and since 1986 the use of both crocidolite and amosite has been banned by legislation. In western Europe and North America as a whole the use of all types of asbestos has declined dramatically since 1980 in the face of widespread public anxiety about environmental health effects. However, the use of asbestos (mainly chrysotile) in the rest of the world has so far been little affected.

Chrysotile fibres are long, white, soft, flexible and often curly but there is some variation in these physical features in fibres from different regions. Crocidolite and amosite fibres are blue and brown, respectively, shorter than those of chrysotile, stiff and straight; in addition, amosite is more brittle and has less tensile strength than the other two (Figure 14.1). Fibrous tremolite is brittle and tends to break down into 'chunky' fragments.

The physical properties that make the asbestos minerals invaluable are: fire resistance, poor conduction of heat and sound; the facility with which chrysotile, and to a lesser extent crocidolite, can be woven into fabrics; resistance to acids (except for chrysotile) and alkalis; and electrical resistance and mechanical strength.

It is sometimes said that asbestos is indestructible, but this is not correct. It is true, in general, that the various asbestos types possess good resistance to heat but at certain temperatures all decompose. Chrysotile breaks down to forsterite (an anhydrous silicate, Mg_2SiO_4) and silicon dioxide (SiO_2) between 800 and 850°C; crocidolite breaks down between 800 and 900°C; amosite, between 600 and 900°C; and anthophyllite, between 850 and 1000°C (Hodgson, 1966). Hence, under industrial and other conditions which generate high temperatures, decomposition will occur. Forsterite is not known to have any harmful effects (see Chapter 16, page 559). The amphiboles also have good weather resistance, but chrysotile is leached of its magnesium by water, and then breaks down and fragments.

Uses of asbestos and sources of exposure

Uses

The manufacture of *asbestos–cement products* consumes the greatest quantity of asbestos fibre. These products, used in the construction industry, are in three main categories: first, corrugated sheeting used for roofing and vertical cladding of structures such as farm buildings, garages and factories; secondly, flat sheeting used for roof tiles, partitioning and doorfacing; thirdly, for pipes and rainwater goods, including gutters and cisterns. The fibre acts as a reinforcing agent. Chrysotile is the predominant fibre, but some amphibole has been used in the past, particularly for pressure pipes, for which crocidolite was considered an essential ingredient because it permitted the more rapid elimination of excess water during manufacture. Fibre is milled to an appropriate size, mixed with cement as a slurry and passed onto a conveyor to make sheeting, or into moulds for making pipes and other shapes. Water is then extruded and the product air cured for some 28 days. The alternative method, more capital intensive and used mainly in North America, utilizes quartz and lime as materials instead of cement, the product then being autoclaved to convert the mixture into calcium silicate. Cases of silicosis have resulted from this production method.

The *floor tiling industry* used to take the next largest quantity of chrysotile. Some 10 to 30 per cent of short fibre acted as a reinforcing agent and filler in asphalt floorings and with organic resins for vinyl tiles. Asbestos has now been largely replaced by organic fibre for this purpose in Europe and North America.

Fibre has been used widely for *insulation and fireproofing*. Low-density asbestos–cement products were made in sections for pipe and boiler covering;

amosite mixed with sodium silicate or light-weight magnesia had a similar use as well as an important place for lining ships' bulkheads. Until the late 1960s, laggers mixed chrysotile or amosite and, occasionally, crocidolite with water by hand and applied the mixture after stripping away pre-existing lagging. Insulation, fire-proofing and sound-proofing were also done by spraying a fibre mixture (crocidolite, chrysotile or amosite with inorganic binders in water) on to walls, ceilings, girders and spandrels of buildings, and ships' bulkheads. This technique has been extensively used in shipbuilding and repair since the middle of the Second World War, but was one of the first processes to be banned in Europe and America owing to the extreme dustiness during application and the friability of the end-product.

Asbestos textiles employ chrysotile, crocidolite to a lesser extent, and sometimes both together; however, crocidolite has not been used in the UK since 1970. Other types of fibre are unsuitable. Fibre freed of extraneous matter may be mixed with cotton, hemp or synthetic fibre; it is carded, spun, woven, braided or plaited, and calendered. Until recent times these were dry and potentially dusty processes. Now, fibre is first blended in a slurry and then extruded into a coagulant to form tough, wet strands which are conveyed to the spinning or other machines. The process continues in the wet state so that dust emission is greatly reduced. Carding is now usually done by an enclosed wet dispersion process. Asbestos textiles have a wide range of uses: for fire-protective clothing, gloves, hoods and leggings, fire barriers, blankets and safety curtains, conveyor belts, brake and clutch linings, wicks for oil heaters and lamps, ropes, flexible tubings, and packings for groutings, autoclaves and ovens. Fire-protective clothing is made from chrysotile only.

Chrysotile is the main constituent (about 80 per cent) of *asbestos paper products* which include millboard, insulating papers, engine gaskets, roofing felts, wall coverings, soldering pads, cooking mats and flooring felt.

Another important application of chrysotile is in *friction materials* – most notably brake linings and facings – which consist of about 60 per cent of fibre in combination with phenolic resins, polymers, graphite, barytes, metals and pigments.

Chrysotile floats have been used in paints and welding rods and to reinforce thermosetting and polypropylene plastics. Machining and grinding asbestos-reinforced plastics may release a small amount of fibre. Chrysotile 'flock' has had an extensive application in filters for wines, beers, drugs and other fluids.

A limited use of crocidolite (but important from the point of view of disease potential) was in the manufacture of respirator filters – especially gas masks during the Second World War. It has also been incorporated into the filter tips of cigarettes in the USA. Chrysotile has found unusual uses as 'snow' in motion picture production, for Christmas decoration and for the manufacture of Santa Claus whiskers.

Anthophyllite has had a much more restricted application, being used as a filler in rubber and plastics. Of least importance are actinolite (which is rare) and fibrous tremolite, but they find some use as fillers and filter materials.

Substitutes

It is possible to substitute other materials for asbestos in most products, but usually at a considerably increased cost, and safety (as with friction materials for automobiles) or durability (with asbestos–cement construction products) cannot be ensured without long processes of product development. Moreover, among the most valuable characteristics of asbestos are its durability, causing it to persist in lung tissue, and fine diameter, which gives a very high surface-to-weight ratio but also renders it respirable. The most successful substitutes are, in most cases, those that possess these same characteristics, and great technological effort is being devoted to synthesize new fibres with even greater durability and surface-to-weight ratio. Thus, there is a real danger that the drive towards substitution may abolish only the name 'asbestos' and not the associated diseases, unless regulatory controls established for asbestos are extended to all respirable fibres.

Sources of exposure

The evidence on past dust levels in the occupational environment has been reviewed by Liddell (1991). The asbestosis risk is relatively low in open-cast mining of chrysotile and, because the serpentine rocks in which it occurs contain no quartz, there is no risk of silicosis. Amphibole asbestos is obtained mainly by underground methods which involve drilling, blasting and shovelling. The related rocks (banded ironstones) contain significant amounts of quartz. Dust is controlled by 'wetting down' methods. The asbestos risk is now low but silicosis may occur.

Long fibre used to be extracted by 'hand-cobbing', that is, gentle hammering to dislodge attached rock; now it is separated from the gangue (the residual rock) by crushing, screening, sieving and air-lifting. In this way seven grades of milled fibre, ranging from that suitable for textiles to that appropriate for cements, roof coatings, floor tiles, plastics and other filler purposes, are produced. These were dusty processes until the late 1940s, but application of wet methods or total enclosure have since effectively reduced pollution of the working environment by milling plants at the mine and by 'fiberizing' processes in the factory.

Bagging of fibre was a dusty operation until the 1960s when the introduction of pressure packing of all fibre types in 'leak-proof' bags of polythene-lined hessian or woven polythene was introduced. Previously, bags consisted of hessian only and were readily damaged in transit resulting in substantial leakage of fibre. Hence, dockers working in the holds of ships and in dockside warehouses were intermittently exposed to a dust hazard and, to a lesser degree, so were truck drivers and loaders. The transport of bags in sealed containers has further reduced this risk.

In 1969, a voluntary ban on the use of crocidolite was agreed by manufacturers, and no crocidolite fibre has been imported into the UK for industrial purposes since 1970. This ban, extended also to amosite, was given legislative backing in the UK in 1986 and, apart from the use of crocidolite for pressure pipes and packings, by the European Community in 1983. The dismantling of old lagging produces large amounts of dust unless specific precautions are taken. Men who built and maintained steam locomotives were often exposed to asbestos lagging materials. Spraying fibre on walls and ceilings was a potential source of high local concentrations of air-borne fibre. Spraying deckheads and bulkheads, lagging and stripping operations, and sweeping up of debris in the confined spaces of ships and submarines have, in the past, all been particularly culpable; in many instances, dust was dispersed for considerable distances from its source (Harries, 1976). As might be expected, shipbreaking was a potential source of high concentrations of dust.

Power drilling and sawing of asbestos board with high-speed tools produces significant quantities of fibre-containing dust, but much of the fibre is captive in cement fragments and of non-respirable dimensions, although some fibres – most of which are shorter than 5 μm – may escape. There is no risk when these operations are carried out on board containing only chrysotile fibre with slow running tools and handsaws in the open air or in well-ventilated areas, and special precautions are not necessary. Continuous runs with power tools, particularly in confined spaces, may produce hazardous dust levels close to the operator's face and extraction equipment, with or without specially designed tools, is required (Asbestos International Association, 1979). Abrasive sanding and grinding of asbestos boards is always dusty and requires exhaust ventilation.

Chrysotile has been used for brake linings and clutch facings from the beginning of the century, nowadays in concentrations up to 60 per cent in a resin-impregnated matrix. At temperatures of 830°C, chrysotile rapidly decomposes to forsterite and, because the temperature at the point of friction in braking normally exceeds 1000°C, little free fibre is released (Anderson, 1987). Several studies have shown that over 99.9 per cent of the original chrysotile is broken down (Williams and Muhlbaier, 1982; Sheehy et al., 1988) and that, of the fibres liberated, less than 1 per cent are longer than 5 μm (Rodelsperger et al., 1986; Sheehy et al., 1988), most being less than 1 μm, although the proportion of longer fibres released from the brakes of large vehicles is higher.

Unexpected sources of past exposure include the operation of machines for twisting asbestos string round welding rods (a dusty job often done by women in the 1930s) and the use of asbestos rope or fibre, either dry or wet, to grout bricks in furnaces and kilns. Because furnace and kiln workers, and some insulation workers in ships who use asbestos materials as well as refractory bricks for lining boilers, are often known as 'bricklayers' their exposure to asbestos may not be suspected. Demolition workers may have been exposed intermittently to an asbestos hazard when breaking up old lagging and other types of insulation.

Men clearing and maintaining exhaust ventilation ducts and duct disposal units in asbestos processing factories may be exposed to high concentrations of dust; also laundry workers may have been potentially at risk from asbestos used in lining rollers and ironing machines, and for insulation.

Paraoccupational exposure

During work done by others in their vicinity, workmen who themselves have never used asbestos materials may have been exposed to it intermittently in varying degree over many years. Important examples of such indirect exposure are maintenance fitters and electricians in asbestos-processing factories; stokers, fitters and others in boiler houses, power stations and ships around whom insulation operations involving stripping, lagging and spraying have been carried out; and plumbers, welders and carpenters who may have been in proximity to insulation being applied.

Domestic exposure

Many vivid descriptions have been recorded of asbestos workers in pre-war days returning home liberally dusted with fibre, and of their hair and clothes being brushed and shaken in the single living room of an artisan's house. There is a paucity of actual measurements, but Nicholson et al. (1980), using gravimetric measurements, found fibre levels to be several times higher in the homes of Newfoundland chrysotile miners than in others in the community. Sawyer (1979) showed that crocidolite could remain air-borne for up to 3 days in a domestic situation, and levels of over 100 fibres/ml (fibres per millilitre of air) have been reported following the shaking of clothes dusted with crocidolite in such circumstances. Certainly, the number of mesotheliomas known to have occurred among families of workers leaves no doubt that considerable exposure must have been experienced (Anderson *et al.*, 1979). High exposure in such cases has recently been confirmed by measurement of the lung fibre burden (Huncharek, Capotorto and Muscat, 1989; Gibbs *et al.*, 1990).

Buildings' exposure

Another type of exposure which has received much attention recently has been that of the occupants of buildings insulated with asbestos products, especially where walls and ceilings have been sprayed, and where low-density pipe and slab insulation has been installed. These types of asbestos installations tend to become friable if damaged or inadequately sealed, and fear of hazardous release of fibre into the atmosphere has resulted in panic removal measures in Europe and North America in the last decade.

However, a number of measurements which have recently been made by transmission electron microscopy (TEM) show these fears to be grossly exaggerated (Health Effects Institute, 1991). Chatfield (1983) found levels of less than 0.001 fibre/ml of asbestos fibres over 5 μm long in 19 buildings containing friable sprayed asbestos (that is, less than one two-hundredth of the occupational exposure limit for amphibole asbestos in the UK and the USA). Burdett and Jaffery (1986) reported similar levels; Gazzi and Crockford (1987) found an average level of 0.0003 fibre/ml in 25 dwellings containing amosite board; Lee (1987) found only 15 fibres of greater than 5 μm in 300 air samples taken from US schools containing friable asbestos. Chesson *et al.* (1990) reported results of samples by the US Environmental Protection Agency of air outside and inside buildings in which asbestos was either absent, present but in good condition, or present and damaged. They found the measured levels and differences small in absolute magnitude, and an analysis of the results by Crump and Farrar (1989) showed no statistically significant differences between any of the locations. At the same time reports from the UK, the USA, Canada and Sweden have all shown that fibre levels may be higher after removal of friable asbestos, even when carried out according to best practice, than before. Moreover, these higher levels may persist for a considerable

time after removal (Burdett, Jaffery and Rood, 1989). Vinyl floor tiles incorporating short fibres as reinforcement do not liberate detectable fibres of greater than 5 μm length in normal use.

Environmental exposure

Asbestos is very widely found in rock formations throughout the world, with chrysotile being the most ubiquitous. A study of the Greenland ice cap revealed the presence of chrysotile in cores dated back to 1750 (Bowes, Langer and Rohl, 1977) and recent air samples taken at the summit of Mont Blanc showed appreciable levels of chrysotile, known to be present in the serpentine belt of the Alps. In the New Idria area of California, levels of more than 1 fibre/ml have been found from natural chrysotile sources (Cooper *et al.*, 1979). In Quebec chrysotile mining towns, levels of 0.008 fibre/ml greater than 5 μm long were found in residential areas (Lebel, 1984), compared with 0.0007 fibre/ml at a control site away from the mines. Comparable figures were reported from Austria near a natural deposit (0.002 fibre/ml) and an asbestos–cement plant (0.005 fibre/ml) (Felbermayer and Ussar, 1980). The Canadian figures are of particular interest because Churg (1986) has shown that they are accompanied by higher lung fibre burdens of both chrysotile and tremolite; despite this, however, there appears to be no resultant increase in asbestos-related disease. Very high levels have been found downwind of tailing dumps at the crocidolite mines in South Africa, up to 0.6 fibre/ml of greater than 5 μm and mesotheliomas are known to have occurred in people whose only exposure was to this environment. No evidence of environmental asbestos-related mesotheliomas was found in a mortality study of residents in the vicinity of a very dusty amosite factory by Hammond *et al.* (1979) or a dockyard (Sheers and Coles, 1980), or in towns in Austria (Neuberger, Kundi and Friedl, 1984) or Switzerland (Rüttner, Schuler and Walchi, 1983) in which large asbestos–cement plants were located. Whilst Newhouse and Thompson (1965) and Bohlig and Hain (1973) both reported higher levels of mesotheliomas in residents living near asbestos factories, the linking of retrospective histories with geographical location involves a simple potential source of error: that part of the history which is forgotten, or unknown, will have a higher probability of involving occupational or domestic exposure in those living near the factory than in those living at a distance; consequently their data are unreliable.

Levels in urban air away from any particular source of industrial asbestos vary from less than 0.0001 fibre/ml to 0.001 fibre/ml of greater than 5 μm length. Chatfield (1983) found slightly higher levels at busy urban intersections, but the average figure remained around 0.0005 fibre/ml – a figure now commonly accepted as a representative outdoor urban level, and recently confirmed by Burdett, Smith and Papanicolopoulos (1989) in a study of levels at an urban road junction. The question has been raised whether the higher fibre levels in urban compared with rural ambient air are due to release of fibres from vehicle brakes. However, in view of the very small release in braking of fibres greater than 5 μm in length, mentioned earlier, it is probable that most industrial fibres come from building and demolition operations, the higher levels in traffic resulting largely from greater air disturbance.

Finally, mention must be made of asbestos fibres in drinking water. Apart from a contribution possible from asbestos cement pipes, virtually all water contains natural asbestos fibres. Their lengths are normally short, with median values of less than 1 μm. Levels in UK drinking water have been found to range from 0 to 11×10^6 (chrysotile) and 0 to 1×10^6 (amphibole) per litre (Commins, 1988).

Asbestos in history

The use of asbestos extends back into prehistory. Anthophyllite was used in Finland as a reinforcing fibre in the preparation of clay pottery as long ago as 2500 BC (Kiviluoto, 1965) and, according to the local Museum of Ethnography, chrysotile in Corsica was put to similar use. Apart from its use in ceramics, chrysotile has been spun and woven into fabric for perhaps as long as 3000 years. An extant Chinese document, the book *Liezhi* from the third century AD, refers to King Zhoumen (about 1000 BC) receiving a fire-rinsed cloth by way of a tribute, and another book of the same period quotes a book *Chou* written in 400 BC which records a similar incident (Liang-ho Su and Zhong-jun Li, 1980). The woven cloth that was cleansed by fire instead of being destroyed appears frequently in ancient literature. It was said to have saved Charlemagne in a desperate situation by impressing an enemy with its apparent magical powers.

In classical literature asbestos is also referred to as *amiantos*, from the Greek ἀμίαντος meaning undefiled – another reference to its propensity to be restored by fire to its original purity. Derivatives from this root have remained in current use in southern Latin languages, whilst 'asbestos' took hold in northern Europe and North America. An early reference is by Strabo (64 BC to AD 19) who refers to the stone produced in Carystos, which is

combed and woven into towels (*Geography* 10, 1). Carystos is in southern Euboea, where asbestos is produced today.

Pliny the Elder in the first century AD describes (*Natural History* 19, 4) how it can, with some difficulty, be woven into cloth, and how this cloth can be cleansed by fire. It was, he said, made into shrouds for royalty which enabled the ashes to be kept separate from the pyre. It came from India and when found rivalled the price of fine pearls. In 1702 a funeral urn, now on display in the Vatican Museum, was found in excavations near the Naevian Gate in Rome. It contained bones and ashes wrapped in asbestos cloth.

Asbestos, or amiantos, is mentioned by many other classical writers, among them Dioscorides (*De Materia Medica* 5, 138) who mentioned cloth woven from mineral mined in Cyprus, and St Augustine (*De Civitate Dei* 21, 5) who described it as a stone obtained from Arcadia which once set alight could never be extinguished. There was, he said, a shrine of Venus with a lamp containing some device constructed from the asbestos stone in which the flame so burned that no storm or rain could extinguish it. Perhaps it was from St Augustine that the eleventh century monastic compiler of the first vernacular English lapidary (B.L. Cotton, 1050) obtained his reference to the stone from Arcadia which, when set on fire, neither water nor wind could put out.

Some manufacture of cloth continued throughout the Middle Ages. A reference to asbestos cloth appears in a Sanskrit work *Lives of Sixty Three Illustrious Persons* from twelfth century India, and Chinese writers continued to refer to it. Marco Polo (1298) gives a convincing description (purporting to be first hand) of the mining and manufacture of cloth from chrysotile in Southern Siberia. A small trade continued through the Middle Ages, and a contemporary account of the siege of Rouen refers to:

The Kingis herauldis and pursuivantis
In cotis of armys amyauntis.

A description of woven Italian chrysotile is found again in 1671 in the *Philosophical Transactions of the Royal Society of London* (vol. VI, no. 72). A hundred years later Canadian chrysotile first appears; in 1752 the young Benjamin Franklin, recently arrived in London and seeking to raise some money, wrote to Sir Hans Sloane offering for sale a purse made of 'Stone Asbestos' which he had obtained from the 'Northern Parts of America'. The woven chrysotile purse is now on show in the Natural History Museum in London, where, curiously, it is labelled 'tremolite'.

Two further references in classical literature may be mentioned. In one, Pliny describes how workers refining minium (probably cinnabar – mercuric sulphide) used to tie bladder-skins over their faces *'ne in respirando pernicialum pulverem trahunt'* – to prevent the inhalation of the poisonous dust (*Natural History* 33, 50). In the other, Strabo (*Geography* 12, 3) describes the employment of incorrigible slaves in the mountain where realgar, or arsenic sulphide, was worked. Because of 'the grievous odour of the ore, the workmen are doomed to a quick death'. Both descriptions have frequently been wrongly quoted as referring to asbestos.

Asbestos: the beginnings of modern industry

The origins of contemporary exploitation of asbestos may be placed early in the nineteenth century, when two Italians carried out some experimental work with chrysotile cloth mined and woven in the area, and were awarded a distinction by Napoleon I. The disturbed political climate of the time seems to have inhibited development for some decades. An Englishman, Richard Lloyd, took out a patent in the USA for packing involving asbestos in 1857, but this does not appear ever to have come into use. Then, in 1866, a Signor Albonico, a native of the North Italian asbestos-bearing area, formed a partnership with a local priest and a nobleman, and obtained mining concessions (Fisher, 1892; Murray, 1990).

By 1871 the Patent Asbestos Manufacturing Company had begun operations at premises in Drummond Street, Glasgow, and a year or two later the 'Italo-English Pure Asbestos Company' of London came into existence, with a factory in Turin. In 1880 these joined to form 'The United Asbestos Company', a year after Bell had begun the manufacture of plaited asbestos packings on a large scale (Anon, 1883).

Canadian chrysotile had been exhibited in London at the International Exhibition of 1862. The discovery of widespread deposits is credited to Fecteau, but mining operations did not begin until 1878, when a total of 50 tons was extracted. From then on, development of both Italian and Canadian deposits was rapid, and search was made for asbestos elsewhere in the world. By the early 1890s specimens had been received from, among other places, Africa and Australia, and a considerable quantity of Russian chrysotile from the Urals had been imported by the United Asbestos Company. At about the same time the exploitation of crocidolite deposits in the Northern Cape of South Africa had begun. In 1890 Oats, a Cornish mining engineer, had been shown a specimen of crocidolite, and 3

years later he had raised support to form the Cape Asbestos Company. Amosite was discovered in 1907 in the Transvaal, and commercial exploitation began 7 years later.

On the manufacturing side, the first addition to plain textile operations was the production of millboard by processes more akin to paper-making, for which credit is give to Corona, the clerical member of the original north Italian trio. There is a report of the use of asbestos in roofing felt in the USA in 1866. Filters and other uses followed, and by 1892 United Asbestos were offering 100 different products for sale. The final developments came in 1900 with the invention by Hatschek in Austria of the process of asbestos–cement manufacture, and the use of asbestos in automotive brake linings in 1906.

Early recognition of health hazards

The first person on record to have reported the ill-effects of inhalation of asbestos dust was Miss Deane, a woman factory inspector (Annual Report of HM Chief Inspector of Factories for 1898). In France an inspector named Auribault (1906) reported 50 deaths in workers in an asbestos weaving textile factory between 1890 and 1895. The first description of asbestosis was by Dr Montague Murray (1907) in evidence to the departmental committee on compensation for industrial diseases. The histological slides of the case he described survived at least to 1970, and showed both diffuse interstitial fibrosis and asbestos bodies (Greenberg, 1982). A perusal of the committee's report makes clear their concern to distinguish between tuberculous phthisis and fibroid or dust phthisis, of which silicosis – 'ganister disease' – was the most commonly encountered.

Concern continued to be expressed at intervals during the next 20 years. Dr Collis, in the Annual Report of the Chief Inspector of Factories for 1910, described 5 deaths in 5 years from a staff of 40 engaged in the production of asbestos insulation mattresses, one stage of which was to beat them flat with a wooden flail. It is of interest that he also mentions the consequent reorganization of the process with exhaust ventilation, and the institution of annual medical examinations. The US Department of Labor published a review of respiratory mortality in dusty trades by Hoffman (1918), in the course of which he comments on the practice of insurance companies to decline asbestos workers 'on account of the assumed health-injurious conditions of the industry'.

The first case of asbestosis to be described fully in the medical literature was by Cooke (1924) who later coined the word asbestosis (Cooke, 1927). Although his original case was complicated by cavitary tuberculosis, the distinction between tuberculosis, silicosis and asbestosis was by now beginning to be clarified, aided also by the demonstration by Beattie in 1912 (Merewether and Price, 1930), in work for the Factory Department, that asbestos inhalation caused fibrosis in animals. A further case, in 1927 (Haddow, 1929) of severe fibrosis of the lungs accepted as being non-tuberculous, resulted in an enquiry being instigated by the Home Office Factory Department. This was carried out by Merewether and Price, whose report (1930) provided the basis for the first regulations to control dust emission in certain processes of asbestos manufacture, to prescribe medical surveillance of employees and compensation for anyone suffering from asbestosis 'to such a degree as to make it dangerous for him to continue to work in the industry'.

During the 1930s attention was drawn to the occurrence of lung cancer – then still an uncommon malignancy – in workers with asbestosis. Credit for the first case report drawing attention to a possible relationship should go to Lynch and Smith (1935), although in the previous year Wood and Gloyne (1934) had published a series of 53 cases of asbestosis, in 2 of which lung cancer was also present. It was, however, in Germany that the relationship was first accepted, whilst doubts remained for a few more years in the UK and even longer in the USA. In the UK, the issue was settled by the Annual Report of the Chief Inspector of Factories for 1947, in which Merewether (1949) recorded that lung cancer was present in 17 per cent of 128 male deaths between 1924 and 1946 from or complicated by asbestosis and reported to the inspectorate. The comparable figure for silicosis was only 1.3 per cent. The seal was set by Doll (1955) who published the first historical cohort mortality study of asbestos workers, and found that the lung cancer standardized mortality ratio (SMR) was greatly increased in workers with asbestosis but not in those without.

Another landmark in the UK was the report in 1950 to the Industrial Injuries Advisory Council that drew attention to the occurrence of asbestosis outside the manufacturing trades scheduled in the 1931 regulation, particularly among laggers.

Mesothelioma, meanwhile, had been the subject of a number of individual case reports, but worldwide recognition of its relationship with asbestos exposure came with the publication of 33 cases, all linked with exposure to crocidolite in South Africa, by Wagner, Sleggs and Marchant (1960). The fascinating story behind this discovery has been related by Wagner (1991). The literature on asbestos and malignancy up to the first comprehensive world conference on asbestos-related disease held in New York in 1964 has been reviewed by Enterline

(1978). A more personal account has been given by Murray (1990) and in letters by Murray and Castleman (1991).

Asbestosis

Incidence and prevalence

Accurate statistics of the incidence and prevalence of asbestosis are few, and are bedevilled by problems of definition of both disease and exposure. Dreessen et al. (1938) studying dust and disease in a South Carolina textile factory had concluded that at dust levels below 5 million particles per cubic foot (5×10^{-6} m.p.p.c.f.) (probably equivalent to between 15 and 30 fibres/ml), new cases of asbestosis would not occur. Smither (1965) gave a detailed account of the lengthening times before the onset of symptoms and disability in employees of an East London factory which operated from 1913. In the early 1930s, exposure (which would have been before the 1931 regulations had taken effect) averaged 7 years (range 1.5 to 19 years) before the onset of certified asbestosis. In the 1940s the average had risen to 10 years; in the 1950s 14.5 years (range 3 to 32 years); and for cases occurring after 1960, 17.5 years (range 4 to 35 years). As Smither pointed out, criteria for certification of asbestosis changed during this time, allowing for earlier acceptance of cases and, thereby, tending to shorten the exposure time, so that the effects of reduction of exposure were, in fact, more pronounced than was evidenced by the figures.

The diagnosis of asbestosis is discussed later (see page 437); for epidemiological purposes the choice of end-points has been between clinical effects (basal inspiratory crackles), radiographic change (defined in terms of ILO subcategories – see Chapter 7) or lung function deficit (taken, at its simplest, as a reduction exceeding 20 per cent under standard for static lung volumes and ventilatory capacity). The British Occupational Hygiene Society (BOHS) Committee on Hygiene Standards (1968) estimated, on the basis of data from an English textile factory, that a 1 per cent risk of developing basal crackles would occur at a cumulative risk of about 112 fibres/ml years and significant radiographic change 130 fibres/ml years. Berry et al. (1979) reduced these estimates, calculating that a 1 per cent risk of crackles would occur at 43, possible asbestosis at 55 and certified asbestosis at 72 fibres/ml years. *Cumulative exposure*, expressed in fibres/ml years, is represented by the product of the average dust level in fibres/ml to which the subject is exposed and the number of years worked at this average level.

Becklake (1983, 1991) demonstrated a tenfold difference in the prevalence of radiographic change ILO subcategory 1/0 or more in relation to cumulative exposure in a small number of studies, permitting a comparison and she discussed possible reasons for this. Differences in fibre type undoubtedly contribute. The solubility, fragmentation and easier clearance of chrysotile, discussed on page 426, compared with the amphiboles would be expected to reduce the continuing lung fibre burden and, hence, reduce the slope of the dose–response line. Weill et al. (1977) and Hughes, Weill and Hammad (1987) have shown that this appears to be true in a comparative study of two asbestos–cement plants, and have shown also the important difference resulting from relatively small proportions of amphibole mixed in with chrysotile. Asbestosis is a disappearing disease, and it is scarcely possible to study this point prospectively. However, if the attributable risk of lung cancer is accepted as an index of the prevalence of asbestosis (a point to be discussed later) the difference between asbestos–cement plants using only chrysotile, and those which used a mixture, becomes very clear (Ohlson and Hogstedt, 1985; Gardner and Powell, 1986).

Whether the dose–response relationship is linear, and whether a *threshold* exists below which no effect is experienced, were considered by the Ontario Royal Commission on Asbestos (1984). Their conclusion was that a linear relationship was consistent with published studies, and that a threshold exists so that asbestosis will not progress to clinical manifestation at or below lifetime occupational exposures of 25 fibres/ml years. This conclusion was endorsed by Doll and Peto in their 1985 review prepared for the UK Health and Safety Executive. Further evidence of a threshold was provided by Churg (1986) who compared the lung fibre burden of long-term residents of a chrysotile mining town (who were not themselves occupationally exposed) with those of a general urban population. He found that amounts of both chrysotile and tremolite fibres greater than 5 µm long were significantly raised in the mining town residents. Nevertheless, several epidemiological studies have failed to find an excess of disease in the town which is attributable to asbestos. Bégin et al. (1987b) found evidence of a tolerance threshold in studies of lavage fluid of sheep exposed to chrysotile. As will be discussed later, this conclusion is to be expected as an understanding of the biological mechanism of asbestosis becomes clearer.

Sluis-Cremer, Hnizdo and du Toit (1990) have published evidence of a threshold for asbestosis in South African amphibole miners as assessed at autopsy. The threshold level was estimated to be 2 fibres/ml years with follow-up as long as 45 years, but the authors list many reasons why exposures were probably underestimated, including the fact that they were based on average fibre concentrations throughout individual mines, and average job rankings, not on individual exposures. Estimates of this type are subject to threshold smoothing problems (which also produce underestimates) to an extreme degree. But the finding of a threshold, with autopsy confirmation, is of considerable interest even if the estimated cumulative exposure level is unreliable.

Pathology

Macroscopic appearances

The external features of the lungs depend on the extent and severity of disease and the degree of diffuse thickening of the overlying pleura. The pulmonary pleura in most cases is thickened, varying from a slight, diffuse loss of translucency (due to a thin layer of fibrosis) to widespread fibrosis (with fusion of pulmonary and parietal layers) which tends to be most evident over the lower half of the lungs.

When the lungs are sliced sagitally, early asbestosis may only be discernible to the touch: the tissues feel firmer and more resilient than normal and the pleural margins and subpleural intralobular septa of the lower lobes stand out prominently (Figure 14.2). With disease of moderate severity these changes are more pronounced and a network of grey-coloured irregular fibrosis is visible in the subpleural regions of the lower lobes and, to a lesser extent, in the middle lobe and lingula to a depth of about 1 to 2 cm. When disease is advanced the lower part of the lungs is pale and greatly indurated, and the interlobular septa are obviously thickened and fibrosed. At this stage irregular fibrosis is coarse and extends more deeply from the pleura and interlobular septa into the lung. Demarcation from adjacent normal lung tissue is often ill-defined in contrast to interstitial fibrosis due to other causes which is usually sharply outlined (Figures 14.2 and 14.3) (see Chapter 15). The fibrosis is distributed mainly in proximity to the diaphragmatic and posterolateral pulmonary pleura of both lower lobes and, to a lesser degree, of the middle lobe and lingula (Figure 14.2). In advanced disease the subpleural zones of the bases of the upper lobes may be involved, in addition to the more extensive fibrosis of the lower lobes. *Reversal of this predominantly basal distribution points to some other lung pathology.* As a rule the extent of fibrosis is roughly equal in both lungs. In the early stages of asbestosis the lungs are of normal size whereas, in advanced disease, they are small, pale and rubbery.

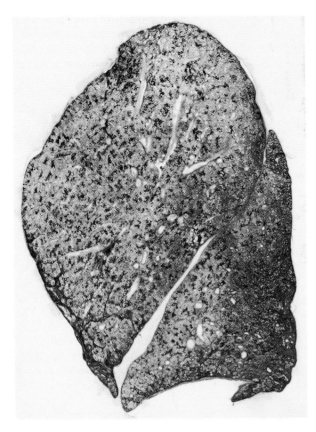

Figure 14.2 Asbestosis of slight-to-moderate degree involving the posterior and basal zones of the lower lobe which is reduced in size, and the lingula and lower part of the upper lobe anteriorly. The fibrosis is limited to the lower half of the lung, does not involve the more central parts of the lobes and cyst formation is absent. The numerous macules are those of 'city dwellers' lung' due to the deceased having lived and worked in London from the 1920s to the early 1950s

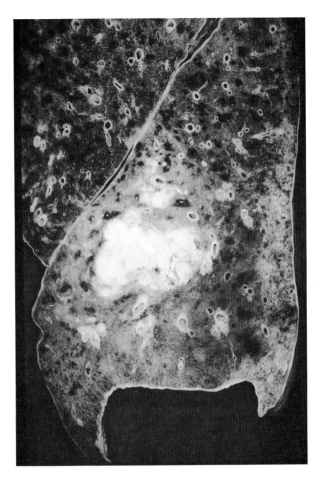

Figure 14.3 Slice of lung from a man, a life-long cigarette smoker, employed for 20 years in a factory processing amosite. It shows moderately severe asbestosis (more advanced than that shown in Figure 14.2) distributed at the periphery of the lower lobe (mostly diffuse) and slight thickening of the pulmonary pleura which is, thus, sharply defined. Note that cystic spaces in the fibrosis are few and very small. Carcinoma is also present in the lower lobe

The fibrotic areas occasionally contain small cysts within a subpleural zone approximately 1 cm in depth but these are few and rarely larger than 3 mm in diameter (Hourihane and McCaughey, 1966). In advanced cases, the cut surface of the lung may have a honeycomb appearance extending irregularly into the lobe well beyond the subpleural layer. Cysts up to 1 cm diameter may also be seen in these areas (Craighead et al., 1982; Churg, 1988a), but these may be due to superimposed non-specific infection (Ashcroft and Heppleston, 1973) or to other causes. (This is discussed further in Chapter 15.)

The hilar lymph nodes show no gross abnormality. Irregular (scar) emphysema of the fibrotic lower lobes is not seen. Panacinar emphysema appears to be remarkably uncommon. Bronchiectasis, if present, is not a consequence of asbestosis which is distributed distal to the bronchi. Silicotic nodules may be found in the lungs of men who worked

crushing and milling ore at asbestos mines and, in the USA, in those of some asbestos–cement workers.

Microscopic appearances

Although some intra-alveolar desquamation occurs, a desquamative fibrosing alveolitis (see Chapter 15, 'cellular pattern', page 507) – a semi-acute disorder – is not a feature of the early stages of asbestosis. A thin reticulin network gradually evolves in relation to damaged alveolar epithelium and envelops cells and asbestos fibres. Collagenous fibrosis then replaces the reticulin fibres until these alveoli are more or less obliterated. Hence, the primary lesion

– the earliest stage identifiable in man – is a plastering of the alveoli from within the lumen of the respiratory bronchioles (Wagner, 1965). Patchy bronchiolitis obliterans may develop. Later the fibrosis spreads peripherally into the alveolar ducts and alveolar walls obliterating many alveoli, especially in the subpleural regions (Gloyne, 1932–33; Caplan et al., 1965; Hourihane and McCaughey, 1966). It is now a diffuse interstitial pulmonary fibrosis (DIPF) (Figure 14.4). In spite of this obliteration the elastic network of alveolar walls is often seen to be intact when elastic tissue stains are used (Webster, 1970). However, in areas where the fibrosis is solid, alveolar architecture is completely replaced by a mass of collagen. Numerous macrophages – some of which contain short asbestos fibres – may be present in neighbouring patent alveoli the walls of which are thickened by fibrosis and cellular infiltration. Cyto- plasmic hyaline material may be present in type I pneumocytes but appears to be a non-specific reaction to injury (Warnock, Press and Churg, 1980).

Asbestos bodies (see page 423) are usually numerous, particularly in the airspaces, but they may also be seen in fibrous tissue. Ashcroft and Heppleston (1973) showed that the concentration of asbestos fibres increases in proportion to the degree of pulmonary fibrosis up to asbestosis of moderate degree, but that no such correlation exists in severe fibrosis which they interpreted as advanced asbestosis.

Microscopically, fibrosis may be found when its presence is not suspected on gross examination (Figure 14.4a). The early pathological changes precede clinical, physiological and radiographic evidence of the disease process. In order that the extent of lung involvement can be properly assessed, an attempt should be made to sample the worst and best areas, and to include central and peripheral portions of all lobes (Churg, 1988a).

There is, unfortunately, no universally agreed system of assessing the degree of asbestosis histologically. However, most pathologists now use either the following schema (Craighead et al., 1982) or a very similar one (Gibbs and Seal, 1982):

Grade 0: no fibrosis is associated with bronchioles.
Grade 1: fibrosis involves wall of at least one respiratory bronchiole with or without extension into the septa of the immediately adjacent layer of alveoli; there must still be a zone of non-fibrotic alveolar septa between adjacent bronchioles.
Grade 2: fibrosis appears as in grade 1, plus involvement of alveolar ducts or two or more layers of adjacent alveoli; there must still be a zone of non-fibrotic alveolar septa between adjacent bronchioles.

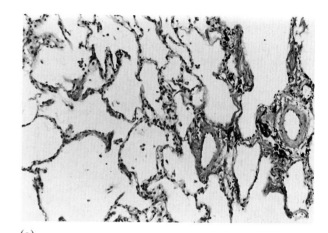

(a)

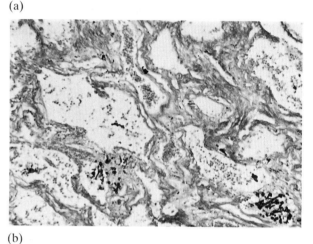

(b)

Figure 14.4 (a) Very early stage of asbestosis showing peribronchiolar fibrosis. The alveolar walls are hardly involved in this stage. (Biopsy: magnification × 150; van Giesen stain). (b) Asbestosis of moderate to severe degree. Collagenous fibrosis is widespread in the alveolar walls and alveolar spaces are partly obstructed. Clusters of whole and fragmented asbestos bodies which, in the right lower quadrant, are incarcerated by fibrosis. (Magnification × 50; van Giesen stain)

Grade 3: fibrosis appears as in grade 2, but with coalescence of fibrotic change such that all alveoli between at least two adjacent bronchioles have thickened fibrotic septa; some alveoli may be obliterated completely.
Grade 4: fibrosis appears as in grade 3, but with formation of new spaces of a size larger than alveoli, ranging up to as much as 1 cm; this lesion has been termed 'honeycombing'. Spaces may or may not be lined by epithelium.

This can be combined with a system of grading extent of fibrosis to obtain a standard method of assessing the degree of asbestosis in the lungs as a whole. Hinson et al. (1973) proposed four grades of extent of lung involvement: none; less than 25 per cent; 25 to 50 per cent; and over 50 per cent. An alternative grading of extent proposed by Craighead records the number of bronchioles involved: none; occasional only; frequent but less than 50 per cent; and more than 50 per cent. Recently, Ashcroft, Simpson and Timbrell (1988) have suggested a new method of estimation using a nine-point scale.

To this should be added a standardized method of quantifying the content of asbestos fibres (see page 425).

Subpleural crescents of apical fibrosis may also be encountered consisting of dense collagen in which asbestos bodies may be found but evidence of tuberculosis is absent. These occur particularly in tall, thin men and may be developmental in origin (Corrin, 1990). More extensive apical fibrosis is known to be associated with ankylosing spondylitis (Hillerdal, 1983), psoriasis (Bourke et al., 1988) and ulcerative colitis (Meadway, 1974). Green and Dimcheff (1974) attributed three cases to asbestos exposure; however, in each case both exposure and lung fibre burden were low and evidence of pathogenesis uncertain. Apical fibrosis is discussed further on page 463.

Necrobiotic nodules of rheumatoid disease are microscopically similar to subcutaneous rheumatoid nodules and lack the striking features of classic Caplan's nodules. They have been found in areas of asbestosis – which may be of minimal amount – and when large may be more fibrotic, although still exhibiting the characteristic cell reaction. Asbestos bodies have been observed in the lungs of all of the few reported cases (Rickards and Barrett, 1958; Tellesson, 1961; Morgan, 1964; Mattson, 1971). However, the nodules are not so clearly related to asbestos dust as they are to coal dust, and it is open to question whether the DIPF in these cases is an expression of rheumatoid disease or of asbestosis. White, Swift and Becklake (1974) failed to detect any relationship between rheumatic complaints and radiographic change in Canadian chrysotile miners.

There is little dust and negligible fibrosis in the hilar lymph nodes, although asbestos fibres may be found when obscuring carbon is removed by incineration.

Asbestos bodies (coated asbestos fibres)

The first clear description of these bodies was by Marchand in Leipzig in 1907, although he did not associate them with asbestos fibres or exposure. In 1927, Cooke drew attention to them in the lungs of asbestos workers, and McDonald suggested that they originated chemically from asbestos (Cooke, 1927; S. McDonald, 1927). Finally, Gloyne (1932) showed the fibre lying in the centre of the body by dissolving the coating in sulphuric acid under dark-ground illumination. Gloyne noted the presence of iron in the coating which was subsequently identified as ferritin by Davis, who also reviewed the history in more detail (1970).

Asbestos bodies (Figure 14.5) begin as a fibre normally more than 10 µm long, part or all of which is enclosed within a macrophage or an aggregation of macrophages forming a giant cell. When first found, the capsule of the asbestos body is quite transparent or colourless, and normally 3 to 5 µm in diameter. In time, the capsule becomes yellowish, darkening to brown as the mucopolysaccharide base takes up ferritin, at which stage it will stain blue with Perl's reagent. Thickening frequently occurs at each end, giving a dumb-bell appearance.

A mature body may persist unchanged for many years, perhaps indefinitely. However, after some years segmentation takes place in an increasing proportion, producing a beaded appearance probably due to transverse cracking and shrinking of the protein coat. This may sometimes be accompanied by fragmentation of the fibre core, resulting in increased numbers of curiously shaped particles which may then be ingested and removed by macrophages (Beattie, 1961).

'Curious bodies', to use Cooke's original name, have been known to occur around non-asbestos cores at least since 1931 (Tylecoat and Dunn). Gross, Cralley and de Treville (1967) pointed out that bodies may develop around a variety of fibres deposited in the lungs and proposed the generic term 'ferruginous bodies'. Churg, Warnock and Green (1979) isolated and examined, with a transmission electron microscope and microprobe analysis, a large number of bodies from non-occupationally exposed subjects. They concluded that most bodies resulting from environmental exposure were asbestos, that their cores were transparent and that they were distinguishable in most cases by light microscope. Non-asbestos cores were either black and very probably carbon, corresponding to the bodies known to occur occasionally in coal miners and those exposed to graphite (see Chapter 13), or a birefringent pale-yellow compound of platy or fibrous sheet-silicate (such as mica, talc and various clays) or of the siliceous bodies of diatoms, in general of low refractive index.

When the central core is asbestos, it is found to be preponderantly amphibole in environmentally exposed people. This was noted by Pooley (1972). Churg and colleagues, in three studies from the general population (Churg and Warnock, 1977, 1979; Churg, Warnock and Green, 1979), examined 600 bodies from over 80 patients and found 98 per cent to have an amphibole core; the remaining 2 per cent appeared to be chrysotile. However, Holden

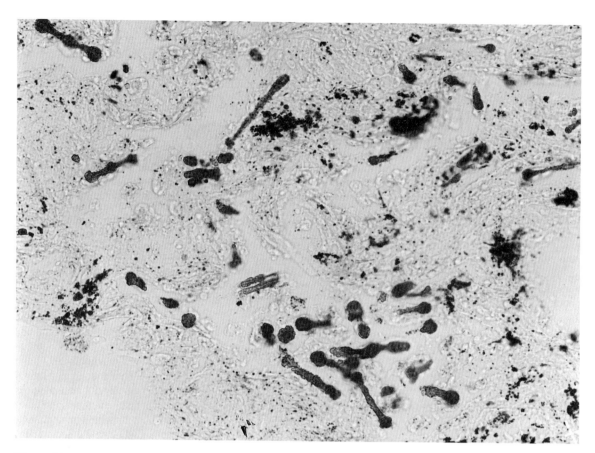

Figure 14.5 Asbestos bodies in an unstained 30-μm section of lung with asbestosis. There are long segmented bodies with lubbed ends and others that are shorter and stumpy. Fragments of bodies are scattered throughout the field in the centre of which a short, partly coated fibre is seen. A few small aggregations of carbon particles are also present. Compare these bodies with coal and graphite bodies which have thick, black cores. (Magnification × 380)

and Churg (1986), in an examination of lungs of chrysotile miners with asbestosis, found that approximately two-thirds of identified cores of bodies examined were around long chrysotile fibres; most of the remainder were actinolite and tremolite, two amphiboles found in chrysotile-bearing rock. The cores were long, with a mean length of 35 μm. As discussed on page 426, chrysotile fibres are preferentially cleared from human lungs, and it is possible that these were preserved from rapid dissolution partly by the coating itself and partly by the interstitial fibrosis which, by being relatively acellular, appears to delay the fragmentation and dissolution of chrysotile (Davis et al., 1986).

Morgan (1980) showed that the probability of a fibre becoming coated increases with its length. Bodies of less than 10 μm long are rarely encountered, whilst for fibres longer than 80 μm the probability of coating is virtually 100 per cent. Morgan and Holmes (1985) reviewed dimensional effects on the formation of bodies. Bodies are formed more readily on fibres of greater diameter. About 10 per cent of fibres visible by the light microscope are coated, irrespective of fibre type, but the proportion of fibres visible will, in the case of crocidolite, be less than one in ten, so that the true proportion of fibres coated is less than 1 per cent, whereas with anthophyllite, which has a greater mean diameter, the true proportion is higher. The proportion of coated fibres increases with increasing lapse of time from last exposure, suggesting that the longer the fibre stays in the lung, the greater the chance that it is coated (Bignon, Sebastien and Bientz, 1979).

Thomson (1965) showed that the probability of finding bodies in the lungs of urban dwellers was high and increased with age. Since that time it has become clear that, if searched for with sufficient diligence, bodies can be found in the lungs of all adults living in cities (Bignon, Sebastien and Bientz, 1979; Churg and Warnock, 1979). They have been found in the lungs of 6 of 17 infants examined (aged 2.5 to 10 months) (Hague, Hernandez and Dillard, 1985). In subjects with large numbers of bodies in their lungs, small numbers may be found in many other organs such as spleen, thyroid and pancreas (Auerbach et al., 1980). Cigarette smoking, perhaps by its adverse effect on lung clearance mechanisms, is associated with higher counts (Churg and Warnock, 1977). Asbestos bodies may be found in the sputum, and may continue to appear more than 30 years after brief exposure (Bignon, Sebastien and Bientz, 1979); they may also appear in the faeces, the protein coat remaining apparently undigested (Gloyne, 1931).

The coating of fibres is probably part of the lung's defence mechanisms and, on the assumption that asbestos bodies are inert and no longer immunogenic, they have been called 'tombstones of asbestos fibres' (Morgan and Holmes, 1980). Vorwald, Durkan and Pratt (1951) found that intratracheal injection of bodies recovered from the lungs of an asbestos worker failed to produce asbestosis experimentally, and McLemore et al. (1981) showed that coated fibres similarly recovered were less toxic to macrophages in vitro than uncoated fibres. If this is also true in vivo, however, it remains to be explained why such a small proportion of long fibres become coated.

Asbestos bodies in post-mortem lung tissue

Asbestos bodies are readily seen by optical microscopy. Early attempts at quantification used smears of lung juice but, because of the inherent inaccuracy, this method has been abandoned for weighed portions of lung tissue. Sampling procedure is important if counts are to be made because the proportion of coated to uncoated fibres may vary by more than an order of magnitude in the same lobe, decreasing from the centre to the periphery (Le Bouffant et al., 1976; Morgan and Holmes, 1984) and between different lobes in the same lung.

High counts may occasionally reveal an unsuspected occupational exposure, but low counts may be encountered in those known to have previous exposure (Dodson et al., 1984, Mollo et al., 1987). The subject is reviewed by Roggli (1990) and by Churg (1988a) who has emphasized the importance for individual laboratories of establishing their own standards for the non-occupationally exposed population owing to the great inter-laboratory variation mentioned earlier.

Lung fibre burdens and the attribution of disease

The three major asbestos-related diseases – diffuse interstitial pulmonary fibrosis, mesothelioma and lung cancer – may all occur independently of exposure to asbestos and, where the occupational history is uncertain or absent, it may be essential to look for quantitative evidence of asbestos in the lungs. The technical problems of recovering mineral fibres from biological material in an accurate and reproducible manner are considerable, and have been reviewed by Davis, Gylseth and Morgan (1986). There is, unfortunately, no standardized method, and inter-laboratory variations may be considerable (Gylseth et al., 1986), so that much care should be taken in the interpretation of individual figures.

Either asbestos bodies or fibres may be counted, and examination may be by either a light or phase contrast optical microscope, or by an electron microscope. All combinations have their disadvantages. Bodies are easier to identify but only a small proportion of the total lung fibre burden becomes coated, varying with the length of fibre. Most bodies examined are found to have an amphibole core, apparently because bodies found on chrysotile do not survive the fragmentation and dissolution of the fibre, because they are readily found in those currently exposed. Optical microscopy cannot discriminate between asbestos and many other fibres; even by phase-contrast microscopy only about 5 to 15 per cent of fibres visible by transmission electron microscopy (TEM) can be seen (that is, those fibres more than 2 μm long and more than 0.2 μm in diameter); and finally, most chrysotile fibres, even when they exceed these dimensions, are not visible. These problems can all be overcome with TEM equipped for energy-dispersive X-ray analysis (EDXA) which can detect and identify almost all fibres. However, the equipment is very expensive, requires considerable expertise and is very time-consuming; moreover, because it is only practicable to count much smaller numbers of fibres, margins of error in the results are correspondingly greater and standards for occupational and environmental exposure are less well established.

Both coated and uncoated fibres may be recovered in vivo from sputum, by bronchoalveolar lavage and in biopsy material.

Asbestos fibres in lung tissue

Disappearing chrysotile, persisting amphibole

In 1965, Wagner and Skidmore found, surprisingly, that in inhalation experiments with rats, chrysotile appeared to be cleared from their lungs more rapidly than amphiboles. Wagner et al. reported further experimental results in 1974 which showed that, whilst the weight of dust of crocidolite, amosite and anthophyllite retained in the lungs showed an approximately proportional increase over 2 years of inhalation, the amount of retained chrysotile appeared to stabilize after 3 months at a much lower level than the amphiboles, and after that deposition was balanced by clearance.

In human lungs, Pooley (1972) and Sebastien et al. (1977) both found less chrysotile than expected in comparison with amphibole. Following this, a series of studies of cases of mesothelioma (J.S.P. Jones et al., 1980; McDonald, McDonald and Pooley, 1982; Wagner et al., 1982a, 1986; Albin et al., 1990a) and asbestosis (Wagner et al., 1982a, 1986) showed that, whereas the lung amphibole burden was increased, that of chrysotile was not. Rowlands, Gibbs and McDonald (1982) looked at the lungs of chrysotile miners, and found approximately as much tremolite as chrysotile, even though the amount of tremolite in the ore, in which it occurs as a contaminant, is extremely small. This finding has since been confirmed by Churg (1986) and Case and Sebastien (1987); both papers at the same time demonstrate that inhabitants of Quebec mining towns have significantly higher levels of chrysotile fibres more than 5 μm long and higher tremolite levels than control populations from other regions, although epidemiological studies have shown no evidence of increased asbestos-related disease in those not occupationally exposed.

Wagner et al. (1988) examined the lung fibre burdens of workers from an East London factory which had used crocidolite, amosite and chrysotile. As well as relating to the presence of disease, amphibole counts related to an approximate index of exposure, whilst chrysotile did not. Similar findings were reported by Albin et al. (1990a).

There was much uncertainty at first over whether this effect was to be attributed mainly to chrysotile being deposited higher in the bronchial tubes and, hence, cleared by the 'ciliary escalator', or whether it dissolved in lung tissue. Jaurand et al. (1976) showed that chrysotile dissolved in lung tissues; this is perhaps not surprising when it is remembered that only the amphiboles are acid resistant, and the acidity inside a macrophage lysosome may be as low as pH 4. (This is a point of considerable importance commercially, and is the reason why crocidolite was specified almost universally prior to the Second World War for insulating coal-fired steam engines, the fumes from which may be very acid.) Moreover, chrysotile is known to lose its magnesium in water or physiological saline, and separates into individual fibrils which easily fragment.

But the question of whether higher deposition or dissolution plays the major role has been settled experimentally. Accurate sizing of length and diameter of inhaled fibres at varying intervals after the end of exposure in rats has shown that, whilst numbers of short amphibole fibres reduce steadily, those of long fibres decline only slowly and the average diameter remains unchanged. With chrysotile, however, the number of long fibres may even increase initially, although the diameter is found to be much less, showing that many fibres have been split into component fibrils; then the number of long fibres reduces rapidly as they fragment transversely (Roggli and Brody, 1984; Roggli, George and Brody, 1987; Davis, 1989).

This work has also settled the apparent anomaly that chrysotile in animal experiments is at least as hazardous as the amphiboles, whereas epidemiological evidence indicates clearly that chrysotile is associated with less disease in human beings. Davis et al. (1978) showed that, in equal weights of UICC (standard) samples of chrysotile, crocidolite and amosite, not only did the chrysotile sample contain approximately twice as many fibres more than 5 μm long as crocidolite and four times as many as amosite, but the ratio of extra long fibres (more than 20 μm) was actually 60 : 6 : 1. This is of particular importance when results with a short-lived species such as the rat are compared with human experience, because the rate of dissolution in lung tissue would be approximately the same for both species, whilst disease processes are more rapid by an order of magnitude. It is clear that, in an examination of the pathogenicity of any fibres, durability in the tissues in relation to lifespan is an essential determinant (Davis, 1989).

Although dissolution of amphibole fibres is not apparent, some clearance probably continues in the long term at a slow rate. Du Toit (1991) and Rendall and Du Toit (1991) have given evidence from both human and animal studies that crocidolite has a half-life in the lungs of about 5 to 6 years.

Quantitative determination as an aid to diagnosis

Ashcroft and Heppleston, in 1973, suggested a method of preparation of lung tissue for counting all fibres by optical microscope and demonstrated that numbers of fibres counted bore some relationship to the severity of interstitial fibrosis when present, up to moderate severity. This method was modified by Whitwell, Scott and Grimshaw (1977) who counted coated and uncoated fibres together, but only of length greater than 6 μm. They showed a difference, with some overlap, in cases of mesothelioma between those with occupational exposure and those without, and demonstrated the much higher levels associated with asbestosis. The value of the technique and some of the difficulties associated with it have been illustrated by Seal (1980). The method, and developments using preparations involving filters rather than the Fuchs–Rosenthal counting chamber which provide permanent preparations, are discussed by Davis, Gylseth and Morgan (1986). Several further series have been reported (for example, Stovin and Partridge, 1982; Rogers,

1983; Roggli, Pratt and Brody, 1986) and certain conclusions have been drawn: namely, that using these methods asbestosis will infrequently be found with less than 10^6 fibres/g dried lung and never below 250×10^3/g. Mesothelioma is associated with lower levels than asbestosis even when occupationally caused, but counts in the latter case will rarely be below 10^5 fibres/g. These figures are, however, quoted as illustrative only; differences in counting methods are considerable and, until they are as standardized as those for estimating air-borne asbestos, any laboratory undertaking them should establish its own standards, and any individual count provided must be accepted as possessing margins of error little short of an order of magnitude.

Where attribution to asbestos is at issue in individual cases (particularly with cases of mesothelioma), useful information may be provided with the transmission electron microscope. Unfortunately, many earlier counts did not separate numbers of short from long fibres. As is now established on epidemiological (Friedrichs and Otto, 1981; McDonald et al., 1989) as well as experimental grounds, it is essential for the diagnosis of asbestos causation to count fibres longer than 5 μm (perhaps longer than 8 μm) if attribution of disease to asbestos is to be confirmed. Because of the lack of standardized methods and considerable differences between individual laboratories (Gylseth et al., 1986), no figures will be listed here and reference should be made to Roggli (1990) and Churg (1988a).

The pathogenesis of asbestosis

Fibre dimensions

The belief that fibre length is important for the pathogenicity of asbestosis has a long history, dating back to King, Clegg and Rae (1946), and has been documented by Davis and Jones (1988). In the 30 years following King's work, a number of experiments demonstrated that, for equivalent weights, long fibres produced a much greater fibrogenic effect than short fibres. The problem was always to obtain specimens of asbestos in sufficient quantity which retained their fibrous characteristics but which were free of fibres greater than a defined length. However, in 1972, Davis was able to show that fibres less than 1 μm long produced almost no reaction in mice by intraperitoneal injection, whereas long-fibre samples produced massive fibrosis. Similar results with fibres less than 5 μm long were obtained by Wright and Kuschner in 1977 using a variety of fibres by intratracheal injection in guinea-pigs. Stanton and Wrench (1972) and Pott, Huth and Friedrichs (1974) were at that time

looking at carcinogenesis following fibre implantation in the pleural and peritoneal cavities of rats. Both found greater activity with the longer fibres, and a theoretical relationship was drawn up combining length and diameter.

Since that time it has been realized that even small proportions of long fibres in short-fibre samples might vitiate conclusions about the latter. Wagner, Griffiths and Hill (1984) drew attention to the dangers, based on their own experience, of drawing conclusions from size distributions and in vitro studies without considering in vivo mechanisms, and suggested that this might account for the pathological effects in other studies apparently attributable to short fibres, for example, those of Kolev (1982). Brown et al. (1986) have also shown that animal studies purporting to show that chrysotile was as hazardous, or more hazardous, than amphiboles have been misleading due to *unequal numbers* of long fibres to which the animals were exposed when these were controlled by *equal mass*. More complete exclusion of long fibres from short-fibre samples has confirmed expectations. Platek et al. (1985) administered short chrysotile (less than 5 μm long) to rats and monkeys, and Davis (1986) administered amosite to rats, both by inhalation; both confirmed the absence of pulmonary fibrosis. A comparable result was obtained by Adamson and Bowden (1987) after lung instillation of crocidolite, and by Wagner (1990) who gave erionite by inhalation. In all cases, animals given the same type of fibre but containing a substantial proportion more than 5 μm long developed the expected interstitial fibrosis, whereas the short fibre produced no more reaction than controls.

Some confirmation is available from human studies. McDonald et al. (1978) showed that miners of cummingtonite–grunerite (the non-fibrous form of amosite) are not subject to the diseases associated with asbestos exposure, and Cooper (1990) has shown that the same is true of other non-fibrous amphiboles. However, the evidence from lung fibre burdens is more important.

Friedrichs and Otto (1981) showed that, when fibre counts made by scanning electron microscopy (SEM) on cases of normal lungs and of spontaneous mesotheliomas were compared with those of asbestos-related disease, the two groups could be reliably differentiated only when fibres longer than 5 μm alone were counted. In a case-control study using TEM, McDonald et al. (1989) showed that only long amphibole fibres (longer than 8 μm) were associated with excess of mesothelioma, and that counts of fibres less than 8 μm long did not contribute to the discrimination.

This almost unassailable evidence that the specific pathogenicity of asbestos fibres only exists at lengths greater than 5 μm (probably greater than 8 μm) is in accord with what is known of the mechanism of fibrogenesis at the cellular level (Mossman

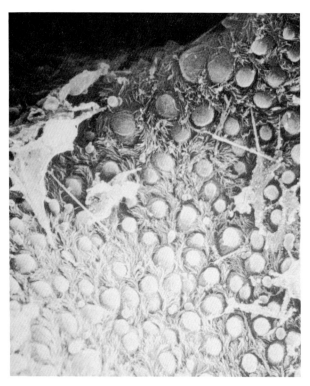

Figure 14.6 Medium power view of a terminal bronchiole showing Clara cells and deposited long amosite fibres. A macrophage is present with several partially phagocytosed fibres (magnification × 800). (Courtesy of Dr K. Donaldson and the Institute of Occupational Medicine)

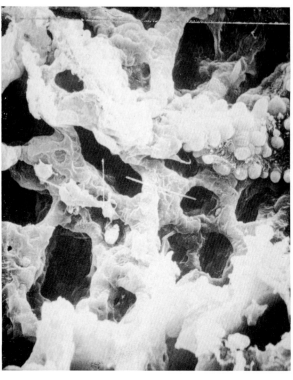

Figure 14.7 Medium power view of the transition zone between a terminal bronchiole and alveolar duct. Ciliated cells and Clara cells of the bronchiolar epithelium are visible. There is also an accumulation of alveolar macrophages on the alveolar surface and long amosite fibres. One macrophage has phagocytosed a fibre (magnification × 810). (Courtesy of Dr K. Donaldson and the Institute of Occupational Medicine)

et al., 1990). The role of the lung macrophage is central in removal by phagocytosis of particles that penetrate beyond the ciliated bronchial epithelium to the respiratory bronchioles and alveoli (Brain, 1988) (Figure 14.6). The different effects of asbestos fibres and quartz particles on the macrophages in the development of asbestosis and silicosis have been shown in several studies. Miller et al. (1978) demonstrated the presence of large numbers of aggregations of mature cells after dusting with crocidolite, indicating that the fibre was non-toxic to the macrophages, and had stimulated them to develop to maturity and recruitment; quartz by contrast displayed a characteristic pattern of toxic effects. Bateman, Emerson and Cole (1980), using diffusion chambers in the mouse peritoneal cavity, showed that macrophages implanted with asbestos produced a diffusible fibrogenic factor that continued apparently throughout a normal macrophage lifespan. Quartz was rapidly toxic.

The role of the macrophage is not merely phagocytic, but also secretory and regulatory (Brain, 1988). The list of cytokines, or peptide regulatory factors,

synthesized by lung macrophages is considerable (Kelley, 1990). Of particular importance in the generation of asbestosis appear to be fibroblast and epithelial growth factors (Lemaire et al., 1986; Brody, 1991), superoxide and other reactive oxygen species (Case et al., 1986; Hansen and Mossman, 1987) and proteolytic enzymes. The production of growth factors is dependent on the stimulus of phagocytosis, and also on the nature of the particles, indigestible materials inducing a more persistent secretion (Bowden, 1987). Macrophages also modulate the production of collagen by fibroblasts (Mossman et al., 1986), a factor which may be relevant to the formation of pleural plaques, especially if pleural macrophages have characteristics differing from those found in the lung (see Chapters 4 and 5).

The probable sequence of events after inhalation of asbestos is that fibres tend to be deposited at bifurcations of respiratory bronchioles and alveolar ducts (Figure 14.7). A chemotactic factor may be produced on alveolar surfaces inducing an accumulation of macrophages (Brody, 1986) (Figure 14.8). Fibres are then rapidly taken up not only by alveolar

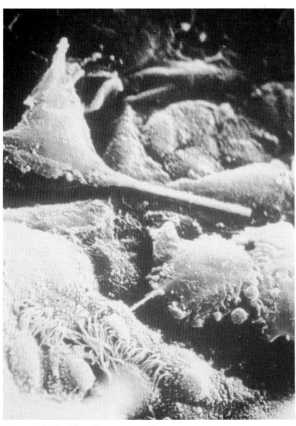

Figure 14.8 Alveolar macrophages at a bronchiolar/alveolar duct junction. The ciliated cells of the bronchiolar epithelium are visible in the foreground and macrophages that have phagocytosed long amosite fibres are present on the alveolar surface (magnification × 2500). (Courtesy of Dr K. Donaldson and the Institute of Occupational Medicine)

macrophages, but also actively by type I epithelial cells and translocated with the action of cellular myofibrils to the interstitial region, where they may be engulfed by the interstitial macrophages (Barry et al., 1983). What follows depends on the intensity and duration of exposure. If the stimulus is sufficient, macrophage recruitment follows in proportion to the inhaled load until saturation is reached, the supply of macrophages deriving at least in part from local proliferation (Bowden, 1987). There is little polymorph activity at this stage.

Fibre clearance then proceeds along the lines discussed in Chapter 3, with concentration of fibres at the periphery of the lungs, probably because this is the direction of lymph flow dictated by the valves (Lauweryns and Baert, 1977), and with short fibres cleared preferentially. Long fibres have repeatedly been shown to be more cytopathic when added to certain cell-lines in vitro (Chamberlain, Brown and Griffiths, 1980; Brown et al., 1986) and this corresponds in vitro with the situation that Kuschner (1987) has vividly described as 'the frustrated macrophage'. Normal phagocytosis involves the engulfing of particles through the invagination of the external cell membrane, forming a phagosome towards which lysosomes migrate to liberate their secretions. With long fibres, ingestion is incomplete and secretions into the phagosome, including proteolytic enzymes and tissue-damaging superoxides, are no longer completely enclosed within the cell, but leak out to affect the adjacent tissues. (See Chapter 1, page 14, for the size range of normal alveolar macrophages.)

To the degree to which the fibre is insoluble – and this, as we have seen, is the major difference between the amphiboles and chrysotile – chronic and, to some extent, lifelong effects are produced on the surrounding tissues. It appears to be the continuing stimulus of indigestible and incompletely phagocytosed particles in macrophages – which, as has been noted, possess a variety of different functions – that results in the final preponderance of fibrosis. A similar situation occurs in reactions to other foreign bodies that remain chemically unaltered in living tissue (Brand, 1986). In parallel with the fibroblast increase, multiplication of alveolar cells, both type I and type II, takes place (Brody, 1986), both from macrophage-derived growth factors and also probably from factors produced by proliferating fibroblasts (Duff, 1989) which, in advanced asbestosis, results in complete disruption of the alveolar architecture (Davis et al., 1986b).

Platelet-derived growth factor (PDGF), originally identified in platelets but now known to be produced by many cell types, appears to be the main cytokine causing fibroblast proliferation (Shaw, 1991; Shaw et al., 1991). Transforming growth factor β (TGFβ), also produced by macrophages, acts on fibroblasts to induce production of fibronectin and procollagen, thereby increasing the extracellular matrix. However, macrophages also produce tumour necrosis factor α (TNFα) and interleukin-1 (IL1) which may initially stimulate fibroblast proliferation, but may also act together to augment production of prostaglandins, so producing the opposite effect. Several other peptide regulatory factors have also been identified which, together with those listed, constitute a complex system of modulation of response to changing situations (see Chapter 4, pages 66 to 68).

The finding by Churg et al. (1989) that the proportion of short fibres in the lungs of chrysotile miners increased with the degree of fibrosis led them to suggest that tremolite fibres less than 5 μm long may contribute to the fibrotic process. However, because short fibres are cleared more readily from normal lung (see Chapter 3, page 42), and because fibrosis delays clearance (Davis et al., 1986b), their observation is exactly what would be expected on the hypothesis that only long fibres are involved in fibrogenesis, and it sheds no light on the pathogenicity of short fibres.

Host response: immunological effects

Differences in susceptibility to asbestos-related disease among workers employed on similar tasks have frequently been commented on, and are familiar to all with experience in the surveillance of asbestos-exposed subjects. Correspondingly, from the early days, there has been a hope of a pre-employment test that would identify the susceptibles.

The increased prevalence of circulating antinuclear antibody (which is not sex dependent) and rheumatoid factor, in individuals with asbestosis but not in asbestos-exposed persons without evidence of asbestosis, raised the possibility that immunological events might participate in pathogenesis, especially as antinuclear antibody (ANA) titres tend to rise slowly with the passage of time (Turner-Warwick and Parkes, 1970; Turner-Warwick, 1977; Lange, 1980). The fact that the characteristics of antinuclear antibody associated with asbestosis are different from those of antinuclear antibody in connective tissue diseases of the lung suggested that its origin and mode of action (if any) are different. The prevalence of non-organ-specific complement-fixing antibodies is not increased above normal in asbestosis as it is in cryptogenic fibrosing alveolitis (Turner-Warwick and Haslam, 1971).

Reduction in the proportion and absolute numbers of circulating T lymphocytes, but not of B lymphocytes, and impairment of T-cell functions have been reported in patients with radiographic evidence of asbestosis (Kang et al., 1974; Kagan et al., 1977a,b; Lange and Skibinski, 1977; Haslam et al., 1978; de Shazo et al., 1983, 1986) (see Chapter 4, 'Lymphocytes and their subpopulations'). However, the Tulane group in the USA found that the decreased numbers of all lymphocyte populations (B, T, T-helper and T-suppressor) were unrelated to the degree of chest radiograph abnormality, cumulative exposure or pulmonary function, and concluded that immunological abnormalities detected in peripheral blood might not be related to the pathogenic process (Bozelka, Jones and de Shazo, 1984). Minor abnormalities of lymphocyte subsets were found in a cross-sectional study of asbestos-exposed workers by Sprince et al. (1991), but the significance of the findings, and whether they have any predictive or diagnostic value, remains uncertain without long-term follow-up. Kagamimori et al. (1984) found a small increase in serum interferon in subjects with asbestosis, and pointed out that a negative correlation has been found in some autoimmune diseases between serum interferon and natural killer cell activity. Robinson et al. (1988) measured γ-interferon release from cells recovered by lavage from subjects suffering from asbestosis; increased release was present in only one-third.

These cytological changes related to the fibrotic response are associated with cutaneous anergy for recall antigens such as tuberculin (purified protein derivative, PPD) and *Candida albicans* (Pierce and Turner-Warwick, 1980). This suggests the possibility of impaired function of one or more components of the cellular immune response. Lymphocyte sensitization to DNA has been shown to occur in some ANA-positive patients with asbestosis – and, also, cryptogenic fibrosing alveolitis – which implies that delayed hypersensitivity may sometimes contribute to lung damage in both diseases (Haslam, Turner-Warwick and Lukoszek, 1975). Indeed, impairment of cell-mediated immunity, as indicated by lack of response to recall antigens, is most pronounced in asbestos workers with asbestosis and circulating ANAs, although it is present to a lesser degree in those without asbestosis but with circulating ANAs (Lange et al., 1978, 1986).

Although depression of cell-mediated immunity has been reported, indicators of humoral immunity have been found to be raised by many investigators, in keeping with raised levels of antinuclear antibody and rheumatoid factor mentioned above. Hyperactivity of B cells with elevation of serum immunoglobulins (Kagan et al., 1977a; Lange, 1980; de Shazo et al., 1986; Anton-Culver, Culver and Kurosaki, 1988) and circulating immune complexes (Doll, Stankus and Barkman, 1983) have been reported in asbestos-exposed workers both in the presence and in the absence of asbestosis. Procollagen III peptide levels have also been found to be raised in bronchial lavage fluid (Bégin et al., 1986) and, less certainly, in serum (Okazaki et al., 1987).

An apparent association between the HLA antigen B27 and asbestosis posed the question that some individuals might be more susceptible than others to the damaging effects of asbestos on the lungs (Merchant et al., 1975; Matej, Lange and Smolnik, 1977). A trend towards an increased frequency of HLA-B27, which was not present in a large number of unaffected asbestos workers and control subjects, had been demonstrated among asbestos workers with radiographic evidence of DIPF. Furthermore, the workers with pulmonary fibrosis and HLA-B27 had a significantly shorter duration of exposure to asbestos than those without this antigen, although the mean profusion score of radiographic opacities was the same in both. But more detailed controlled studies have not shown any statistical difference in the prevalence to HLA-B27 in those with asbestosis and the controls (Evans, Lewinsohn and Evans, 1977; Gregor et al., 1979; Huuskonen, Tiilikainen and Alanko, 1979). Although Darke, Wagner and McMillan (1979) found this phenotype twice as frequently in dockyard workers with asbestosis as in those without, theirs was not a case-control study. There was also a suggestion that HLA-B5, apparently more common in individuals who do not develop asbestosis, may play a protective role (Evans, Lewinsohn and Evans, 1977) as may HLA-B18 (Huuskonen, Tiilikainen and Alanko, 1979).

However, the general conclusion from controlled studies is that there is no significant or consistent difference in the frequency of HLA phenotypes on the A, B and C loci in people with asbestosis compared with control subjects. Bégin et al. (1987a) using 53 phenotypes of the HLA-A, -B, -C and -DR antigens found no significant change in their frequency between subjects with asbestosis and controls. They concluded, with Turner-Warwick (1979), that is is not possible on present evidence to identify individuals who may have an undue susceptibility or resistance to developing asbestosis.

To summarize, then, all the positive results so far found have been inconstant, unpredictable and uninterpretable in the clinical context. One has to agree with de Shazo et al. (1986) that they are probably epiphenomena unrelated to the disease causation, and with Bégin et al. (1987a) that individual differences in response may relate better to lung structure or lung function than to immunogenic factors. For the individual patient, immunological tests are of no diagnostic significance.

Liddell and Miller (1983) make the distinction between *protection* factors – such as those which may have shielded the 188 Thetford miners over 60 years old still at work after 40 years' exposure to fibre levels exceeding 100 fibres/ml to the extent that only 52 per cent had an abnormal chest radiograph – and *vulnerability* factors, such as those responsible for more than 10 per cent of the women who assembled gas masks in Canada for only a short period subsequently succumbing to mesothelioma. Vulnerability appears to be particularly important for mesothelioma, where a simple dose–response relationship with cumulative exposure probably does not apply. Becklake et al. (1983) have found evidence that a shorter trachea and a narrower transthoracic diameter may increase susceptibility to asbestosis, although probably not to pleural plaques (Delfino, Ernst and Bourbeau, 1989), whilst Bégin, Masse and Sebastien (1989) have shown that individual capacity for alveolar dust clearance may be important (see Chapter 3). Possible familial predisposition to mesothelioma and pleural plaques is discussed later. Familial idiopathic pulmonary fibrosis (Bitterman et al., 1986) is a condition in which alveolar macrophages appear spontaneously to release mediators stimulating fibroblast growth; whilst this is of great interest for the pathogenesis of asbestosis, its relevance to vulnerability, if any, still needs to be elucidated (see Chapter 15).

Clinical features

Neither symptoms nor physical signs are pathognomonic as they are found in DIPF due to a variety of other causes (see Chapter 6).

Symptoms

These are of insidious onset and the time-lag between their first being noticed by the patient and the patient's earliest past exposure to asbestos varies considerably; in some cases it may be so long that patients have forgotten that they had worked in contact with asbestos, emphasizing the need for direct questioning when taking an occupational history.

As a rule, the most important symptom is breathlessness on effort, slight at first, being experienced only on undue effort, and then increasing in severity until finally it may be present at rest. In most cases this increase occurs slowly over a period of many years, and in some there may be very little change over a decade. When breathlessness has become at least moderate in degree, some patients complain of chest tightness and inability to breathe in deeply and, in some cases, to yawn due (as in advanced DIPF) to substantially increased stiffness – or reduced compliance – of the lungs. A proportion of patients, however, never complain of breathlessness.

Cough is absent in early disease, but is present in the later stages of most, although not all, cases. It is usually 'dry' or productive of only small quantities of viscid mucoid sputum. This may be difficult to raise and thus provoke paroxysms of coughing. Paroxysms may also be related to effort. But some patients with advanced asbestosis have remarkably little cough.

Sputum, when present, is usually mucoid and tends to be raised in the first 2 hours after rising in the morning. Cough and sputum throughout the day appear to be exceptional rather than the rule (Elmes, 1966), except when they occur in relation to smoking.

Haemoptysis is not caused by asbestosis. When it does occur, complicating bronchial carcinoma may be responsible and must be sought. Similarly, chest pain is not a feature of asbestosis, although it may result from concomitant diffuse pleural thickening. However, poorly localized aching, tightness of the chest or transient, sharp pains are sometimes complained of by patients with severe dyspnoea and may arise from overtaxed intercostal and other chest wall muscles. It must be remembered that persistent pain may be the first evidence of carcinoma of the lung or malignant mesothelioma of the pleura. Lassitude is not uncommon in advanced disease.

Physical signs

Clubbing of fingers and toes is an inconstant sign. It is present in varying severity in approximately half the cases of more advanced asbestosis and less often in those with mild disease. It may or may not increase as fibrosis progresses. Rapid onset or worsening of existing clubbing may signal the presence of complicating bronchial carcinoma. Hypertrophic pulmonary osteoarthropathy is rarely, if ever, seen in uncomplicated asbestosis.

Clubbing is deemed to be present when the hyponychial angle is 195 degrees or more. Using this measurement, Huuskonen (1978) recorded clubbing in 32 per cent of 133 cases of asbestosis of all grades of severity: in 22 per cent with ILO category 1/0 to 1/1 irregular opacities and in 55 per cent with category 2/3 or higher. Coutts et al. (1987b) found it to be indicative of an adverse prognosis.

Equilateral impairment of expansion affecting the lower chest wall occurs with advancing disease. Measurement of expansion from full inspiration, around the maximum circumference of the chest each time the patient is examined is a helpful index of progression but, of course, has no diagnostic value. When disease is slight expansion is usually 'normal' (that is, about 2.5 inches (6.3 cm) or more) but, when advanced, may be reduced to 0.5 inch (1.2 cm) or less. Some reduction occurs naturally with age. This sign is only of value in following individual patients and, due to its wide variability, has no relevance in epidemiological surveys.

Inspiratory crackles, the most important physical sign, are discussed in Chapter 6. They are heard bilaterally, early in the development of the disease, patchily in the basal regions of the lower lobes, usually posteriorly but often first in the lower axillae, and sometimes in the middle lobe and lingular regions. At this stage they are of a fine, crisp quality (that is, high pitched, about 700 Hz), are unaltered by cough and may only be heard at the end of full inspiration especially after a short period of breath-holding at low lung volume. They often precede respiratory symptoms and may antedate abnormality of routine lung function tests and chest radiographs. As fibrosis progresses, fine to medium quality crackles (about 400 Hz) are present throughout inspiration but not in expiration, and gradually become bilaterally widespread in the lower lobes, middle lobe and lingula; they are rarely heard anteriorly over the upper lobes. In the presence of bilateral diffuse thickening of the pleura, they may be difficult to detect due to impairment of sound conduction and, possibly, to reduction in expansion of the lungs. A consistent feature of the crackles of any DIPF is their persistent and repetitive pattern in each respiratory cycle. Crackles in many other lung diseases may be provoked or discharged by coughing, are often present in expiration and are frequently coarser or lower pitched (about 250 Hz).

One study (referred to already in Chapter 6, page 154) has shown that in patients with diffuse interstitial lung disease, diagnosed both clinically and by biopsy, bilateral fine crackles were present in about 60 per cent of cases of asbestosis and fibrosing alveolitis (DIPF) and in 40 per cent of cases of extrinsic allergic alveolitis, but less often in patients with sarcoidosis, chronic bronchitis and emphysema (Epler, Carrington and Gaensler, 1978).

Wheezes and rhonchi are not caused by asbestosis but are present concurrently in some cases, usually in bronchitic smokers. Pleural friction may sometimes be heard, especially at the lung bases, and may be related to the development of diffuse pleural fibrosis.

Loss of weight is not a feature and, although it may occur in advanced disease, it should prompt suspicion of carcinoma of the lung. Central cyanosis may be seen in advanced disease, usually after effort, and is made worse in the presence of coexistent airflow obstruction. The signs of pulmonary heart disease – cor pulmonale – may follow.

A high rate of pulmonary tuberculosis was observed before 1950 in subjects with asbestosis, but in recent years its frequency has been no higher than in the general population (Buchanan, 1965; Enterline, 1965; Smither, 1965). The earlier findings were merely a reflection of the greater prevalence of tuberculosis in the working urban population of that period. There is no evidence that asbestosis or asbestos exposure predispose to the development of tuberculosis, a finding in accord with what is now known of the pathogenesis of asbestosis, because the fibre differs from silica in the absence of a direct toxic effect on macrophages (Miller et al., 1978; Bateman, Emerson and Cole, 1980). Bronchiectasis was occasionally described in the past in association with advanced asbestosis, but is now rarely seen.

Investigations

Sputum

In general, examination of sputum for asbestos bodies is of no practical value because their presence merely confirms exposure to asbestos in people with a known occupational history but does not prove the existence of asbestos-related disease; also, vice versa, their absence does not indicate freedom from such disease. However, the findings of these bodies may be of some help in cases where both the clinician and patient are in doubt as to whether a past occupation involved asbestos exposure. Both Sluis-Cremer (1965) and Bignon, Sebastien and Bientz (1979) found a relationship between numbers of asbestos bodies in sputum and exposure. The latter showed that asbestos may be found in sputum more than 30 years after the end of exposure even where this has been brief or at a low level; they also identified uncoated fibres by TEM. Not all specimens, however, contained bodies even in exposed subjects, and this inconsistency was confirmed by Gupta and Frost (1981) who examined sputa from 5000 subjects for the Johns Hopkins Lung Project. Thirty-three per cent of formerly heavily exposed asbestos workers, 8 per cent of lightly exposed, 1 per cent with some history of exposure and 0.2 per cent of smokers with none produced sputum that contained bodies. Sebastien et al. (1984) found ferruginous bodies seven times more frequently in the mesothelioma villages of central Turkey than in the unaffected neighbouring villages. Sebastien et al. (1988a) also found a relationship between macrophages and bodies formed around tremolite cores in the sputum of vermiculite miners and their cumulative exposure. The application of such investigations, however, would appear to be limited.

Bronchoalveolar lavage

Bronchoalveolar lavage (BAL) has received much attention in recent years for the investigation of asbestos-related interstitial lung disease (Rebuck and Brande, 1983; Rubino, 1986; Donaldson and Brown, 1993). Asbestos bodies in the recovered fluid may be counted by light microscope; a finding of more than 1 body/ml is rare in those not occupationally exposed (De Vuyst et al., 1987; Sebastien et al., 1988b). However, they are a marker only of exposure and not of disease, and are not a reliable guide to cumulative exposure (Xaubet et al., 1986) (see Chapter 4, 'Bronchoalveolar lavage in the investigation of occupational lung disorders').

Changes in the cell content of recovered fluid may occasionally be of help in the differential diagnosis of asbestosis (Turner-Warwick and Haslam, 1986). Normally, the total cell content increases; within the total, macrophage proportions may fall below 90 per cent whilst neutrophils, lymphocytes and eosinophils may all increase, characteristically to proportions of the order of 8 per cent, 4 per cent and 1 to 2 per cent respectively in confirmed asbestosis, although with considerable variability (Robinson et al., 1986). The increase in neutrophils helps to distinguish asbestosis and silicosis from extrinsic allergic alveolitis. Subpopulations among the increased lymphocytes have been investigated by Gellert et al. (1986b), but no clear differences have emerged. As in sputum and lung parenchyma, fibres may be identified by

TEM in lavage fluid (Gellert et al., 1986a) and within recovered macrophages (Johnson et al., 1986). Bégin et al. (1983b) have followed changes in BAL fluid in sheep corresponding to the progression of asbestosis. Several groups have also looked at the protein content of the fluid, and Bégin et al. (1986, 1987b) have found evidence, from enzyme changes, of a threshold of tolerance for chrysotile.

In summary, it may be said that this invasive procedure, not without risk in subjects whose lungs are already compromised, has added much of research interest but is seldom of help to individual asbestos-exposed subjects. Its use as a method of washout, comparable to that in alveolar proteinosis, has been discussed by Bignon, Sebastien and Bientz (1979), who point out that only 1 per cent of the total lung burden is likely to be in position within the alveolar or bronchiolar lumen where it would be accessible to be removed.

Gallium-67 scan

This technique has been used as an aid to diagnosis (Bégin et al., 1983b; Rubino, 1986), and increased gallium uptake has been demonstrated in established disease. However, its value for early diagnosis remains to be established (see Chapter 7, 'Inflammatory activity studies', page 201).

Erythrocyte sedimentation rate

This is sometimes raised in individuals with moderate-to-advanced asbestosis in the absence of any other evident disease. The significance of this finding remains to be explained.

Serology

The association of ANAs and rheumatoid factors (RFs) with asbestosis has already been discussed on page 430. Apart from the different characteristics of ANAs in asbestosis compared with connective tissue disease of the lungs, it is of no diagnostic assistance.

Lung function

Physiological tests reveal only the abnormal patterns of function that characterize diffuse interstitial fibrosis (fibrosing alveolitis) from any cause. For practical purposes, the most important tests are those that determine the lung volumes (TLC, RV, FRC and VC), ventilatory capacity (FEV, FVC) and gas transfer (T_{LCO}). A very early abnormality of lung function appears to be an increase in static elastic pressure (decreased compliance).

However, consistent impairment of vital capacity (VC) in the absence of significant airflow obstruction or other chronic chest disease reflects reduction of compliance and is the most sensitive routine test for the early detection of asbestosis (Thomson, Pelzer and Smither, 1965; Gandevia, 1967; Becklake et al., 1970) and correlates better with dust exposure than T_{LCO} (Becklake, Rossiter and McDonald, 1972).

Vital capacity and T_{LCO} do not, however, appear to be more sensitive than radiographic changes in detecting slight or early asbestosis (Becklake et al., 1970; Weill, Waggenspack and Bailey, 1973; Weill et al., 1975). Weill et al. (1977) suggested that crocidolite exposure causes significantly smaller lung volumes and lower forced expiratory flow rates and T_{LCO} values than chrysotile exposure, a finding which is no doubt related to the greater tendency of the amphiboles to cause progressive asbestosis. No clear decrease in T_{LCO} was observed with increasing exposure in Canadian chrysotile miners and millers (McDonald et al., 1974). Although, on the basis of pathology, a decline in the transfer factor should be an important index of interstitial fibrosis, the variability to which it is subject reduces its usefulness in individual cases.

In the early stages of the disease, slight hyperventilation may occur on effort due to hypoxaemia resulting from reduction in gas transfer in the absence of any abnormality of lung function tests at rest or of radiographic changes. With increased fibrosis, the changes in function in a majority of sufferers are those of the restrictive syndrome (see Chapter 2). Total lung capacity (TLC) and forced vital capacity (FVC) are diminished but residual volume (RV) is either only slightly changed (so that RV/TLC is increased) or decreased. VC, FVC and forced expiratory volume (FEV) are reduced – and to a severe degree when disease is advanced – but the FEV/FVC ratio is usually normal or greater than normal.

Airflow obstruction when present is usually mainly related to cigarette smoking and coexistent chronic obstructive bronchitis. However, attention in recent years has been focused on the presence of small airways' disease and accompanying airflow obstruction independent of smoking. This was suggested by Muldoon and Turner-Warwick (1972) and Fournier-Massey and Becklake (1975). A great difficulty has been that any changes due to asbestos effects are small in comparison with those due to cigarette smoking (Becklake et al., 1982; Siracusa et al., 1983; Kilburn, Warshaw and Thornton, 1986). Bégin et al. (1983a) studied 17 lifelong non-smokers who had worked in chrysotile mines and mills for an average of 28 years. Seven were diagnosed as having asbestosis; these subjects all had typical restrictive patterns of lung function, but more detailed tests, including measurement of transpulmonary pressure

and pressure and flow–volume curves, suggested that an increase in airways' resistance was present at low lung volumes, although expiratory flow rates were maintained as a result of the decreased compliance, as had been suggested earlier by Jodoin et al. (1971). In the 10 subjects without asbestosis, no significant differences from controls were found in standard tests, and only minimal dysfunction of the peripheral airways possibly limiting airflow at very low lung volume was found on one of the more complex tests. Non-smoking shipyard workers with asbestos exposure were also studied by Mohsenifar et al. (1986); they found that 13 out of 45 workers had reduced maximum mid-half flow rate (MMFR), but, unfortunately, the extent of exposure to asbestos and possible toxic fumes was not well documented, and the choice of controls open to criticism.

The effects of mineral dusts in the causation of bronchitis are discussed in Chapter 11. Wright and Churg (1985) compared the lungs of 36 long-term chrysotile miners with an equal number of controls matched for age and smoking. They found more fibrosis around the terminal bronchioles proximal to respiratory bronchioles than could be accounted for by smoking, as well as considerably more around the respiratory bronchioles. They considered, however, that these lesions were a reaction to mineral dust in general and not specific to asbestos. In another study, Churg (1983) compared the lung fibre burden of nine miners with this type of airways' disease but without interstitial fibrosis with that of nine others matched for age, smoking and exposure without histological evidence of airways' disease. A small difference in fibre concentrations between the groups was found, but it was suggested that other factors may be involved. Copes, Thomas and Becklake (1985) found a relationship between both bronchitis and airways' obstruction to cigarette smoking and dust load independently; Ernst et al. (1987) found that symptoms of wheezing and breathlessness were related primarily to smoking and evidence of hyperactive airways antedating exposure. Agostoni et al. (1987), in evaluating the complaint of dyspnoea in asbestos-exposed subjects seeking compensation, found that only 26 per cent had a respiratory cause and of these over three-quarters were smokers.

The conclusion is that whilst asbestos undoubtedly produces changes in the terminal bronchioles, these may be non-specific and comparable to those produced by other mineral dusts. The functional changes they produce are minimal in the absence of interstitial fibrosis and likely to be swamped in smokers by the tobacco effect, or by pre-existing airway hyperreactivity. The cornerstone of lung function testing in the diagnosis of asbestosis is still constituted by indices of lung volumes and gas transfer.

Once the diagnosis of asbestosis is established, progress of the disease can be adequately assessed at subsequent re-examination by VC, FVC and FEV. Decline in VC and FVC values greater than that due to the normal ageing effect with a normal FEV/FVC ratio indicates progress of fibrosis. Such a decline may continue in workers exposed to amphibole asbestos after removal from exposure even in the absence of clinical asbestosis (Ohlson et al., 1985).

Radiographic appearances

As described in Chapter 7, posteroanterior (PA) and suitably angled right and left anterior oblique views should be taken in all new cases of suspected asbestosis. Good technique is of paramount importance. By contrast with silicosis and coal pneumoconiosis, the appearances of asbestosis are predominant in the lower halves of the lung fields. This, however, is also true in some cases of DIPF due to other causes.

The earliest abnormalities are usually found in both lower zones near the costophrenic angles and may be verified more easily by anterior oblique views than by the standard PA films (Figure 14.9). The first perceptible changes consist of more fine vessel opacities than are normal in these regions with thickening of the vascular markings where they branch and divide. Linear opacities which look like extensions of vascular markings may reach the periphery, often crossing over each other to give a net-like appearance (Figure 14.10). Initially the opacities are tenuous and difficult to define with confidence, but they become progressively thicker and, when few, may resemble Kerley 'B' lines although often they do not reach the pleura. Another early abnormality consists of minute bead-like opacities, 1 to 2 mm in diameter, close to distal branches of the pulmonary arteries in the costophrenic angles (Fletcher and Edge, 1970) (Figure 14.10c).

As asbestosis progresses, linear and irregular opacities become thicker and spread into the middle zones but rarely reach the upper zones (Figure 14.11). The appearance of basal interstitial fibrosis is normally symmetrical or almost so, but may be more prominent on one side. This may be due to a more extensive general opacity caused by diffuse pleural thickening on that side. It is never unilateral.

The ILO U/C International Classification of Radiographs (1980) (see Chapter 7) codifies irregular opacities as categories s, t and u according to a crude scale of thickness. But there is greater difficulty in assigning these categories than is the case with categories p, q and r and, hence, more observer disagreement.

The costophrenic and cardiophrenic angles are frequently obliterated. Diffuse pleural thickening which usually takes the form of an ill-defined haze in both middle and lower zones (sometimes more on one side than the other) is commonly present (see Figure 14.11). When it is advanced, evidence of basal intrapulmonary fibrosis may be obscured on standard radiographs but is usually demonstrable by using increased voltage and anterior oblique views. The heart outline may be blurred due to superimposition of fibrosis of the parietal pericardium, lungs and pleura (so-called 'shaggy heart'), but this appearance is exceptional and non-specific. As fibrosis advances the area of the lung fields often diminishes due to fibrotic contraction. The line of the lesser fissure shifts downwards and there may be crowding of the vascular pattern in the lower zones (Figure 14.12). In far advanced asbestosis, enlargement of the heart and proximal pulmonary artery shadows due to pulmonary hypertension may be seen.

Differential diagnosis of small irregular opacities must include age and cigarette smoking, the radiological effects of which are discussed in the next section, crowding of the vasculature in the lung bases due to poor inspiration, and obesity. These are all conditions liable to lead to a mistaken diagnosis of asbestos-related disease, and similar small opacities may arise from a number of other unrelated diseases. An independent re-evaluation by three expert radiologists of the radiographs of 439 subjects, suspected in one survey of having asbestos-related disease, found valid radiographic evidence in only 11 (2.5 per cent) (Reger et al., 1990).

In difficult cases, and where the lung fields are obscured by pleural fibrosis, a great advance in diagnostic possibilities has resulted from the recent development of high-resolution computed tomography (see Chapter 7, 'Computed tomography'). Two features are looked for in early asbestosis: first, the normal gravity effect of increased perfusion in the dependent part of the lung is abolished (Figure 14.13); secondly, a variety of subpleural and transpulmonary bands and an appearance of honeycombing may be seen (Figure 14.14) (Gamsu, Alberle and Lynch, 1989). Some post-mortem validation has been attempted by Akira et al. (1989) who, however, suggested that prospective studies on much larger numbers are required before complete reliability can be placed on the interpretation of some of the apparent abnormalities found. This note of caution has been echoed by Friedman et al. (1990), particularly in relation to subpleural curvilinear lines.

Round opacities (up to about 2 cm diameter) indicative of rheumatoid necrobiotic nodules have been described in asbestos workers with and without accompanying evidence of asbestosis. They may closely resemble typical Caplan's lesions (see Figure 13.35) (Rickards and Barrett, 1958; Tellesson, 1961; Morgan, 1964; Mattson, 1971;

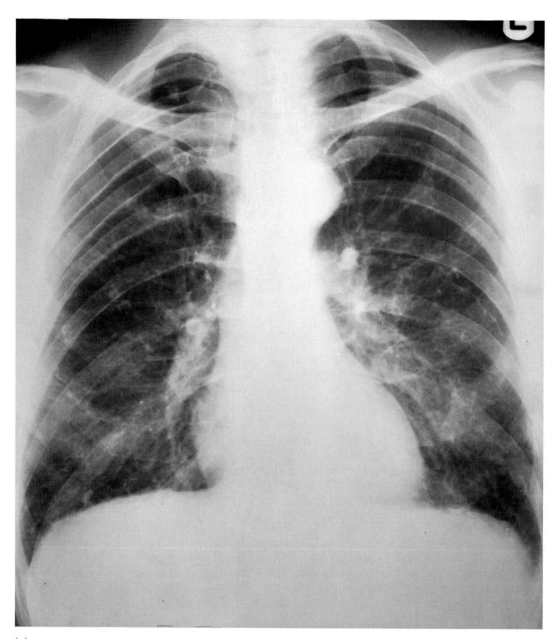

(a)

Figure 14.9 Appearances of clinically early asbestosis (DIPF). (a) Fine irregular opacities (category s) in both lower zones especially the costophrenic angles (b) and (c). Small calcified pleural plaques are also present and are most clearly demonstrated in the 45 degree anterior oblique views. Note: hyaline plaques (arrowed) in the left lower zone of the left anterior oblique view (that is, right lung field). No diffuse pleural thickening evident and costophrenic angles are sharply defined. Insulation worker, aged 52, with 50 years' intermittent exposure to asbestos. No respiratory symptoms; ballroom dancer. Fine persistent inspiratory crackles in both lower lobes. Lung function: slight reduction of TLC, T_L and K_{CO}

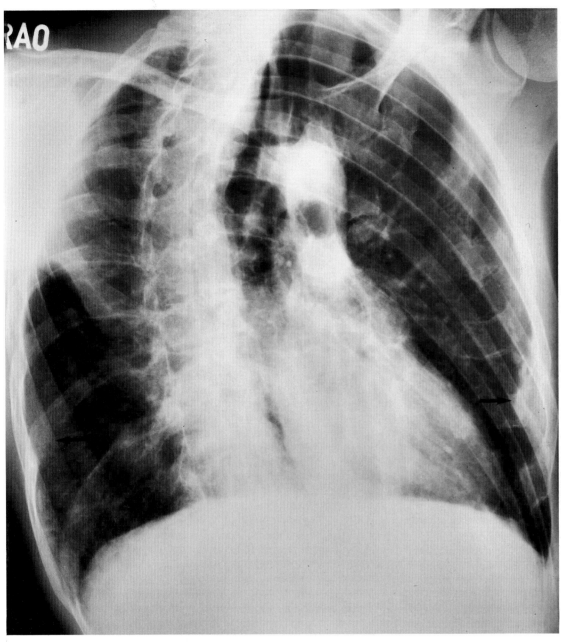

(b)

Figure 14.9 *Continued*

Greaves, 1979). But these appearances are evidently rare and their significance in relation to asbestosis uncertain (see Chapter 5, page 121).

Diagnosis

Asbestosis possesses no pathognomonic clinical, physiological or radiological features. Hence,

given evidence of past occupational asbestos exposure the diagnosis of asbestosis rests first upon establishing the clinical features described above and, secondly, upon excluding DIPF due to other causes or to disease that may simulate it. Asbestos bodies in the sputum or radiographic evidence of bilateral pleural plaques may confirm exposure but do not establish the existence of asbestosis; equally their absence does not exclude it (see also Chapter 15).

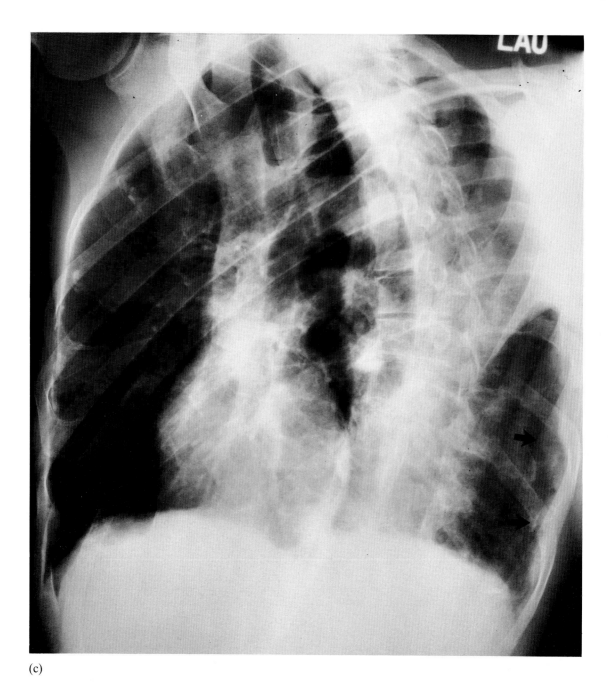

(c)

Figure 14.9 *Continued*

Clinical criteria

Abnormal physical signs

Persistent, bilateral, basal late-inspiratory crackles of high-to-medium frequency which occur early in the evolution of the disease are the important sign that is only exceptionally absent. Coarse quality crackles in inspiration and expiration suggest some other disease. Finger clubbing has no discriminatory value because it is observed in only some cases of asbestosis and occurs with a variety of diseases including DIPF due to other causes (see Chapter 6).

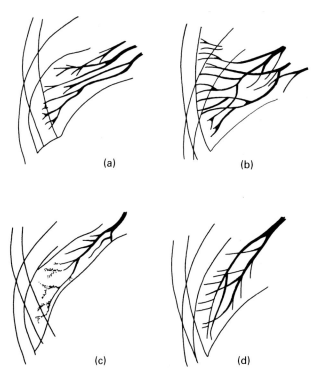

Figure 14.10 Diagram showing the various radiographic patterns of early asbestosis. (a) More small vessel markings than is normal; (b) vessel markings tend to be thickened where they branch and divide, an appearance occasionally seen in normal chests. Vessels may have the same calibre over the peripheral 2 or 3 cm and extend to the pleural margin. Branches cross giving a coarse net-like appearance; (c) fine, 'nodular' opacities 1 to 2 mm in diameter accompanying the smaller peripheral vessels; (d) horizontal linear pattern resembling Kerley 'B' lines. Some of these lines are continuous with vessel markings and do not reach the pleural margin. (Reproduced with permission from Fletcher and Edge, 1970)

Abnormalities of lung function

Significant reduction of TLC, VC, FVC and $T_{L}CO$ with or without lightly increased RV. Gas transfer coefficient (K_{CO}) is usually, but not always, reduced. These parameters are not necessarily equally impaired.

Radiographic abnormalities

The important points are: (1) the appearance and distribution of the abnormalities; and (2) their mode of development and progression. Involvement of the upper zones is rarely seen and then only when the lower and mid-zone changes are far advanced. In many cases there is evidence of bilateral, diffuse thickening of the pleura. Progression may occur

slowly over a number of years, and at some point may cease (see Figure 14.12). Severe hyperinflation may occasionally compress the lower parts of the lungs sufficiently to give a superficial resemblance to bilateral, diffuse, intrapulmonary, basal fibrosis. Other pneumoconioses are sometimes seen in asbestos-exposed workers (Figures 14.15 and 14.16).

In general, it may be said that a diagnosis of clinical asbestosis in a live subject requires an adequate history of exposure to asbestos and symptoms of effort dyspnoea, together with appropriate abnormalities in at least two of these three categories. Criteria for the attribution of disease to asbestos exposure have been discussed by the medical advisory panel of the Asbestos International Association (McCullagh et al., 1982), the American Thoracic Society (Murphy et al., 1986) and the Council on Scientific Affairs of the American Medical Association (AMA, 1984).

The influence of smoking on non-malignant asbestos-related disease

The malign influence of smoking on the incidence of lung cancer in subjects with asbestosis was established with the study by Selikoff, Hammond and Churg in 1968. It has, however, taken longer to clarify the situation with regard to asbestosis itself and pleural change. A substantial number of papers from several different countries have reported cigarette smoking to be associated with an increased prevalence of radiological small opacities (e.g. McMillan, Pethybridge and Sheers, 1980; Viallat and Boutin, 1980; Weiss, 1984, 1988a, 1991; Lerman et al., 1986; Kasuga et al., 1987; Hnizdo and Sluis-Cremer, 1988; Barnhart et al., 1990; Ducatman, Withers and Young, 1990), but whether this represents a true increase in asbestosis has been disputed.

The problem arises because of the pathological changes created independently by smoking. Auerbach et al. (1963) and Auerbach, Garfinkel and Hammond (1974) described interstitial fibrosis together with thickening of bronchiolar and arteriolar walls and rupture of alveolar walls in males in a large autopsy series; very little was present in non-smokers, and there was a strong dose–response relationship between most of these changes and the number of cigarettes smoked per day. Comparable changes were confirmed in a series of experiments in dogs (Cross et al., 1982) and rats (Heckman and Dalbey, 1982). In a study of asbestos-related lung pathology, Wagner et al. (1982a) found that whilst the interstitial fibrosis in diagnosed asbestosis was graded mild in 46 per cent, moderate in 39 per cent and severe or gross in 14 per cent, mild fibrosis was also present in 70 per cent and moderate fibrosis in

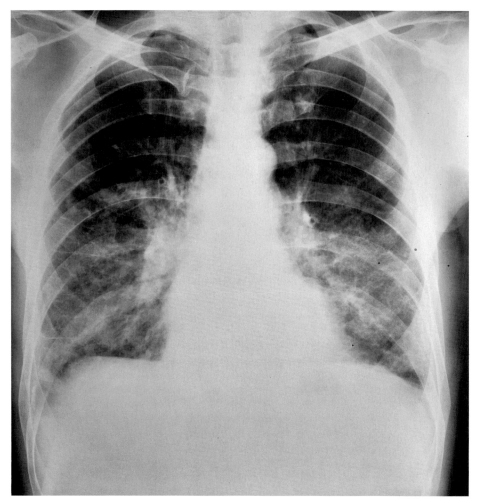

(a)

Figure 14.11 Moderately advanced asbestosis: category t irregular opacities. Note: (1) freedom of the upper zones in the PA and 45 degree right anterior oblique view (b); (2) presence of slight bilateral diffuse pleural thickening and loss of costophrenic angles; (3) calcified plaques in both lower zones in the oblique view that are not evident in (a). Insulation worker for 34 years, aged 59 years. Moderate dyspnoea after climbing 14 steps. Persistent medium inspiratory crackles in both lower lobes, middle and lingula; none in the upper lobes. Lung function: moderately severe restriction and impairment of T_L with slight reduction of K_{CO}

20 per cent of unexposed male industrial workers serving as controls. Smoking was not controlled for, but the great majority in both series were smokers. Johansson et al. (1987) found an association between smoking and interstitial fibrosis in their non-exposed controls. Adesina et al. (1990) analysed the lungs of males who had died suddenly having previously lived in a clean air environment and not employed in dusty trades. They found a significant association between smoking and fibrosis of terminal bronchioles.

Whether smoking-related changes would give rise to radiographic opacities has been disputed by Kilburn (1981) but there is now abundant evidence that they do. McDonald, Gibbs and Oakes (1984) reported an incidence of 20 per cent for males over 40 used as non-asbestos-exposed controls; Epstein et al. (1984) reported a 9 per cent incidence in older males with no history of dust exposure. Glover et al. (1980) and Nemeth et al. (1986) also reported a positive incidence, although at lower levels. Carilli, Kotzen and Fisher (1973) showed that women over

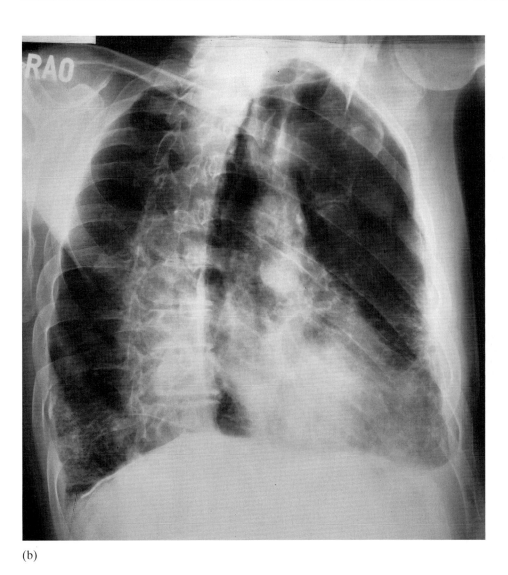

(b)

Figure 14.11 *Continued*

35 could be identified on their chest radiograph as smokers or non-smokers with an accuracy exceeding 60 per cent. Weiss (1988a), in an analysis of his own data, showed a dose–response for radiographic changes suggesting diffuse pulmonary fibrosis rising to a prevalence of 20 per cent in subjects who had smoked more than a pack a day for over 20 years. Kilburn et al. (1986b) suggested that smoking did not cause small opacities; however, in their study the prevalence was 3.7 per cent in men without direct occupational asbestos exposure and of average age 50 years; since only 60 per cent were smokers this would be equivalent to 6.1 per cent in smokers if all the changes were due to this cause.

Cigarette smoking by itself, therefore, is a cause of radiographic small opacities, and may be assumed to have an additive effect on the radiographic changes due to asbestosis. There is some uncertainty about whether it has an additional direct effect rendering the smoker more liable to asbestosis. Smoking is known to inhibit long-term particle clearance (Bohning, Atkins and Cohn, 1982) and to increase long-term retention (Churg and Wiggs, 1987) (see Chapter 3). Animal experiments have shown that exposure to cigarette smoke increased the long-term retention of crocidolite in rats, but not of chrysotile or synthetic mineral fibre (Muhle et al., 1989), presumably due to the dissolution of these fibres which is known to occur. Tron et al. (1987) have shown that smoke worsens airways' and parenchymal disease induced by amosite in guinea-pigs. In this study they confirmed previous work from the same laboratory showing that smoke exposure increased retention of amosite administered by intratracheal injection, and also that it increased the penetration of fibres into the bronchiolar walls. In

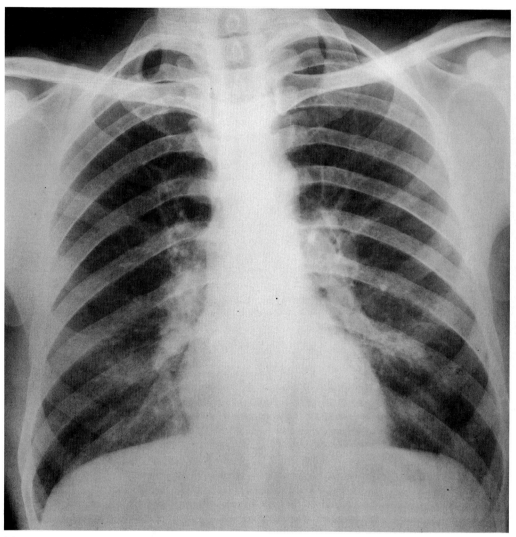

(a)

Figure 14.12 Progression of asbestosis over 20 years. Operator of disintegrator and crusher of crude asbestos fibre filler 1956 to 1959. (a) 1957, no evident abnormality. (b) 1969, slight to moderate asbestosis: cateory s. Note: clear upper zones, and minimal evidence of diffuse pleural thickening. Asbestosis with many asbestos bodies confirmed by biopsy. Clinically: persistent fine pan-inspiratory crackles in both lower lobes, middle lobe and lingula with moderate restrictive and gas transfer defects. (c) 1978, advanced disease (category t/u). Note downward displacement of lesser fissure; evidence of diffuse pleural thickening with obliteration of the costophrenic angles, indefinite ('shaggy') cardiac outline and clear upper zones. Severe respiratory disability

producing these and other changes, cigarette smoke appeared to act synergistically with asbestos. As was to be expected, progression of radiographic changes after removal from heavy exposure was found in several series to be greater in smokers than in non-smokers (Rubino et al., 1979a; Rossiter, Heath and Harries, 1980; Suoranta et al., 1982; Gaensler, Jederlinic and McLoud, 1990).

However, narrowing of airways which can result from inflammation or mucus hypersecretion produces more proximal deposition (Lippman, Yeates and Albert, 1980) and, hence, may reduce penetration of fibre to the alveoli (see Chapter 3). In human subjects, two studies have failed to find significant evidence of interaction between smoke and fibre (Samet et al., 1979; Hnizdo and Sluis-Cremer, 1988).

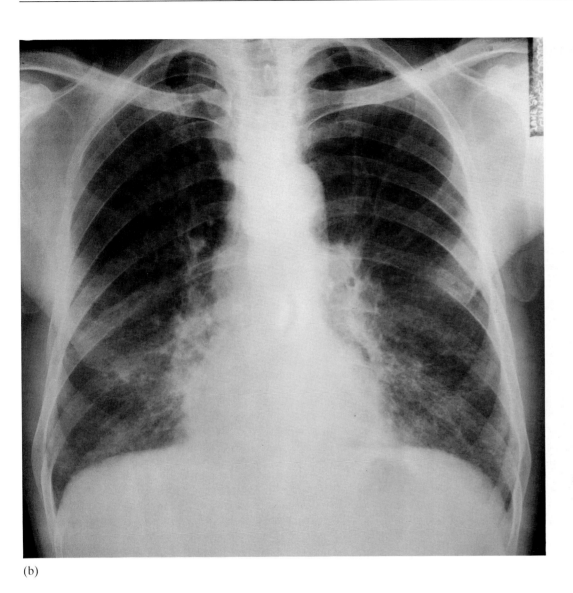

(b)

Figure 14.12 *Continued*

The details of their interaction in human beings are, therefore, not fully established, although that there is some potentiation and not merely an additive radiographic effect can hardly be doubted in view of the strength of the association demonstrated in so many cohorts. Certainly, any future study of asbestosis prevalence should take cumulative smoking effects into account.

Pleural change has been found, in most series, not to be associated with smoking. This has been the case even when in the analysis no distinction has been made between pleural plaques and diffuse pleural thickening and despite the known associations between cigarette smoking, respiratory infection and pleuritic inflammation (for example, Rossiter and Harries, 1979; Lilis et al., 1986; Kasuga et al., 1987; Marshall and Stein, 1990). Contrary

findings have been reported by Viallat and Boutin (1980), Weiss, Levin and Goodman (1981), Baker, Dagg and Greene (1985), who did not find any excess pleural disease related to cigarette smoking in the absence of significant asbestos exposure, and McMillan, Pethybridge and Sheers (1980), who looked at a sample of the same cohort as Rossiter and Harries (1979) and came to the opposite conclusion. Andrion, Pira and Mollo (1984) found a higher incidence of pleural plaques in an unselected autopsy population among smokers than among non-smokers in men, but not in women. The difference remained even when those with a probable occupational exposure were excluded, although occupational histories were retrospective; in view of the absence of any higher incidence in women, there may have been some undetected asbestos exposure.

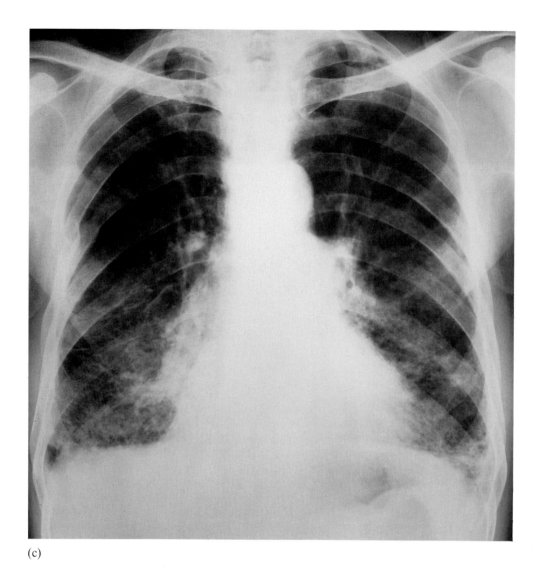

(c)

Figure 14.12 *Continued*

Of major importance in regard to any aetiological relationship with pleural plaques is the time factor, because duration from first exposure has the major influence on prevalence. This is well illustrated in the numerical figures given by Weiss; ex-smokers appeared to have double the incidence of plaques shown by current smokers, but the average duration since first exposure was 32 years compared with 24. The issue can probably only be settled by a series sufficiently large to control adequately for both smoking and duration from onset of exposure.

Progression

Progression of asbestosis after removal from exposure is normally slow and by no means invariable.

Radiographic follow-up studies of chrysotile miners in Corsica (Viallat et al., 1983), Italy (Rubino et al., 1979a) and Quebec (Becklake et al., 1979) all found that the probability of progression was related to the radiographic category at the termination of exposure which, in turn, was related to cumulative exposure. Among Quebec miners those with less than 2 years' exposure had no excess of radiographic small opacities and none had appeared after an average follow-up of 17 years, whilst of those with more than 2 years' exposure (average 14 years) and the same duration of follow-up, 12 per cent progressed by two or more ILO subcategories. Among Italian miners with mean exposure of 23 years and follow-up of 12 years after leaving the mines, 8 per cent of those with a radiograph of category 0/0 or 0/1 on leaving showed small opacities on their later film (the 'attack rate'), whilst 39 per cent of those whose 'leaving'

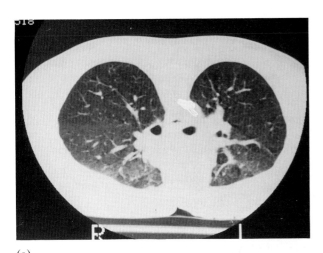

(a)

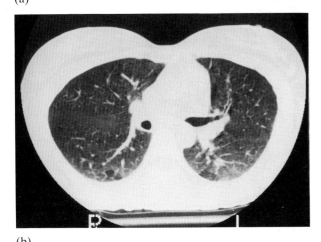

(b)

Figure 14.13 CT scan of normal lung thin slice, prone and supine, demonstrating gravity-dependent perfusion. (Courtesy of Dr D. Hansell)

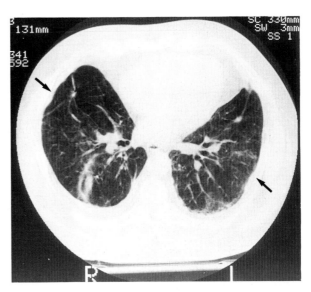

Figure 14.14 CT scan of diffuse pleural thickening and parenchymal involvement. (Courtesty of Dr D. Hansell)

films were already abnormal showed evidence of progression. The sample of Corsican miners studied had the heaviest mean exposure of 27 years, and the mean follow-up period after exposure ended was 16 years. Among these men there was an 'attack rate' of 39 per cent for those whose last film at work was normal, whilst 63 per cent of those who were 1/1 or higher initially showed progression. Heavier smoking was a feature of the progressors but did not provide the whole explanation. Cordier, Theriault and Provencher (1984) also looked at Quebec miners with low level exposure. Their subjects had cumulative exposures varying from 7 fibres/ml years to 3000 fibres/ml years and were followed for an average period of 20 years; 2.1 per cent showed small opacities of 1/0 or more, but this did not correlate with any index of exposure, and was identical with a referent group of office workers in the same industry, of whom 2.1 per cent (1/48) also had small opacities.

Because the fate of chrysotile in the lungs differs from that of amphiboles, it may be anticipated that the progression of interstitial fibrosis would also differ. Cookson et al. (1986a,b) reported on a 30-year radiographic follow-up of Australian crocidolite miners. The authors calculated that definite radiographic signs of asbestosis resulted from a median cumulative exposure of 91 fibres/ml years (although this figure may require substantial upward revision; Rogers, 1990) and appeared at a median time of 14 years after starting work (range 2 to 34 years). Twenty-five per cent of their sample remained in category 0 by the end of the period. Of those rated as category 1 within 5 years of the onset of their first exposure, 50 per cent had progressed to category 2, 15 years later. Moreover, progression continued over the period of follow-up. Of those with small opacities, only 4 per cent did not progress by at least one subcategory in the last 10 years. However, the authors made no adjustment for age or smoking. These results were also based on applicants for compensation and, therefore, likely to include a higher proportion of progressors; based on a random sample of all the former workers at this crocidolite mine, the authors found more than twice as many cases who had radiographic small opacities 1/0 or higher but who had not applied for compensation.

A comparable study of mainly amphibole miners in South Africa was undertaken by Sluis-Cremer and Hnizdo (1989). They found age to be the strongest predictor of progression, with exposure and smoking having smaller but significant effects. Among men followed for at least 12 years, in those aged under 30 years at the time of their first chest

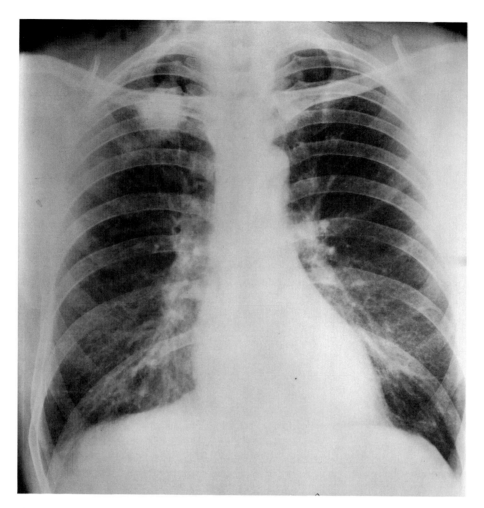

Figure 14.15 Coal pneumoconiosis with PMF in right upper zone and slight to moderate asbestosis (1980). Coal miner at the 'dump end' of a coal conveyor underground for five and a half years (1936 to 1942). Very dusty conditions. 1961 to 1968: fitter assembling asbestos cement panels in a power station; however, chief exposure occurred in the earlier years of this period when he was in proximity to asbestos insulation workers. Open lung biopsy revealed coal pneumoconiosis, mild asbestosis and moderate numbers of asbestos bodies in 30-μm sections

radiograph, the average progression was only 0.3 of a subcategory, whereas in those aged 35 to 44 years, the average progression was 1.8.

As with chrysotile, the general finding was that progression was faster in those with higher cumulative exposures and in those in whom small opacities appeared after a shorter than average interval from first exposure.

For men employed in the manufacture of asbestos–cement (mainly chrysotile but also with a small amount of amphibole), Jones et al. (1980) looked at changes over a 6-year period. They found, as expected, that the probability of progression of asbestosis increased with increasing average and cumulative dust exposures. It was also higher in men with higher initial profusions of small opacities,

but this effect was to be expected since such subjects would tend to have higher cumulative exposures. They commented that few cases of progression were observed in men with less than 20 years' exposure but did not provide detailed figures. A further study of the same cohort (Jones et al., 1989) confirmed a relationship between probability of progression of radiographic category and cumulative exposure, and the greater probability of progression if small opacities were present at the onset of the 10-year observation period. During this time, 13 per cent showed progression of small opacities, the probability being higher in men working in the one of the two plants in which some crocidolite was used.

Other series have related to subjects with mixed exposures in various trades. Gaensler, Jederlinic and

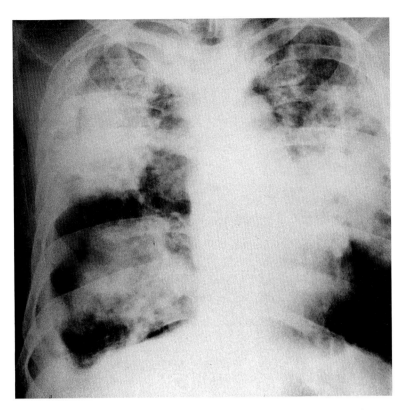

Figure 14.16 Radiograph of silicosis in a young miner with about 10 years' high dust exposure in a North Cape (S. Africa) crocidolite mine. In addition to the large opacities, smaller round opacities are present as well as evidence of extensive diffuse pleural thickening over the right lung. (Reproduced with permission from Solomon et al., 1971)

McLoud (1990) followed up 1764 workers from shipyards and manufacturing plants over 11 years. They found progression, defined as an increase of two ILO subcategories, occurred in 13 per cent, although for men over 50 years of age with more than 20 years exposure before the start of the follow-up period, 30 per cent showed progression. Initial readings of 1/1 or higher had a worse prognosis than those in lower categories, and they also found that progression was significantly more common in smokers. Shipyard workers were also looked at by Rossiter, Heath and Harries (1980) over a 9-year period from 1965, when strict control over air-borne dust was first enforced; during that time the proportion of laggers and sprayers radiologically greater than category 1/0 increased from 4 to 24 per cent but no estimate was given of cumulative exposures. A notable feature of this series was that no progression to 1/1 was recorded among non-smokers.

Suoranta et al. (1982), Gregor et al. (1979) and Barnes (1986) studied subjects already diagnosed as suffering from asbestosis. Suoranta looked at radiographic change over 4 years and found progression of at least one subcategory in one-third of the 85 patients examined. Progression was related to initial category – only 13 per cent of subjects in category 1/1 or less progressed, compared with 66 per cent with an initial score of more than 1/1. Smokers also fared worse than non-smokers, as did sprayers, who were the only subjects in the cohort who had heavy exposure to crocidolite. Gregor et al. (1979) reported on 119 subjects with asbestosis attending the UK Pneumoconiosis Medical Panel for compensation purposes. Progression occurred more frequently in those with higher initial category scores, and the percentage increased with increasing duration of observation. However, after 7 years only one-third had progressed. A comparable series which included some of the same subjects was studied by Coutts et al. (1987a). They followed 164 patients for an average of 7.5 years; 66 died during this time but of the 98 survivors only 37 showed evidence of progression, which was more frequent in those rated 1/0 or more at the first examination. These authors suggested that an early active stage was in many cases followed by a non-progressive stage. Barnes found that 36 out of 72 subjects diagnosed as having asbestosis but whose radiograph did not exceed 0/1 had moved up by at least one subcategory after a mean period of 8 years.

To summarize, from these studies it appears that progression of radiographic category is related first to cumulative exposure and to the fibre type – chrysotile or amphibole. Duration of exposure prior to the appearance of small opacities is negatively correlated with progression probability: the shorter the duration the greater the likelihood of subsequent further progression. Speed of onset largely reflects cumulative exposure, but also involves the element of individual susceptibility. For those whose main exposure has been to amphibole asbestos, the probability is very high that once asbestosis has been diagnosed, progression of at least one ILO subcategory will occur despite removal from further exposure, although the change may take many years to become manifest. For those exposed mainly to chrysotile, however, progression is much less probable. As with crocidolite, the probability increases with both increasing cumulative exposure and the higher profusion of small opacities on the ILO scale recorded at the onset of the observation period following removal from exposure. The duration of the period of exposure is also relevant, but even when this covers many years, only a small proportion of those less than 1/1 at the onset are likely to progress. Almost all studies found that smoking is an important additional risk factor, so that ceasing to smoke is a major therapeutic option. Age is also an additional independent determinant of small opacities (Epstein et al., 1984; Seaton, Louw and Cowie, 1986), even in non-smokers (Ghio, Renzetti and Crapo, 1990). In series with mixed exposures, intermediate rates of progression have been found, mostly of the order of magnitude of about 40 per cent over 10 years for subjects rated 1/1 or more at the onset of observation (see Figure 14.12).

No therapy has hitherto been available to halt progression. Systemic corticosteroids have been tried in occasional cases, particularly where progression has been unusually rapid in relation to exposure, but without sufficient benefit to outweigh the adverse effects. Recently, however, two possibilities have appeared. Glutathione is a known extracellular antioxidant which has been shown to be deficient in cryptogenic fibrosing alveolitis; a preliminary trial of glutathione administered by aerosol has been carried out (Borok et al., 1991) and, should a more extended trial demonstrate therapeutic benefit in that disease, an extension to asbestosis would be warranted. An alternative approach centres around platelet-derived growth factor B (PDGF-B) – a peptide regulatory factor produced by macrophages, and perhaps the most important cytokine involved in producing the fibrotic response, converting chronic inflammation into lung fibrosis. If macrophage production of PDGF-B can be inhibited, progression of asbestosis may be prevented (Shaw, 1991) (see Chapter 4, 'Therapeutic approaches', pages 90 to 93).

Prognosis

The outlook for subjects diagnosed as having radiographic small opacities or actual asbestosis has been studied by several authors. Liddell and McDonald (1980) related radiographic abnormalities to subsequent mortality. Relative risks of death were considerably higher in the presence of both small opacities and pleural change, this increase being present over the range of possible asbestos-related diseases as well as those not normally associated. Cumulative dust exposures, however, were also higher in those with radiographic abnormalities, as was the level of cigarette smoking, and it is probable that the level of relative risk was influenced by abnormalities directly related to smoking.

Berry (1981) studied the mortality of people certified by the UK Pneumoconiosis Medical Panel as suffering from asbestosis between 1952 and 1976, graded according to their clinical condition. Thirty-nine per cent of deaths were due to lung cancer, 9 per cent to mesothelioma and 20 per cent to asbestosis. The rates of all these diseases increased with the percentage assessed disability, and for a man certified at the age of 55 Berry calculated that life expectancy would be reduced by 3, 5, 8 or 12 years in relation to assessments of 10 per cent, 20 per cent, 30 to 40 per cent and 50 per cent or above. The percentage of assessed disability, however, would be influenced by morbidity from causes additional to asbestosis, such as the effects of smoking and ischaemic heart disease. Coutts et al. (1987a) studied a smaller group of similar subjects but related mortality to radiographic change and other clinical variables. The main causes of death were closely comparable to those found by Berry: 29 per cent of deaths were from lung cancer, 10 per cent from mesothelioma and 19 per cent from non-malignant respiratory disease. Cases certified as having asbestosis, but with category 0 for small opacities, had no increase in overall mortality, although lung cancer incidence was increased, and the authors suggested that the diagnosis may be in doubt in the absence of radiographic evidence of small opacities. Vital capacity, diffusion capacity (T_L) and FEV were studied, but only FEV, as a percentage of predicted value, was related to mortality risk, again emphasizing the relevance of smoking. Finger clubbing had an adverse prognostic significance unrelated to other factors (Coutts et al., 1987b). Huuskonen (1978) also found that mortality in Finnish subjects diagnosed as having asbestosis had an important relationship with smoking. Their exposure was heavy, the diagnosis being made an average of 22 years from first exposure, and 42 per cent actually died from asbestosis, whilst 32 per cent died of lung cancer. No mesotheliomas were recorded. However, although the average survival time of smokers was 7 and 17 years for men over and under 50 years at the time of diagnosis, more than half the non-smokers were still alive at the end of the follow-up, with survival times exceeding 14 and 25 years respectively.

Benign asbestos pleural disease

Introduction

The focus of clinical interest in asbestos-related disease has changed progressively with the reduction in exposure. After the recognition of asbestosis as a disease to be distinguished first from pulmonary tuberculosis and then from silicosis, reduction in exposure and early removal of incipient cases led to improved survival rates; this, in turn, led to an increase in proportional mortality from lung cancer as milder cases survived long enough to develop a malignancy. The same process in recent years has led to greater interest in the benign pleural diseases: in particular differentiation between diffuse pleural thickening, originating in the pulmonary layer, and circumscribed thickening (or plaques) of the parietal pleura, and the discovery of asbestos-related pleural effusions.

Gloyne, in 1933 (Gloyne, 1932–33), drew attention to the finding of hyaline plaques at autopsy in association with asbestosis, and pleural calcification was noted by several authors during the same decade (Selikoff, 1965). Jacob and Bohlig (1955) listed pleural calcification as a radiographic outcome of asbestos exposure in their large-scale study of asbestos workers, and Kiviluoto, in 1965, described the occurrence of endemic calcification in Finland. By 1966, Elmes had pointed to the need to distinguish radiologically between circumscribed hyaline fibrosis in the parietal pleura and diffuse pleural thickening which he related to underlying parenchymal disease. At the same time Eisenstadt (1965) described asbestos-related benign pleural effusion.

Hyaline plaques of the parietal pleura

These are discrete, circumscribed, usually bilateral raised areas of fibrosis (often partially calcified) on the inner surface of the rib cage, and on the diaphragm (Figures 14.17 and 14.18).

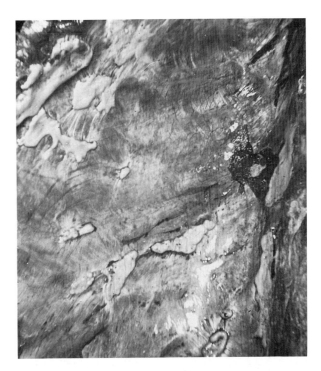

Figure 14.17 Post-mortem appearances of hyaline plaques of the parietal pleura (sternum to left, paraverterbral gutter to right). They are flat, irregular in outline, sharply demarcated, smooth, shiny and raised a few millimetres above the adjacent pleural surface. The substernal and paravertebral lesions are elongated in the vertical axis; the contour of some of the others is roughly parallel with the ribs

Prevalence

The reported prevalence of plaques varies widely according to a number of factors: (1) whether in occupationally or environmentally exposed populations; (2) whether derived from post-mortem or radiographic evidence; (3) the methodological standards of radiological studies (Rossiter, Browne and Gilson, 1988); (4) whether calcified or non-calcified plaques only are reported; and (5) the particular type of fibre involved among those occupationally exposed. The prevalence in surveys of calcified plaques is particularly dependent on the length of follow-up, and isolated figures have little meaning out of context. However, a reasonable generalization is that between a third and a half of all those occupationally exposed to asbestos containing some amphibole and followed up for a minimum of 30 years will be found to have calcified plaques. After a follow-up of 20 years a smaller proportion, between 5 and 15 per cent, may be expected to show uncalcified plaques. Results from a number of studies are listed by Jarvholm et al. (1986).

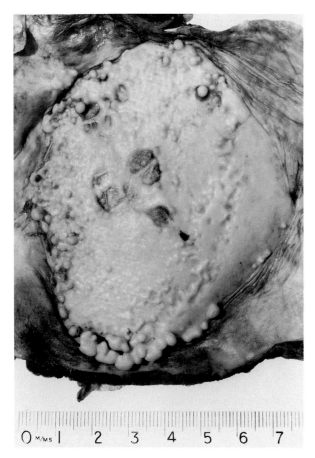

Figure 14.18 Hyaline plaques over the central tendon of the diaphragm. It is sharply circumscribed, raised above the surface and exhibits both flat and nodular features. On section it was substantially calcified. These lesions (which are invariably bilateral) seen end-on in standard chest radiographs produce densely radio-opaque arcs

Excluding surveys of areas with endemic pleural calcification, which will be considered below, the small number of general autopsy series specifying plaques all contain a proportion without identifiable asbestos exposure. An overall prevalence of plaques of 39 per cent was found in two urban populations (one of which was an anthophyllite mining community) in Finland (Meurman, 1966). Prevalences of 11, 12 and 33 per cent were found in London, Glasgow and Copenhagen respectively (Hourihane, Lessof and Richardson, 1966; Roberts, 1971; Francis et al., 1977).

Andrion, Pira and Mollo (1984) found plaques at autopsy in 53 per cent of men over 50 years with a history of occupational exposure, compared with 30 per cent in men without. An independent relationship with cigarette smoking was also suggested. Of women over 50 years old without an occupational history, approximately 8 per cent had plaques. Subjects with plaques were graded according to whether the total area was less or greater than 50 cm; whereas numbers in each grade were approximately equal in exposed men over 50 years, in the non-exposed fewer than one-fifth were in the larger category. Churg (1982) compared the lung fibre burdens of 29 patients with plaques at autopsy with 25 controls selected because they had had no occupational exposure. A history of asbestos exposure was obtained for 16 of the 29 with plaques, and this correlated well with an increase in numbers of larger amphibole (but not chrysotile) fibres in the lung. The remaining patients had counts of long amphibole fibres much closer to the control group. Counts of chrysotile and non-commercial amphibole fibres did not differ significantly between cases and controls.

As both hyaline and calcified plaques must be sufficiently dense to be visible on the standard chest radiograph, their prevalence in radiographic surveys is lower than in post-mortem surveys. Only 15 per cent of the cases of plaques observed *post mortem* by Hourihane, Lessof and Richardson (1966) were detected during life. Wain, Roggli and Foster (1984), in 25 consecutive autopsy cases of plaques without asbestosis, found that only 28 per cent had identifiable pleural change on standard radiographs taken prior to death. They list other studies with sensitivities varying from 8 to 40 per cent. Rubino et al. (1980) comment, not surprisingly, that the proportion was much higher for cases with large plaques (mostly those with known occupational exposure) than for those with small. In 20 per cent of their series, plaques were diagnosed where none was found at autopsy, giving a specificity of 80 per cent. The prevalence of plaques at autopsy is affected by the same factors as radiographic surveys.

Dose–response

Sheers and Templeton (1968), in their survey of dockyard workers, found that the prevalence of plaques increased with intensity of exposure. Using four grades, prevalence increased from 1.5 per cent in the lowest exposure group to 24 per cent in the highest. Others have reported similar findings, including Mollo et al. (1983), on the basis of autopsy findings. However, there is evidence that the relationship is not simply linear between cumulative dose and response. Occurrences such as the typical bilateral plaques, seen on the radiograph of a doctor whose only exposure was a weekly half-day visit to the medical room of an amosite manufacturing plant over the preceding 30 years, are familiar to all with experience of examinations of an asbestos-exposed population. Stronger evidence has been provided by R. Jones et al. (1980) who found that whilst the radiographic appearance of asbestosis and diffuse pleural thickening were related to cumulative exposure in their study of asbestos–cement workers, the appearance of plaques was directly related only to time from first exposure.

In this respect, plaques follow the pattern of mesothelioma (see later) rather than the diseases of the lung – asbestosis and lung cancer – both of which appear to be related more directly to cumulative exposure. As Mollo et al. (1983) stated 'plaques may be absent in subjects with definite and long occupational exposure, while severe lesions can be observed in non-exposed people. Therefore, plaques. . . may be a useful indicator of exposure to asbestos in population studies; however, their validity in individual cases observed in pathological routine is more limited'. Becklake et al. (1979), looking at radiographic changes after cessation of exposure, could not relate pleural increase to any measure of exposure, and Rockoff et al. (1987) found a weaker relationship with exposure for plaques than for diffuse thickening. Gibbs (1979) found the correlation between presence and degree of calcification and cumulative exposure was negligible ($r = 0.09$), but this was influenced by the fact that the incidence of plaques was negligible in certain areas.

Of particular importance is the fact that bilateral plaques and asbestosis (intrapulmonary fibrosis) do not necessarily occur in conjunction. The post-mortem study of 56 cases of pleural plaques by Hourihane, Lessof and Richardson (1966) showed microscopic evidence of asbestosis in only 24 cases (43 per cent) although asbestos bodies were present in the lungs of all. A similar observation was made by Cartier (1965) who found microscopic asbestosis in 29 per cent of pleural plaque cases. In one radiographic study of asbestos workers with hyaline plaques, evidence of asbestosis was detectable in 46 per cent (Navratil and Dobias, 1973). The present author's own experience indicates a corresponding lack of correlation between the presence of plaques and evidence of asbestosis both pathologically and clinically. Implications of this interesting situation are discussed further under 'Pathogenesis'.

Pathology

Macroscopic appearances

Asbestos-related lesions are bilateral, although not always of equal degree, and consist of elevated areas of hyaline fibrosis, a few millimetres to 1 cm thick, which are well circumscribed, of irregular shape with a smooth, polished, slightly convex, ivory-coloured surface that resembles articular cartilage (Figure 14.17). Some are multinodular (Figure 14.18) (the nodules having a mamillated appearance) and others consist of a combination of both forms. When removed they can be bent like leather.

They are distributed irregularly on the inner surface of the rib cage chiefly in the mid-zones anteriorly, laterally and posteriorly – but by no means equally – and tend to follow rib lines, although they are often spread at right angles across one or more intercostal spaces. When very advanced they fuse into large cuirass-like sheets. Their other common locations are along the paravertebral gutters and over the central tendons of the diaphragm. However, they do not occur at the thoracic apices, in the costophrenic sulci or in the mediastinum but are sometimes found in the pleura over the left cardiac border. Irregular areas of calcification of greater or lesser extent are frequently present in the plaques. Fusion of plaques with the pulmonary pleura rarely occurs so that the lungs move over them unimpeded during respiration. Any adhesions that may be present are in areas away from the plaques and only exceptionally are they involved in widespread pleural symphysis.

Plaques may also occur very occasionally in the pulmonary pleura (Rous and Studený, 1970) and very rarely on the peritoneal surface of the liver (Andrion, Pira and Mollo, 1983).

Microscopic appearances

Plaques consist almost entirely of avascular, acellular, laminated collagen fibres arranged parallel to the surface, with hyaline changes, but a few spindle-shaped fibroblasts may be found between the fibres. The appearances resemble 'basket-weave', but in the mamillary nodules the arrangement is concentric like the rings of an onion. In some plaques the fibres stain predominantly for elastic tissue rather than for collagen and may be 'pseudoelastic fibres' due to changes in the composition of collagen (Roberts, 1971). Dystrophic calcification is present in central areas where collagen has undergone degeneration. The surface is usually acellular but, at an early stage of development, appears to be covered by a mesothelial cell lining (Thomson, 1970). The deepest parts show fibroblastic activity with collections of lymphocytes and plasma cells, and there is some vascularity.

Fibres and asbestos bodies have been found in both normal parietal pleural tissue and plaques, and papers concerned with this aspect have been listed by Sebastien et al. (1979). These authors, in a detailed study using electron microscopy, confirmed the report by Le Bouffant et al. (1976) that lung parenchymal retention is not a good indicator of pleural retention. They found that many pleural samples even in heavily exposed subjects contained no detectable fibre, and what fibre was found was almost all short chrysotile, both in plaques and in normal tissue. Only 1 subject out of 29 had a significant amount of amphibole in the tissue examined.

Pathogenesis

As Churg (1988a) has emphasized, basket-weave lamination of collagen which constitutes the typical plaque is not specific to asbestos, but is one reaction of the pleura to a variety of insults, which include trauma, exposure to titanium (Garabrant et al., 1987; Churg and DePaoli, 1988) and possibly infection, particularly tuberculous (Hourihane, Lessof and Richardson 1966; Rous and Studený, 1970). In these circumstances the plaques are normally unilateral and small. The possible relationship between smoking and plaques has been discussed earlier. Bilateral pleural plaques are associated with exposure to all types of asbestos. However, the following questions remain to be answered: Is there some other causal agency? Why are the lesions virtually confined to the parietal pleura and irregular in shape? Why do plaques and asbestosis so often occur independently? Why does the dose–response for the diseases of the parietal pleura – plaques and mesothelioma – appear to differ from that for diseases of the lung parenchyma – asbestosis and lung cancer?

Calcified plaques have been observed in individuals in agricultural communities with no occupational exposure to asbestos, notably in what has been called 'the Central European arc of pleural pathology' extending from Finland (Kiviluoto, Meurman and Hakama, 1979) through Russia (Ginzburg et al., 1970), Czechoslovakia (Rous and Studený, 1970), Austria (Haider and Neuberger, 1981), Bulgaria (Burilkov and Michailova, 1970) and north-west Greece (Bazas et al., 1981) to south-east Turkey (Yazicioglu et al., 1980). In one such community in Czechoslovakia, they were also found in cattle in the same area (Rous and Studený, 1970).

It is of particular interest in this connection that, in the Canadian (Quebec) chrysotile mining complex, calcified plaques were found to be very common in workers in four mines, rare in those in four other mines and absent among men in yet another large mine which is not far distant from the rest (Cartier, 1965). These observations raise the possibility that chrysotile may not be the causal agent. A recent study of 15 689 men in the Quebec industry suggests that pleural calcification is related to tremolite or some other contaminant of chrysotile ore, present in some mines (for example, Thetford) but not in others (Gibbs, 1979). A small study of environmental pleural plaques in the Thetford area has also suggested a role for tremolite (Churg and DePaoli, 1988).

In a tobacco-growing region of Bulgaria where pleural plaques are endemic among the human population, soil samples demonstrated the presence of small amounts of anthophyllite, tremolite and sepiolite derived from outcropping rocks (Burilkov and Michailova, 1970). Tremolite has also been demonstrated in the soil of the areas of north-west Greece (Bazas et al., 1981; Langer et al., 1987), south-east Turkey (Yazicioglu et al., 1980) and Austria (Haider and Neuberger, 1981), where endemic pleural calcification occurs. Tremolite has also been identified as a contaminant of chrysotile in both north-east Corsica (Boutin et al., 1989) and Cyprus (McConnochie et al., 1989) in the regions surrounding the mines. In Finland the predominant amphibole in the soil of such areas is anthophyllite. Tremolite occurs as a contaminant in varying proportions in the Quebec mines, and appears in the lungs of miners at autopsy (Rowlands, Gibbs and McDonald, 1982). In the South African crocidolite mines, crocidolite itself is almost certainly the aetiological agent for the extensive pleural calcification seen. This is confirmed by the experience of manufacturing industry, where a high proportion of subjects exposed to crocidolite or amosite develop plaques, whereas these are uncommon in those exposed only to chrysotile. Fibre solubility in the lungs and pleural tissues appears, therefore, to play an important role; in agreement with this is the extensive pleural calcification which is endemic in Karain and the surrounding area in Turkey, where the association is with the non-asbestos, but equally insoluble, zeolite fibre erionite.

But, assuming that amphibole asbestos is responsible for most pleural plaques, the route by which the fibres reach the parietal pleura is not yet fully established or, indeed, whether they reach the pleura at all. The alternatives that have been considered are direct passage across the pleural cavity, passage via the lymphatics and passage of mediators only, produced by the fibre–macrophage interaction. The earlier theories, and some objections to each, have been reviewed by Hillerdal (1980). It has been suggested that sharp fibres in the lungs penetrate the pulmonary pleura during respiration and pass directly into the parietal layer, possibly causing traumatic microhaemorrhages and fibrin deposition (Heard and Williams, 1961; Thomson, 1970). Although this hypothesis is compatible with plaques being sited predominantly where respiratory excursions are greatest, plaque formation does not appear to be preceded by episodes of inflammatory disease or fibrinous exudates (Meurman, 1968), and adhesions between plaques and the pulmonary pleura are absent. It is possible that they may gain access via lymphatic vessels. Fibres that reach the superior and inferior tracheobronchial lymph nodes may pass via the anterior bronchomediastinal lymphatic vessels to the retrosternal lymph nodes and via the posterior vessels to the internal intercostal lymph nodes; from these sites they gain direct access to the intercostal lymphatic vessels that run along the upper and lower margins of the intercostal spaces below the surface of the pleura (von Hayek, 1960). Although this entails passage through

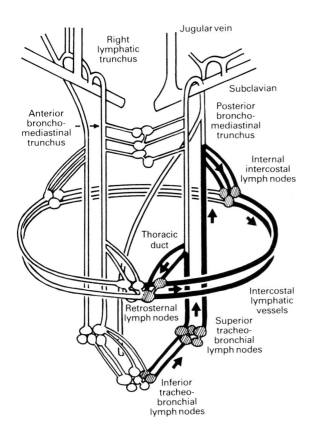

Right lymphatic trunchus

Jugular vein

Subclavian

Anterior broncho-mediastinal trunchus

Posterior broncho-mediastinal trunchus

Internal intercostal lymph nodes

Thoracic duct

Intercostal lymphatic vessels

Retrosternal lymph nodes

Superior tracheo-bronchial lymph nodes

Inferior tracheo-bronchial lymph nodes

Figure 14.19 Diagram of the thoracic lymphatic system. The hypothetical routes by which dust particles may be transported is shown by black vessels and arrows. (Adapted, with permission, from Taskinen, Ahlman and Wiikeri, 1973)

valves against the direction of normal flow, it is evidently possible, because coal dust can be demonstrated in these vessels in cases of coal pneumoconiosis (Taskinen, Ahlman and Wiikeri, 1973) and may be due to a 'suction pump' action during inspiration (Figure 14.19). A similar process could operate in the network of lymphatic vessels in the diaphragm.

The passage of mediators only has been suggested due to the rarity with which fibre penetration of the internal elastic lamina underlying the visceral pleura can be found (Dodson and Ford, 1985; Davis, 1989), whereas vacuolization and cystic hyperplasia can regularly be found in the mesothelial cells overlying collections of amphibole fibres in the lung adjacent to the internal lamina (Figures 14.20 and 14.21).

It is probable that all these hypotheses apply, each being responsible for one of the three pleural pathological states of plaque, mesothelioma and diffuse thickening with or without effusion, and all of which may occur in the same individual. The problem is to reconcile facts that include: that anthophyllite and, also, perhaps, coarse tremolite rarely cause mesotheliomas, but produce plaques in a high proportion of exposed subjects; the occurrence of peritoneal mesotheliomas; that plaques and pleural effusion may coexist in the same subjects; and that amphibole fibres are rarely detected in the pulmonary pleura, but experimental evidence suggests that considerable numbers are required to initiate a mesothelioma.

It has been noted that, even when fibres are abundant in the lungs, they are absent or very hard to find (Hourihane, 1964) in the pleural space or

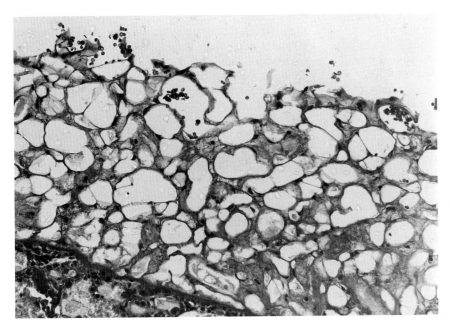

Figure 14.20 Area of degenerative visceral pleural surface of a rat lung 18 months after the end of exposure to long-fibre chrysotile. Many tissue spaces have been formed in a matrix of loose connective tissue, and these are lined with flattened cells of mesothelial type. The occurrence of this pleural metaplasia is related to the presence of advanced interstitial fibrosis in the lung and is common where patches of the parenchymal lesion have reached the surface (magnification × 245; haematoxylin and eosin). (Reproduced with permission from Davis, 1989)

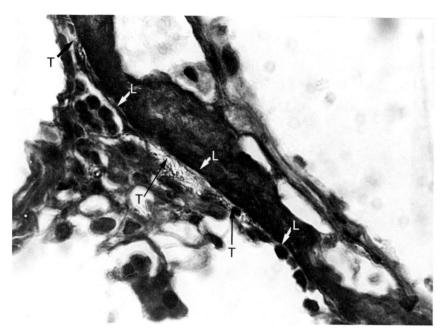

Figure 14.21 Areas from the surface of rat lungs treated with tremolite dust as seen by light microscopy with an oil immersion lens. Outside the internal elastic lamina of the lung (L), delineated by Weigert's elastin stain, is an area of vesicular pleural hyperplasia. Closely apposed to the inside of the lamina are deposits of tremolite fibres (T) (magnification × 480). (Reproduced with permission from Davis, 1989)

pulmonary pleura itself. This has been confirmed by recent animal studies using electron microscopy. Davis (1989) found virtually no fibre penetration of the internal elastic lamina of the visceral pleura even when fibres were abundant adjacent to it (Figure 14.21). Dodson and Ford (1985) observed fibres in the subpleural alveoli at all time periods from 2 hours to 3 months after intratracheal inoculation but, again, they never appeared to cross the internal elastic lamina. Holt (1983), confirming the migration of fibre towards the pleura (Morgan, Evans and Holmes, 1977), demonstrated the occasional passage of a fibre-bearing macrophage through the visceral pleura, and Viallat et al. (1986) found short fibres in the pleural space, after intratracheal injection of chrysotile. These observations are concordant with autopsy studies in human beings by Sebastien et al. (1979) in which they regularly found short chrysotile fibres in the parietal pleura, but only rarely amphibole fibres even when the latter had been the predominant occupational exposure.

The evidence therefore suggests, if we ignore the short chrysotile fibres as being non-pathogenic in the present context, that occasional amphibole fibres may cross the pleural space. The common sites for pleural plaques overlie the intercostal lymphatic pathways, but also coincide closely with

the sites of the Kampmeier foci (Herbert, 1986) which contain aggregates of macrophages, specialized mesothelial cells and stomata (Wang, 1975), the function of which appears to be to take up cells and large particles from the pleural space (Moalli et al., 1987). It is suggested that the rare insoluble amphibole fibre, too long to be transported onwards by macrophages, lodges in this region and causes, through the stimulus of mediators produced either by macrophages or the mesothelial cells themselves (Whitaker, Papadimitriou and Walters, 1982), the characteristic plaque reaction.

Sahn and Antony (1984) showed that injection of asbestos into the pleural cavity of healthy rabbits resulted in the development of pleural plaques following an exudative effusion, whereas in rabbits that had been made neutropenic the effusion was followed by pleural fibrosis. The latter reaction appeared to result from the failure of the neutropenic rabbits to develop an influx of macrophages. Both macrophages and healthy mesothelial cells (Herbert, 1986) possess considerable fibrinolytic activity, and it is probable that this accounts for the absence of adhesions and evidence of acute inflammatory response after the passage of very small numbers of fibres across the pleural space.

Damaged mesothelial cells, however, lose their capacity for fibrinolysis. Both Davis (1989), and

Dodson and Ford (1985), in the experiments cited above, noted areas of vacuolization, vesicular hyperplasia and degeneration in the visceral mesothelium overlying accumulations of fibre in the adjacent lung parenchyma. They, and Shore, Daughaday and Spilberg (1983), attribute these changes to the effect of mediators released by alveolar macrophages, and the resultant effusion, fibrosis and obliteration of the pleural space, found by Sahn and Antony (1984), could have its parallel in human experience. Diffuse pleural thickening and benign effusions usually occur in subjects with considerable cumulative exposure; more, that is, than seems to be necessary to initiate a plaque although not always so much as to be accompanied by asbestosis. Diffuse thickening has been shown to develop in subjects with pre-existing plaques (Miller, 1993), confirming two different modes of pathogenesis. The development of these types of pleural disease will be considered in more detail in the next two sections.

Neither of these models can, however, satisfactorily explain the development of peritoneal mesotheliomas, or the apparent paradox that coarse amphibole fibres, such as anthophyllite, readily produce plaques, and produce mesotheliomas by direct implantation in animal experiments, but rarely cause mesotheliomas in man (Tuomi et al., 1989). These, and other findings such as the proportionally greater effect of erionite by inhalation than by implantation (Davis, 1989), can only be readily explained by lymphatic transport of the fibre wholly or partially engulfed by macrophages (Harmsen et al., 1985) and the concomitant filtration effect (Oberdorster, Morrow and Spurny, 1988). They will be considered further in the section on mesothelioma.

There remains the question of whether genetic or immunological influences play any part. An increased frequency of plaques in close relations has been noted by Kiviluoto (1965), Rous and Studený (1970), Gibbs (1979) and Baris (1987), but it is not certain whether this merely represents common environmental rather than genetic factors. It may, however, be relevant that a similar situation exists for mesothelioma (Browne, 1983a). A hypothesis that immunological factors were important in the genesis of plaques was put forward by Kagan et al. (1977b) but support has not been forthcoming. Investigations into the prevalence of circulating ANAs and RFs in subjects with plaques, but without asbestosis, has not revealed any increase (Stansfield and Edge, 1974).

Clinical features

Whether calcified or not, pleural plaques alone are symptomless; dyspnoea, chest pain, abnormal physical signs and impairment of lung function are absent (Leathart, 1968; Lumley, 1977). In the absence of accompanying radiographic evidence of diffuse intrapulmonary fibrosis (asbestosis), regional lung function is normal. It has been suggested that, when they are very extensive, widely calcified and cuirass-like, there may be some restriction on movement of the chest wall with a mild degree of breathlessness on effort and restriction of ventilation. However, Ohlson et al. (1985) and McLoud et al. (1985) found no difference in respiratory function in subjects with or without plaques. Jarvholm and Sanden (1986) found a small impairment in men with plaques, but decided that the volume occupied even by large plaques was too small to affect results, and suggested that subclinical fibrosis was a more probable explanation. Schwartz et al. (1990) also found a small decrement in function associated with plaques after controlling for radiographic evidence of fibrosis, but accepted the possibility that those with plaques (who had a slightly longer exposure history) might have more DIPF within each category than those with normal pleura. Several other reports have appeared which are in agreement that, when large populations are studied, mean figures for lung volumes show a small but statistically significant deficit for those with plaques (Bourbeau et al., 1990; Brochard et al., 1993). Whether this is a true effect of plaques, however, remains uncertain because in addition to the explanations given by Jarvholm and Sanden, and by Schwartz et al., the difficulty in distinguishing between plaques and diffuse thickening is a further source of confounding. Because these cannot always be reliably differentiated, even by high-resolution CT, when confined to the lateral chest wall, most series classify any radiographic pleural thickening without obliteration of the costophrenic angle as plaques, and thereby include some cases of diffuse thickening (McLoud et al., 1985).

Radiographic appearances

Plaques are not visible radiographically until the thickness of their fibrous tissue or amount of calcium deposition is sufficiently radiodense. In many cases, therefore, they are not detected during life. However, the better the radiological technique and vigilance of the observer, the more likely they are to be seen. Hyaline plaques are demonstrated best by films taken at about 120 kV and calcified plaques by films taken at about 80 kV. In addition, right and left, 45 degree, anterior oblique views are an important complement to the PA film, for the detection and delineation of plaques both on the chest wall and diaphragm because they display many of them tangentially at maximum radiodensity which the PA film may fail to do (Anton, 1968) (see Chapter 7, page 167).

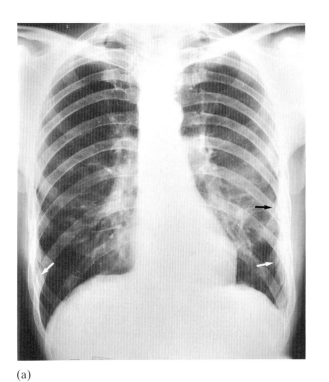

(a)

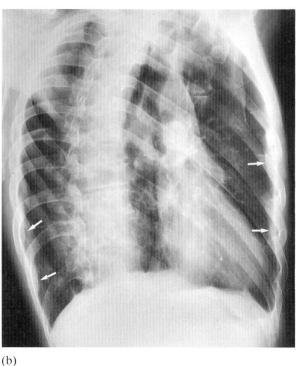

(b)

Figure 14.22 Mild hyaline plaque formation visible on both costal margins in the mid and lower zones. (a) The ill-defined haze in the left mid-zone is due to a plaque seen *en face* (see diagram). (b) Some of the plaques are shown in sharper relief when tangential to the X-ray beam in the right anterior oblique view. Calcifications are not evident in any of the lesions. No evidence of DIPF in either film. Insulation worker for 18 years before and after the Second World War

On the standard PA film, uncalcified plaques appear as ill-defined misty opacifications of the middle or lower zones of the lung fields when they lie at right angles, *en face*, to the X-ray beam; when they are more or less parallel to the beam, they appear as slightly to moderately protuberant linear or ovoid opacities along the costal or diaphragmatic margins, rarely extending vertically more than four interspaces, and not involving the apices or costophrenic angles (Fletcher and Edge, 1970; Sargent et al., 1978). As a rule these appearances are fairly obvious but slight *en face* haziness and small peripheral opacities (which have a tendency to be contiguous with and run along subcostal rims in the lower mid-zones) may easily be missed if the lung fields are not scrutinized systematically and oblique views omitted (Figure 14.22). 'Companion shadows' along the lateral chest walls caused by muscular interdigitations and the serratus anterior muscle or by folds of extrapleural costal fat, although uncommon, must be carefully distinguished from uncalcified plaques; they are usually bilateral, but not necessarily symmetrical, and their

similarity on the two sides is evident (see Chapter 7 for fuller discussion).

Calcified plaques *en face* have an irregular, unevenly dense and sometimes dramatic pattern ('holly leaf') which has neither a segmental nor a lobar distribution thus indicating their extrapulmonary site (Figures 14.23 and 14.24). Peripherally, they are seen as very opaque, usually discontinuous lines along the chest wall, diaphragm or cardiac border. In many cases, however, the opacities are small and easily overlooked (especially in too-white films) unless they are systematically sought. They are sometimes seen in the absence of any evidence of plaques on the chest wall. Care must be taken not to mistake calcified costal cartilages for plaques – in particular, when these are seen through the shadow of the diaphragm.

Bilateral calcified plaques may occasionally draw attention to unspecified (if mild) past asbestos exposure (Figure 14.25). However, it must also be emphasized that the appearances of both hyaline and calcified plaques can result from causes other than asbestos exposure (Figure 14.26).

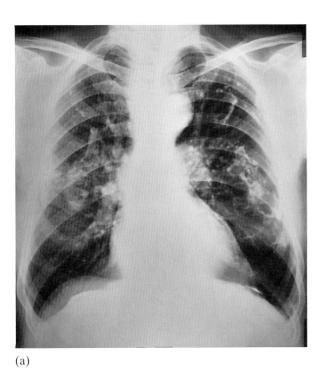

(a)

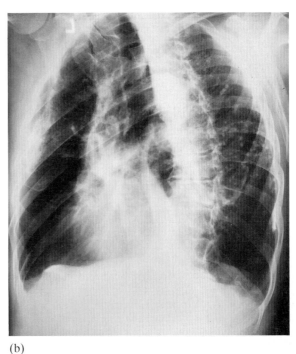

(b)

Figure 14.23 Bilateral calcified pleural plaques on chest walls and diaphragm. (a) Note irregular outline and variable density of the large lesion seen *en face* and the rim of calcification along the left cardiac border. The small rounded lesions also represent calcification in plaques and are not intrapulmonary. (b) The large plaque in the right lung field on the PA film is seen end-on against the chest wall (left field). No evidence of DIPF in either film. Ex-insulation worker (1925 to 1932) aged 65. No crackles in lungs. Lung function: severe airflow obstructions and hyperinflation only

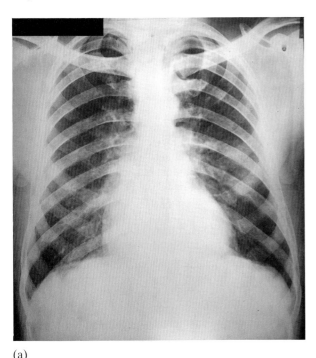

(a)

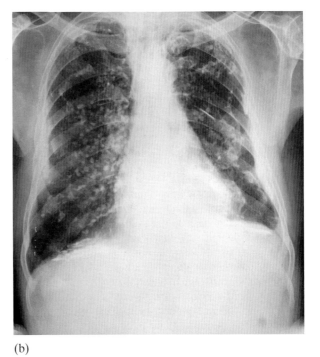

(b)

Figure 14.24 Development of widespread calcified plaques of different patterns in costal and diaphragmatic parietal pleura over 25 years: (a) 1948, (b) 1973. Asbestos insulation worker 40 years. Died aged 70. *Post mortem*: confirmed parietal pleural plaques. Gross evidence of intrapulmonary fibrosis absent but mild asbestosis demonstrated microscopically with numerous asbestos bodies

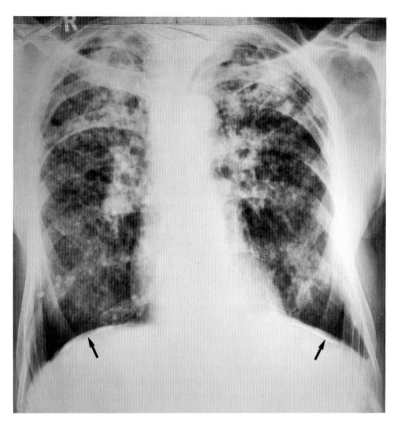

Fgure 14.25 Category 3rA silicosis in a crusher and grinder of flint and ochre ore for 8 years. This work was done on the same site as an asbestos-processing factory. Subsequently odd jobs brought him into close proximity with various parts of this factory for 20 years. Note the dense linear opacities indicative of calcifications in both leaves of the diaphragm (arrowed). Biopsy of lung 10 years before death showed numerous asbestos bodies and confirmed silicosis. *Post mortem*: calcified plaques present in both leaves of diaphragm and smaller plaques on the costal surfaces, but no asbestosis

Diagnosis

During life this rests entirely on radiographic evidence. Asbestos-related plaques are always bilateral but by no means of equal extent. Bilateral pleural calcification may also be the result of old tuberculous disease, empyema, traumatic haemothorax or other causes, but such changes are generally unilateral. Whether calcified or not plaques are distinguished by their sharp outline, when viewed tangentially, and by their absence from the costophrenic angles and apices of the lung fields. By contrast, diffuse pleural thickening is often ill-defined and irregular, irrespective of the angle from which it is viewed, and the costophrenic sulci are regularly obliterated.

Computed tomography is capable of detecting plaques in the lateral pleura which are invisible on conventional radiographs and may be useful in individual cases (Figure 14.27). But, as mentioned in

Chapter 7 (pages 168 and 194), a comparison of CT with four-view radiographs (PA, lateral and obliques), in a series of 127 asbestos workers, found the latter superior in detecting changes in the diaphragm and costophrenic angle (Bégin et al., 1984). However, high-resolution CT (HRCT) is helpful in diagnosing subpleural fat (a cause of wrong diagnosis in 10 to 20 per cent of patients thought to have plaques on plain radiography – Friedman et al., 1990) and prominent serratus anterior or external oblique muscles. Plaques in the paravertebral site are also better displayed by HRCT, on which, however, they may be mimicked by paravertebral veins (Friedman et al., 1990).

Prognosis and complications

Plaques themselves have no effect on life expectancy and are not known to give rise to any complications.

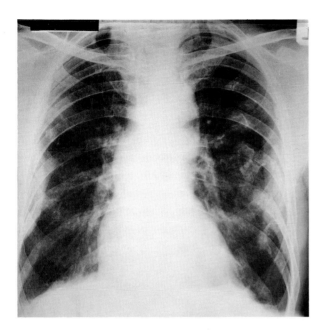

Figure 14.26 Bilateral hyaline and calcified plaques in a coal miner. No occupational exposure to asbestos. Such appearances may follow the resolution of bilateral pneumothoraces

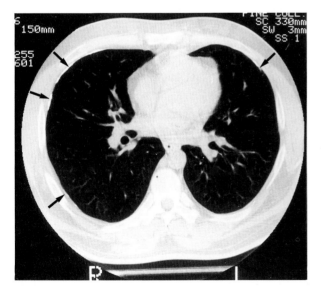

Figure 14.27 CT scan showing pleural plaques – calcified and hyaline. Lung is otherwise normal. (Courtesy of Dr D. Hansell)

In subjects followed radiologically, plaques may be observed to increase in size over a period of years in a proportion of subjects before becoming static. De Klerk et al. (1989b) reported no progress of plaques after the initial diagnosis in their cases; their diagnostic criteria may, however, have influenced this finding. Calcification may be first detected 10 or more years later and progresses in extent with age. Sheers (1979), following 256 dockyard workers with pleural changes over a period of 9 years found that, excluding those who developed an additional abnormality, only one-fifth of simple plaques increased in extent during this time, whilst rather more had begun to show evidence of calcification. Where calcification had been present initially, two-thirds showed an increase in extent of the calcified shadow.

It has been suggested that there may be evidence of an increase in lung cancer in individuals with pleural plaques. But the problem has always been to allow for the confounding effect of high exposures which tended to occur in the groups with plaques, and it is acknowledged that, in the studies of shipyard workers by Fletcher (1972) and Edge (1979), the effect could be readily explained by greater asbestos exposure. Gibbs (1979), after controlling for exposure, found that the mortality experience of Quebec chrysotile miners with plaques was the same as those without; a Finnish study failed to find any association between plaques and excess lung cancer (Kiviluoto, Meurman and Hakama, 1979) as did a study of Devonport dockyard employees (Sheers, 1979). Wain, Roggli and Foster (1984) carried out a study of consecutive autopsy cases with plaques but without asbestosis and found no increase in prevalence of lung cancer over controls, a finding identical to that of Thiringer et al. (1980). Harber, Mohsenifar and Oven (1987) also found that plaques were not an independent factor for asbestos-associated malignancy. However, perhaps most telling is the absence of excess mesotheliomas and lung cancers detected in any area of endemic plaques except Turkey, where the tremolite is believed to be of finer diameter. The reasons for this lie in the mode of pathogenesis. Although a malignant mesothelioma, which apparently arose from the surface of a plaque, has been reported (Lewinsohn, 1974), there is no evidence to suggest that plaques are precursors of this tumour and, indeed, Hourihane, Lessof and Richardson (1966) observed that plaques appeared to halt the continuous spread of tumour on the pleural surface where they coexisted.

Benign pleural effusion

After Eisenstadt (1965) reported a case of recurrent and otherwise unexplained bilateral effusion in an asbestos-exposed worker, several small series were published during the following decade suggesting that benign pleural effusion should be added to the established list of asbestos-related diseases. The initial difficulty was that diagnosis could only be made by exclusion of the other known causes, and because most collections of pleural effusions unrelated to asbestos exposure include a percentage, usually of the order of 5 to 10 per cent, in which no cause can be established (Chretien and Hirsch, 1983; Herbert 1986), asbestos could only be identified as an aetiological agent, on epidemiological grounds, by demonstrating an increased incidence.

This has now been established both among unselected clinic series and occupational studies. Mårtenssen et al. (1987) followed 99 females and 235 males with pleural effusions referred to the university clinic at Gothenburg because of previous inconclusive findings. All had chest radiographs, blood, sputum, pleural fluid and tissue analyses and a minimum 3-year follow-up. A definite cause was found in all except 7 of the 99 females, but 64 of the 235 males (27 per cent) were undiagnosed. Forty-two out of the 64 (66 per cent) gave a history of occupational exposure to asbestos, compared with 44 per cent of controls, and only two out of the seven females (29 per cent). In both exposed and non-exposed the effusion was blood-stained in about half of the cases, and eosinophils were present in a fifth. Hillerdal (1981), following up 891 patients with plaques and significant asbestos exposure in a general population, noted otherwise unexplained effusions in 22 (2.5 per cent). A positive diagnostic point was the presence of converging linear shadows or rounded atelectases.

Epler, McLoud and Gaensler (1982) found a prevalence of effusions of 4.7 per cent in a survey of 1135 exposed factory and shipyard workers, compared with 1 per cent among a control series. Nineteen cases (1.6 per cent) were attributable to known causes, leaving 35 cases (3.1 per cent) which fulfilled similar criteria to those of Mårtensson et al. (1987) and, in the absence of alternative explanations, were deemed to be due to asbestos. Lemenager et al. (1985) found 6 cases of pleural effusion (1.6 per cent) using similar criteria among 380 factory workers.

Lilis, Lerman and Selikoff (1988), examining nearly 3000 insulators with more than 30 years' asbestos exposure, obtained a definitive history of effusion in 20 (0.7 per cent). However, a feature of all the prevalence studies was that most effusions attributed to asbestos exposure were small; less than 20 per cent of those detected exceeded 500 ml. Epler, McLoud and Gaensler (1982) noted an increase in prevalence in their series with increasing exposure, and calculated annual incidence rates of 9 per 1000 employees with exposure graded high, 4 per 1000 graded medium and 1 per 1000 graded low.

Clinical features

Robinson and Musk (1981) noted pleuritic pain in two-thirds of their patients, but in prevalence surveys a majority of cases are found to be symptom free, with only the minority of larger effusions presenting with shortness of breath. A blood-stained effusion is found in about half the cases, irrespective of size, and in a smaller percentage the effusion is eosinophilic. The ESR is often, but not always, raised. Occasionally on presentation the effusion may be bilateral.

There is a clear impression among occupational physicians who have experience both of industrial groups exposed only to chrysotile and to amphibole or mixed fibres, that asbestos effusions, as for other pleural disease, are less common with chrysotile. One physician has seen no effusions in 6000 routine radiographs of workers exposed to low levels of chrysotile over a 6-year period, although in a small number obliteration of the costophrenic angle has been noted to have taken place between routine examinations (T.P. Goffe, 1988, personal communication).

Whilst most reported cases of asbestos pleural effusion have occurred late in subjects with prolonged exposure, both Robinson and Epler noted a small number appearing within 10 years of first exposure. The common progression to diffuse pleural thickening suggests a less effective host defence. However, a pleural effusion cannot be regarded as an alternative to plaques as a reaction to asbestos exposure, because both are frequently present at the same time, or alternatively either may develop before the other (Miller, 1993).

Prognosis

Asbestos-related effusions usually reabsorb spontaneously within a few months. Occasionally the radiograph may then revert to normal, but more often the costophrenic angle becomes blunted, with thickening of the visceral pleural. Due to this, and to the fact that so many effusions are small and asymptomatic, it is possible that the blunting of the angle which is often found to have taken place between one routine examination and the next is usually the sequel of an undetected effusion (particularly as an effusion has to exceed 200 ml to be detected radiologically). About one in every three or four subjects experiences a recurrence of the initial effusion, either on the same or the opposite side, and a small number may have multiple recurrences.

A proportion of subjects with loss of the costophrenic angle will have no further reaction, whilst others will develop widespread diffuse pleural thickening. This occurred in about half of the cases of Epler, McLoud and Gaensler (1982), but exposure appears to have been heavy, because more than 50 per cent were graded 1/0 or more for parenchymal small opacities. The proportion in other series was smaller, and development appears to depend on continued exposure, fibre type and host response.

Diffuse pleural thickening

Incidence

There are many causes of diffuse pleural thickening and, as with benign effusions, diagnosis of the asbestos-related disease is by elimination. Clarification, therefore, has had to wait on the evidence of surveys, aided, perhaps, by the great reduction in tuberculosis, formerly the most common cause. McLoud et al. (1985) found otherwise unexplained diffuse pleural thickening in 6.3 per cent of 1373 subjects occupationally exposed to asbestos compared with 0.1 per cent in a control group of university employees. Only in less than a quarter of these did it appear to be due to fibrotic extension to the pleura from asbestosis, and in two-thirds (4.2 per cent of all subjects) there was evidence of a previous effusion diagnosed either by paracentesis or by serial radiographs showing the sudden blunting of the costophrenic angle. This compared with a prevalence of pleural plaques of 16.5 per cent. Bohlig and Calavrezos (1987) studied 1204 German workers with at least 1 year's asbestos exposure. Prevalence of plaques (18 per cent) was very similar, but obliteration of the costophrenic angle was present in only 24 (2 per cent). However, they found diffuse pleural thickening of the middle and lower zones in 60 per cent of their exposed subjects and in 15 per cent of a non-exposed control population.

Other prevalence studies include that of Lemenager et al. (1985) who found a prevalence of 6 per cent of costophrenic angle obliteration (preceded in a quarter of the cases by an effusion) with no identifiable cause except their asbestos exposure, which averaged 22 years; Sheers and Templeton (1968) also found a prevalence of plaques of 21 per cent and of extensive diffuse pleural thickening in 5 per cent of the heavily exposed group of dockyard workers.

The British Thoracic and Tuberculosis Association and the MRC Pneumoconiosis Unit (1972) undertook a survey of patients with pleural abnormalities attending chest clinics, to find out in what proportion past exposure to asbestos was likely to be a factor. The increase in proportions of asbestos-exposed subjects over controls as assessed for the survey samples was small and not significant, leading to the conclusion that asbestos exposure was not an important cause of pleural change. Unfortunately, this survey suffered from three handicaps: first, pleural plaques, the most likely type to show a relationship with asbestos exposure, were not separately distinguished; secondly, cases with unilateral obliteration of the costophrenic angle were excluded (another group more likely to show a relationship); and, thirdly, the area chosen had little asbestos manufacturing or user industry. Consequently, the survey provides no information on the incidence of disease in the occupationally exposed.

Albeda et al. (1982) reviewed the chest radiographs of over 800 consecutive patients admitted to a hospital: 6.2 per cent had bilateral pleural thickening and, of these, 67 per cent had a history of asbestos exposure; when known non-asbestos aetiologies were excluded, the percentage increased to 81 per cent. Hillerdal (1981), in his clinic series referred to above, found progressive diffuse pleural thickening in 27 of his patients, in addition to 84 with obliteration of a costophrenic angle and a further 22 with pleural effusions, in all cases believed to be due to asbestos exposure. This incidence of 133 cases compared with 827 with pleural plaques, giving a ratio of approximately 1 : 6, was intermediate between that found by McLoud et al. (1985) and Bohlig and Calavrezos (1987).

Pathology and pathogenesis

In the early stages all that may be seen macroscopically is a slight diffuse loss of translucency, due to a thin layer of fibrosis over the lower half of the lungs. At a later stage, and where there has been resolution of an effusion, fibrosis is more widespread, with fusion of the visceral and parietal pleural layers (Sluis-Cremer and Webster, 1972). Occasionally this may develop into a thick layer 1 cm or more in depth covering the whole lung. Microscopically, the typical basket-weave fibrous structure may be seen with focal lymphatic connections (Stephens et al., 1987). But at times, unlike plaques, the fibrous layer may also be vascularized and consist of irregular bundles of non-hyalinized fibrous tissue (Craighead et al., 1982).

Thickening of the interlobar fissures is another manifestation of diffuse pleural thickening. Normally, the lesser (horizontal) interlobar fissure is the most readily seen, and is detectable in up to 50 per cent of normal radiographs in an unexposed population, the rate depending on radiological technique and the positioning of the patient. Solomon et al. (1979) used a standard film for reference, and found that the prevalence of thickened fissures increased from 2 per cent in amphibole miners with less than 7 years' exposure to 25 per cent with more than 15 years' exposure. Prevalence also increased with age as an independent variable. Rockoff et al. (1987)

graded fissures from 0 to 3, the lowest category (normal) being less than 0.5 mm throughout. Dose–response was evident only in the categories with thickening of more than 1 mm. Using lateral as well as PA radiographs, thickening of more than 1 mm of either the major or minor fissures was present in 55 per cent of their exposed subjects, compared with 16 per cent in the non-exposed control group. It was present in 85 per cent of subjects with asbestosis but only in 45 per cent of those without.

It is of interest that Rockoff et al. found a closer relationship with cumulative exposure for diffuse thickening than for plaques. This is in accord with the suggested pathogenesis. Subpleural accumulation of fibre would normally be directly related to cumulative exposure to amphibole and, hence, to the probability of degenerative changes in the overlying visceral pleura, whilst the rare penetration of individual fibres through the elastic lamina and across the pleural space appears less predictable and may, perhaps, depend more upon individual susceptibility.

Clinical effects

Unlike pleural plaques, diffuse thickening has been shown in several studies to have a potentially adverse effect on lung function which is exerted through its corset-like effect on the respiratory movements of the chest wall. As with plaques, however, the difficulty arises in separating the specific effects from those of early or radiologically undetectable asbestosis; this becomes a particular problem with diffuse thickening when, as commonly happens, it obscures the parenchyma in the radiograph.

Lumley (1977) did not demonstrate beyond doubt the decline in lung function which he attributed to pleural thickening. However, Wright et al. (1980), in a small number of subjects all but one of whom had CT scans, were able to show more convincingly that diffuse pleural fibrosis with normal lung parenchyma results in lowered lung volumes and gas transfer factor (TLCO), but a raised transfer coefficient (KCO). Compatible findings were reported in a large number of cases by McGavin and Sheers (1984) and McLoud et al. (1985) who confirmed their diagnosis with more detailed investigation, including serial films and histology. Schwartz et al. (1990), having controlled for age, smoking and category of radiographic small opacities, found that both plaques and diffuse thickening were associated with a reduction in the FVC but not in the FEV$_1$/FVC ratio, loss from diffuse thickening being twice that from plaques, although both might have been exaggerated by the presence of more interstitial fibrosis than in the controls.

Hillerdal (1984) determined the ESR in a number of patients with plaques, diffuse pleural thickening or diffuse interstitial fibrosis, or a combination of these. His conclusion was that only diffuse pleural thickening, particularly if bilateral, commonly resulted in a raised sedimentation rate. Pain is often complained of, and was an accompaniment of diffuse thickening in a fifth of the cases described by Lemenager et al. (1985).

Progression and prognosis

Unfortunately, few studies have distinguished between plaques and diffuse thickening in reporting on rates of attack (that is, first appearance of a pleural lesion) and progression following removal from exposure. Among chrysotile miners and millers, Becklake et al. (1979) found 20 per cent showed an increase in pleural abnormality in a follow-up period averaging 17 years, of whom 17 per cent experienced new lesions and the remaining 3 per cent progression of an existing lesion. Viallat and Boutin (1980) reported similar findings in Corsican miners; at the end of exposure 6.5 per cent had bilateral pleural changes, a percentage which rose to 27 per cent after 16 years' follow-up. Crocidolite miners were studied by de Klerk et al. (1989b); in men applying for pneumoconiosis compensation, approximately 50 per cent developed evidence of pleural disease, mainly diffuse. The main progression of the lesion occurred early after its first appearance, and no progression took place more than 15 years after the onset. Barnes (1986), following applicants for compensation over an average of 7.6 years, found the prevalence of diffuse thickening increased from 15 to 22 per cent during this period; this is in accord with Rossiter, Heath and Harries (1980) who found an increase of 11 per cent 9 years after removal from exposure. Suoranta et al. (1982) looked only at workers with asbestosis, and found that 28 per cent progressed during 4 years of observation; among those in whom asbestosis had progressed, 50 per cent showed an increase in pleural thickening compared with less than 20 per cent among those whose asbestosis was static. Finally Sheers (1979) found 11 new cases (1.1 per cent) of diffuse pleural thickening among 971 dockyard workers during the 11 years after the end of exposure. He also looked at mortality and found no excess of lung cancer compared with men with normal radiographs, and no increased incidence of mesothelioma when compared with men diagnosed as having pleural plaques.

Summarizing these observations, in men heavily exposed to asbestos and followed up for more than 15 years, about 20 per cent will be found to develop diffuse pleural thickening with or without accompanying parenchymal abnormality; most will have

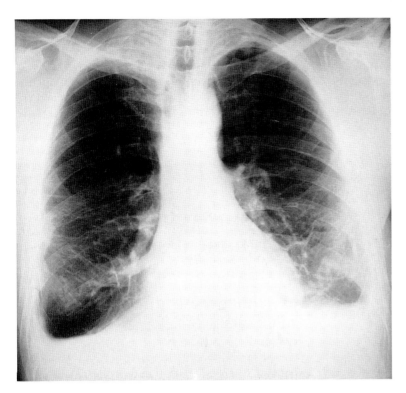

Figure 14.28 Bilateral diffuse pleural thickening: 52-year-old male who had worked for 34 years in the asbestos–cement industry. Many pleural streaks are visible. Parenchymal change is concealed by pleural shadow, but is probably not severe. Lung function showed a restrictive defect

occurred early in the observation period and the prevalence is much higher in subjects with progressing asbestosis. No evidence has appeared to suggest that diffuse pleural thickening in itself is likely to predispose to malignancy.

Diagnosis

Diffuse pleural fibrosis is a regular sequel of trauma and inflammation, and long-standing tuberculous pleurisy or empyema may be followed by gross thickening. It is, therefore, a much less specific indication of asbestos aetiology than plaques even in those who have been occupationally exposed. Other causes of diffuse thickening, with or without a preceding effusion, include other granulomatous diseases, rheumatoid and other autoimmune diseases, and a wide variety of drugs.

The pattern of asbestos-related pleural thickening was investigated by Bohlig and Calavrezos (1987), who compared its presence in 1204 workers with 622 controls. Their conclusions were that bilateral symmetrical involvement of the middle zone was the most frequent sequel of asbestos exposure. Apical pleural thickening (defined as more than 5 mm in thickness) was discussed by Hillerdal (1990), who found it was present in only 40 of 1600 subjects with asbestos-related pleural change. In all but one of the cases, it was part of a generalized pleural thickening which was progressive in all cases followed over 5 years. This is in contrast to two cases reported by Oliver and Neville (1988) in which thickening was confined to the apical region, and for which there appeared no good reason to attribute it to their minimal asbestos exposure. Hillerdal found that the correlation with exposure was poor, and suggested that his cases were examples of a serous 'pleuroparenchymatous lesion'.

These last points are important. Cryptogenic bilateral fibrosing pleuritis has been described by Buchanan et al. (1988) and this may be one variant of the 'pachypleurites cryptogeniques' of Clavier et al. (1976), and of the 'hyalinosis complicata' referred to in writings from eastern Europe (Navratil et al., 1986) and of sclerosing fibrosis (Kittredge, 1974). Buchanan identified two groups: those presenting with effusions progressing to diffuse thickening but retaining normal lung parenchyma, and those without effusion who had additional infiltration of the lung. The parallel with asbestos-related disease is of interest. In rapidly progressing cases, it certainly seems that an abnormal host response is the major factor, and the presence of asbestos either acts as a trigger or is merely coincidental. The three cases of progressive pericardial fibrosis in subjects with only a 'moderate degree of asbestos exposure' reported by Davies, Andrews and Jones (1991) would appear to fall into this category.

Radiology

Indications of asbestos aetiology in cases of bilateral diffuse pleural thickening are the presence of fissural lines and numerous linear opacities (Zivy, 1981), together with 'infolding' and 'pseudotumour' formation (Blesovsky, 1966; Mintzer and Cugell, 1982; Hillerdal, 1989). These, however, are only present at an advanced stage.

Differences to be sought include the following (Fletcher and Edge, 1970; Sargent et al., 1984).

Diffuse pleural thickening

The costophrenic angle is obliterated in a majority of cases (Figure 14.28). In profile, the medial margin may be sharp, widening inferiorly and becoming more tapered superiorly. *En face*, it may appear as a veil-like shadow without perceptible borders, and may obscure the borders of the heart and diaphragm. The margin may be relatively concave at the point of fusion with the obliterated costophrenic angle.

Pleural plaques

Pleural plaques do not normally involve apices or costophrenic angles. The onset may be unilateral, but later they are usually bilateral but asymmetrical.

In profile, a sharply outlined convex medial surface will be seen, giving a lobulated appearance when multiple.

On a PA film, a plaque will usually be seen partly in profile and partly *en face*; the shadow will then fade as it passes posteromedially.

As indicated earlier, plaques must be distinguished from subpleural fat pads. These are normally of symmetrical and midthoracic distribution, do not obliterate the costophrenic angles – although fat pads are sometimes present in the cardiophrenic angles – and often cause the apical pleura to appear thickened (Gluck et al., 1972). The serratus anterior muscle may also cause a lateral haze in the region of the fifth and sixth ribs which is not infrequently queried as intrathoracic disease (Collins, Brown and Batia, 1983). Where doubt arises on a PA film, the

issue will usually be settled by oblique films. Occasional cases may require HRCT for a final decision; the sensitivity is undoubtedly superior, although misinterpretation and over-diagnosis may still arise (Friedman et al., 1990). (These important normal variants are discussed in Chapter 7, under 'The soft tissues'.)

Asbestos-related malignant disease

The pathogenesis of asbestos-related malignancy

A great amount of time and money has been expended in an effort to demonstrate carcinogenic properties in asbestos. But being chemically inert has always been one of its industrial virtues, and, perhaps as a natural consequence, asbestos has proved not to be a mutagen. Much ingenuity has been exercised in in vitro studies to induce malignant transformation, but most merely produce cell or chromosomal damage and the remainder do not appear to have direct application to exposure in human beings (Mossman et al., 1990; Voytek et al., 1990). Nearly all fail to explain the lack of effect of fibres of less than 5 µm in length, why the carcinogenicity appears to be a general property of a range of fibres of different chemical composition, why durability is a prerequisite (Pott, 1987), or why the pathological effects are limited to three, namely interstitial fibrosis, lung cancer and mesothelioma. Asbestos was, however, shown to be capable of acting as a classic tumour promoter (Topping and Nettlesheim, 1980), although classic tumour promotion is associated with a threshold below which no response occurs.

Parallel with this research, an understanding of the importance of the macrophage has taken place, demonstrating its essential role as an intermediary in the pathogenesis of all asbestos-related disease, and showing the search for direct carcinogenic effects of asbestos to be misconceived. Incomplete ingestion of long asbestos fibres, resulting in the liberation of macrophage mediators, including proteolytic enzymes, superoxide tissue damaging agents and growth promotion factors, into the adjacent tissues was discussed earlier in connection with the genesis of interstitial fibrosis (pages 428–429).

The next step, the transition from tissue damage and growth promotion to malignant transformation, is one for which there is abundant experimental evidence. Scar cancers, the development of malignant change adjacent to chronic granulomatous tissue, have been recognized for a very long time, particularly in relation to the lung (Spencer, 1985), but the tendency has been to regard this as being too rare a phenomenon to be applicable to asbestos-related disease. This view fails to recognize the peculiar chronicity of the fibre–macrophage interaction, particularly with indestructible amphibole fibre. That inert foreign bodies can cause malignancy – the Oppenheimer effect or solid-state carcinogenesis – is established; this effect also probably results from macrophage action (Brand, 1986). In the case of heavy asbestos exposure, there is chronic continuing stimulation of both fibroblast and epithelial proliferation. Chronic tissue proliferation is now accepted as a major factor in oncogenesis, 'mitogenesis leading to mutagenesis' (Ames and Gold, 1990; Cohen and Ellwein, 1990), by multiplying the potential for copying errors arising in DNA, and perhaps by defeating the normal mechanism whereby the original DNA is preserved at stem-cell division and the copy, which may contain errors, passes to the expendable daughter cell. This sequence is well established in oncology (Cairns, 1975; Slack, 1986; Editorial, 1989; Browne, 1991a). Destruction of normal tissue architecture, particularly in the case of lung epithelium, appears also to be an important element in predisposing to malignancy (Cairns, 1975), and the transition has been demonstrated experimentally in asbestos-exposed rats (Wagner, Berry and Timbrell, 1973; Davis et al., 1986a).

The similarity between asbestos-related diffuse interstitial pulmonary fibrosis (DIPF) and that of cryptogenic fibrosing alveolitis must not be overlooked. It has been shown by Turner-Warwick et al. (1980) and others that cryptogenic fibrosing alveolitis also carries a high risk of lung cancer. The DIPF in this disease is also macrophage mediated, with the production of a comparable excess of growth factors and other cytokines (Du Bois, 1990) and resultant fibrosis accompanied by disorganized proliferation of alveolar epithelium.

In the pleura and peritoneum, the target organ on which the fibre acts is almost certainly the subserosal stem cell (Davis, 1979; Editorial, 1989). The experiments listed in the discussion on the pathogenesis of asbestosis also failed to produce any excess mesotheliomas or lung tumours with fibres less than 5 μm long, even with direct intrapleural or peritoneal injection, and even with erionite which has appeared to have the greatest potency for producing mesothelioma. The absence of persisting inflammation after the peritoneal injection of short crocidolite fibre has been demonstrated by Moalli et

al. (1987). Inflammation appears to be a prerequisite for tumour induction by direct injection (Stanton, Layard and Tegeris, 1981; Suzuki and Kohyama, 1984), and Davis (unpublished observation) has found that more mesotheliomas are produced for a given quantity of fibre if it is injected into the peritoneum in divided doses (thereby creating more inflammation) than if it is injected as a single dose. The chronic inflammation is initiated and organized by macrophages following their incomplete ingestion of long fibres and is accompanied by the production of excess growth factors in the manner outlined earlier (page 429). Its persistence with long but not short fibres has been demonstrated by Moalli et al. (1987), and Goodglick and Kane (1990), involving the same mechanism as that by which asbestosis is produced. Finally, the inflammatory response of implanted fibre and its progress towards malignant change has been traced by TEM in the rat omentum (Friemann et al., 1987; Hill, Edwards and Cathew, 1990; Friemann, Muller and Pott, 1990).

Diffuse malignant mesothelioma of pleura and peritoneum

The early recognition of asbestos-related mesothelioma was obscured by doubts about the very existence of mesothelioma itself. The early literature, reviewed by Robertson (1924), included a reference to a possible case description in a 15-year-old boy by Lieutaud in 1767, and many probable cases throughout the nineteenth century, of which, in the light of present knowledge, those of E. Wagner (1870) appear to be the earliest in which confidence can be placed. But Robertson himself did not believe there was such an independently identifiable tumour, and his doubts were shared by Willis (1960) in his influential textbook.

Nevertheless, the diagnosis of 'endothelioma' continued to be made, and a link with asbestos was suggested by Wedler in 1943. Subsequently sporadic cases (reviewed by Enterline, 1978) were published and the diagnosis appeared on the death certificates of many more asbestos workers, but the link was not firmly established until the report of 33 cases among people with industrial or environmental contact with crocidolite in the north-west Cape Province of South Africa (Wagner, Sleggs and Marchand, 1960).

Prevalence and incidence

Data on mesothelioma cases in the UK are entered on a mesothelioma register, which is based on death certificate data supplemented by information from regional cancer registers, the Department of Health and Social Security and the Health and Safety Executive. For 1984, 535 deaths from mesothelioma were recorded in men and 82 in women. These figures represent death rates of 20 and 3 per million respectively (Jones, Smith and Thomas, 1988). In the following 5 years numbers have continued to increase, deaths from mesothelioma in 1989 totalling 853. The ratio of pleural to peritoneal sites has been approximately 10 : 1 in males and 5 : 1 in females.

Figures for the USA are available based on a 10 per cent sample of the population. For the years 1973–1984 the death rate for males was 11.4 per million per year and for females 2.8, with pleural to peritoneal ratios 9 : 1 and 2 : 1 (Spirtas et al., 1986; Connelly et al., 1987). Comparable figures for Denmark (Andersson and Olsen, 1985) and Canada (McDonald, 1985) have also appeared.

An important feature of the published figures is the age-adjusted incidence rates. The UK pattern is shown in Figure 14.29 which demonstrates no increase in incidence for females under 55 years and for males under 45 years over the last 20 years. A similar picture appears in the US, Canadian and Danish data. This finding has implications both for the effect of environmental exposures and background levels of mesothelioma incidence, discussed below.

Pleural : peritoneal ratio

A wide range of ratios between these two sites for mesothelioma has appeared in published series (Browne and Smither, 1983). Two factors make comparison difficult: misdiagnosis particularly in relation to peritoneal cases, and differing proportions of occupational to background cases, because in most but not all series of occupationally related mesotheliomas pleural cases predominate, whereas in background cases it is probable that the ratio approximates to 2 : 1.

The reasons for the differing proportions within industrial populations are uncertain. In a detailed examination of one large industrial series, Browne and Smither (1983) found that peritoneal cases were slightly more likely to have had higher levels of exposure for longer periods than the pleural cases, but the differences were not great. The clearest relationship was with era. Cases with first exposure prior to 1920 had a 1 : 5 pleural-to-peritoneal ratio;

this showed a continuous change over four subsequent time periods, until those exposed after 1951 had a 3 : 1 pleural predominance. It was suggested that the high levels of other dusts present in the earlier years may have predisposed to peritoneal cases by an effect on lymphatic drainage; this would particularly apply where interstitial fibrosis at the lung bases might disrupt the normal pattern of drainage to the periphery of the lung and onward to regional lymph nodes, and divert flow through diaphragmatic lymphatics.

The other major series in which peritoneal have exceeded pleural cases, the North American insulation workers, also included high levels of mixed dust and of asbestosis (Ribak et al., 1988) and found differences comparable to those from the East London factory, although a cohort effect was not looked for. In series with lower average exposures, and particularly those in which exposure has been to chrysotile with small proportions of amphibole, mesotheliomas, when occurring, have been almost invariably pleural (Albin et al., 1990b).

The influence of fibre type

Differences in the liability of fibre types to cause mesothelioma were already evident by the mid-1960s and a voluntary ban by UK manufacturers ended the use of crocidolite in Britain in 1969. Since then the major difference between chrysotile and the amphiboles has been confirmed beyond reasonable doubt in epidemiological and experimental studies (Dunnigan et al., 1988).

The epidemiological evidence is clear-cut (McDonald and McDonald, 1987a; Langer and Nolan, 1989; Liddell, 1989; McDonald and McDonald, 1991) and, because mesothelioma is a rare tumour in the non-occupationally exposed, differences in cohorts may be most easily assessed by differences in proportional mortality. In chrysotile miners and millers two studies have shown this to be 0.3 per cent (Rubino et al., 1979b; McDonald et al., 1980) whilst in crocidolite miners the figure was 3.9 per cent (Armstrong et al., 1988) and in vermiculite–tremolite miners 2.4 per cent (McDonald et al., 1986). In textile manufacture, proportional mortality for chrysotile workers was 0 (Weiss, 1977) and 0.2 (McDonald et al., 1983a), whilst in a comparable factory where crocidolite and amosite were also used the figure was 1.6 per cent (McDonald et al., 1983b). In manufacture of friction materials no mesotheliomas were found in a factory using only chrysotile (McDonald et al., 1984), whereas in a factory in which a small amount of crocidolite was used proportional mortality was 0.6 per cent (Berry and Newhouse, 1983; Newhouse and Sullivan, 1989). No mesotheliomas occurred in three asbestos–cement plants

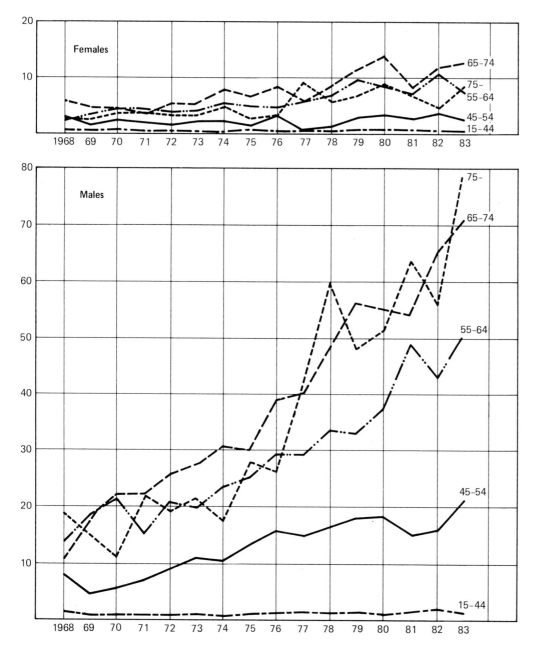

Figure 14.29 Mesothelioma age- and sex-specific death rates (per million), the United Kingdom and Ireland (total pleural and peritoneal). (Reproduced with permission from Jones, Smith and Thomas, 1988)

using only chrysotile (Gardner and Powell, 1986), whereas all asbestos–cement cohorts of workers exposed to appreciable quantities of amphiboles have included some deaths from mesothelioma, ranging from 1 per cent (Neuberger and Kundi, 1990) to 15.7 per cent (Finkelstein, 1984). Finally, among women assembling gas masks in three factories using crocidolite filter pads, proportional mortalities were 16 per cent (McDonald and

McDonald, 1978), 10 per cent (J.S.P. Jones et al., 1980) and 2.3 per cent (Acheson et al., 1982); however, at a factory where only chrysotile pads were used, only one mesothelioma occurred among 177 deaths and this woman was believed to have worked previously in a factory assembling crocidolite pads (Acheson et al., 1982).

Studies of lung fibre burdens are also strongly indicative of a difference between amphiboles and chrysotile. The evidence concerning the persistence of long amphibole fibres in human lungs and the disappearance of chrysotile has been discussed above, and studies of mesothelioma cases and controls have shown that in occupationally exposed cases there has been a considerable excess in amphibole fibre retained in the lungs, but not of chrysotile. In the case of chrysotile miners (Rowlands, Gibbs and McDonald, 1982; Churg et al., 1984) and certain textile (Sebastien et al., 1989) and asbestos–cement workers (Albin et al., 1990a), considerable quantities of fibrous tremolite have been found in the lungs at autopsy despite the fact that it only appeared as a contaminant and probably never exceeded a concentration of 1 per cent of the total fibre. As a consequence, the possibility has been raised that tremolite has been responsible for the small number of cases of mesothelioma in chrysotile workers. The evidence has been reviewed by Churg (1988b) and McDonald et al. (1988), who both concluded that some of these mesotheliomas, but not necessarily all, may have been produced by the contaminating tremolite.

Much of the objection to regarding chrysotile as less likely to cause mesotheliomas than the amphiboles has arisen out of a misinterpretation of experimental data. Animal experiments appeared to show that when equal amounts of chrysotile and crocidolite were administered by inhalation or by implantation, the former produced at least as many and possibly rather more tumours than the latter. However, dosage was by equal weight of fibre. The work of Stanton (1973) and Pott (1978) has shown the importance of fibre dimensions and when fibre numbers in the relevant size range were looked at by electron microscopy (Davis et al., 1978), it was found that the number of fibres in the chrysotile sample were many times – more than two orders of magnitude in one recent study (Coffin et al., 1988) – that of crocidolite per unit mass. Experimental evidence, discussed earlier (page 427) in relation to the pathogenesis of asbestosis, has shown that fibres shorter than 5 μm are little or no more pathogenic than particulate dust, confirming the importance of counting only numbers of long fibres in assessing tumour genesis.

Within the amphibole group, there is a definite gradient of risk from crocidolite, through amosite, to anthophyllite. Liddell (1989) found a proportional mortality of 6.6 per cent for cohorts exposed only to crocidolite and 2.9 per cent for amosite; anthophyllite was thought at one time not to have produced any mesotheliomas, but some cases (probably due to this fibre) have recently been reported (Tuomi et al., 1989). A similar gradient appears in injected animals, and is almost certainly related to fibre diameters.

Short-term in vitro studies have shown that fibre length is important for exerting a toxic effect on macrophages (Forget et al., 1986), and also on epithelial cells, perhaps because longer fibres overlap cell boundaries and lie on the cell surfaces instead of becoming membrane bound and passing into the cell (Jaurand, 1989). However, in addition to immediate effects, durability is important. Pott (1987) has recently suggested that for a fibre to be classed as fibrogenic it should, in addition to its dimensional characteristics, also be capable of persisting in tissue for more than 3 years. As discussed in the next section, although solubility in tissue is likely to be the same in rat as in human tissues, the time taken for tumour to develop is less than one-tenth in the rat, so that the solubility of chrysotile could, perhaps, affect the rat and yet dissolve in human tissue before the stage of production of disease is reached.

The latent period

A feature of asbestos-related mesothelioma is the long interval between first exposure to asbestos and the onset of symptoms. Because the duration of illness is brief, it is customary to take the time from first exposure to death as the latent period. In series with adequate follow-up, the mean latent period is consistently between 35 and 40 years. Latent periods of less than 20 years are unusual, and *the shortest latent period in an industrial cohort is 14 years* (Browne, 1983b). Occasional cases are reported with shorter periods, but on investigation evidence of earlier exposure, or none, can usually be identified, for example, the maintenance worker in the series of Peto et al. (1985) with an apparent 10-year latency who was found at autopsy to have calcified plaques – evidence of much earlier exposure; or the case reported by Booth and Weaver (1986) which subsequent correspondence revealed to have probably been spontaneous. Unfortunately, it is often impossible to obtain a complete early history and, consequently, reliance must be placed only on evidence from fully documented cohorts. In keeping with this, the youngest person known to have died of mesothelioma in the erionite area around Karain where exposure would have begun at birth was over 20 years old (Y.I. Baris, 1991, personal communication).

An interesting aspect of the latent period is the finding in animal experiments involving implantation of asbestos or other fibres in the pleura or peritoneum (Brand, 1986; Pott, 1987; Davis, 1989; Hill, Edwards and Cathew, 1990) that, as the dose of fibre is reduced, the latent period before the appearance of tumours lengthens, so that, below a certain critical level, the latent period extends beyond the animal's natural lifespan, and no tumour is produced. This is in accord with the mechanism of pathogenesis outlined on page 470, because increased fibre numbers result in a quantitative increase in macrophage numbers and consequent cytokine production. There is a suggestion, in the few studies that provide relevant information, that the same may be true for workers exposed to asbestos. This would require that the dose reaching the pleura or peritoneum be proportional to the inhaled dose, for which there is no evidence either for or against. If true, however, it would have important implications for environmental or low-dose occupational exposures.

Tumours with long latency periods are found normally not to develop host rejection responses because of their inability to express tumour-associated transplantation antigens, and this has been shown to be the case in both human and rat asbestos-related mesotheliomas (Whitaker, Papadimitriou and Walters, 1982).

Mesothelioma unrelated to asbestos exposure

Due to the universality of asbestos in the environment, from natural deposits as well as human activities, and because it can always be found in human lungs at autopsy if looked for diligently, the suggestion has been made that all cases of mesothelioma may be caused by asbestos or other mineral fibres. If this were true it would be unique among tumours, because there is no other tumour to which only one single cause is invariably ascribed. However, there are several reasons for rejecting the suggestion: *first*, mesothelioma occurs in a wide range of vertebrates both wild and domesticated, from fish and chickens to monkeys and leopards (Ilgren and Wagner, 1991); *secondly*, mesothelioma has occurred at all ages from infancy onwards (Mirabella, 1986; Fraire et al., 1988; Lin-Chu, Lee and Ho, 1989; Kane, Chahinian and Holland, 1990), and because no mesothelioma caused by environmental fibre in Turkey has been found in residents under the age of 20 years (in keeping with the minimum latent period established in occupationally exposed cases), these childhood cases must fall into the spontaneous category; and *finally*, the flat pattern of annual incidence for adults under 45 years shown in the UK, the USA and Denmark, and for women in Canada, is evidence that the greatly increased use of amphibole asbestos since the 1940s has not been the cause of environmentally related mesothelioma.

Evidence for a separate frequency distribution of mesothelioma cases among subjects with no identifiable asbestos exposure was found by Hirsch et al. (1982) in France and by Peto, Henderson and Pike (1981) in Los Angeles. Characteristics of these groups, additional to an absent history of exposure, were a more nearly equal sex ratio, a younger average age, and a longer survival period from first symptoms to death. This was also found by Law et al. (1983). The frequency of spontaneous mesothelioma has been estimated to be about 1 or 2 per million per year, or about 1 or 2 in every 10 000 deaths (McDonald and McDonald, 1987a).

Mesothelioma has developed after exposure to a variety of non-fibrous agents (Peterson, Greenberg and Buffler, 1984; Pelnar, 1988). In human beings, these include ionizing radiation, a variety of chemicals, and chronic inflammatory lung disease (Hillerdal and Berg, 1985); in animals, they include viruses, hormones and other drugs. A possible occupational cause may exist among sugarcane workers as cane residue may be fibrous (Newman, 1986), and in furniture workers (Minder and Vader, 1988). Environmental exposure to the non-asbestos fibrous zeolite, erionite, as a cause of mesothelioma, is now well established through the pioneer observations of Baris (Baris et al., 1987) (see Chapter 16).

Dose–response

The paucity of information on dose in cases of occupational mesothelioma has the result that it is impossible to derive an accurate model relating risk to quantitative measures of dust exposure. However, there are several indications that no simple formula will give a complete picture.

Peto suggested that, analogous with the situation of continuing cigarette smokers, mesothelioma risk for exposed workers rises proportionally to the third or fourth power of time from first exposure (Peto, Seidman and Selikoff, 1982). This implies continuing exposure, because it is known that risk for cigarette smokers declines after ceasing to smoke, and is justified in the case of workers exposed to amphibole on the grounds that the inhaled fibre is retained in the lungs for life. (Consequently, it should be noted that it cannot, therefore, apply to chrysotile.) The Peto formula is: mesothelioma incidence $= b \times t^{3.2}$ (subsequently amended to $b \times (t - 10)^{3.2}$ to take account of the latent period; Hughes and Weill, 1986) where t is time since first exposure and b is a constant varying with cumulative exposure and, perhaps, fibre type.

The formula has been applied to give expected rates for five industrial series without, it must be said, any very impressive agreement, although a reasonable fit was obtained with UK naval dockyard workers (Sullivan, Lam and Rossiter, 1988) and for environmental erionite exposure in Karain (Saracci et al., 1982). But the implication of the constant *b* is that, for a given time since first exposure, a linear relationship exists between dose and risk. There is much evidence that this is not the case. Both J.S.P. Jones et al. (1980) and Enterline, Hartley and Henderson (1987) commented that no simple relationship appeared between risk and duration of exposure or cumulative dose in their series. The same was also true of Barking (UK) workers (Browne, 1983a). There are two indications that the process by which fibre inhalation influences the development of mesothelioma occurs for most subjects soon after the onset of exposure (even allowing for the fact that if risk is proportional to the third or fourth power of time, later exposures will contribute correspondingly less to risk than previously). First, an examination of series for which the data are available shows that the average latency time is approximately the same for both short-term and long-term workers (Browne and Smither, 1983; Mowe et al., 1984; Peto et al., 1985). Secondly, with heavy exposures there appears to be little or no further increase in relative risk after 2 years' exposure (Seidman, Selikoff and Hammond, 1979; Browne, 1983a; Armstrong et al., 1988). These findings may be related to the effect of dose on the latent period, discussed earlier.

In addition, it is probable that a threshold exposure exists below which there is no risk of mesothelioma both for animals and human beings (Ilgren and Browne, 1991; Liddell, 1993). An exposure as brief as 3 weeks has been reported; this involved very heavy exposure spinning crocidolite in 1927 (Browne, 1983a) and, recently, a mesothelioma has occurred in a gas-mask worker who is reported to have been employed in this work for only 2 weeks in 1942 (Jones, 1987; Jones, 1990, personal communication) but her lung fibre burden of crocidolite was very high, being close to the median count by the same laboratory for unselected cases of occupational mesothelioma. In other series of pure amphibole exposure (Seidman, Selikoff and Hammond, 1979; Hobbs et al., 1980), and in the other Nottingham gas-mask workers (Jones et al., 1980) no case has resulted from less than 5 months' exposure; similarly, in other series, the briefest recorded exposures have been 3 months (Hughes, Weill and Hammad, 1987) and 5 fibres/ml years (Neuberger and Kundi, 1990) (as defined earlier, page 416). Considerably higher levels of tremolite have been found in the lungs of residents of Thetford (Canada) (Churg, 1986; Sebastien et al., 1989) and those of chrysotile textile workers without any apparent increase in the mesothelioma rate. A mortality study with 20 to 50 years' follow-up of workers exposed to low-dose crocidolite found no mesotheliomas among 247 deaths (Newhouse et al., 1988). In implantation experiments in animals both Davis (1989) and Pott (1987) have found that a minimum number of long fibres – of the order of 100 000 – is required to produce mesothelial tumours. It is probable that a certain threshold intensity of exposure must be passed in addition to a total cumulative threshold. This is consistent with the probable pathogenesis.

Pathogenesis

Reasons for believing that mesothelioma arises from fibre reaching the parietal pleural and peritoneal tissues via the lymphatic system were given in discussion of the pathogenesis of pleural disease (page 452). Hence, there are two separate aspects of pathogenesis, both of which need clarification: the passage of the fibre to the mesothelial tissues, and the action of the fibre when it reaches the target site.

Most fibres probably pass through the lymphatic system wholly or partially ingested by macrophages (Corry, Kulkarni and Lipscomb, 1984; Harmsen et al., 1985). Their passage is influenced first by their dimensions. It is probable that the maximum length and diameter of fibres able to make the passage are low (Oberdorster, Morrow and Spurny, 1988). Timbrell (1990) gave evidence to suggest that the difference in mesothelioma risk between crocidolite, amosite and anthophyllite depends on the proportions of fibres less than 0.1 μm in diameter. He related this to Stanton's (1973) finding that the mesothelioma-producing potential of asbestos in implantation experiments appeared to depend on decreasing fibre diameter as well as on increasing length. However, as Peto (1989) pointed out, in a given weight of fibre, thicker diameters imply smaller numbers and, if the likelihood of tumours is a function of fibre numbers over a certain length, no deduction can be made from Stanton's work about relative pathogenicity of different fibre diameters. Timbrell's evidence regarding the critical fibre diameter of less than 0.1 μm is, therefore, probably to be interpreted as being related to the passage of fibres through the lymphatic system to the parietal pleura.

The passage of fibres is probably influenced by the state of macrophage activation. Whilst the passage of short fibres may be facilitated by complete ingestion by macrophages, it is probable that longer fibres may be retained in the interstitial lung tissue and the regional lymph nodes when ingestion is incomplete. It follows that passage of fibres more than 8 μm long through the regional nodes to the parietal pleura or peritoneum may only take place when the lung macrophages are swamped by a high concentration of fibre either through inadequate activation, or where this has been depressed – for example by intercurrent infection.

Large quantities of fibre have not been found in the parietal pleura, and most of what is found has been short chrysotile. However, in 1 case out of the 29 studied by Sebastien et al. (1979), significant quantities of amosite were found, and smaller quantities in other cases, whilst Dodson et al. (1990) found amphibole fibres, 8 per cent of which were more than 10 μm in length in pleural plaques from shipyard workers. Yet quite small quantities of an insoluble fibre may be sufficient to cause malignant change if the fibres become embedded in optimum sites. Unlike epithelial cells which have evolved to sustain continuing trauma, mesothelial cells are not normally exposed to chronic insult, and can be shown experimentally to be much more readily transformed than those of the epithelium.

Once it reaches the target tissue of submesothelial stem cells, inflammatory and ultimately malignant change may follow (Friemann, Muller and Pott, 1990; Hill, Edwards and Cathew, 1990) through the mechanism discussed earlier (see page 465).

It is a noteworthy feature of mesothelioma that even the heaviest exposures have caused the proportional mortality to exceed 10 per cent in only two series, in both of which numbers were relatively small (McDonald and McDonald, 1987a). It is known that mesothelioma occurs significantly more frequently in first-degree relations but not in spouses, suggesting an inherited susceptibility. This appears to be true of both asbestos- and erionite-related and spontaneous cases (Browne, 1983a; Baris, 1987; Hammar et al., 1989; Dawson et al., 1992). No specific chromosomal abnormality has been implicated although chromosome 3 rearrangement has been found in a considerable proportion (Gibas et al., 1986), and an abnormality associated with the short arm of chromosome 7 appeared to be an adverse prognostic factor (Tiainen et al., 1989). It is possible that the tailing off of cases after 35 years reported by Seidman, Selikoff and Gelb (1986) reflects this elimination of susceptibles rather than a failure of the Peto formula.

Cigarette smoking is not an additional risk factor for mesothelioma (Berry, Newhouse and Antonis, 1985; Muscat and Wynder, 1991).

Pathology

Asbestos-associated mesothelioma is invasive and highly malignant. A localized fibrous tumour of the pleura which has been termed 'benign' is also recognized; this is neither of mesothelial origin nor related to asbestos exposure. More recently, other less malignant forms of peritoneal mesothelioma

have been described, including multicystic mesothelioma (Weiss and Tavassoli, 1988) and well-differentiated papillary mesothelioma (Daya and McCaughey, 1990). These tumours are probably unrelated to asbestos exposure, and their recognition is important for the approach to both therapy and prognosis. The remainder of this chapter is concerned with the much more frequently encountered malignant mesothelioma.

Macroscopic features

The pleural tumour is ivory-white, grey or yellow, sometimes with reddish striae, and it varies in extent from a hard sheet about 0.5 to 1.0 cm thick covering a limited part of the surface of the lung, with some tendency to spread into interlobar fissures, to a thick softer mass totally encasing one lung and invading it in lobulated fashion (Figure 14.30). All lobes of the lung are then greatly compressed and may be virtually obliterated. Both the pulmonary and the parietal pleurae are involved and frequently there is massive direct invasion along interlobar and interlobular fissures, into and around the pericardium and, sometimes, the contralateral pleura and the liver. The cut surface of the tumour may be glutinous (due to the production of hyaluronic acid); in places there may be necrotic cavities. It must be emphasized, however, that these gross appearances are not diagnostic. The peritoneal tumour presents similar gross post-mortem appearances which may vary from a confluent mass enclosing most of the abdominal organs to multiple nodules of the intestines, peritoneum and other organs (Entiknap and Smither, 1964). A variable amount of glutinous ascitic fluid is often present. Invasion of the gut wall beyond the muscularis propria is rare (Hourihane, 1964). In some instances the liver and spleen may be encased by a thin layer of growth and in others the peritoneal cavity is obliterated and the viscera completely engulfed by the tumour.

Spread of both pleural and peritoneal tumours to local lymph nodes (hilar, mediastinal or abdominal) is fairly common. Distant metastatic deposits may occur in about half the cases of mesotheliomas in either site (Roberts, 1976; Whitwell and Rawcliffe, 1971; Kannerstein and Churg, 1977; Edge and Choudhury, 1978); in the contralateral lung, pericardium, heart, peritoneum, kidneys, suprarenals, liver, spleen, brain, pancreas and skeleton from pleural tumours; in liver, suprarenals, pleura, lung and pericardium from peritoneal tumours. Secondary invasion of pleura or peritoneum occurs by direct extension through the diaphragm (Thomson, 1970), and it is sometimes impossible to determine in which cavity the tumour originated. There is no clear association between histological

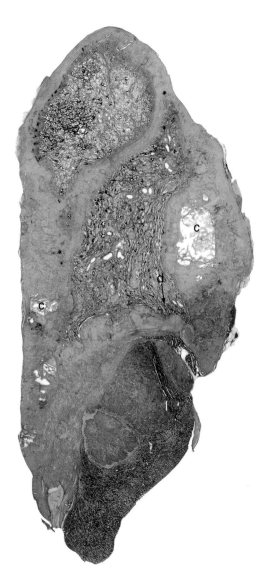

Figure 14.30 Malignant mesothelioma of the pleura of the right lung in a man exposed to an asbestos hazard for 18 months, 25 years before his death. Note the encasement and compression of the lung by the tumour, its extensions into the fissures with necrotic cavities (c) in the tumour mass. The tumour has spread through the diaphragm (d) into the liver (1)

type and a propensity to blood-borne or lymph-borne metastasis (Roberts, 1976). Extension of the pleural tumour in the chest wall may cause rib erosion, and invasion of aspiration needle tracks and thoracotomy incisions is apt to occur.

Microscopic features

Characteristically mesothelial tumours are pleomorphic. At one extreme the appearances closely resemble adenocarcinoma and, at the other, fibrosarcoma. Electron microscopy shows that typical and atypical epithelial and mesenchymal cells (which appear similar in ultrastructure to fibroblasts) are connected by a variety of transitional forms suggesting that malignant mesothelioma cells can differentiate into a number of different cell lines (Suzuki, Churg and Kannerstein, 1976; Gormley et al., 1980).

Three distinct histological patterns are recognized:

1. Tubulopapillary type (predominantly epithelial).
2. Sarcomatous type (predominantly mesenchymal).
3. Mixed type.

But it must be emphasized that the classification refers to the predominant cell type; the more diligent the search, the more frequently will all cell types be found. No difference in cell type has been established between asbestos-exposed and non-exposed cases (Wright and Sherwin, 1984). Most pleural series show approximately twice as many epithelial as sarcomatous cases, with the proportion of mixed types occupying an intermediate position. In peritoneal tumours sarcomatous histology is less common.

Tubulopapillary type

This consists predominantly of serpiginous, glandular tubules lined by regularly ordered, low columnar or cuboid cells with a few mitotic figures; in some places the cells are flat and in others appear as branching papillary projections covering a fine core of reticulin (Figure 14.31). In general, this is the most common type of mesothelioma and, in many cases, is very difficult to distinguish from adenocarcinoma of lung, breast, stomach, pancreas, prostate or ovary if the primary tumour is not identified.

Sarcomatous type

The pattern varies from that of a very cellular fascicular fibrosarcoma with uniform spindle cells, but sometimes with rounded cells of near-epithelial appearances, to virtually acellular masses of collagen fibres (Figure 14.32). Cell nuclei tend to be regular and mitotic figures are few. The acellular form may closely resemble a benign fibrous pleural plaque in places and extensive search of the tumour may be necessary before its sarcomatous character is identified.

Secondary fibrosarcoma, particularly fibromyosarcoma of the uterus, must be excluded.

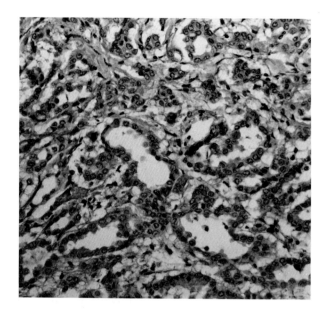

Figure 14.31 Malignancy mesothelioma of tubulopapillary type (see text for description). Magnification × 380; haematoxylin and eosin stain. (By courtesy of Dr J.C. Wagner)

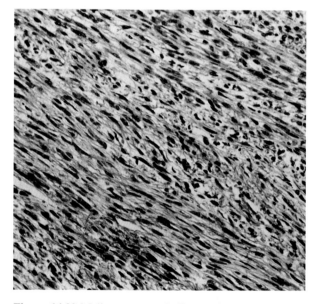

Figure 14.32 Malignant mesothelioma of sarcomatous type. Cellular fibrosarcomatous appearance. Note small spindle-shaped clefts (see text). Magnification × 380; haematoxylin and eosin stain

Mixed type

This is a mixture of the other two types although one is usually predominant. Widespread examination of the tumour and metastatic deposits (for example, in local lymph nodes) may be necessary before its mixed nature is evident.

Electron microscopy

The ultrastructure of mesothelioma has been explored by electron microscopy in an effort to discover features specific to that tumour (Wang, 1973; Davis, 1979; Dewar et al., 1987; Warhol, 1987). In practice, however, the results have been variable and many pathologists have found them of little help in differential diagnosis (Churg, 1988a). Reactive mesothelial cells cannot be distinguished from mesothelioma by electron microscopy.

Staining reactions

Many malignant mesotheliomas produce a mucinous substance, hyaluronic acid, which it was hoped would help to identify them positively. It is chiefly extracellular and stains blue with Alcian blue and Hale's colloidal iron but not with periodic acid–Schiff (PAS) or mucicarmine. By contrast, adenocarcinomas often produce an intracellular mucin which is usually PAS positive but occasionally gives the Alcian blue reaction. The application of these stains before and after removing the mucoid substance with the enzyme hyaluronidase may cause reversion of previously positive Alcian blue and colloidal iron reactions to negative. Unfortunately, this is not consistent and is least helpful in those cases that are microscopically the most difficult. However, in many cases the PAS test is negative in mesothelioma sections which are pre-digested by the enzyme diastase (DPAS test), whereas a strongly positive reaction within cell cytoplasm and mucin in the lumina of neoplastic glands favours adenocarcinoma.

The introduction of immunohistochemical techniques has led to a considerably improved discrimination between mesothelioma and adeno-carcinoma, the most commonly used antigens being carcinoembryonic antigen (CEA) and keratin. The former is usually absent in mesothelioma and present in pulmonary adenocarcinoma. Antibodies to cytokeratin are normally present with both types of tumour, but Al-Izzi, Thurlow and Corrin (1989) have shown that there is normally no reaction with localized fibrous tumour of the pleura. Other tumour antigens are also available (Gibbs et al., 1985), but the variation in results in different hands (Churg, 1988a) is evidence that no standardized diagnostic technique is yet available. Even among pathologists experienced in the problems of mesothelioma diagnosis, neither certainty nor unanimity is achieved in all cases. Although the situation has improved since 1973 when McCaughey and Oldham reported 'gross disagreement' over histological diagnosis between three such observers in nearly 20 per cent of cases, disagreement or major uncertainty still exists in about 5 to 10 per cent of

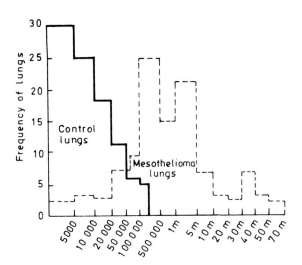

Figure 14.33 Comparison of asbestos fibre content of lungs from mesothelioma and normal control series. (Reproduced, with permission, from Whitwell, Scott and Grimshaw, 1977)

cases. Among pathologists with less experience in diagnosis of this tumour, the uncertainty is much greater. Wright et al. (1984) reviewed all cases of malignant mesothelioma diagnosed by Los Angeles County pathologists from 1972 to 1979. Adequate specimens were obtained for review in 162 cases, or 120 if cases where the original pathologist was uncertain are excluded. Of these only 42 (35 per cent) were classified by the experienced pathologist as definite, probable or possible mesotheliomas; the remainder were all classified as tumours of a different origin, although in 24 (20 per cent) the possibility of mesothelioma could not be excluded.

Lung fibre burden

Whitwell, Scott and Grimshaw (1977) carried out counts of lung fibres greater than 6 μm long by optical microscopy (thereby counting mainly amphibole fibres) on 100 consecutive cases of pleural mesothelioma. Seven had no history of asbestos exposure, and the count in all cases was below 40 000 fibres/g dried lung. Of the remaining 93 cases, almost all with a known history of exposure, 87 (94 per cent) had more than 50 000 fibres/g. Twenty-three of these also had asbestosis, and all had counts in excess of 1 million fibres/g, whereas the average of those without asbestosis was between 500 000 and 1 million fibres/g. Of 100 controls, 85 had less than 50 000 fibres/g (Figure 14.33).

This pattern of lung fibre burden has been found in other surveys since that time, with occupationally exposed cases of mesothelioma falling for the most part between those with no occupational exposure (less than 30 000 fibres/g) and those with asbestosis (more than 1 million fibres/g). But, more recently, electron microscope studies have revealed that the increase over control levels is restricted to amphibole fibres; it has been repeatedly shown that the lung chrysotile content is no greater in cases than in controls (McDonald and McDonald, 1987a; Churg, 1988a). Churg (1988b) reviewed the evidence of fibre burdens in chrysotile miners and concluded that, in the small number of cases of mesothelioma recorded, exposure was very heavy, to the extent of both accumulating an appreciable burden of tremolite and causing concomitant asbestosis.

As was discussed earlier for asbestosis, the use of lung fibre burdens to decide whether individual cases of mesothelioma are likely to have been caused by asbestos is bedevilled by inter-laboratory differences and the absence of any standard methodology.

Asbestosis and mesothelioma

As might be expected from what has been said previously, a proportion of mesotheliomas occurs at levels of cumulative exposure to amphibole asbestos insufficient to cause asbestosis. Among Barking (UK) workers 86 per cent were found to have some interstitial fibrosis at autopsy (Browne and Smither, 1983), the severity being slightly higher among peritoneal than among pleural cases. There was evidence also of a high proportion among American insulators (Lilis et al., 1987). Exposure levels in both these cohorts, however, tended to be heavy. Where average levels were much lower, but subject to occasional peaks, as in dockyard work (Sheers and Coles, 1980), the dissociation of mesothelioma from asbestosis is readily seen. The lowest estimated cumulative exposure on record resulting in a mesothelioma appears to be of the order of 5 fibres/ml years in a woman exposed to crocidolite in an asbestos–cement pipe-making department (Ilgren and Browne, 1990; Neuberger and Kundi, 1990). This may be contrasted with the generally accepted figure of 25 fibres/ml years below which clinical asbestosis will not be seen.

Summary of diagnostic microscopy

A definitive diagnosis of malignant mesothelioma cannot be made during life or *post mortem* other than by microscopy. Tissue for biopsy must be sufficiently large to permit, if possible, different features of the tumour to be identified. But even with adequate material, in many cases the diagnosis during life can only be putative.

At post-mortem, a thorough search for a possible primary growth (which may be minute) is necessary. Willis (1973), in emphasizing the difficulties involved, asserted: 'No tumour, whatever its structure, can be regarded as a primary coelomic one until the most painstaking and exhaustive search of all viscera has failed to disclose a primary epithelial growth.' Although some pathologists may regard this as too sweeping a statement, it is desirable to bear it in mind as a general rule. Peritoneal tumours are more likely to be wrongly diagnosed as malignant mesotheliomas in women than in men due to the range of potentialities of cells in the female pelvis (Kannerstein and Churg, 1977).

Clinical features

Symptoms

The pleural tumour

In the great majority of cases the presenting symptoms are breathlessness on exertion or pain. Breathlessness, when the first symptom, is almost always due to the development of a pleural effusion, although later it may result from the expansion of the tumour, and may progress until it is present at rest. Pain tends to be of heavy, nagging quality unrelated to movement or respiration, may become severe due to involvement of intercostal nerves, and may be referred to the abdomen or the ipsilateral shoulder. Occasionally, local invasion of the brachial plexus may cause pain, paraesthesiae and muscular weakness (with wasting) on the ulnar side of the ipsilateral arm.

Lassitude, malaise and loss of weight are rarely early symptoms but are the rule later. In the absence of pre-existing chronic bronchitis or other lung disease, cough is not a troublesome feature but, when the growth is advanced, it may be productive due to complicating respiratory infection. Haemoptysis does not occur. Some patients complain of distressing night sweats.

Because of the gradual onset of symptoms, there is usually an interval of some 3 or 4 months between the patient first experiencing them and seeking medical advice (Elmes and Simpson, 1976). In the late stage of the disease, dysphagia may be present due to oesophageal involvement.

The peritoneal tumour

Again, the onset of symptoms may be insidious. At first there is a poorly localized abdominal discomfort with loss of appetite and weight and, in some instances, constipation; however, painless, diffuse swelling of the abdomen with increasing abdominal girth may be the first symptom. In about one-third of cases, symptoms of intermittent upper or lower intestinal obstruction occur, which may or may not be associated with colicky pain. Ultimately, however, the symptoms of complete obstruction are usual.

Physical signs

The pleural tumour

When first seen the patient is usually in good general health but later when the disease is advanced he is ill, emaciated and dyspnoeic at rest.

Unilateral signs of pleural effusion or thickening are frequently present to a greater or lesser degree. The chest wall may be tender or painful on palpation, and in advanced disease is flattened and immobile. Palpable or visible tumour masses may be present particularly after thoracotomy or needling of the chest. Signs of mediastinal shift to the opposite side are infrequent and are usually associated with rapidly developing effusion and dyspnoea. For reasons that are not clear, the tumour occasionally presents with an ipsilateral spontaneous pneumothorax but this is not often detectable clinically. Pericardial friction is sometimes heard due to extension of the tumour into the sac.

Finger clubbing is seldom seen. It was observed in 9.5 per cent of cases by Elmes and Simpson (1976) who also noted an occasional case of hypertrophic pulmonary osteoarthropathy.

When invaded by tumour the liver may be palpable well below the costal margin but is not often tender. There is rarely any clinical evidence of local lymph node metastasis or signs of superior mediastinal obstruction. The features of Horner's syndrome on the side of the tumour are occasionally seen with impaired sweating of the face and sometimes of the shoulder, arm and hand of that side due to invasion of the paravertebral sympathetic nerve chain (Stanford, 1976).

The peritoneal tumour

Abnormal signs are often absent on initial examination but soon some diffuse abdominal fullness is evident and the signs of ascites may be present. Later the abdomen is much distended and its girth may increase rapidly; at this stage firm masses are

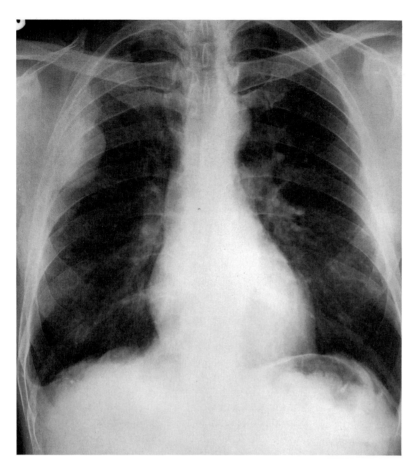

Figure 14.34 Appearances of localized malignant mesothelioma of pleura in a 65-year-old man who had worked as a steam locomotive boiler maker for 45 years. Asbestos insulation frequently carried out in his vicinity. Erosion of right first, second, third and forth ribs evident 4 months later. *Post mortem*, naked eye: tumour mass enclosed most of right lung. Microscopy: mesothelioma confirmed; no evidence of asbestosis but moderate number of asbestos bodies present in 30-μm lung sections

usually palpable by direct or bimanual palpation, although it is not possible to relate these to any abdominal organ. The patient is now ill and emaciated. Jaundice is not seen.

Investigations

Radiographic appearances

Although yielding no pathognomonic signs, the chest radiograph is the most informative of the routine investigations.

The pleural tumour
The most important changes are as follows:

1. Irregular, lobulated, well-demarcated, protuberant opacities which line part or all of one inner chest wall and extend to a greater or lesser degree into the lung field, sometimes surrounding it completely. Dense elongated opacities due to the spread of tumour along the greater or lesser fissures may be seen. At an early stage, the opacities may be indistinguishable from those of pleural plaques but they are unilateral (Figures 14.34 and 14.35). Occasionally, the appearance of a hilar mass is predominant.

2. A unilateral pleural effusion above which lobular opacities along the costal margin or near the hilum may be discernible. Some cases present the appearances of diffuse irregular pleural thickening with crowding of ribs, scoliosis and mediastinal shift towards the affected side. Ultimately the hemithorax may be completely opaque.

3. Exceptionally, the signs of pleural infiltration, discrete tumour deposits or the pattern of malignant lymphangitis in the lung on the opposite

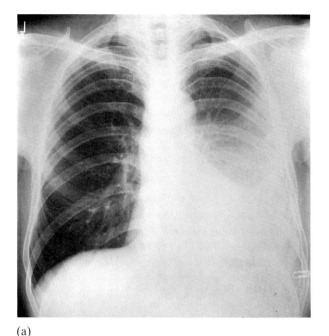

(a)

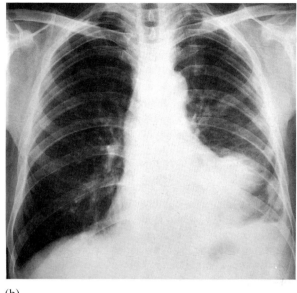

(b)

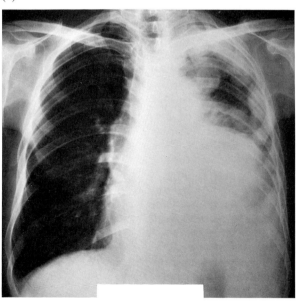

(c)

Figure 14.35 Stages in the development of a diffuse malignant pleural mesothelioma. Asbestos insulation worker 29 years. (a) March, 1972: left pleural effusion; (b) July, 1972: massive opacities localized to left lower zone; (c) December, 1972: widespread massive, lobulated opacities. Right lung field normal throughout. *Post mortem*, naked eye: left lung surrounded by soft, lobulated, partly necrotic tumour mass. Deposits of tumour within the lung, hilar lymph nodes and liver. Microscopy: mesothelioma of mixed type. Minimal asbestosis and moderate numbers of asbestos bodies

side may occur late in disease. Computed tomography may provide useful information in a proportion of cases, particularly where the tumour outline is obscured by an effusion (Kreel, 1981; Whitley, 1987). (See Chapter 7 for further discussion on the relevance of computed tomography and other imaging techniques in this respect.)

The peritoneal tumour
The signs of bilateral calcified pleural plaques or of DIPF (asbestosis) may be present in the chest film. Occasionally, there is evidence of invasion of the pleura on one or both sides in advanced disease. In some cases, however, there is no abnormality. Radiology of the abdomen, when associated with a history of asbestos exposure and evidence of small or large bowel obstruction (with or without ascites), displacement of intra-abdominal structures by soft tissue masses or diffuse extrinsic indentation of the bowel with submucosal infiltration and encapsulation shown by barium meal or enema suggests the possibility of a mesothelioma (Young and Reddy, 1980). As with

pleural disease, computed tomography may sometimes be helpful.

Biopsy of tumour tissue and cytology of effusion

This may be necessary especially to exclude other types of growth that may be amenable to treatment. The number of correct diagnoses increases with the amount of tissue obtained, but is still relatively small. Elmes and Simpson (1976) found that the diagnosis of mesothelioma was correct in 26 per cent of needle specimens, 38 per cent of thoracotomy specimens and 70 per cent of surgical excision specimens. In considering the use of these techniques, the propensity for mesothelial tumours to advance along needle tracks and thoracotomy scars has to be borne in mind; in fact, 80 per cent of palpable masses of the tumour in the chest wall have been related to these sites (Elmes and Simpson, 1976).

Examination of aspirated fluid is normally undertaken routinely, and both cytology and chemistry may contribute towards a diagnosis of mesothelioma. Raised hyaluronic acid levels in effusions provide an indication of mesothelioma in a proportion of cases. With cytology the finding of cell aggregates is a distinctive feature; certain other morphological characteristics may be present, as well as characteristic staining reactions (Whitaker and Shilkin, 1984). For this purpose all available fluid should be sent to the laboratory to give a maximum cell volume. Many diagnostic difficulties remain, however, of which the difficulty in distinguishing reactive mesothelium is prominent. Combined with needle biopsy, Whitaker and Shilkin (1984) were able to make a diagnosis in 80 per cent of cases. However, as Herbert (1984) pointed out, two methods of probable diagnosis do not add up to one certainty, and the best compromise between minimal intervention with inadequate diagnosis and major surgery in a terminally ill patient will often be provided by thoracoscopy.

In the case of the peritoneal tumour, laparotomy is usually unavoidable in the endeavour to obtain a definite diagnosis and the need to exclude treatable disease. Here also the tumour may infiltrate through incisions.

Examination of sputum

Asbestos bodies, if found, will alert the clinician to the possibility of malignant mesothelioma if a history of past exposure to the mineral has not been elicited. Mesothelial cells are *not* found.

Diagnosis
During life

Important suggestive features are as follows:

1. A history of exposure to amphibole asbestos, with a latent period of 20 years or more since first exposure.
2. Insidious onset of symptoms and good general health in the early stage of the disease with raised ESR.
3. No clinical evidence of lymphadenopathy or other forms of metastasis.
4. The appearances of the chest radiograph and, if necessary, computed tomography.

Post-mortem

1. In most cases the tumour exhibits the gross features described previously which, although suggesting its identity, can be caused by other neoplasms – for example, metastasis from renal carcinoma (Taylor et al., 1987).
2. A searching necropsy fails to reveal a primary growth of which the suspected mesothelioma could be a metastatic deposit.
3. The microscopic criteria described earlier are satisfied.

Differential diagnosis

Clinically, this includes all causes of subacute or chronic unilateral pleural effusion, chronic pleural thickening and the exclusion of any suspicion of a primary growth elsewhere. Bronchial carcinoma may be most difficult to differentiate as it is common and, at times, may present unusual features. Sputum cytology, bronchoscopy and bronchography are uninformative in mesothelioma.

Pleural disease of insidious onset in individuals over middle age should cause the diagnosis of malignant mesothelioma to be considered. However, a history of asbestos exposure must not be allowed to close the mind to the more likely possibility of some other disease. The most important goal, however, is to distinguish it from benign or treatable malignant disease.

Prognosis

The outlook is almost invariably rapidly fatal. Elmes and Simpson (1976) found that the average period between the onset of symptoms and death was 16 months in the case of pleural tumours and 9 months with peritoneal tumours; similar figures have been found in a number of series since then. Longer survival was found in patients with epithelial histology by Brunner et al. (1982) and Adams et al. (1986), but not by Law et al. (1984), Solomons (1984), Chailleux et al. (1988) or Pillgram-Larsen et al. (1984). All larger series contain a small number of cases with longer survival times, about 5 per cent surviving beyond 5 years, but some of these cases may represent the more benign variants (Daya and McCaughey, 1990) referred to on page 471. Law et al. (1983) and Hirsch et al. (1982) both found evidence of longer survival for patients with no history of asbestos exposure.

As the disease advances there is increasing weight loss and, in the case of pleural tumours, progressive dyspnoea, and often severe and intractable chest pain. Death usually occurs from respiratory failure or bronchopneumonia, but occasionally as a result of invasion of the pericardium causing haemorrhage and tamponade. With peritoneal tumours there is malnutrition and electrolyte imbalance resulting from anorexia and frequent vomiting and, in some cases, progressive ascites. Complete intestinal obstruction is common terminally, but bronchopneumonia may supervene before this happens.

Treatment

Aspiration of intrathoracic fluid at regular intervals relieves breathlessness. Initially, this may be required at intervals that are as frequent as every 1 to 2 weeks, but later only occasionally as fluid accumulates. However, increasing thickness and hardness of the tumour mass may ultimately make aspiration impossible. Chemical pleurodesis – for example, by the instillation of talc (Chailleux et al., 1988) or mepacrine (Pillgram-Larsen et al., 1984; Tattersall and Boyer, 1990) – may reduce, or eliminate, the need for repeated paracentesis.

Brunner et al. (1982) reported survival of more than 5 years in 7 patients (6 per cent) out of 123, of whom 93 were treated surgically, but this does not differ significantly from results in untreated cases. Law et al. (1984) felt that surgery may have produced some palliative benefit but no increased survival except, possibly, in one case with a localized sarcomatous type of tumour. Chemotherapy has also given disappointing results in pleural disease. Brunner et al. had evidence of remission in only 3 of 78 patients treated. Both Law et al. and Pillgram-Larsen et al. found no objective evidence of benefit and Adams et al. (1986) reported that the results of treatment were discouraging.

Markman et al. (1986) reported on the use of intracavitary cisplatin – an alkylating cytotoxic drug. Only one out of eight patients with pleural disease showed any clinical response, and then only briefly. Nine out of thirteen patients with peritoneal tumours, however, showed some response, although toxic effects were considerable. The median survival of the non-responding patients was only 4 months whilst that of the responders was more than 18 months, partly, no doubt, from the inclusion of those patients who would have had longer survival without treatment. Lederman et al. (1987) treated six patients with peritoneal malignancies with surgical 'debulking' followed by various combinations of chemotherapy and, then, whole abdomen irradiation. All were still alive 6 to 62 months after completion of treatment, but the average age was only 33 years and no details of diagnosis were given. Radiotherapy in other hands has proved uniformly disappointing. It is of interest that the only long survivor in the series by Law et al. (1984) treated with radiotherapy was also a young woman with no history of asbestos exposure. It is clear, therefore, that, except under controlled conditions in research units, treatment of diffuse malignant mesothelioma is essentially only palliative.

Lung cancer

The early recognition that asbestos exposure might increase the risk of lung cancer was discussed on page 419. Buchanan (1965) gave figures showing how, among those certified as suffering from asbestosis for compensation, deaths from lung cancer increased steadily from 0 to 56 per cent between 1920 and 1960. Hammond, Selikoff and Churg (1965) also drew attention to the high proportion of lung cancer deaths among insulators, and it was apparent that, in absolute numbers, lung cancer had become the most important asbestos-related cause of death. Two reasons were offered for the progressive increase in the proportion of subjects with asbestosis dying of lung cancer: first, that this happened in parallel with the increase in lung cancer in the general population which followed, with a 25-year time lag, the great increase in cigarette smoking that started just before the First World War; and, secondly, that the effect of the 1931 asbestos regulations in the UK had been to detect those developing asbestosis at an early stage and remove them from further exposure, thereby enabling them to survive long enough to develop lung cancer.

Standardized mortality ratios (SMRs) for 37 male and 13 female cohorts have been listed and summarized by McDonald and McDonald (1987b). Of these, 30 male and 9 female cohorts had SMRs for lung cancer in excess of 120.

Fibre type

The attempt to compare the effects of different asbestos fibres has met with many difficulties, some of which have been discussed earlier in connection with asbestosis. Nevertheless, a comparison of lung cancer SMRs in those exposed only to chrysotile with those exposed to amphibole or mixtures of both clearly demonstrates the lesser hazard of exposure to chrysotile (McDonald and McDonald, 1987b), a conclusion reinforced by more recent studies (Gardner and Powell, 1986; Hughes, Weill and Hammad, 1987; Newhouse and Sullivan, 1989; Neuberger and Kundi, 1990).

Four circumstances have obscured the major difference in lung cancer hazard between these two types of asbestos fibre (as, indeed, they have with the other related diseases). Two have been discussed earlier in relation to the pathogenesis of asbestosis and mesothelioma, namely, the misinterpretation of animal and in vitro experiments through using equivalent weights of fibres instead of numbers more than 5 µm long, and of ignoring the effects of chrysotile dissolution in lung tissue. The third is that, until lung fibre burden studies were carried out by electron microscopy, the major effects of small additions of amphibole to chrysotile in manufacturing processes were not realized. The consequences of this have been especially unfortunate for the understanding of mesothelioma risk.

The fourth circumstance has had particular importance for lung cancer risk assessment. Mortality studies of three asbestos textile factories have revealed a very high lung cancer incidence compared with most other asbestos manufacturing industries and, even more strikingly, with mining (McDonald et al., 1983a, b; Peto et al., 1985). Several hypotheses were advanced to explain the difference, the most favoured until recently being the greater average fibre length of chrysotile required for textiles than for reinforcing purposes in asbestos–cement and friction materials. This, however, was refuted by the finding that average fibre lengths (and tremolite content – another explanation offered) in the lungs of the textile workers were not significantly different from those of chrysotile miners whose estimated risk, dose for dose, was only one-fifth (Sebastien et al., 1989). Another hypothesis has now emerged which seems likely to be correct but awaits experimental confir-

mation: mineral oil sprays, of a kind now known to be carcinogenic, were used to control the dust in the American textile factories and it was suggested by McDonald and McDonald (1987b) that this might account for the increase in risk, either by a direct effect or by delaying the dissolution of the chrysotile. Support for this hypothesis comes from the third textile factory, at Rochdale, where Peto et al. (1985) had already commented on the fact that lung cancer ratios in those exposed after 1950 had not fallen correspondingly to a fall in dust levels. Enquiries have revealed that an oil spray was introduced in this factory also from 1950 to 1970 (S. Holmes, 1990, personal communication). Exposure to oil sprays in cable making (in the absence of asbestos) has been shown to cause both interstitial fibrosis and a greatly increased incidence of lung cancer (Ronneberg, Anderson and Skyberg, 1988).

Whatever confounding factor in these textile factories is ultimately established, it is clear from the evidence of other cohorts that chrysotile exposure by itself has a lower lung cancer risk than amphibole. This conclusion is in keeping with the known lesser risk of asbestosis discussed earlier, and the pathogenesis outlined later.

Dose–response

During the 1970s mortality studies began to appear that included estimates of individual exposures. Almost all such studies suggested a linear relationship between cumulative dose and risk of lung cancer at high levels of exposure (Figure 14.36). Extrapolation to very low doses followed, at first as a convenience but then as a popular article of faith, despite the acknowledged statistical illegitimacy of this procedure (as distinct from interpolation) and

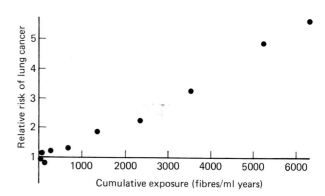

Figure 14.36 Relative risk of lung cancer in Quebec chrysotile miners and millers as a function of cumulative exposure. At very high levels of cumulative exposure, the relative risk of lung cancer appears to be linear

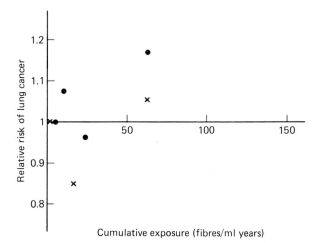

Figure 14.37 Quebec miners and millers: when levels of cumulative exposure below 300 fibre/ml years are examined, the linear relative-risk relationship disappears, both when calculated by SMR (x x) and by case-control methods (• •). Two-thirds of the cohort are included in this category. (Data from Liddell, McDonald and Thomas, 1977)

despite the biological absurdity of the assumption that the body has no defence against inhaled fibre at any level, however low, and, most reprehensibly, without close examination of the actual evidence (Figure 14.37).

One other flaw in extrapolation of the dose–response back to zero exposure is that in almost no cohort study does the line pass through the origin (McDonald, 1990). This merely suggests that an inappropriate standard for lung cancer in the general population was chosen, and the difficulty can be overcome by using relative risk (Liddell and Hanley, 1985). On this basis, and omitting the textile cohorts for the reason given in the preceding section, calculation of the increase in relative risk for each fibre/ml year of cumulative exposure gives figures from 0 to 0.001, the latter representing an increase of 0.1 per cent in relative risk of lung cancer for each year worked at a dust level of 1 fibre/ml, the risk increasing directly with increased exposure levels.

However, these calculations, although they may be helpful for assessing risk at high exposure levels, do not correspond with the available data at lower levels (Figure 14.36). Such evidence as exists is more compatible with the existence of a threshold below which relative risk of lung cancer is not raised (Browne, 1986b). In addition to the series listed in that study, further studies have been published (Browne, 1991b) that show no increase in relative risk at low exposure levels (Neuberger and Kundi, 1990), in addition to follow-up studies of two previously described cohorts – a UK friction materials

factory (Newhouse and Sullivan, 1989) and the Australian crocidolite miners (de Klerk et al., 1989a) – where no increased risk of lung cancer was found in those employed for less than 2 years. All these series taken together show an impressively consistent threshold-type pattern. This would be entirely in keeping with what is now known about pathogenesis, and the dependence of increased risk upon the presence of asbestosis. Epidemiological evidence is, perhaps, not sensitive enough to provide a conclusive answer to the question of whether a threshold for lung cancer exists, but further support has recently come from two studies designed specifically to test the hypothesis: both found that risk of lung cancer only increased in cohort members with signs of pre-existing asbestosis (Hughes and Weill, 1991; Sluis-Cremer and Bezuidenhart, 1989, 1990). Both studies also provided strong evidence that the presence of asbestosis was a determinant of lung cancer risk independent of exposure. Confirmation also comes from another interesting and important approach by Vacek and McDonald (1990, 1991). Doubts have always been felt about the use of cumulative exposures for the assessment of risk, equating, as they do, long exposures at low intensity with short, high-intensity exposures. Vacek and McDonald analysed intensity separately from duration for four cohorts, and found evidence in each case of a level of exposure below which no increased risk of lung cancer was found.

Pathogenesis

The question of whether increased lung cancer in asbestos workers was due to a direct effect of the fibre itself or whether it was a consequence of asbestosis, the latter disease 'preparing the soil for the occurrence of cancer' as Merewether expressed it, was raised in the 1930s. The first cohort mortality study (Doll, 1955) showed an increased lung cancer SMR only in men with asbestosis, and the prevailing view, that diffuse interstitial fibrosis was a prerequisite for the increase in lung cancer, was not seriously challenged until the 1970s. Then, the demonstration of a linear relationship between cumulative exposure at high levels and risk of lung cancer led to extrapolation of risk to levels of exposure at which no asbestosis occurred.

However, research into the mechanism of fibre carcinogenesis, discussed on pages 464–465, has established that the primary effect is on the macrophage, and that it is only when the inhaled dose of long fibres exceeds a certain level that the regulatory capacity of the macrophage to maintain the balance of cytokines is destroyed.

Pathogenesis and epidemiology, accordingly, both indicate the existence of a level of asbestos fibre exposure below which no increased risk of lung cancer occurs. Non-occupational support for this threshold is provided by the finding of higher tremolite and chrysotile levels in the residents of mining towns without any detectable increase in lung cancer (or DIPF or mesothelioma) (Churg, 1986; Case and Sebastien, 1987). Other evidence, deriving from a number of sources including pathology and animal experiments, points in the same direction (Browne, 1986a). It is particularly relevant that lung histology in two of the larger cohorts of asbestos-exposed workers – American insulators and East London factory workers – has shown that lung cancer was associated with asbestosis in 90 per cent of cases (Newhouse, Berry and Wagner, 1985; Kipen et al., 1987). The threshold of exposure below which clinical evidence of asbestosis would not appear has been put conservatively at 25 fibres/ml years (Ontario, 1984; Doll and Peto, 1985). Epidemiological evidence suggests a slightly higher exposure threshold for increased lung cancer risk (Browne, 1986b). Kipen et al. (1987) proposed that, because 18 per cent of their series showed no radiological evidence of asbestosis, such chest radiographs should not be used as evidence against asbestos causation. However, Weiss (1989) has demonstrated that if allowance is made for the number of lung cancers to be expected in the cohort unrelated to asbestos exposure, the excess corresponds well with the number of men with positive radiological evidence of asbestosis.

Pathology

Asbestos workers have the same liability to develop lung cancer proportional to their smoking habits as others in their community. If they also have asbestosis, there is no way in which those whose malignancy has developed solely as a result of their smoking can be distinguished from those in whom asbestosis has made a contribution.

When groups of exposed subjects are studied, however, two features of the asbestos-related tumours have been suggested: first a reversal of the usual upper : lower lobe ratio and, secondly, an increase in the proportion of adenocarcinomas to other types. In the general population, the ratio of upper to middle and lower lobe tumours is approximately 2 : 1 (Byers, Vena and Rzepka, 1984), whereas studies of lung cancers in subjects with asbestosis show a reversal with ratios of up to 1 : 4 (Whitwell, Newhouse and Bennett, 1974; Weiss, 1988b). Because asbestosis normally begins and predominates in the lower lobes, this finding is to be expected from the pathogenesis.

More controversial, and perhaps less important, is the increase in the proportion of adenocarcinomas compared with other histological types. The issue has been confused by the inclusion in some series of all asbestos workers, whereas it is relevant *only* to workers with asbestosis. Attention has been particularly drawn to this because scar tumours have been held to be predominantly adenocarcinomatous. Hourihane and McCaughey (1966) and Hasan, Nash and Kazemi (1978) found a higher than expected number of adenocarcinomas among subjects with asbestosis, and Whitwell, Newhouse and Bennett (1974) and Newhouse, Berry and Wagner (1985) both found a higher proportion of adenocarcinomas among lung cancers associated with asbestosis than among those without. The comparison is complicated, however, by the increase in the proportion of adenocarcinomas in the general population in recent years (Vincent, Pickren and Lane, 1977). Bronchoalveolar epithelium is a very labile tissue endowed with multipotential properties (Spencer, 1985) and because acknowledged asbestos-related cancers clearly do appear in all the histological types for reasons that are not understood, any difference in proportions, if it exists, is not of obvious relevance.

Cigarette-smoking and asbestos-related lung cancer

Since the high incidence of lung cancer in the early cohorts of asbestos workers was noted, there has been speculation over whether asbestos acted synergistically with smoking. Saracci (1977) outlined three modes of interaction. First, asbestos and smoking might act independently, so that their effects were additive: if asbestos causes a 5 per cent increase in risk and smoking a 10 per cent increase for given levels of exposure, then the increased risk to a smoking asbestos worker at these levels would be approximately 15 per cent. The second possibility is a multiplicative effect, whereby the addition of smoking to asbestos exposure produces an effect in proportion: if the same risks of 5 per cent and 10 per cent are assumed, the increased risk to the smoking asbestos worker becomes 50 per cent. The third possibility is that asbestos alone is not carcinogenic, but acts in conjunction with smoking to increase the latter risk. Early on Selikoff and his colleagues, who carried out pioneer work on this subject, believed the third to be the model, but showed later, when larger numbers were available (non-smokers being relatively rare among asbestos workers), that asbestos did have an independent effect (Hammond, Selikoff and Seidman, 1980).

The available data, together with the difficulty of obtaining accurate information about past smoking habits, were analysed by Berry, Newhouse and Antonis (1985). These confirm the independent effect of asbestos but show some heterogeneity over the strength of the effect. This is to be expected, partly because of small numbers – no series other than Canadian miners and millers had more than five cases among non-smokers – but mainly due to the fact that, as the asbestos relative risk only increases when asbestosis is present, the results will depend crucially on the proportion of such cases in the total workforce. However, it is probable that the combined effect of *asbestosis* and smoking is more than additive. Among cases of asbestosis certified for compensation 3 out of 32 non-smokers (11 per cent) died of lung cancer compared with 43 per cent of smokers (Berry, 1981).

The way in which cigarette smoking and asbestos exert their combined effect has also been investigated, and a favoured solution has been the adsorption of the carcinogens in cigarette smoke onto the fibre, which enables them to be retained and carried into bronchial epithelium to facilitate their effects. Doubt has been cast on this by the demonstration that the quantities involved would be too small to overcome the defensive enzyme systems (Gerde and Scholander, 1989) and by the absence of any smoking effect on mesothelioma incidence, because adsorbed carcinogens should exert a similarly adverse effect on the mesothelium (Roe, 1988). In any case, the enhanced carcinogenic effect is amply explained by the effect of excessive growth factors, secreted by the macrophages after incomplete ingestion of long fibres, on an epithelium already unstable and undergoing early transformation from the action of cigarette smoke carcinogens.

Other malignant disease

Some early cohort mortality studies suggested that SMRs for malignancies other than of the lung and mesothelium were raised in asbestos workers. These cohorts included a considerable proportion of subjects exposed before 1950 to high levels of airborne dust. Specific organs were singled out, but Goldsmith (1982) reviewing 11 cohorts found no evidence for other site specificity and thought that systemic carcinogenesis was a more probable explanation, perhaps as a result of immunological impairment from excessive lung fibre burdens suggested by Turner-Warwick and Parkes (1970). Peto (1989) has also commented on the fact that relative risks for virtually all sites except lung cancer and mesothelioma increase at an equal pace. A large number of mortality studies recently published, however, give no support to any specific or systemic effects other than lung cancer and mesothelioma. Although the hypothesis of immunological impairment remains a possibility in conditions of gross dust overload and poor nutrition, such as prevailed in some situations prior to the Second World War, a more probable explanation is that the use of national mortality rates for comparison with employees in dusty trades coming, in those days, predominantly from social classes 4 and 5 was inappropriate.

Laryngeal cancer

The main difficulty in assessing an asbestos effect on the incidence of laryngeal cancer arises due to the major confounding effects of alcohol, tobacco and social class. The SMR for UK publicans in 1971 was 367 and for barmen in 1951 (the latest figure available) was 500. In 1971 also the SMR in the lowest social class was three times that of the highest (Logan, 1982). Moreover, dusty trades and the construction and lagging industries have always tended to have a high labour turnover, with a greater proportion of single men having an atypical lifestyle resulting in higher SMRs for violence, suicide and lung cancer, and higher tobacco and alcohol consumption.

Few studies of laryngeal cancer in asbestos workers have been controlled adequately for these confounding factors. Recent reviews by Chan and Gee (1988), Edelman (1989), Liddell (1990), and Muscat and Wynder (1992) show that, when such studies are examined critically, there is no support for a specific causal relationship with asbestos exposure. Like a variety of other materials, however, asbestos may have a non-specific irritant effect (Parnes, 1990).

Gastrointestinal cancer

Hammond, Selikoff and Churg (1965) reported to the 1964 New York conference that 29 deaths from cancer of the gastrointestinal tract had occurred among their group of insulation workers, whereas only 9.7 were to be expected from US national rates. This was followed by other early studies which suggested an increase in gastrointestinal (East London factory workers) or stomach (Canadian miners and millers) cancers, and the belief became implanted that asbestos was also responsible for this class of malignancies. However, since that time a large number of studies have shown no increase. Edelman (1988) identified 32 cohorts of asbestos workers with data on gastrointestinal cancer incidence. No consistent pattern could be seen, and nine SMRs were significantly less than 1 ($P<0.05$) compared with ten significantly greater. Where groups of exposed workers were compared with non-exposed, no significant difference was found, and where dose–response calculations were possible no consistent increase in risk was seen with increasing exposure.

As with laryngeal cancer, confounding effects are considerable. Cancer of the oesophagus and pancreas are definitely related to smoking (in the UK the relative risk of oesophageal cancer in smokers is three times that of non-smokers) and the former also to social class (relative risk class 5 to class 1 is 1.7 in the UK and >2 in the USA). For stomach cancer the difference in relative risk between classes is even more extreme: 2.9 : 1 between classes 5 and 1 in the UK, whilst even within class 3 manual workers had a 50 per cent greater risk than non-manual workers. Similarly, in the USA white males with less than 8 years' education had a relative risk of 2.2 compared with college graduates (Logan, 1982). It is also of interest that other studies have shown higher rates of stomach cancer in a wide range of dusty trades (Wright et al., 1988).

Frumkin and Berlin (1988) showed that if asbestos cohorts were separated into those with lung cancer SMRs above and below 200, the combined SMR for stomach cancer would be found to be moderately raised in the former group and normal in the latter. However, they also found a significant difference in non-asbestos-related mortality between the two groups; this is evidence that the confounding effects listed above were operative in the high lung-cancer SMR cohorts, and against the possibility of a true causal relationship. Peto (1989) pointed out that where lung cancer relative risks have been substantially raised, so also have those of virtually all other sites, again casting doubt on any specific relationship between asbestos and gastrointestinal cancer.

Despite demonstrations that a small number of ingested fibres can be recovered from the gastrointestinal lymph (Sebastien, Masse and Bignon, 1980) and urine (Guillemin et al., 1989), animal experiments have consistently failed to show any effect of ingested asbestos on gastrointestinal malignancies, and the same negative result has come from epidemiological studies of asbestos in drinking water (Commins, 1988; MacRae, 1988).

The data relating to colorectal cancer, in the 21 cohorts where this has been listed separately, have been reviewed by Weiss (1990). The summary SMR for all cohorts was 0.97, with no dose–response relationship in the two studies from which this could be deduced. Urogenital cancer risks in relation to asbestos exposure have been reviewed by Edelman (1992), who found the evidence conflicting and insufficient to enable any conclusion to be reached. Short asbestos fibres, identified by Guillemin et al. (1989), were present in the urine of both exposed workers and controls in approximately equal numbers.

The conclusion, therefore, is that the data provide no evidence of a specific relationship between asbestos and gastrointestinal malignancy.

Lymphoproliferative disorders

A number of case reports have been published linking asbestos exposure to lymphatic or haematological malignancies. Kagan and Jacobson (1980) gave details of 13 assorted cases and reviewed a number of others previously reported. Ross et al. (1982) reported a case-control study purporting to show a relationship between asbestos exposure and non-Hodgkin's lymphoma of the gastrointestinal tract, but this was found after reading to each subject a list of potentially hazardous substances, and consequently must be taken as only hypothesis forming; publication was followed by a case-control study from Sweden (Bengtsson, Hardell and Eriksson, 1982) suggesting that exposure to other chemicals coincidentally was a more likely cause. Some further support for this came from Dolan, Levine and Dolan (1983), who found seven cases of small cleaved follicular central cell lymphomas in plumbers; investigation again suggested chemicals rather than asbestos as the possible common factor, as did another study by Olsson and Brandt (1983).

Ross's cases did not appear, with one exception, to have been heavily exposed to asbestos, and the relationship with the disease was equally strong for malaria, known for its adverse effects on the immune system. The 13 cases reported by Kagan and Jacobson (1980), however, had all been heavily exposed: two had mesotheliomas and nine others had asbestosis, and they discussed the possibility that the lymphomas resulted from some form of chronic immunological stimulation. However, as they pointed out, cases were referred to them from a wide area due to their known interest, and it was not possible to determine whether this number exceeded expectations.

On the basis of evidence that B-cell hyperactivity and elevation of serum immunoglobulins have been found in some asbestos workers, Schwartz et al. (1988) undertook a case-control study of chronic lymphoid leukaemia (CLL) and multiple myeloma and asbestos exposure. No evidence of any relationship with multiple myeloma appeared, but a small excess risk of CLL could not be ruled out. A previous case-control study of CLL (Linet et al., 1987) had not shown any excess risk for asbestos exposure, and on the data given by Schwartz et al., exposures did not appear to have been high, thus making confounding factors even more probable as the explanation for their finding.

The seven cases reported by Robinson, Lemen and Wagoner (1979) were from a population for which the expectation was only 3.3. But in the four large cohorts for which lymphoproliferative disorders were separately classified, Enterline, Hartley and Henderson (1987) found 9 cases with 10.8 expected (leukaemias observed 3, expected 5.4), Hughes, Weill and Hammad (1987) found 16 cases with 20.6 expected, Puntoni et al. (1979) found 12 with 11.1 expected, and Selikoff, Hammond and Seidman (1979) found 16 lymphomas with 20.1 expected and 15 leukaemias with 13.1 expected.

The epidemiological evidence, therefore, is against a direct relationship between asbestos exposure and the development of either lymphoma or leukaemia.

Skin corns

Asbestos corns (or warts) were a common feature in workers handling asbestos fibres and textiles until recent years. They are callosites on the dorsal and palmar surfaces of the hands (especially the knuckles and finger tips) and on the forearms. They consist of pronounced thickening and hyperkeratosis of the surface epithelium with some fibrosis of the dermis, round cell infiltration and occasional foreign body giant cells in the papillary layer (Alden and Howell, 1944; Schwartz, Tulipan and Birmingham, 1957). Asbestos fibres are invariably present, amphiboles apparently being more culpable than chrysotile. They do not ever appear to have been associated with local malignancy of the skin.

The corns, which may be tender on pressure, persist for years unless the spicules of fibre are removed. The workers usually learn to do this themselves. Although uncommon today they are still seen occasionally but, apart from drawing attention to asbestos exposure, are of no importance.

Tremolite

R.N. Jones, Hans Weill and W. Raymond Parkes

Tremolite, of course, is an amphibole asbestos mineral (see Appendix I) that, in general, has been of negligible commercial value and its importance as a risk to health given limited attention in the past. However, because it occurs, in varying degree, as an accessory mineral – or 'impurity' – in chrysotile, vermiculite and talc deposits and, thus, may be present in their respective commercial forms, its biological significance has attracted much attention in recent years.

As for other types of asbestos, tremolite occurs naturally, in both asbestiform (fibrous) and non-asbestiform (cleavage fragment) habits, the latter being much the more common (see Appendix I). The biological implications of the two habits raise the same fundamental questions of pathogenesis as do the other amphiboles and require similar critical appraisal (see earlier in this chapter and Chapter 5).

For these reasons it is discussed as a separate section.

Epidemiological evidence

Epidemiological information concerning tremolite as a potential health risk comes, therefore, from studies of workers occupationally exposed as a consequence of tremolitic contamination of ores (chrysotile, vermiculite and talc), and of residents of certain regions in Turkey where exposures result from naturally occurring deposits, from the contamination of road-building materials and from dust carried into streets from the land by heavy rains.

Chrysotile

Since some chrysotile deposits contain tremolite, it has been suggested that the relatively few mesothelioma cases among chrysotile workers may actually have been caused by fibrous tremolite (Churg, 1988b). Because tremolite is present in small and variable amounts in chrysotile ore, supporting evidence for the role of tremolite comes primarily from mineralogical analyses of lungs of chrysotile workers. These studies have found that the most important difference between mesothelioma cases and matched controls is the tremolite content, indicating differing tremolite exposure. However, owing to the extensive elimination of chrysotile from the lung, over time, there may have been greater differences (between cases and controls) in their previous chrysotile exposure than the lung burden analyses indicate.

Consequently, currently available population-based data do not allow definite conclusions concerning the relative roles of tremolite and chrysotile in causing cancer among chrysotile workers.

Vermiculite (see Chapter 16)

Workers from two vermiculite mines have been studied: one in Libby, Montana, studied by two independent groups of researchers (McDonald et al., 1986; McDonald, Sebastien and Armstrong, 1986; Amandus and Wheeler, 1987), and one in South Carolina (McDonald et al., 1988). Ores from both mines were contaminated with tremolite, but exposure levels and the amount of contamination were lower in South Carolina.

There was considerable overlap in the two Libby cohorts (members were required to have worked for at least a year for both studies), and overall results were similar. Exposure estimates (in fibres/ml) were based on measurements in the 1970s using the membrane filter method, and on trends in measurements made in the past using the midget impinger method.

In the McDonald et al. (1988) study, in which mean length of employment was 8.7 years, there were excess pneumoconioses (eight cases), four cases of mesothelioma, and an excess lung cancer risk (observed/expected = 23/9.4 = 2.45).

In both studies, lung cancer risk was related to estimated cumulative exposure, and the slopes of the dose–response relationships, although not identical, were reasonably similar. Based on these, 50 years of mine exposure to 0.1 fibre/ml would result in an increase in lung cancer risk of approximately 5 per cent (an SMR of 105).

Because of the non-fibrous nature of vermiculite, and the finding of pneumoconioses and elevated lung cancer rates, tremolite was interpreted to be the causative agent. Additionally, the morbidity studies (McDonald, Sebastien and Armstrong, 1986; Amandus et al., 1987) found evidence of fibrotic effects, including small discrete opacities, pleural thickening and pleural calcification.

Taken together, these studies constitute important evidence that tremolite exposures result in respiratory health consequences similar to other forms of asbestos, including lung cancer and mesothelioma. The South Carolina cohort was too small (194), and exposure levels too low, for significant excess cancer risk to have been demonstrated (McDonald et al., 1988).

Talc (see Chapter 16)

A proportional mortality study of several New York mines with tremolite contamination (Kleinfeld et al., 1967; Kleinfeld, Messite and Zaki, 1974) noted an excess in lung cancer risk among miners with at least 15 years of employment. In view of the potential problems of all proportional mortality studies, the fact that New York lung cancer rates during 1950 to 1959 were 29 per cent higher than US rates, and the lack of smoking information, these findings were considered uncertain.

Employees of a New York talc mine initially believed not to contain any abestiform minerals were the subjects of three published reports; in one, ore samples were found to contain asbestiform minerals, including tremolite, and to be similar to that from other New York mines. All three studies reported an overall excess of lung cancer (Brown, Dement and Wagoner, 1979; Stille and Tabershaw, 1982; Lamm et al., 1988). In the first two of these studies, no attempt was made to relate lung cancer risk to employment duration or cumulative exposure, although in the Brown et al. study, the expected relationship with time since hire was found. In the third study, the overall excess lung cancer risk occurred primarily among workers employed less than a year, although period of follow-up was not considered. This finding in short-term employees is of doubtful significance, because several epidemiological studies of other exposures have observed a higher risk among short-term workers than among longer-term, and it has been suggested that short-term workers may differ from other workers in ways related to cancer risk, possibly including personal lifestyles.

A study of 392 miners who had worked for at least a year in Vermont talc mines, in which the ore was reported to be *free* of asbestos contamination (Selevan et al., 1979), found an excess lung cancer risk, although a study of millers did not, even though millers were believed to have had higher exposure levels. The authors mentioned several potential influencing factors for which no information was available; these include radon exposure, smoking and the possibility that miners may have been employed previously in a talc mine in the region which was closed, but which had tremolite contamination.

A study of a large cohort ($n = 2000$) of Italian talc miners (Rubino et al., 1976) employed for at least 1 year found no evidence of excess cancer risk. The ore is reputed to be one of the purest anywhere, although analyses of the ore found a small amount of tremolite. An observed pneumoconiosis risk was attributed by the authors to silica exposure.

Lung burden studies

Limited information is available on the tremolite content of human lung in occupationally or environmentally exposed populations, or on the fibres to which various populations have been exposed, but the data which do exist indicate that both fibre concentration and fibre size can be correlated with disease patterns. Because chrysotile tends to disappear rapidly from lung, the typical lung of a chrysotile miner will contain more tremolite than chrysotile, even though tremolite constitutes only a few per cent of the ore (Churg and Wiggs, 1986; McConnochie et al., 1987). Tremolite is also seen in substantial amounts in the lungs of South Carolina chrysotile asbestos textile workers, although in a lower ratio to chrysotile (Green et al., 1986; Pooley and Mitha, 1986; Sebastien et al., 1989). In the Quebec mining and milling population, the concentration of tremolite in workers with asbestosis is, overall, markedly increased compared to those with no parenchymal disease. In both the Quebec mining and milling population, and the South Carolina textile workers, there is a good correlation between the concentration of tremolite per gram lung tissue and the degree of interstitial fibrosis (asbestosis) (Green et al., 1986; Churg et al., 1989); there is also, however, a reasonably strong correlation between chrysotile concentration and severity of fibrosis (Green et al., 1986; Churg et al., 1989), and these data do not indicate whether tremolite or chrysotile is more important in this process.

Compared to the incidence in workers heavily exposed to amosite or crocidolite, there have been relatively few mesotheliomas in the Quebec chrysotile mining population. Although analysis shows that occasional cases from the mining regions have amosite and crocidolite in their lungs (particularly workers from the region of the town of Asbestos – Case and Sebastien, 1987), most of the cases, and especially those from the region of Thetford Mines, contain only tremolite and chrysotile, the former in larger amounts than the latter (Churg et al., 1984), indicating that one or both of these fibres is the agent inducing mesothelioma. It may be important that the median tremolite content of the lungs of the Quebec workers with mesothelioma is higher than that of those with asbestosis, in contrast to the situation in workers with heavy exposure to amosite or crocidolite, where mesothelioma is associated with far lower lung burdens than asbestosis (Churg and Wright, 1989).

Studies of the lungs of Quebec miners indicate that some of the tremolite has the form of cleavage fragments of irregular diameter (which are not fibrogenic), rather than asbestiform fibres. Churg et al. (1989) found that both mean length and mean aspect ratio of tremolite showed significant, though weak, negative correlation with grade of fibrosis, that is, the more advanced the fibrosis, the greater the proportion of both shorter and thicker fibres, suggesting the inclusion of many cleavage fragments. This might be taken to imply that cleavage fragments possess fibrogenic potential. However, Churg's observation is not new; Morgan and Holmes (1980) pointed out that it is, in fact,

consistent with established findings that only long fibres are fibrogenic, but that fibrosis impairs clearance of insoluble particles in general.

Tremolite exposure from ambient air has been documented by lung analysis in various environmentally exposed populations. Tremolite, similar to other amphiboles, appears to accumulate readily in lungs at all exposure levels, and is the most commonly encountered amphibole fibre in the lungs of urban dwellers in North America (Churg and Wiggs, 1986). Here again, the fibre is a short, low-aspect ratio mineral (actually considerably shorter than the fibres seen in chrysotile miners), which is probably derived from chrysotile ore (Churg and Wiggs, 1986).

Studies of the lungs of residents of the Quebec mining townships of Asbestos (Case and Sebastien, 1987) and Thetford Mines/Black Lake (Churg, 1986; Case and Sebastien, 1987, 1989; Case, 1988), who have not been employed in the mines, provide additional information. Analysis of lung asbestos content in the latter shows that these lungs contain approximately as much tremolite as chrysotile (Churg, 1986; Case and Sebastien, 1987, 1989; Case, 1988), even though the ambient chrysotile level is several hundredfold higher than the ambient tremolite level (Sebastien et al., 1986). Fibre burden is significantly correlated both with distance of domicile from the mines, and with time lived in the mining region (Case, 1988; Case and Sebastien 1989). Even greater burdens are found in those who have household contact exposure because a close relative works in the mining and milling industry (Case, 1988). In residents of Asbestos, however, there is no tremolite excess, presumably because the ambient tremolite concentration (0.0002 fibres/ml) is much less than in Thetford Mines (0.0015 fibres/ml) (Sebastien et al., 1986).

This fibre burden is apparently occasionally associated with pleural plaques. Plaques were seen in 7 of 72 cases studied (Case and Sebastien, 1987), particularly in individuals such as farmers who encounter dust from soil (Churg and DePaoli, 1988), although there is no epidemiological evidence that either chrysotile or tremolite at this exposure level produces an excess of lung cancer or mesothelioma.

When populations are environmentally exposed to longer, and usually much higher aspect ratio, tremolite, mesotheliomas appear. Yazicioglu et al. (1980) reported a population in Turkey, and Constantopoulos and colleagues (Constantopoulos et al., 1985; Langer et al., 1987) a population in Greece, with substantial incidences of mesothelioma and exposure to long fibres with aspect ratio greater than 50. It has also been suggested that long tremolite fibres are responsible for some of the mesotheliomas seen in people other than chrysotile miners in North America (McDonald, 1988). The exact role of length versus aspect ratio is uncertain, because several apparently environmentally induced mesotheliomas have been reported from an area of Corsica, where the tremolite fibres in the lung are fairly long (probably on average as long as the amosite fibres seen in the lungs of shipyard and insulation workers in North America), but the aspect ratio is considerably lower (Magee et al., 1986).

These studies suggest that long, and probably high aspect ratio, tremolite fibres behave much like other amphiboles of comparable size, and are of particular concern because they apparently induce mesothelioma. The data also appear to indicate that tremolite of fairly low aspect ratio, probably in fairly low concentrations, is capable of causing pleural plaques. However, because the populations with exposure to this type of mineral have also had extremely high chrysotile exposure, which is not well reflected in mineral analyses of lung content, the role of chrysotile versus tremolite in the production of disease cannot be clearly sorted out.

Animal investigations

There is a limited number of studies of animals exposed to tremolite, and these studies are beset with difficulties in definition of the exact mineral used, primarily because tremolite appears in both 'asbestiform' and 'cleavage fragment' forms. There is debate concerning these mineralogical distinctions and, in many of the experiments, fibre size, length and shape are incompletely characterized (see Appendix I).

Smith (1973, 1974) and Smith et al. (1979) found that a commercial New York talc sample containing 50 per cent very large diameter tremolite (1 μm mean diameter) produced no tumours when injected into the pleural cavity of hamsters. However, mesotheliomas were produced with what are described as long and thin or 'asbestiform fibres' from other samples of 'tremolitic talc'. Unfortunately, the exact fibre sizes are not provided, and it is impossible to determine whether these samples would be properly classified as asbestiform.

The most important and widely cited studies in regard to tremolite are those by Stanton and colleagues (Stanton and Wrench, 1972; Stanton et al., 1977; Stanton, Layard and Tegeris, 1981; Harington, 1981). Using a large number of different types of mineral fibres implanted in rat pleural cavities, they showed that fibre carcinogenesis was related to fibre size, shape and durability, rather than to chemical composition. Although they found that fibres longer than 8 μm and less than 0.25 μm in diameter were, in general, the most carcinogenic,

they did observe a very high incidence of tumours with tremolite, which, in fact, was much shorter and broader. Their data suggest that tremolite fibres greater than 4 μm in length and with a diameter of less than 1.5 μm are highly carcinogenic when implanted into the pleural cavity of rats.

Wagner et al. (1982b) tested three samples of tremolite. A sample prepared from a South Korean rock which was about 80 per cent fibrous, with about one-third of the fibres longer than 8 μm and most less than 0.6 μm in diameter, produced mesotheliomas in 30 per cent of animals. By contrast, two other samples which had fewer fibres failed to produce any tumours.

Davis et al. (1985) tested an asbestiform Korean tremolite in an inhalation experiment, and found 2 mesotheliomas and 16 carcinomas in 40 animals. No tumours were seen in the controls. Their data indicate that approximately 60 per cent of the fibres were shorter than 4 μm and thicker than 0.25 μm, and 90 per cent had diameters of less than 1 μm. The authors noted that the tremolite was one of the most carcinogenic materials they had used.

These data raise the question of whether some of the original animal studies of chrysotile toxicity by inhalation may have been influenced by the presence of tremolite. Wagner, Griffiths and Munday (1987) noted that, although no tremolite was found in the original chrysotile fibre samples and fibres taken from dusting chambers using UICC chrysotile A and a fine Quebec chrysotile, re-analysis of the lung burdens of exposed rats clearly indicated the presence of tremolite fibre. Langer and Nolan (1987) were also unable to find tremolite in any specimen of Quebec chrysotile, even though studies of the lungs of both miners and those living in the neighbourhood of miners clearly indicate the presence of large quantities of tremolite (Case and Sebastien, 1989). Thus, the lung has the ability to concentrate tremolite, and to what extent effects ascribed in animal studies to chrysotile are really effects of tremolite is as yet unclear (Wagner, Griffiths and Munday, 1987; Davis, 1988; Davis and McDonald, 1988).

In summarizing the animal studies, it is clear that tremolite produces mesotheliomas and carcinomas in experimental animals, and that it is a powerful mesothelial carcinogen in these test systems. There do not appear to be any reliable data in the literature which are specifically informative with regard to the differences in the biological effect of tremolite cleavage fragments compared to asbestiform tremolite.

Although substantial uncertainties persist, unquestioned health effects of tremolite asbestos have been demonstrated in both human beings and animals. These effects are identical to those produced by other forms of asbestos. Even accepting a mineralogical distinction between asbestiform and non-asbestiform (cleavage fragments) tremolite mineral particles, beyond fibre dimension and tissue durability, this does not *per se* constitute evidence for biological effect distinctions.

References

Acheson, E.D., Gardner, M.J., Pippard, E.C. and Grime, L.P. (1982) Mortality of two groups of women who manufactured gas masks from chrysotile and crocidolite asbestos: a 40 year follow-up. *Br. J. Ind. Med.* **39**, 344–348

Adams, V.I., Unni, K., Muhm, J.R., Jett, J.R., Ilstrup, D. and Bernatz, P. (1986) Diffuse malignant mesothelioma of the pleura. *Cancer* **58**, 1540–1551

Adamson, I. and Bowden, D.H. (1987) Response of mouse lung to crocidolite. Minimal fibrotic reaction to short fibres. *J. Pathol.* **152**, 99–107

Adesina, A.M., Vallyathan, V., McQuillen, E.N., Weaver, S.O. and Craighead, J.E. (1990) Bronchiolar inflammation and fibrosis associated with smoking: morphological and cross-sectional population analysis. *Am. Rev. Respir. Dis.* **143**, 144–149

Agostoni, P., Smith, D., Schoene, R., Robertson, T. and Butler, J. (1987) Evaluation of breathlessness in asbestos workers. *Am. Rev. Respir. Dis.* **134**, 812–816

Akira, M., Yamamoto, S., Yokoyama, K. et al. (1989) Asbestosis: high-resolution CT-pathologic correlation. *Radiology* **176**, 389–394

Albeda, S.M., Epstein, D.M., Gefton, W.B. et al. (1982) Pleural thickening : its significance and relationship to asbestos dust exposure. *Am. Rev. Respir. Dis.* **126**, 621–624

Albin, M., Johansson, L., Pooley, F.D., Jakobsson, K., Attewell, R. and Mitha, R. (1990a) Mineral fibres, fibrosis, and asbestos bodies in tissue from deceased asbestos cement workers. *Br. J. Ind. Med.* **47**, 767–774

Albin, M., Attewell, R., Jakobsson, K., Johansson, L. and Welinder, H. (1990b) Mortality and cancer morbidity in cohorts of asbestos cement workers and referents. *Br. J. Ind. Med.* **47**, 602–610

Alden, H.S. and Howell, W.M. (1944) The asbestos corn. *Archs Dermatol. Syph.* **49**, 312–314

Al-Izzi, M., Thurlow, N.P. and Corrin, B. (1989) Pleural mesothelioma of connective tissue type, localised fibrous tumour of the pleura, and reactive submesothelial hyperplasia. An immuno-histochemical comparison. *J. Pathol.* **158**, 41–44

Amandus, H.E. and Wheeler, R. (1987) The morbidity and mortality of vermiculite miners exposed to tremolite–actinolite: Part II. Mortality. *Am. J. Ind. Med.* **11**, 15–26

Amandus, H.E., Althouse, R., Morgan, W.K.C., Sargent, E.N. and Jones, R.N. (1987) The morbidity and mortality of vermiculite miners exposed to tremolite–actinolite: Part III. Radiographic findings. *Am. J. Ind. Med.* **11**, 27–37

AMA, Council on Scientific Affairs (1984) A physician's guide to asbestos related diseases. *J. Am. Med. Assoc.* **252**, 2593–2597

Ames, B.N. and Gold, L.S. (1990) Too many rodent carcinogens: mitogenesis increases mutagenesis. *Science* **249**, 970–971

Anderson, A.E. (1987) Brake system performance. *Proceedings of Symposium on Fibres in Friction Materials*, Asbestos Institute, Montreal

Anderson, H.A., Lilis, R., Daum, S.M., Fischbein, A.S. and Selikoff I.J. (1979) Asbestosis among household-contacts of asbestos factory workers. *Ann. NY Acad. Sci.* **330**, 387–399

Andersson, M. and Olsen, J.H. (1985) Trend and distribution of mesothelioma in Denmark. *Br. J. Cancer* **51**, 699–705

Andrion, A., Pira, E. and Mollo, F. (1984) Pleural plaques at autopsy, smoking habits and asbestos exposure. *Eur. J. Respir. Dis.* **65**, 125–130

Andrion, A., Pira, E. and Mollo, F. (1983) Peritoneal plaques and asbestos exposure. *Archs Pathol. Lab. Med.* **107**, 609–610

Anon (1883) Asbestos and its applications. *Engineer* June 22, 467–468

Anton, H.C. (1968) Multiple pleural plaques. Part 1. *Br. J. Radiol.* **41**, 341–348

Anton-Culver, H., Culver, B. and Kurosaki, T. (1988) Immune response in shipyard workers with x-ray abnormalities consistent with asbestos exposure. *Br. J. Ind. Med.* **45**, 464–468

Armstrong, B.K., de Klerk, N.H., Musk A.W. and Hobbs, M.S.T. (1988) Mortality in miners and millers of crocidolite in Western Australia. *Br. J. Ind. Med.* **45**, 5–13

Asbestos International Association (1979) *Asbestos Cement Products*. Health and Safety Publication. Recommended Control Procedure No. 2 (RCP 2)

Ashcroft, T. and Heppleston, A.G. (1973) The optical and electron microscopic determination of pulmonary asbestos fibre concentration and its relation to the human pathological reaction. *J. Clin. Pathol.* **26**, 224–234

Ashcroft, T., Simpson, J.M. and Timbrell, V. (1988) Simple method of estimating severity of pulmonary fibrosis on a numerical scale. *J. Clin. Pathol.* **41**, 467–470

Auerbach, O., Garfinkel, L. and Hammond, E.C. (1974) Relation of smoking and age to findings in the lung parenchyma. *Chest* **65**, 29–35

Auerbach, O., Conston, A., Garfinkel, L., Parks, V., Kaslow, H. and Hammond, E.C. (1980) Presence of asbestos bodies in organs other than the lung. *Chest* **77**, 133–137

Auerbach, O., Stout, A.P., Hammond, E.C. and Garfinkel, L. (1963) Smoking habits and age in relation to pulmonary changes. *N. Engl. J. Med.* **269**, 1045–1054

Auribault, M. (1906) Note sur l'hygiene et la securite des ouvriers dans les filatures et tissage d'amiante. *Bull. Insp. Trav.* **14**, 120–132

Baker, E.L., Dagg, T. and Greene, R.E. (1985) Respiratory illness in the construction trades. *J. Occup. Med.* **27**, 483–489

Baris, Y.I. (1987) *Asbestos and Erionite-related Chest Diseases*, Department of Chest Diseases, Hacettepe University, Ankara

Baris, Y.I., Simonato, L, Artvinli, M. et al. (1987) Epidemiological and environmental evidence of the health effects of exposure to erionite fibres. *Int. J. Cancer* **39**, 10–17

Barnes, R. (1986) Progression of radiographic changes in asbestos workers and ex-workers. *J. Soc. Occup. Med.* **36**, 9–12

Barnhart, S., Thornquist, M., Omenn, G.S., Goodman, G., Feigl, P. and Rosenstock, L. (1990) The degree of roentgenographic parenchymal opacities attributable to smoking among asbestos-exposed subjects. *Am. Rev. Respir. Dis.* **141**, 1102–1106

Barrett, J.C., Lamb, P.W. and Wiseman, R.W. (1989) Multiple mechanisms for the carcinogenic effects of asbestos and other fibres. *Environ. Health Perspect.* **81**, 81–89

Barry, B.E., Wong, K.C., Brody, A.R. and Crapo, J.D. (1983) Reaction of rat lungs to inhaled chrysotile asbestos. *Expl Lung Res.* **5**, 1–21

Bateman, E., Emerson, R. and Cole, R. (1980) The use of diffusion chambers to examine the effects of mineral dusts. In: *The In Vitro Effects of Mineral Dusts* (eds R.C. Brown, I.P. Gormly, M. Chamberlain and R. Davies), Academic Press, London, pp. 289–296

Bazas, T., Bazas, B., Kitas, D. et al. (1981) Pleural calcification in north west Greece. *Lancet* **2**, 254

Beattie, J. (1961) The asbestos body. In: *Inhaled Particles and Vapours I* (ed. C.N. Davis), Pergamon Press, Oxford, pp. 434–442

Becklake, M.R. (1983) Occupational lung disease – past record and future trend. *Clin. Invest. Med.* **6**, 305–317

Becklake, M. (1991) The epidemiology of asbestosis. In: *Mineral Fibers and Health* (ed. D. Liddell and K. Miller), CRC Press, Boca Raton, FA, pp. 103–119

Becklake, M.R., Rossiter, C.E. and McDonald, J.C. (1972) Lung function in chrysotile asbestos mine and mill workers of Quebec. *Arch. Environ. Health* **24**, 401–409

Becklake, M.R., Fournier-Massey, G., McDonald, J.C., Siemiatycki, J. and Rossiter, C.E. (1970) Lung function in relation to chest radiographic changes in Quebec asbestos workers. In: *Proceedings of the International Conference, Johannesburg, 1969* (ed. H. Shapiro), Oxford University Press, Cape Town, pp. 223–261

Becklake, M.R., Liddell, F.D.K., Manfreda, J. and McDonald, J.. (1979) Radiological changes after withdrawal from asbestos exposure. *Br. J. Ind. Med.* **36**, 23–28

Becklake, M., Thomas, D., Liddell, D. and McDonald, J.C. (1982) Follow-up respiratory measurements in Quebec chrysotile miners. *Scand. J. Work Environ. Health* **8**, 105–110

Becklake, M., Toyota, B., Stewart, M., Hanson, R. and Hanley, J. (1983) Lung structure as a risk factor in adverse pulmonary responses to asbestos. *Am. Rev. Respir. Dis.* **128**, 385–388

Bégin, R., Masse, S. and Sebastien, P. (1989) Alveolar dust clearance capacity as determinant of individual susceptibility to asbestosis. *Ann. Occup. Hyg.* **33**, 279–282

Bégin, R., Cantin, A., Berthiaume, Y., Boileau, R., Peloquin, S. and Masse, S. (1983a) Airway function in lifetime non-smoking older asbestos workers. *Am. J. Med.* **75**, 631–638

Bégin, R., Rola-Pleszczynski, M., Masse, S. et al. (1983b) Assessment of asbestosis in the sheep model by bronchoalveolar lavage. *Thorax* **38**, 449–457

Bégin, R., Boctor, M., Bergerov, D. et al. (1984) Radiographic assessment of pleuropulmonary disease in asbestos workers. *Br. J. Ind. Med.* **41**, 373–383

Bégin, R., Martel, M., Desmarais, Y. et al. (1986) Fibronectin and procollagen levels in bronchoalveolar lavage of asbestos-exposed human subjects and sheep. *Chest* **89**, 237–243

Bégin, R., Menard, H., Decarie, F. and St-Saveur, A. (1987a) Immunogenetic factors as determinants of asbestosis. *Lung* **165**, 159–163

Bégin, R., Masse, S., Rola-Plezczynski, M., Boctov, M. and Drapeau, G. (1987b) Asbestos exposure dose – bronchoalveolar milieu response in asbestos workers and the sheep model. *Drug Chem. Toxicol.* **10**, 87–103

Bengtsson, N., Hardell, L. and Eriksson, M. (1982) Asbestos exposure and malignant lymphoma. *Lancet* **2**, 1463

Berry, G. (1981) The mortality of workers certified by pneumoconiosis medical panels as having asbestos disease. *Br. J. Ind. Med.* **38**, 130–137

Berry, G. and Newhouse, M.L. (1983) Mortality of workers manufacturing friction materials using asbestos. *Br. J. Ind. Med.* **40**, 1–7

Berry, G., Newhouse, M.L. and Antonis, P. (1985) Combined effect of asbestos and smoking on mortality from lung cancer and mesothelioma in factory workers. *Br. J. Ind. Med.* **42**, 12–18

Berry, G., Gilson, J.C., Holmes, S. Lewinsohn, H.C. and Roach, S.A. (1979) Asbestosis : a study of dose–response relationships in an asbestos textile factory. *Br. J. Ind. Med.* **36**, 98–112

Bignon, J., Sebastien, P., and Bientz, M. (1979) Review of some factors relevant to the assessment of exposure to asbestos dusts. In: *The Use of Biological Specimens for Assessment of Human Exposure to Environmental Pollutants* (ed. Berlin), Nijhoff, The Hague, pp. 73–108

Bitterman, P., Rennard, S., Keogh, B., Wewers, M., Adelberg, S. and Crystal, R. (1986) Familial idiopathic pulmonary fibrosis. *N. Engl. J. Med.* **314**, 1343–1347

BL Cotton (1050) British Library manuscript, Cotton Tiberius A III, mid-eleventh century. 101v–102v

Blesovsky, A. (1966) The folded lung. *Br. J. Dis. Chest* **60**, 19–22

Bohlig, H. and Calavrezos, A. (1987) Development, radiological zone patterns and importance of diffuse pleural thickening in relation to occupational exposure to asbestos. *Br. J. Ind. Med.* **44**, 673–681

Bohlig, H. and Hain, E. (1973) Cancer in relation to environmental exposure. In: *Biological Effects of Abestos* (ed. P. Bogovski), IARC Scientific Publications No. 8, Lyon, pp. 217–221

Bohning, D.E., Atkins, H.L. and Cohn, S.H. (1982) Long term particle clearance in man. *Ann. Occup. Hyg.* **26** 259–271

Booth, S.J. and Weaver, E.J.M. (1986) Mesothelioma shortly after brief exposure to asbestos. *Lancet* **1**, 435; 746; 1094

Borok, Z., Buhl, R., Grimes, C.J. et al. (1991) Effect of glutathione aerosol on oxidant–antoxidant imbalance in idopathic pulmonary fibrosis. *Lancet* **338**, 215–216

Bourbeau, J., Ernst, P., Chrome, J., Armstrong, B. and Becklake, M.R. (1990) The relationship between respiratory impairment and asbestos-related abnormality in an active work force. *Am. Rev. Respir. Dis.* **142**, 837–842

Bourke, S., Campbell, J., Henderson, R.F. and Stevenson, R.D. (1988) Apical pulmonary fibrosis in psoriasis. *Br. J. Dis. Chest* **82**, 444–446

Boutin, C., Viallat, J.., Steinbauer, J., Gaudichet, A. and Dufour, G. (1989) Pleural plaques and environmental asbestosis in North Corsica. In: *Non-occupational Exposure to Mineral Fibres* (eds J. Bignon, J. Peto and R. Saracci), IARC publications 90, Lyon, pp. 406–410

Bowden, D.H. (1987) Macrophages, dust and pulmonary diseases. *Expl Lung Res.* **12**, 89–107

Bowes, D.R., Langer, A.M. and Rohl, A.N. (1977) Nature and range of mineral dusts in the environment. *Phil. Trans. R. Soc. London* **286**, 593–610

Bozelka, B., Jones, R. and de Shazo, R. (1984) Is the immune system a contributing factor to the pathogenesis of asbestosis? *Semin. Respir. Med.* **5**, 289–299

Brain, J.D. (1988) Lung macrophages: how many kinds are there? What do they do? *Am. Rev. Respir. Dis.* **137**, 507–509

Brand, K.G. (1986) Fibrotic scar cancer in the light of foreign body tumorigenesis. In: *Silica Silicosis and Cancer* (eds D.F. Goldsmith, D.M. Winn and C.M. Shy), Praeger, New York, pp. 281–286

British Occupational Hygiene Society (1968) Hygiene standards for chrysotile asbestos dust. *Ann. Occup. Hyg.* **11**, 47–69

British Thoracic and Tuberculosis Association and the MRC Pneumoconiosis Unit (1972) A survey of pleural thickening : its relation to asbestos exposure and previous pleural disease. *Envir. Res.* **5**, 142–151

Brochard, P., Ivvatsubo, Y., Pairon, J., Larde, D. and Ameille, J. (1993) Plaques pleurales asbestoseqnes et fonction respiratoire. In: *Proceedings of the 8th International Conference on Occupational Lung Disease* (eds J. Hurych, M. Lesage and A. David), Czech Medical Society, Prague pp. 274–281.

Brody, A.R. (1986) Pulmonary cell interactions with asbestos fibres. *Chest* **89**, 1555–1595

Brody, A.R. (1991) Asbestos-induced proliferation of pulmonary bronchiolar cells. In: *Asbestos-related Cancer* (ed. M. Sluyser), Ellis Horwood, Chichester, pp. 191–206

Brown, D., Dement, J.M. and Wagoner, J.K. (1979) Mortality patterns among miners and millers occupationally exposed to asbestiform talc. In: *Dusts and Disease* (eds R. Lemen and J.M. Dement), Pathotox, Illinois, pp. 357–363

Brown, G.M., Cowie, H., Davis, J.M.G. and Donaldson, K. (1986) In vitro assays for detecting carcinogenic mineral fibres. *Carcinogenesis* **7**, 1971–1974

Browne, K. (1983a) Asbestos-related mesothelioma: epidemiological evidence for asbestos as a promoter. *Arch Environ. Health* **38**, 261–266

Browne, K. (1983b) The epidemiology of mesothelioma. *J. Soc. Occup. Med.* **33**, 190–194

Browne, K. (1986a) Is asbestos or asbestosis the cause of the increased risk of lung cancer in asbestos workers? *Br. J. Ind. Med.* **43**, 145–149

Browne, K. (1986b) A threshold for asbestos-related lung cancer. *Br. J. Ind. Med.* **43**, 556–558

Browne, K. (1991a) Asbestos-related malignancy and the Cairns hypothesis. *Br. J. Ind. Med.* **48**, 73–76

Browne, K. (1991b) A threshold for asbestos-related lung cancer. In: *Asbestos-related Cancer* (ed. M. Sluyser), Ellis Horwood, Chichester, pp. 218–240

Browne, K. and Smither, W.J. (1983) Asbestos-related mesothelioma: factors discriminating between pleural and peritoneal sites. *Br. J. Ind. Med.* **40**, 145–152

Brunner, J., Sordillo, P., Magill, G. and Golbey, R. (1982) Malignant mesothelioma of the pleura. *Cancer* **49**, 2431–2435

Buchanan, D.R., Johnston, I.D.A., Kerr, I.H., Hetzel, M.R., Corrin, B. and Turner-Warwick, M. (1988) Cryptogenic bilateral fibrosing pleuritis. *Br. J. Dis. Chest* **82**, 186–193

Buchanan, W.D. (1965) Asbestosis and primary intrathoracic neoplasms. *Ann. NY Acad. Sci.* **132**, 507–518

Burdett, G.J. and Jaffery, S. (1986) Asbestos concentrations in public buildings. *Ann. Occup. Hyg.* **30**, 185–199

Burdett, G.J., Jaffery, S. and Rood, A.P. (1989) Airborne asbestos fibre levels in buildings. In: *Non-occupational Exposure to Mineral Fibres* (eds J. Bignon, J. Peto and R. Saracci), IARC Scientific Publication 90, Lyon, pp. 277–290

Burdett, G.J., Smith, J.J. and Papanicolopoulos, C.D. (1989) Airborne asbestos fibre levels in buildings and their impact on risk management. In: *Symposium on Health Aspects of Exposure to Asbestos in Buildings* (ed. J.D. Spengler), Harvard University Energy and Environmental Policy Centre, Cambridge, MA, pp. 235–266

Burilkov, T. and Michailova, L. (1970) Asbestos content of the soil and endemic pleural asbestosis. *Environ. Res.* **3**, 443

Byers, T.E., Vena, J.E. and Rzepka, T.F. (1984) Predilection of lung cancer for the upper lobes: an epidemiological enquiry. *J. Natl Cancer Inst.* **72**, 1271–1275

Cairns, J. (1975) Mutation selection and the natural history of cancer. *Nature* **255**, 197–200

Caplan, A., Gilson, J.C., Hinson, K.F.W., McVittie, J.C. and Wagner, J.C. (1965) A preliminary study of observer variation in the classification of radiographs of asbestos-exposed workers and the relation of pathology and X-ray appearances. *Ann. NY Acad. Sci.* **132**, 379–386

Carilli, A.D., Kotzen, L.M. and Fischer, M.J. (1973) The chest roentgenogram in smoking females. *Am. J. Respir. Dis.* **107**, 103–106

Cartier, P. (1965) Discussion on pleural plaques. *Ann. NY Acad. Sci.* **132**, 387–388

Case, B. (1988) Microanalytic classification of environmental exposure in a chrysotile mining region. *Am. Rev. Respir. Dis.* **137**, (Part 2), A94

Case, B.W. and Sebastien, P. (1987) Environmental and occupational exposures to chrysotile asbestos: a comparative microanalytic study. *Archs Environ. Health* **42**, 185–191

Case, B. W. and Sebastien, P. (1989) Fiber levels in lung and correlation with air samples. *Mineral Fibres in the Non-occupational Environment*, IARC, Lyon, pp. 207–218

Case, B.W., Michael, P.C., Padilla, M. and Kleinerman, J. (1986) Asbestos effects on superoxide production. *Environ. Res.* **39**, 299–306

Chailleux, E., Dabouis, G., Pioche, D. et al. (1988) Prognostic factors in diffuse malignant mesothelioma. *Chest* **93**, 159–162

Chamberlain, M., Brown, R.C. and Griffiths, D.M. (1980) The correlation between the carcinogenic effects in vivo and the cytopathic effects in vitro of mineral dusts. In: *The In Vitro Effects of Mineral Dusts* (eds R.C. Brown, I.P. Gormly, M. Chamberlain and R. Davies), Academic Press, London, pp. 345–349

Chan, C.K. and Gee, J.B.L. (1988) Asbestos exposure and laryngeal cancer. *J. Occup. Med.* **30**, 23–27

Chatfield, E. (1983) *Measurement of asbestos fibre concentrations in ambient atmospheres.* Report prepared for the Ontario Royal Commission on matters of health and safety arising from the use of asbestos

Chesson, J., Hatfield, J., Schultz, B., Dutrow, E. and Blake, J. (1990) Airborne asbestos in public buildings. *Environ. Res.* **51**, 100–107

Chretien, J. and Hirsch, A. (1983) *Diseases of the Pleura*, Masson, Paris

Churg, A. (1982) Asbestos fibres and pleural plaques in a general autopsy population. *Am. J. Pathol.* **109**, 88–96

Churg, A. (1983) Asbestos fibre content of the lungs in patients with and without asbestos airways disease. *Am. Rev. Respir. Dis.* **127**, 470–473

Churg, A. (1986) Lung asbestos content in long-term residents of a chrysotile mining town. *Am. Rev. Respir. Dis.* **134**, 125–127

Churg, A. (1988a) 1. Non-neoplastic diseases caused by asbestos; 2. neoplastic asbestos-induced diseases. In: *Pathology of Occupational Lung Disease* (eds A. Churg and F.H.Y. Green), Igaku-Shoin, New York, pp. 213–325

Churg, A. (1988b) Chrysotile, tremolite and malignant mesothelioma in man. *Chest* **93**, 621–628

Churg, A. (1991) Analysis of lung asbestos content. *Br. J. Ind. Med.* **48**, 649–652

Churg, A. and dePaoli, L. (1988) Environmental pleural plaques in residents of a Quebec chrysotile mining town. *Chest* **94**, 58–60

Churg, A. and Warnock, M.L. (1977) Correlation of quantitative asbestos body counts and occupation. *Archs Pathol. Lab. Med.* **101**, 629–634

Churg, A.M. and Warnock, M.L. (1979) Analysis of the cores of ferruginous (asbestos) bodies from the general population III Patients with environmental exposure. *Lab. Invest.* **40**, 622–626

Churg, A. and Wiggs, B. (1986) Fiber size and number in workers exposed to processed chrysotile asbestos, chrysotile miners, and the general population. *Am. J. Ind. Med.* **9**, 143–152

Churg, A. and Wiggs, B. (1987) Mineral particles in the lungs of urban male smokers. *Environ. Res.* **42**, 121–129

Churg, A. and Wright, J.L. (1989) Fiber content of lung in amphibole vs chrysotile-induced mesothelioma. *Mineral Fibres in the Non-occupational Environment*, IARC, Lyon

Churg, A.M., Warnock, M.L. and Green, N. (1979) Analysis of the cores of ferruginous (asbestos) bodies from the general population. II True asbestos bodies and pseudoasbestos bodies. *Lab. Invest.* **40**, 31–38

Churg, A., Wiggs, B., dePaoli, L., Kampe, B. and Stevens, B. (1984) Lung asbestos content in chrysotile workers with mesothelioma. *Am. Rev. Respir. Dis.* **130**, 1042–1045

Churg, A., Wright, J.L., dePaoli, L. and Wiggs, B. (1989) Mineralogic correlates of fibrosis in chrysotile miners and millers. *Am. Rev. Respir. Dis.* **139**, 891–896

Clavier, J., Daniel, C., Kerbrat, G. and Quilland, A. (1976) Pachypleurites cryptogeniques. *Le Poumon et le Coeur* **32**, 295–298

Coffin, D.L., Palekar, L.D., Cook, P.M. and Creason, J.P. (1988) *Comparative mesothelioma induction in rats by asbestos and non-asbestos mineral fibres.* EPA Report no. 600/D-88/189. US EPA, Research Triangle Park, NC27711

Cohen, S. and Elwein, L. (1990) Cell proliferation in carcinogenesis. *Science* **249**, 1007–1011

Collins, J.D., Brown, R.K. and Batia, P. (1983) Asbestosis and the serratus anterior muscle. *J. Am. Med. Assoc.* **75**, 296–300

Commins, B. (1988) *Abestos fibres in drinking water,* Commins Associates, Altwood Close, Maidenhead SL6 4PP, UK

Connelly, R.R., Spirtas, R., Myers, M.H., Percy, C.L. and Fraumeni, J.F. (1987) Demographic patterns for mesothelioma in the US. *Am. J. Ind. Med.* **9**, 397–407

Constantopoulos, S.H., Goudevenos, J.A., Saratzi, N., Langer, A., Selikoff, I.J. and Moutsopoulos, H.M. (1985) Metsovo lung: pleural calcification and restrictive lung function in Northwestern Greece. Environmental exposure to mineral fiber as etiology. *Environ. Res.* **38**, 319–333

Cooke, W.E. (1924) Fibrosis of the lungs due to the inhalation of asbestos dust. *Br. Med. J.* **2**, 147

Cooke, W.E. (1927) Pulmonary asbestosis. *Br. Med. J.* **2**, 1024–1025

Cookson, W., De Klerk, N., Musk, A., Armstrong, B., Glancy, J. and Hobbs, M. (1986a) Prevalence of radiographic asbestosis in crocidolite miners at Wittenoom. *Br. J. Ind. Med.* **43**, 450–457

Cookson, W., De Klerk, N., Musk, A., Armstrong, B., Glancy, J. and Hobbs, M. (1986b) The natural history of abestosis in former crocidolite workers of Wittenoom. *Am. Rev. Respir. Dis.* **133**, 994–998

Cooper, W.C. (1990) Epidemiologic studies of mining populations exposed to non-asbestiform amphiboles. *Proceedings of the Seventh International Pneumoconioses Conference,* Pittsburgh. DHSS (NIOSH) publications 90–108; vol. 1, pp. 831–834

Cooper, W.C., Murchio, J., Popendorf, W. and Wenk, H.R. (1979) Chrysotile asbestos in a California recreational area. *Science* **206**, 685–688

Copes, R., Thomas, D. and Becklake, M. (1985) Temporal patterns of exposure and non-malignant pulmonary abnormality in Quebec chrysotile workers. *Archs Environ. Health* **40**, 80–87

Cordier, S., Theriault, G. and Provencher, S. (1984) Radiographic progression in a group of chrysotile miners exposed to low asbestos dust concentrations *Br. J. Ind. Med.* **41**, 384–388

Corrin, B. (1990) *The Lungs,* Vol. 5 *Systemic Pathology,* 3rd edn (ed. W. St C. Symmers), Churchill Livingstone, Edinburgh, pp. 429–430

Corry, D., Kulkarni, P. and Lipscomb, M. (1984) The migration of bronchiolar macrophages into hilar lymph nodes. *Am. J. Pathol.* **115**, 321–328

Coutts, I., Gilson, J.C., Kerr, I.H., Parkes, W.R. and Turner-Warwick, M. (1987a) Mortality in cases of asbestosis diagnosed by a pneumoconiosis medical panel. *Thorax* **42**, 111–116

Coutts, I., Gilson, J.G., Kerr, I.H., Parkes, W.R. and Turner-Warwick, M. (1987b) The significance of finger clubbing in asbestosis. *Thorax* **42**, 117–119

Craighead, J.E., Abraham, J.L., Churg, A. et al. (1982) The pathology of asbestos-associated diseases: diagnostic criteria and proposed grading schema. *Archs Pathol. Lab. Med.* **106**, 544–596

Cross, F.T., Palmer, R.F., Filipy, R.E., Dagle, G. and Stuart, B. (1982) Carcinogenic effects of radon daughters, uranium ore dust and cigarette smoke in beagle dogs. *Health Phys.* **42**, 33–52

Crump, K.S. and Farrar, D.B. (1989) Statistical analysis of data on airborne bodies collected in an EPA survey of public buildings. *Reg. Toxicol. Pharm.* **10**, 51–62

Darke, C., Wagner, M.M.F. and McMillan, G.H. (1979) HLA-A and B antigen frequencies in an asbestos exposed population with normal and abnormal radiographs. *Tissue Antigens* **13**, 228–232

Davies, D., Andrews, M.I.J. and Jones, J.S.P. (1991) Asbestos-induced pericardial effusion and constrictive pericarditis. *Thorax* **46**, 429–432

Davis, J.M.G. (1970) Further observations on the ultrastructure and chemistry of the formation of asbestos bodies. *Expl Mol. Pathol.* **13**, 346–358

Davis, J.M.G. (1972) The fibrogenic effect of mineral dusts injected into the pleural cavity of mice. *Br. J. Expl Pathol.* **53**, 190–204

Davis, J.M.G. (1979) The histopathology and ultrastructure of pleural mesotheliomas produced in the rat by injection of crocidolite. *Br. J. Expl Pathol.* **60**, 642–652

Davis, J.M.G. (1986) The pathogenicity of long versus short fibre samples of amosite. *Br. J. Expl Pathol.* **67**, 415–430

Davis, J.M.G. (1988) Commentary: on the statement by Jacques Dunnigan. *Am. J. Ind. Med.* **14**, 629–630

Davis, J.M.G. (1989) Mineral fibre cacinogenesis: experimental data relating to the importance of fibre type, size deposition, dissolution and migration. In: *Non-occupational Exposure to Mineral Fibres* (eds J. Bignon, J. Peto and R. Saracci), IARC Scientific Publications 90, Lyon, pp. 33–45

Davis, J.M.G. and Jones, A.D. (1988) Comparison of the pathogenicity of long and short fibres of chrysotile asbestos in rats. *Br. J. Expl Pathol.* **69**, 717–737

Davis, J.M.G. and McDonald, J.C. (1988) Low level exposure to asbestos: is there a cancer risk? (Editorial) *Br. J. Ind. Med.* **45**, 505–508

Davis, J.M.G., Gylseth, B. and Morgan, A. (1986) Assessment of mineral fibres from human tissue. *Thorax* **41**, 167–175

Davis, J.M.G., Beckett, S.T., Bolton, R.E., Collings, P. and Middleton, A.P. (1978) Mass and number of fibres in the pathogenesis of asbestos-related lung disease in rats. *Br. J. Cancer* **37**, 673–688

Davis, J.M.G., Addison, J., Bolton, R.E., Donaldson, K., Jones, A.D. and Miller, B.G. (1985) Inhalation studies on the effects of tremolite and brucite dust. *Carcinogenesis* **6**, 667–674

Davis, J.M.G., Bolton, R., Brown, D. and Tully, H.E. (1986) Experimental lesions in rats corresponding to advanced human asbestosis. *Expl Mol. Pathol.* **44**, 207–221

Daya, D. and McCaughey, W. (1990) Well-differentiated papillary mesothelioma of the peritoneum. *Cancer* **65**, 292–296

Dawson, A., Gibbs, A., Browne, K., Pooley, F. and Griffiths, M. (1992) Familial mesothelioma: details of 17 cases with histopathology and mineral analysis. *Cancer* **170**, 1183–1187

De Klerk, N.H., Armstrong, B.K., Musk, A.W. and Hobbs, M.S.T. (1989a) Cancer mortality in relation to measures of occupational exposure to crocidolite at Wittenoom Gorge. *Br. J. Ind. Med.* **46**, 529–536

De Klerk, N.H., Cookson, W.O., Musk, A.W., Armstrong, B.K. and Glancy, J.J. (1989b) Natural history of pleural thickening after exposure to crocidolite. *Br. J. Ind. Med.* **46**, 461–467

De Shazo, R., Hendrick, D., Diem, J. et al. (1983) Immunologic aberrations in asbestos-cement workers. *J. Allergy Clin. Immunol.* **72**, 454–461

De Shazo, R., Daul, C., Morgan, J. et al. (1986) Immunologic investigations in asbestos-exposed workers. *Chest* **89**, 162S–165S

De Vuyst, P., Dumortier, P., Moulin, E. Yourassowsky, N. and Yernault, J. (1987) Diagnostic value of asbetos bodies in bronchoalveolar lavage fluid. *Am. Rev. Respir. Dis.* **136**, 1219–1224

Delfino, R., Ernst, P. and Bourbeau, J. (1989) Relationship of lung geometry to peural abnormalities in insulation workers exposed to asbestos. *Am. J. Ind. Med.* **15**, 417–426

Dewar, A., Walente, M., Ring, N.P. and Corrin, B. (1987) Pleural mesothelioma of epithelial type and pulmonary adenocarcinoma: an ultrastructural and cytochemical comparison. *J. Pathol.* **152**, 309–316

Dodson, R.F. and Ford, J.O. (1985) Early response of the visceral pleural following asbestos exposure. *J. Toxicol. Environ. Health* **15**, 673–686

Dodson, R., Greenberg, D., Williams, M., Cora, C., O'Sullivan, M. and Hurst, G. (1984) Asbestos content in lungs of occupationally and non-occupationally exposed individuals. *J. Am. Med. Assoc.* **252**, 68–71

Dodson, R.F., Williams, M.G., Corn, C.J., Brollo, A. and Bianchi, C. (1990) Asbestos content of lung tissue, lymph tissue, lymph nodes and pleural plaques from former shipyard workers. *Am. Rev. Respir. Dis.* **142**, 843–847

Dolan, B.P., Levine, A.M. and Dolan, D.C. (1983) Small cleaved follicular centre cell lymphoma: seven cases in California plumbers. *J. Occup. Med.* **25**, 613–615

Doll, N.J., Stankus, R.P. and Barkman, W. (1983) Immunopathogenesis of asbestosis, silicosis and coal workers' pneumoconiosis. *Clin. Chest Med.* **4**, 3–14

Doll, R. (1955) Mortality from lung cancer in asbestos workers. *Br. J. Ind. Med.* **12**, 81–86

Doll, R. and Peto, J. (1985) *Effects on Health of Exposure to Asbestos.* HMSO, London

Donaldson, K. and Brown, G.M. (1993) Bronch0alveolar lavage in the assessment of the cellular response to fibre exposure. In: *Fibre Toxicology* (ed. D. Warheit), Academic Press, New York

Dreessen, W.C., Dallavalle, J.M., Edwards, T.I. et al. (1938) *A Study of Asbestosis in the Asbestos Textile Industry*, Public Health Bulletin No. 241. US Govt printing office, Washington

Du Bois, R.M. (1990) Advances in our understanding of the pathogenesis of fibrotic lung disease. *Respir. Med.* **84**, 185–187

Du Toit, R.S.J. (1991) An estimate of the rate at which crocidolite asbestos fibres are cleared from the lung. *Ann. Occup. Hyg.* **35**, 433–438

Ducatman, A.M., Withers, B.F. and Yang, W.N. (1990) Smoking and roentgenographic opacities in US Navy asbestos workers. *Chest* **97**, 810–813

Duff, G.W. (1989) Peptide regulatory factors in non-malignant disease. *Lancet* **1**, 1432–1434

Dunnigan, J., Churg, A., Becklake, M., Craighead, J., Roggli, V., McDonald, J.C. and Davis, J.M.G. (1988) Linking chrysotile asbestos with mesothelioma. *Am. J. Ind. Med.* **14**, 205–209, 235–249, 629–630

Edelman, D.A. (1988) Exposure to asbestos and the risk of gastro-intestinal cancer. *Br. J. Ind. Med.* **45**, 75–82

Edelman, D.A. (1989) Laryngeal cancer and occupational exposure to asbestos. *Int. Archs Occup. Environ. Health* **61**, 223–227

Edelman, D.A. (1992) Does asbestos exposure increase the risk of urogenital cancer? *Int. Archs Occup. Environ. Health* **63**, 469–475

Edge, J.R. (1979) Incidence of bronchial carcinoma in shipyard workers with pleural plaques. *Ann. NY. Acad. Sci.* **330**, 289–294

Edge, J.R. and Choudhury, S.L. (1978) Malignant mesothelioma of the pleura in Barrow-in-Furness. *Thorax* **33**, 26–30

Editorial (1989) Stem cells in neoplasia *Lancet* **1**, 701–702

Eisenstadt, H.B. (1965) Benign asbestos pleurisy. *J. Am. Med. Assoc.* **192**, 419–421

Elmes, P.C. (1966) The epidemiology and clinical features of asbestosis and related diseases. *Postgrad. Med. J.* **42**, 623–635

Elmes, P.C. and Simpson, M.J.C. (1976) The clinical aspects of mesothelioma. *Q.J. Med.* **45**, 427–449

Enterline, P.E. (1965) Mortality among asbestos workers in US *Ann. NY Acad. Sci.* **132**, 165–176

Enterline, P.E. (1978) *Asbestos and Cancer: The First 30 Years.* Pittsburgh, P.E. Enterline

Enterline, P.E., Hartley, J. and Henderson, V. (1987) Asbestos and cancer: a cohort followed up to death. *Br. J. Ind. Med.* **44**, 396–401

Entiknap, J.B. and Smither, W.J. (1964) Peritoneal tumours in asbestosis. *Br. J. Ind. Med.* **21**, 20–31

Epler, G.R., Carrington, C.B. and Gaensler, E.A. (1978) Crackles (râles) in the interstitial pulmonary diseases. *Chest* **73**, 333–339

Epler, G.R., McLoud, T.C. and Gaensler, E.A. (1982) Prevalence and evidence of benign asbestos pleural effusion in a working population. *J. Am. Med. Assoc.* **247**, 617–622

Epstein, D.M., Miller, W.T., Bresnitz, E.A., Levine, M. and Gefter, W. (1984) Application of ILO classification to a population without industrial exposure. AJR *Am. J. Roentgenol.* **142**, 53–58

Ernst, P., Shapiro, S., Dales, R. and Becklake, M. (1987) Determinants of respiratory symptoms in insulation workers. *Br. J. Ind. Med.* **44**, 90–95

Evans, C.C., Lewinson, H.C. and Evans, J.M. (1977) Frequency of HL-A antigens in asbestos workers with and without pulmonary fibrosis. *Br. Med. J.* **1**, 603–605

Felbermeyer, W. and Ussar, M.B. (1980) Environmental pollution by weathering of asbestos cement sheets. Institut für Unweltzschultz und Emissionsfragen. Research report A 8700. Leoben, Austria.

Finkelstein, M.M. (1894) Mortality among employees of an Ontario asbestos-cement factory. *Am. Rev. Respir. Dis.* **129**, 754–761

Fisher, A.J. (1892) The mining, manufacture and uses of asbestos. *Trans Institute of Marine Engineers* **4**, 5–22

Fletcher, D.E. (1972) A mortality study of shipyard workers with pleural plaques. *Br. J. Ind. Med.* **29**, 142–145

Fletcher, D.E. and Edge, J.R. (1970) The early radiological change in pulmonary and pleural asbestosis. *Clin. Radiol.* **21**, 355–365

Forget, G., Lacroix, M.J., Brown, R.C., Evans, P.H. and Scrois, P. (1986) Response of perfused macrophages to glass fibres. Effect of exposure duration and fibre length. *Environ. Res.* **39**, 124–135

Fournier-Massey, G. and Becklake, M.R. (1975) Pulmonary function profiles in Quebec asbestos workers. *Bull. Physio-Pathol. Respir.* **11**, 429–445

Fraire, A.E., Cooper, S., Greenberg, S.D., Buffler, P. and Langston, C. (1988) Mesothelioma of childhood. *Cancer* **62**, 838–847

Francis, D., Jussuf, A., Mortensen, T., Sikjare, B. and Viskum, K. (1977) Hyaline pleural plaques and asbestos bodies in 198 randomized autopsies. *Scand. J. Respir. Dis.* **58**, 193–196

Friedman, A.C., Fiel, S.B., Radecki, P.D. and Lev-Toaff, A.S. (1990) Computed tomography of benign pleural and pulmonary parenchymal abnormalities related to asbestos exposure. *Semin. Ultrasound, CT and MR* **11**, 393–408

Friedrichs, K.H. and Otto, H. (1981) Fibres in human lung dust samples: a scanning electron microscope study. *Am. Ind. Hyg. Assoc. J.* **42**, 150–156

Friemann, J., Muller, K.M. and Pott, F. (1990) Mesothelial proliferation due to asbestos and man-made fibres. *Pathol. Res. Pract.* **186**, 117–123

Friemann, J., Voss, B., Weller, W. and Muller, K. (1987) Asbestos induced fibrosis in the omentum of rats. *Virchows Arch. [A]* **411**, 403–408

Frumkin, H. and Berlin, J. (1988) Asbestos exposure and gastrointestinal malignancy. *Am. J. Ind. Med.* **14**, 79–95

Gaensler, E.A., Jederlinic, P.J. and McLoud, C. (1990) Progression of asbestosis. *Proceedings of the Seventh International Pneumoconioses Conference*, Pittsburgh. DHSS (NIOSH) Publication no. 90-108, pp. 386–392

Gandevia, B. (1967) Pulmonary function in asbestos workers : a three year follow-up study. *Am. Rev. Respir. Dis.* **96**, 420–427

Gamsu, G., Aberle, D.R. and Lynch, D. (1989) Computed tomography in the diagnosis of asbestos-related thoracic disease. *J. Thorac. Imag.* **4**, 61–67

Garabrant, D.H., Fine, L.J., Oliver, C., Bernstein, L. and Peters, J. (1987) Abnormalities of pulmonary function and pleural disease among titanium metal production workers. *Scand. J. Environ. Health* **13**, 47–51

Gardner, M.J. and Powell, C.A. (1986) Mortality of asbestos-cement workers using almost exclusively chrysotile fibre. *J. Soc. Occup. Med.* **36**, 124–126

Gazzi, D. and Crockford, G.W. (1987) Indoor asbestos levels on a housing estate. *Ann. Occup. Hyg.* **31**, 429–439

Gee, J.B.L. (1980) Cellular mechanisms in occupationl lung disease. *Chest* **78**, 384–387

Gellert, A.R., Kitajewska, J., Uthayakumar, S., Kirkham, J.B. and Rudd, R.M. (1986a) Asbestos fibres in bronchoalveolar lavage fluid from asbestos workers. *Br. J. Ind. Med.* **43**, 170–176

Gellert, A.R., Macy, M.G., Uthayakumar, S., Kirkham, J.B. and Rudd, R.M. (1986b) Lymphocyte subpopulations in bronchoalveolar lavage fluid in asbestos workers. *Am. Rev. Respir. Dis.* **132**, 824–828

Gerde, P. and Scholander, P. (1989) Adsorption of PAH on to asbestos. In: *Non-occupational Exposure to Mineral Fibres*, (eds J. Bignon, J. Peto and R. Saracci), IARC Scientific Publications 90, Lyon, pp. 140–148

Ghio, A.J., Renzetti, A.D. and Crapo, R.O. (1990) ILO (1980) classification and the association of small opacities with ageing. *Proceedings of the Seventh International Pneumoconiosis Conference*, Pittsburgh. DHSS (NIOSH) Publications no. 90-108, pp. 1336–1339

Gibas, Z., Li, F.P., Antman, K.H., Bermal, S., Stahel, R. and Sandberg, A.A. (1986) Chromosome changes in malignant mesothelioma. *Cancer Genet. Cytogenet.* **20**, 191–201

Gibbs, A.R. and Seal, R.M.E. (1982) Occupational lung disorders, II. Silicate Pneumoconioses. In: *Atlas of Pulmonary Pathology*, MTP Press, Lancaster, p. 91

Gibbs, A.R., Harach, R., Wagner, J.C. and Jasani, B. (1985) Comparison of tumour markers in malignant mesothelioma and pulmonary adenocarcinoma. *Thorax* **40**, 91–95

Gibbs, A.R., Griffiths, M., Pooley, F. and Jones, J.S.P. (1990) Comparison of fibre types and size distributions in lung tissues of paraoccupational and occupational cases of malignant mesothelioma. *Br. J. Ind. Med.* **47**, 621–626

Gibbs, G.W. (1979) Aetiology of pleural calcification. *Archs Environ. Health* **2**, 76–83

Ginzburg, E.A., Shilova, M.V., Korneeva, M.U. et al. (1970) The pleural form of non-occupational asbestosis. *Klin. Med. (Mosk.)* **12**, 55–60

Glover, J.R., Bevan, C., Cotes, J.E. et al. (1980) Effects of exposure to slate dust in North Wales. *Br. J. Ind. Med.* **37**, 152–162

Gloyne, S.R. (1931) Presence of asbestos bodies in faeces in a case of pulmonary asbestosis. *Tubercle* **12**, 158–159

Gloyne, S.R. (1932) The asbestos body. *Lancet* **1**, 1351–1355

Gloyne, S.R. (1932–3) The morbid anatomy and histology of asbestosis. *Tubercle* **14**, 445–451; 493–497; 550–558

Gluck, M.C., Twigg, H.L., Ball, M.F. et al. (1972) Shadows bordering the lung in normal and obese persons. *Thorax* **27**, 232–238

Goldsmith, J.R. (1982) Asbestos as a systemic carcinogen. *Am. J. Ind. Med.* **3**, 341–348

Goodglick, L.A. and Kane A.B. (1990) Cytotoxicity of long and short crocidolite asbestos fibres in vivo and in vitro. *Cancer Res.* **50**, 5153–5163

Gormley, L.P., Bolton, R.E., Braun, G., Davis, J.M.G. and Donaldson, K. (1980) Studies on the morphological patterns of asbestos induced mesotheliomas in vivo and in vitro. *Carcinogenesis* **2**, 219–231

Greaves, I.A. (1979) Rheumatoid 'pneumoconiosis' (Caplan's syndrome) in an asbestos worker: a 17 years' follow-up. *Thorax* **34**, 404–405

Green, F.H.Y., Harley, R., Vallyathan, V., Dement, J., Pooley, F. and Althouse, R. (1986) Pulmonary fibrosis and asbestos exposure in chrysotile asbestos textile workers: preliminary results. *Accompl. Oncol.* **1**, 59–68

Green, R.A. and Dimcheff, D.G. (1974) Massive bilateral upper lobe fibrosis secondary to asbestos exposure. *Chest* **65**, 52–55

Greenberg, M. (1982) The Montague Murray Case. *Am. J. Ind. Med.* **3**, 351–356

Gregor, A., Parkes, W.R. du Bois, R. and Turner-Warwick, M. (1979) Radiographic progression of asbestosis. *Ann. NY Acad. Sci.* **330**, 147–156

Gross, P., Cralley, L.J. and de Treville, R.T.P. (1967) 'Asbestos' bodies: their non-specificity. *Am. Ind. Hyg. Assoc. J.* **28**, 541–542

Guillemin, M.P., Litzistorf, G. and Buffat, P.A. (1989) Urinary fibres in occupational exposure to asbestos. *Ann. Occup. Hyg.* **33**, 219–234

Gupta, P.K. and Frost, J.K. (1981) Cytologic changes associated with asbestos exposure. *Semin. Oncol.* **8**, 283–289

Gylseth, B., Churg, A., Davis, J.M.G. et al. (1986) Analysis of asbestos fibres and asbestos bodies in tissue samples from human lung. *Scand. J. Work Environ. Health* **11**, 107–110

Haddow, A.C. (1929) Clinical aspects of pulmonary asbestosis. *Br. Med. J.* **2**, 580–581

Hague, A.K., Hernandez, J.C. and Dillard, E.A. (1985) Asbestos bodies found in infant lungs. *Archs Path. Lab. Med.* **109**, 212

Haider, M. and Neuberger, M. (1981) *Pleural plaques and asbestos exposure*, Research Report 2/81, Federal Ministry of Health and Environmental Protection, Vienna

Hammar, S.P., Bockus, D., Remington, F., Friesman, S. and Lazerte, G. (1989) Familial mesothelioma: a report of two families. *Human Pathol.* **20**, 107–112

Hammond, E.C., Selikoff, I.J. and Churg, J. (1965) Neoplasia among insulation workers in the US with special reference to intra-abdominal neoplasia. *Ann. NY Acad. Sci.* **132**, 519–525

Hammond, E.C., Selikoff, I.J. and Seidman, H. (1980) Asbestos exposure, cigarette smoking and death rates. *Ann. NY Acad. Sci.* **330**, 473–490

Hammond, E.C., Garfinkel, L., Selikoff, I.J. and Nicholson, W.J. (1979) Mortality experience of residents in the neighbourhood of an asbestos factory. *Ann. NY Acad. Sci.* **330**, 417–422

Hansen, K. and Mossman, B.T. (1987) Generation of superoxide from alveolar macrophages exposed to asbestiform and non-fibrous particles. *Cancer Res.* **47**, 1681–1686

Harber, P., Mohsenifar, Z. and Oven, A. (1987) Pleural plaques and asbestos-associated malignancy. *J. Occup. Med.* **29**, 641–644

Harington, J.S. (1981) Fiber carcinogenesis: epidemiologic observations and the Stanton hypothesis (Guest Editorial). *J. Natl Cancer Inst.* **67**, 977–988

Harries, P.G. (1976) Experience with asbestos disease and its control in Great Britain's naval dockyards. *Environ. Res.* **11**, 261–267

Harmsen, A.G., Muggenburg, B.A., Snipes, M.B. and Bice, D.E. (1985) The role of macrophages in particle translocation from lungs to lymph nodes. *Science* **230**, 1277–1281

Hasan, F.M., Nash, G. and Kazemi, H. (1978) Asbestos exposure and related neoplasia. *Am. J. Med.* **65**, 649–654

Haslam, P., Turner-Warwick, M. and Lukoszek, A. (1975) Antigen-nuclear antibody and lymphocyte responses to nuclear antigens in patients with lung disease. *Clin. Expl Immunol.* **20**, 379–395

Haslam, P., Lukoszek, A., Merchant, J.A. and Turner-Warwick, M. (1978) Lymphocyte responses to phytohaemagglutinin in patients with asbestosis and pleural mesothelioma. *Clin. Expl Immunol.* **31**, 178–188

Health Effects Institute (1991) *Asbestos in Public and Commercial Buildings.* Health Effects Institute – Asbestos Research. Cambridge, MA, vol. 4, pp. 13–70

Heard, B.E. and Williams, R. (1961) The pathology of asbestosis with reference to lung function. *Thorax* **16**, 264–281

Heckman, C.A. and Dalbey, W.E. (1982) Pathogenesis of lesions induced in rat lung by chronic tobacco smoke inhalation. *J. Natl Cancer Instit.* **69**, 117–129

Herbert, A. (1984) The diagnosis of malignant mesothelioma. *J. Pathol.* **143**, 145–146

Herbert, A. (1986) Pathogenesis of pleurisy. *Thorax* **41**, 176–189

Hill, R.J., Edwards, R.E. and Cathew, P. (1990) Early changes in the pleural mesothelium following intrapleural inoculation of the mineral fibre erionite and the subsequent development of mesotheliomas. *J. Expl Pathol.* **71**, 105–118

Hillerdal, G. (1980) The pathogenesis of pleural plaques. *Eur. J. Respir. Dis.* **61**, 129–138

Hillerdal, G. (1981) Non-malignant asbestos pleural disese. *Thorax* **36**, 669–675

Hillerdal, G. (1983) Ankylosing spondylitis lung disease – an underdiagnosed entity? *Eur. J. Respir. Dis.* **64**, 437–441

Hillerdal, G. (1984) Asbestos related pleuropulmonary lesions and the ESR. *Thorax* **39**, 752–758

Hillerdal, G. (1989) Rounded atelectasis. Clinical experience with 74 patients. *Chest* **95**, 836–841

Hillerdal, G. (1990) Pleural and parenchymal fibrosis mainly affecting the upper lung lobes in persons exposed to asbestos. *Respir. Med.* **84**, 129–134

Hillerdal, G. and Berg, J. (1985) Malignant mesothelioma secondary to chronic inflammation and old scars. *Cancer* **55**, 1968–1972

Hinson, K.F.W., Otto, H., Webster, I. and Rossiter, C.E. (1973) Criteria for the diagnosis of grading asbestosis. In: *Biological Effects of Asbestos* (eds P. Bogovski, J.C. Gibson, V. Timbrell and J.C. Wagner), IARC Scientific Publication no. 8, Lyon, pp. 54–57

Hirsch, A., Brochard, P., de Cremoux, H. et al. (1982) Features of asbestos-exposed and unexposed mesothelioma. *Am. J. Ind. Med.* **3**, 413–422

Hnizdo, E. and Sluis-Cremer, G.K. (1988) Effects of tobacco smoking on the presence of asbestosis at post mortem and on the reading of irregular opacities. *Am. Rev. Respir. Dis.* **138**, 1207–1212

Hobbs, M.S.T., Woodward, S., Murphy, B., Musk, A.W. and Elder, J.E. (1980) The incidence of pneumoconiosis mesothelioma and respiratory cancer in men engaged in mining crocidolite. In: *Biological Effects of Mineral Fibres* (ed. J.C. Wagner), Lyon, IARC Scientific Publications no. 30, pp. 615–625

Hodgson, A.A. (1966) *Fibrous Silicates. Lecture series 1965*; 4. Royal Society of Chemistry, London

Hodgson, A.A. (1977) Nature and paragenesis of asbestos minerals. *Philos. Trans. R. Soc. Lond. [Biol.]* **286**, 611–624

Hoffman, F.L. (1918) Mortality from respiratory diseases in dusty trades. *US Bureau of Labour Statistics Bulletin* **231**, 178

Holden, J. and Churg, A. (1986) Asbestos bodies and the diagnosis of asbestosis in chrysotile workers. *Envir. Res.* **39**, 232–236

Holmes, S. (1965) Developments in dust sampling and counting techniques in the asbestos industry. *Ann. NY Acad. Sci.* **132**, 289–297

Holt, P.F. (1983) Translocation of inhaled dust to the pleura. *Environ. Res.* **31**, 212–220

Hourihane, D. O'B. (1964) The pathology of mesotheliomata and an analysis of their association with asbestos exposure. *Thorax* **19**, 268–278

Hourihane, D. O'B. and McCaughey, W.T.E. (1966) Pathological aspects of asbestosis. *Postgrad. Med. J.* **42**, 613–622

Hourihane, D. O'B., Lessof, L. and Richardson, P.C. (1966) Hyaline and calcified pleural plaques as an index of exposure to asbestos. A study of radiological and pathological features of 100 cases with a consideraion of epidemiology. *Br. Med. J.* **1**, 1069–1074

Hughes, J.M. and Weill, H. (1986) Asbestos exposure – quantitative assessment of risk. *Am. Rev. Respir. Dis.* **133**, 5–13

Hughes, J.M. and Weill, H. (1991) Asbestosis as a precursor of asbestos-related lung cancer: results of a prospective mortality study. *Br. J. Ind. Med.* **48**, 229–233

Hughes, J.M., Weill, H. and Hammad, Y. (1987) Mortality of workers employed in two asbestos cement manufacturing plants. *Br. J. Ind. Med.* **44**, 161–174

Huncharek, M., Capotorto, J.V. and Muscat, J. (1989) Domestic asbestos exposure, lung fibre burden and pleural mesothelioma in a housewife. *Br. J. Ind. Med.* **46**, 354–355

Huuskonen, M.S. (1978) Clinical features, mortality and survival of patients with asbestosis. *Scand. J. Work Environ. Health* **4**, 265–274

Huuskonen, M.S., Tiilikainen, A. and Alanko, K. (1979) HLA-B18 antigens and protection from pulmonary fibrosis in asbestos workers. *Br. J. Dis. Chest* **73**, 253–259

Ilgren, E.B. and Browne, K. (1991) Asbestos-related mesothelioma: evidence for a threshold in humans and animals. *Regul. Toxicol. Pharmacol.* **13**, 116–132

Ilgren, E.B. and Wagner, J.C. (1991) Background incidence of mesothelioma: animal and human evidence. *Regul. Toxicol. Pharmacol.* **13**, 133–149

Jacob, G. and Bohlig, H. (1955) Roentgenological complications in pulmonary asbestosis. *Fortschr. Roentg.* **83**, 515–525

Jarvholm, B. and Sanden, A. (1986) Pleural plaques and respiratory function. *Am. J. Ind. Med.* **10**, 419–426

Jarvholm, B., Arvidsson, H., Bake, B., Hillerdal, G. and Westion, C-G. (1986) Pleural plaques – asbestos – ill health. *Eur. J. Respir. Dis.* (suppl. 145) **68**, 1–59

Jaurand, M.C. (1989) Particulate-state carcinogenesis: a survey of recent studies on the mechanisms of action of fibres. *Non-occupational Exposure to Mineral Fibres* (eds J. Bignon, J. Peto and R. Saracci), IARC Scientific Publication no. 90, Lyon, pp. 54–73

Jaurand, M., Goni, J., Jeaunot, P., Sebastien, P. and Bignon, J. (1976) Solubilite du chrysotile in vitro et dans le poumon humaine. *Rev. fr. Mal. Respir.* **4** (suppl. 2), 111–120

Jodoin, G., Gibbs, G.W., Macklem, P.T., McDonald, J.C. and Becklake, M.R. (1971)Early effects of asbestos exposure on lung function. *Am. Rev. Respir. Dis.* **104**, 525–535

Johansson, L.G., Albin, M., Jakobsson, K.M., Welinder, H., Ranstam, P. and Attewell, R. (1987) Ferruginous bodies and pulmonary fibrosis in dead low to moderately exposed asbestos cement workers: histological examination. *Br. J. Ind. Med.* **44**, 550–558

Johnson, N.F., Haslam, P., Dewar, A., Newman Taylor, A.J. and Turner-Warwick, M. (1986) Identification of inorganic dust particles in bronchoalveolar lavage macrophages. *Archs Environ. Health* **41**, 133–144

Jones, J.S.P. (1987) *Pathology of the Mesothelium*, Springer-Verlag, Berlin, p. 239

Jones, J.S.P., Smith, P.G., Pooley, F.D., Berry, G. and Sawle, G.V. (1980) The consequences of exposure to asbestos dust in a wartime gas mask factory. In: *Biological Effects of Mineral Fibres* (ed. J.C. Wagner), IARC Scientific Publication no. 30, Lyon, pp. 537–554

Jones, R., Smith, D.M. and Thomas, G. (1988) Mesothelioma in Great Britain in 1968–83. *Scand. J. Work Environ. Health* **14**, 145–152

Jones, R., Diem, J., Glindmeyer, H., Weill, H. and Gilson, J. (1980) Progression of asbestos radiographic abnormalities. In: *Biological Effects of Mineral Fibres* (ed. J.C. Wagner), IARC Scientific Publication no. 30, Lyon, pp. 537–544

Jones, R., Diem, J.E., Hughes, J.M., Hammad, Y.Y., Glindmeyer, H.W. and Weill, H. (1989) Progression of asbestos effects: a prospective longitudinal study of chest radiographs and lung function. *Br. J. Ind. Med.* **46**, 97–105

Kagamimori, S., Watanabe, M., Kubota, M. et al. (1984) Serum interferon levels and natural killer cell activity in patients with asbestosis. *Thorax* **39**, 65–66

Kagan, E. and Jacobson, R.J. (1980) Lymphoid and plasma cell malignancies : asbestos-related disorders of long latency. *Am. J. Clin. Pathol.* **80**, 14–20

Kagan, E., Solomon, A., Cochrane, J.C., Kuba, P., Rocks, P.H. and Webster, I. (1977a) Immunological studies of patients with asbestosis. II studies in circulating lymphoid cell numbers and humoral immunity. *Clin. Expl Immunol.* **28**, 268–275

Kagan, E., Solomon, A., Cochrane, J.C., Beissner, E.I., Gluckman, J., Rocks, P.H. and Webster, I. (1977b) Immuno-logical studies of patients with asbestosis. I studies of cell-mediated immunity. *Clin. Expl Immunol.* **28**, 261–267

Kane, M.J., Chahinian, A.P. and Holland, J.F. (1990) Malignant mesothelioma in young adults. *Cancer* **65**, 1449–1455

Kang, K.Y., Sera, Y., Okochi, T. and Yamamura, Y. (1974) T lymphocytes in asbestosis. *N. Engl. J. Med.* **291**, 735–736

Kannerstein, M. and Churg, J. (1977) Peritoneal mesothelioma. *Human Pathol.* **8**, 83–94

Kasuga, H., Mikami, R., Tamoura, M., Miyazaki, T. and Narita, N. (1987) Effects of smoking on asbestos-related pulmonary and pleural changes. *Jap. J. Ind. Health* **29**, 191–195

Kelley, J. (1990) Cytokines of the lung. *Am Rev. Respir. Dis.* **141**, 76–788

Kilburn, K.H. (1981) Cigarette smoking does not produce or enhance the radiologic appearance of pulmonary fibrosis. *Am. J. Ind. Med.* **2**, 305–308

Kilburn, K., Warshaw, R. and Thornton, J.C. (1986) Asbestosis, pulmonary symptoms and functional impairment in shipyard workers. *Chest* **88**, 254–259

Kilburn, K.H., Lilis, R., Anderson, H.A., Miller, A. and Warshaw, R. (1986) Interaction of asbestos, age and cigarette smoking in producing radiographic evidence of diffuse pulmonary fibrosis. *Am. J. Med.* **80**, 377–381

King, E.J., Clegg, J.W. and Rae, V.M. (1946) Effects of asbestos on the lungs of rabbits. *Thorax* **1**, 188–197

Kipen, H.M., Lilis, R., Suzuki, Y., Valciukdas, J.A. and Selikoff, I.J. (1987) Pulmonary fibrosis in asbestos insulation workers with lung cancer. *Br. J. Ind. Med.* **44**, 96–100

Kittredge, R.D. (1974) The many facets of sclerosing fibrosis. *AJR Am. J. Roentgenol.* **122**, 288–298

Kiviluoto, R. (1965) Pleural plaques and asbestos. *Ann. NY Acad. Sci.* **132**, 235–239

Kiviluoto, R., Meurman, L.O. and Hakama, M. (1979) Pleural plaques and neoplasia in Finland. *Ann. NY Acad. Sci.* **330**, 31–33

Kleinfeld, M., Messite, J. and Zaki, M.H. (1974) Mortality experi-ences among talc workers: a follow-up study. *J. Occup. Med.* **16**, 345–349

Kleinfeld, M., Giel, C.P. , Majeranowski, J.F. and Zaki, M.H. (1967) Mortality among talc miners and millers in New York State. *Archs Environ. Health* **14**, 663–667

Kolev, K. (1982) Experimentally induced mesothelioma in white rats in response to intraperitoneal administration of amorphous crocidolite. *Environ. Res.* **29**, 123

Kreel, L. (1981) Computed tomography in mesothelioma. *Semin. Oncol.* **8**, 302–312

Kuschner, M. (1987) The effects of MMMF on animal systems: some reflections on their pathogenesis. *Ann. Occup. Hyg.* **31**, 791–797

Lamm, S.H., Levine, M.S., Starr, J.A. and Tirey, S.L. (1988) Analysis of excess lung cancer risk in short-term employees. *Am. J. Epidemiol.* **127**, 1202–1209

Lange, A. and Skibinski, G. (1977) T and B cells and delayed-type skin reactions in asbestos workers. *Scand. J. Immunol.* **6**, 720

Lange, A., Smolik, R., Chmielarczyk, W., Garncarek, D. and Gielgier, Z. (1978) Cellular immunity in asbestosis. *Archs Immunol. Ther. Exp.* **26**, 899–903

Lange, A., Garmcarek, D., Tomeczko, J. et al. (1986) Outcome of asbestos exposure with respect to skin reactivity. *Environ. Res.* **41**, 1–13

Lange, A. (1980) An epidemiological survey of immunological abnormalities in asbestos workers. *Environ. Res.* **22**, 162–183

Langer, A.M. and Nolan, R.P. (1987) The properties of chrysotile asbestos as determinants of biological activity: variations in cohort experience and disease spectra as related to mineral properties. *Accompl. Oncol.* **1** (2), 30–51

Langer, A.M. and Nolan, R.P. (1989) Fibre type and mesothelioma risk. In: *Symposium on Health Effects of Exposure to Asbestos in Buildings* (ed. J. Spengler), Harvard University Energy and Environmental Policy Centre, Cambridge, MA, pp. 91–140

Langer, A.M., Nolan, R.P., Constantopoulos, S.A. and Moutsopoulos, M. (1987) Association of Metsovo lung and pleural mesothelioma with exposure to tremolite-containing whitewash. *Lancet* **1**, 965

Lauweryns, J.M. and Baert, J.H. (1977) Alveolar clearance and the role of the pulmonary lymphatics. *Am. Rev. Respir. Dis.* **115**, 625–683

Law, M.R., Ward, F.G., Hodgson, M. and Heard, B.E. (1983) Evidence for longer survival of patients with pleural mesothe-lioma without asbestos exposure. *Thorax* **38**, 744–746

Law, M.R., Gregor, A., Hodson, M.E., Bloom, H.J.G. and Turner-Warwick, M. (1984) Malignant mesothelioma of the pleura: a study of 52 treated and 64 untreated patients. *Thorax* **39**, 255–259

Le Bouffant, I., Bruyere, S., Martin, J.C., Tichoux, G. and Normand, C. (1976) Quelques observations sur les fibres d'amiante et les formations mineral diverse rencontrees dans les poumons asbestosiques. *Rev. Fr. Mal. Resp.* **4** (suppl. 2), 121–140

Leathart, G.L. (1968) Pulmonary function tests in asbestos workers. *Trans. Soc. Occup. Med.* **18**, 49–55

Lebel, J. (1984) *Review of fibre concentrations in Quebec asbestos mining towns.* Quebec Asbestos Mining Association, Quebec

Lederman, G.S., Recht, A., Herman, T., Osteen, R., Corson, J. and Antman, K. (1987) Long-term survival in peritoneal mesothelioma. *Cancer* **59**, 1882–1886

Lee, R.J. (1987) *The Constant Study Revisited.* Energy Technology Consultants, Monroeville, PA

Lemaire, I., Beaudouin, H., Masse, S. and Grondin, C. (1986) Alveolar macrophage stimulation of lung fibroblast growth in asbestos-induced pulmonary fibrosis. *Am. J. Pathol.* **122**, 205–211

Lemenager, J., Raffaelli, C., Letourneux, M. et al. (1985) Atteintes pleurales et retentissement fonctionnel de l'asbestose. *La Presse Medicale* **14**, 1462–1464

Lerman, Y., Selikoff, I.J., Lillis, R., Seidman, H. and Gelb, S. (1986) Clinical findings among asbestos workers in US: influences of cigarette smoking. *Am. J. Ind. Med.* **10**, 449–458

Lewinsohn, H.C. (1974) Early malignant changes in pleural plaques due to asbestos exposure: a case report. *Br. J. Dis. Chest* **68**, 121–127

Liang-ho Su and Zheng-jun Li (1980) Researches on the records about asbestos in ancient Chinese literature. *Proceedings of the Fourth International Conference on Asbestos*, Turin

Liddell, D. (1991) Asbestos in the occupational environment. In: *Mineral Fibers and Health* (ed. D. Liddell and K. Miller), CRC Press, Boca Raton, FA, pp. 103–119

Liddell, F.D.K. (1989) Epidemiological observations on mesothelioma and their implications for non-occupational exposure to asbestos. In: *Symposium on Health Aspects of Exposure to Asbestos in Buildings* (ed. J.D. Speagler), Harvard University Energy and Environmental Policy Centre, Cambridge, MA, pp. 47–70

Liddell, F.D.K. (1990) Laryngeal cancer and asbestos. *Br. J. Ind. Med.* **47**, 289–291

Liddell, F.D.K. (1993) Health effects of historical exposures to asbestos. In: Health Risks from Exposure to Mineral Fibres (ed. G.W. Gibbs, J. Dunnigan, M. Kido and T. Higashi), Captus University Publications, Ontario, pp. 49–65

Liddell, F.D.K. and Hanley, J.A. (1985) Relations between asbestos exposure and lung cancer SMRs in occupational cohort studies. *Br. J. Ind. Med.* **42**, 389–396

Liddell, F.D.K. and McDonald, J.C. (1980) Radiological findings as predictors of mortality in Quebec asbestos workers. *Br. J. Ind. Med.* **37**, 257–267

Liddell, F.D.K. and Miller, K. (1983) Individual susceptibility to inhaled particles. *Scand. J. Work Environ. Health* **9**, 1–8

Liddell, F.D.K., McDonald, J.C. and Thomas, D.C. (1977) Methods of cohort analysis: appraisal by application to asbestos mining. *J.R. Statist. Soc.* **140**, 469–491

Lilis, R., Lerman, Y. and Selikoff, I.J. (1988) Symptomatic benign pleural effusions among asbestos insulation workers. *Br. J. Ind. Med.* **45**, 443–449

Lilis, R., Lerman, Y., Selikoff, I.J., Seidman, H. and Gelb, S. (1986) Asbestosis: interstitial pulmonary fibrosis and pleural fibrosis: influence of cigarette smoking. *Am. J. Ind. Med.* **10**, 459–470

Lilis, R., Ribak, J., Suzuki, Y., Penner, L., Bernstein, N. and Selikoff, I.J. (1987) Non-malignant chest x-ray changes in patients with malignant mesothelioma. *Br. J. Ind. Med.* **44**, 402–406

Linet, M.S., Stewart, W.F., Van Natta, M.L., McCaffrey, L.D. and Szklo, M. (1987) Comparison of methods for determining occupational exposure in a case-control interview study of chronic lymphatic leukaemia. *J. Occup. Med.* **29**, 136–142

Lin-Chu, M., Lee, Y.J. and Ho, M.Y. (1989) Malignant mesothelioma in infancy. *Archs Pathol. Lab. Med.* **113**, 409–411

Lippman, M., Yeates, D.B. and Albert, R.E. (1980) Deposition, retention and clearance of inhaled particles. *Br. J. Ind. Med.* **37**, 337–362

Logan, W.P.D. (1982) *Cancer Mortality by Occupation and Social Class 1851–1971.* IARC and OPCS. HMSO, London

Lumley, K.S. (1977) Physiological changes in asbestos pleural disease. In: *Inhaled Particles 4* (ed. W. Walton), Pergamon, Oxford, pp. 781–788

Lynch, K.M. and Smith, W.A. (1935) Pulmonary asbestosis: carcinoma of the lung in asbesto-silicosis. *Am. J. Cancer* **24**, 56–64

McCaughey, W.T.E. and Oldham, P.E. (1973) Diffuse mesotheliomas: observer variation in histological diagnosis. In: *Biological Effects of Asbestos* (ed. P. Bogovski), IARC Publications no. 8, Lyon

McConnochie, K., Simonato, L., Mevrides, P., Christofides, P., Pooley, F.D. and Wagner, J.C. (1987) Mesothelioma in Cyprus: the role of tremolite. *Thorax* **42**, 342–347

McConnochie, K., Simonato, L., Mevrides, P., Christofides, P., Mitha, R. and Wagner, J.C. (1989) Malignant mesothelioma in Cyprus. In: *Non-occupational Exposure to Mineral Fibres* (eds J. Bignon, J. Peto and R. Saracci), IARC Scientific Publication 90, Lyon

McCullagh, S.F., Aresini, G., Browne, K. et al. (1982) Criteria for the diagnosis and considerations in the attribution of lung cancer and mesothelioma to asbestos exposure. *Int. Archs Occup. Environ. Health* **49**, 357–361

McDonald, A.D. and McDonald, J.C. (1978) Mesothelioma after crocidolite exposure during gas mask manufacture. *Environ. Res.* **17**, 340–346

McDonald, A.D. and McDonald, J.C. (1987a) Epidemiology of malignant mesothelioma. In: *Asbestos-related Malignancy* (eds K. Antman and J. Aisner), Grune & Stratton, Orlando, FA, pp. 31–55

McDonald, A.D. and McDonald, J.C. (1987b) Epidemiology of asbestos-related lung cancer. In: *Asbestos-related Malignancy* (eds K. Antman and J. Aisner), Grune & Stratton, Orlando, FA, pp. 57–79

McDonald, A.D., McDonald, J.C. and Pooley, F. (1982) Mineral fibre content of lung in mesothelial tumours in N. America. In: *Inhaled Particles V* (ed. W.H. Walton), Pergamon, Oxford, pp. 417–422

McDonald, A.D., Fry, J.S., Woolley, A.J. and McDonald, J.C. (1983a) Dust exposure and mortality in an American chrysotile textile plant. *Br. J. Ind. Med.* **40**, 361–367

McDonald, A.D., Fry, J.S., Woolley, A.J. and McDonald, J.C. (1983b) Dust exposure and mortality in an American factory using chrysotile, amosite and crocidolite in mainly textile manufacture. *Br. J. Ind. Med.* **40**, 368–374

McDonald, A.D., Fry, J.S., Woolley, A.J. and McDonald, J.C. (1984) Dust exposure and mortality in an American chrysotile friction products plant. *Br. J. Ind. Med.* **41**, 151–157

McDonald, J.C. (1985) Health implications of environmental exposure to asbestos. *Envir. Health Persp.* **62**, 319–328

McDonald, J.C. (1988) Tremolite, other amphiboles, and mesothelioma. *Am. J. Ind. Med.* **14**, 247–249

McDonald, J.C. (1990) Cancer risks due to asbestos and man-made fibres. In: *Recent Results in Cancer Research*, Vol. 120 (ed. P. Band), Springer-Verlag, Berlin, pp. 122–131

McDonald, J.C. and McDonald, A. (1991) Epidemiology of mesothelioma. In: *Mineral Fibers and Health* (eds. D. Liddell and K. Miller), CRC Press, Boca Raton, FA, pp. 103–119

McDonald, J.C., Gibbs, G.W. and Oakes, D. (1984) Radiographic response to cumulative chrysotile exposure. Paper presented to the 21st International Congress on Occupational Health, Dublin 1984 (abstract)

McDonald, J.C., Sebastien, P. and Armstrong, B. (1986) Radiological survey of past and present vermiculite miners exposed to tremolite. *Br. J. Ind. Med.* **43**, 445–449

McDonald, J.C., Becklake, M.R., Gibbs, G.W., McDonald, A.D. and Rossiter, C.E. (1974) The health of chrysotile asbestos mine and mill workers of Quebec. *Archs Environ. Health* **28**, 61–68

McDonald, J.C., Gibbs, G.W, Liddell, F.D. and McDonald, A.D. (1978) Mortality after long exposure to cummingtonite-grunerite. *Am. Rev. Respir. Dis.* **118**, 271–277

McDonald, J.C., Liddell, F.D.K., Gibbs G.W., Eyssen, G.E. and McDonald, A.D. (1980) Dust exposure and mortality in chrysotile mining. 1910–1975. *Br. J. Ind. Med.* **37**, 11–24

McDonald, J.C., McDonald, A., Armstrong, B. and Sebastien, P. (1986) Cohort study of vermiculite miners exposed to tremolite. *Br. J. Ind. Med.* **43**, 436–444

McDonald, J.C., McDonald, A.D., Sebastien, P. and Moy, K. (1988) Health of vermiculite miners exposed to trace amounts of fibrous tremolite. *Br. J. Ind. Med.* **45**, 630–634

McDonald, J.C., Armstrong, B., Case, B., Doell, D., McCaughey, W.T.E., McDonald, A.D. and Sebastien, P. (1989) Mesothelioma and asbestos fibre type. *Cancer* **63**, 1544–1547

McDonald, S., (1927) Histology of pulmonary asbestosis. *Br. Med. J.* **2**, 105–1026

McGavin, C.R. and Sheers, G. (1984) Diffuse pleural thickening in asbestos workers. *Thorax* **39**, 604–607

McLemore, M., Roggli, V., Marshall, M., Lawrence, C., Greenberg, D. and Stevens, P. (1981) Comparison of phagocytosis of uncoated versus coated asbestos fibres by cultured human macrophages. *Chest* **50**, 39S–42S

McLoud, T.C., Woods, B.O., Carrington, C.B., Epler, G. and Gaensler, E.A. (1985) Diffuse pleural thickening in an asbestos-exposed population. AJR *Am. J. Roentgenol.* **144**, 9–18

McMillan, G.H., Pethybridge, R.J. and Sheers, G. (1980) Effects of smoking on attack rates of pulmonary and pleural lesions related to exposure to asbestos dust. *Br. J. Ind. Med.* **37**, 268–272

MacRae, K.D. (1988) Asbestos in drinking water and cancer. *J. R. Coll. Physns* **22**, 7–10

Magee, F., Wright, J.L., Chan, N., Lawson, L. and Churg, A. (1986) Malignant mesothelioma caused by childhood exposure to long-fiber low aspect ratio tremolite. *Am. J. Ind. Med.* **9**, 529–533

Marchand, F. (1907) Uber eigentumliche Pigmentkristalle in den lungen. *Ver. Deutsch. Path. Gesell.* **10**, 223–228

Marco Polo (1298) *The Travels of Marco Polo*, Penguin, London, pp. 88–90

Markham, M., Cleary, S., Pfeifle, C. and Howell, S. (1986) Cisplatin administered by the intracavitary route as treatment for malignant mesothelioma. *Cancer* **58**, 18–21

Marshall, E.G. and Stein, E.C. (1990) Respiratory morbidity among plumbers and pipefitters associated with past asbestos exposure. *Proceedings of the Seventh International Pneumoconiosis Conference*, Pittsburgh. DHSS (NIOSH) publications no. 90-108, 1, 334

Mårtensson, G., Hagberg, S., Petterson, K. and Thiringer, G. (1987) Asbestos pleural effusion: a clinical entity. *Thorax* **42**, 646–651

Matej, H., Lange, A. and Smolnik, R. (1977) HLA antigens in asbestosis. *Archs Immunol. Ther. Exp.* **25**, 489–491

Mattson, S.B. (1971) Caplan's syndrome in association with asbestos. *Scand. J. Respir. Dis.* **52**, 153–161

Meadway, J. (1974) Ulcerative colitis, colitic spondylitis and associated apical pulmonary fibrosis. *Proc. R. Soc. Med.* **67**, 324–325

Merchant, J.A., Klouda, P.T., Soutar, S.A., Parkes, W.R., Lawler, S.D. and Turner-Warwick, M. (1975) The HL-A system in asbestos workers. *Br. Med. J.* **1**, 189–191

Merewether, E.R.A. (1949) Annual Report, Chief Inspector of Factories, 1947. HMSO, London

Merewether, E.R.A. and Price, C.W. (1930) *Report on Effects of Asbestos on the Lungs and Dust Suppression in the Asbestos Industry*. HMSO, London

Meurman, L. (1966) Asbestos bodies and pleural plaques in a Finnish series of autopsy cases. *Acta Pathol. Microbiol. Scand.* suppl. 181

Meurman, L.O. (1968) Pleural fibrocalcific plaques and asbestos exposure. *Environ. Res.* **2**, 30–46

Miller, A. (1993) The advent of asbestos-related pleural thickening on pleural plaques. In: *Proceedings of the 8th International Conference on Occupational Lung Disease* (eds J. Hurych, M. Lesage and A. David), Czech Medical Society, Prague

Miller, K., Webster, I., Handfield, R.M. and Skikne, M.I. (1978) Ultra-structure of the lung in the rat following exposure to crocidolite and quartz. *J. Partic.* **124**, 39–44

Minder, C.E. and Vader, J-P. (1988) Malignant pleural mesothelioma among Swiss furniture workers. *Scand. J. Work Environ. Health* **14**, 252–256

Mintzer, R.A. and Cugell, D.W. (1982) The association of asbestos-induced pleural disease and rounded atelectasis. *Chest* **81**, 457–460

Mirabella, F. (1986) Mesothelioma in children. *Folia Oncol.* **9**, 71–81

Moalli, P.A., McDonald, J.L. Goodglick, L.A. and Kane, A.B. (1987) Acute injury and regeneration of the mesothelium in response to asbestos fibres. *Am. J. Pathol.* **128**, 426–445

Mohsenifar, Z., Jasper, A.J., Mahrer, T. and Koerner, S. (1986) Asbestos and airflow limitation. *J. Occup. Med.* **28**, 817–820

Mollo, F., Andrion, A., Pira, E. and Barocelli, M.P. (1983) Indicators of asbestos exposure in autopsy routine. Pleural plaques and occupation. *Med. Lav.* **74**, 137–142

Mollo, F., Andrion, A., Belles, D. and Bertoldo, E. (1987) Screening of autopsy populations for previous occupational exposure to asbestos. *Archs Environ. Health* **42**, 44–50

Montague Murray, H. (1907) Evidence in: *Report of the departmental committee on compensation for industrial diseases*. HMSO, London, pp. 127–128

Morgan, A. (1980) Effect of length on the clearance of fibres from the lung and on body formation. In: *Biological Effects of Mineral Fibres* (ed. J.C. Wagner), IARC Scientific Publications 30, Lyon, pp. 329–335

Morgan, A. and Holmes, A. (1980) Concentrations and dimensions of coated and uncoated asbestos fibres in human lungs. *Br. J. Ind. Med.* **37**, 25–32

Morgan, A. and Holmes, A. (1984) The distribution and characteristics of asbestos fibres in the lungs of Finnish anthophyllite workers. *Environ. Res.* **33**, 62–75

Morgan, A. and Holmes, A. (1985) The enigmatic asbestos body. *Environ. Res.* **38**, 283–292

Morgan, A., Evans, J.C. and Holmes, A. (1977) Deposition and clearance of inhaled fibrous minerals in the rat. Studies using radioactive tracer techniques. In: *Inhaled Particles IV* (ed. W.H. Walton), Pergamon, Oxford, pp. 259–272

Morgan, W.K.C. (1964) Rheumatoid pneumoconiosis in association with asbestosis. *Thorax* **19**, 433–435

Mossman, B.T. and Gee, J.B.L. (1989) Asbestos-related diseases. *N. Engl. J. Med.* **320**, 1721–1730

Mossman, B.T., Gilbert, R., Doherty, S.B., Shatos, M., Marsh, J. and Cutroneo, K. (1986) Cellular and molecular mechanisms of asbestosis. *Chest* **89**, 1605–1615

Mossman, B.T., Bignon, J., Corn, M., Seaton, A. and Gee, J.B.L. (1990) Asbestos: scientific developments and implications for public policy. *Science* **247**, 294–301

Mowe, G., Gylseth, B., Hartveit, F. and Skang, V. (1984) Occupational asbestos exposure, lung-fibre concentration and latency time in malignant mesothelioma. *Scand. J. Work. Environ. Health* **10**, 293–298

Muhle, H., Bellmann, B., Spurny, K. and Pott, F. (1989) Inhalation experiments on retention and lung clearance of asbestos in combination with cigarette smoking. In: *Biological Interaction of Inhaled Mineral Fibres and Cigarette Smoke* (ed. A.P. Wehner), Batelle, Columbus, OH, pp. 183–194

Muldoon, B.C. and Turner-Warwick, M.W. (1972) Lung function studies in asbestos workers. *Br. J. Dis. Chest* **66**, 121–132

Murphy, R.L., Becklake, M.R., Brooke, S. et al. (1986) The diagnosis of non-malignant diseases related to asbestos. *Am. Rev. Respir. Dis.* **134**, 363–368

Murray, R. (1990) Asbestos – a chronology of its origins and health effects. *Br. J. Ind. Med.* **47**, 361–365

Murray, R. and Castleman, B.I. (1991) Asbestos and cancer; history and public policy. Letters to the editor. *Br. J. Ind. Med.* **48**, 427–432

Muscat, J.E. and Wynder, E.L. (1991) Cigarette smoking, asbestos exposure and malignant mesothelioma. *Cancer Res.* **51**, 2263–2267

Muscat, J.E. and Wynder, E.L. (1992) Tobacco, alcohol, asbestos and occupational risk factors for laryngeal cancer. *Cancer* **69**, 2244–2251

Navratil, M. and Dobias, J. (1973) Development of pleural hyalinosis in lung from studies of persons exposed to asbestos dust. *Environ. Res.* **6**, 455–472

Navratil, M., Moravkova, K., Gafronova, M. and Hruska, F. (1986) The fate of men with pleural hyalinosis. *Pracovni Lekarstvi* **38**, 433–437

Nemeth, L., Tolnai, K., Hovanyl, E. et al. (1986) Frequency, sensitivity and specificity of roentgenographic features of slight and moderate asbestos-related disease. *Fortsch. Roentg.* **144**, 9–16

Neuberger, M. and Kundi, M. (1990) Individual asbestos exposure, smoking and mortality. *Br. J. Ind. Med.* **47**, 615–620

Neuberger, M., Kundi, M. and Friedl, H.P. (1984) Environmental asbestos exposure and cancer mortality. *Archs Environ. Health* **39**, 261–265

Newhouse, M.L. and Sullivan, K.R. (1989) A mortality study of workers manufacturing friction materials. *Br. J. Ind. Med.* **46**, 176–179

Newhouse, M.L. and Thompson, H. (1965) Mesothelioma of pleura and peritoneum following exposure to asbestos in the London area. *Br. J. Ind. Med.* **22**, 261–269

Newhouse, M.L., Berry, G. and Wagner, J.C. (1985) Mortality of factory workers in East London 1933–80. *Br. J. Ind. Med.* **42**, 4–11

Newhouse, M.L., Matthews, G., Sheikh, K., Knight, K.L., Oakes, D. and Sullivan, K.R. (1988) Mortality of workers at acetylene production plants. *Br. J. Ind. Med.* **45**, 63–69

Newman, R.H. (1986) Fine biogenic fibres in sugar cane: a possible hazard. *Ann. Occup. Hyg.* **30**, 365–370

Nicholson, W.J., Rohl, A.N., Weisman, I. and Selikoff, I.J. (1980) Environmental asbestos concentrations. In: *Biological Effects of Mineral Fibres* (ed. J.C. Wagner), IARC Scientific Publication 30, Lyon, pp. 713–721

Oberdorster, G., Morrow, P.E. and Spurny, K. (1988) Size dependent lymphatic short term clearance of amosite fibres in the lung. In: *Inhaled Particles V* (ed. J. Dodgson), Pergamon, Oxford, pp. 149–156

Ohlson, C-G. and Hogstedt, C. (1985) Lung cancer among asbestos-cement workers. A Swedish cohort study. *Br. J. Ind. Med.* **42**, 397–402

Ohlson, C-G., Bodin, L., Rydman, T. and Hogstedt, C. (1985) Ventilatory decrements in former asbestos cement workers. *Br. J. Ind. Med.* **42**, 612–616

Okazaki, I., Marayama, K., Kobayashi, Y., Lilis, R. and Suzuki, Y. (1987) Serum type III procollagen peptide: indicator for pulmonary fibrosis. *Am. J. Ind. Med.* **11**, 439–446

Oliver, R.M. and Neville, E. (1988) Progressive apical pleural fibrosis. *Br. J. Dis. Chest* **82**, 439–443

Olsson, H. and Brandt, L. (1983) Asbestos exposure and non-Hodgkin's lymphoma. *Lancet* **1**, 588

Ontario (1984) Royal Commission on matters of health and safety arising from the use of asbestos in Ontario. Ontario Ministry of the Attorney General, Toronto

Parnes, S.M. (1990) Asbestos and cancer of the larynx : is there a relationship? *Laryngoscope* **100**, 254–260

Pelnar, P.V. (1988) Further evidence of non-asbestos-related mesothelioma. *Scand. J. Work Environ. Health* **14**, 141–144

Peterson, J.T., Greenberg, S.D. and Buffler, P.A. (1984) Non-asbestos related malignant mesothelioma. *Cancer* **55**, 1968–1972

Peto, J. (1989) Fibre carcinogenesis and environmental hazards. In: *Non-occupational Exposure to Mineral Fibres* (eds J. Bignon, J. Peto and R. Saracci), IARC Scientific Publication 90, Lyon, pp. 457–470

Peto, J., Henderson, B.E. and Pike, M.C. (1981) Trends in mesothelioma incidence in the United States. In: *Banbury Report 9: Quantification of Occupational Cancer.* Cold Spring Harbour Laboratory, New York, pp. 51–72

Peto, J., Seidman, H. and Selikoff, I.J. (1982) Mesothelioma mortality in asbestos workers: implications for models of carcinogenesis and risk assessment. *Br. J. Cancer* **45**, 124–135

Peto, J., Doll, R., Hermon, C., Binns, W., Clayton, R. and Goffe, T. (1985) Relationship of mortality to measures of environmental asbestos pollution in an asbestos textile factory. *Ann. Occup. Hyg.* **29**, 305–355

Pierce, R. and Turner-Warwick, M. (1980) Skin tests with tuberculin (PPD), *Candida albicans* and *Trichophyton* spp. in cryptogenic fibrosing alveolitis and asbestos-related lung disease. *Clin. Allergy* **10**, 229–237

Pillgram-Larsen, J., Urdal, L., Smith Meyer, R. and Birkeland, S. (1984) Malignant pleural mesothelioma. *Scand. J. Thor Cardiovasc. Surg.* **18**, 69–73

Platek, S.F., Groth, D.E., Ulrich, C.E. et al. (1985) Chronic inhalation of short fibres. *Fund. Appl. Toxicol.* **5**, 327–340

Pooley, F.D. (1972) Electron microscope characteristics of inhaled chrysotile asbestos fibre. *Br. J. Ind. Med.* **29**, 146–153

Pooley, F.D. and Mitha, R. (1986) Fiber types, concentrations and characteristics found in lung tissues of chrysotile-exposed cases and controls. *Accompl. Oncol.* **1**, 1–11

Pott, F.D. (1978) Some aspects on the dosimetry of the carcinogenic potency of asbestos and other fibrous dusts. *Staub-Reinhalt. Luft* **38**, 486–490

Pott, F. (1987) The fibre as a carcinogenic agent. *Zentralbl. Bakteriol. MikroBiol. Hyg.* **184**, 1–23

Pott, F., Huth, F. and Friedrichs, K.H. (1974) Tumorigenic effect of fibrous dusts in experimental animals. *Environ. Health Perspect.* **9**, 313–315

Pott, F., Roller, M., Ziem, U. et al. (1989) Carcinogenicity studies on natural and man-made fibres with the intraperitoneal test in rats. In: *Non-occupational Exposure to Mineral Fibres* (eds J. Bignon, J. Peto and R. Saracci), IARC Scientific Publication no. 90, Lyon, pp. 277–290

Puntoni, R., Vercelli, M., Merlo, F., Valerio, F. and Santi, L. (1979) Mortality among shipyard workers in Genoa. *Ann. NY Acad. Sci.* **330**, 353–377

Rebuck, A.S. and Brande, A. (1983) Bronchoalveolar lavage in asbestosis. *Archs intern Med.* **143**, 950–952

Reger, R.B., Cole, W.S., Sargent, E.N. and Wheeler, P.S. (1990) Cases of alleged asbestos-related disease: a radiologic re-evaluation. *J. Occup. Med.* **32**, 1088–1090

Rendall, R.E.G. and Du Toit, R.S.J. (1991) The retention and clearance of glass fibre and different varieties of asbestos (Abstract). *Proceedings, Seventh International Symposium on Inhaled Particles*, Edinburgh, Sept. 1991

Ribak, J., Lilis, R., Suzuki, Y., Penner, L. and Selikoff, I.J. (1988) Malignant mesothelioma in a cohort of asbestos insulation workers. *Br. J. Ind. Med.* **45**, 182–187

Rickards, A.G. and Barrett, G.M. (1958) Rheumatoid lung changes associated with asbestosis. *Thorax* **13**, 185–193

Roberts, G.H. (1971) The pathology of parietal pleural plaques. *J. Clin. Pathol.* **24**, 348–353

Roberts, G.H. (1976) Distant visceral metastasis in pleural mesothelioma. *Br. J. Dis. Chest* **70**, 246–250

Robertson, H.E. (1924) Endothelioma of the pleura. *J. Cancer Res.* **8**, 317–375

Robinson, B.W.S. and Musk, A.W. (1981) Benign asbestos pleural effusion. *Thorax* **36**, 895–900

Robinson, B., Rose, A., James, A., Whitaker, D. and Musk, A. (1986) Alveolitis of pulmonary asbestosis. *Chest* **90**, 396–402

Robinson, B., Rose, A., Hayes, A. and Musk, A.W. (1988) Increased pulmonary gamma interferon production in asbestosis. *Am. Rev. Respir. dis.* **138**, 278–83

Robinson, C.F., Lemen, R.A. and Wagoner, J.K. (1979) Mortality patterns among workers employed in an asbestos textile friction and packing products manufacturing facility. In: *Dusts and Diseases* (ed. J.M. Dement and R. Lemen), Pathotox, Illinois, pp. 131–143

Rockoff, S.D., Kagan, E., Schwartz, A., Kriebel, D., Hix, W. and Rohatgi, P. (1987) Visceral pleural thickening in asbestos exposure: the occurrence and implications of thickened inter-lobar fissure. *J. Thorac. Imag.* **2**, 58–66

Rodelsperger, K., Jahn, H., Bruckel, B., Mauke, J., Paur, R. and Woitowitz, H.J. (1986) Asbestos dust exposure during brake repair. *Am. J. Ind. Med.* **10**, 63–72

Roe, F.J.C. (1988) Biological interactions: important things we do not know. In: *Biological Interaction of Inhaled Mineral Fibres and Cigarette Smoke* (ed. A.P. Wehner), Battelle Press, Columbus, Ohio, pp. 1–14

Rogers, A.J. (1983) Mineral fibre content of human lung tissue as an index of past exposure to asbestos types. *Occup. Health Aust. NZ* **5**, 55–61

Rogers, A.J. (1990) Cancer mortality and exposure to crocidolite. *Br. J. Ind. Med.* **47**, 286–287

Roggli, V.L. (1990) Human disease consequences of fibre exposure: a review of human lung pathology and fibre burden data. *Environ. Health Perspect.* **88**, 295–303

Roggli, V. and Brody, A. (1984) Changes in numbers and dimensions of chrysotile fibres in the lungs of rats following short-term exposure. *Expl Lung Res.* **7**, 133–147

Roggli, V.L., George, M.H. and Brody, A.R. (1987) Clearance and dimensional changes of crocidolite asbestos fibres isolated from lungs of rats following short term exposure. *Environ. Res.* **42**, 94–105

Roggli, V., Pratt, P. and Brody, A. (1986) Asbestos content of lung tissue in asbestos associated diseases. *Br. J. Ind. Med.* **43**, 18–28

Ronneberg, A., Andersen, A. and Skyberg, K. (1988) Mortality and incidence of cancer among oil exposed workers in a Norwegian cable manufacturing company 1953–84. *Br. J. Ind. Med.* **45**, 595–601

Ross, R., Dworsky, R., Nichols, P. et al. (1982) Asbestos exposure and lymphomas of the gastrointestinal tract and oral cavity. *Lancet* **2**, 118–120

Rossiter, C.E. and Harries, P.G. (1979) UK Naval dockyards asbestosis study. *Br. J. Ind. Med.* **36**, 281–291

Rossiter, C.E., Browne, K. and Gilson, J.C. (1988) International classification trial of AIA set of 100 radiographs of asbestos workers. *Br. J. Ind. Med.* **45**, 538–543

Rossiter, C.E., Heath, J.R. and Harries, P.G. (1980) Royal Naval dockyards asbestosis research project. *J. R. Soc. Med.* **73**, 337–344

Rous, V. and Studený, J. (1970) Aetiology of pleural plaques. *Thorax* **25**, 270–284

Rowlands, N., Gibbs, G.W. and McDonald, A. (1982) Asbestos fibres in the lungs of chrysotile miners and millers. *Ann. Occup. Hyg.* **26**, 411–415

Rubino, G. (1986) Bronchoalveolar lavage and Gallium Scintigraphy in the evaluation of the occupational interstitial lung diseases. *Am. J. Ind. Med.* **9**, 393–395

Rubino, G.F., Newhouse, M., Murray, R., Scansetti, G., Piolatto, G. and Aresini, G. (1979a) Radiologic changes after cessation of exposure among chrysotile abestos miners in Italy. *Ann. NY Acad. Sci.* **330**, 157–161

Rubino, G.F., Piolatto, G., Newhouse, M.L., Scansetti, G., Aresini, G.A. and Murray, R. (1979b) Mortality of chrysotile asbestos workers at the Balangero mine. *Br. J. Ind. Med.* **36**, 187–194

Rubino, G.F., Scansetti, G., Pira, E. et al. (1980) Pleural plaques, and lung asbestos bodies in the general population. In: *Biological Effects of Mineral Fibres* (ed. J.C. Wagner), IARC Scientific Publication 30, Lyon, pp. 545–551

Ruttner, J.R., Schuler, G. and Walchi, P. (1983) Todesfalle im Umfeld einer Schweizer Asbestindustrie. *Soz. Praventifmed.* **28**, 262–263

Sahn, S.A. and Antony, V.B. (1984) Pathogenesis of pleural plaques. *Am. Rev. Respir. Dis.* **130**, 884–887

Samet, J.M., Epler, G.R., Gaensler, E.A. and Rosner, B. (1979) Absence of synergism between exposure to asbestos and cigarette smoking in asbestosis. *Am. Rev. Respir. Dis.* **121**, 75–82

Saracci, R. (1977) Asbestos and lung cancer: an analysis of the epidemiological evidence on the asbestos-smoking interaction. *Int. J. Cancer* **20**, 323–331

Saracci, R., Simonato, L., Baris, Y.I., Artvinli, M. and Skidmore, J. (1982) The age-mortality curve of endemic pleural mesothelioma in Karain. *Br. J. Cancer* **45**, 147–149

Sargent, E.N., Gordonson, J., Jacobson, G., Birnbaum, W. and Shaub, M. (1978) Bilateral pleural thickening: a manifestation of asbestos dust exposure. *AJR Am. J. Roentgenol.* **131**, 579–585

Sargent, E.N., Boswell, W.D., Rolls, P.W. et al. (1984) Subpleural fat pads in patients exposed to asbestos. *Radiology* **153**, 272–277

Sawyer, R.N. (1979) Indoor asbestos pollution. *Ann. NY Acad. Sci.* **330**, 579–585

Schwartz, D.A., Fuortes, L.J., Galvin, J.R. et al. (1990) Asbestos-induced pleural fibrosis and impaired lung function. *Am. Rev. Respir. Dis.* **141**, 321–326

Schwartz, L., Tulipan, L. and Birmingham, D.J. (1957) *Occupational Diseases of the Skin*, 3rd ed, Kimpton, London, p. 846

Schwartz, P.A., Vaughan, T.L., Heyer, N.J. et al. (1988) B cell neoplasms and occupational asbestos exposure. *Am. J. Ind. Med.* **14**, 661–671

Seal, R.M.E. (1980) Current views on pathological aspects of asbestosis. The unresolved questions and problems. In: *Biological Effects of Mineral Fibres* (ed. J.C. Wagner), IARC Scientific Publication 30, Lyon, pp. 217–226

Seaton, A., Louw, S.J. and Cowie, H.A. (1986) Epidemiologic studies of Scottish oil shale wokers. *Am. J. Ind. Med.* **9**, 409–421

Sebastien, P., Masse, R. and Bignon, J. (1980) Recovery of ingested asbestos fibres from the gastrointestinal lymph of rats. *Environ. Res.* **22**, 201–216

Sebastien, P., Fondimare, A., Bignon, J., Monchaux, G., Desbordes, J. and Bonnand, G. (1977) Topographic distribution of asbestos fibres in human lung in relation to occupational and non-occupational exposure. In: *Inhaled Particles IV* (eds W.H. Walton and B. McGovern), Pergamon, Oxford, pp. 435–444

Sebastien, P., Janson, X., Bonnard, G. et al. (1979) Translocation of asbestos fibres through respiratory tract and gastrointestinal tract according to fibre type and size. In: *Dusts and Disease* (eds R. Lemen and J.M. Derwent), Pathotox, Illinois, pp. 65–85

Sebastien, P., Bignon, J., Baris, Y.I., Awad, L. and Petit, G. (1984) Ferruginous bodies in sputum as an indication of exposure to airborne mineral fibres in Cappadocia. *Archs Environ. Health* **39**, 18–23

Sebastien, P., Plourde, M., Robb, R. et al. (1986) *Ambient Air Asbestos Survey in Quebec Mining Towns. Part 2 – main study.* Environment Canada Report 5/AP/RQ-2E

Sebastien, P., Armstrong, B., Case, B., Barwick, H., Keskula, H. and McDonald, J.C. (1988a) Estimation of amphibole exposure from asbestos body and macrophage counts in sputum. In: *Inhaled Particles VI* (ed. J. Dodgson), Pergamon, Oxford, pp. 195–201

Sebastien, P., Armstrong, B., Monchaux, G. and Bignon, J. (1988b) Asbestos bodies in bronchoalveolar lavage fluid and in lung parenchyma. *Am. Rev. Respir. Dis.* **137**, 75–78

Sebastien, P., McDonald, J.C., McDonald, A.D., Case, B. and Harley, R. (1989) Respiratory cancer in chrysotile textile and mining industries: exposure inferences from lung analysis. *Br. J. Ind. Med.* **46**, 180–187

Seidman, H., Selikoff, I.J. and Gelb, S.K. (1986) Mortality experience of amosite asbestos factory workers. *Am. J. Ind. Med.* **10**, 479–514

Seidman, H., Selikoff, I.J. and Hammond, E.C. (1979) Short term asbestos work exposure and long term observation. *Ann. NY Acad. Sci.* **330**, 61–89

Selevan, S.G., Dement, J.M., Wagoner, J.K. and Froines, J.R. (1979) Mortality patterns among miners and millers of non-asbestiform talc: preliminary report. In: *Proceedings of the Conference on Occupational Exposures to Fibrous and Particulate Dust and their Extension into the Environment, 1977, Washington DC* (eds R. Lemen and J.M. Dement). Pathotox, Park Forest South, Illinois, pp. 379–388

Selikoff, I.J. (1965) The occurrence of pleural calcification among asbestos insulation workers. *Ann. NY Acad. Sci.* **132**, 351–367

Selikoff, I.J., Hammond, EC. and Churg, J. (1968) Asbestos exposure, smoking and neoplasia. *J. Am. Med. Assoc.* **204**, 106–112

Selikoff, I.J., Hammond, E.L. and Seidman, H. (1979) Mortality experience of insulation workers in the US and Canada. *Ann. NY Acad. Sci.* **330**, 91–116

Shaw, R.J. (1991) The role of lung macrophages at the interface between chronic inflammation and fibrosis. *Respir. Med.* **85**, 267–274

Shaw, R.J., Benedict, S.H., Clark, R.A.F. and King, T.E. (1991) Pathogenesis of pulmonary fibrosis in interstitial lung disease. *Am. Rev. Respir. Dis.* **143**, 167–173

Sheehy, J.W., Todd, W.F., Cooper, T.C. and Van Waganen, H.D. (1988) Evaluation of brake drum service controls at Cincinnati Bell maintenance factory. *Government Reports, Announcements and Index*, issue 10

Sheers, G. (1979) Asbestos-associated disease in employees of Devonport dockyard. *Ann. NY Acad. Sci.* **330**, 281–287

Sheers, G. and Coles, R. (1980) Mesothelioma risks in a naval dockyard. *Archs Environ. Health* **35**, 276–282

Sheers, G. and Templeton, A.R. (1968) Effects of asbestos in dockyard workers. *Br. Med. J.* **3**, 574–579

Shore, B.L., Daughaday, C. and Spilberg, I. (1983) Benign asbestos pleurisy in the rabbit. *Am. Rev. Respir. Dis.* **128**, 481–485

Siracusa, A., Fiore, M., Scielzo, R. et al. (1983) Small airways disease after short term occupational exposure. *Med. Lav.* **74**, 13–22

Slack, J.M.W. (1986) Epithelial metaplasia and the second anatomy. *Lancet* **2**, 268–271

Sluis-Cremer, G.K. (1965) Asbestosis in South Africa. *Ann. NY Acad. Sci.* **132**, 215–234

Sluis-Cremer, G.K. and Bezuidenhart, B.N. (1989) Relation between asbestosis and bronchial cancer in amphibole asbestos miners. *Br. J. Ind. Med.* **46**, 537–540

Sluis-Cremer, G.K. and Beduizenhart, B.N. (1990) Relation between asbestosis and bronchial cancer in amphibole asbestos miners (letter) *Br. J. Ind. Med.* **47**, 215–216

Sluis-Cremer, G.K. and Hnizdo, E. (1989) Progression of irregular small opacities in asbestos miners. *Br. J. Ind. Med.* **46**, 846–852

Sluis-Cremer, G.K. and Webster, I. (1972) Acute pleurisy in asbestos exposed persons. *Environ. Res.* **5**, 380–392

Sluis-Cremer, G.K., Hnizdo, E. and du Toit, R.S.J. (1990) Evidence for an amphibole asbestos threshold exposure for asbestosis assessed by autopsy in South African asbestos miners. *Ann. Occup. Hyg.* **34**, 443–451

Smith, W.E. (1973) Asbestos, talc and nitrites in relation to gastric cancer. (Under the heading: 'Industrial Hygiene Summary Reports', a category meant for '. . . brief comments derived from daily activities'.) *Am. Hyg. Assoc. J.* **34**, 227–228

Smith, W.E. (1974) Experimental studies on biological effects of tremolite talc on hamsters. *Proceedngs of the Symposium on Talc. US Bureau of Mines*, Washington DC, A. Goodwin, Information Circular #8639, pp. 43–48

Smith, W.E. and Hubert, D.D. (1974) The intrapleural route as a means for estimating carcinogenicity. *Experimental Lung Cancer: Carcinogenesis and Bioassays*, International symposium held at the Battelle Seattle Research Center, Seattle, June 23–26, 1974. Springer-Verlag, New York, pp. 92–101

Smith, W.E., Hubert, D.D., Sobel, H.J. and Marquet, E. (1979) Biologic tests of tremolite in hamsters. *Dusts and Disease. Proceedings of the Conference on Occupational Exposures to Fibrous and Particulate Dusts and their Extension into the Environment.* Pathotox, Park Forest South, Illinois, pp. 335–339, 341–355

Smither, W.J. (1965) Secular changes in asbestosis in an asbestos factory. *Ann. NY Acad. Sci.* **132**, 166–181

Solomon, A., Goldstein, B., Webster, I. and Sluis-Cremer, G.K. (1971) Massive fibrosis in asbestosis. *Environ. Res.* **4**, 430–439

Solomon, A., Irwig, L.M., Sluis-Cremer, G.K. et al. (1979) Thickening of interlobar fissures. Exposure response relationships in crocidolite and amosite miners. *Br. J. Ind. Med.* **36**, 195–198

Solomons, K. (1984) Malignant mesothelioma – clinical and epidemiological features. *S. Afr. Med. J.* **66**, 407–412

Spencer, H. (1985) *Pathology of the Lung*, 4th ed. Pergamon, Oxford

Spirtas, R., Beebe, G.W., Connelly, R.R. et al. (1986) Recent trends in mesothelioma incidence in the US. *Am. J. Ind. Med.* **9**, 397–407

Sprince, N.L., Oliver, L.C., McLoud, T.C., Eisen, E.A., Christiani, D.C. and Ginns, L.C. (1991) Asbestos exposure and asbestos-related pleural and parenchymal disease: associations with immune imbalance. *Am. Rev. Respir. Dis.* **143**, 822–828

Stanford, F. (1976) Sympathetic nerve involvement with mesothelioma of the pleura. *Br. J. Dis. Chest* **70**, 134–137

Stansfield, D. and Edge, J.R. (1974) Circulating rheumatoid factor and antinuclear antibodies in shipyard workers with pleural plaques. *Br. J. Dis. Chest* **68**, 166–170

Stanton, M.F. (1973) Some aetiological considerations of carcinogenesis. In: *Biological Effects of Asbestos* (eds P. Bogovski, J. C. Gibson, V. Timbrell and J.C. Wagner), IARC Scientific Publication 8, Lyon, pp. 289–294

Stanton, M.F. and Wrench, C. (1972) Mechanisms of mesothelioma induction with asbestos and fibrous glass. *J. Natl Cancer Inst.* **48**, 797–821

Stanton, M.F., Layard, M. and Tegeris, A. (1981) Relation of particle dimension to carcinogenicity in amphibole asbestoses and other fibrous minerals. *J. Natl Cancer Inst.* **65**, 967–975

Stanton, M.F., Layard, M., Tegeris, A., Miller, E., May, M. and Kent, E. (1977) Carcinogenicity of fibrous glass: pleural response in the rat in relation to fiber dimension. *J. Natl Cancer Inst.* **58**, 587–597

Stephens, M., Gibbs, A.R., Pooley, F.D. and Wagner, J.C. (1987) Asbestos induced diffuse pleural fibrosis. *Thorax* **42**, 583–588

Stille, W.T. and Tabershaw, I.R. (1982) The mortality experience of upstate New York talc workers. *J. Occup. Med.* **24**, 480–484

Stovin, P. and Partridge, P. (1982) Pulmonary asbestos and dust content in E. Anglia. *Thorax* **37**, 185–192

Sullivan, K.R., Lam, T.H. and Rossiter, C.E. (1988) HM Naval Bases: mesothelioma and time since first employment. *Ann. Occup. Hyg.* **32**, 491–496

Suoranta, H., Huuskonen, M.S., Zitting, A. and Juntunsu, J. (1982) Radiographic progression of asbestosis. *Am. J. Ind. Med.* **3**, 67–74

Suzuki, Y., Churg, J. and Kannerstein, M. (1976) Ultrastructure of human malignant diffuse mesothelioma. *Am. J. Pathol.* **85**, 241–251

Suzuki, Y. and Kohyama, N. (1984) Malignant mesothelioma induced by asbestos and zeolite in the mouse peritoneal cavity. *Environ. Res.* **35**, 277–292

Taskinen, E., Ahlman, K. and Wiikeri, M. (1973) A current hypothesis of the lymphatic transport of inspired dust to the parietal pleura. *Chest* **64**, 193–196

Tattersall, N.H.N. and Boyer, M.J. (1990) Management of malignant pleural effusions. *Thorax* **45**, 81–82

Taylor, D.R., Page, W., Hughes, D. and Vaighese, G. (1987) Metastatic renal cell carcinoma mimicking pleural mesothelioma. *Thorax* **42**, 901–902

Tellesson, W.G. (1961) Rheumatoid pneumoconiosis (Caplan's syndrome) in an asbestos worker. *Thorax* **16**, 372–377

Thiringer, G., Blanquist, N., Brolin, I. and Mattson, S. (1980) Pleural plaques in chest X-rays of lung cancer patients and matched controls. *Eur. J. Respir. Dis.* (Suppl .107) **61**, 119–222

Thomson, J.G. (1970) The pathogenesis of pleural plaques. In: *Pneumoconiosis. Proceedings of the International Conference*, Johannesburg, 1969 (ed. H.A. Shapiro), Oxford University Press, Cape Town, pp. 138–141

Thomson, J.G. (1965) Asbestos and the urban dweller. *Ann. NY Acad. Sci.* **132**, 196–214

Thomson, M.L., Pelzer, A.M. and Smither, W.J. (1965) The discriminant value of pulmonary function tests in asbestosis. *Ann. NY Acad. Sci.* **132**, 421–436

Tiainen, M., Tammilento, L., Rantonen, J., Tuomi, T., Mattson, K. and Knuutila, S. (1989) Chromosomal abnormalities and their correlations with asbestos exposure and survival in mesothelioma patients. *Br. J. Cancer* **60**, 618–626

Timbrell, V. (1990) Review of the significance of fibre size in fibre-related lung disease. *Ann. Occup. Hyg.* **33**, 483–505

Topping, D.C. and Nettlesheim, P. (1980) Two-stage carcinogenesis studies with asbestos in Fischer 344 rats. *J. Natl Cancer Inst.* **65**, 627–630

Tron, V., Wright, J.L., Harrison, N., Wiggs, B. and Churg, A. (1987) Cigarette smoking makes airway and early asbestos-induced lung disease worse in the guinea pig. *Am. Rev. Respir. Dis.* **136**, 271–275

Tuomi, T., Segerberg-Konttinen, M., Tammilento, L., Tossavainen, L.A. and Vanhala, E. (1989) Mineral fibre concentration in lung tissue of mesothelioma patients in Finland. *Am. J. Ind. Med.* **16**, 247–254

Turner-Warwick, M. (1977) Immune reactions in pulmonary fibrosis. *Schweiz. Med. Wochenschr.* **107**, 171–175

Turner-Warwick, M. (1979) HLA phenotypes in asbestos workers. *Br. J. Dis. Chest* **73**, 243–244

Turner-Warwick, M. and Haslam, P. (1971) Antibodies in some chronic fibrosing lung diseases. *Clin. Allergy* **1**, 83–95

Turner-Warwick, M. and Haslam, P. (1986) Clinical applications of bronchoalveolar lavage. *Br. J. Dis. Chest* **80**, 105–121

Turner-Warwick, M. and Parkes, W.R. (1970) Circulating rheumatoid and anti-nuclear factors in asbestos workers. *Br. Med. J.* **3**, 492–495

Turner-Warwick, M., Lebowitz, M., Burrows, B. and Johnson, A. (1980) Cryptogenic fibrosing alveolitis and lung cancer. *Thorax* **35**, 496–499

Tylecote, F.E. and Dunn, J.S. (1931) Case of asbestos-like bodies in the lungs of a coal miner who had never worked in asbestos. *Lancet* **2**, 632–633

Vacek, P.M. and McDonald, J.C. (1990) Effect of intensity in asbestos cohort exposure-response analyses. In: *Occupational Epidemiology* (ed. H. Sakurai), Elsevier Science, Amsterdam, pp. 189–193

Vacek, P.M. and McDonald, J.C. (1991) Risk assessment using exposure intensity: an application to vermiculite mining. *Br. J. Ind. Med.* **48**, 543–547

Viallat, J.R. and Boutin, C. (1980) Radiographic changes in chrysotile mine and mill ex-workers in Corsica. *Lung* **157**, 155–163

Viallat, J.R., Boutin, C., Pietri, J. and Fonderai, J. (1983) Late progression of radiographic changes in Canari chrysotile mine ex-workers. *Archs Environ. Health* **38**, 54–58

Viallat, J.R., Rayband, F., Pssarel, M. and Boutin, C. (1986) Pleural migration of chrysotile fibres after intratracheal injection in rats. *Archs Environ. Health* **41**, 282–286

Vincent, R.G., Pickren, J.W. and Lane, W.W. (1977) The changing histopathology of lung cancer. *Cancer* **39**, 1647–1655 von Hayek, H. (1960) *The Human Lung* (trans. V.E. Krahl), Hafner, New York

Vorwald, A.J., Durkan, T.M. and Pratt, P.C. (1951) Experimental studies of asbestosis. *Archs Ind. Hyg. Occup. Med.* **3**, 1–43

Voytek, P., Anver, M., Conley, J. and Anderson, E. (1990) Mechanisms of asbestos carcinogenicity. *J. Am. Coll. Toxicol.* **9**, 541–550

Wagner, E. (1870) Das tuberkelahnliche Lymphadenon. *Arch. Heilk.* **11**, 495–525

Wagner, J.C. (1965) The sequelae of exposure to asbestos dust. *Ann. NY Acad. Sci.* **132**, 691–695

Wagner, J.C. (1990) Significance of the fibre size of erionite. *Proceedings of the Seventh International Pneumoconiosis Conference*, Pittsburgh. DHSS (NIOSH) Publication 90-108, vol. 2, pp. 835–839

Wagner, J.C. (1991) The discovery of the association between blue asbestos and mesotheliomas and the aftermath. *Br. J. Ind. Med.* **48**, 399–403

Wagner, J.C. and Skidmore, J.W. (1965) Asbestos dust deposition and retention in rats. *Ann. NY Acad. Sci.* **132**, 77–86

Wagner, J.C., Berry, G. and Timbrell, V. (1973) Mesothelioma in rats after innoculation with asbestos and other materials. *Br. J. Cancer* **28**, 173–185

Wagner, J.C., Griffiths, D.M. and Hill, R.J. (1984) The effect of fibre size on the in vivo activity of UICC crocidolite. *Br. J. Cancer* **49**, 453–458

Wagner, J.C., Griffiths, DM and Munday, D.E. (1987) Recent investigations in animals and humans. *The Biological Effects of Chrysotile* (ed. J.C. Wagner), *Accomplishments in Oncology* 1(2), 11–120

Wagner, J.C., Sleggs, C.A. and Marchand, P. (1960) Diffuse pleural mesothelioma. *Br. J. Ind. Med.* **17**, 260–271

Wagner, J.C., Berry, G., Skidmore, J.W. and Timbrell, V. (1974) The effects of inhalation of asbestos in rats. *Br. J. Cancer* **29**, 252–269

Wagner, J.C., Pooley, F., Berry, G. et al. (1982a) A pathological and minerological study of asbestos-related deaths in the UK in 1977. *Ann. Occup. Hyg.* **26**, 423–430

Wagner, J.C., Chamberlain, M., Brown, R.C. et al. (1982b) Biological effects of tremolite. *Br. J. Cancer* **45**, 352–360

Wagner, J.C., Moncrieff, C., Coles, R., Griffiths, D. and Munday, D. (1986) Correlation between fibre content of the lungs and disease in naval dockyard workers. *Br. J. Ind. Med.* **43**, 391–395

Wagner, J.C., Newhouse, M., Corrin, B., Rossiter, C. and Griffiths, D. (1988) Correlation between fibre content of the lung and disease in East London asbestos factory workers. *Br. J. Ind. Med.* **45**, 305–308

Wain, S.L., Roggli, V.L. and Foster, W.L. (1984) Parietal pleural plaques, asbestos bodies and neoplasia. *Chest* **86**, 707–713

Wang, N-S. (1973) Electron microscopy in the diagnosis of pleural mesotheliomas. *Cancer* **31**, 1046–1054

Wang, N-S. (1975) The preformed stomas connecting the pleural cavity and the lymphatics in the parietal pleura. *Am. Rev. Respir. Dis.* **111**, 12–19

Warhol, M.J. (1987) Electron microscopy in the diagnosis of mesothelioma. In: *Asbestos-related Malignancy* (eds K. Antman and J. Aisner), Grune and Stratton, London, pp. 201–221

Warnock, M.L., Press, M. and Churg, A. (1980) Further observations on cytoplasmic hyaline in the lung. *Human Pathol.* **11**, 59–65

Webster, I. (1970) The pathogenesis of asbestosis. In: *Pneumoconiosis. Proceedings of the International Conference, Johannesburg, 1969* (ed. H.A. Shapiro), Oxford University Press, Cape Town, pp. 117–119

Wedler, H.W. (1943) Asbestos und lungenkrebs. *Dtsch. Med. Wochenschr.* **69**, 575–576

Weill, H., Waggenspack, C. and Bailey, W. (1973) Radiographic and physiologic patterns amongst workers engaged in manufacture of asbestos cement products. *J. Occup. Med.* **15**, 248–252

Weill, H., Zisking, M.M., Waggenspack, C. and Rossiter, C.E. (1975) Lung function consequences of dust exposure in asbestos cement manufacturing plants. *Archs Environ. Health* **30**, 88–97

Weill, H., Rossiter, C.E., Waggenspack, C., Jones, R.N. and Ziskind, M.M. (1977) Differences in lung effects resulting from chrysotile and crocidolite exposure. In: *Inhaled Particle IV* (eds W.H. Walton and B. McGovern), Pergamon, Oxford, pp. 789–796

Weiss, S.W. and Tavassoli, F. (1988) Multicystic mesothelioma. *Am. J. Surg. Pathol.* **12**, 737–746

Weiss, W. (1977) Mortality of a cohort exposed to chrysotile asbestos. *J. Occup. Med.* **19**, 737–740

Weiss, W. (1984) Cigarette smoke, asbestos and small irregular opacities. *Am. Rev. Respir. Dis.* **130**, 293–301

Weiss, W. (1988a) Smoking and pulmonary fibrosis. *J. Occup. Med.* **30**, 33–39

Weiss, W. (1988b) Lobe of origin in the attribution of lung cancer to asbestos. *Br. J. Ind. Med.* **45**, 544–547

Weiss, W. (1989) Pulmonary fibrosis in asbestos insulation workers with lung cancer. *Br. J. Ind. Med.* **46**, 430

Weiss, W. (1990) Asbestos and colorectal cancer. *Gastroenterology* **99**, 876–884

Weiss, W. (1991) Cigarette smoking and small irregular opacities. *Br. J. Ind. Med.* **48**, 841–844

Weiss, W., Levin, R. and Goodman, L. (1981) Pleural plaques and cigarette smoking in asbestos workers. *J. Occup. Med.* **23**, 427–430

Whitaker, D. and Shilkin, K. (1984) Diagnosis of pleural malignant mesothelioma in life – a practical approach. *J. Pathol.* **143**, 147–175

Whitaker, D., Papadimitriou, J. and Walters, M. (1982) The mesothelioma and its reactions: a review. *CRC Crit. Rev. Toxic.* **10**, 81–144

White, F.M., Swift, J. and Becklake, M.R. (1974) Rheumatic complaints and pulmonary response to chrysotile dust inhalation in the mines and mills of Quebec. *Can. Med. Assoc. J.* **111**, 533–535

Whitley, N.O. (1987) Computed tomography and malignant mesothelioma. In: *Asbestos-related Malignancy* (eds K. Antman and J. Aisner), Grune and Stratton, London, pp. 265–299

Whitwell, F. and Rawcliffe, R.M. (1971) Diffuse malignant pleural mesothelioma and asbestos exposure. *Thorax* **26**, 6–22

Whitwell, F., Newhouse, M.L. and Bennett, D.R. (1974) A study of the histological cell types of lung cancer in workers suffering from asbestosis in the United Kingdom. *Br. J. Ind. Med.* **31**, 298–303

Whitwell, F., Scott, J. and Grimshaw, M. (1977) Relationship between occupations and asbestos-fibre content of the lungs in patients with pleural mesothelioma, lung cancer and other diseases. *Thorax* **32**, 377–386

Williams, R.L. and Muhlbaier, J.L. (1982) Asbestos brake emissions. *Envir. Res.* **29**, 70–82

Willis, R.A. (1960) *Pathology of Tumours*, 3rd ed., Butterworths, London

Willis, R.A. (1973) *The Spread of Tumours in the Human Body*, 3rd ed., Butterworths, London, pp. 56–60

Wood, W.B. and Gloyne, S.R. (1934) Pulmonary asbestosis. *Lancet* **2**, 1383–1385

Wright, G.W. and Kuschner, M. (1977) The influence of varying lengths of glass and asbestos fibres on tissue response in guinea pigs. In: *Inhaled Particles IV* (eds W.H. Walton and B. McGovern), Pergamon, Oxford, pp. 455–472

Wright, J.L. and Churg, A. (1985) Severe diffuse small airways abnormalities in long term chrysotile miners. *Br. J. Ind. Med.* **42**, 556–559

Wright, P.H., Hanson, A., Kreel, L. and Capel, L.H. (1980) Respiratory function changes after asbestos pleurisy. *Thorax* **35**, 31–36

Wright, W.E. and Sherwin, R.P. (1984) Histological types of malignant mesothelioma and asbestos exposure. *Br. J. Ind. Med.* **41**, 514–517

Wright, W.E., Sherwin, R.P., Dickson, E.A., Bernstein, L., Fromm, J.B. and Henderson, B.E. (1984) Malignant mesothelioma: incidence asbestos exposure and reclassification of histology. *Br. J. Ind. Med.* **41**, 39–45

Wright, W.E., Bernstein, L., Peters, J.M., Garabrant, D.H. and Mack, D.M. (1988) Adenocarcinoma of the stomach and exposure to occupational dust. *Am. J. Epidemiol.* **128**, 64–73

Xaubet, T., Rodriguez-Rosin, R., Bombi, J., Marin, A., Roca, J. and Agasti-Vidal, A. (1986) Correlation of bronchoalveolar lavage and clinical and functional findings in asbestosis. *Am. Rev. Respir. Dis.* **133**, 848–854

Yazicioglu, S., Ibcayto, R., Balci, K. et al. (1980) Pleural calcification, pleural mesotheliomas and bronchial cancers caused by tremolite dust. *Thorax* **35**, 564–569

Young, J.R. and Reddy, E.R. (1980) Peritoneal mesothelioma. *Clin. Radiol.* **31**, 243–247

Zivy, P. (1981) *Pulmonary and Pleural Radiology of Workers Exposed to Asbestos.* Publications Essentilles, Paris

15

An approach to the differential diagnosis of asbestosis and non-occupational diffuse interstitial pulmonary fibrosis

W. Raymond Parkes

Introduction

Diffuse pulmonary fibrosis may be predominantly intra-alveolar or interstitial, of known or unknown cause and, if known, of occupational or non-occupational origin (Table 15.1). It is the result of inflammation of the lower respiratory tract which involves not only (and mainly, in most instances) alveoli (that is, alveolitis), but also alveolar ducts, respiratory bronchioles and, often, membranous bronchioles (Dunnill, 1990). When its cause is not known it is referred to either as *idiopathic diffuse interstitial pulmonary fibrosis* (DIPF) or *cryptogenic fibrosing alveolitis* (CFA). Because DIPF represents a common end-result of many different causes of pulmonary damage, it is frequently impossible to determine its origin pathologically. However, clinically, there are usually valuable clues in the individual patient's history, in the mode of evolution, distribution and progression of the fibrosis, and often in the association of relevant non-pulmonary disease.

As Jones (1991) has rightly pointed out, there are two criteria for the clinical diagnosis of asbestosis: a history of occupational exposure to asbestos that is consistent with a substantial risk of developing asbestosis, and the presumed absence of confounders that can cause or simulate DIPF. He

believes that the clinician should 'be able to identify a history so weak that it fails to satisfy the exposure criterion' as well as identifying the presence of potential confounders in the process of reaching a sound clinical diagnosis of asbestosis. Unfortunately, however, experience, on the whole, indicates that this is far from the case. Thus, this chapter ponders some of the difficulties that exist in distinguishing the DIPF of asbestosis from confounders of non-occupational origin, and the implications of these difficulties. It is, as pointed out in Chapter 6, imperative that the distinction is made as quickly as possible so that, on the one hand, the patient is spared unnecessary, and possibly intrusive, investigations and, on the other, that appropriate therapy for treatable disease is administered without delay.

Injurious agents can reach the pulmonary parenchyma by three routes (Figure 15.1):

1. The airways (inhaled micro-organisms, dusts and chemicals) with consequent damage mainly to the alveolar epithelium.
2. The pulmonary circulation with resultant injury chiefly to the capillary endothelium (circulating micro-organisms, immune complexes, therapeutic drugs and 'shock'), but some ingested chemicals (such as paraquat) which reach the lungs in this way primarily affect the alveolar epithelium.

Table 15.1 Some causes of diffuse interstitial pulmonary fibrosis (DIPF)

1. Lone DIPF
   (a) *Inhaled materials*

Micro-organisms	Viruses; bacteria (including *Legionella pneumophila*); fungi	⎫
Secretions of chronic upper respiratory tract sepsis		⎬ Organized pneumonia
Chemical	Refluxed gastric contents; oily nasal drops	⎭
Inorganic	Asbestos / Beryllium metal and compounds / Cobalt ('hard metal') / Aluminium / Mercury vapour / Nickel-carbonyl (?)	
Organic	Fungal proteins / Avian proteins / Other foreign proteins / Hairsprays (?)	

   (b) *Blood-borne (ingested or parenteral materials)*

   Medications* (toxicity or hypersensitivity):

Acebutalol	Methotrexate
Amiodarone	Methysergide
Bischloroethylnitrosourea	Mitomycin
Bleomycin	Nitrofurantoin
Busulphan	Practolol
Carmustines	Procainamide
Chlorambucil	Procarbazine
Cyclophosphamide	Penicillamine
Gold salts	Sulphasalazine
Melphalan	Vincristine

   Other Paraquat

   (c) *Ionizing radiation* Localized or diffuse. Fibrosis not evident for months or years after therapy
   (d) *Chronic interstitial oedema* Chronic left ventricular failure / Chronic renal failure
   (e) *Idiopathic (syn.* cryptogenic fibrosing alveolitis)

2. Associated systemic disease

   CTD/CVD† ⎰ Rheumatoid disease / Systemic sclerosis and its variants / Systemic lupus erythematosus / Polymyositis/dermatomyositis ⎱

   Sjögren's disease / Sarcoidosis / Histiocytosis X / Neurofibromatosis / Polyarteritis nodosa / Inflammatory bowel disease (ulcerative colitis; Crohn's disease) (see Chapter 6, page 140) / Idiopathic pulmonary haemosiderosis / Hyperglobulinaemic renal tubular acidosis

3. Familial pulmonary fibrosis

*See Bedrossian (1982); Castle (1985); Cooper, White and Matthay (1986) †CTD: connective tissue disorders. CVD: collagen vascular disorders..

3. Directly from outside (ionizing radiation – in particular therapeutic X-rays).

The site or region of the initial attack is likely to determine the form and distribution that the ultimate fibrosis will take. Fibrosis may, on the one hand, be predominantly intra-alveolar due to organization of unresolved bacterial, eosinophilic or chemical pneumonia, and to unknown (idiopathic) causes or, on the other, mainly involve the interstitial compartment. Experimentally, Brentjens et al. (1974) showed that, if immune complexes were inhaled, they were deposited first on the alveolar basement membrane but, if injected intravenously, were deposited first on the basement membrane of the capillary endothelium. For example, microvascular disease seems to be the basic disorder in systemic sclerosis (Jayson, 1983) and may well be so in idiopathic DIPF (CFA) associated with other connective tissue disorders (CTDs) (Turner-Warwick, 1988). Inhaled particles, fumes and gases tend to be distributed more in the upper halves of the lungs than the lower although, in some respects, fibrous particles tend to behave differently (see Chapter 3). By contrast, blood-borne agents are more likely to be concentrated in the lower halves of the lungs where, under normal circumstances, blood flow and capillary perfusion are substantially greater than in the upper halves (West, 1979).

Pathology and aetiology of DIPF

The basic pathological changes are parenchymal damage, inflammation (including sarcoid granulomas and interstitial exudates) and fibrosis. There are several variants of interstitial pneumonia and fibrosis, the histological features and differing terminologies of which are well known (Liebow, 1975) and, therefore, not described in detail here. The dominant cells may be alveolar macrophages (so-called 'desquamative interstitial pneumonia' – DIP) or lymphocytes ('usual interstitial pneumonia' – UIP). Whether or not these represent different pathogenic processes is uncertain. Although the severity of cellular infiltration varies and fibrosis occurs at different stages in the evolution of the disease and progresses at different rates in different patients, the histological appearances can be simply and practically categorized into three patterns: cellular, mixed and fibrotic. The *cellular pattern*, consisting of large collections of macrophages in the alveolar spaces with a smaller number of neutrophils, eosinophils and lymphocytes, desquamation of type I cells, and minimal fibrosis of alveolar walls, corresponds to Liebow's DIP. The *mixed pattern* (intermediate) consists of

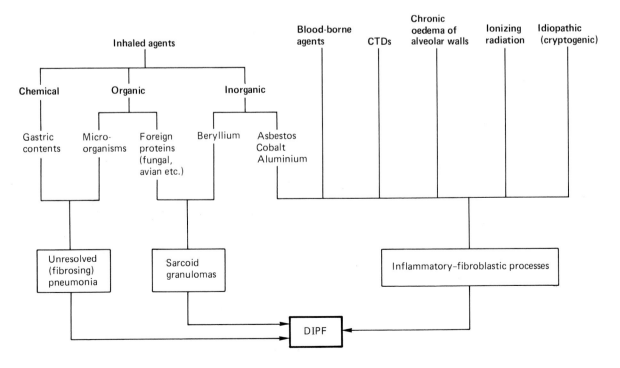

Figure 15.1 Schema of pathogenic pathways of DIPF

large collections of inflammatory cells with more fibrous thickening of alveolar walls. The *fibrotic stage* is composed of mats of dense collagen fibres replacing many alveoli, cystic spaces lined by bronchiolar epithelium and variable numbers of inflammatory cells in the airspaces and interstitium – DIPF (Heard, 1984). The often-employed term 'usual interstitial pneumonia' is considered by Spencer (1985) to be 'meaningless' as there is no indication of what should be regarded as the 'unusual form'; similarly, according to Crystal et al. (1984), it should not be used as a substitute for DIPF. In the early stages of asbestosis a cellular pattern, although common in experimental animals (Bégin et al., 1983), is only occasionally seen in human disease, and cellular remnants adjacent to the fibrosis, or elsewhere in the lung, are usually absent.

As Table 15.1 shows, there is a large array of agents from various sources – air-borne, aspirated or blood-borne – and a number of systemic disorders that are known to cause DIPF. The relationship to connective tissue disorders and inflammatory bowel disease is mentioned in Chapter 6 (see 'Connective tissue disorders'). It is worth emphasizing that, although DIPF induced by therapeutic drugs is uncommon, it is sufficiently frequent to merit routine enquiry into past and present details of medication, and consideration in differential diagnosis.

The possibility that idiopathic DIPF might be caused by exposure to environmental dusts has, at times, been suggested without any substantiation. But the observation by Johnston et al. (1990) that mortality from CFA is higher in the central parts of England and Wales than elsewhere in the country prompted these authors to speculate that environmental causes may be involved. Furthermore, from a small, well-conducted, case-control study of 40 patients, Scott, Johnston and Britton (1990) found a significant association with atmospheric dusts (in particular, metals and wood), work with cattle and living in houses heated by wood fires, and also, that atopy may be an additional risk factor. Notably, however, it was not associated with coal, sand or stone dusts, cigarette smoking or social class.

Idiopathic DIPF can also be familial – that is, genetically determined. Reiser and Last (1986) have remarked that '. . . what is striking is not that there are so many agents that can potentially induce pulmonary fibrosis, but that the lung has such capabilities for recovery'. They suggested that pulmonary fibrosis may be considered 'as the end result of a process in which the balance of normal injury/repair mechanisms is disrupted. There is clearly no single "fibrogenic event". Rather, there seem to be a number of places where disruption of balance/repair processes may begin... Loss of

Table 15.2 Host factors that may influence development of DIPF

Genetic
1. Dimensions and branching angles of airways (see Chapter 1)*
2. Number and size of alveoli (see Chapter 1)*
3. Ciliary function in airways (mucociliary clearance – see Chapter 3)*
4. Familial idiopathic DIPF (similar cytological features in unaffected relatives)
5. Other determinant genes (see Chapter 4):
   (a) Rheumatoid arthritis and other connective tissue disorders
   (b) Neurofibromatosis
   (c) Non-familial idiopathic DIPF associated with HLA phenotypes (?)
6. Phenotypically distinct subpopulations of alveolar macrophages (Campbell, Poulter and Du Bois, 1986)
7. Susceptibility to accumulation of fibrin in alveoli and interstitium (Chapman, Allen and Stone, 1986)

Acquired
1. Abnormality of upper respiratory tract with shift from nasal to oral breathing (see Chapter 3)*
2. Failure of control of fibroblast proliferation by alveolar macrophages (Elias et al., 1985)
3. Persistent local inflammation resulting in dominant clones of collagen-producing fibroblasts (Jordana et al., 1988)
4. Selective deficiency of immuoglobulin subclasses (chronic suppuration – see Chapter 6)

*Factors that affect the dose, distribution or retention in the lungs of inhaled aerosols.

control may occur at the genetic level, leading to the destructive alveolitis that is the apparent precursor of fibrosis'. Thus, in spite of there being diverse causes, the natural history of DIPF (that is, whether or not fibrosis develops and, if it does, its extent and rate of progress), undoubtedly appears to be influenced by host factors. This notion is underscored by similarities and differences, not only in the lungs' response to a wide variety of fibrogenic stimuli, but also in their response to the same stimulus. 'Even if the initiating events differ, is there any sort of final common pathway to fibrosis? Although some fibrogenic agents may provoke similar sequences of early cellular events, if we survey pulmonary fibrosis as a whole it seems unlikely that there is any point, except at the very late stages of fibrosis, where pathways may actually converge' (Reiser and Last, 1986). Table 15.2 indicates some of the host factors that may operate. In addition, evidence that pathways of collagen deposition may differ in different forms of fibrosis has now emerged (Laurent, 1986; Du Bois, 1990) (see Chapter 4, 'Genetic control of immune responses').

Although ultrastructural studies suggest that *initial* pathogenic events are similar in idiopathic DIPF and in asbestosis (Corrin et al., 1985), there is reason to believe that they may be distinct because local T-lymphocyte-mediated immune responses are apparently involved in the former (Campbell et al., 1985; Kradin et al., 1986; Meliconi et al., 1990), but not in the latter (Bégin et al., 1983).

Familial idiopathic DIPF, which follows an autosomal dominant pattern with variable penetrance, is clinically and morphologically indistinguishable from non-familial idiopathic DIPF and has the same antecedent pattern of macrophage and neutrophil accumulations. Bronchoalveolar lavage (BAL) studies have shown that about half the clinically normal members of families in whom this disorder has occurred have increased numbers of similarly activated alveolar macrophages as their affected relatives (Bitterman et al., 1986). In one family, in which there were three definite and two probable cases in three generations, susceptibility appeared to be segregated with Gm allotypes on chromosome 14, but not with HLA antigens on chromosome 6 (Musk et al., 1986). Non-familial, idiopathic DIPF is, apparently, associated with HLA-B and HLA-D alleles (Evans, 1976; Varpela et al., 1979), HLA-DR2 being particularly linked with linear and 'cystic honeycombing' radiographic patterns (Libby et al., 1983), in contrast to asbestosis in which there is no positive or negative association with these phenotypes (Bégin et al., 1987). There is some evidence to suggest that the expression of class II antigens in type I and type II pneumocytes in idiopathic DIPF, although not specific, may be relevant to pathogenesis in that these cells may be recognized as autoantigenic by sensitized T lymphocytes (Kallenberg et al., 1987) (see Chapter 4, 'MHC-linked genes'). Furthermore, patients with non-familial fibrosis appear to be susceptible to accumulation of fibrin in alveolar spaces and the interstitium during the cellular phase of the disease (Chapman, Allen and Stone, 1986).

Findings such as these suggest the possibility that genetically susceptible individuals may fail to control inflammatory and immunological processes provoked in the lungs by many different types of insult (Bitterman and Crystal, 1980). Thus, it can be envisaged that, apart from the influence of other possible factors (such as those listed in Table 15.1), individuals with similar occupational exposures to fibrogenic agents may react differently with regard to the development, severity and progression of fibrosis. In short, the question of susceptibility – or, alternatively, 'resistance' – to acquiring or developing any of these disorders has particular relevance to differential diagnosis. This is discussed from the standpoint of asbestosis in particular. It is interesting that Vorwald, in 1950,

noted that: 'Only a minor proportion of all persons exposed to toxic dusts [under similar conditions] develop pulmonary disease', but he was unable to offer a satisfactory explanation.

Circumstances affecting the diagnosis of asbestosis

Even with satisfactory evidence of occupational exposure to asbestos, the clinical and histopathological diagnosis of asbestosis is not as simple as is often supposed. There are probably at least four reasons for this:

1. Over the last 50 years or more many pulmonary pathologists have noted an increased prevalence of idiopathic DIPF in the general population (Spencer, 1985). Although this may, in part, be the consequence of better recognition, an important explanation is thought to result from an increasing incidence of organization of pneumonic exudates coincident with a rapidly expanding, but often inadequate, use of antibacterial agents since the 1940s (Auerbach, Mims and Goodpasture, 1952). During the same period, viral ('atypical') pneumonias with fibrotic sequelae have also increased. Whatever the causes, a substantial and increasing number of deaths due to idiopathic DIPF occurred in England and Wales between 1979 and 1988. The annual total mortality rose considerably over the age of 45 years, doubling from 336 to 702 – in all a total of 5135 deaths, 60 per cent of which were in men (Johnston et al., 1990). A significant diagnostic miscoding of idiopathic DIPF, that is, underdiagnosis, has also been found among patients admitted to hospital (Johnston et al., 1991). Interestingly, descriptions of idiopathic DIPF – excluding, perhaps, 'cirrhosis of the lung' – first described by Rindfleisch in 1897 – do not seem to appear in most standard textbooks of respiratory disease until about the beginning of the 1950s at least (see review by Livingstone et al., 1964).
2. Coincidentally the prevalence and severity of asbestosis has decreased substantially owing to increasingly effective measures of dust suppression rather than to a shorter period of 'follow-up' in later exposed individuals (Figure 15.2). It is now rarely recorded as the primary cause of death (Davis, 1984; Gaensler, Jederlinic and McLoud,

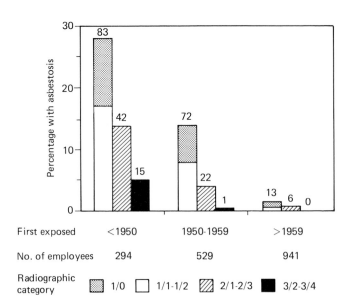

Figure 15.2 Prevalence and profusion of irregular small opacities at last visit (1988) of 1764 employees seen during industrial surveys. There were 254 (14.4 per cent) with presumed asbestosis. The prevalence decreased from 47.6 per cent for those first exposed before 1950 to 18.0 per cent for 1950–1959, and was only 2.0 per cent for those first exposed during 1959–1987. Exclusion of 1/0 readings would have reduced these three figures to 36.4 per cent, 10.2 per cent and 0.6 per cent respectively. (Reproduced, with permission, from Gaensler, Jederlinic and McLoud, 1990 and DHHS (NIOSH) Publications)

1990). However, with hindsight many cases of 'asbestosis' reported or recorded from the 1920s to the early 1950s appear to be examples of some other disease – in particular tuberculosis, bilateral localized or diffuse bronchiectasis, pulmonary fibrosis secondary to chronic bronchial sepsis, and sarcoidosis (for example, Seiler, 1928; Ellman, 1933; Wyers, 1949). The most notable is one of the earliest reports – often quoted as an historical turning-point in the recognition of asbestosis – of 'fibrosis of the lungs' in a young female asbestos worker being attributed, *post mortem*, to asbestos, although the radiographic and pathological features were those of advanced fibrocavernous tuberculosis (Cooke, 1924; Cooke and Hill, 1927). It is of interest that the decisive factor leading to this conclusion was the finding of 'large, solid, angular particles' in the lungs, similar to particles found in the workplace dust. One may wonder, in view of the known possibility of diagnostic miscoding, whether all the cases in more recent studies of asbestosis reported in the journals are, in fact, asbestosis.

3. Other causes of DIPF may be misinterpreted as asbestosis because some may have clinical, radiographic and pathological features that, to some extent, resemble it. But even those cases in which there is little resemblance may often be wrongly interpreted as asbestosis. Important differences that exist between asbestosis and DIPF from other causes are discussed in more detail later.

4. The susceptibility of some individuals to developing DIPF is also well known to apply to asbestosis. Many workers, similarly and even heavily exposed to asbestos, have remained unaffected lifelong whereas others, with relatively low levels of exposure, have been affected (Liddell and Miller, 1983). Furthermore, among those who develop asbestosis, progression occurs in some but not in others – the majority. It is likely that the susceptibility of individuals to develop DIPF varies according to the type of insult suffered by the lungs and its route of access (airways or blood stream) and, if multiple insults occur, susceptibility to each of these will be dissimilar. Thus, workers with significant past exposure to asbestos who do not develop asbestosis may, nevertheless, be open to pulmonary fibrosis from some other cause.

In practice, difficulty arises when patients with diffuse pulmonary fibrosis have a history of occupational exposure to asbestos or when asbestos bodies are found in the sputum, BAL fluid or microsections of the lung because the diagnosis of asbestosis is then usually made often in the face of discordant evidence – one aspect of a common defect in diagnostic thinking referred to already in Chapter 6. This is reinforced by an uncritical acceptance of the rule-of-thumb that the association of asbestos bodies with fibrosis proves that the fibrosis is asbestosis (see 'The problem of asbestos bodies', page 528).

Extrapulmonary disorders associated with DIPF

An association of bilateral pulmonary fibrosis with chronic, recurrent aspiration of matter from gastro-oesophageal reflux or oronasal sepsis is more common than is generally recognized (see Chapter 6). DIPF also occurs in 20 to 25 per cent of cases of sarcoidosis (Crystal et al., 1984) and in about 30 per cent of individuals with rheumatoid arthritis (Roschmann and Rothenberg, 1987) anteceding the development of clinical arthritis by a number of years in some 15 per cent of cases (Payne, 1984); it develops within 4 years of the onset of arthropathy in 70 per cent of cases and, when it precedes it, the joints are involved within 3 years (Turner-Warwick and Courtenay-Evans, 1977).

In systemic sclerosis 46 per cent of patients are affected by DIPF (Rowell, 1985), in polymyositis about 9 per cent (Salmeron, Greenberg and Lidsky, 1981), in mixed connective tissue disease (in which two or more of these CTDs overlap) 19 per cent (Prakash, Luthra and Divertie, 1985), and in systemic lupus erythematosus up to 6 per cent (Eisenberg, 1982). The pulmonary fibrosis of systemic sclerosis is, however, in part frequently contributed to by occult aspiration from oesophagopharyngeal reflux due to related oesophageal dysfunction (Johnson et al., 1989). Some 20 per cent of individuals with neuro-fibromatosis – an autosomal dominant trait with a frequency of about 1 : 3000 (Riccardi, 1981) – develop DIPF over the age of 30 years (Webb and Goodman, 1977); it is important that, in a number of patients, when first seen, cutaneous neurofibromas may be few and of slight degree, and that multiple 'café-au-lait' areas may be the only clinical evidence of the disease.

Thus, the association of DIPF with this multiplicity of disorders, which in themselves are not rare, is fairly common and the presence of any one of them in an asbestos worker should raise the possibility that the pulmonary disease may not be asbestosis. However, although the radiographic appearances of idiopathic and other forms of DIPF may, in some cases, resemble asbestosis, their individual histological features often differ (see 'Microscopic appearances').

The differential diagnosis of asbestosis and other forms of fibrosis can, therefore, be usefully considered from two points of view: comparative clinical and radiographic features, and comparative pathological features.

Comparative clinical and radiographic features

Clinical features

Symptoms

The earliest symptom of idiopathic DIPF and asbestosis is breathlessness on exertion, the rate of

development of which depends upon the pace of progression of the underlying process: in asbestosis, it is more gradual and insidious, and may never be severe. An irritating, non-productive, persistent cough, fairly common early in idiopathic DIPF, is unusual in asbestosis until it is fairly advanced. These symptoms vary in severity in other forms of DIPF.

Physical signs

Clubbing of the fingers, often severe ('drum-stick' appearance), occurs in some 60 to 70 per cent of cases of idiopathic DIPF, but is inconstant in asbestosis, being found in some cases of advanced, but rarely of milder, disease; when present, the clubbing is not severe. This may reflect differences in the genetics of pulmonary fibrosis (see Chapter 6, 'Digital clubbing'). Clubbing is seldom associated with other forms of DIPF.

As noted in Chapter 6 ('Digital vasculitis'), the signs of Raynaud's disease, or digital vasculitis, are present in a proportion of cases of idiopathic DIPF either 'lone' or combined with systemic sclerosis, polymyositis, rheumatoid arthritis or systemic lupus erythematosus but not with asbestosis, other than coincidentally. The association is particularly high in systemic sclerosis and its variants, and is an early manifestation in most cases (Rowell, 1985). Whatever its cause it appears to differ from that of the pulmonary fibrosis in that it does not improve with treatment by corticosteroids whereas the fibrosing stages of DIPF may; it does, however, respond to immunosuppressant therapy (Turner-Warwick, 1988).

The diagnostic importance of the timing and acoustic quality of crackles in the respiratory cycle on auscultation, and their distribution in the lungs is discussed at length in Chapter 6 ('Abnormal (adventitious) intrapulmonary sounds').

Physiology

There are differences in the emphasis of physiological abnormality. In idiopathic DIPF, gas transfer is much reduced whilst pulmonary mechanics may be fairly well preserved, whereas in asbestosis, changes in mechanics tend to occur at a fairly early stage, but reduction in gas transfer is less severe (see 'Clinicopathological differences').

Radiographic features

Distribution

The overall pattern of distribution in the lung fields of opacities consistent with DIPF is a valuable pointer towards diagnosis, but when the appearances are predominant in both lower zones differentiation may become difficult. The relationship of smoking to the presence of irregular opacities is discussed in Chapter 7 ('Factors that influence the interpretation of radiographs') and Chapter 14 ('The influence of smoking on non-malignant asbestos-related disease').

Although tuberculous fibrosis is usually distributed in the upper zones, irregular, asymmetrical opacities in the middle and lower zones are not uncommon. Fibrosis due to recurrent aspiration is seen most frequently in the upper and middle zones of the right lung field but is often confined to the lower zones of one or both fields (that is, middle lobe, lingula or lower lobes); if bilateral, it is usually asymmetrical. Enquiry into the patient's habitual sleeping posture confirms that the more affected lung is dependent, although almost symmetrical, basal involvement may be seen in those who habitually sleep on their backs (Figure 15.3). Fibrotic sarcoidosis, beryllium disease, extrinsic allergic alveolitis and histiocytosis X favour the upper and middle zones, but, in some cases, an inverse distribution is seen (Figure 15.4). The distribution is probably most closely akin to that of asbestosis in idiopathic DIPF ('lone' or in association with CTD), familial fibrosis and fibrosis associated with neurofibromatosis; appearances caused by chronic left ventricular failure may be similar. However, there are important distinguishing features. In idiopathic and many other forms of DIPF both costophrenic angles visualized by standard posteroanterior (PA) films are, in most cases, sharp and clear, and the degree and distribution of abnormality in the two lung fields, frequently dissimilar (see Figures 15.5 to 15.8). The appearances of multiple cysts ('honeycombing') are common, often prominent (Figure 15.9) with intervening confluent opacification, but the signs of calcified pleural plaques or diffuse pleural fibrosis are absent, although, occasionally, they may be coincidental. By contrast, in asbestosis, both costophrenic angles are usually blunted (an abnormality that may be slight and not necessarily symmetrical, and has to be sought carefully in PA and oblique views in full aspiration) or obliterated by pleural fibrosis in more advanced disease where it may extend along the costal margins as far as the mid-zone regions. The pulmonary fibrosis is bilaterally similar in distribution, mainly affecting the lower zones, and absent in the upper zones; 'honeycombing' is not evident or is of very slight degree. However, bilateral calcified plaques are present in about one-third of cases (see Chapter 14). These various features are compared diagrammatically in Figure 15.10.

The differences between idiopathic DIPF and asbestosis are clearly demonstrated, in most cases,

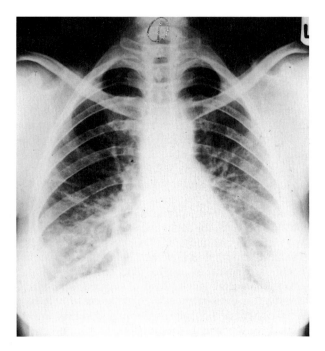

Figure 15.3 Diffuse, bilateral, basal pulmonary fibrosis due to prolonged recurrent oesophagopharyngeal reflux and aspiration in a woman with Barrett's oesophagus. When occupational exposure to asbestos is elicited in such cases of aspiration fibrosis, asbestosis may be (and has been) wrongly diagnosed. 'Barrett's oesophagus' is a columnar cell-lined oesophagus caused by chronic gastro-oesophageal reflux. (Courtesy of Mr Ronald Belsey, FRCS)

by high-resolution CT scans (see Chapter 7) (Hansell and Kerr, 1991), and they correlate well with the respective pathological features.

1. The appearances of idiopathic DIPF are more widespread and often extend to sections at the level of the carina or higher. They are frequently present anteriorly and in the upper lobes. Asymmetrical distribution is common; cysts are numerous and often large; there may be areas of confluent opacification which correspond, pathologically, to tracts of solid fibrosis, and demarcation from normal lung is usually sharp. Diffuse pleural thickening is absent. A crescentic, subpleural distribution of these appearances concentrated mainly in the posterobasal segments of the lower lobes is virtually pathognomonic (Figure 15.11) (Strickland and Strickland, 1988).
2. The appearances of asbestosis are limited to the lower regions of the lungs, usually well below the carina, and are maximal subpleurally; an anterior distribution is uncommon and generally less than

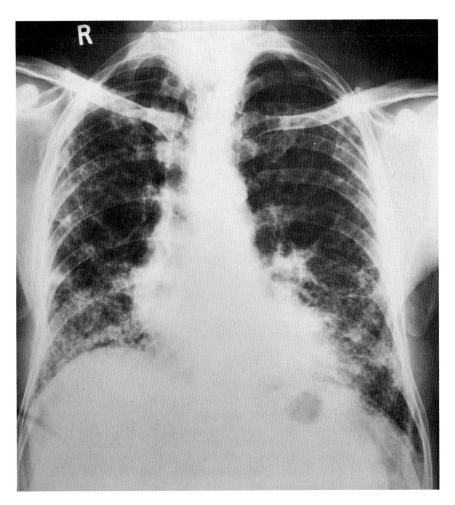

Figure 15.4 Irregular opacities with cystic appearances in all zones, particularly the lower. *History*: labourer in demolition industry (1946 to 1974) with paraoccupational exposure to asbestos insulation work for 4 years in the 1950s. He bred budgerigars for 12 years and illness developed in 1973. *Clinically*: coarse inspiratory and expiratory crackles in all lobar regions; persistent inspiratory 'squawks' in left upper lobe region. Avian precipitins present. *Lung function*: severe restrictive and gas transfer defects. *Post mortem*: gross appearances of multiple small air cysts ('bosselation') on surface of pulmonary pleura. Extensive well-demarcated DIPF subpleurally and centrally with numerous cysts 0.2 to 2 cm diameter in lung slices; more pronounced in the lower than in the upper halves of the lungs. *Microscopy*: highly vascularized DIPF with coarse 'honeycombing' and, in places, cellular components in alveolar spaces and interstitium. No granulomas; occasional asbestos bodies in 30-μm sections. *Diagnosis*: avian extrinsic allergic alveolitis (bird fanciers' lung). Radiographic distribution of disease in the lung fields is not typical (see Chapter 20). Asbestosis diagnosed during life

the posterior distribution; distribution, in the main, is symmetrically equal; cysts are usually inconspicuous but, when present, are few and small, and confluent opacification is absent; demarcation from normal lung is ill-defined; and

subpleural linear opacities and diffuse thickening of the pleura, of variable degree, are common (Figure 15.12). The crescentic, subpleural distribution of idiopathic DIPF is either ill-defined or absent.

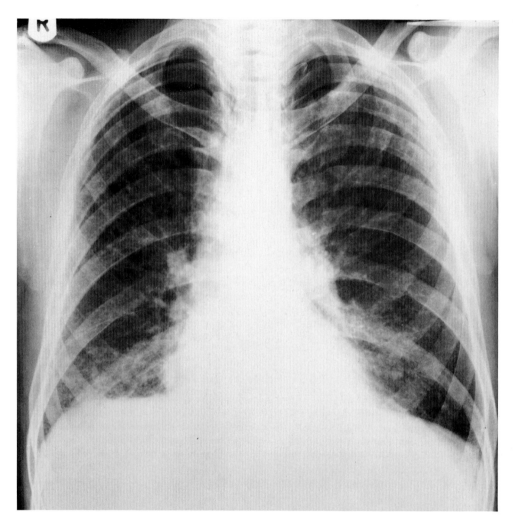

Figure 15.5 Irregular opacities mainly in lower zones, but also seen to a lesser degree in upper zones. Note: clear costophrenic angles, and no diffuse pleural thickening. *History*: docker and stevedore, 1939 to 1949, handling asbestos cargoes intermittently. *Clinically*: onset of dyspnoea on exertion 20 years after leaving docks; persistent medium to coarse crackles in mid and late inspiration in both lower lobe regions and, anteriorly, in upper lobe regions; no arthrophathy or skin lesion. RF and ANA negative. *Diagnosis*: idiopathic DIPF (see Figure 15.17)

Since this chapter was written, a comparative study by Al-Jarad et al. (1992) of patients with CFA and asbestosis using high-resolution CT has very largely confirmed these differentiating features.

Progression

The mode of development and evolution, or progression, of disease that is well documented by sequential changes in chest radiographs provides the important, complementary key to radiographic differentiation. As pointed out in Chapter 14 the onset of asbestosis is gradual and progression either

very slow or absent. For some years past, progression appears to have been no more common among those who have continued to be exposed to asbestos at low levels than among those in whom exposure has ceased (Gaensler, Jederlinic and McLoud, 1990). In other types of DIPF, however, speed of onset and progression is much more variable, and often rapid (see Figures 15.6 and 15.9). Aspiration fibrosis may develop fairly quickly (especially after an episode of aspiration pneumonia) but, even when less dramatic in onset, it is, in many cases, gradually progressive (Pearson and Wilson, 1971; Iverson, May and Samson, 1973). The fibrosis of chronic sarcoidosis, beryllium disease and extrinsic allergic

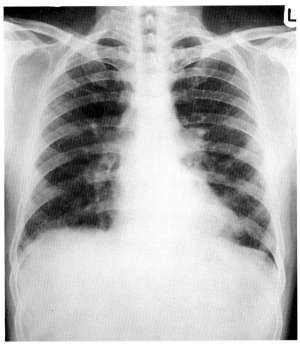

(a)

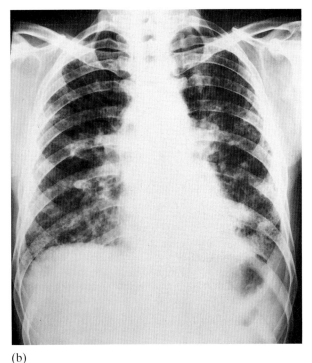

(b)

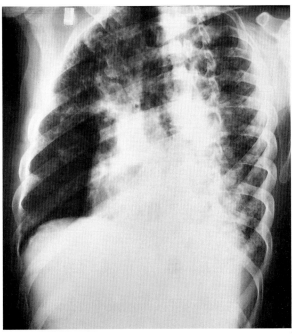

(c)

Figure 15.6 (a) 1974, irregular opacities in all zones (some breathlessness on exertion noted a year previously). Note involvement of right upper zone. (b) 1977, significant progression: coarse, irregular opacities in all zones with some cystic appearances. (c) Left 45 degree anterior oblique view (same day) confirms widespread distribution and, particularly, the prominent involvement of the right upper lobe; note that much of the right lower zone is relatively free of opacities. Plumber and pipe-fitter for 25 years; intermittent paraoccupational proximity to insulation workers; kept a budgerigar for 6 years. *Clinically*: coarse inspiratory crackles in all lobar areas. No arthropathy. Circulating RF and avian precipitins absent. Lung biopsy: DIPF with diffuse immunofluorescent staining by IgG; occasional asbestos bodies. *Post mortem*: naked eye: multiple small ('hobnail') air blebs on pulmonary pleura. Widespread patches of DIPF in all lobes especially in more central zones with numerous cysts from 2 to 7 mm in diameter. Right upper lobe particularly affected. *Microscopically*: DIPF with bronchiolectasis, smooth muscle hyperplasia and occasional asbestos bodies. *Diagnosis*: idiopathic DIPF, but asbestosis considered during life

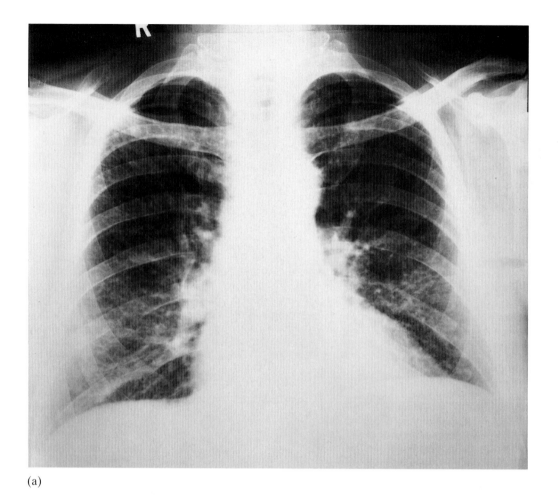

(a)

Figure 15.7 1975: (a) fine irregular opacities in both lower zones and coarse irregular opacities in right upper zone; however, note absence of opacities in the costophrenic angles in the left anterior oblique view (b). Appearances developed slowly over 8 years following onset of rheumatoid arthritis 2 years earlier. Machinist milling and turning asbestos-containing brake linings from 1967 to 1977. Fibre count very low in work area in latter years. *Clinically*: transient, coarse, inspiratory crackles in both lower lobes. Moderate restrictive and gas transfer defects with low *K*CO. Moderately severe rheumatoid arthritis with subcutaneous nodules. Lung biopsy: fibrosing 'alveolitis' of predominantly mural type with prominent lymphoid follicular hyperplasia; no asbestos bodies. *Post mortem*: 4 years later (see Figure 15.18). *Diagnosis*: 'rheumatoid lung', but asbestosis diagnosed during life in spite of the clinicopathological evidence

alveolitis progresses at varying speed; however, chronic farmers' and bird fanciers' lung are not always progressive. Idiopathic DIPF, and that associated with CTDs, with the notable exception of systemic sclerosis, is frequently rapid both in onset and progression; although some patients survive 10 years or more, many succumb in about 5 years. This relatively aggressive behaviour is in sharp contrast to asbestosis as Figure 15.6 exemplifies (see Chapter 14 for comparison with asbestosis).

Thus, mode of onset, radiographic distribution and rate of progression assist greatly in differential diagnosis and should always be carefully considered. It cannot be too strongly emphasized that past clinical details and chest radiographs should be obtained whenever possible for the perspective they provide on the natural history of the disease. It is not uncommon to find that the subsequent evolution of radiographic changes turns out not to conform with an initial diagnosis of asbestosis. This state of affairs

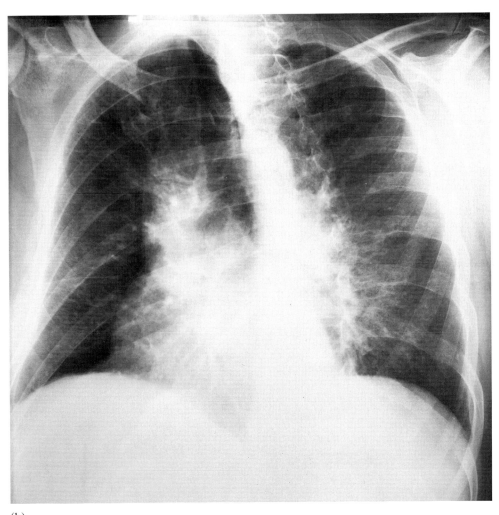

(b)

Figure 15.7 *Continued*

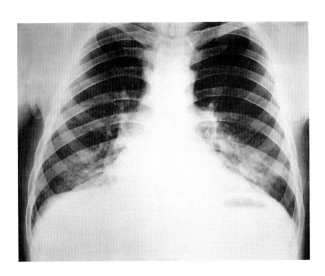

Figure 15.8 Asymmetrical, bilateral, basal, irregular opacities associated with moderately advanced, multiple neurofibromatosis (von Recklinghausen's disease). No diffuse pleural thickening and costophrenic angles clear. Machinist in an asbestos processing factory. *Clinically*: no abnormal physical signs in the lungs. *Physiology*: lung volumes within normal limits but some reduction in T_L and K_{CO}. Diagnosed as asbestosis. *Pathological features*: those of cystic DIPF with some hyperplasia of smooth muscle adjacent to distal airways and of the neurilemmal (Schwann) cells of periarterial nerves. Occasional groups of asbestos bodies. Glomus-like structures may be present in small pulmonary artery branches in some cases. These changes may occur in patients with focal cutaneous hyperpigmentation ('café-au-lait' spots) only

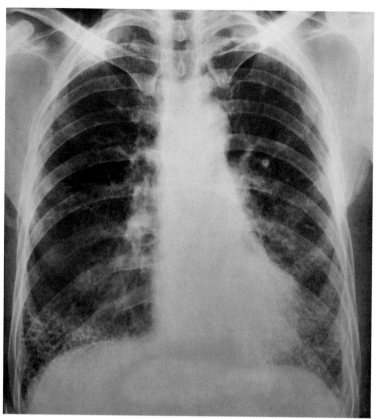

(a)

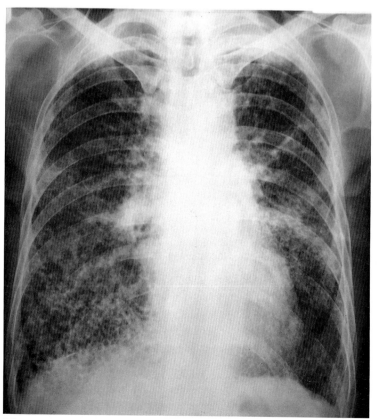

(b)

Figure 15.9 (a) 1972) and (b) 1974: coarse DIPF pattern with multiple 'cystic' appearances involving all zones in (b). No diffuse pleural thickening but small calcified plaque in right hemidiaphragm. The costophrenic angles are clear. The changes occurred within 2 years, 30 years after the patient left the asbestos industry in which he worked as a disintegrator and mill operator of unprocessed fibre from 1938 to 1940. *Clinically*: persistent coarse crackles throughout inspiration (also heard at mouth) and early in expiration in all lobar regions. *Post mortem*: see Figure 15.19. *Diagnosis*: idiopathic DIPF, although asbestosis diagnosed during life

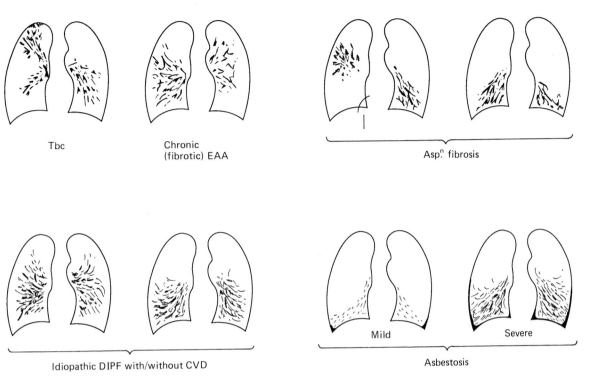

Tbc

Chronic (fibrotic) EAA

Asp.^{n} fibrosis

Idiopathic DIPF with/without CVD

Mild

Severe

Asbestosis

Figure 15.10 Typical radiographic distributions of diffuse pulmonary fibrosis due to different causes. (Arrow indicates segment of gas-filled stomach in cardiophrenic angle – an occasional tell-tale sign of hiatus hernia)

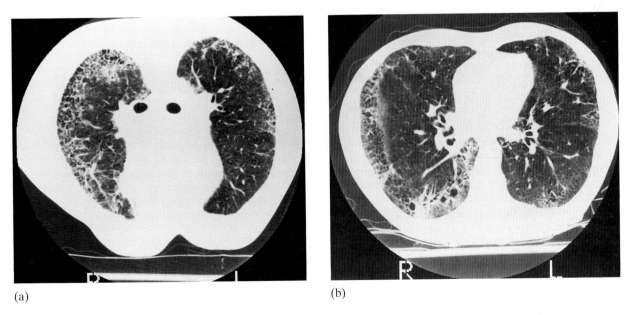

(a)

(b)

Figure 15.11 Appearances of idiopathic DIPF on high-resolution CT in two cases. (a) Prone position; section just below the carina. Widespread fibrosis of asymmetrical, crescentic, mainly subpleural distribution extending deeply into the lungs on the right with extensive anterior involvement, more than the left. Sharp demarcation from normal lung. Numerous, fairly large cysts, many located immediately adjacent to the pleura (especially in the right lung), causing irregularities that give the pathological appearances of bosselation. Note: absence of pleural thickening. Vessels appear as dense, curvilinear opacities. (b) Supine position; mid-thoracic level. Patchy, fairly dense, mainly peripheral fibrosis of crescentic, asymmetrical distribution. Sharply demarcated from normal lung. Anterior regions of both lungs involved. Numerous cysts of vaying size, some large. No pleural thickening. (Courtesy of Dr B. Strickland)

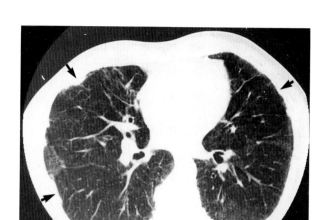

(a)

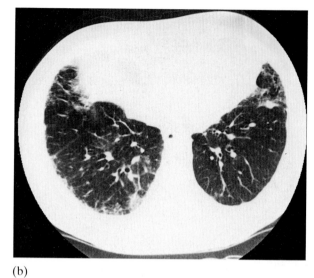

(b)

Figure 15.12 Appearances of asbestosis on high-resolution CT in two cases. (a) Supine position: bilateral subpleural DIPF posteriorly, to a lesser degree laterally and slight anteriorly; extension into the lung limited; no clear demarcation from normal lung; cysts few and small; bilateral, localized pleural plaques (some arrowed). (b) Supine position: predominantly subpleural distribution in lower lobes with more involvement of anterior regions than in (a). The linear and reticular changes show poor demarcation from normal parenchyma. Cysts are very few and small; there is some diffuse bilateral thickening of the pleura and occasional, subpleural, linear opacities. (Courtesy of Dr B. Strickland)

will probably be encountered more often as asbestosis becomes less prevalent and less severe.

Over the last two to three decades, the latent period between the commencement of significant occupational exposure to asbestos and the first clinical evidence of asbestosis is likely to be well in excess of 15 years (Murphy, 1986). Exceptions may occur following unusually heavy exposure, but these have, in general, been rare since the 1960s. DIPF that first becomes apparent 15 to 20 years *after* exposure ceased is unlikely to be asbestosis. Thus, in spite of the difficulty that may sometimes exist, in the clinical setting, of assessing whether past exposure has been sufficient to cause fibrosis, the chronology of the development of DIPF in relation to the beginning and end of exposure may hold an important clue as to whether the fibrosis is likely to be asbestosis or some other disorder. In this respect it is of interest that, in their longitudinal radiological study of 1974 asbestos workers which ended in 1988, Gaensler, Jederlinic and McLoud (1990) did not find a single case of 'significant asbestosis' among those first exposed since 1960 (see Figure 15.2). Unfortunately in the UK, radiographs more than 8 years old are, by general policy, destroyed, and it is to be hoped that some practical system of 'storage of images', such as those discussed in Chapter 7 (page 203) will be developed and, thus, enable suitable records to be kept for many years.

Comparative pathological features

Macroscopic appearances

In many cases of DIPF – *excluding those of asbestosis* which is described in Chapter 14 – the surface of the pulmonary pleura is studded, especially in advanced disease, with multiple small, soft, 'hobnail' or 'cobblestone' protuberances (bosselation) caused by underlying cysts and resembling cirrhotic liver. Diffuse thickening of the pulmonary pleura is, in general, absent – in contrast to asbestosis, in which pleural fibrosis is usual; however, exceptions to this sometimes occur in cases of rheumatoid disease, systemic lupus erythematosus and systemic sclerosis.

When cut (in sagittal slices 1 to 2 cm thick, if possible), the lung with non-occupational DIPF shows an irregular pattern of light or dark grey to brown-coloured fibrosis which, although predominant in either its upper or lower half, involves the rest of the lung to a greater or lesser degree. In some instances the middle third of the lung is most affected. Fibrosis is usually patchy in distribution and, although present subpleurally, is on the whole more prominent deeper in the lobes. Its distribution is frequently dissimilar in location and degree in the two lungs. These differences are, of course, well displayed in the chest radiographs. Blackening of

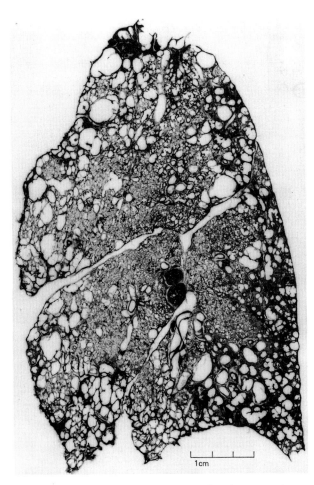

Figure 15.13 Paper-mounted section showing extensive, non-pigmented, idiopathic DIPF with multiple cysts up to about 12 mm in diameter, involving all lobes. Note the clear demarcation between the affected areas and adjacent normal lung, the tendency for the largest cysts to be away from the periphery and the absence of fibrosis of the pulmonary pleura. There was no occupational risk

the fibrotic areas, due to accumulated carbon, is sometimes seen. In general, there is a sharp demarcation between the fibrotic areas and adjacent normal lung (Figure 15.13). Where there is pleural bosselation, only a thin rim of fibrosis separates cysts from the pleura (Figure 15.14). Honeycomb cysts, varying from 2 to 15 mm or more in diameter, may also be present in the areas of fibrosis except where there this is most dense; they are bilateral but not necessarily equally, so may be localized or widespread, and larger cysts are more apt to occur away from the immediate periphery of the lobes (Heppleston, 1956) (see Figure 15.13).

The DIPF of chronic extrinsic allergic alveolitis has a similar variability of distribution and honeycomb formation, although with a tendency to preponderance in the upper halves of the lungs. In some areas it may be confluent, forming large, irregular masses which are more central than peripheral. Thickening of the pulmonary pleura is frequent but not often prominent so that, in advanced disease, bosselation may be present in affected areas.

In asbestosis, even when clinically undetectable, the pulmonary pleura is invariably diffusely thickened, if only to a slight degree, as indicated by loss of translucency or a diffuse 'milky' appearance; bosselation is absent. In more advanced disease there is often partial or complete symphysis with thickened parietal pleura. The essence of the DIPF of asbestosis is that it is sited peripherally in the lower lobes, middle lobe and lingula. Only occasionally, in advanced disease, does it involve the more central zones of these lobes. Its demarcation from normal lung, unlike idiopathic DIPF, is usually ill-defined. Cysts are uncommon but, when present, rarely exceed about 3 mm in diameter and are few in number; multiple large cysts (or coarse 'honeycombing') are not a feature of asbestosis (see Figure 15.15 and see also Figures 14.2 and 14.3).

Evaluation of these gross appearances of lung slices is greatly enhanced by impregnating them with barium sulphate using Heard's technique which is discussed in Appendix III.

It is widely believed that asbestosis, when advanced, does not differ from other forms of end-stage DIPF – apart, that is, from the microscopic presence of asbestos bodies; indeed, the American Thoracic Society has stated officially that the appearance 'most frequently observed in asbestosis is a combination of both diffuse fibrosis and honeycombing' (Murphy, 1986). The foregoing considerations, however, suggest that this is not so, and that this pattern of disease in asbestos workers [as illustrated, for example, by Craighead (1982) in figures in which honeycombing is prominent and by many other authors] represents some pathology other than asbestosis. Indeed, Davis (1984) has also proposed that prominent honeycombing favours another diagnosis.

Microscopic appearances

This brief account is concerned with DIPF other than asbestosis, the histology of which is discussed in Chapter 14.

Alveolar walls are thickened by collagen fibrosis with obliteration of alveolar spaces in some areas. The is a relative increase in type I and a decrease in typer III collagen in well-established disease but, in the earlier stages, the ratio of type III to type I is reversed and is reflected in an increased concentration of type III procollagen peptide in the serum (Laurent, 1986). Large numbers of lymphocytes and plasma cells may be present in the alveolar walls and there are many macrophages in airspaces

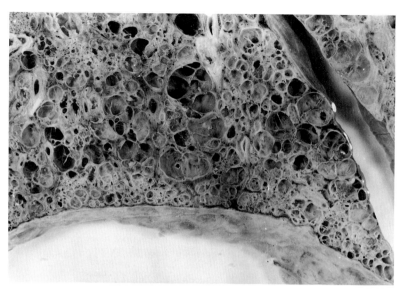

Figure 15.14 Detail of advanced idiopathic DIPF with severe honeycombing. Diffuse thickening of the pleura with some bosselation. Barium sulphate preparation showing anterior base of lower lobe. (Courtesy of Professor B.E. Heard)

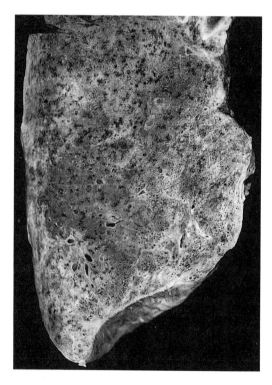

Figure 15.15 Slice of lung showing advanced asbestosis posteriorly, basally and anteriorly in lower lobe. For the most part demarcation between fibrosis and normal lung is ill-defined, and cysts are absent. A few dilated bronchi are seen. Note: diffuse thickening of parietal pleura. *Occupation:* 1957–1969: asbestos insulation sprayer, often in confined spaces. *Post mortem:* 4274 × 10^6 amosite fibres/g and 10 990 × 10^6 crocidolite fibres/g dried lung tissue

adjacent to the fibrosis. Where the fibrosis is uniformly black, the individual has usually been exposed to carbon in some form (for example, soot, coal, graphite) and macrophages in the vicinity are often laden with black pigment that is usually carbon but that may also be related (at least in part) to pigment from cigarette smoke. The blackening suggests that the fibrosis occurred in an already dusty or pigmented lung containing dust-laden macrophages.

Involvement of bronchioles is very variable. Many are narrowed by inflammation and a smaller number obliterated by fibrosis (Watters et al., 1987). Cystic dilatation – 'honeycombing' – of respiratory bronchioles, alveolar ducts and some alveoli is common. Coincident inflammation of more proximal membranous bronchioles is present in some cases (Heard, 1984). Unlike emphysema, honeycomb cysts have no crossing strands and are partly lined by cuboidal, ciliated or non-ciliated columnar epithelium. An important factor in their formation, other than fibrosis, appears to be collapse of alveoli with denuded walls and their subsequent permanent apposition, adhesion and coalescence (so-called *collapse-induration*) (Katzenstein, 1985; Burkhardt, 1989). Thus, fibrosis and collapse-induration may occur to a differing degree in different disease processes (Figure 15.16).

Proliferation of smooth muscle in large or small bundles is often present to a varying degree in the fibrotic areas as a lattice work among the cysts, or in parallel groups beneath the pulmonary pleura, and also in the walls of vessels, especially those of the lymphatics (Liebow, Loring and Felton, 1953;

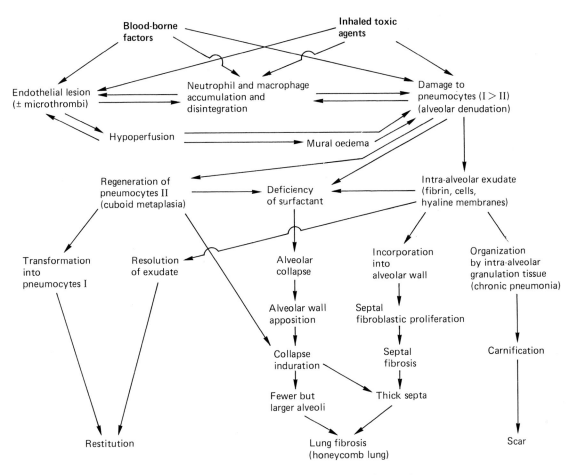

Figure 15.16 Putative schema of the pathogenesis of fibrosing alveolitis. At the top, noxious agents are shown with their possible actions on endothelium, pneumocytes or phagocytes as sites of initial damage. Below, the subsequent progression of lesions through various intermediary steps, some of them interdependent, leading to protraction and formation of vicious cycles (for example, mediated through hypoperfusion) is demonstrated. The possible outcomes, restitution, lung fibrosis or scar formation, are presented at the bottom. (Reproduced, with permission, from Burkhardt, 1989)

Heppleston, 1956; Herbert et al., 1962; Davies et al., 1966; Ovenfors et al., 1980) (Figure 15.17). Fibroblasts with structural and functional properties intermediate between those of typical fibroblasts and smooth muscle cells (that is, *myofibroblasts*), which arise from resident fibroblasts, have been described in many clinical disorders that are characterized by prominent fibrosis in a variety of organs, including the lungs (Seemayer, Schürch and Lagacé, 1981). Indeed, fibroblasts are a heterogeneous, phenotypical family some of which are capable of undergoing muscular differentiation to a degree unsuspected on morphological analysis, although demonstrable by immunological techniques (Skalli et al., 1989); for

example, fibroblasts in systemic sclerosis, express α-smooth muscle actin, and their distribution coincides with the localization of the fibrotic process in the lungs (Sappino et al., 1990). Cytokines possessing growth-promoting activity elaborated by macrophages, lymphocytes or platelets are known to influence the induction of fibrosis (Rifkin and Moscatalli, 1989) (see Chapter 4, 'Type IV hypersensitivity', page 76 and Figure 4.5). Quantitative and qualitative variation in cytokine production probably regulates the phenotypical differences of fibroblasts and, thus, of their biological behaviour in different circumstances (Skalli et al., 1989); there is evidence, in vitro, that various growth factors modulate features of myoid

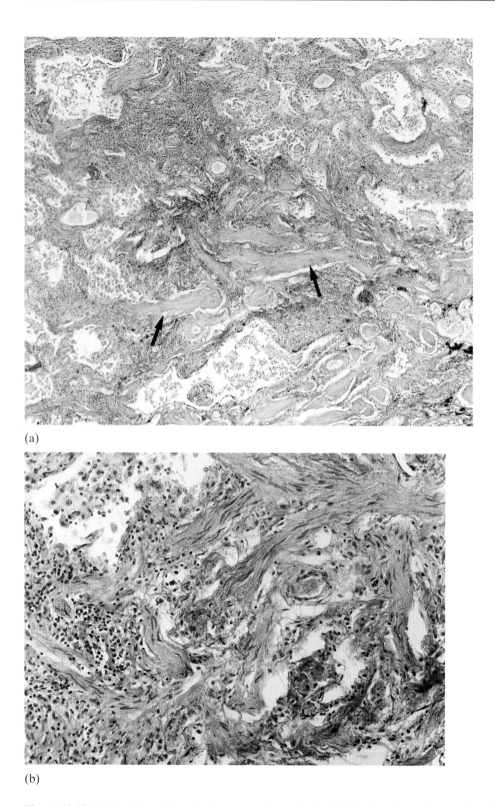

(a)

(b)

Figure 15.17 DIPF with well-marked muscular hyperplasia. (a) Bands of smooth muscle cells are especially prominent in the central area of the field (arrows). Note fibrosis of alveolar walls, the cellularity and multiple cysts, and the lymphoid aggregation in the left upper quadrant; no granulomas. Occasional asbestos bodies in multiple 30-μm sections, but not in this (magnification × 60). (b) Enlarged view of bands of hyperplasic smooth muscle from the same lung (magnification × 240). *Gross appearance*: bosselation of the pulmonary pleura; no pleural thickening; widespread, patchy DIPF in all lobes (especially upper right), including their central zones, with multiple cysts 2 to 7 mm in diameter (see Figure 15.5). *Diagnosis:* idiopathic DIPF

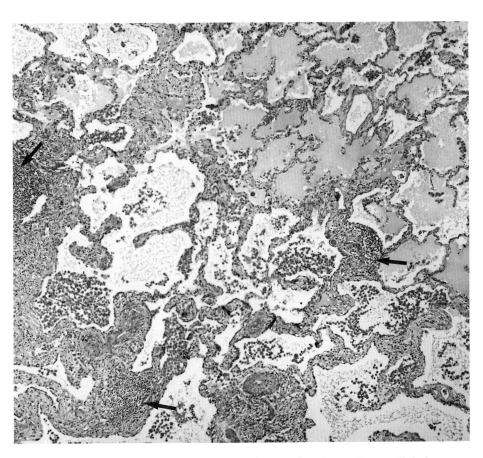

Figure 15.18 DIPF with lymphoid hyperplasia (arrowed) and prominent cellularity. Patchy, moderate fibrosis of alveolar walls. Occasional cysts; no granulomas; no asbestos bodies seen in multiple 30-μm sections (magnification × 60). *Gross appearances*: slight, diffuse thickening of the pleura with moderate bosselation. Widespread, well-demarcated DIPF in all lobes, but sparing extreme base of lower lobes. 'Honeycomb cysts' from 2 to 10 mm diameter (see Figure 15.7)

differentiation in fibroblasts (Rubbia et al., 1989). Electron microscopic studies show that normal myofibroblasts can assume the characteristics of smooth muscle cells (Evans, Kelley and Adler, 1980), and when these occur in areas of fibrosis they are frequently distant from their normal locations. Hyperplasia of these cells is particularly prominent in some genetically determined forms of DIPF such as tuberous sclerosis and neurofibromatosis, and is common in the DIPF of rheumatoid disease and systemic sclerosis, and in many cases of 'lone' idiopathic DIPF. Thus, the development and degree of ectopic smooth muscle hyperplasia in DIPF appear to be related to the cause, or nature, of the fibrosis. Smooth muscle hyperplasia, therefore, is not a feature that is common to all forms of DIPF.

Lymphocytic infiltration and *lymphoid hyperplasia* – often in follicular form and sometimes with germinal centres – may also be seen. In some instances these may represent a survival from the antecedent cellular pattern of disease in which such changes are common (Scadding and Hinson, 1967; Heard, 1984). They are, however, a feature of DIPF associated with rheumatoid arthritis and often prominent adjacent to airways – 'follicular bronchitis or bronchiolitis' (Yousem, Colby and Carrington, 1985) (Figure 15.18), and there appears to be a higher prevalence of such hyperplasia in the interstitial disease of systemic sclerosis than in lone idiopathic DIPF (Harrison et al., 1991). Lymphoid hyperplasia may also be found in the DIPF of systemic lupus erythematosus. It is absent in idiopathic DIPF (see Chapter 4, 'Type IV hypersensitivity').

Elastic tissue, either as single strands or dense tangled masses, may often be prominent due, partly, to compaction of normal elastic tissue resulting from

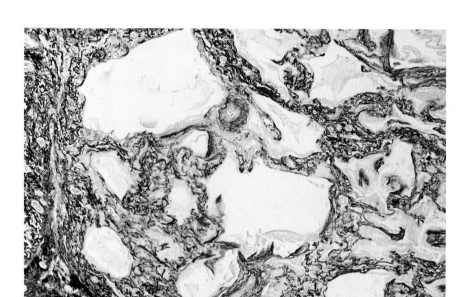

Figure 15.19 Severe DIPF with substantial increase of elastic fibres (dense wavy lines) and cystic bronchiolectasis heavily infiltrated by plasma cells in places; occasional groups of asbestos bodies in some 30-μm sections; no granulomas. (magnification × 60; elastic van Giesen stain). *Gross appearances*: slight diffuse thickening of pulmonary pleura. Severe, well-demarcated DIPF in all lobes with numerous thick-walled cysts 2 to 10 mm diameter involving right lung more than left (see Figure 15.9)

collapse and to obliteration of alveolar spaces and respiratory bronchioles; however, in areas where it is denser, the excess is probably the result of active hyperplasia – 'elastosis' (Heppleston, 1956) (Figure 15.19).

The DIPF of neurofibromatosis appears to be similar to DIPF in general with prominent muscular hyperplasia. But in some cases hyperplasia of neurilemmal cells in the intrapulmonary nerves, particularly in periarterial branches, and glomus-like structures in small branches of the pulmonary veins are seen (Spencer, 1985).

Fibrosis following chemical pneumonia and aspiration of gastric contents tends to be intra-alveolar rather than interstitial.

In sarcoidosis and chronic beryllium disease, active granulomas or whorled scars of healed lesions may persist in the lungs and hilar lymph nodes, but are absent in well-established chronic extrinsic allergic alveolitis.

Bronchiolitis obliterans, incidentally, is sometimes a pathological complication of irradiation pneumonitis (Kaufman and Komorowski, 1990), and it may also occur in association with the uncommon disorder cryptogenic organizing pneumonitis (COP) which, essentially, is an intra-alveolar fibrosis although bronchiolitis obliterans and interstitial fibrosis are present in some cases (Davidson et al., 1983; Bellomo et al., 1991; Woodhead and du Bois, 1991). Bronchiolitis obliterans organizing pneumonia (BOOP) is the common, but less satisfactory, synonym for this disorder (Corrin, 1992).

By contrast, the histological features of asbestosis differ in some important respects from the foregoing descriptions. Proliferation of smooth muscle and lymphoid hyperplasia are absent and, although there may be some compaction of elastic fibres in fibrotic alveolar walls, it is scanty (Heard and Williams, 1961); also active hyperplasia (elastosis) does not seem to occur. Furthermore, there are no accumulations of lymphocytes or plasma cells which are present in the active (desquamative) cellular pattern of idiopathic DIPF. In more advanced asbestosis, most of the respiratory and some membranous bronchioles in the affected areas are obliterated and, eventually, much of the lobule may be occupied by dense collagen (Spencer, 1968; Heard, 1984). This may, perhaps, account for cystic dilatations being small or absent (Spencer, 1968).

There are, in short, three pathways in the development of DIPF: (1) proliferation of fibroblasts and deposition of collagen in the interstitium; (2) alveolar collapse and apposition of alveolar septa; and (3) incorporation of intra-alveolar exudates into alveo-

Table 15.3 Comparison of pathological features of different types of DIPF

	Idiopathic (cryptogenic)	*Chronic extrinisic allergic 'alveolitis' (hypersensitivity pneumonia)*	*Asbestosis*
GROSS FEATURES			
Diffuse thickening of pulmonary pleura	Uncommon (unless infected)	Fairly common	Very common
Multiple pleural cysts ('bosselation')	Common	Fairly common	Absent
Distribution in lung: predominantly 'lower zones' (i.e. lower lobes, middle lobe and lingula)	Uncommon except in cryptogenic disease	Uncommon Usually 'upper and mid-zones' (upper lobes). Generalized in severe disease	Invariable Lower part of upper lobes affected in advanced disease
Lobar distribution: peripheral (subpleural) vs central	Peripheral usual but may be slight. Central zones of upper and lower lobes commonly involved. Peripheral zone spared in some cases	Peripheral and central zone involvement usual	Peripheral invariable More central involvement unusual
Demarcation from normal lung	Well-defined; sharp	Well-defined	Ill-defined
Honeycomb cysts	Common (2–15 mm diameter or more)	Common (2–15 mm diameter or more)	Uncommon (seldom more than 3 mm diameter)
MICROSCOPIC FEATURES			
Asbestos bodies in lung	Absent if no exposure to asbestos	Absent if no exposure to asbestos	Numerous (i.e. readily found)
Smooth muscle proliferation	Fairly common; may be pronounced	Infrequent	Absent
Follicular lymphoid hyperplasia	Common in SLE and rheumatoid disease	Fairly common	Absent
Elastin apparent increase due to compaction or real increase due to hyperplasia	Often prominent especially when fibrosis severe	Fairly common especially when fibrosis severe	Exceptional and mild
Features of desquamative fibrosing 'alveolitis' (DIP) in adjacent lung	Occasional	Rare	Absent
Sarcoid-type granulomas Lungs Lymph nodes	Absent; occasionally seen in fibrotic sarcoidosis and chronic beryllium disease	Usually absent but sometimes remnant follicular scars seen	Absent

lar walls (Katzenstein, 1985; Burkhardt, 1989). The relative contribution of each of these is likely to vary according to the underlying causation, resulting in qualitative differences in the degree of severity and zonal distribution; collapse-induration 'probably contributes decisively' to honeycomb cyst formation (Burkhardt, 1989) by causing 'enlargement of adjacent airspaces by a traction-type phenomenon' (Katzenstein, 1985). These differences could also explain the different characteristics of crackles, discussed in Chapter 6, which may occur in asbestosis and other forms of DIPF, and account for qualitative differences in the degree of impairment of pulmonary mechanics.

Clinicopathological differences

The existence of differences in degree of parenchymal involvement is supported by the clinicopathological observations of Agusti et al. (1988), who found that, despite careful matching of subjects with the two disorders (including a similar degree of resting ventilatory impairment), those with idiopathic DIPF have a 'dramatic fall' of PaO_2 during exercise whereas those with asbestosis do not. They suggested that the difference is related to underlying morphology 'which probably includes more airways disease and less pulmonary vascular involvement or a different degree of interstitial fibrotic change or both, in asbestosis'. Likewise, Cookson, Musk and Glancy (1984) found that, 'despite pathological, functional and radiographic similarities, lung function for a given degree of radiographic parenchymal abnormality is better in subjects with asbestosis than in subjects with cryptogenic fibrosing alveolitis. . .'. Destruction of the vascular bed and other vascular abnormalities are often seen in acute and chronic interstitial pneumonia (DIPF) (Katzenstein, 1985), and it is possible that larger arterial vessels are involved in idiopathic DIPF (Turner-Warwick, 1988; Yousem, 1990) than in asbestosis.

Consequently, asbestosis, on the one hand, and idiopathic and other forms of DIPF, on the other, differ in a number of important respects (some of the pathological features of which are summarized in Table 15.3); asbestosis is not, as is widely believed, identical to other forms of 'end-stage' fibrosis *apart from* the presence of asbestos bodies and fibres. Some discussion of this important topic therefore seems relevant.

The problem of asbestos bodies

For many years the association of asbestos bodies with diffuse pulmonary fibrosis in histological sections has been considered to be a necessary criterion for the fibrosis to be diagnosed as asbestosis, as is exemplified by this statement of the American Thoracic Society:

> The presence of . . . . asbestos bodies in the presence of interstitial fibrosis is mandatory for the pathological diagnosis of asbestosis   (Murphy, 1986)

and also, conversely, from another source, by:

> . . . . a definite diagnosis of asbestosis cannot be made in cases that show characteristic fibrosis that is, consistent with asbestosis in the absence of asbestos bodies, even in a patient with a history of exposure.
> (Craighead, 1982)

Although both these statements are correct confusion and misdiagnosis have often been, and continue

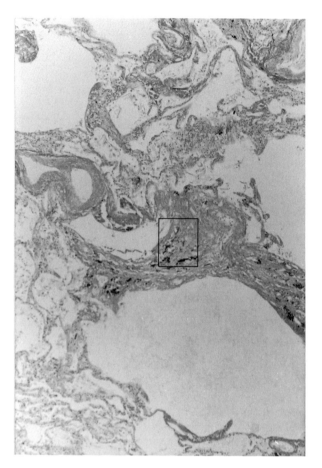

(a)

Figure 15.20 Female: died in 1983 aged 66. 1939 to 1946: manufacture of asbestos insulation mattresses. History of hiatus hernia with episodic oesophagopharyngeal reflux from mid-1950s. Surgical repair 1965 and 1971, but reflux continued clinically and on X-ray imaging. 1958: dyspnoea on exertion. From late 1960s: troublesome cough, purulent sputum and gradually worsening dyspnoea. *Chest radiographs*: 1958 to 1965 considered normal; 1970, a few irregular opacities in right upper zone; 1971, widespread fibrosis in right upper and left midzones; 1972, asbestosis seriously considered but idiopathic DIPF diagnosed and prednisolone prescribed. *Post mortem*: tracts of dense fibrosis in both upper lobes – lateral and posterior segments on right, lingula on left; limited fibrosis apex of right lower lobe. *Histology report*: 'severe interstitial fibrosis associated with many asbestos bodies'. (a) Section from right upper lobe showing DIPF with cyst formation (magnification × 60).

to be, caused by the presence of asbestos bodies being taken as *incontrovertible* proof that fibrosis cannot be other than asbestosis. This situation seems to have arisen from a simple logical error:

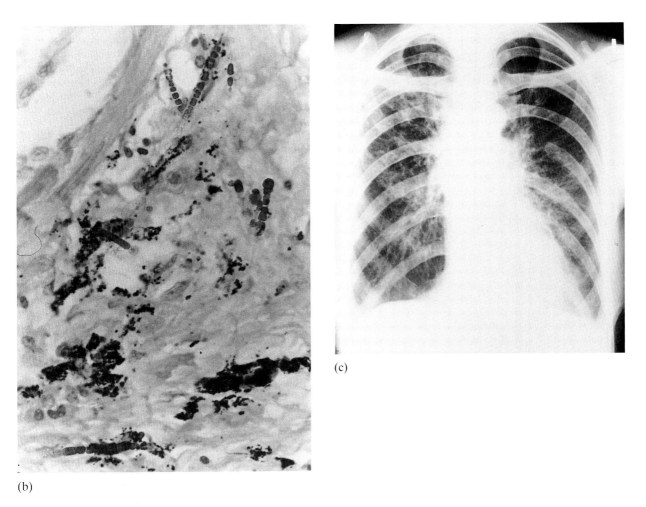

(b)

(c)

Figure 15.20 *(contd)* (b) Higher power of area of rectangle shows a number of asbestos bodies in the fibrotic area (magnification × 300). (c) This film (1979) shows fairly coarse, irregular opacities of right upper and mid-zones (a common distribution of aspiration fibrosis) and left mid-zone. (Absence of posterior segment of left seventh rib due to hernia repair operation.) *Diagnosis*: aspiration fibrosis diagnosed *post mortem* as asbestosis because of the presence of bodies. Aspiration as a possible cause of the pulmonary disease was not considered at any time during life or *post mortem*

that the assertion 'asbestos bodies must be present for the pathological diagnosis of asbestosis' is taken to exclude the possibility that 'fibrosis associated with asbestos bodies is not necessarily asbestosis'. Thus, uncritical acceptance of the implied equation 'diffuse pulmonary fibrosis + asbestos bodies = asbestosis' in the face of contradictory clinical or other evidence will inevitably lead to the wrong diagnosis. The American Thoracic Society dictum,

> Even in the absence of a history of asbestos exposure, the presence of several or more asbestos bodies in areas of extensive interstitial fibrosis is sufficient evidence for a morphological diagnosis of asbestosis.
> (Murphy, 1986)

tends to support such risky reasoning.

It is now acknowledged that DIPF with some resemblance to asbestosis can occur in asbestos workers due to any of the causes just considered (Seal, 1980; Davis, 1984; Gaensler, Jederlinic and Churg, 1991). The fact that only some of those exposed, even heavily, actually develop asbestosis implies that the remaining workers, for one reason or another, are relatively resistant or 'protected'. However, this does not exclude the possibility of the latter developing some unrelated fibrotic disorder to which they may well be as susceptible as they are resistant to asbestosis.

Asbestos fibres and bodies are present in the lungs of occupationally exposed persons who do not have asbestosis as well as in the lungs of those who do; although only slightly more than 1 per cent of

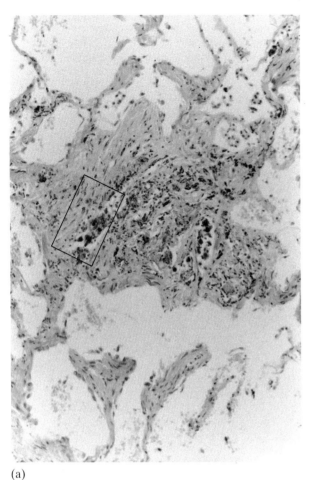

(a)

Figure 15.21 Male, died aged 68. 1951 to 1954: asbestos manufacture – beater floor operative and felter. From 1970: observation for quiescent, treated pulmonary tuberculosis. Despite radiographic appearances of bilateral, dense fibrosis of the upper lobes, but none of DIPF, asbestosis was diagnosed clinically. *Post mortem*: coarse fibrosis of apical region of both upper lobes with thickening of the pulmonary pleura. No fibrosis in lower zones. *Histology*: dense fibrosis of upper lobes with some asbestos bodies in 30-μm sections. No DIPF in middle or lower lobes. Occasional Langhans' cells but no acid-fast bacilli or active tuberculous lesions seen. (a) Section near the periphery of fibrotic area in right upper lobe (magnification × 150). (b) Higher magnification of area within rectangle shows a few intact asbestos bodies and fragments within the fibrosis (magnification × 300). (c) Radiograph showing fibrosis with some contraction of both upper lobes, but no appearances elsewhere consistent with DIPF. *Pathologist's diagnosis*: 'asbestosis of mainly apical distribution'

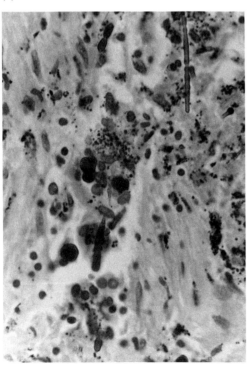

(b)

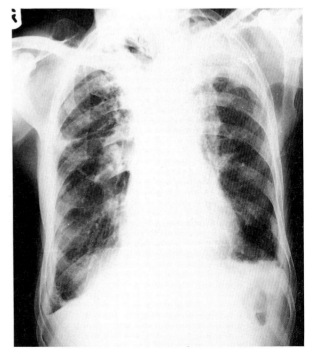

(c)

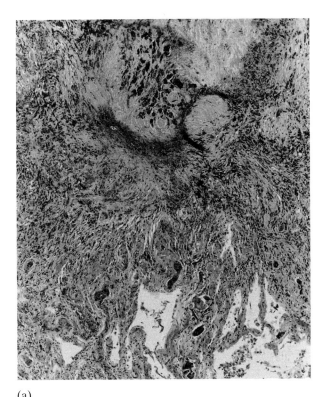

(a)

Figure 15.22 Male, died aged 65. 1945 to 1947: coal miner. 1947 to 1950: tunneller (granite). 1962 to 1974: asbestos board manufacture. *1975*: silicosis diagnosed. *Post mortem* (*1985*): multiple, partly pigmented, silicotic nodules. *Histology*: silicotic ('mixed dust fibrosis' type) lesions confirmed. Asbestos bodies present in the periphery of many of these lesions. (a) Lesion from right upper lobe (magnification × 75). (b) Asbestos bodies and fragments in the peripheral zone of fibrotic nodule (arrow). Entrapment of bodies by silica-induced fibrosis (magnification × 180). (c) Detail of bodies in arrowed area (magnification × 750)

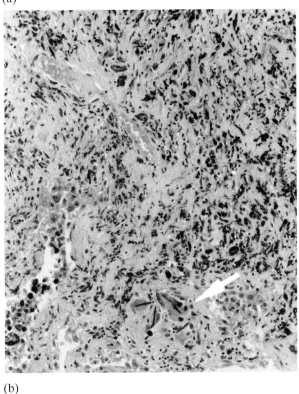

(b)

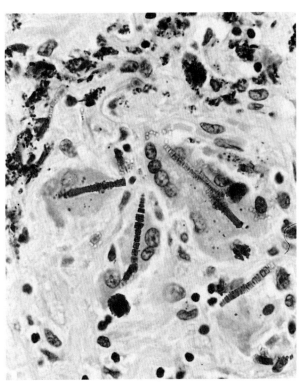

(c)

fibres become coated, asbestos bodies, entire or fragmented, are usually not difficult to find on careful examination of a number of sections from different locations in the lungs, whether or not fibrosis is present. The burden of asbestos – chiefly amphibole – correlates roughly with the severity of asbestosis, that is, there is wide variation (Davis, Gylseth and Morgan, 1986). In part, this may be due to differences in the susceptibility of exposed individuals to developing asbestosis, but fibre counts in lungs of patients with severe asbestosis may appear lower than in those with little fibrosis, even if the total number of fibres in both instances is the same. This is because counts are usually expressed as the number of fibres *per gram dried lung*, and the proportion of solid tissue (dried weight) is much greater in lungs with advanced fibrosis (Davis, Gylseth and Morgan, 1986). Bodies tend to form on amphibole fibres that are more than 20 μm in length; the longer the fibre the more apt it is to be coated (Morgan and Holmes, 1985).

As already mentioned in Chapter 3, asbestos bodies, like fibres (which, optically, are less easily seen), are apt, because of their length, to be poorly cleared from areas of fibrosis – *irrespective of its cause* – and to be trapped as the fibrosis advances (Timbrell, 1982; Vincent et al., 1985). Consequently, they are seen as clusters in surviving airspaces and discretely within fibrotic areas.

In this light it is evident that asbestos bodies do not provide certain proof that asbestos is the cause of the fibrosis with which they are associated.

It is not difficult to find asbestos bodies in fibrosis that is clearly not asbestosis (as well as in that which resembles it) in the lungs of individuals who have had occupational exposure to asbestos. Some examples are illustrated in Figures 15.20 to 15.22 with the relevant details in the accompanying legends. The inappropriate diagnoses in the first two of these cases emphasize the necessity of considering all aspects – past and present – of each case with great care when the appearances and distribution of fibrosis bear a resemblance to asbestosis, for example, idiopathic DIPF. However, it is not uncommon for pathologists, if uncertain of the nature of the fibrosis in a given case, to resolve the diagnostic difficulty by stating that (as it is often put) there are 'sufficient numbers' of asbestos bodies in the fibrotic areas to indicate a causal relationship – that is, asbestosis. In biopsy material, a corollary is sometimes added to the effect that, if the patient has some other disease, the presence of asbestos might have contributed to its fibrogenic effect. Such reasoning is flawed because:

1. 'A sufficient number of asbestos bodies' is a subjective evaluation, the significance of which is questionable in these circumstances and, by itself, hardly justifiable as an index of causality. The

notion of 'sufficient numbers' has to be based on comparison with some acceptable laboratory standard (see Chapter 14, 'Asbestos bodies in post-mortem lung tissue'.)
2. Although it is conceivable that asbestos may contribute to the pathogenesis of DIPF caused by some other non-occupational agency, for the most part, such dual causality is conjectural and, in any case, probability would suggest that it is a rare event.

Clearly, the root cause of this (often needless) dilemma is the mistaken, touchstone-like, significance usually attributed to the asbestos body – an error that can prove to be a will-o'-the-wisp luring the observer into the marshes of misdiagnosis.

Conclusions

This chapter has sought to emphasize the care that should be exercised in appraising the relevance of a history of occupational exposure to asbestos and the finding of asbestos bodies in association with pulmonary fibrosis, before a diagnosis of asbestosis is confidently accepted or rejected. This is as important for the prompt diagnosis of treatable disease as for the identification of asbestosis. From biopsy analysis of a large number of thoracic surgical cases with asbestos exposure, Gaensler, McLoud and Carrington (1985) concluded that: '. . .when there are atypical clinical features or when first exposure was less than 15 years ago, the operation [thoracotomy] may lead to unexpected diagnoses of treatable disorders'. In most instances, however, it should be possible to establish this without resort to biopsy. As has been shown, there are many clinical and radiographic features that can resolve the differential diagnosis.

In making a histopathological diagnosis of asbestosis the following points should, whenever possible, be taken into account:

1. Clinical evidence of systemic or other disease that can cause pulmonary fibrosis.
2. The clinical behaviour of the pulmonary disease especially its rate of development and radiographic distribution, and appearances on high-resolution CT.
3. Whether numbers of asbestos bodies are compatible with a burden of fibres that can cause asbestosis, according to acceptable individual laboratory standards (see Chapter 14).
4. That the gross and microscopic appearances are consistent with asbestosis as described.

5. That the association of prominent smooth muscle, lymphoid hyperplasia or elastosis with DIPF suggests the likelihood of some other disorder even if asbestos bodies are present.

It is conceivable that, in the foreseeable future, some form of *specific* marker for asbestosis will be found. Until then the significance of asbestos bodies in fibrotic lungs requires to be critically evaluated, in the diagnostic process.

References

Agusti, A.G.N., Roca, J., Rodriguez-Roisin, R., Xaubet, A. and Augusti-Vidal, A. (1988) Different patterns of gas exchange response to exercise in asbestosis and idiopathic pulmonary fibrosis. *Eur. Respir. J.* **1**, 510–516

Al-Jarad, N., Strickland, B., Pearson, M.C., Rubens, M.B. and Rudd, R.M. (1992) High resolution computed tomographic assessment of asbestosis and cryptogenic fibvrosing alveolitis: a comparative study. *Thorax* **47**, 645–650

Auerbach, S.H., Mims, O.M. and Goodpasture, E.W. (1952) Pulmonary fibrosis secondary to pneumonia. *Am. J. Pathol.* **28**, 69–81

Bedrossian, C.W.M. (1982) Pathology of drug-induced lung diseases. *Sem. Resp. Med.* **4**, 98–106

Bégin, R., Rola-Pleszczynski, S., Massé, S., Lemaire, I., Sirois, P., Boctor, M., Nadeau, D., Drapeau, G. and Bureau, M.A. (1983) Asbestos-induced lung injury in the sheep model: the initial alveolitis. *Environ. Res.* **30**, 195–210

Bégin, R., Menard, H., Décarie, F. and St-Sauveur, A. (1987) Immunogenetic factors as determinants of asbestosis. *Lung* **165**, 159–163

Bellomo, R., Finaly, M., McLaughlin, P. and Tai, E. (1991) Clinical spectrum of cryptogenic organising pneumonitis. *Thorax* **46**, 554–558

Bitterman, P.B. and Crystal, R.G. (1980) Is there a fibrotic gene? *Chest* **78**, 549–550

Bitterman, P.B., Rennard, S.I., Keogh, B.A., Wewers, M.D., Adelberg, S. and Crystal, R.G. (1986) Familial idiopathic pulmonary fibrosis. *N. Engl. J. Med.* **314**, 1343–1347

Brentjens, J.R., O'Connel, D.W., Pawlowski, I.B., Hsu, K.C. and Andres, G.A. (1974) Experimental immune complex disease of the lung. The pathogenesis of a laboratory model resembling certain interstitial lung disease. *J. Expl. Med.* **140**, 105–125

Burkhardt, A. (1989) Alveolitis and collapse in the pathogenesis of pulmonary fibrosis. *Am. Rev. Respir. Dis.* **140**, 513–524

Campbell, D.A., Poulter, L.W. and Du Bois, R.M. (1986) Phenotypic analysis of alveolar macrophages in normal subjects and in patients with interstitial lung disease. *Thorax* **41**, 429–434

Campbell, D.A., Poulter, L.W., Janossy, G. and Du Bois, R.M. (1985) Immunohistological analysis of lung tissue from patients with cryptogenic fibrosing alveolitis suggesting local expression of immune hyper-sensitivity. *Thorax* **40**, 405–411

Castle, W.M. (1985) Drugs and fibrotic reactions – Part II. *Adverse Drug React. Bull.* **114**, 424–427

Chapman, H.A., Allen C.L. and Stone, O.L. (1986) Abnormalities in pathways of alveolar fibrin turnover among patients with interstitial lung disease. *Am. Rev. Respir. Dis.* **133**, 437–443

Cooke, W.E. (1924) Fibrosis of the lungs due to the inhalation of asbestos dust. *Br. Med. J.* **2**, 147

Cooke, W.E. and Hill, C.F. (1927) Pneumoconiosis due to asbestos dust. *J.R. Microsoc. Soc.* **48**, 232–238

Cookson, W.O.C.M., Musk, A.W., and Glancy, J.J. (1984) Asbestosis and cryptogenic fibrosing alveolitis: a radiological and functional comparison *Aust. N Z J. Med.* **14**, 626–630

Cooper, J.A.D., White, D.A. and Matthay, R.A. (1986) Drug-induced pulmonary disease. Part 1. Cytotoxic drugs. *Am. Rev. Respir. Dis.* **133**, 321–340; Part 2. Non-cytotoxic drugs *Am. Rev. Respir. Dis.* **133**, 488–505

Corrin, B. (1992) Bronchiolitis obliterans organizing pneumonia. A British view. *Chest* **102** (suppl.), 7S

Corrin, B., Dewar, A., Rodriguez-Roisin, R. and Turner-Warwick, M. (1985) Fine structural changes in cryptogenic fibrosing alveolitis and asbestosis. *J. Pathol.* **147**, 107–119

Craighead, J.E. (Chairman of Committee) (1982) The pathology of asbestos-associated diseases of the lungs and pleural cavities: diagnosis criteria and proposed grading system. Report of Pneumoconiosis Committee of the College of American Pathologists and the National Institute for Occupational Safety and Health. *Arch. Pathol. Lab. Med.* **1906**, 544–596

Crystal, R.G., Bitterman, P.B., Rennard, S.I, Hance, A.J. and Keogh, B.A. (1984) Interstitial lung diseases of unknown cause (two parts). *N. Engl. J. Med.* **310**, 154–166, 285–244

Davies, D., McFarlane, A., Darke, C.S. and Dodge, O.G. (1966) Muscular hyperplasia ('cirrhosis') of the lung and bronchial dilations as features of chronic diffuse fibrosing alveolitis. *Thorax* **21**, 272–289

Davis, J.M.G. (1984). The pathology of asbestos related disease. *Thorax* **39**, 801–808

Davis, J.M.G., Gylseth, B. and Morgan, A. (1986) Assessment of mineral fibres from human lung tissue. *Thorax* **41**, 167–175

Du Bois, R.M. (1990) Advances in our understanding of the pathogenesis of fibrotic lung disease. *Respir. Med.* **84**, 185–187

Dunnill, M.S. (1990) Pulmonary fibrosis. *Histopathology* **16**, 321–329

Eisenberg, H. (1982) The interstitial lung diseases associated with the collagen-vascular disorders. *Clin. Chest Med.* 565–578

Elias, J.A., Rossman, M.D., Zurier, R.B. and Daniele, R.P. (1985) Human alveolar macrophage inhibition of lung fibroblast growth. A prostaglandin-dependent process. *Am. Rev. Respir. Dis.* **131**, 94–99

Ellman, P. (1933) Pulmonary asbestosis: its clinical, radiological and pathological features and associated risk of tuberculous infection. *J. Ind. Hyg.* **15**, 165–183

Evans, C. (1976) HLA antigens in diffuse fibrosing alveolitis. *Thorax* **31**, 483

Evans, J.N., Kelley, J. and Adler, K.B. (1980) Contractile properties of parenchymal tissue in pulmonary fibrosis. International Colloquium on Pulmonary Fibrosis, February, 1980. University of London

Gaensler, E.A., Jederlinic, P.J. and Churg, A. (1991) Idiopathic pulmonary fibrosis in asbestos-exposed workers. *Am. Rev. Respir. Dis.* **144**, 689–696

Gaensler, E.A., Jederlinic, P.J. and McLoud, T.C. (1990) Radiographic progression of asbestosis with and without continued exposure. In *VIIth International Pneumoconiosis Conference (NIOSH-ILO)*. DHHS (NIOSH) Publication No. 90-108, Part 1, September 1990, pp. 386–392

Gaensler, E.A., McLoud, T.C. and Carrington, C.B. (1985) Thoracic surgical problems in asbestos-related disorders. *Ann. Thorac. Surg.* **40**, 82–96

Hansell, D.M. and Kerr, I.H. (1991) The role of high resolution computed tomography in the diagnosis of interstitial lung disease. *Thorax* **46**, 77–84

Harrison, N.K., Myers, A.R., Corrin, B., Soosay, G., Dewar, A., Black, C.M., Du Bois, R.M. and Turner-Warwick, M. (1991) Structural features of interstitial lung disease in systemic sclerosis. *Am. Rev. Respir. Dis.* **144**, 706–713

Heard, B.E. (1984) Quantitative pathology of interstitial lung disease. *Semin. Respir. Med* **6**, 20–30

Heard, B.E. and Williams, R. (1961) The pathology of asbestosis, with reference to lung function. *Thorax* **16**, 264–281

Heppleston, A.G. (1956) The pathology of honeycomb lung. *Thorax* **11**, 77–93

Herbert, F.A., Nahurias, B.B., Gaensler, E.A. and MacMahon, H.E. (1962) Pathophysiology of interstitial pulmonary fibrosis. *Archs Intern. Med.* **110**, 628–648

Iverson, L.I.G., May, I.A. and Samson, P..C. (1973) Pulmonary complications of benign esophageal disease. *Am. J. Surg.* **126**, 223–228

Jayson, M.I.V. (1983) Systemic sclerosis – a microvascular disorder? *J. R. Soc. Med.* **76**, 635–642

Jederlinic, P.J., Churg, A. and Gaensler, E.A. (1987) Idiopathic pulmonary fibrosis in asbestos exposed persons. *Am. Rev. Respir. Dis.* **135** (2nd part), A347

Johnson, D.A., Drane, W.E., Curran, J., Catteau, E.L., Ciarleglio, C., Khan, A., Cotelingham, J. and Benjamin, S. (1989) Pulmonary disease in progressive systemic sclerosis. A complication of gastroesophageal reflux and occult aspiration? *Archs Intern. Med.* **149**, 589–593

Johnston, I.D.A., Britton, J.R., Kinnear, W.J.M. and Logan, R.F.A. (1990) Rising mortality from cryptogenic fibrosing alveolitis. *Br. Med. J.* **301**, 1017–1021

Johnston, I.D.A., Bleasdale, C., Hind, C.R.K. and Woodcock, A.A. (1991) Accuracy of diagnostic coding of hospital admissions for cryptogenic fibrosing alveolitis. *Thorax* **46**, 589–591

Jones, R.N. (1991) The diagnosis of asbestosis. *Am. Rev. Respir. Dis.* **144**, 477–478

Jordana, M., Schulman, J., McSharry, C., Irving, L.B., Newhouse, M.T., Jordana, G. and Gauldie, J. (1988) Heterogenous proliferative characteristics of human adult lung fibroblast lines and clonally derived fibroblasts from control and fibrotic tissue. *Am. Rev. Respir. Dis.* **137**, 579–584

Kallenberg, C.G.M., Schilizzi, B.M., Beaumont, F., de Leij, L., Poppema, S. and The T.H. (1987) Expression of class II major histocompatibility complex antigens on alveolar epithelium in interstitial lung disease: relevance to pathogenesis of idiopathic pulmonary fibrosis. *J. Clin. Pathol.* **40**, 725–733

Katzenstein, A.A. (1985) Pathogenesis of 'fibrosis' in interstitial pneumonia. An electron microscopic study. *Human Pathol.* **16**, 1015–1024

Kaufman, J. and Komorowski, R. (1991) Bronchiolitis obliterans. A new clinico-pathological complication of irradiation pneumonitis. *Chest* **97**, 1243–1244

Kradin R.L., Divertie, M.B., Colvin, R.B., Ramirez, J., Ryu, J., Carpenter, H.A. and Bhan, A.K. (1986) Usual interstitial pneumonitis is a T-cell alveolitis. *Clin. Immun. Immunopathol.* **40**, 224–235

Laurent, G.J. (1986) Lung collagen: more than scaffolding. *Thorax* **41**, 418–428

Libby, D.M., Gibofsky, A., Fotino, M., Waters, S.J. and Smith, J.P. (1983) Immunogenetic and clinical findings in idiopathic pulmonary fibrosis. *Am. Rev. Respir. Dis.* **127**, 618–622

Liddell, D. and Miller, K. (1983) Individual susceptibility to inhaled particles. A methodological essay. *Scand. J. Work Environ. Health.* **9**, 1–8

Liebow, A.A. (1975) Definition and classification of interstitial pneumonias in human pathology. *Progr. Respir. Dis.* **8**, 1–33

Liebow, A.A., Loring, W.E. and Felton, W.L. (1953). The musculature of the lungs in chronic pulmonary disease. *Am. J. Pathol.* **29**, 885–911

Livingstone, J.L., Lewis, J.G., Reid, L. and Jefferson, K.E. (1964) Diffuse interstitial pulmonary fibrosis. *Q. J Med.* **23**, 71–103

Meliconi, R., Lalli, E., Borzi, R.M., Galavotti, V. and Gasbarrini, G. (1990) Idiopathic pulmonary fibrosis: can cell mediated immunity markers predict clinical outcome? *Thorax* **45**, 536–540

Morgan, A. and Holmes, A. (1985) The enigmatic asbestos body: its formation and significance in asbestos–related ·disease. *Environ. Res.* **38**, 283–292

Murphy, R.L. (Chairman of Committee) (1986) The diagnosis of nonmalignant diseases related to asbestos. Official statement of the American Thoracic Society, March, 1986. *Am. Rev. Respir. Dis.* **134**, 363–368

Musk, A.W., Zilko, P.J., Manners, P., Kay, P.H. and Kamboh, M.I. (1986) Genetic studies in familial fibrosing alveolitis. Possible linkage with immunoglobulin allotypes (Gm). *Chest* **89**, 206–210

Ovenfors, C-O., Dahlgren, S.E., Ripe, E. and Ost, A. (1980) Muscular hyperplasia of the lung: a clinical, radiographic and histopathological study. AJR *Am. J. Roentgenol.* **135**, 703–712

Payne, C.R (1984) Pulmonary manifestations of rheumatoid arthritis. *Br. J. Hosp. Med.* **32**, 192–197

Pearson, J.E.G. and Wilson, R.S.E. (1971) Diffuse pulmonary fibrosis and hiatus hernia. *Thorax* **26**, 300–305

Prakash, W.B.S., Luthra, H.S. and Divertie, M.B. (1985) Intrathoracic manifestations of mixed connective tissue disease *Mayo Clin. Proc.* **60**, 813–821

Reiser, K.M. and Last, J.A. (1986) Early cellular events in pulmonary fibrosis. *Exp. Lung Res.* **10**, 331–355

Riccardi, V.M. (1981) Von Recklinghausen neurofibromatosis. *N. Engl. J. Med.* **305**, 1617–1627

Rifkin, D.B. and Moscatelli, D. (1989) Recent developments in the cell biology of basic fibroblast growth factor. *J. Cell Biol.* **109**, 1–6

Rindfleisch, G.E. (1897) Uber Cirrhosis Cystica Pulmonum *Zentrabl. Allg. Path. Anat.* **8**, 864–865

Roschmann, R,A, and Rothenberg, R.J. (1987) Pulmonary fibrosis in rheumatoid arthritis: a review of clinical features and therapy. *Semin. Arthritis Rheum.* **16**, 174–185

Rowell, N.R. (1985) Systemic sclerosis. The Watson Smith Lecture 1984. *J. R. Coll. Physns Lond.* **19**, 23–30

Rubbia, L., Sappino, A-P., Hansson, H.K.K. and Gabbiani, G. (1989) Action of different cytokines on actin isoform expression on fibroblasts *in vitro* (abstract). *Experientia* **45**, A49

Salmeron, G., Greenberg, D. and Lidsky, M.D. (1981) Polymyositis and diffuse interstitial lung disease. A review of the pulmonary histopathologic findings. *Archs Intern. Med.* **141**, 1005–1010

Sappino, A-P, Masouyé, I., Saurat, J-H. and Gabbiani, G. (1990) Smooth muscle differentiation in scleroderma fibroblastic cells. *Am. J. Pathol.* **137**, 585–591

Scadding, J.G. and Hinson, K.F.W. (1967) Diffuse fibrosing alveolitis (diffuse interstitial fibrosis of the lungs). Correlation of histology at biopsy with prognosis. *Thorax* **22**, 291–304

Scott, J., Johnston, I.D.A. and Britton, J.R. (1990) Aetiology of cryptogenic fibrosing alveolitis: a case-control study of environmental dust exposure. *Thorax* **45**, 783

Seal, R.M.E. (1980) Current views on pathological aspects of asbestosis (the unresolved questions and problems). In *Biological Effects of Mineral Fibres* (ed. J.C. Wagner) Vol. 1. Scientific Publication No. 30. IARC, Lyon, pp. 217–235

Seemayer, T.A., Schürch, W. and Lagacé, R. (1981) Myofibroblasts in human pathology. *Human Pathol.* **12**, 491–492

Seiler, H.E. (1928) A case of pneumoconiosis. Result of the inhalation of asbestos dust. *Br. Med. J.* **2**, 982

Skalli, O., Schürch, W., Seemayer, T., Lagacé, R., Montandon, D., Pittet, B. and Gabbiani, G. (1989) Myofibroblasts from diverse pathologic settings are heterogenous in their content of actin isoforms and intermediate filament proteins. *Lab. Invest.* **60**, 275–285

Spencer, H. (1968) Chronic interstitial pneumonia. In *The Lung* (A.A. Liebow and D.E. Smith, eds) Williams and Wilkins, Baltimore, pp. 142–143

Spencer, H. (1985) *Pathology of the Lung* 4th ed. Pergamon Press, Oxford and New York

Strickland, B. and Strickland, N.H. (1988) The value of high definition narrow section computed tomography in fibrosing alveolitis. *Clin. Radiol.* **39**, 589–594

Timbrell, V. (1982) Deposition and retention of fibres in the human lung. *Ann. Occup. Hyg.* **26**, 347–369

Turner-Warwick, M. (1988) Some connective tissue disorders of the lung. *Postgrad. Med. J.* **64**, 497–504

Turner-Warwick, M. and Courtenay-Evans, R. (1977) Pulmonary manifestations of rheumatoid disease. *Clin. Rheum. Dis.* **3**, 549–564

Varpela, E., Tiilikainen, A., Varpela, M. and Tukiainen, P. (1979) High prevalences of HLA-B15 and LHA-DW6 in patients with cryptogenic fibrosing alveolitis. *Tissue Antigens* **14**, 68–71

Vincent, J.A., Johnston, A.M., Jones, A.D., Bolton, R.E. and Addison, J. (1985) Kinetics of deposition and clearance of inhaled minerals dusts during chronic exposure. *Br. J. Ind. Med.* **42**, 707–715

Vorwald, A.J. (1950) Variation in individual susceptibility to industrial dusts inhaled into the lungs. *Am. Rev. Tuberc.* **62**, 13–21

Watters, L.C., Schwarz, M.I., Cherniack, R.M., Waldron, J.A., Dunn, T.L., Stanford, R.E. and King, T.E. (1987) Idiopathic pulmonary fibrosis. Pretreatment broncho-alveolar lavage cellular constituents and their relationships with histopathology and clinical response to therapy. *Ann. Rev. Respir. Dis.* **135**, 696–704

Webb, W.R., and Goodman, P.C. (1977) Fibrosing alveolitis in patients with neurofibromatosis. *Radiology* **122**, 289–293

West, J.B. (1979) *Respiratory Physiology: The Essentials*, 2nd ed. Williams and Wilkins, Baltimore

Woodhead, M.A. and Du Bois, R.M. (1991) Bronchiolitis obliterans, cryptogenic pneumonitis and BOOP. *Resp. Med.* **85**, 177–178

Wyers, H. (1949) Asbestosis. *Postgrad. Med. J.* **25**, 631–638

Yousem, S.A. (1990) The pulmonary pathologic manifestations of the CREST syndrome. *Human Pathol.* **21**, 467–474

Yousem, S.A., Colby, T.V. and Carrington, C.B. (1985) Follicular bronchitis/bronchiolitis. *Human Pathol.* **16**, 700–706

16

Disease related to non-asbestos silicates

Robert N. Jones, Hans Weill and W. Raymond Parkes

'Talc' pneumoconiosis

Although the mineral talc has a precise definition, the word 'talc', as applied to ores and their subsequent products, is a generic term that can encompass mixtures of differing composition. Commercial talcs range from high grades of purity, containing over 95 per cent talc proper, down to 'industrial' grades that contain 50 per cent or more impurities. Some of those impurities (see following section) have significant effects on the lung.

Talc pneumoconiosis was first described by Thorel in 1896, 11 years before the first published description of asbestosis. Unfortunately, many subsequent writers have not actually described their materials except as talc, with the result that much of the clinical and experimental literature is difficult to interpret and apply. The term 'talcosis' could be applied to several diseases with more specific radiographic and pathological appearances, and is probably best avoided because it implies a single entity. Talc pneumoconiosis has the same liability, and so perhaps should be written 'talc pneumoconioses' in any general discussion.

The various talcs can produce several distinctive radiographic appearances: a nodular or quasi-nodular (stellate opacities) pattern resembling silicosis or mixed dust fibrosis, including, in some cases, large opacities; a diffuse linear interstitial pattern, simulating asbestosis; or a combination of nodular and linear patterns in the same radiograph. Three histological lesions occur: *quasi-nodular fibrosis, diffuse interstitial fibrosis* and *foreign body granulomas*. A vasculocentric granulomatous process results from intravenous injection. The composition of an inhaled talc is likely to be the major determinant of the appearance and biological behaviour of the resulting pneumoconiosis.

Definition and mode of occurrence of talc

Talc is a hydrated magnesium silicate with the formula $Mg_3Si_4O_{10}(OH)_2$, although calcium, aluminium and iron are always present in variable amounts. It occurs in sheets that readily cleave and break down to form flat flaky plates and, to a lesser degree, short rolled sheets. It is usually formed in one of two ways: either by low-grade thermal metamorphism of siliceous dolomites or by hydrothermal alterations – frequently accompanied by dynamic metamorphism – of magnesium-rich ultrabasic rocks (see Appendix I). In consequence, other minerals are almost invariably present in association with talc. These include serpentines (usually antigorite but, rarely, chrysotile), cholorites, quartz, magnesite, calcite and the amphiboles tremolite and anthophyllite. Magnesium silicate mineral remnants such as olivine, enstatite and diopside may also be present. According to the geographical area of origin, therefore, talc deposits exhibit a wide variety of mineral assemblages which differ in occurrence and proportion. This is exemplified in Tables 16.1 and 16.2. Intergrowths of tremolite and anthophyllite, usually in prismatic crystalline form, may be intimately associated with talc, but in some geological regions (notably New York State) which appear to be uncommon, if not exceptional, they may occur in true fibrous (that is, asbestos) form and persist after one processing. High-purity (high-grade) white talcs from the Italian Alps, Pyrenees, China and India were formed from siliceous dolomite and dolomite limestones, and contain little or no quartz, although this mineral may be encountered in small amounts in the mining of Italian talc. Domestically produced Norwegian talc is, however, of fairly low grade, and usually contains chlorite, magnesite and, possibly, non-

Table 16.1 Typical mineralogical composition of some commercial grades of talc

	Weight per cent†					
	1	2	3	4	5	6
Talc	95	90	89	50	49	45
Chlorite	3	4	8	49	15	12
Magnesite	–	0.6	–	–	31	37
Dolomite	1	0.8	–	Trace	–	4
Tremolite	–	–	–	–	Trace	–
Serpentine	–	–	–	–	*	–
Quartz	–	Trace	Trace	Trace	–	–
Opaques	–	–	–	Trace	Trace	Trace
Percentage reflectance	94	89	84	70	70	64

*Serpentine identified by X-ray diffraction but included by thermogravimetry in chlorite figure. Mineralogical compositions obtained by X-ray diffractometry; weight percentages derived from thermogravimetric data. Percentage reflectance gives an indication of whiteness.
†1 Chinese talc – cosmetic grade.
2 Italian (Pinerolo) talc – cosmetic grade.
3 French (Luzenac) talc – high quality.
4 French (Luzenac) talc – industrial grade.
5 Norwegian talc – industrial grade.
6 Unst talc (Shetland) – industrial grade.
Reproduced by courtesy of Dr H.E. Highley and HMSO.

Table 16.2 Varieties of commercial 'talc' from New York State (Gouverneur District)

	1	2	3	4	5	6	7	8	9	10
Tremolite	68	98	17	–	78	38	29	15	88	46
Anthophyllite	–	–	20	–	–	–	45	78	4	39
Talc	–	1	63	–	4	–	–	7	1	5
Serpentine*	–	1	–	80	18	54	26	–	4	4
Quartz	31	–	–	–	–	–	–	–	2	4
Others	1	–	–	20	–	8	–	–	1	2

*Either massive or fibrous.
Figures indicate percentage composition.
Dashes indicate no determination made.
By courtesy of Johns-Manville Research and Engineering Center, New Jersey.

fibrous tremolite and trace amounts of quartz. The 'talc' from the famous mines of St Lawrence County in New York State frequently contains as much as 50 per cent or more of tremolite, with less than 25 per cent talc, and significant amounts of anthophyllite and quartz occur in some samples (Weiss and Boettner, 1967). In these deposits, a significant proportion of both tremolite and anthophyllite is of true fibrous habit. The variable composition of some New York State 'talc' samples is shown in Table 16.2. Californian (Death Valley) 'talc' is associated with non-fibrous tremolite, quartz, serpentine and calcite. Talc from the Vermont area, however, is associated with magnesite and dolomite, and there are no asbestos minerals; quartz is either absent or present in trace amounts (Boundy et al., 1979). Canadian 'talc', which comes mainly from the Madoc district of Ontario, has a similar geological origin to that of St Lawrence County, and contains considerable quantities of tremolite and dolomite, and some quartz which may remain in variable amount in the final product. In the UK, only a small quantity of impure (low-grade) talc is produced in the Shetlands, and this has decreased in recent years due to its previous use in the roof felting industry being much restricted.

Low-grade talcs, therefore, may contain in excess of 50 per cent impurities, and significant amounts of quartz, tremolite and anthophyllite (of prismatic or fibrous habit according to origin) may be present in some. Where talc is associated with substantial quantities of tremolite and anthophyllite, it is often known as *asbestine*. The presence of chrysotile is rare, although it occurs occasionally as a result of intrusion in some low-grade talcs. But *sepiolite* fibres (also anhydrated magnesium silicate), which are occasionally found in talc samples, may be mistaken for chrysotile, as they have a very similar

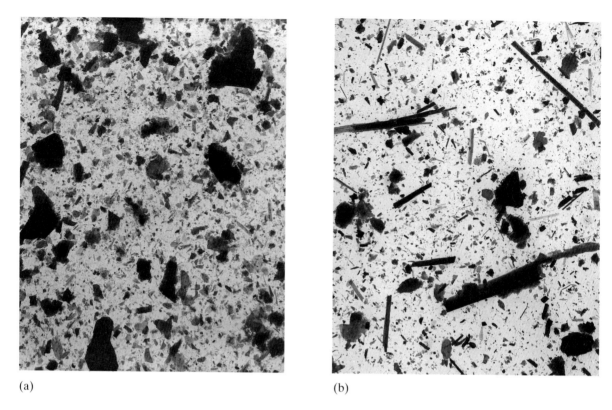

(a)   (b)

Figure 16.1 (a) Talc plates, good quality cosmetic talc. (b) Talc plates and tremolite, the acicular crystals and fibres of which are evident by their long axes. This is typical of industrial grade talc used in the USA. Electron micrographs, magnification × 5000. (By courtesy of Johns-Manville Research and Engineering Center, New Jersey)

microscopic appearance, and can only be differentiated by sophisticated analytical methods (Pooley and Rowlands, 1977).

Under the light microscope, talc appears as flat, angular, polygonal plates (that is, platy, non-fibrous talc), and occasionally as short 'fibres' that are, in fact, rolled talc sheets, whereas tremolite and anthophyllite both consist of prismatic and acicular crystals and, occasionally, true fibres. The term 'fibrous' talc, therefore, is only applicable to 'talc' in which these amphiboles occur in asbestiform habit and are predominant (Figure 16.1). Talc and tremolite are strongly birefringent, but anthophyllite is only weakly so. However, electron microscopy and diffraction, and X-ray diffraction, are needed for positive identification. The inability of light and phase contrast microscopy to distinguish rolled talc plates and talc shards from asbestos fibres must be borne in mind when considering the total fibre content of industrial talcs (Boundy *et al.*, 1979).

'Steatite' is the term used to describe the massive, fine-grained (cryptocrystalline) variety of talc, which is often referred to as french chalk; 'soapstone' is a term loosely applied to impure talcose rocks containing variable amounts of talcs and other minerals.

Pyrophyllite (see Appendix I) is sometimes wrongly referred to as 'talc' in industry. It is a hydrated aluminosilicate with very similar properties to talc although, except in its purest form, it contains quartz in abundance. Hence, the term 'talc' should be confined to the description of a mineral containing at least 95 per cent platy talc with no amphibole and negligible quartz content. It is important to reiterate that, with the exception of such regions as New York State and Madoc, Ontario, tremolite and anthophyllite in talc occur mainly in prismatic crystalline form, and not in fibrous form; it is also important to emphasize that statements such as 'talc is closely related to asbestos', often seen in medical and public health literature, are most misleading.

Most of the talc used for industrial purposes in the UK prior to and since the Second World War has come from Norway, France, China and Italy. However, during the war, all these sources of supply were cut off, and were apparently replaced mainly by Canadian and, possibly, some American 'talc'. The use of these talcs, which contain substantial quantities of fibrous tremolite and anthophyllite, may have had an influence on the type of pneumoconiosis that has been sporadically observed in some 'talc'-exposed workers in the UK since the Second World War. After 1970, imports of 'tremolitic talc' into the UK have been recorded separately, and only small amounts have been used.

Uses of talc

The valuable qualities of talc in industry are its extreme softness, whiteness (when pure), good hiding power, high surface area, high slip or lubricating power, chemical inertness, low electrical and heat conductivity, oil adsorption properties and high refractoriness. Because of this great versatility, talc in a variety of grades is put to a large number of industrial uses, but only the most common are referred to. In the UK, the greatest consumption of talc occurs in the paint, pharmaceutical and cosmetics industries.

Paints

High-grade talc is used in the paint industry as a filler and inert extender because of its whiteness and laminar form, but 'fibrous talc' (asbestine) is also widely employed because its good suspending powers reduce settling in the can, and it also increases the mechanical strength of paint films. However, it appears that the term 'asbestine' is also being used in the paint industry in the UK for some grades of talc which do not contain fibrous minerals (Highley, 1974). The paint industry is the main consumer of tremolitic 'talc' in the UK.

Cosmetic and pharmaceutical industries

High-grade talcs are used in large quantities in these industries, for example, face powders, talcum powders, other cosmetic preparations and dermopaediatric powders, and for polishing tablets. The particle size of good cosmetic grade talc lies between 0.3 and 50 μm (Hamer, Rolle and Schelz, 1976), but only a fraction of the particles are of respirable size. Quartz and other harsh minerals should be absent or only present in trace amounts and, apart from chlorite, which, as a holder of perfume, may be acceptable, the only impurity should be calcium sulphate. But this level of purity may not always exist in poor quality preparations (see 'Industrial applications'). The best cosmetic talcs come from Italy, China and Vermont (USA). Talc used in the British cosmetic industry is specifically controlled for asbestos minerals, whether of fibrous habit or not (Phillipson, 1980).

Ceramics

Both talc and steatite are employed in small amounts in the ceramics industry, for a variety of purposes. Talc mixed with clay and alumina, and fired at 1250 to 1400°C forms *cordierite* (a pseudo-hexagonal crystalline, aluminum magnesium iron silicate), which is used for such things as coil forms, fuse cores, rheostat blocks, fire bars, electrical insulators, and the manufacture of saggers and other types of refractory kiln equipment. Steatite, together with ball clay and a barium carbonate flux, fired between 1200 and 1350°C, is widely employed in electronic ceramics, for example, in condenser end-plates, stand-off insulators, valve holder bases, valve electrode spacers and panel bushes. In the USA, but not in the UK, talc is used as a substitute for feldspar in the manufacture of earthenware bodies, especially for wall tiles and dinnerware.

Roof felting industry

Here, the lubricating properties of talc are used for dusting roofing felts to prevent the layers sticking when rolled, and to increase resistance to fire and weather. Low-grade talcs are employed but, in the UK, they have recently been largely replaced by silica sand.

Rubber industry

Again, the lubricating properties are exploited as a dusting agent to prevent adhesion of the rubber in the moulds and to provide smooth extrusion, but, in recent years, this use has declined considerably. Talc is also used as a filler in hard rubber goods, such as accumulator cases and valves (which may require grinding, hence the term ' rubber-grinder'), in cable manufacture and as an inert filler in some plastic polypropylene compounds. Small quantities of 'tremolitic talc' are employed for these purposes in the UK.

Fertilizer industry

Significant amounts of low-grade talc are used as an anti-caking agent in the manufacture of fertilizers.

Refractory materials

Low-grade talc is used as a refractory filler for moulds and cores in both ferrous and non-ferrous castings.

Paper industry

Due to its whiteness, good retention and ability to improve the gloss, opacity and brightness of paper, talc may be substituted for china clay as a coater and filler of paper. Although this use is very small in the UK, it is increasing rapidly in the USA due to the availability of a 'micronized' talc, in which particle size ranges from 5 μm to less than 0.5 μm (Roe, 1975).

Textile industry

Finely ground french talc is used for 'loading' and bleaching cotton sacks, cordage, string and rope.

Miscellaneous

Talc is used as a dusting agent for glass moulds and as a polishing medium for chocolate, peanuts, rice and chewing gum; until the 1950s, it was employed to dust moulds for the manufacture of lead accumulator plates before coating. It is also used as a carrier for insecticides, in oil adsorption treatment of leather, for dusting of furs and in shoe manufacture to prevent the adherence of layers of leather.

Sources of exposure

Mining is carried out by both open-pit and underground methods. The milling operations involve jaw and roll crushers, screen and pebble mills. Cases of diffuse interstitial pulmonary fibrosis have been recorded in miners and millers of New York State 'talc' (Siegel, Smith and Greenburg, 1943; Greenburg, 1947; Kleinfeld et al., 1964a). Bagging of the milled material is also a potential risk.

Radiographic appearances consistent with silicosis have been reported in Italian talc miners, mainly with medium-size rounded small opacities (ILO category q) (Pettinati et al., 1964), but the quartz content falls progressively during milling and preparation for factory use, in which there appears to be no risk of silicosis (Dettori, Scansetti and Gribaudo, 1964). Some workers milling and bagging high-grade, allegedly quartz-free, talc in the Hamata area of Egypt have, however, been found to have either 'nodular' or conglomerate opacities (El-Ghawabi, El-Samra and Mehasseb, 1970).

Industrial applications

Exposure to fibrous tremolite, and to quartz in industries normally using low-grade talc, probably occurred to some extent in the UK during the Second World War due to substitution by Canadian and American 'talc' and pyrophyllite, and stocks may have continued for some years after the war. Recent analysis of imported bulk talc samples in powder and rock form, by means of X-ray diffraction, thermal gravimetric and differential thermal analysis, and electron microprobe analysis, has shown that the major contaminating minerals are chlorite, carbonates and quartz, with tremolite in only a minority, although in one sample tremolite was the major mineral phase, apparently in fibrous form (Pooley and Rowlands, 1977).

Exposure has occurred (1) in the roof felting and shingle industry, where talc is distributed liberally on the felt surfaces prior to rolling to prevent adhesion, and may be used as a filler in asphalt coating; (2) in the rubber industry, where the powder is blown onto the tacky rubber surface (for example, during extrusion of tubes and sheets) or dusted onto rubber goods before storage; (3) in the mouldings of accumulator plates; (4) in leather finishing; and (5) in preparing the mix for electric ceramics, tiles and refractory kiln bodies. In all these processes, only low-grade talc is required and, therefore, accessory minerals may be present. It should be noted that, before and during the Second World War, women worked in the rubber trade, especially in tyre extrusion, and were probably exposed to considerable quantities of mixed dust.

Talc heated at temperatures greater than 1000°C (as is required in the manufacture of some ceramics) yields *clinoenstatite* (a prismatic magnesium silicate) and cristobalite, which is strongly fibrogenic (see Appendix I and Chapter 12). However, in this form, it gives rise to little dust. Exposure to tremolite and anthophyllite, probably mostly in non-fibrous form, may occur in the manufacture of some types of paints.

Talc employed in the manufacture of cosmetic, toilet and pharmaceutical talcum powder is normally of high purity. However, X-ray diffraction analysis of 21 powders obtained through retail channels in the USA showed that few consisted of pure talc. Quartz, ranging from 2 to 5 per cent, was found in eight, and in a single sample was 35 per cent. Detectable amounts of 'fibrous' tremolite and anthophyllite were reported to be present in ten, and chrysotile in two; other mineral phases identified were platy serpentine, chlorite, pyrophyllite, mica and carbonate minerals (Rohl et al., 1976). It should, however, be pointed out that overlap of diffraction peaks of chlorite – commonly present in talc – and chrysotile make identification of the latter difficult or impossible unless other analytical methods are used (see Appendix V).

Strict specifications to ensure high purity of cosmetic talc have recently been laid down by the Toilet Preparations Federation in the UK, and the Cosmetic Toiletry and Fragrance Association in the

USA, and methods of characterizing talc for this purpose have been described (Hamer, Rolle and Schelz, 1976).

Millman (1947) recorded the case of a man, with small discrete radiographic opacities interpreted as indicative of pneumoconiosis (although this was not proven), who had spent years in a cosmetic factory weighing, mixing and sifting talc containing less than 0.5 per cent crystalline silica. In the USA, apart from the cosmetic industry, much of the industrial 'talc' used has probably been fibrous.

Because talc is expensive, substitutes for filler and low-grade dusting applications are used in a variety of processes, and have been for some years. In the UK, especially during and after the Second World War, one of the most important of these was powdered slate, which contains significant quantities of quartz, and a china clay byproduct, which contains small amounts of quartz and mica, has been employed in the roof felting industry. Such substitutes have often been loosely referred to by the workers in the UK as 'french chalk'. But, apart from substitution, ground flint and silica sands have been used as surfacing materials for some roof felts, and asbestos has been exploited as an asphalt filler to produce a fire- and weather-resistant material. These points may need to be borne in mind when evaluating a past occupational risk.

Epidemiology

There have been very few controlled epidemiological studies of the incidence and prevalence of pneumoconiosis in workers exposed to industrial talc, although, since 1896, many cases of disease resembling either silicosis or asbestosis have been reported (Hildick-Smith, 1976).

In 1970, a study of 39 men mining and milling talc containing fibrous tremolite and anthophyllite for a mean period of 16.2 years (ranging from 11 to 22 years) in New York State discovered only one man (2.6 per cent) with radiographic changes consistent with pneumoconiosis, whereas among 35 men with a similar mean period of exposure at a neighbouring talc mining and milling plant (presumably similar mineralogically) examined in 1964, 12 (34 per cent) had radiographic evidence of pneumoconiosis. The average dust count in 1970 at the first plant (in which dust controls were installed at the start of operations in 1948) was 18 million particles per cubic foot (18 m.p.p.c.f.) of talc with an average of 43 fibres/ml longer than 5 μm; in the second plant, the average count carried out in 1969 was 23 m.p.p.c.f., with an average of 159 fibres/ml longer than 5 μm. Hence, although dust control reduced the incidence of pneumoconiosis in the first plant, the fibre count was still excessively high. It was thus concluded that fibrous tremolite and anthophyllite

are less fibrogenic than other asbestos types at comparable dust exposures (Kleinfeld, Messite and Langer, 1973).

In a group of 70 mine employees producing cosmetic grade talc (free of amphiboles and quartz), compared with a matched control group of agricultural workers, there was no evidence of pneumoconiosis, and ventilatory function tests in the two were similar; however, an increase of phlegm production was noted in those talc miners who smoked (Hildick-Smith, 1977). A later study of New York State talc miners and millers showed that respiratory symptoms were only slightly more prevalent than in a control population of 'potash miners', although ventilatory function was significantly decreased, and the presence of 'pleural thickening' and calcification was greater than in the controls (Gamble, Fellner and Dimeo, 1979).

In 299 talc miners from Montana, North Carolina and Texas, there was no association between exposure and reduced lung function. Two were found to have ILO category 1 rounded small opacities (Gamble, Greife and Hancock, 1982).

A group of 116 Vermont talc workers included 12 with small opacities of category 1/0 or greater. Follow-up 1 year later on 103 workers showed apparent accelerated loss of ventilatory function, although this did not correlate with exposure (Wegman et al., 1982). Mortality statistics of talc miners and millers in New York State showed that pulmonary heart disease was a significant complication of pneumoconiosis in the early 1960s, but this was reduced by half in the later period 1965 to 1969; the number of deaths was, in fact, very small – 9 compared with 4 – but over the period 1940 to 1969 it was recorded as responsible for 29 of a total of 108 deaths. The overall proportional mortality from carcinoma of the lung for this period (1940 to 1969) was approximately four times that expected, and was more predominant in the age group at 60 to 79 years than in that at 40 to 59 years; however, in the years 1965 to 1969 it was approximately the same as the generally expected rate. However, data of smoking habits were not available, and expected mortality was calculated from all deaths among white males in the USA in 1955 (Kleinfeld, Messite and Zaki, 1974) (see 'Complications' later).

In Italy, Rubino et al. (1976, 1979) compared the causes of death among men who had worked for more than 1 year between 1920 and 1950 mining and milling Piedmont talc (which, in its natural state, is pure and is used in the cosmetic and pharmaceutical industries), with mortality among agricultural workers with similar social and economic conditions in a neighbouring area, and also with expectation of death in the Italian male population. The miners were exposed to dust containing about 5 per cent crystalline silica, whereas the millers were exposed to a content of about 0.5 per cent, and to a lower

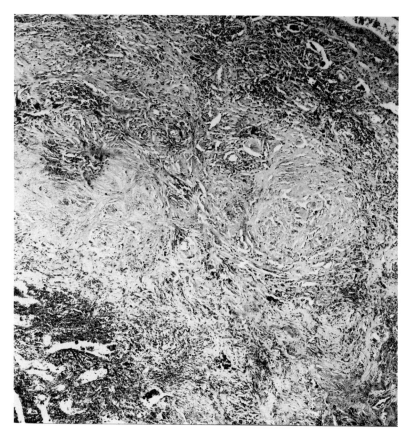

Figure 16.2 Ill-defined nodular lesions in a rubber worker exposed for many years to 'talc' dust. The fibrosis is relatively acellular and shows only a weak concentric pattern of typical silicotic nodules. Magnification × 55; H & E stain

total dust concentration. An excess mortality due to silicosis and silicotuberculosis occurred in the miners, but there was no increase in mortality from lung cancer in either the miners or the millers. A cohort mortality study of 655 white male New York talc miners and millers showed no significant elevation of death rates from all causes, respiratory cancers or non-malignant respiratory disease (Stille and Tabershaw, 1982). Elevated rates were found in the subset with other occupations prior to starting talc work.

The mortality experience of silica- and talc-exposed workers making ceramic plumbing fixtures ('sanitary porcelain') was examined in a cohort of 2055 men in three US plants (Thomas and Stewart, 1987). 'Montana steatite talc', presumed to contain no asbestiform fibres, was used to dust moulds in the cast shop, and excess mortality from lung cancer was associated with the casting process, which also involved exposures to crystalline silica. More than a third of the lung cancer deaths in those with 'non-fibrous talc exposure' occurred within 5 to 14 years from first exposure, which

raises the question of latency. There are other findings that need explanation: a deficiency of tuberculosis deaths despite appreciable silica exposure and deaths from pneumoconiosis (that is, silicosis) in the whole cohort; a fall in non-malignant respiratory disease rates with increasing duration and time from first exposure to 'non-fibrous talc', whereas these death rates rose with longer duration and time from first exposure to silica. The absence of smoking data detracts from this study, as does the lack of dust measurements and analyses. The purported association cannot be considered adequately established.

Hence, epidemiological studies, in general, indicate that prolonged industrial exposure to cosmetic grade talc is not associated with the development of pneumoconiosis or cancer of the lung, although exposure to industrial grade talc (depending upon its composition) may result in silicosis, 'mixed dust fibrosis' (see Chapter 12) and diffuse interstitial pulmonary fibrosis. The question of lung cancer in talc workers exposed to fibrous tremolite and anthophyllite is considered in Chapter 14.

Pathology

Macroscopic appearances

Fibrous adhesions of the pleural surfaces are often present, and in some cases may be dense, and hyaline and calcified plaques have been observed in the diaphragmatic, mediastinal and costal parietal pleura in cases in which there may have been a significant exposure to 'fibrous talc' (Kleinfeld et al., 1963). The cut surfaces of the lung reveal one of two different patterns of fibrosis. One kind shows ill-defined nodules somewhat larger than silicotic nodules (but lacking their compact concentric arrangement) or the appearances of 'mixed dust fibrosis' (see Chapter 12), with the individual elements usually scattered throughout the lungs, although with some partiality for their middle zones. Some confluence of these lesions, which are grey, grey–white or sometimes greenish in colour, may occur (McLaughlin, Rogers and Dunham, 1949); occasionally, there are large coalescent fibrotic masses, some of which may contain ischaemic cavities similar to those seen in the progressive massive fibrosis (PMF) of coal pneumoconiosis (Hunt, 1956) (see Chapter 13). Typical silicotic nodules are also sometimes seen when there has been exposure to industrial talc containing significant quantities of quartz. In the other pattern, the appearances are identical to those of asbestosis: they are predominant in the lower halves of the lungs and are usually accompanied by some diffuse thickening of the pulmonary pleura. Both the nodular and diffuse patterns of fibrosis are sometimes present in the same lung.

Patchy, diffuse interstitial fibrosis and large conglomerate areas of fibrosis have been described with intravenous injection of talcs from dissolved tablets (Crouch and Churg, 1983).

Microscopic appearances

The primary reaction to talc mine dust in the human lung consists of an accumulation of macrophages around blood vessels in the vicinity of respiratory bronchioles, with the formation of small, stellate lesions which contain some reticulin fibres, but negligible collagen. Numerous acicular or platy particles which are strongly birefringent under crossed polaroid filters are present in and adjacent to the lesions both within and outside macrophages (Schepers and Durkan, 1955a). Talc particles in the lungs indicate exposure to a talc-containing mineral, but are not necessarily proof of talc-associated disease. If the majority of the particles are greater than 5 μm in diameter, the possibility of intravenous injection of talc-contaminated drugs should be considered (Abraham and Brambilla, 1979).

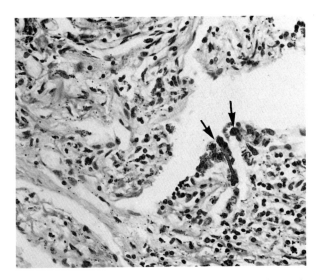

Figure 16.3 Slight DIPF with pronounced cellularity and tremolite or anthophyllite bodies (arrowed). Elsewhere acellular DIPF with occasional small 'honeycomb' cysts was present (not seen in this field). Polarized light revealed numerous, strongly birefringent platy particles. Exposure to mixed 'talc' materials for 30 years. Magnification × 285; H & E stain (See Figure 16.7 for radiographic appearances in this case)

Three distinct types of lesions may subsequently occur:

1. Ill-defined nodular lesions.
2. Diffuse interstitial pulmonary fibrosis.
3. Foreign body granulomas.

Ill-defined nodular lesions These consist of irregular, acellular collagenous tissue (Figure 16.2), which in places may show incomplete whorling identical to the arrangement of immature silicotic nodules, and is associated with a relatively high quartz content in the lungs. Often the lesions have the irregular stellate form of a 'mixed dust fibrosis' and, similarly, they appear to represent a modification of the silicotic reaction by talc (see Chapter 12). Likewise, they vary considerably in size, and may ultimately form large confluent masses. Numerous macrophages containing birefringent particles surround the lesions, and these particles are readily identifiable within the lesions. Sometimes there are necrotic areas of amorphous, finely granular material which colours yellow with van Giesen's stain (Hunt, 1956). Adjacent endarteritis with intimal hyperplasia is common.

Diffuse interstitial pulmonary fibrosis (DIPF) This originates around respiratory bronchioles, and has the same appearance as asbestosis; many alveolar spaces are obliterated in advanced disease, but in some areas there may be pronounced infiltration of

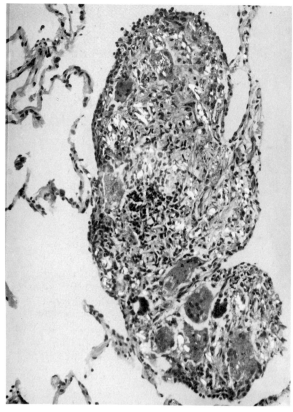

(a)

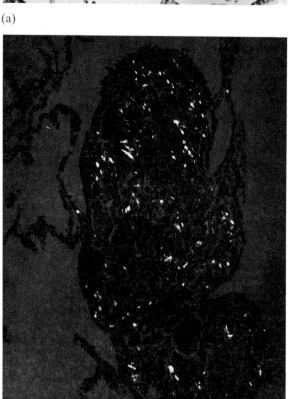

(b)

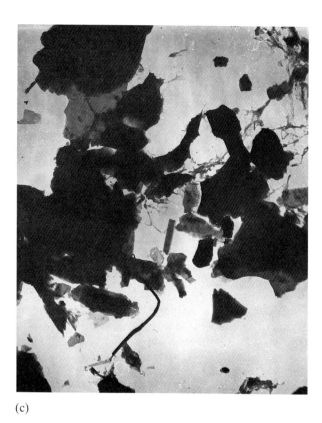

(c)

Figure 16.4 (a) Foreign body granuloma in a worker exposed to talc dust in the rubber industry for 10 years. Note the cellularity and giant cells, and the normality of the adjacent alveolar walls. No asbestos bodies found. Magnification × 240; (b) Polarized light demonstrates the presence of birefringement talc plates. (c) Electron micrograph of the lesion: talc and mica-like plates. Magnification × 3000. (Courtesy of Drs Steel and F.D. Pooley.) (See Figure 16.6 for radiographic appearances)

alveolar walls by macrophages containing birefringent talc particles, and in others they lie free within the walls. Endarteritis may be present. 'Ferruginous bodies', which are identical to asbestos bodies (but have been misleadingly called 'talc bodies'), are readily found in and adjacent to the fibrosis, and are demonstrated by the same techniques (see Chapter 14; they may contain asbestiform tremolite or anthophyllite (Figure 16.3). The bodies are also sometimes seen in small numbers, in some cases with ill-defined nodular lesions; this may imply past exposure to fibrous tremolite or to some other asbestos mineral. Schepers and Durkan (1955a) found that, when the tremolite asbestos content of the lung ash from talc miners was low, such bodies were sparse. Ferruginous bodies formed on talc and other sheet silicate minerals are distinguishable from asbestos bodies under light microscopy, by morphology and core colour (Churg and Green, 1988).

Foreign body granulomas These may also occur in variable degree in association with ill-defined nodular disease and diffuse interstitial pulmonary fibrosis; rarely, they are the only lesions (Figure 16.4). They consist of macrophages, epithelioid cells and foreign body giant cells, all of which contain doubly refractile particles of talc, and asteroid bodies may be observed in some giant cells (Kleinfeld et al., 1963). A reported case of multiple sarcoid-type granulomas in a man who cleaned factory ventilators in which 'talc' dust was deposited seems to have been one of coincidental sarcoidosis (Miller et al., 1971).

Birefringent polygonal particles in and around all these lesions can be identified as platy talc crystals, and the fibrous particles as tremolite or anthophyllite, by combining electron microscopy, differential thermal analysis, thermal gravimetric analysis and X-ray diffraction (Pooley and Rowlands, 1977). Many talc plates lie sideways to the line of vision and, by light microscopy, may give the impression of particles of fibrous habit. Talc crystals visible by the light microscope vary from 0.5 to 5 μm in size, but many may be less than 0.5 μm, and thus can only be identified by electron microscopy; however, it is improbable that 'submicron' particles occur in the lungs in the absence of larger particles.

Analysis of the lungs of talc miners and millers in New York State showed that those with the ill-defined nodular types of lesions contained considerable quantities of talc and small amounts of quartz, but little tremolite or anthophyllite, whereas those with DIPF contained large quantities of fibrous tremolite, and occasionally anthophyllite, in addition to talc (Schepers and Durkan, 1955a). Vallyathan and Craighead (1981) found focal fibrosis in Vermont talc miners and millers with short durations of exposure, and confluent areas of diffuse fibrosis in those with longer exposures. Death was the direct result of lung disease in only one of their seven cases, and three of six with recent radiographs taken *ante mortem* had no radiological evidence of pneumoconiosis (see Chapter 14, 'Tremolite').

The three distinctive lesions of 'talc' pneumoconiosis may occur alone or in various combinations in individuals according to the composition of the dusts to which they were exposed, but none of these lesions possesses any pathognomonic features.

Pathogenesis

Schepers and Durkan (1955a) postulated that talc modifies the reaction of the lungs to quartz. This is supported by their observation in experimental animals that the fibrogenic effect of quartz when combined with talc appears to be reduced, although granulomatous lesions and fibrosis may result – that is, a 'mixed dust fibrosis' (Schepers and Durkan, 1955b).

In general, among the many investigations of 'talc' that have been conducted in animals, rarely has the precise nature of the mineral used been specified, its particle size indicated or the details of administered doses defined. However, two important studies have furnished this information precisely. Wehner et al. (1977) exposed hamsters to the inhalation of high-grade cosmetic talc consisting of 95 per cent (w/w) platy talc and trace quantities of carbonates, chlorite and rutile, but no quartz or amphiboles; the mass mean aerodynamic diameter of the particles was 6 μm. Total doses up to nearly 2000 times those to which babies are exposed during toilet care had no effect on survival or the degree of histopathological change compared with control animals. In short, no fibrosis or increased incidence of neoplasia in the lungs was observed. Wagner et al. (1977) exposed rats to inhalation of high-grade talc consisting of 95 per cent talc, 3 per cent chlorite, 1 per cent carbonate minerals and 0.5 per cent quartz (w/w) in doses which, at their highest level, exceeded those used by Wehner et al. (1977) about threefold. A slight degree of respiratory bronchiolar fibrosis, which was little more than that in the control animals, was found, and there was no excess of tumour. By contrast, talc calcined at 1200°C produces intense collagen fibrosis in animals due, possibly, to the presence of cristobalite (Luchtrath and Schmidt, 1959) (see 'Industrial applications').

Pure talc particles 0.3 to 10 μm in size are apparently capable of penetrating the cell membrane, but not the nuclear membranes of fibroblasts in culture (Henderson et al., 1975). What significance this may have – if any – in human disease remains to be elucidated.

Foreign body granulomas are caused by talc itself. They have been observed in the peritoneum, fallopian tubes and ovaries contaminated by talc from surgical glove dusting powder (German, 1943; Roberts, 1947), and following intraperitoneal injection in animals (Blümel, Piza and Zischka-Konorsa, 1962). They may also occur, although rarely, in human lungs as a result of the inhalation of pure talc (Moskowitz, 1970) (Figure 16.4), and are found after the intravenous injection of talc (Hopkins and Taylor, 1970; Smith, Graf and Silverman, 1978). Birefringent talc crystals may be seen in such lesions through crossed polarizers.

Calcified pleural plaques, which seem to occur only in those 'talc' workers exposed to fibrous 'talc' and asbestine, are probably due to contaminating fibrous amphibole or some extraneous asbestos exposure.

Summary

'Talc' pneumoconiosis is an enigma. Indeed, whether pneumoconiosis attributable to the inhalation of pure talc really occurs is uncertain.

Explanations of the various types of lung disease associated with occupational exposure to the heterogeneous dusts referred to as 'talc' (or french chalk) may be tabulated as follows:

1. Nodular silicosis or 'mixed dust fibrosis' may be due to:
   (a) quartz contamination of talc: for example, in talc mining and in low-grade talcs used in industry;
   (b) quartz or some other form of crystalline silica in additional minerals used in the same industrial processes (see page 540);
   (c) Cristobalite in calcined talc in certain processes.
2. Diffuse interstitial pulmonary fibrosis may be due to:
   (a) association of asbestiform tremolite or anthophyllite with talc – mainly encountered in mining, and occasionally in the use of low-grade industrial talcs, but otherwise rarely;
   (b) use of an asbestos mineral in the same process for which talc is used: for example, as a filler for asphalt in some roofing felts (see page 540).
3. Foreign body granulomas: these appear to be caused by inhaling pure platy talc, but are rare. There is no convincing evidence that subsequent fibrosis occurs. They are common in intravenous exposures, and may then be associated with severe fibrosis.

The finding of birefringent talc plates in the lungs does not establish a causal relationship with associated disease except, perhaps, in the case of foreign body granulomas.

Clinical features

Symptoms

There may be no symptoms for years, but ultimately dyspnoea on effort, often with cough and sputum, is complained of in many cases, and is more commonly associated with advancing diffuse interstitial pulmonary fibrosis-type disease than the ill-defined nodular form. Dyspnoea in the latter is usually found in individuals with radiographic evidence of large confluent masses and related scar emphysema. Symptoms tend to develop after 15 to 20 years of exposure to industrial talc dust. Occasionally, when dust concentrations have been very high, severe dyspnoea has developed within about 2 years with rapidly progressive 'nodular'-type disease (Alivisatos, Pontikakis and Terzis, 1955). The chief symptoms associated with foreign body granulomas alone are usually progressive dyspnoea and unproductive cough, which may be of mild or severe degree.

Physical signs

There are no abnormal physical signs either in the early stages or in many cases of the later stages of predominantly 'nodular' disease. When large confluent masses are present, chest expansion and breath sounds may be locally reduced.

In disease of the diffuse fibrotic type, the range of abnormal physical signs is the same as that observed in asbestosis and some other forms of bilateral basal DIPF (see Chapters 14 and 15).

In the case of lone granulomatous disease, abnormal signs may be absent or there may be widespread fine, late, inspiratory crackles.

Investigations

Lung function

The 'nodular' form of the disease – as in the case of silicosis – causes little if any abnormality in its early stages, but later a restrictive defect develops with decreased compliance, ventilation–perfusion imbalance, impaired gas transfer and hypoxia on effort with oxygen desaturation. In advanced cases, oxygen desaturation may be present at rest (Alivisatos, Pontikakis and Terkis, 1955). In the diffuse fibrotic form, the functional abnormalities are similar to those seen in asbestosis. In general, abnormal values are appreciably greater in people with diffuse fibrosis who have been exposed to 'tremolitic talc' than in those with 'nodular' disease (Kleinfeld et al., 1964a,b), although the correlation between functional abnormalities and the radiographic appearances is poor, and impairment of the same parameters of lung function which mark the earliest stages of asbestosis has been observed before radiographic evidence of this type of 'talc' pneumoconiosis is apparent (Kleinfeld et al., 1965).

In foreign body granulomatous disease, static lung volume and compliance may be reduced and gas transfer (TL) diminished. This may only be evident after exercise, or may be present at rest, with significant reduction in systemic arterial oxygen (PaO$_2$).

Radiographic appearances

As might be anticipated from the different types of lesions associated with 'talc' minerals, the appearances of 'talc pneumoconioses' vary widely. This diversity is emphasized in a recent review (Feigin, 1986), but is evident from any survey of older articles.

Nodular   This consists either of opacities some 3 to 5 mm in diameter, identical to those of silicosis or of appearances similar to 'mixed dust fibrosis' (see Chapter 12). These changes sometimes favour the

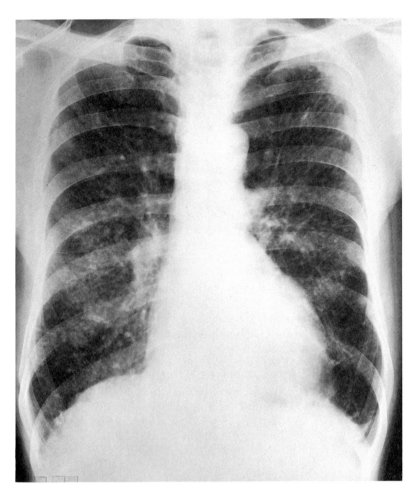

Figure 16.5 Discrete silicotic-type opacities (category q) in a machine operator and cutter in the roof felting industry. Constant use of 'french chalk'. Microscopy: poorly formed silicotic nodules (similar to Figure 16.2) and small areas of DIPF with occasional whole and fragmented asbestos bodies

middle lung fields, but may be distributed throughout all zones (Figure 16.5). There are large opacities similar to those of silicotic conglomerations or coal PMF, which may show evidence of cavity formation (Hunt, 1956; Kipling and Bech, 1960). One such case was associated with rheumatoid arthritis and microscopic features of rheumatoid activity in the lung lesions.

Exceptionally, very small, widely disseminated opacities (about 2 to 3 mm in diameter), similar to the miliary lesions of sarcoidosis or tuberculosis, and due to multiple foreign body granulomas, may be seen (Figure 16.6).

Diffuse interstitial pulmonary fibrosis   The features are the same as those of asbestosis (see Chapter 14, pages 440–441) (Figure 16.7).

Mixed   Both types of appearance may occur in combination. This is probably uncommon, and other causes of diffuse fibrosis should be considered before attributing it to fibrous tremolite or anthophyllite – in particular, exposure to other asbestos minerals.

Pleural   There may evidence of diffuse, bilateral pleural thickening with obliteration of the costophrenic angles. Bilateral calcified plaques are occasionally associated with exposure to talc containing fibrous tremolite or anthophyllite, or to some other unrelated asbestos mineral (Kleinfeld et al., 1963; Yazicioglu et al., 1980).

Diagnosis

This rests upon the past occupational history and a known exposure to 'talc', and on the appearances of the chest radiograph. However, it is often impossible to obtain precise details of the type (or types) of

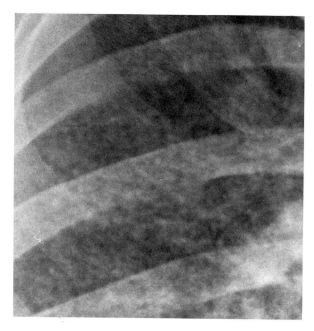

Figure 16.6 Faint miliary opacities due to multiple foreign body granulomas in a rubber worker exposed to talc powder (see Figure 16.4). Similar appearances present throughout both lung fields. Unchanged during 5 years' observation. No clinical stigmata of sarcoidosis. Kveim test negative. Serum calcium and protein normal. Tuberculin test positive; cultures of *Mycobacterium tuberculosis* negative. No evidence of drug addiction

'talc' used in industry 20 or more years ago, although this is sometimes available from the manufacturer's or supplier's records. It should be borne in mind that a worker may speak of having handled 'french chalk' (talc), when in fact the material may have been powdered slate or a china clay byproduct, and that some industries which employed talc may also have used asbestos- or quartz-containing minerals (as, for example, in roofing felt manufacture). It is also to be remembered that women have sometimes been exposed to industrial grade talc in various industries (chiefly rubber) in the past.

The diagnosis can be made in the majority of cases without lung biopsy but, if this proves necessary, sufficient tissue should be taken (preferably by thoracotomy) not only to enable adequate demonstration of the pathology, but for positive mineral identification. The differential diagnosis lies chiefly between quiescent tuberculosis, silicosis or some unrelated type of DIPF and, in the case of the granulomatous type of disease, sarcoidosis.

After death, and in particular in cases encountered for the first time, the diagnosis is made virtually certain by the combination of an accurate history of industrial exposure, the presence of one or more of the pathological entities described, and

of numerous highly birefringent, platy and acicular particles and, in some cases, of ferruginous bodies, especially in those with DIPF. If the ocupational history is uninformative, positive identification of the minerals may be necessary. However, it should be recalled that the identification of talc proper serves only as a marker of exposure.

Prognosis

As a rule, 'talc' pneumoconioses tend to progress very slowly even after exposure to the dust has ceased and, although a variable degree of respiratory disability may occur, life expectancy appears rarely to be significantly shortened. However, in those cases where there is massive confluent fibrosis or extensive DIPF, pulmonary heart disease may ultimately cause death in congestive heart failure. However, as indicated under 'Epidemiology', this is a rare event, although death may result from respiratory failure, especially when there is concurrent lung disease.

Occasionally, when there has been exposure to very high concentrations of 'talc' dust, progression to advanced massive fibrosis with severe respiratory disability occurs within a few years, due almost certainly to a high quartz content (Alivisatos, Pontikakis and Terzis, 1955).

Complications

In general, there is no evidence that 'talc' pneumoconioses predispose to the development of tuberculosis, although they may when there has been exposure to industrial talc with a high quartz content. Colonization by opportunist mycobacteria or aspergilli may occur in advanced disease.

Rheumatoid 'talc' pneumoconiosis does not seem to have been described, but Hunt's (1956) case was an example, as later re-examination of the microsections confirmed, of typical rheumatoid nodules.

The question of cancers in relation to exposures to some talcs has been mentioned under 'Epidemiology', and relevant discussion is to be found in the section on tremolite in Chapter 14. An IARC working group has concluded that there is inadequate evidence for the carcinogenicity of talc to experimental animals or human beings, except for the latter in whom talcs containing (that is, contaminated by) asbestiform fibres, are deemed to be sufficient evidence of carcinogenicity (IARC, 1987).

An association between 'talc' pneumoconiosis and coronary artery disease in talc miners in the USA has been suggested (Nash and Nash, 1978), but requires epidemiological investigation. At present, there is no evidence of a causal relationship.

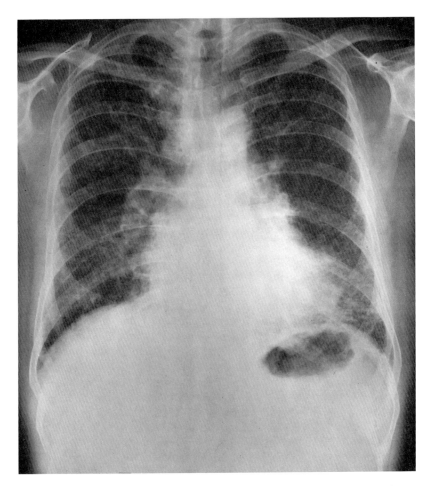

Figure 16.7 Widespread DIPF in a man who weighed, mixed and bagged high-grade talc powders from many sources for 30 years. Post-mortem microscopy indicated the presence of tremolite (see Figure 16.3). No arthropathy or connective tissue disease. Rheumatoid factor negative

Although talc crystals have been found in ovarian carcinomas, there is nothing to indicate that they were the cause of the tumour (Henderson et al., 1971; Henderson, Hamilton and Griffiths, 1979), but investigation of the problem continues.

Treatment

In general, no treatment is effective apart from that required for concurrent lung disease or, in the case of advanced pneumoconiosis, for congestive heart failure or respiratory failure. However, when the pneumoconiosis consists of foreign body granulomas, a substantial, if not complete, regression appears to be possible with large daily doses (40 to 60 mg) of prednisolone (Moskowitz, 1970; Smith, Graf and Silverman, 1978). Whether or not such improvement is permanent remains to be established, but it indicates that lung biopsy is justifiable in individuals whose chest radiographs suggest the granulomatous type of disease. Steroids may be used empirically in respiratory failure associated with recent intravenous exposure, and spontaneous radiographic and clinical improvement has even been noted in a few such cases.

Prevention

Dust suppression measures have been applied to the mining, crushing and milling of talc for some years past. Finely milled talc has a particle size which may range from 0.5 to 25 μm. Exhaust ventilation and enclosure of dusty processes have been introduced into most large industries, but some small factories or workplaces may still be dusty. In circumstances where efficient dust suppression cannot be applied, respirators are required. Good housekeeping is essential to prevent dust accumulation, and monitoring of air-borne dust in the worker's breathing zone is desirable.

A detailed record of the type and source of talc, and of other relevant non-talc minerals used in an industrial setting, should be kept.

Threshold limit values recommended by the American Conference of Governmental Industrial Hygienists (1988) take into account the different biological effects of the non-fibrous and fibrous forms of 'talc', that is, talc proper, tremolite asbestos and anthophyllite.

Pneumoconiosis associated with other silicates

Kaolin (china clay)

Description of disease

The disease manifests as mainly nodular or massive fibrosis of the lungs associated with past exposure to kaolin dust, which is apparently free of accessory quartz or contains small amounts.

Nature and origin of kaolin

China clay, or kaolin as it is internationally known, consists predominantly of the mineral *kaolinite*, which is a hydrated aluminosilicate (approximate composition $Al_2O_3 \cdot 2SiO_2 \cdot 2H_2O$) with a platy, pseudo-hexagonal, non-fibrous morphology under the electron microscope (Beutelspacher and van der Marel, 1968).

Kaolinite is formed by the hydrothermal alteration of aluminosilicates such as feldspars in granites (as in Cornish china clay), by residual weathering of granites, and by erosion of kaolinized granite and its subsequent deposition (as in the large sedimentary kaolin deposits in some of the eastern states of the USA). Hence, these clays may contain a wide variety of mineral impurities in their natural state. Cornish china clay consists of 10 to 40 per cent kaolinite, the residue being mainly quartz, mica and feldspar; Georgia South Carolina kaolin contains 85 to 95 per cent kaolinite, the remainder being largely quartz and a variety of other silicates.

Although commercial kaolins contain very little quartz, the raw material from which they are produced may contain appreciable amounts. For example, in Cornwall, 3.7 tonnes of coarse, mainly quartz, sand are produced for each tonne of china clay. Consequently, 'raw' kaolin is always processed in some way to improve its properties for the intended use.

Cornish kaolin is obtained by means of directing a high-pressure jet of water onto the walls of the open pit, and subjecting the resultant slurry to differential sedimentation in water, so that impurities such as grit, sand and mica are removed while the kaolin remains suspended. This differential settling is enhanced by hydrocyclones and centrifuges. The water is largely removed by the use of filter presses, and the resultant filtrate ('filter cake') transferred to drying kilns. Moisture content is thus reduced to about 10 per cent, and the clay residue is either shovelled or conveyed on a moving belt to storage hoppers. Spray drying of high-grade clays is increasingly being used. It is then either bagged mechanically (but, until recent years, this was done by hand shovel) or bulk-loaded into trucks for transportation. Increasingly, kaolin is transported in slurry form. Some quartz may remain in the lower-grade clays.

In the USA, the clay is obtained in moist lumps by opencast mining and, following dispersion in water, is piped as a slurry through degritting and segregating units. Beneficiation is done by dry or wet methods. Lower quality kaolin is produced by the dry method, which includes air flotation to remove grit. The wet method, which produces grades of kaolin with uniform properties, has been more extensively and highly developed in recent years. Here, the clay is passed as a slurry through various refining processes to apron, drum, rotary or spray driers and then, in the dried state, to pulverizers.

There is an increasing demand for calcined kaolins with strong open aggregates and improved brightness and hardness. By controlling the nature and composition of the feedstock and the basic firing schedule (maximum temperature, its duration and rate of increase above 400°C), a range of materials with different properties and uses is produced. Most kaolin is calcined at temperatures below those at which mullite is formed (see 'Mullite', later). However, if subjected to high temperatures (around 1500°C), Cornish clay converts to mullite but, due to its high alkali content, forms a glass and not cristobalite (see Appendix I, page 850).

Uses of kaolin

Kaolin has many industrial applications. It is used as a filler to give body to paper pulp, for coating paper to produce a smooth surface, for the manufacture of ceramics, including earthenware, porcelain, bone china, sanitary ware and wall tiles. Residual kaolin is used for these purposes in the UK, and secondary kaolin of high purity in the USA. Kaolin also has important uses: (1) as a filler and extending agent in rubber, paints, inks, plastics and insecticides; (2) in the manufacture of refractory bricks, crucibles, saggars and glass; and (3) a refractory grog is produced by calcining it at high temperatures. It is employed as a mild abrasive in soaps and tooth-pastes, and as a stiffener of textiles. Kaolin of high purity and small particle size is used for medicinal and cosmetic purposes.

Sources of exposure

Exposure has occurred mainly in the china-clay industry. After the clay left the driers, all parts of the process some years ago were dusty; although ventilation and enclosure methods now do much to reduce the dust, brushing clay spilled from convey-ors, cleaning driers, bagging and bulk loading may still be dusty activities (Sheers, 1964).

Other sources of significant exposure have been, and may still be, found in the manufacture of paper, rubber and plastics. In the pottery and fireclay industries, kaolinitic clays, when heated to around 1470°C form cristobalite from silica that is exsolved from mullite formed at lower temperatures, and is fully crystallized; thus, cristobalite-containing dust may be produced. Exposure may also occur to dusts of other minerals, such as flint, feldspar, graphite and quartzite sand.

It is of interest that silicosis due to quartz and cristobalite associated with kaolin has been reported in the Missouri firebrick industry. The cristobalite probably originated from pulverization for re-use of previously fired bricks (Lesser, Zia and Kilburn, 1978) (see Chapter 12, 'Refractory ceramics').

Prevalence

In a radiographic survey of 553 Cornish kaolin-processing workers, evidence of pneumoconiosis was found in 9 per cent (Sheers, 1964) and, among 1130 similar workers in Georgia, in 3.7 per cent (Edenfield, 1960). Of 914 processing workers in Ayyat, United Arab Republic, 6 had pneumoconio-sis – 2 with confluent masses (Warraki and Herant, 1963). Oldham (1983) reported that 22.6 per cent of Cornish china-clay workers had abnormal radio-graphs (ILO category >0/1), with 1.1 per cent having large opacities according to at least one of three readers. The overall prevalence of pneumoconiosis was 9.2 per cent of 459 kaolin workers in Georgia (USA) (Kennedy et al., 1983). Sepulveda et al. (1983) found abnormal radiographs in 8 of 65 US kaolin workers with 5 or more years of exposure.

Duration of exposure to the dust was apparently significant in the Cornish workers studied by Sheers,

in that 23 per cent of those exposed to high dust concentrations in milling, bagging and loading for more than 15 years had pneumoconiosis by contrast with 6 per cent of men similarly exposed for 5 to 15 years. Among all 553 workers, there were 12 (2.2 per cent) with confluent masses, and 30 (5.4 per cent) with ILO category 2 or 3 opacities (Sheers, 1964). In the workers studied by Oldham (1983), average dust levels had a strong effect on radio-graphic prevalence; two jobs were so dusty that the average worker would be expected to reach ILO category 2 by the end of a working lifetime. In a more recent study of this industry, detailed histories of past occupation, not available in earlier reports, revealed that *china stone* milling yielded the highest incidence of pneumoconiosis greater than ILO category 1 – category 2 to 3 in workers over 40 years of age. However, the process was discontinued in the early 1970s and, in men exposed since 1971, this effect has been absent (Ogle, Rundle and Sugar, 1989). As noted in Appendix I (page 861), china stone may contain up to 25 per cent quartz and, thus, its effect in the lungs tends to be progressively fibrogenic after exposure has ceased. Over the same period, exposure to kaolin dust of high purity in the 'attritor' mills, of all occupations in the industry, has had the greatest effect on radiographic category, but this has barely reached category 1. Since 1971, therefore, the average worker in any part of the industry is unlikely to develop category 1 pneumo-coniosis during a full working life (Ogle, Rundle and Sugar, 1989).

In the survey of Kennedy et al. (1983), duration of exposure greater than 15 years, and age greater than 55 years, were the significant correlates with radiographic abnormality.

Pathology

Macroscopic appearances

The pulmonary pleura of lungs containing massive lesions is usually thickened.

Lesions that simulate immature silicotic nodules have been found in some cases (Lynch and McIver, 1954; Hale et al., 1956), but as a rule there are dust macules similar to those of coal pneumoconiosis, although of a greyish hue. Massive confluent lesions, which favour the upper parts of lungs, are well circumscribed, grey to blue–grey in colour and, although firm to the touch, are not as hard as conglomerate silicotic masses.

Microscopic appearances

Numerous dust-laden macrophages and extracellu-lar dust particles are present around bronchiolar

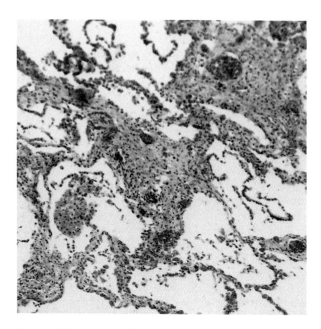

Figure 16.8 Section of lung from a china-clay worker showing nodular lesions consisting of many macrophages and other cells, and some collagenous fibrosis. Limited fibrosis in some alveolar walls. Magnification × 40; H & E stain. (Courtesy of Dr J.C. Wagner)

arteries, and fill adjacent alveolar spaces. Proliferation of reticulin fibres supports both cells and dust particles.

Nodules and massive confluent lesions consist of randomly distributed collagenous fibres, some of which are hyalinized, and large quantities of dust in similar fashion to the PMF of coal and carbon pneumoconiosis; they are infiltrated and surrounded by innumerable dust-laden macrophages. Evidence of tuberculosis does not seem to have been found (Hale et al., 1956; Edenfield, 1960), but obliterative endarteritis is prominent in the vicinity of the lesions, and is responsible for the necrosis that is sometimes observed in them. Lapenas et al. (1984) found confluent lesions composed mainly of kaolinite aggregates, traversed by randomly oriented and relatively narrow fibrous bands, in the lungs of five kaolin workers in Georgia. Macules and large fibrotic nodules were found, but collagen was not abundant and was not of the whorled appearance of silicotic nodules.

Lynch and McIver (1954) noted conspicuous fibrosis of alveolar walls in one of their cases, a photomicrograph of which is consistent with DIPF. A slight degree of DIPF with much cellular infiltration, including dust-containing macrophages, has also been observed in a few cases of Cornish china-clay workers, both in the presence and absence of nodular or massive fibrotic lesions (K.F.W. Hinson, 1972, personal communication; J.C. Wagner, 1972, personal communication) (Figure 16.8).

Analysis of lung dust in a Cornish case revealed a large amount of kaolin and about 1 per cent quartz; in a case from Georgia with confluent masses, the lungs contained some 98 per cent kaolin and no trace of quartz. The size of kaolin particles in the Cornish case ranged from 1.0 to 2.0 μm, and in the case from Georgia from 0.5 to 1 μm (Hale et al., 1956). The lungs from the five Georgia cases of Lapenas et al. (1984) contained no silica by analytical scanning electron microscopy (SEM) or X-ray diffractometry.

Lung tissue samples from 42 autopsy cases of Cornish china-clay and china-stone workers were subjected to mineralogical and pathological analyses by Wagner et al. (1986). A high content of kaolinite was associated with DIPF, whereas high silica content was associated with nodular fibrosis.

Kaolinite is weakly birefringent.

Pathogenesis

The question is whether kaolin is wholly or partly responsible for these lesions, or whether other causative factors are involved.

Although it has been claimed that some quartz always accompanies particles of kaolin (Policard and Collet, 1954), only trace to undetectable amounts, as just noted, have been reported in lungs containing large quantities of kaolin; however, there are not many reports of sensitive lung analysis. This is analogous to the situation in carbon and coal pneumoconiosis. The high concentrations of dust experienced by some workers, and the predominantly small size and low density of kaolin particles, favour the deposition of dust in the lungs. Incidentally, it should be remembered that some cristobalite, and also β-quartz, is formed when kaolinite is heated to temperatures in excess of 950°C (see page 251).

Tuberculous infection has been suggested as the factor which, in combination with kaolin dust, determines the development of these lesions (Edenfield, 1960). Although this has not been evident in human disease, fibrotic lesions have been produced in the lungs of experimental animals by a combination of kaolin and chromogenic opportunist mycobacteria (Byers and King, 1959) or *Mycobacterium tuberculosis* (var. *muris*) (Byers, King and Harrison, 1960).

Most experimental observations have shown that kaolinite alone does not cause collagenous fibrosis in the lungs of rats or guinea-pigs (Kettle, 1934; King, Harrison and Nagelschmidt, 1948; Attygalle et al., 1954; Schmidt and Luchtrath, 1958; Goldstein and Rendall, 1970), although a mild degree was reported in rats by Martin, Daniel and Le Bouffant (1977); however, kaolinite does provoke a diffuse accumulation of cells – including giant cells – in the alveolar walls and spaces and there is some aggregation of cells with slight proliferation of supporting reticulin fibres, but no nodulation. By contrast, combinations of kaolinite and quartz give rise to pronounced collagen fibrosis (Schmidt and Luchtrath, 1958).

Kaolin particles actively adsorb antigens, and are known to be a good adjuvant to immune reactions. Thus, it has been proposed that antigen attached to retained dust particles might localize an antigen–antibody reaction (Vigliani and Pernis, 1958). There is, however, no evidence that this occurs in human beings, although analysis of the protein composition of the hyaline tissue of massive fibrosis in a Cornish china-clay worker showed it to be rich in globulins (73 per cent) and relatively low in collagen content (27 per cent) (Vigliani and Pernis, 1958).

After phagocytosis by human and guinea-pig alveolar macrophages in vitro, kaolinite particles are apparently capable of causing the release of lysosomal and cytoplasmic marker enzymes (Davis, Mortara and Green, 1975), but are only significantly cytotoxic when not coated with serum protein as they are in vivo (Low, 1978).

Morgan (1983) concluded that the circumstantial evidence strongly favours kaolinite as a sufficient cause of kaolin pneumoconiosis, without it necessarily being the only factor in individual cases, and with reservations about the importance of its effects on lung function.

Summary

The pathogenesis of kaolin pneumoconiosis is far from clear. It may be due – if kaolinite alone is responsible – to the effect of a large dust load in the lungs, as has been thought to be the case in pure carbon pneumoconiosis (see Chapter 13), but it is possible that quartz, tuberculous infection or, occasionally, cristobalite, plays a significant role (at least in some cases); immunological factors may also be involved, although this remains speculative. The cytotoxic and fibrogenic potential of kaolinite alone, however, appears to be extremely low.

Clinical features

Symptoms

There are no symptoms associated with discrete lesions, but breathlessness on effort, cough and sputum may be present when there are confluent masses, and in some of these cases disability is severe (Edenfield, 1960). There is no conclusive evidence that disability was caused by pneumoconiosis attributed to kaolin in the English cases reported by Sheers (1964).

Physical signs

The same conditions apply as in the case of coal and carbon pneumoconiosis (see Chapter 13).

Investigations

Lung function

Kaolin pneumoconiosis in 5 of 65 Georgia workers was associated with lower FEV_1 and FVC, as were years of work in the processing area (where average dust level in 1981 was 1.74 mg/m^3) (Altekruse et al., 1984). The ratio FEV_1/FVC remained unchanged, indicating a restrictive tendency, but the mean values for each test were normal in the entire group. In the large cohort studied by Oldham (1983), pneumoconiosis was associated with significant reduction of vital capacity, although duration of exposure was not a significant determinant after allowing for radiographic status. Kennedy et al. (1983) found significant reduction of ventilatory function only in cases with large opacities, and stated that 'Clinical impairment of pulmonary function does not occur except in advanced cases, and appears to be mild even in these'. Data from the same study were later re-examined (Baser et al., 1989), and a decrement in FVC was found in one of the two plants – that with the higher adjusted odds ratio for pneumoconiosis. The 65 kaolin workers studied by Sepulveda et al. (1983) were reported to have significantly lower FEV_1 and FVC values than did a comparison group.

Radiographic appearances

These are similar to the range of abnormal opacities seen in coal pneumoconiosis. Some cases with confluent masses have signs of bullous emphysema (Hale et al., 1956). Predominance of irregular small opacities was found on radiographs *ante mortem* in the cases with high lung kaolinite burdens (see 'Pathology' above) in Cornish workers (Wagner et al., 1986).

Prognosis

In the absence of masses, the prognosis for health and lifespan appears to be normal but, when masses are present, slowly increasing respiratory disability occurs; pulmonary heart disease may develop and ultimately cause death.

Treatment

No treatment, other than for concurrent lung disease, is effective.

Prevention

In the kaolin industry, wet methods, exhaust ventilation, enclosure of some sections, and vacuum cleaning of the factory floor and other surfaces where dust accumulates are standard practice in the UK, and similar measures apply in the USA. Control of dust in the bagging areas, however, is difficult.

Ball clays and stoneware clays

Ball clays consist essentially of kaolinite and, like china clay, they originated by natural decomposition of feldspathic rocks, but were subsequently transported from their site of origin by rivers. During this journey, the ratio of quartz to kaolin increased on account of loss of clay, so that a larger quantity of quartz is present than in primary china clay.

These clays are mined by opencast and underground methods in Dorset and Devon in the UK, and in Tennessee and Kentucky in the USA. The 'crystalline silica' content of Devon and Dorset ball clays has been reported to range from 5 to 30 per cent (Thomas, 1952; Patterson and Murray, 1975). Their main use is for china- or whiteware, sanitary pottery ware and electrical porcelain, refractory products and porcelain enamel slips.

Pneumoconiosis has occurred among workers milling and preparing these clays (Thomas, 1952) and, due to their fairly high quartz content, it is of silicotic type, although poorly formed immature silicotic nodules may be present. The clinical features and radiographic appearances are similar to those of silicosis.

Mullite

This aluminium silicate ($3Al_2O_3 \cdot 2SiO_2$) in its natural form is, as indicated in Appendix I, an exceedingly rare mineral. However, its synthetic counterpart has important applications, chiefly as a refractory material. It is manufactured by fusion, or sintering, of carefully controlled qualities and quantities of raw materials such as kaolin, alumina and silica in an electric arc furnace, or by calcining sillimanite, kyanite or andalusite at temperatures of 1700°C or more. Any excess silica present changes to cristobalite or to a glassy phase. Impurities which are apt to occur in the glass phase can be detrimental to the refractoriness of the material. Thus, the production of synthetic mullite requires a chemical recipe that contains about 72 per cent Al_2O_3 and is as close as possible to the theoretical formula ($3Al_2O_3 \cdot 2SiO_2$)

of pure crystalline mullite (Power, 1985) (see Appendix I, Figure A.2).

Fused mullite refractories are produced from grains of selected size bound together by high alumina bonding agents and fired to shape. They are highly resistant to high temperatures, to spalling, cracking and flame damage, and to corrosive chemicals (Power, 1985).

Mullite occurs as weakly birefringent crystals of long prismatic habit in the form of laths or needles (upon which ferruginous bodies may form in the lungs), but not in fibrous form, as has been suggested in some medical reports. Single particles from pulverized fuel ash ranged from 1.2 to 1.9 μm in length and from 0.09 to 0.31 μm in diameter in one report (Golden et al., 1982), and from 1.0 to 4.9 μm (94 per cent) in length with an average aspect ratio of 19 : 1 in another (Churg, 1983), well within the phagocytic capability of alveolar macrophages; but those formed by prolonged cooling of synthetic mullite may be considerably larger.

In a study of workers from a London asbestos factory, Wagner et al. (1988) found no evident correlation between asbestosis, pulmonary carcinoma complicating asbestosis, or malignant mesothelioma and the presence of mullite in the lungs. A report from Australia (Musk et al., 1980), however, attributed scattered pulmonary granulomas and variable fibrosis to mullite in a worker exposed to dust from a reclaimed and dried residue of alunite [$KAl_3(SO_4)_2(OH)_6$] used for cat litter. The authors did not explain how a crystalline aluminium silicate (mullite) was the chief constituent of a residue of potassium aluminium sulphate. The alunite, worked between 1944 and 1949 to produce potassium sulphate (K_2SO_4), is the main ingredient (60 per cent) of a feldspathic sediment derived from granitic rocks of the district, the remainder consisting of 21 per cent quartz and 19 per cent aluminium silicates (Essen, 1926). This was calcined (temperature not known) to yield K_2SO_4. If the temperature was in excess of 1000°C, mullite would have been formed, but it was probably not sufficient to form cristobalite (see Appendix I). Subsequently, Musk et al. (1988) described slight radiographic and physiological changes, consistent with the effects of smoking, in 4 of 32 workers in the industry, but no indication of pneumoconiosis; they also showed that instillation of the mullite dust in the lungs of hamsters produced no adverse effects. Accordingly, they retracted their earlier suggestion of a causal relationship between mullite and pulmonary fibrosis. The pathogenesis of their original case is uncertain; sarcoidosis is a possibility.

Although Seal (1980) and Golden et al. (1982) speculated that mullite might have caused pulmonary fibrosis in three of their cases, this was hardly justifiable because asbestos fibres were present in all.

It can be concluded that mullite does not cause pulmonary fibrosis. Fibrosis of lungs in which it is found may have been caused by quartz, cristobalite (with which it is often associated) or asbestos. The presence of mullite, therefore, should prompt thorough appraisal of the industrial processes and environment to which the worker was exposed.

Uses

Synthetic mullite has a wide and important application in refractory castables, mortars, high alumina bricks, foundry mouldings, and in the construction of kilns, furnaces and hearth burner blocks. It is also employed in electric insulators, ceramic bodies and as a filler in plastics.

Presence in the lungs

Due to its formation during high-temperature combustion of coal as a decomposition product of kaolinite and illite in the non-coal mineral fraction of bituminous coals, mullite is abundant in furnace ash, and this, undoubtedly, accounts for its presence in the lungs of insulation and other workers at coal-fired power stations and boiler houses (see Chapter 13). The use of pulverized fuel ash as a filler in the manufacture of some asbestos cement products may also explain the not infrequent finding of mullite in the lungs of those who have made or used these materials.

Fuller's earth

Very few cases of pneumoconiosis supposedly caused by these clays have been reported, and most of these were incompletely studied.

The geological identities of 'fulling' clays and important differences in their terminology are referred to in Appendix I (page 851). 'Fuller's earth' may refer to fine-grained *calcium montmorillonite clays* or *bentonite* (see 'Bentonite', next), and to *attapulgite* (palygorskite) clays, which are mineralogically unrelated to the montmorillonites, but possess similar adsorptive properties.

Large deposits of calcium montmorillonite occur in the UK at Redhill, Surrey, Woburn in Bedfordshire and near Bath, Somerset (where production ceased in 1979), and in the USA in Arkansas, Mississippi and Illinois. In Georgia and Florida deposits of attapulgite are extensively worked.

Fuller's earth is mined by opencast (tractor-scrapers and dragline excavators) and underground mining methods. It is dried in rotary driers and graded into a granular or fine powder by air flotation or elutriation. Until recently, the vicinity of driers, mills and bagging areas was very dusty.

The quartz content of Redhill fuller's earth is extremely low, except in intercalated sand layers, and is about 0.8 per cent of the milled product, with only a trace amount in elutriated fractions which have a particle size of less than 5 µm (Bramwell, Leech and Dunstall, 1940). By contrast, quartz is more abundant in the Illinois montmorillonite deposits (Grim, 1933) and, although it may be present in mill dust, it is largely removed by the subsequent air flotation processes. However, appreciable amounts of quartz – up to about 20 per cent – may be found in some deposits.

The highly adsorbent property of fuller's earth enables it to remove grease and oily material with great efficiency. It has a wide variety of uses: to clarify mineral, vegetable and animal oils; in refining mineral oils; as a carrier for herbicides and insecticides; as an adsorbent of alkaloids and vitamins; as a binder in foundry sands; as a filtering agent; as a stabilizing agent in emulsion paints; and as a filler in cosmetics, mud packs, toilet and baby powders.

Only three post-mortem studies appear to have been recorded, and these were upon men who had been exposed to Nutfield fuller's earth. The fundamental lesions are round, firm – but not hard – black 'nodules', varying from 2 to 7.5 mm in diameter, with more in the upper than in the lower parts of the lungs (Campbell and Gloyne, 1942; Tonning, 1949; Sakula, 1961); in one case they tended to run into small confluent masses in the upper lobes. Hilar lymph nodes are black.

The lesions are situated mainly around bronchiolovascular bundles, and consist of aggregations of macrophages containing brownish particles, some of which are extracellular; they are enmeshed by a network of reticulin fibres. Foreign body giant cells are absent. There is, therefore, a close resemblance to the lesions of kaolin pneumoconiosis and the non-collagen macules of coal pneumoconiosis. Reticulin proliferation, but little collagenous fibrosis, is present in the nodules, with some extension into contiguous alveolar walls as has been described (Tonning, 1949). Numerous birefringent particles may be seen in the nodules (Sakula, 1961), and are probably montmorillonite, which is moderately birefringent. X-ray and electron diffraction studies in Sakula's (1961) case showed the patterns of montmorillonite, but no evidence of quartz.

In a radiological survey of 49 fuller's earth workers in Illinois, there were 2 workers (apparently occupied mainly in milling and bagging) whose films showed large confluent shadows indistinguishable from those that occur in coal miners and some cases of silicosis. No post-mortem examinations were done (McNally and Trostler, 1941). Discrete opacities were also observed in a small group of fuller's earth workers in Germany, but various proportions of quartzite sand had been added to the clay in the past, and there was also a significant content of naturally occurring quartz (Gärtner, 1955).

It is possible that montmorillonite may cause pneumoconiosis in some cases, but quartz was probably the decisive factor in the Illinois and German cases. Tuberculous infection has not been observed. The problem of pathogenicity remains unsolved, as post-mortem studies have been so few, and recorded animal experiments have been inconclusive and not related to the lungs (McNally and Trostler, 1941; Campbell and Gloyne, 1942). If fuller's earth (calcium montmorillonite) does possess fibrogenic potential, it would seem to be of very low order.

A retrospective cohort mortality study of 2302 attapulgite miners and millers disclosed an excess of lung cancers in white men and a deficit of lung cancers in non-white men (Waxweiler et al., 1988). No smoking data were available, and the lung cancer risks were not generally influenced by intensity or duration of dust exposure, or by time since first exposure. A sample of long-fibred Spanish (Torrejon) attapulgite produced pleural mesotheliomas after intrapleural injection in rats, but short-fibred Spanish attapulgite was not carcinogenic after inhalation or intrapleural injection (Wagner, Griffiths and Munday, 1987a). Short attapulgite fibres (mean length, 0.77 μm) failed to produce tumours after pleural injection (Jaurand et al., 1987). An IARC working group concluded that there was limited evidence for carcinogenicity of attapulgite to animals and insufficient evidence of its carcinogenicity to human beings (IARC, 1987).

In general, fuller's earth pneumoconiosis, which is evidently rare, appears to occur only after long exposure to high concentrations of 'fuller's earth' dust; it is represented by small, discrete, low-density opacities (which occasionally show some tendency to confluence) mainly in the upper halves of the lungs. It runs a benign course, and does not shorten life expectancy. Respiratory disability without radiographic evidence of pneumoconiosis has been reported in some fuller's earth workers, and was apparently due to non-specific chronic airways' obstruction.

Exposure to fuller's earth in industrial processes and from cosmetic preparations is most probably harmless.

Bentonite

Bentonite consists of fine-grained clays containing not less than 85 per cent montmorillonite. The name originates from the occurrence of such clays at Fort Benton in Wyoming in the USA: it is, in fact, sodium montmorillonite with high swelling properties, which has a greater capacity for water adsorption and cation exchange than other plastic clays. Similar clays are found in Italy, Greece, Spain and elsewhere.

The bentonite clays were deposited as air-borne volcanic ash, and later subjected to alteration by sea and ground water. All bentonites contain mineral impurities of varying type and quantity, which include kaolinite, cristobalite and other forms of crystalline silica. The Wyoming clay is associated with sandstone and siliceous shale, and is reported to have a 'crystalline silica' content varying from less than 1 per cent to about 23 per cent (Phibbs, Sundin and Mitchell, 1971).

Mining is carried out by the opencast method, which is not a source of dust hazard, and the clay is then crushed and milled. Crushing and milling is carried out indoors, and is a very dusty process. After crushing, the clay is dried in oil-fired cylindrical driers. The 'crystalline silica' in air-borne and settled mill-dust has been found to consist of 'appreciable amounts of cristobalite' (Phibbs, Sundin and Mitchell, 1971), which was almost certainly formed by high-temperature conversion of quartz during the volcanic period, and not by the heat of the driers, which does not exceed about 800°C. Bentonite from Wyoming (the world's largest producer) is imported into the UK in the crude form, and milled and processed here.

The main uses of bentonite are in oil-well drilling muds and oil refining, as a bonding material for foundry sands, in various adsorbents, in insecticides and fungicides, in ceramics, as a fire retardant, and also as a filtering agent (especially in clarifying wine), in cosmetics and animal feeds, as a slurry to make tunnel and dam foundations impermeable to water, as a suspension agent for drilling fresh water muds, and as a lubricant in sinking piles and caissons.

Bentonite itself is not fibrogenic in the lungs of experimental animals, but causes local accumulation of large cells with foamy cytoplasm, which stain strongly positive with periodic acid–Schiff, and a mild proliferation of reticulin. When mixed with quartz, however, collagen fibrosis occurs, but is not as severe as that produced by quartz alone (Timar, Kendrey and Juhasz, 1966).

Pneumoconiosis reported in bentonite millers developed fairly rapidly, was disabling and, in some cases, fatal (Phibbs, Sundin and Mitchell, 1971). It is undoubtedly due to the crystalline silica content – chiefly cristobalite – of the clay. In short, it is silicosis. Pneumoconiosis does not seem to have been reported in relation to other types of exposure to bentonite, but vigilance would seem to be advisable in some of its uses.

Sepiolite and meerschaum

These are two varieties of hydrous magnesium silicate that are structurally related to the amphiboles. Sepiolite has an earthy, clay-like form and meerschaum ('sea foam') a compact nodular form. Both consist of lath-like particles and short fibres associated with crystalline silica. Particles of sepiolite are more elongated and axially parallel than those of meerschaum (Beutelspacher and van der Marel, 1968) (see Appendix I, 'Palygorskite (attapulgite) and sepiolite').

Sepiolite has many uses similar to bentonite, but it is also used as a suspending agent for cosmetics and paints, as a colour holder in copying papers and for toughening epoxy resins. Meerschaum has a limited use in the manufacture of decorative pipes, cigar and cigarette holders, and ornamental objects.

Neither form of this mineral appears to be associated with the development of a pneumoconiosis. However, it has been suggested that sepiolite in the soil of a tobacco-growing region of south-eastern Bulgaria may be responsible for calcified pleural plaques encountered there (Burilkov and Michailova, 1972) (see page 452). No dust-induced pleural lesions were found in 63 Turkish sepiolite trimmers; although radiographic pulmonary fibrosis was described in 10 of them, there was no relationship to parameters of sepiolite exposure, and exposures to asbestiform tremolite and fibrous zeolites were suspected (Baris, Sahin and Erkan, 1980).

An IARC working group has determined that there is inadequate evidence of the carcinogenicity of sepiolite to animals, and no data to evaluate its carcinogenicity to human subjects (IARC, 1987).

The mica group

This group is referred to in Appendix I (page 846). Its most important members in industry are *muscovite*, *phlogopite* and *vermiculite*.

Unmanufactured mica is classed either as sheet mica or scrap and flake mica.

Muscovite is the best sheet mica. It occurs as large laminated crystals or 'books or leaves' in granitic pegmatite, which is rich in quartz. Its main sources are the Bihar and Madras areas of India, Brazil and West Africa. Phlogopite, a lesser source of sheet mica, is found in pegmatite-rich sedimentary rocks, which also contain quartz. Its largest resources are in Canada and the Malagasy Republic.

Scrap and flake mica were originally the poor quality remainders from the milling and processing of sheet mica, but, due to increased industrial demand, smaller size mica crystals and flake mica have been mined for this purpose from pegmatite, schist and clay deposits since early in this century. Hence, they are likely to contain variable amounts of quartz.

After mica from the mines has been crushed, washed and screened, it has, since the mid-1960s, been reduced to a high degree of purity by the use of acid cationic or alkaline anionic–cationic flotation methods. Previously, small amounts of contaminating minerals were likely to have been present.

Uses

Sheet mica is used for electrical insulators; for vacuum tubes and capacitors in the electronics industry, in the windows of furnaces and as a liner for the gauge glass of high-pressure steam boilers, and as splittings cemented by an organic or inorganic binder into sheets that are hot-pressed and cut, milled or stamped into a variety of shapes for many purposes.

Scrap and flake mica are employed in oil-well drilling, in the manufacture of roofing felt to prevent adhesion and improve weather-proofing, in the protective coatings of cables and welding rods, as a filler in asphalt products, cements and acoustic plastics, and, in very fine mesh, for paints and other decorative materials. *Biotite*, which was previously employed to a minor degree in the crushed state as a filler and coating in the rubber and roof felt industries, is now rarely, if ever, used.

Clinical and pathological considerations

Muscovite

Pneumoconiosis is rarely caused by exposure to dust of the mica group of minerals alone. Certainly, silicosis has occurred in Indian muscovite miners in Bihar, owing to the high quartz content of associated pegmatite rocks (Government of India Ministry of Labour, 1953, 1956), and this remains a potential risk. When crude mica is crushed and milled, quartz is usually present in the dust, and is not separated out until the later stages of refinement. However, remarkably little radiographic evidence of silicosis was found in one survey of muscovite and pegmatite miners in North Carolina (Dressen et al., 1940), although in another survey of 79 men in the same region who milled mica, which was not thought to contain 'crystalline silica', 7 were reported to have evidence of pneumoconiosis (Vestal, Winstead and Joliot, 1943).

Very few workers exposed to mica dust have been reported to have radiographic appearances consistent with a pneumoconiosis and, of these, the abnormalities have usually been of a minor order, and other causes not excluded. A radiographic survey of 61 workers processing muscovite with less than 1 per cent crystalline silica showed no clear evidence of pneumoconiosis (Heimann et al., 1953). Radiographic appearances consistent with diffuse interstitial pulmonary fibrosis were observed in one muscovite grinder in North Carolina (Dressen et al., 1940), and evidence of pleural calcification on chest films has been regarded in some cases as being due to mica (Smith, 1952; Kleinfeld, 1966), but in these the possibility of additional exposure to asbestos minerals (including fibrous tremolite) was not excluded.

Diffuse pigmented fibrosis was found at autopsy in the lungs of a man who had prolonged exposure to dusting powders in the rubber industry; the fibrotic areas contained numerous birefringent crystals (the mica minerals, incidentally, are all strongly birefringent), which on X-ray diffraction proved to be biotite, and 'crystalline silica' was absent (Vorwald, 1960). Due to the variety of mineral dusts to which this man could have been exposed, Vorwald concluded that there was considerable 'uncertainty' that biotite was responsible, and he was unable to eliminate other possible causes.

Pimental and Menezes (1978) reported the case of a woman exposed to muscovite dust for 7 years during grinding and packing operations, who suddenly developed respiratory symptoms for the first time after a 'common cold'. Two years later, fine inspiratory crackles were present in both lungs, and the chest radiograph showed 'bilateral reticulomicronodular shadows and some nodular densities in the left lower lobe'. After 3 years, she died in respiratory failure. Post-mortem examination revealed extensive areas of 'diffuse fibrosis' with honeycombing. Microscopically, alveolar walls were thickened and contained collagen fibres and muscovite particles, and sarcoid-type granulomas were present in the liver. However, the features of this case suggest sarcoidosis rather than a pneumoconiosis.

Davies and Cotton (1983) reported radiographic evidence of nodular pneumoconiosis in two men who ground and packed mica. Post-mortem examination in one case (death was due to ischaemic cardiomyopathy) showed a mixed nodular and diffuse fibrosis, and mineral analysis showed 9 per cent muscovite by dry lung weight, with no other mineral present.

The literature of mica pneumoconiosis was tabulated and interpreted by Skulberg et al. (1985). Of the total 66 cases reported to that date, 26 were regarded as possibly caused by mica alone; only 6 cases were diagnosed by 'clinical examination, radiography, and lung biopsy or autopsy results', and in 1 case the purity of mica exposure was questioned by the reporting authors. After also reviewing the experimental studies, Skulberg et al. concluded:

Present knowledge does not exclude the possibility that pure mica may cause pneumoconiosis in man. Probably there is a causal relationship, but a definite such relationship is difficult to establish.

Due to the fact that the micas are strongly birefringent and, therefore, readily visible by polarized light, they may be wrongly regarded as the cause of coexistent lung disease in individuals with occupational exposures.

The majority of observers have shown that muscovite, biotite and sericite in the lungs of experimental animals produce only local macrophage accumulations with mild reticulin proliferation (King, Gilchrist and Rae, 1947; Tripsa and Rotura, 1966; Goldstein and Rendall, 1970), and the changes are those of a foreign body response to an inert dust, which resolves in about 12 months (Vorwald, 1960). Intratracheal injection of 50 mg muscovite in rats results in alveolar lipoproteinosis after 84 days, and very slight collagen formation after 290 days, but not in acellular collagenized lesions (Kaw and Zaidi, 1973; Martin, Daniel and Le Bouffant, 1977). Hence, the micas evidently do not cause a fibrotic pneumoconiosis in animals. There is also no evidence of macrophage cytotoxicity or collagenous fibrosis in the tracheobronchial lymph nodes of guinea-pigs, followed at intervals for 1 year after intratracheal injection of muscovite, although there is some reticulin accumulation (Shanker et al., 1975).

The available evidence (which has rarely included satisfactory details of past occupational dust exposures and differential diagnosis), therefore, suggests that mica has relatively low fibrogenic potency.

Vermiculite

This is the name given to a family of micaceous magnesium–aluminium silicates derived from hydrothermally altered biotite. The group is often classed with the clay minerals. Vermiculite is flaky, of light weight, and has the property of expanding – or 'exfoliating' – to some 12 times its original size when heated. It is obtained in various parts of the world (especially in the USA) by opencast mining, after which the ore is crushed and transported generally in the unheated (that is, unexpanded) form, which is less bulky than the expanded form. When received by the expanding plant, prepared vermiculite is subjected to a furnace temperature of about 1100°C, cooled, passed over separators to remove any impurities and packed in paper bags.

Expanded vermiculite is a good lightweight thermal insulator, is fireproof and resists decomposition, and has the properties of a mineral sponge.

Its uses in industry include insulation granules for industrial and domestic buildings, as an aggregate for fireproof concrete, refractory bricks and pipe-lagging and, combined with gypsum, for fireproof building plasters; it is also used in soil conditioners, fertilizers and pesticides. Hence, expanded vermiculite is a valuable substitute for the asbestos minerals. In 1984, Lockey et al. reported an unusual prevalence of pleural abnormalities, especially pleurisy with effusion, in fertilizer plant workers handling vermiculite contaminated with fibrous tremolite. McDonald, Sebastien and Armstrong (1986) reported a radiological survey of 244 current and past workers from the Montana mine that was the source of that vermiculite. Pulmonary (9.1 per cent) and pleural (15.9 per cent) abnormalities were found, with a dose–response relationship for lung opacities similar to that of chrysotile miners and millers. Amandus et al. (1987), in a parallel survey of the same working population, found lung and pleural abnormalities in 9.8 and 15.2 per cent, respectively. McDonald et al. (1986) also studied the mortality of 406 men employed in this mine before 1963: mesothelioma was the cause of death in 2.4 per cent (4/165 deaths), and respiratory cancer mortality was significantly elevated (observed/expected = 2.45). In relation to estimated exposures, these rates were higher than those observed in chrysotile mining. In a different cohort drawn from the same mine, Amandus and Wheeler (1987) found significant elevation of lung cancer rates (standardized mortality ratio, SMR = 223), and two mesotheliomas.

McDonald et al. (1988) found no significant elevation of lung cancer mortality and no deaths from mesothelioma in a small cohort of South Carolina workers of a vermiculite mine minimally contaminated with tremolite. Eighty-six current or recent workers included four with lung small opacities and seven with pleural thickening, rates not different from those of non-exposed controls and much lower than in the Montana miners. Hessel and Sluis-Cremer (1989) studied 172 South African workers mining and processing vermiculite that was contaminated by little, if any, tremolite; symptoms were no greater than in controls, lung function values were comparable, and only two vermiculite workers had radiographic small opacities, both in ILO category 1.

The epidemiology thus incriminates tremolite contamination of vermiculite ore as the cause of excess morbidity and mortality in miners, and morbidity in users, of the Montana vermiculite. Effects of tremolite are considered separately in Chapter 14.

Vermiculite does not cause fibrosis of the lungs in animals (Goldstein and Rendall, 1970), nor malignant mesothelioma after intrapleural injection in rats (Hunter and Thompson, 1973).

Some other natural silicates

Olivine

'Olivine' is a generic term for a group of orthosilicate minerals, which consist essentially of magnesium-rich forsterite (Mg_2SiO_4) and iron-rich fayalite (Fe_2SiO_4). They are mined by open-cast and underground methods, and then dry-crushed. Crushed olivine has been widely used as a substitute for quartz since the 1930s. It is employed: for a variety of refractory materials such as firebricks, heat resistant concrete, ceramic bodies for saggars, insulators and sparking plugs; in foundry moulds, paints and parting powders (to replace quartz sands); and in the production of magnesia (MgO). The refractory properties are due mainly to forsterite.

There is, apparently, no record of olivine causing pneumoconiosis in human lungs and, in the rat lung, forsterite causes only a minimal foreign body reaction and no fibrosis (King et al., 1945; Governa, Durio and Comai, 1979). Indeed, it was introduced as a substitute for flint and silica sands to eliminate silicosis in foundries. Forsterite is the chief breakdown product of asbestos when subjected to high temperatures, such as those generated in brake shoes during braking (see Chapter 14).

Anhydrous aluminium silicates

These consist of *andalusite*, *kyanite* and *sillimanite*, which have the same formula ($Al_2O_3 \cdot SiO_2$) but different crystal structures. They occur in different metamorphic rocks, such as gneisses and schists. Sillimanite is found mainly in the form of long, acicular crystals which shatter readily, and as aggregates of wispy fibres with interlaced and interlocked quartz, and other minerals that are not removed by beneficiation. Kyanite occurs as long, thin, blade-like crystals (Bennett and Castle, 1975).

These minerals are invaluable for the manufacture of high-grade refractories, which are chemically inert under acidic or basic conditions and capable of withstanding higher temperatures than fireclay bodies. Hence, they are used in the manufacture of porcelains for laboratory ware, sparking plugs and thermocouple tubing, and in special alumina–silica refractory bricks and mortars when high resistance to wear and temperature is required.

The raw ores are calcined at about 1550°C for 24 hours, dry-crushed and then milled with water in cylindrical mills. The resulting slip is mixed with varying amounts of clay for processing whatever type of ware is required. Formed brick and tiles are dried and again fired at different temperatures. The calcination and crushing processes are potentially dusty. Calcination at this temperature converts these minerals to mullite (see earlier), cristobalite and glass. However, the quantity of cristobalite formed depends upon the amount of alkaline or other fluxes (naturally associated with the minerals or added) present, because these favour its conversion to the glassy phase. If there is much glass formation, little or no cristobalite may be produced. Thus, according to the circumstances, there may be variable amounts of cristobalite in 'respirable' dust. Some corundum may also be formed (see Chapter 18).

There appear to be no authentic cases of pneumoconiosis caused by these silicates on record. The minimal abnormality of chest radiographs reported by Middleton (1936) in 4 out of 15 sillimanite workers whom he examined is of doubtful significance, but small, irregular fibrotic nodules were described by Gärtner and van Marwyck (1947) in the lungs of a sillimanite furnace worker and attributed to mullite. In fact cristobalite is likely to have been responsible (see Appendix I).

Goldstein and Rendall (1970) showed that, in animals, uncalcined sillimanite causes localized accumulations of cells, with some loose reticulin formation but no collagen, although slight fibrosis was described by Jötten and Eickhoff (1944). There were no lesions of a silicotic type.

Summary

Exposure to the dust of these clay minerals when calcined may, under certain conditions, give rise to a silicosis hazard from cristobalite, so that regular medical surveillance and analysis of air-borne dust in the manufacture of alumina refractories is desirable. In their uncalcined form, however, there is no convincing evidence that andalusite, kyanite or sillimanite cause pneumoconiosis.

Wollastonite

This is a monocalcium silicate ($CaSiO_3$) which is found in contact-metamorphic deposits of limestones and in igneous rocks. Hence, it is sometimes associated with quartz. It occurs in acicular and fibrous forms, the aspect ratio of the 'fibres' usually being about 7:1 or 8:1 (Elevatorski, 1975). It is moderately birefringent. Its chief source is the USA, but it is also mined in Mexico, Finland and Kenya.

Wollastonite has only been exploited for industrial use since 1952. It is most extensively employed in the ceramic industry to improve the mechanical properties of the ware, and as an important substitute for sand and flint in the prevention of silicosis (see page 292). It is also widely used in paints to increase weather resistance and reduce oil absorption. As it possesses a high resistance to heat, it is assuming importance as a substitute for asbestos minerals in insulation, mainly as mineral wool made into tiles, boards and blankets.

Owing to the fibrous or semi-fibrous habit of this mineral, it is important to know if it is likely to offer any hazard to health, even though its molecular structure is different from the asbestos minerals. Shasby et al. (1979) examined 104 mine and mill workers in the USA by respiratory questionnaire, physical examination, lung function tests and chest radiographs. They found no association between respiratory symptoms and increasing exposure; no significant abnormalities of ventilatory capacity, TLC or gas transfer function; and no radiographic evidence of pleural plaques or of irregular opacities suggestive of DIPF. A follow-up (1976 to 1982) study of this mine and mill showed no worsening of radiographs; a greater longitudinal decline in peak flow was found in workers with higher dust exposure (Hanke et al., 1984). Huuskonen et al. (1983) thought that 'slight lung fibrosis' was seen on the radiographs of 14 out of 46 workers in a Finnish limestone–wollastonite quarry, and that lung function tests indicated a possibility of small airways' disease. In experimental animals, wollastonite has activated complement but failed to decrease macrophage viability (Warheit, Hill and Brody, 1984), and has produced slight fibrogenic effects in comparison to asbestos (Wozniak et al., 1986).

Wollastonite seems to have little potential for causing lung fibrosis.

Zeolites

These are a family of hydrated aluminium silicates with sodium and calcium as their principal bases. They occur in vesicular cavities and fissures in basic lavas (or tuffs), and may be associated with small quantities of other silicates and quartz. However, for commercial purposes, they are obtained by quarrying sedimentary volcanic deposits originally formed in fresh water and marine environments. Of the many different species (more than 35) the most important commercially are chabazite, erionite (which has a needle-like form), faujasite and mordenite, which consists of ultrathin submicroscopic fibres (Mumpton, 1975).

They possess remarkable adsorptive properties, so that they have been used increasingly during the last decade as ion exchange systems, gas purifiers in adsorption, and other molecular sieves for the separation and collection of radioactive wastes, in petroleum refining, animal feeds and agricultural products. They are also employed in pozzolanic cements and concrete, as dimension stone, as fillers for paper and, after calcination at about 1300°C, for lightweight aggregates.

There appears to be no credible report of pneumoconiosis caused by occupational exposure to these minerals. However, interest has recently been focused on them following the observation of calcified pleural plaques and malignant pleural mesothelioma in agricultural populations, with no evident contact with asbestos minerals, in the central uplands of Turkey. Although the plaques do not shorten life expectancy, malignant mesothelioma is said to account for about 50 per cent of deaths in two villages. Diffuse pleural fibrosis has also been observed. Both villages stand on volcanic rock, which is used for building. This rock contains a submicroscopic, fibrillar zeolite, which is also found in the soil and street dust (Baris et al., 1978a, b; Baris, Artvinli and Sahin, 1979). A preliminary study has demonstrated the presence of a fairly large number of long fibres (probably erionite), 75 per cent of which are less than 0.25 µm in diameter (Pooley, 1979). Environmental levels were so low as to raise doubts initially about an aetiological role (Baris et al., 1981). However, animal studies, including using the inhalational route, have confirmed very high potency of erionite (in samples from Oregon as well as Turkey) to produce pleural mesotheliomas (Wagner et al., 1985). Increased risks of lung cancer and malignant peritoneal mesothelioma in some Turkish villages have been related to their higher proportions of erionite fibre in air-borne dust (Baris et al., 1987).

It is of interest that many buildings of the Mayan regions in southern Mexico have been found to be constructed of zeolite blocks with a high mordenite content, and that the same tuff is still being quarried today in Oaxaca for use in local buildings. Early ranch houses in the American West were built of locally quarried erionite (Mumpton, 1975). Fibrous zeolites are sufficiently widespread and abundant to warrant close monitoring of any heavily exposed population, in light of the carcinogenicity of some of these materials.

Synthetic (man-made) mineral fibres

Since the later 1890s, a variety of synthetic mineral fibres (generally known as man-made mineral fibres

or MMMFs) have been increasingly used for thermal and acoustic insulation, in textiles and for plastic reinforcement; latterly, their use has expanded further in the substitution of asbestos minerals. This has raised the question as to whether synthetic fibres cause pneumoconiosis or malignancy in human beings, in view of the fact that fibrous particles of less than 2.5 µm in diameter – irrespective of their chemical composition – have been shown to cause malignant tumours in animals when introduced directly into their pleural or peritoneal cavities.

Synthetic mineral fibres fall into the following main groups:

slag or rock wools (also called mineral wool)
glass wools
continuous filament glass
ceramic fibres

The mineral wools are made from melts of specific argillaceous limestones and smelter slags, sometimes with the addition of wollastonite or kaolinite; glass wool (or fibreglass) is made from different types of silicate glass (Hill, 1977). They are all glassy minerals which, unlike the asbestos minerals, are amorphous silicates. Diameters of ordinary glass fibres are usually greater than 3 µm, but may vary down to diameters of less than 1 µm. 'Melts' at a temperature of 1000 to 1500°C are 'fiberized' by drawing, blowing or centrifugal methods (Klingholz, 1977). The diameters and lengths of fibres differ according to the use for which they are required, and are manufactured to a controlled 'nominal' (specified) diameter. Continuous filament glass for textiles and reinforcement of plastics and similar materials has a large diameter ranging from 12 to 20 µm, and only a very small number of 'respirable' fibres occur in the process. For insulation (which forms the major part of commercial production), fibres are usually about 6 µm in diameter, but a proportion (8 per cent or less) may be smaller than 3 µm in diameter. Fibres less than 1 µm in diameter may be produced for aerospace applications and for certain limited specialized purposes (such as high efficiency filters), but they represent only about 1 per cent of world production (Hill, 1978). Ceramic fibres have special uses dependent on their remarkable resistance to heat, such as in the aerospace industry, and are called refractory fibres; significant use did not begin until the 1970s and they are usually made of silica, alumina and other metal oxides. They have diameters of 2 to 3 µm and, of the synthetic mineral fibres (MMMFs), are the most durable in lung tissue, having very slow clearance rates.

MMMFs are commonly coated with a binder, which is usually a biologically inert, fully polymerized, thermosetting resin. They have also been

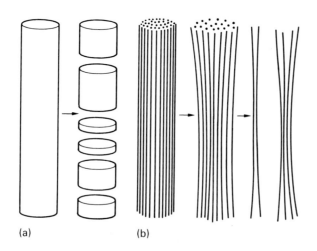

Figure 16.9 Mode of fracture of (a) synthetic and (b) asbestos fibres compared. (Adapted from Klingholz, 1977)

coated with mineral oil to reduce dust emissions and to serve as a lubricant between fibres to improve handling properties. Unlike asbestos fibres, which split longitudinally into numerous fibrils of much smaller diameter, MMMFs break transversely into shorter fragments with the same diameter (Assuncao and Corn, 1975) (Figure 16.9).

Silicon carbide fibres are discussed in Chapter 11, and carbon fibres in Chapter 13.

Sources of exposure

Dust is generated during handling of the various wools, in insulation operations and in sawing, grinding and cutting board containing these fibres. Such operations cause fibre breakage, which may give rise to some particles small enough to remain air-borne for a short time. However, it has been shown that chamfering, cutting and machining of calcium silicate insulating board reinforced with glass fibre, with the exhaust ventilation switched off, produces air-borne fibres with an average length of 100 μm and an almost uniform diameter of 12 μm. Fibres of these dimensions have a high setting velocity, are quickly removed from the air-borne dust, and are unlikely to reach the lower respiratory tract (Hounam, 1973). If inhaled, they will be deposited in the upper respiratory tract (see Chapter 3).

The average range of concentration of 'respirable' fibres evolved during the manufacture of continuous filament and insulation wools is, in general, reported to be about 0.03 to 0.2 fibres/ml (Hill, 1977). In a study of the exposure of employees to mineral wool fibres in five US plants producing synthetic fibres, the size and length distributions of the fibres were found to be remarkably consistent, in spite of differences in

the manufacturing and handling processes. About 80 per cent of the fibres were less than 50 μm in length, and about 10 per cent less than 10 μm in length. Approximately 50 per cent were less than 3 μm in diameter, but very few less than 1 μm in diameter. Compared with a similar study of fibrous glass manufacture, the overall air-borne concentrations of both types of fibre were of the order of 0.1 to 0.3 fibres/ml, of which the 'respiratory' fraction (fibres less than 3 μm in diameter) accounted for about 50 per cent (Esmen et al., 1979). Exposure levels of MMMFs in the course of insulation activities in the construction trades and secondary production use may exceed the primary manufacturing exposures. This is particularly true of fine diameter glass and ceramic fibres whose concentrations may range up to 10 or more fibres/ml (Head and Wagg, 1980; Schneider, 1984).

Effects on the lungs

Slag and rock wools have been produced since the late 1840s, and glass wool since about 1930, yet no clearly authenticated cases of causally related lung disease have been reported, even though fibres of 'respirable' dimensions have been present in most products since manufacture began (Klingholz, 1977). Two cases of acute respiratory infections, and a third with bronchiectasis, were attributed to fibre-glass exposure, but without satisfactory proof (Hill, 1977). The presence of glass fibres in the lungs in such cases does not, of course, establish a pathogenic relationship.

Epidemiological studies have provided additional information. Radiological surveys of workers with long periods of exposure in the rock and slag wool industry (Carpenter and Spolyar, 1945), the fibreglass industry (Wright, 1968; Nasr, Ditcheck and Scholtens, 1971), the glass and rock wool industry, and in insulation work (Keane and Zavon, 1966; Hill et al., 1973), have not revealed any evidence of pneumoconiosis. Similarly, investigation of respiratory symptoms and lung function in workers exposed to fibreglass and glass and rock wools have not identified any abnormality attributable to them (Bjure, Soderholm and Widimsky, 1964; Utidjian and de Treville, 1970; Hill et al., 1973). A study of 1028 men having median employment length of 18 years, and working in seven fibrous glass and mineral wool plants in the USA, assessed chest radiographic findings by the ILO classification and pulmonary function. Correlations were sought with reconstructed individual estimates of fibre exposure. Small opacities on chest radiograph were found to be low level and in low prevalence. Probability of small opacities increased with age and smoking. However, after these variables were taken into account, small opacities were also found to be

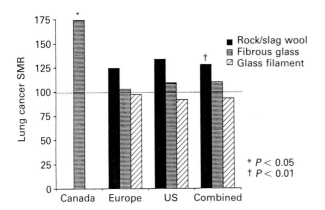

Figure 16.10 SMRs of lung cancer by plant type

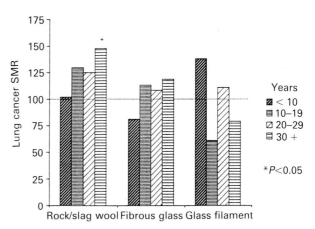

Figure 16.11 SMRs of lung cancer by time in years since hire (three cohorts combined)

related to exposure to fine diameter fibres, and to level of exposure. At a follow-up survey 7 years later, the same authors found no radiographic, symptomatic or functional effects of MMMF exposure (Weill et al., 1983; Hughes et al., 1993).

Post-mortem examination of the lungs of individuals exposed to fibreglass for 16 to 32 years, compared with the lungs of unexposed control urban subjects, showed no evidence of fibrosis or tissue response which could be attributed to the glass dust. Furthermore, the quantity and dimension of fibres present in the fibreglass workers' lungs were similar to those in the 'control' lungs, suggesting that any glass fibres deposited in the workers' lungs over the years were largely removed by the normal clearance mechanisms (Gross, 1976).

Fibres from the 'wools' may cause some irritation of the nose and throat, with sneezing, but itching of the skin of the hands, wrists, neck, waist and ankles is the most irksome complaint among workers unaccustomed to handling these materials. This is due to the mechanical effects of superficially embedded fibres, and not to skin sensitization. The unpolymerized resins, amines and hardeners in the coating of finished fibres are not reactive (Hill, 1977).

The recent evidence dealing with MMMF exposure and carcinogenic risk is extensively documented (World Health Organization, 1987, 1988; IARC, 1988). This evidence comes primarily from three major cohort studies: in Europe (Simonato et al., 1987), the USA (Enterline et al., 1987) and Canada (Shannon et al., 1987). The European and US cohorts were very large: 22 000 workers in 13 plants and 16 700 workers in 17 plants, respectively. On present evidence, there is not likely to have been excess work-related mortality from non-malignant respiratory disease, although the US study showed slightly raised rates for this category. Also there were no excess mortality rates from non-respiratory cancers, and no risk of mesothelioma

found. However, an excess lung cancer risk was found in rock/slag wool manufacturing in the US and European studies, which was statistically significant when the studies were combined (Figure 16.10). There were slight excesses in fibrous glass production (non-significant) in the two larger studies, and a statistically significant excess in the smaller (2500 workers) Canadian study. No excess lung cancer risk was found in workers making glass filament, and no mortality data are available in ceramic fibre manufacturing.

Although these studies provide little evidence that lung cancer risk is related to individually estimated cumulative levels of fibre exposure *within* any of these industrial cohorts, limited evidence of an exposure-related lung cancer risk emerges from the following findings. First, when lung cancer standardized mortality ratios (SMR) are examined by segment of the industry, for the three cohorts combined, in relation to time since hire, a significant excess is found after 30 years in rock/slag wool production (Figure 16.11). A non-significant excess was found for 10 to 19 and 20 to 29 years after hire, and no excess for less than 10 years. A small, but non-significant, excess was found for workers in fibrous glass production 10 or more years after hire. No sensible pattern of risk in relation to time of hire was found in glass filament manufacturing. Secondly, the gradient of lung cancer risk is consistent with the gradient of fibre concentrations *across* sectors of the industry, that is, decreasing measured fibre levels in rock/slag wool, glass wool and continuous filament glass manufacturing, consistent with a dose–response relationship (Doll, 1987).

The European study results found that the excess lung cancer risk was most prominent in those employed in the 'early technological phase' (controlling for follow-up time), suggesting the possibility that other respiratory carcinogens (for example, those associated with bitumen and mineral oil) may be responsible, but this finding, by year of hire, was not confirmed in the US study. Whilst the observed lung cancer risk may have been occupationally related, the role of MMMFs is still open to question.

Experimental observations

As has already been indicated elsewhere, the dimensions of fibres rather than their chemical composition appear to be the important factors in their ability to induce lung disease. It was reported early on that neither uncoated nor plastic-coated glass fibres inhaled or injected via the intratracheal route into rats, guinea-pigs, rabbits and monkeys caused pulmonary fibrosis (Schepers and Delahant, 1955; Schepers, 1959). Later observations have shown that the inhalation by rats and hamsters of glass fibres, with an approximate diameter of 0.5 μm and approximate length range of 5 to 20 μm, caused neither fibrosis nor malignancy in the lungs or pleural surfaces, irrespective of whether the fibres are coated (with resin or starch-like binders) or uncoated; also, in spite of heavy exposure, little glass dust is found in the lungs, apparently as a result of its rapid clearance (Gross, 1976). The lack of fibrogenicity reported in these studies may have been the result of either the coarse dimensions of the fibres used, which preclude pulmonary deposition, or the substantial ball milling to which the fibres were subjected, thus destroying their fibrous properties. Another major difficulty encountered in comparing results obtained from different studies is due to the wide range of criteria employed by the authors to define fibrosis and neoplasm histologically.

In an attempt to standardize such procedures, McConnell et al. (1984) described an 8-point grading system for fibrosis and 4 classifications for lung tumours that were later used by a panel of 11 pathologists to evaluate the health effects of both natural and synthetic mineral fibres. Wagner et al. (1982) used these criteria in an investigation where rats were exposed to fibrous dust clouds of Swedish rock wool without binder, English 'ordinary' glass wool with and without binders, and American 'very fine' glass wool without binder. These investigators also used comminution techniques that would reduce the fibres to the appropriate length range without destroying their fibrous properties. The same panel evaluated the tissue samples developed in this study. Inhalation of MMMFs induced mild degrees of fibrosis in the following descending order: very fine fibres, rock wool, glass wool with binder and glass wool without binder. Adeno-carcinomas were seen in one animal from both the

'very fine fibres' group and from the 'glass wool with binder' group. Glass wool without binder yielded one case of adenoma and one of broncho-alveolar hyperplasia. Exposure to rock wool resulted in one case of bronchoalveolar hyperplasia, one benign adenoma and another with some malignant features.

The fibrogenicity of the very fine fibrous glass was further confirmed by the production of fibrosis, morphologically similar to that produced by asbestos, in baboons (Goldstein, Webster and Rendall, 1984). Davis and his co-workers (1984) reported on the toxic properties of ceramic fibres, a new type of MMMF introduced commercially in the 1950s. The fibres were administered to rats by inhalation. They found that ceramic fibres induced fibrosis and malignant pulmonary tumours, as well as peritoneal mesothelioma. One case of mesothelioma was also reported in hamsters by Smith et al. (1987). The authors also noticed that fibrous glass and slag wool fibres recovered from animal lungs were highly etched, but they did not observe any etching of the ceramic fibres. These findings may reflect the greater degree of durability of ceramic fibres reported by Hammad et al. (1988).

In a recent experiment with rats, lasting 17 to 19 days, in which glass fibres of 1.5 μm mean diameter, and either 5 μm or 60 μm in length, were instilled via the trachea, little difference was found in the clearance rates of long versus short fibres, although short fibres were successfully engulfed by macrophages and transported to the lymph nodes, whereas long fibres were not. Long fibres caused well-demarcated, foreign body granulomas containing numerous giant cells and glass fibres, but neither long nor short fibres provoked any fibrosis. A few short fibres were seen in the lymph nodes of animals exposed only to long fibres (Bernstein, Drew and Kuschner, 1980). Earlier, Wright and Kuschner (1977) found mild local DIPF 2 years after intratracheal injection of short fibres – about 5 μm. However, intratracheal instillation is non-physiological and, compared with inhalation, causes excessively high local concentrations of fibres.

The situation is very different when fibres are introduced directly into the coelomic 'cavities' of animals. Experiments in which glass fibres, ranging from less than 5 μm to more than 10 μm in length, and less than 2.5 μm in diameter, were implanted in the pleural or peritoneal 'spaces' of rats have resulted in sarcomatous tumours classed as mesotheliomas – although the criteria for this diagnosis are not always given (Stanton and Wrench, 1972; Wagner, Berry and Timbrell, 1973; Pott, Huth and Friedrich, 1974). Stanton et al. (1977) have since investigated 17 fibrous glasses of diverse type and dimensions by introducing them into the pleural 'spaces' of rats, and shown that, as the diameter of the fibres is reduced below 1.5 μm, and their length increased above 8 μm, the yield of 'pleural sarcoma' increases; when all the fibres are shorter than 8 μm, they are inactivated by phagocytosis, and no statistically significant excess of tumour occurs. Under similar circumstances, fibres of asbestos and synthetic aluminium silicate, as well as glass fibres, also possess tumour-producing potential if they are thinner than 0.5 μm and longer than 10 μm or 20 μm (Maroudas, O'Neill and Stanton, 1973; Wagner, Berry and Timbrell, 1973). However, the induction of small numbers of malignant tumours (classed as mesotheliomas) in rats by intrapleural inoculation of such diverse non-fibrous substances as ultrafine non-crystalline silicon dioxide, barium sulphate, aluminium oxide and powdered glass (Stanton and Wrench, 1972; Wagner, Berry and Timbrell, 1973) suggests that neither the fibrous form nor a particular chemical composition is essential for the production of malignancy in this animal species. Such implantation experiments are not likely to have any relevance to human pathology for the following reasons:

1. The direct introduction of glass fibres (or other substances) into the pleural or peritoneal cavities of animals bypasses the normal defence mechanisms, and is in no way analogous to their normal mode of entry into the human body; the numbers of fibres implanted is almost certainly greatly in excess of any accumulation – assuming that this occurs – that might conceivably result from inhalation.
2. The animal used almost exclusively in these experiments has been the rat, in which it is known that sarcomatous tumours can be readily induced in different anatomical sites by the surgical implantation of a variety of chemically dissimilar solids due, it is postulated, to so-called 'solid-state surface' oncogenesis (Bischoff and Bryson, 1964; Brand, 1975).

Summary

1. There continues to be insufficient evidence to conclude that occupational exposure to MMMFs produces a pneumoconiosis.
2. No cases of mesothelioma in human beings have been attributable to MMMF exposure.
3. Excess lung cancer risk may have resulted from past exposures in MMMF manufacturing, although the evidence is incomplete with regard to incrimination of the fibre exposures. On the basis of the mixed animal and human evidence, the IARC (1988) has classified rock or slag wool, fibrous glass and ceramic fibres as 'possible human carcinogens' (group 2B). Continuous glass filaments were found not to be classifiable, and are therefore placed in group 3.

References

Abraham, J.L. and Brambilla, C. (1979) Particle size for differentiation between inhalation and injection pulmonary talcosis. *Am. Rev. Respir. Dis.* **119** (suppl.), 196

Alivisatos, G.P., Pontikakis, A.E. and Terzis, B. (1955) Talcosis of unusually rapid development. *Br. J. Ind. Med.* **12**, 43–49

Altekruse, E.B., Chaudhary, B.A., Pearson, M.G. and Morgan, W.K.C. (1984) Kaolin dust concentrations and pneumoconiosis at a kaolin mine. *Thorax* **39**, 436–441

Amandus, H.E. and Wheeler, R. (1987) The morbidity and mortality of vermiculite miners exposed to tremolite–actinolite: Part II. Mortality. *Am. J. Ind. Med.* **11**, 15–26

Amandus, H.E., Althouse, R., Morgan, W.K.C., Sargent, E.N. and Jones, R.N. (1987) The morbidity and mortality of vermiculite miners exposed to tremolite–actinolite: Part III. Radiographic findings. *Am. J. Ind. Med.* **11**, 27–37

American Conference of Governmental Industrial Hygienists (1988) *Threshold Limit Values and Biological Exposure Indices for 1988–1989.* American Conference of Governmental Industrial Hygienists, Cincinnati, OH

Anderson, F.G., Selvig, W.A., Baur, G.S., Colbassani, P.J. and Bank, W. (1956) *Composition of Perlite*, Report of Investigations 5199. US Bureau of Mines, Washington DC

Assuncao, J. and Corn, M. (1975) The effects of milling on diameters and lengths of fibrous glass and chrysotile asbestos fibres. *Am. Ind. Hyg. Assoc. J.* **36**, 811–819

Attygalle, D., Harrison, C.V., King, E.H. and Mohanty, G.P. (1954) Infective pneumoconiosis. 1. The influence of dead tubercle bacilli (BCG) on the dust lesions produced by antracite, coal mine dust, and kaolin in the lungs of rats and guinea pigs. *Br. J. Ind. Med.* **11**, 245–259

Baris, Y.I., Artvinli, M. and Sahin, A.A. (1979) Environmental mesothelioma in Turkey. *Ann. NY Acad. Sci.* **330**, 423–432

Baris, Y.I., Sahin, A.A. and Erkan, M.L. (1980) Clinical and radiological study in sepiolite workers. *Archs Environ. Health* **35**, 343–346

Baris, I., Elmes, P.C., Pooley, F.D. and Sahin, A. (1978a) Mesotheliomas in Turkey. *Thorax* **33**, 538

Baris, Y.I., Sahin, A.A., Ozesmi, M., Kerse, I., Ozen, E., Kolacan, B., Altinors, M. and Goktepeli, A. (1978b) An outbreak of pleural mesothelioma and chronic fibrosing pleurisy in the village of Karain Urgup in Anatolia. *Thorax* **33**, 181–192

Baris, Y.I., Saracci, R., Simonato, L., Skidmore, J.W. and Artvinli, M. (1981) Malignant mesothelioma and radiological chest abnormalities in two villages in central Turkey. An epidemiological and environmental investigation. *Lancet* **1**, 984–987

Baris, I., Simonato, L., Artvinli, M., Pooley, F., Saracci, R., Skidmore, J. and Wagner, C. (1987) Epidemiological and environmental evidence of the health effects of exposure to erionite fibres: a four-year study in the Cappadocian region of Turkey. *Int. J. Cancer* **39**, 10–17

Baser, M.E., Kennedy, T.P., Dodson, R., Rawlings, W., Rao, N.V. and Hoidal, J.R. (1989) Differences in lung function and prevalence of pneumoconiosis between two kaolin plants. *Br. J. Ind. Med.* **46**, 773–776

Bennett, P.J. and Castle, J.E. (1975) Kyanite and related minerals. In *Industrial Minerals and Rocks*, 4th ed. (ed. S.F. Lebond), American Institute of Mining, Metallurgical and Petroleum Engineers, New York, pp. 729–736

Bernstein, D.M., Drew, R.T. and Kuschner, M. (1980) Experimental approaches to exposure to sized glass fibers. *Environ. Health Perspect.* **34**, 47–57

Beutelspacher, H. and van der Marel, H.W. (1968) *Atlas of Electron Microscopy of Clay Minerals and Their Admixtures*, Elsevier, Amsterdam, London and New York

Bischoff, F. and Bryson, G. (1964) Carcinogenesis through solid state surfaces. *Progr. Expl. Tumour Res.* **5**, 85–133

Bjure, J., Soderholm, B. and Widimisky, J. (1964) Cardiopulmonary function studies in workers dealing with asbestos and glass wool. *Thorax* **19**, 22–27

Blümel, G., Piza, F. and Zischka-Konorsa, W. (1962) Tierexperimentelle Untersuchungen der Gerwerbereaktion auf Starke-und Talkumpuder nach intraperitonealer Anwendung. *Wiener Klin. Wochenschr.* **74**, 12–13

Boundy, M.G., Gold, L., Martin, K.P. Jr and Burgess, W.A. (1979) Occupational exposure to non-asbestiform talc in Vermont. In: *Dusts and Disease* (eds R. Lemen and J.M. Dement), Pathotox, Illinois, pp. 365–378

Bramwell, A., Leech, J.G.C. and Dunstall, W.S. (1940) Montmorillonite in fuller's earth. *Geo. Mag.* **77**, 102

Brand, K.G. (1975) Foreign body induced sarcomas. In: *Cancer I* (ed. F.F. Becker), Plenum Press, New York and London, pp. 485–510

Burilkov, T. and Michailova, L. (1972) Uber den sepiolitgehalt des bodens in gebieten mit endomischen pleuraverkalkungen. *Int. Arch. Arbeitsmed.* **29**, 95–101

Byers, P.D. and King, E.J. (1959) Experimental and infective pneumoconiosis with coal, kaolin and mycobacteria. *Lab. Invest.* **8**, 647–664

Byers, P.D., King, E.J. and Harrison, C.V. (1960) The effect of triton, a surface active polyoxethylene ether, on experimental infective pneumoconiosis. *Br. J. Expl. Path.* **41**, 472–477

Campbell, A.H. and Gloyne, S.R. (1942) A case of pneumonoko-niosis due to the inhalation of fuller's earth. *J. Pathol. Bacteriol.* **54**, 75–79

Carpenter, J.L. and Spolyar, L.W. (1945) Negative chest findings in a mineral wool industry. *J. Indiana Med. Assoc.* **38**, 389–390

Churg, A. (1983) Nonasbestos pulmonary mineral fibres in the general population. *Environ. Res.* **31**, 189–200

Crouch, E. and Churg, A. (1983) Progressive massive fibrosis of the lung secondary to intravenous injection of talc. A patho-logic and mineralogic analysis. *Am. J. Clin. Path.* **80**, 520–526

Davies, D. and Cotton, R. (1983) Mica pneumoconiosis. *Br. J. Ind. Med.* **40**, 22–27

Davis, G.S., Mortara, M. and Green, G.M. (1975) Lysosomal enzyme release from human and guinea alveolar macrophages during phagocytosis. *Clin. Res.* **23**, 346A (abstract)

Davis, J.M.G., Addison, J., Bolton, R.E., Donaldson, K., Jones, A.D. and Wright, A. (1984) The pathologic effects of fibrous ceramic aluminum silicate glass administered to rats by inhala-tion or peritoneal injection. *Biological Effects of Man-made Mineral Fibers*, Vol. 2, World Health Organization, Regional Office for Europe, Copenhagen, pp. 303–322

Dettori, G., Scansetti, G. and Gribaudo, C. (1964) 'Relievi sull' uiquinamento ambientale nell' industria del talco. *Med. Lav.* **55**, 453–455

Doll, R. (1987) Symposium on MMMF, Copenhagen, October, 1986: overview and conclusions. *Ann. Occup. Hyg.* **31**(4B), 805–819

Dressen, W.C., Dallavalle, J.M., Edwards, T.I. and Sayers, R.C. (1940) *Pneumoconiosis among Mica and Pegmatite Workers*, Health Bulletin No. 250, US Public Health Service, Washington DC

Edenfield, R.W. (1960) A clinical and roentgenological study of kaolin workers. *Archs Environ. Health* **1**, 392–406

El-Ghawabi, S.H., El-Samra, G.H. and Mehasseb, H. (1970) Talc pneumoconiosis. *J. Egyptian Med. Assoc.* **53**, 330–340

Elevatorski, E.A. (1975) Wollastonite. In: *Industrial Minerals and Rocks*, 4th edn (ed. S.F. Lebond), American Institute of Mining, Metallurgical and Petroleum Engineers, New York, pp. 1227–1233

Enterline, P.E., Marsh, G.M., Henderson, V. and Callahan, C. (1987) Mortality update of a cohort of U.S. Man-made mineral fibre workers. *Man-made Mineral Fibres in the Working Environment*, Vol. 31 (ed. W.H. Walton), Pergamon Press, Oxford and New York, pp. 625–656

Esmen, N., Corn, M., Hammad, Y., Whittier, D. and Kotsko, N. (1979) Summary of measurements of employee exposure to airborne dust and fiber in sixteen facilities producing man-made mineral fibers. *Am. Ind. Hyg. Assoc. J.* **40**, 108–117

Essen, A.G.D. (1926) Alunite Salt Lake deposits, Campion, Avon District. *Ann. Rep. Min. W. Aust.* 125–128

Feigin, D.S. (1986) Talc: understanding its manifestations in the chest. AJR *Am. J. Roentgenol.* **146**, 295–301

Gamble, J.F., Fellner, W. and Dimeo, M.J. (1979) An epidemio-logical study of a group of talc workers. *Am. Rev. Respir. Dis.* **119**, 741–753

Gamble, J., Greife, A. and Hancock, J. (1982) An epidemiologi-cal–industrial hygiene study of talc workers. *Ann. Occup. Hyg.* **26**, 841–859

Gärtner, H. (1955) Die Bleicherde-Lunge. *Arch. Gewerbepath. Gewerbehyg.* **13**, 508–516

Gärtner, H. and von Marwyck, C. (1947) Lugenfibrose durch Sillimanit. *Dtsch. Med. Wochenschr.* **72**, 708–710

German, W.M. (1943) Dusting powder granulomas following surgery. *Surg. Gynecol. Obstet.* **76**, 501–507

Golden, E.B., Warnock, M.L., Hulett, L.D. and Churg, A.M. (1982) Fly ash lung: a new pneumoconiosis. *Am. Rev. Respir. Dis.* **125**, 108–112

Goldstein, B. and Rendall, R.E.G. (1970) The relative toxicities of the main classes of minerals. In: *Pneumoconiosis. Proceedings of the International Conference, Johannesburg, 1969* (ed. H.A. Shapiro), Oxford University Press, Cape Town, pp. 429–434

Goldstein, B., Webster, I. and Rendall, R.E.G. (1984) Changes produced by inhalation of glass fibre in non-human primates. *Biological Effects of Man-made Mineral Fibres*, Vol. 2, World Health Organization, Regional Office for Europe, Copenhagen, pp. 272–285

Governa, M., Durio, G. and Comai, M. (1979) Changes in rat lung produced by olivine dust inhalation. *Pathologica* **71**, 745–753

Government of India Ministry of Labour (1953) *Silicosis in Mica Mining in Bihar*, Report No. 3, Office of the Chief Adviser Factories

Government of India Ministry of Labour (1956) *Silicosis among Hand Drillers in Mica Mining in Bihar*, Report No. 12, Office of the Chief Adviser Factories

Greenburg, L. (1947) The dust exposure in tremolite talc mining. *Yale J. Biol. Med.* **19**, 481–501

Grim, R.E. (1933) Petrography of fuller's earth deposits, Olmstead, Illinois, with a brief study of non-Illinois earths. *Econ. Geol.* **238**, 344–363

Gross, P. (1976) The biological categorization of inhaled fiber-glass dust. *Archs Environ. Health* **31**, 101–107

Hale, L.W., Gough, J., King, E.J. and Nagelschmidt, G. (1956) Pneumoconiosis of kaolin workers. *Br. J. Ind. Med.* **13**, 251–259

Hamer, D.H., Rolle, F.R. and Schelz, J.P. (1976) Characterization of talc and associated minerals. *Am. Ind. Hyg. Assoc. J.* **37**, 296–304

Hammad, Y., Simmons, W., Abdel-Kader, H., Reynolds, C. and Weill, H. (1988) Effect of chemical composition on pulmonary clearance of man-made mineral fibers. *Ann. Occup. Hyg.* **32** (suppl. 1, Inhaled Particles VI), 769–779

Hanke, W., Sepulveda, M.J., Watson, A. and Jankovich, J. (1984) Respiratory morbidity in wollastonite workers. *Br. J. Ind. Med.* **41**, 474–479

Head, I.W.H. and Wagg, R.M. (1980) A survey of occupational exposure to man-made mineral fibre dust. *Ann. Occup. Hyg.* **23**, 235–258

Heimann, H., Moskowitz, S., Iyer, C.R.H., Gupta, M.N. and Mankiker, N.S. (1953) Note on mica dust inhalation. *Archs Ind. Hyg. Occup. Med.* **8**, 531–532

Henderson, W.J., Hamilton, T.C. and Griffiths, K. (1979) Talc in normal and malignant ovarian tissue. *Lancet* **1**, 499

Henderson, W.J., Joslin, C.A.F., Turnbull, A.C. and Griffiths, K. (1971) Talc and carcinoma of the ovary and cervix. *J. Obstet. Gynaec. Br. Commonwealth* **78**, 266–272

Henderson, W.J., Blundell, G., Richards, R., Hext, P.M., Volcani, B.E. and Griffiths, K. (1975) Ingestion of talc particles by cultured lung fibroblasts. *Environ. Res.* **9**, 173–178

Hessel, P.A. and Sluis-Cremer, G.K. (1989) X-ray findings, lung function, and respiratory symptoms in black South African vermiculite workers. *Am. J. Ind. Med.* **15**, 21–29

Highley, D.E. (1974) *Talc*, Mineral Dossier No. 10, Mineral Resources Consultative Committee, HMSO, London

Hildick-Smith, G.Y. (1976) The biology of talc. *Br. J. Ind. Med.* **33**, 217–229

Hildick-Smith, G.Y. (1977) Talc – recent epidemiological studies. *Inhaled Particles IV* (eds W.H. Walton and B. McGovern), Pergamon Press, Oxford, pp. 655–664

Hill, J.W. (1977) Health aspects of man-made mineral fibers. A review. *Ann. Occup. Hyg.* **20**, 161–173

Hill, J.W. (1978) Man-made mineral fibers. *J. Soc. Occup. Med.* **28**, 134–141

Hill, J.W., Whitehead, W.S., Cameron, J.D. and Hedgecock, G.A. (1973) Glass fibers: absence of pulmonary hazard in production workers. *Br. J. Ind. Med.* **30**, 174–179

Hopkins, G.B. and Taylor, D.G. (1970) Pulmonary talc granulomatosis. *Am. Rev. Respir. Dis.* **101**, 101–104

Hounam, R.F. (1973) *Investigations of Airborne Dust produced during the Machining of Glass Fiber Reinforced Calcium Silicate, Insulating Board and "Marinite" Asbestos Reinforced Board*, Report by Health Physics and Medical Division, Atomic Energy Research Establishment, Harwell, UK

Hughes, J.M., Jones, J.N., Glindmeyer, H.W., Hammad, Y.Y. and Weill, H. (1993) Follow-up study of workers exposed to man made mineral fibres. *Br. J. Ind. Med.* **50**, 658–667

Hunt, A.C. (1956) Massive pulmonary fibrosis from inhalation of talc. *Thorax* **11**, 287–294

Hunter, B. and Thompson, C. (1973) Evaluation of the tumorigenic potential of vermiculite by intrapleural injection in rats. *Br. J. Ind. Med.* **30**, 167–173

Huuskonen, M.S., Tossavainen, A., Koskinen, H., Zitting, A., Korhonen, O., Nickels, J., Korhonen, K. and Vaaranen, V. (1983) Wollastonite exposure and lung fibrosis. *Environ. Res.* **30**, 291–304

IARC (1987) Silica and some silicates. *IARC Monographs on the Evaluation of the Carcinogenic Risk of Chemicals to Humans*, Vol. 42, IARC, Lyon, pp. 185–224

IARC (1988) Man-made mineral fibres and radon. *IARC Monographs on the Evaluation of the Carcinogenic Risk of Chemicals to Humans*, Vol. 43, IARC, Lyon

Jaurand, M.C., Fleury, J., Monchaux, G., Nebut, M. and Bignon, J. (1987) Pleural carcinogenic potency of mineral fibers (asbestos, attapulgite) and their cytotoxicity on cultured cells. *J. Natl Cancer Inst.* **79**, 797–804

Jötten, K.W. and Eickhoff, W. (1944) Lungenveränderungen durch Sillimanistaub. *Arch. Gewerbepath. Gewerbehyg.* **12**, 223–232

Kaw, J.L. and Zaidi, S.H. (1973) Effect of mica dust on the lungs of rats. *Expl. Pathol.* **8**, 224–231

Keane, W.T. and Zavon, M.R. (1966) Occupational hazards of pipe insulators. *Archs Environ. Health* **13**, 171–184

Kennedy, T., Rawlings, W. Jr, Baser, M. and Tockman, M. (1983) Pneumoconiosis in Georgia kaolin workers. *Am. Rev. Respir. Dis.* **127**, 215–220

Kettle, E.H. (1934) Infective pneumoconiosis: infective silicatosis. *J. Pathol. Bacteriol.* **38**, 201–208

King, E.J., Gilchrist, M. and Rae, M.V. (1947) Tissue reaction to sericite and shale dusts treated with hydrochloric acid: an experimental investigation. *J. Pathol. Bacteriol.* **59**, 324–327

King, E.J., Harrison, C.V. and Nagelschmidt, G. (1948) Effect of kaolin on the lungs of rats. *J. Pathol. Bacteriol.* **60**, 435–440

King, E.J., Rogers, N., Gilchrist, M., Goldschmidt, V.W. and Nagelschmidt, G. (1945) The effect of olivine on the lungs of rats. *J. Pathol. Bacteriol.* **57**, 488–491

Kipling, M.D. and Bech, A.D. (1960) Talc pneumoconiosis. *Trans. Assoc. Ind. Med. Offrs* **10**, 85–93

Kleinfield, M. (1966) Pleural calcifications as a sign of silicatosis. *Am. J. Med. Sci.* **251**, 215–224

Kleinfeld, M., Messite, J. and Langer, A.M. (1973) A study of workers exposed to asbestiform minerals in commercial talc manufacture. *Environ. Res.* **6**, 132–143

Kleinfeld, M., Messite, J. and Zaki, M.H. (1974) Mortality experiences among talc workers: a follow-up study. *J. Occup. Med.* **16**, 345–349

Kleinfeld, M., Giel, C.P., Majeranowski, J.F. and Messite, J. (1963) Talc pneumoconiosis. *Archs Environ. Health* **7**, 101–115

Kleinfeld, M., Giel, C.P., Majeranowski, J.F. and Shapiro, J. (1964a) Pulmonary ventilatory function in talcosis of the lung. *Dis. Chest* **46**, 592–598

Kleinfeld, M., Giel, C.P., Shapiro, J., Kooyman, O. and Swencicki, R. (1964b) Lung function in talc workers. *Archs Environ. Health* **9**, 559–566

Kleinfeld, M., Giel, C.P., Shapiro, J. and Swencicki, R. (1965) Effect of talc dust inhalation on lung function. *Archs Environ. Health* **10**, 431–437

Klingholz, R. (1977) Technology and production of man-made mineral fibers. *Ann. Occup. Hyg.* **20**, 153–159

Lapenas, D., Gale, P., Kennedy, T., Rawlings, W. Jr and Deitrich, P. (1984) Kaolin pneumoconiosis. Radiologic, pathologic, and mineralogic findings. *Am. Rev. Respir. Dis.* **130**, 282–288

Lesser, M., Zia, M. and Kilburn, K.H. (1978) Silicosis in kaolin workers and firebrick makers. *South. Med. J.* **71**, 1242–1246

Lockey, J.E., Brooks, S.M., Jarabek, A.M., Khoury, P.R., McKay, R.T., Garson, A., Morrison, J., Wiot, J. and Spitz, H.B. (1984) Pulmonary changes after exposure to vermiculite contaminated with fibrous tremolite. *Am. Rev. Respir. Dis.* **129**, 952–958

Low, R.B. (1978) Effects of kaolinite on amino acid transport in incorporation into protein by rabbit pulmonary alveolar macrophages. *Am. Rev. Respir. Dis.* **117**, suppl. (abstract), 243

Luchtrath, H. and Schmidt, K.G. (1959) Uber Talkum und Steatit, ihre Beziehungen zum Asbest Sowie ihre Wirhung beim intrachealer Tierrersuch an Ratten. *Beitr. Silikosforsch.* **61**, 1–60

Lynch, K.M. and McIver, F.A. (1954) Pneumoconiosis from exposure to kaolin dust. *Am. J. Pathol.* **30**, 1117–1127

McConnell, E.E., Wagner, J.C., Skidmore, J.W. and Moore, J.A. (1984) A comparative study of the fibrogenic and carcinogenic effects of UICC Canadian chrysotile B asbestos and glass microfibre (JM 100). *Biological Effects of Man-made Mineral*

Fibers, Vol. 2, World Health Organization, Regional Office for Europe, Copenhagen, pp. 234–250

McDonald, J.C., Sebastien, P. and Armstrong, B. (1986) Radiological survey of past and present vermiculite miners exposed to tremolite. *Br. J. Ind. Med.* **43**, 445–449

McDonald, J.C., McDonald, A.D., Armstrong, B. and Sebastien, P. (1986) Cohort study of mortality of vermiculite miners exposed to tremolite. *Br. J. Ind. Med.* **43**, 436–444

McDonald, J.C., McDonald, A.D., Sebastien, P. and Moy, K. (1988) Health of vermiculite miners exposed to trace amounts of fibrous tremolite. *Br. J. Ind. Med.* **45**, 630–634

McLaughlin, A.I.G., Rogers, E. and Dunham, K.C. (1949) Talc pneumoconiosis. *Br. J. Ind. Med.* **6**, 184–194

McNally, W.D. and Trostler, I.S. (1941) Severe pneumoconiosis caused by inhalation of fuller's earth. *J. Ind. Hyg. Toxicol.* **23**, 118–126

Maroudas, N.G., O'Neill, C.H. and Stanton, M.F. (1973) Fibroblast anchorage in carcinogenesis by fibers. *Lancet* **1**, 807–809

Martin, J.C., Daniel, H. and Le Bouffant, L. (1977) Short and long-term experimental study of the toxicity of coal-mine dust and some of its constituents. In *Inhaled Particles IV* (eds W.H. Walton and B. McGovern). Pergamon Press, Oxford, pp. 361–370

Middleton, E.L. (1936) Industrial pulmonary disease due to the inhalation of dust. *Lancet* **2**, 59–64

Miller, A., Teirstein, A.S., Bader, M.E., Bader, R.A. and Selikoff, I.J. (1971) Talc pneumoconiosis. Significance of sublight microscopic mineral particles. *Am. J. Med.* **50**, 395–402

Millman, N. (1947) Pneumoconiosis due to talc in the cosmetic industry. *Occup. Med.* **4**, 391–394

Morgan, W.K.C. (1983) Kaolin and the lung. *Am. Rev. Respir. Dis.* **127**, 141–142

Moskowitz, R. (1970) Talc pneumoconiosis: a treated case. *Chest* **58**, 37–41

Mumpton, F.A. (1975) Commercial utilization of natural zeolites. *Industrial Minerals and Rocks*, 4th edn (ed. S.J. Lebond), American Institute of Mining, Metallurgical and Petroleum Engineers, New York, pp. 1262–1274

Musk, A.W., Greville, H.W. and Tribe, A.E. (1980) Pulmonary disease from occupational exposure to an artificial aluminium silicate used for cat litter. *Br. J. Ind. Med.* **37**, 367–372

Musk, A.W., Beck, B.D., Greville, H.W., Brain, J.D. and Bohannon, D.E. (1988) Pulmonary disease from exposure to an artificial aluminium silicate: further observations. *Br. J. Ind. Med.* **45**, 246–250

Nash, D.T. and Nash, S.D. (1978) Talcosis and coronary artery disease. *Mt Sinai J. Med. NY* **45**, 265–270

Nasr, A.N.M., Ditchek, T. and Scholtens, P.A. (1971) The prevalence of radiographic abnormalities in the chest of fiberglass workers. *J. Occup. Med.* **13**, 371–376

Ogle, C.J., Rundle, E.M. and Sugar, E.T. (1989) China clay workers in the south west of England: analysis of chest radiograph readings, ventilatory capacity, and respiratory symptoms in relation to type and duration of occupation. *Br. J. Ind. Med.* **46**, 261–270

Oldham, P.D. (1983) Pneumoconiosis in Cornish clay workers. *Br. J. Ind. Med.* **40**, 131–137

Patterson, S.H. and Murray, H.H. (1975) Clays. In *Industrial Minerals and Rocks*, 4th edn, (ed. S.J. Lebond), American Institute of Mining, Metallurgical and Petroleum Engineers, New York, pp. 519–595

Pettinati, L., Coscia, G.C., Francia, A. and Ghemi, F. (1964) Aspetti radiologie clinici della pneumoconiosi nell' industria estrattiva del talco. *Med. Lav.* **55**, 58–63

Phibbs, B.P., Sundin, R.E. and Mitchell, R.S. (1971) Silicosis in Wyoming betonite workers. *Am. Rev. Respir. Dis.* **103**, 1–17

Phillipson, I.M. (1980) Talc quality. *Lancet* **1**, 48

Pimentel, J.C. and Menezes, A.P. (1978) Pulmonary and hepatic granulomatous disorders due to the inhalation of mica dusts. *Thorax* **33**, 219–227

Policard, A. and Collet, A. (1954) Etude experimentale des effets pathologique du kaolin. *Schweiz. Z. Allg. Path. Bakt.* **17**, 320–325

Pooley, F.D. (1979) Evaluation of fiber samples taken from the vicinity of two villages in Turkey. In: *Dusts and Disease* (eds R. Lemen and J.M. Dement), Pathotox, Illinois, pp. 41–44

Pooley, F.D. and Rowlands, N. (1977) Chemical and physical properties of British talc powders. In: *Inhaled Particles IV* (eds W.H. Walton and B. McGovern), Pergamon Press, Oxford, pp. 639–646

Pott, F. Huth, F. and Friedrich, K.H. (1974) Tumorigenic effect of fibrous dusts in experimental animals. *Environ. Health Perspect.* **9**, 313–315

Power, T. (1985) Fused minerals – the high purity, high performance oxides. *Ind. Min.* **214**, 37–57

Roberts, G.B.S. (1947) Granuloma of the fallopian tube due to surgical glove talc. Siliceous granuloma. *Br. J. Surg.* **34**, 417–423

Roe, L.A. (1975) Talc and pyrophyllite. In *Industrial Minerals and Rocks*, 4th edn (ed. S.J. Lebond), American Institute of Mining, Metallurgical and Petroleum Engineers, New York, pp. 1127–1147

Rohl, A.N., Langer, A.M., Selikoff, I.J., Tordini, A., Klimentidis, R., Bowes, D.R. and Skinner, D.L. (1976) Consumer talcums and powders: mineral and chemical characterization. *J. Toxicol. Environ. Health* **2**, 255–284

Rubino, G.F., Scansetti, G., Piolatto, G. and Romano, C.A. (1976) Mortality study of talc miners and millers. *J. Occup. Med.* **18**, 186–193

Rubino, G.F., Scansetti, G., Piolatto, G. and Gay, G. (1979) Mortality and morbidity among talc miners and millers in Italy. In: *Dusts and Disease* (eds R. Lemen and J.M. Dement). Pathotox, Illinois, pp. 357–363

Sakula, A. (1961) Pneumoconiosis due to fuller's earth. *Thorax* **16**, 176–179

Schepers, G.W.H. (1959) Pulmonary histologic reactions to inhaled fiberglass–plastic dust. *Am. J. Pathol.* **35**, 1169–1183

Schepers, G.W.H. and Delahant, A.B. (1955) An experimental study of the effects of glass wool on animal lungs. *Archs Ind. Health* **12**, 276–279

Schepers, G.W.H. and Durkan, T.M. (1955a) The effects of inhaled talc-mining dust on the human lung. *Archs Ind. Health* **12**, 182–197

Schepers, G.W.H. and Durkan, T.M. (1955b) An experimental study of the effects of talc dust on animal tissue. *Archs Ind. Health* **12**, 317–328

Schmidt, K.G. and Luchtrath, H. (1958) Die Wirkung von frischen und gebranntem Kaolin auf die Lunge und das Bauchfell von Ratten. *Beitr. Silikosforsch.* **58**, 1–37

Schneider, T. (1984) Review of surveys in industries that use MMMF. *Biological Effects of Man-made Mineral Fibres. Proceedings of a WHO/IARC Conference, Copenhagen, Denmark, April 20–22, 1982*, Vol. 1. World Health Organization, Regional Office for Europe, Copenhagen, pp. 178–190

Seal, R. (1980) Current views on pathological aspects of asbestosis. The unresolved questions and problems. In: *Biological Effects of Mineral Fibres* (ed. J.C. Wagner), Vol. 1. International Agency for Research on Cancer, pp. 217–235

Sepulveda, M.J., Vallaythan, V., Attfield, M.D., Piacitelli, L. and Tucker, J.H. (1983) Pneumoconiosis and lung function in a group of kaolin workers. *Am. Rev. Respir. Dis.* **127**, 231–235

Shanker, R., Sahu, A.P., Dogra, R.K.S. and Zaidi, S.H. (1975) Effect of intratracheal injection of mica dust on the lymph nodes of guinea pigs. *Toxicology* **5**, 193–199

Shannon, H.S., Jamieson, E., Julian, J.A., Muir, D.C.F. and Walsh, C. (1987) Mortality experience of Ontario glass fibre workers – extended follow-up. In: *Man-made Mineral Fibres in the Working Environment* (ed. W.H. Walton), Vol. 31. Pergamon Press, Oxford and New York, pp. 657–662

Shasby, D.M., Petersen, M., Hodous, T., Boehlecke, B. and Merchant, J. (1979) Respiratory morbidity of workers exposed to wollastonite through mining and milling. *Dusts and Disease* (eds R. Lemen and J.M. Dement), Pathotox, Illinois, pp. 251–256

Sheers, G. (1964) Prevalence of pneumoconiosis in Cornish kaolin workers. *Br. J. Ind. Med.* **21**, 218–225

Siegal, W., Smith, R.A. and Greenburg, L. (1943) The dust hazard in tremolite talc mining including roentgenological findings in talc workers. AJR *Am. J. Roentgenol.* **49**, 11–29

Simonato, L., Fletcher, A.C., Cherrie, J.W., Anderson, A., Bertuzzi, P., Charnay, N., Claude, J., Dodgson, J., Esteve, J., Frentzel-Beyme, R., Gardner, M.J. and Jensen, O. (1987) The International Agency for Research on Cancer historical cohort study of MMMF production workers in seven European countries: extension of the follow-up. *Ann. Occup. Hyg.* **31**(4B), 603–623

Skulberg, K.R., Glyseth, B., Skaug, V. and Hanoa, R. (1985) Mica pneumoconiosis – a literature review. *Scand. J. Work Environ. Health.* **11**, 65–74

Smith, A.R. (1952) Pleural calcification resulting from exposure to certain dusts. *Am. J. Roentgenol.* **67**, 375–382

Smith, D.M., Ortiz, L.W., Archuleta, R.F. and Johnson, N.F. (1987) Long-term health effects in hamsters and rats exposed chronically to man-made vitreous fibers. *Ann. Occup. Hyg.* **31**, 731–754

Smith, R.H., Graf, M.S. and Silverman, J.F. (1978) Successful management of drug-induced talc granulomatosis with corticosteroids. *Chest* **73**, 552–554

Stanton, M.F. and Wrench, C. (1972) Mechanisms of mesothelioma induction with asbestos and fibrous glass. *J. Natl Cancer Inst.* **48**, 797–821

Stanton, M.F., Layard, M., Tegeris, A., Miller, E., May, M. and Kent, E. (1977) Carcinogenicity of fibrous glass: pleural response in the rat in relation to fiber dimension. *J. Natl Cancer Inst.* **58**, 587–597

Stille, W.T. and Tabershaw, I.R. (1982) The mortality experience of upstate New York talc workers. *J. Occup. Med.* **24**, 480–484

Thomas, R.W. (1952) Silicosis in the ball-clay and china-clay industries. *Lancet* **1**, 133–135

Thomas, T.L. and Stewart, P.A. (1987) Mortality from lung cancer and respiratory disease among pottery workers exposed to silica and talc. *Am. J. Epidemiol.* **125**, 35–43

Thorel, C. (1896) Die Specksteinlunge. *Beitr. Path. Anat.* **20**, 85–101

Timar, M., Kendrey, G. and Juhasz, Z. (1966) Experimental observations concerning the effects of mineral dust on pulmonary tissue. *Med. Lav.* **57**, 1–9

Tonning, H.O. (1949) Pneumoconiosis from fuller's earth. *J. Ind. Hyg. Toxicol.* **31**, 41–45

Tripsa, R. and Rotura, G. (1966) Recherches experimentales sur la pneumoconiose provoquee par la poussierre de mica. *Med. Lav.* **57**, 493–500

Utidjian, H.M.D. and de Treville, R.T.P. (1970) Fibrous glass

manufacturing and health reports of an epidemiological study. *Proceedings of the 35th Annual Meeting of the Industrial Health Foundation, Pittsburgh*, Industrial Health Foundation, pp. 10–18

Vallaythan, N.V. and Craighead, J.E. (1981) Pulmonary pathology in workers exposed to nonasbestiform talc. *Human Pathol.* **12**, 28–35

Vestal, T.F., Winstead, J.A. and Joliot, P.V. (1943) Pneumoconiosis among mica and pegmatite workers. *Ind. Med. Surg.* **12**, 11–14

Vigliani, E.C. and Pernis, B. (1958) Immunological factors in the pathogenesis of the hyaline tissue of silicosis. *Br. J. Ind. Med.* **15**, 8–14

Vorwald, A.J. (1960) Diffuse fibrogenic pneumoconiosis. *Ind. Med. Surg.* **29**, 353–358

Wagner, J.C., Berry, G. and Timbrell, V. (1973) Mesotheliomata in rats after inoculation with asbestos and other materials. *Br. J. Cancer* **28**, 173–185

Wagner, J.C., Griffiths, D.M. and Munday, D.E. (1987a) Experimental studies with palygorskite dusts. *Br. J. Ind. Med.* **44**, 749–763

Wagner, J.C., Griffiths, D.M. and Munday, D.E. (1987b) Recent investigations in animals and humans. In *The Biological Effects of Chrysotile* (ed. J.C. Wagner), *Accomplishments in Oncology* 1(2), 11–120

Wagner, J.C., Berry, G., Cooke, T.J., Hill, R.J., Pooley, F.D. and Skidmore, J.W. (1977) Animal experiments with talc. In: *Inhaled Particles IV* (eds W.H. Walton and B. McGovern), Pergamon Press, Oxford, pp. 647–652

Wagner, J.C., Chamberlin, M., Brown, R.C., Berry, G., Pooley, F.D., Davies, R. and Griffiths, D.M. (1982) Biological effects of tremolite. *Br. J. Cancer* **45**, 352–360

Wagner, J.C., Skidmore, J.W., Hill, R.J. and Griffiths, D.M. (1985) Erionite exposure and mesotheliomas in rats. *Br. J. Cancer* **51**, 727–730

Wagner, J.C., Pooley, F.D., Gibbs, A., Lyons, J., Sheers, G. and Moncrieff, C.B. (1986) Inhalation of china stone and china clay dusts: relationship between the mineralogy of dust retained in the lungs and pathological changes. *Thorax* **41**, 190–196

Wagner, J.C., Newhouse, M.L., Corrin, B., Rossiter, C.E.R. and Griffiths, D.M. (1988) Correlation between fibre content of the lung and disease in east London asbestos factory workers. *Br. J. Ind. Med.* **45**, 305–308

Warheit, D.B., Hill, L.H. and Brody, A.R. (1984) In vitro effects of crocidolite asbestos and wollastonite on pulmonary macrophages and serum complement. *Scanning Electron Microscopy (Part 2)*, 919–926

Warraki, S. and Herant, Y. (1963) Pneumoconiosis in china clay workers. *Br. J. Ind. Med.* **20**, 226–230

Waxweiler, R.J., Zumwalde, R.D., Ness, G.O. and Brown, D.P. (1988) A retrospective cohort mortality study of males mining and milling attapulgite clay. *Am. J. Ind. Med.* **13**, 305–315

Wegman, D.H., Peters, J.M., Boundy, M.G. and Smith, T.J. (1982) Evaluation of respiratory effects in miners and millers exposed to talc free of asbestos and silica. *Br. J. Occup. Med.* **39**, 233–238

Wehner, A.P., Zwicker, G.M., Cannon, W.C., Watson, C.R. and Carlton, W.W. (1977) Inhalation of talc baby powders by hamsters. *Food Cosmet. Toxicol.* **15**, 121–129

Weill, H., Hughes, J.M., Hammad, Y.Y., Glindmeyer, H.W., Sharon, G. and Jones, R.N. (1983) Respiratory health in workers exposed to man-made vitreous fibers. *Am. Rev. Respir. Dis.* **128**, 104–112

Weiss, B. and Boettner, E.A. (1967) Commercial talc and talcosis. *Archs Environ. Health* **14**, 304–308

World Health Organization (1987) Man-made mineral fibers in the working environment. *Ann. Occup. Hyg.* **31**(4B)

World Health Organization (1988) *Man-made Mineral Fibres*, Environmental Health Criteria 77, International Programme on Chemical Safety, World Health Organization, Geneva

Wozniak, H., Wiecek, E., Tossavainen, A., Lao, I. and Koakowski, J. (1986) Comparative studies of fibrogenic properties of wollastonite, chrysotile and crocidolite. *Med. Pr.* **37**, 288–296

Wright, G.W. (1968) Airborne fibrous glass particles. Chest roentgenograms of persons with prolonged exposure. *Archs Environ. Health* **16**, 175–181

Wright, G.W. and Kuschner, M. (1977) The influence of varying lengths of glass and asbestos fibers on tissue response in guinea pigs. *Inhaled Particles IV* (eds W.H. Walton and B. McGovern), Pergamon Press, Oxford, pp. 455–472

Yazicioglu, S., Ilcayto, R., Balci, K., Sayli, B.S. and Yorulmaz, B. (1980) Pleural calcification, pleural mesotheliomas and bronchial cancers caused by tremolite dust. *Thorax* **35**, 564–569

17

Beryllium disease

W. Jones Williams

Introduction

Beryllium disease is a multisystem disorder caused by dusts, fumes or mists of beryllium metal or its salts but, because their most common and important mode of entry into the body is the respiratory tract, their effects are predominantly pulmonary. It has two forms: an acute, non-specific, chemical tracheo-bronchopneumonia and a chronic, epithelioid, granulomatous disorder which ends in diffuse fibrosis capable of causing severe respiratory disability.

Although uncommon, with the increasing use of beryllium in a variety of industries, the disease continues to be of medical importance.

Beryllium and its compounds

Metallic beryllium and its compounds are extracted from bertrandite ($4BeO \cdot 2SiO_2 \cdot H_2O$) and beryl ore

Table 17.1 Occupations at risk

Metal and alloy workers
Ceramic manufacturing
Electronic industry:
   Transistors
   Heat sinks
   X-ray windows
Space and atomic engineering:
   Rocket fuels
   Heat shields
Laboratory workers
Extraction from ore
Fluorescent lamps (ceased in 1950)

($3BeO \cdot Al_2O_3 \cdot 6SiO_2$). The end-product of acid extraction – beryllium hydroxide – is then reduced and sold as beryllium oxide powder, pure beryllium metal or compounded to form a variety of alloys, particularly BeCu. A main source is in the USA but it is also produced in Brazil, South America, South Africa, China, Madagascar, Ruanda and Zimbabwe.

First consideration will be given to the occupations at risk, highlighting the major groups (Table 17.1).

Beryllium metal and alloy workers

These workers constitute a major group of potential beryllium disease. Pure beryllium metal rapidly oxidizes, particularly in humid conditions with formation of the light, easily respirable, toxic beryllium oxide. Metal and alloy machining, welding, grinding, heating, melting and other fabrication processes readily produce dangerous respirable particles.

The beryllium alloys have a very wide application in modern technology: beryllium–copper is used extensively in the electrical and electronics industries, in computers and the couplings of underwater cables, in strong non-sparking tools for use under conditions where there is risk of explosion, and in the moving parts of engines. Beryllium–nickel is employed for dies and drill bits, and many components requiring high resistance to wear and extreme heat. Beryllium–aluminium possesses greater toughness and resilience than aluminium.

Reclamation of scrap metals is also a potential source because, in many cases, the operators are unaware of the presence of beryllium (Balmes, Cullen and Robins, 1984) which may be released in the refinery of precious metals (Cullen et al., 1987).

Ceramic workers

Beryllium oxide is used in refractory ceramics such as crucibles and a wide variety of technical ceramics for the electronics industry, in microwave windows and with metallic beryllium in metal ceramics – or *cermets* (that is, materials consisting of a ceramic heat-bonded to a metal) – in rocket motor parts and nose-cones, and in the manufacture of the blading of jet engines.

Space and atomic engineering

Beryllium has important uses in the construction of space vehicles, space mirrors and satellite antennae, and as a reflector to increase neutron flux in atomic reactors. It is employed as a rocket fuel because it contains more energy per unit volume than any other solid and chemically stable material. Analysis of rocket exhaust products has indicated the presence of about 50 per cent beryllium oxide, 40 per cent fluoride, remainder being mainly chloride (Robinson et al., 1968). However, apparently this fuel is not activated until the rocket is outside the earth's atmosphere. Static firing of rocket motors for research purposes is done either in enclosures, in which the exhaust is scrubbed and filtered, or in desert areas under favourable meteorological conditions with the operators sealed off from the atmosphere and with subsequent decontamination of affected areas (W.R. Maxwell, 1971, personal communication).

The metal, when bombarded with α-particles, is an important source of neutrons in nuclear reactors and, because of its low neutron-absorbing capacity, is an excellent moderator and reflector of neutrons.

Laboratory workers

The use of beryllium compounds by laboratory workers – chemists and physicists – has occasionally caused disease (Agate, 1948; McCallum, Rannie and Verity, 1961); cleaning exhaust ventilation ducts, dust collectors, cyclones and high-efficiency filters for air-scrubbing in dry beryllium processes and the replacing of filters are also potential sources of significant exposure.

Fluorescent lamp workers

The manufacture and use of beryllium phosphors in fluorescent and neon lighting tubes were responsible for many cases of disease in the past. Established about 1940 and active until 1950 or thereabouts, this industry caused about half the recorded cases of chronic beryllium disease in the USA up to 1966 (Hardy, Rabe and Lorch, 1967), many cases not being manifest until some 10 years after exposure ceased. All stages of manufacture were potentially dangerous because phosphor dust containing beryllium oxide was released from natural and accidental spillage. Breakage of fluorescent tubes by accident or deliberately during disposal also gave rise to dust. Limited use of beryllium oxide in phosphor powder mixtures apparently still continues, however, for certain types of specialized electronic equipment. Beryllium silicate, which may contain about 0.5 per cent beryllium oxide as an impurity, is employed to coat high-energy cathode ray tubes for radar and similar installations, and appears to have been used in Italy for fluorescent lamps until 1967 (Ambrosi et al., 1968).

Although most of these processes and operations have been subjected to rigorous industrial hygiene controls for many years, the possibility of hazardous contamination exists wherever beryllium and its compounds are used.

Small-scale accidents in the laboratory or factory are the most important potential causes of exposure, for example, breakdown of dust and fume control systems, or rupture of storage containers, can cause sudden high level contamination of a factory's atmosphere. Today, therefore, plant maintenance personnel and workers in specialized ceramic and engineering industries are those most likely to develop disease, although the possibility, even if remote, of large-scale exposures from (for example) accidental activation of rocket fuel before or shortly after 'take-off', or from release of beryllium from nuclear reactors, exists.

As a general principle, it should be noted that because particles of beryllium metals or its compounds are so very light (atomic weight of beryllium = 9.013), they may remain air-borne for prolonged periods, and strict methods of suppression of dust and fume are essential.

Neighbourhood and other non-occupational exposure

Despite original fears and claims that populations living 'down-wind' of beryllium factories may be affected, the majority were probably family contacts exposed to contaminated clothing (Lieben and Metzner, 1959; Sussman, Lieben and Cleland, 1959; Newman and Kreiss, 1992).

Regulations are still in force to prevent air pollution, though some of the world's largest factories deny the existence of any such cases. However, although a highly exceptional event, a disaster at a nuclear processing plant in Kazakhstan in the USSR in September 1990 caused widespread atmospheric contamination by beryllium oxide.

Mantles of gas camping lanterns may consist of nitrates of thorium, cerium and beryllium on rayon fabric. During the first few minutes after lighting a new mantle, significant amounts of beryllium oxide (about 200 µg) are emitted into the air and may also be deposited on the inner surface of the lantern cap (Griggs, 1973).

Acute beryllium disease

General

Acute beryllium disease was originally described in Germany by Weber and Englehardt (1933) and later in the USA by Van Ordstrand, Hughes and Carmody (1943). It is caused very largely by the soluble salts and its severity is determined by intensity of exposure. Although rarely seen today, except for accidental massive contamination, sporadic cases still occur (Hooper, 1981).

Non-respiratory disease includes conjunctivitis, corneal ulceration, allergic blepharitis and allergic contact dermatitis. Beryllium fluoride is chiefly responsible, beryllium sulphate and ammonium beryllium fluoride being less active.

Respiratory disease follows excessive, usually accidental, exposure to dusts, fumes or mists. Transient rhinitis, tracheitis and bronchitis of varying severity, according to the degree of exposure, occur and are due almost entirely to soluble salts. Chemical pneumonia results from inhalation of the less soluble salts and of beryllium oxide fume which consists of particles capable of reaching the alveoli. After massive exposure it occurs within 72 hours and follows a fulminant course; with lower concentrations it may be of insidious and slow development but is classified as 'acute' if it occurs within 12 months (Tepper, Hardy and Chamberlin, 1961).

Acute chemical pneumonia occurred chiefly in the beryllium extraction industry but is now unlikely to be encountered apart from the rare accidental and unexpected conditions referred to earlier.

It is important to note that, although acute disease usually resolves completely, either spontaneously or as a result of corticosteroid treatment, it occasionally progresses to chronic disease with a reported American incidence of 17 per cent (Sprince and Kazemi, 1983). Five cases are known

in the UK (Jones Williams, 1993), of which two are noteworthy, in progressing directly from acute to chronic disease (Rees, 1979).

Symptoms and signs

In acute disease, depending upon the magnitude of exposure, there is irritation of the nose and pharynx with copious mucoid nasal discharge and mild epistaxis, paroxysmal cough, sometimes with blood-stained sputum, a burning, tight sensation in the chest and moderate breathlessness on effort. These symptoms commence within about 72 hours of heavy exposure. There may be low-grade fever, central cyanosis and widespread inspiratory crackles throughout the lung fields. In people who have worked with soluble acid salts there may also be irritation of the eyes and, in some cases, an itching, burning skin rash of exposed parts of the body, without respiratory symptoms. When the onset is slower, or subacute (usually within a few weeks of first exposure), there is a cough of gradually increasing severity which is frequently paroxysmal and small quantities of sputum that may be blood-stained, progressively increasing breathlessness on exertion, and pronounced lassitude with anorexia and weight loss. If these symptoms persist for more than 12 months the disease is said to be chronic.

Lung function

The functional abnormalities of acute disease are the same as those found in pneumonia or pulmonary oedema and consist of hypoxaemia and hypercapnia resulting from uneven distribution of ventilation and perfusion and airways' obstruction. The severity of these changes depends upon the extent of the disease. Unless resolution is incomplete and the disease becomes chronic, function subsequently returns to normal.

Radiographic appearances

Abnormal changes in the lung fields lag behind the symptoms and clinical signs by 1 to 3 weeks. Serial films show the development, first of a diffuse haziness and then of widespread, large, ill-defined opacities similar to those of pulmonary oedema or acute, bilateral pneumonia which correlate with areas of consolidation (Figure 17.1). As the patient

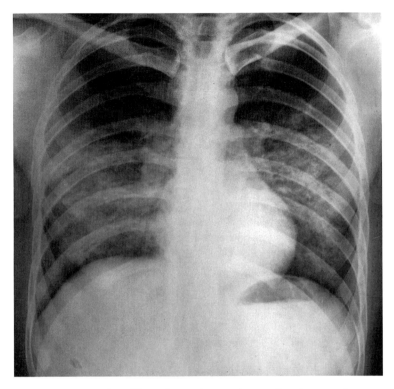

Figure 17.1 Acute beryllium disease in a male metallurgist: complete recovery and radiographic clearing. (By courtesy of Dr Harriet Hardy)

recovers the opacities clear and, in most cases, the appearances return to normal in a few months.

Pathology

Macroscopic appearances

In fatal cases, the lungs are heavy and have a firm, liver-like consistency. The pleura is not thickened although there may be some recent deposition of fibrin. Their cut surfaces have a pink to blue–grey colour, and a frothy, often blood-stained, fluid can be expressed from them. The trachea, bronchi and bronchioles are oedematous and red, and may contain haemorrhagic exudates. The hilar and bronchopulmonary lymph nodes are enlarged. (Hazard, 1959; Sprince, Kazemi and Hardy, 1976).

Microscopic appearances

There is an acute tracheobronchitis and pneumonitis. The lungs show non-specific, acute, interstitial pneumonitis often with massive, sometimes blood-stained, oedema, and associated desquamative

changes and hyaline membrane formation.

Although occasional giant cells may be observed, granulomas are uniformly absent (Freiman and Hardy, 1970).

The only abnormality to be found in the lungs of people who have recovered from the illness may be a very slight excess of connective tissue elements (Vorwald, 1966).

There is nothing characteristic in any of these appearances which are also seen in other chemical pneumonias.

Outside the lungs, centrilobular necrosis of the liver and coagulative necrosis of bone marrow have also been reported (Tepper, Hardy and Chamberlain, 1961).

Diagnosis

The diagnosis of acute nasopharyngitis, tracheobronchitis or pneumonitis depends mainly upon the recognition that a toxic beryllium compound has been inhaled – usually 1 to 2 days before the onset of the symptoms. Other features supporting the diagnosis are low fever and rapid loss of weight. As already described, the appearances of the chest radiograph are in no way characteristic and laboratory tests cannot distinguish this disease from pneumonic disease due to other causes, except in the negative sense that evidence of bacterial or viral infection is lacking. Blood counts, erythrocyte sedimentation rate (ESR), serum protein levels and urinalysis do not help as they show no significant abnormality (Tepper, Hardy and Chamberlin, 1961).

Treatment

Acute disease must be treated immediately with rest and prednisone 60 to 80 mg daily. If it is of fulminant type, oxygen – preferably under positive pressure – will be necessary. Antibiotic agents are not indicated except in the event of secondary infection.

Prognosis

Recovery within 1 to 6 months is the rule in the majority of cases but fulminant disease (usually associated with accidental exposure) carries a risk of death in some 7 per cent of cases (Tepper, Hardy and Chamberlin, 1961). Episodes of pneumonitis may recur, however, following recovery if the subject is re-exposed to beryllium and, as has been described, a proportion of individuals may later develop chronic disease without further exposure to beryllium.

Occasionally, evidence of acute disease in the chest radiograph may persist for almost a year before finally disappearing.

Chronic beryllium disease

Chronic beryllium disease is completely different from acute disease. It was first described by Hardy and Tabershaw in 1946 as an insidious illness occurring after long and variable periods of exposure of up to 20 years (Hardy and Chamberlin, 1972). Although primarily affecting the lungs, other organs may be involved and, with the commonly found evidence of sensitization (see 'Immunological aspects', page 585), it is considered to be a systemic disease.

Symptoms and signs

In chronic disease symptoms develop insidiously, commonly within a month to some 5 years – rarely as much as 25 years – after last exposure, but as previously stated they may become established after the patient has partly recovered from acute disease. The most common symptom is dyspnoea on exertion which, in some cases, is the only symptom. The next most common symptom is an irritating, usually unproductive, cough that is worse in the mornings and after exertion, and may be paroxysmal (suggesting involvement of small to medium-sized bronchi), and ending in retching and vomiting; it is possible that this may be due to granulomas in bronchial walls (Tepper, Hardy and Chamberlin, 1961). Occasionally there is mucoid, or less often purulent, sputum, although haemoptysis has been recorded. In cases of advanced disease, progressive weight loss is a common finding, accompanied by malaise, lassitude, anorexia and arthralgia. However, progression of the symptoms of early disease is prevented, and those of advanced disease alleviated, by steroid treatment (see 'Treatment'). Sudden worsening of dyspnoea, sometimes with chest pain, may be caused by spontaneous pneumothorax (see page 581).

Chronic disease may, however, be symptomless or associated with only slight cough and mild breathlessness on effort but, as noted earlier, sudden exacerbation can occur in relation to respiratory infection, surgery, pregnancy or re-exposure to beryllium compounds.

In cases of mild chronic disease there may be no abnormal signs but, in more advanced disease, finger clubbing is present in about 20 per cent of cases (Stoeckle, Hardy and Weber, 1969); there may be central cyanosis and pleural friction with persistent inspiratory crackles and, occasionally, inspiratory 'squawks' (which predominate in the upper or lower parts of the lungs according to the distribution of the disease) in some cases. In uncomplicated disease the liver is sometimes slightly enlarged, but not tender.

During exacerbation or rapid progression of chronic disease there may be fever up to about 38.9°C (102°F) with rigors, and in advanced disease there may be signs of congestive heart failure; this is uncommon today.

Lung function

The abnormalities seen in chronic disease are in no way specific; they may occur equally in sarcoidosis, extrinsic allergic alveolitis and cryptogenic fibrosing alveolitis (CFA). In the early stages reduction in gas

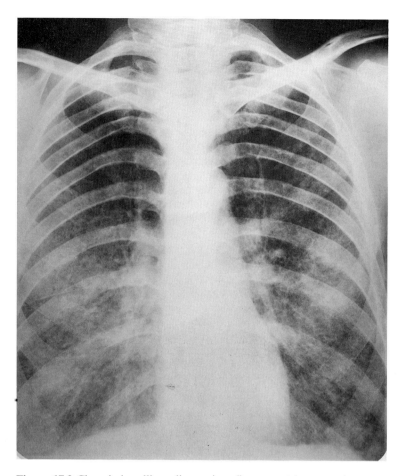

Figure 17.2 Chronic beryllium disease in a fluorescent lamp worker: widespread small and large ill-defined opacities in middle and lower zones

transfer, arterial hypoxaemia – especially on effort – and increase in alveolar–arterial oxygen tension difference are present. These changes are probably due mainly to multiple granulomas and cellular infiltration of alveolar walls because they can be reversed significantly by steroid treatment. With more advanced disease, when a varying amount of nodular or diffuse fibrosis can be expected, combined 'restrictive' and gas transfer defects, the degree of which reflects the severity of the disease, are present. They are unaffected by steroids. Gas transfer tends to deteriorate less over the years than other functional parameters (Andrews, Kazemi and Hardy, 1969).

Obstruction or reduction of airflow, apparently unrelated to smoking, has been noted in a minority of patients with chronic beryllium disease and in sarcoidosis (Andrews, Kazemi and Hardy, 1969; McCarthy and Sigurdson, 1978). This may be due to granulomatous infiltration and fibrosis affecting both proximal and distal airways, and to reduced elastic recoil.

Patients with both restrictive and obstructive defects have more hypoxaemia and greater respiratory disability over a 5-year period than those with a predominantly gas transfer defect (Andrews, Kazemi and Hardy, 1969).

Spontaneous improvement in hypoxaemia and the alveolar–arterial oxygen tension difference has been reported over a 3-year period in 13 of 20 workers (who had not changed their smoking habits) following a substantial reduction in peak air concentrations of beryllium in their factory environment during that time (Sprince et al., 1978). Whether this was due to resolution of granulomas as a result of reduced exposure is uncertain, but possible.

Radiographic appearances

In a review of 60 cases (Stoeckle, Hardy and Weber, 1969) pulmonary densities were classified as granu-

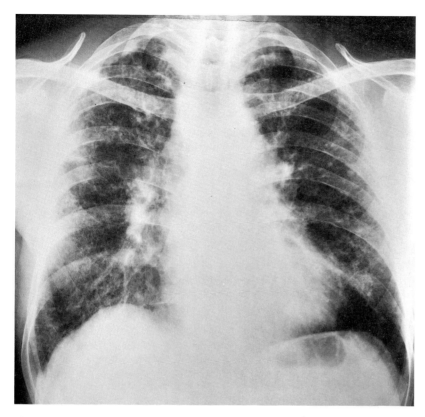

Figure 17.3 Chronic beryllium disease in a foundry worker exposed to beryllium metal: multiple extensive dense opacities with pleural thickening

lar (up to 1 mm), nodular (1 to 5 mm) and linear. The most common presenting pattern was a bilateral admixture of all three (58 per cent) (Figure 17.2), followed by 32 per cent with nodular pattern alone and 10 per cent with only granular features. Although these initial findings may persist unchanged for up to 15 years, the majority develop increasing linear shadowing with ultimate gross fibrosis. In contrast to sarcoidosis, it is exceptional for the changes to regress spontaneously. They may, however, respond to steroid treatment. Evidence of gross fibrosis may occur as early as 1 year from diagnosis. The changes are often prominent in the upper zones with development of cystic change and/or gross emphysema (Figure 17.3). These changes may be associated with pleural thickening (10 per cent) and development of pneumothorax (17 per cent).

Moderate hilar gland enlargement is not uncommon and was reported in 24 of 76 cases (34 per cent) was bilateral in 20 and associated with pulmonary changes (Hasan and Kazemi, 1974). In the same series 4 cases presented with bilateral hilar lymphadenopathy alone, and Sprince, Kazemi and Hardy (1976) reported 2 in 858 cases. Such cases may easily be confused with sarcoidosis.

Both pulmonary and hilar gland calcification have been reported (Weber, Stoeckle and Hardy, 1965; Stoeckle, Hardy and Weber, 1969) and attributed to calcium deposition in hyalinized nodules. However, in the author's experience this has no histological basis and certainly cannot be attributed to the presence of microscopic calcified Schaumann bodies. There is, however, one unique case of a patient who coughed up small lung 'stones' containing beryllium (Weber, Stoeckle and Hardy, 1965). Many of the reported cases may well have had a concomitant silica exposure and should, therefore, be treated with caution.

In conclusion, although essential for diagnosis and to monitor the course of disease, these radiographic features are in no way pathognomonic.

Pathology

Macroscopic appearances

The visceral pleura is thickened and there may be extensive adhesions with the parietal pleura. In some cases multiple, thick-walled blebs – 'honeycomb

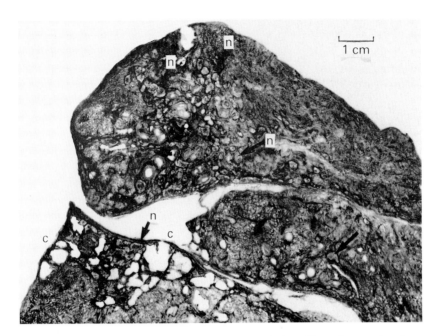

Figure 17.4 Paper-mounted lung section of chronic beryllium disease showing nodular lesions (n) with honeycomb cystic changes (c) and extensive diffuse fibrosis

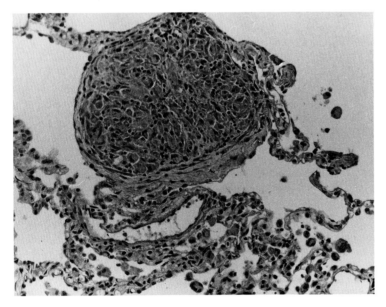

Figure 17.5 Sarcoid-like granulomas with alveolitis (magnification ×150)

lung' – are present on the lung surfaces. The lungs are heavy and their cut surfaces reveal ares of grey–white diffuse fibrosis which is usually present in all lobes although, in some cases, only parts of the lungs are affected. Thick-walled cysts – up to 1 cm or more in diameter – are often associated with the fibrotic areas, and scattered fibrotic nodules which may reach 3 cm in diameter, are occasionally found (Figure 17.4). No particular distribution appears to be favoured. The hilar lymph nodes are usually only slightly enlarged but exceptions to this are seen. None of these features is pathognomonic.

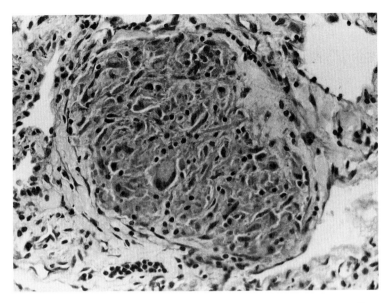

Figure 17.6 Details of granuloma showing epithelioid cells, giant cells and admixed lymphocyte (magnification ×300)

Microscopic appearances

The appearances are those of non-specific interstitial inflammation and epithelioid cell granulomas (Figure 17.5). The alveolar wall infiltration by lymphocytes and histiocytes is a constant, and often prominent, finding and is of value in distinguishing beryllium disease from sarcoidosis (see below). In a useful analysis it was shown that the severity of interstitial change correlates with a worse prognosis (Freiman and Hardy, 1970).

Granulomas are diffusely scattered in the interstitium, in the septa, peribronchial, subpleural and perivascular regions and occasionally in the walls of blood vessels. Although the source of beryllium is air-borne, they are not confined to the peribronchial regions. The granulomas consist of epithelioid cells, often fusing to form Langhans-type, and occasionally foreign-body-type, giant cells admixed with often numerous lymphocytes (Figure 17.6). Epithelioid cells are now proven to be from bone-marrow-derived monocytes and, thus, of macrophage lineage (Van Furth et al., 1980). They are, however, morphologically distinguished from macrophages by showing a predominance of synthesizing rather than phagocytic cells. They show prominent Golgi complexes, they are rich in rough endoplasmic reticulum and they contain numerous mucoprotein-containing vesicles (James and Jones Williams, 1974); it was suggested, at the time, that the secretory products, lymphokines and monokines, may be important in the formation and persistence of granulomas. The importance of T lymphocytes in the development of granulomas has

been well demonstrated in experimental beryllium-induced granulomas (Maceira, Fukuyama and Epstein, 1984) and in the identical granulomas of sarcoidosis where Munro et al. (1987) showed that the majority of intermingled lymphocytes are T-helper cells, whereas T-suppressor and antigen-presenting dendritic cells are conspicuous at the periphery. Plasma cells and eosinophils are not a feature. Central necrosis is unusual and in its absence the granulomas are indistinguishable from those of sarcoidosis, tuberculosis and extrinsic allergic alveolitis (Jones Williams, 1977). A few cases may show extensive necrosis which may reflect a high dosage or possible excessive sensitization (Izumi et al., 1976). Fusion of granulomas may result in nodules up to 2 cm in diameter associated with dense hyalinized collagen deposition. This is distinguished from caseation by persistence of reticulin fibres and from silicotic fibrosis, by absence of birefringent silica crystals and whorled pattern.

A variety of cell inclusions are common in the granulomas, notably Schaumann bodies (Figure 17.7). Schaumann bodies consist of central birefringent crystals of calcite surrounded by calcium-, phosphate- and iron-impregnated mucoglycoprotein conchoidal bodies (Jones Williams, 1960) and many contain beryllium (Jones Williams and Wallach, 1989). Unfortunately, although common in chronic beryllium disease (62 per cent of 52 cases), they are not pathognomonic as they are also found in 88 per cent of cases of sarcoidosis, and in 6 per cent of cases of tuberculosis (Jones Williams, 1960). Star-shaped asteroid bodies in epithelioid and giant cells are also common to beryllium disease, sarcoidosis

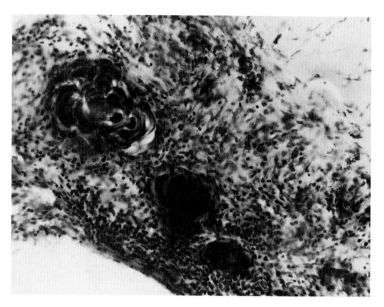

Figure 17.7 Schaumann bodies (magnification ×250)

and tuberculosis. Both Schaumann and asteroid bodies are considered to be of endogenous origin resulting from activated cells and thus not of aetiological significance.

It must be emphasized that granulomas are not pathognomonic of beryllium disease because morphologically, on light and electron microscopy, histochemistry and enzyme content, they are identical with those of sarcoidosis, extrinsic allergic alveolitis and even Crohn's disease (Jones Williams, 1958; Jones Williams and Williams, 1967; Williams, Jones Williams and Williams, 1969; James and Jones Williams, 1974). A real distinction can only be made by the detection of beryllium in the lesions (Jones Williams and Kelland, 1986; Jones Williams and Wallach, 1989) (see 'Tissue and urine analysis', page 583).

End-stage fibrosis is manifested by gross distortion of airspaces with consequent honeycomb (cystic) change. Granulomas are infiltrated by fibroblasts with consequent replacement by reticulin and collagen. Often it is only the persistence of Schaumann bodies that assists in detection of previous granulomatous disease. Pleural fibrosis is not uncommon and is often associated with pneumothorax (Tepper, Hardy and Chamberlin, 1961).

Extrapulmonary manifestations

Granulomas may also be found in the skin, cervical, intrathoracic and abdominal lymph nodes, the liver, spleen, pancreas, kidneys, suprarenal glands, bone marrow, skeletal muscle, and central nervous system; there is also some evidence that the myocardium may occasionally be involved (Sprince, Kazemi and Hardy, 1976). Skin granulomas may precede lung disease and, unlike those seen in sarcoidosis, may ulcerate (Jones Williams et al., 1988). An apparently unique case of chronic beryllium ulceration of a finger followed by extensive local lymphatic spread and later by granulomas of the lungs has been reported; the beryllium content at all the sites involved was high (Jones Williams and Kilpatrick, 1974). Although skin granulomas are usually due to intradermal implantation of beryllium salts, they may occasionally follow respiratory exposure. Stoeckle, Hardy and Weber (1969) found 4 examples among 60 cases of respiratory exposure only, and 2 cases have recently been reported in the UK (McConnochie et al., 1988). Other than the very occasional presence of isolated kidney granulomas, renal calculi associated with hypercalcaemia have also been reported (Tepper, Hardy and Chamberlin, 1961; Stoeckle, Hardy and Weber, 1969). Ocular, salivary glands, peripheral lymph nodes and neural involvement, together with lupus pernio, have not been described in chronic beryllium disease so that their absence is useful in the distinction from sarcoidosis (see page 583).

Complications

Other than massive respiratory failure, following acute exposure, pulmonary heart disease accounts for the vast majority of deaths in the USA from chronic disease (Stoeckle, Hardy and Weber, 1969). Similarly, in the UK series, when incidental causes – mainly ischaemic heart disease – were excluded, all died from pulmonary heart disease (Jones Williams, 1993).

Spontaneous pneumothorax

A fairly common complication, spontaneous pneumothorax has been observed in about 15 per cent of cases; it may be recurrent and bilateral and, in some cases, is the immediate cause of death.

Carcinogenicity

Despite the fact that inhalation of a variety of beryllium compounds causes lung cancer in animals (Reeves, Deitch and Vorwald, 1967), evidence in human beings is unconvincing. A number of authors (Infante, Wagoner and Sprince, 1980; Mancuso, 1980; Wagoner, Infante and Bayliss, 1980) have claimed a marked increase of lung cancer in beryllium process workers, but the data are considered suspect and largely to be discounted (US Public Health Service, 1988). In a series of 76 cases reported to the US Registry between 1966 and 1974, 4 developed lung cancer (Hasan and Kazemi, 1974). However, more detailed analysis of the US Registry confirmed a twofold increased incidence: 28 in a total of 689 patients with both acute and chronic disease (Steenland and Ward, 1991). The majority occurred in acute cases suggesting a dose relationship. The incidence appears to be unrelated to smoking. There are no known cases to date in the UK Registry (Jones Williams, 1993) (see Chapter 19, page 656 and Table 19.3).

Treatment

Before any treatment is instigated the patient must be removed from the offending source and warned against any further exposure.

Administration of corticosteroids is associated with a significant reduction in mortality and increased survival (Hardy, Rabe and Lorch, 1967), although it is difficult to be certain whether this is wholly due to their influence or partly to other causes (Freiman and Hardy, 1970).

When chronic disease is first diagnosed, prednisolone should be commenced at an initial dose of 15 to 30 mg daily or 30 to 60 mg on alternate days and later adjusted according to progress (Stoeckle, Hardy and Weber, 1969). This usually causes a reduction of symptoms and serum globulins, improvement in general health, gas transfer and, in some cases, in radiographic appearances. If treatment is started early progression of fibrosis may seem to be arrested, but deterioration of lung function is not always prevented. However, no controlled trials of corticosteroid treatment appear to have been done due, no doubt, to the comparative rarity of the disease and ethical principles involved, but, in sarcoidosis, such trials indicate that steroids have no significant effect on long-term results (James and Jones Williams, 1985).

When corticosteroids are discontinued there may, in some patients, be prolonged remission. In others, symptoms and abnormalities of lung function and chest radiographs reassert themselves, in which case life-long maintenance of these drugs may be advisable, although the rationale of such treatment is questionable.

The effect of chloroquine and immunosuppressant drugs which appear to cause temporary improvement in some sarcoidosis cases (James and Jones Williams, 1985) does not seem to have been reported in beryllium disease.

Chelating agents – such as aurintricarboxylic acid (ATA) and ethylenediamine tetraacetic acid (disodium edetate or EDTA) – are ineffective.

Supportive treatment of pulmonary heart disease, congestive heart failure and respiratory failure may ultimately be required.

Local skin granulomatous lesions require early and complete excision which in the UK experience appears to be curative (Jones Williams et al., 1988).

Prognosis

Prognosis in the individual cannot be predicted with certainty and different patterns of evolution of the disease occur, any one or all of which may be observed in the same patient.

The minority of individuals who experience no symptoms and in whom the only evidence of disease, apart from beryllium assay and biopsy, is the chest radiograph may remain asymptomatic for a decade or more (Tepper, Hardy and Chamberlin, 1961), but, at any time, symptoms and impairment of lung function may develop without evident change in the radiographic appearances.

The majority of people have symptoms and the impaired pattern of lung function, described already, to the point of being slightly or moderately disabled although able to lead a fairly normal life for years. However, should exacerbation of disease occur it is usually followed by an increase in disability. When exacerbations are accompanied by fever and rigors the prognosis tends to be poor (Tepper,

Hardy and Chamberlin, 1961). Severely disabling disease is of very variable duration – from about 1 to 20 years in corticosteroid-treated patients (Hardy, Rabe and Lorch, 1967). It may end in death from respiratory failure and pulmonary heart disease which, in some cases, may be precipitated by repeated episodes of spontaneous pneumothorax.

Although corticosteroids have a substantial ameliorating effect upon the course of chronic disease, complete resolution, either spontaneous or as a result of treatment, has not been reliably reported. However, if it is not understood that long periods of remission occur in some cases, these may be interpreted as a 'cure' and, although some reduction of discrete radiographic opacities may occur during corticosteroid treatment, this is never complete and the opacities tend to reappear when it is stopped.

Epidemiology

It is difficult to get a figure for number of workers at risk as none is available for the UK. Estimates for the USA have dropped from 30 000 in 1970 to a present figure of approximately 10 000 (NIOSH, 1985), the majority being beryllium alloy workers engaged in the aircraft, electronic and nuclear industries. Other than accidental exposure to breaking up of old fluorescent tubes (Karkinen-Jaaskelainen et al., 1982), beryllium phosphors have ceased to be a hazard.

The most valuable source of information, started by Dr Harriet Hardy, is the *US Beryllium Case Registry* in which most known cases have been recorded since 1952 (Hardy, 1955; Peyton and Worcester, 1959; Hardy, Rabe and Lorch, 1967; Hasan and Kazemi, 1974; Sprince and Kazemi, 1980). There are now over 900 cases in the US Registry, based at the National Institute for Occupational Safety and Health (NIOSH), Cincinnati (Eisenbud and Lisson, 1983); 224 acute cases are on record, mostly resulting from accidental transient exposure, but no new cases are documented after 1968. More than half of the 560 occupationally exposed chronic cases worked in the fluorescent lamp industry but, since 1949, the majority have been metal and alloy workers.

Of 76 new cases added to the *US Beryllium Case Register* since 1966, 53 were men and 23 women which contrasts with the preponderance of women in the late 1940s following employment during the Second World War; the average age of onset in both sexes tended to be younger – the mean age for both

being 46 years whereas prior to 1949 the mean age for men was 53 years and, for women, 52 years. Delay in onset of disease was much shorter in cases developing after 1949 than in those developing prior to 1949. In the majority of those reported before 1949, the period was over 10 years, whereas in most of those reported after this date it was under a year, in spite of the fact that the beryllium levels to which the subject had been exposed were considerably lower than in the pre-1949 group. This paradox is explained by an increased awareness of the disease and effectiveness of diagnosis by physicians, and the limitation of exposure to defined industries in later years.

There has been considerable doubt about the validity of so-called down-wind neighbourhood cases (page 572). A total of 14 cases is recorded in the USA (Eisenbud and Lisson, 1983), 13 occurring before 1950 living within three-quarters of a mile of a poorly controlled production plant, which was closed in 1948. There have been no reported cases in the UK. Although the risks are remote, regulations controlling emission standards are still in force.

There is also a *UK Beryllium Case Registry* (Jones Williams, Noseworthy and Williams, 1980; Jones Williams, 1985) with a present total of 59 cases including 5 with acute lung disease and 7 with skin lesions alone (Jones Williams, 1993). However, it is virtually certain that an unknown number have not been included and may remain undiagnosed.

There are five examples of acute disease, four of which progressed over a period of up to 13 years to chronic disease. Two are noteworthy: following an acute exposure from metal fume exposure in 1975, they directly progressed to chronic disease (Rees, 1979) and are the last known cases to occur in the UK. Twenty-five of the UK chronic cases are known to have died, the majority (21) from pulmonary heart disease due to progressive pulmonary fibrosis as noted in the US series (Stoeckle, Hardy and Weber, 1969).

There is little to suggest any genetic predisposition to beryllium disease. In the US Registry there were only six families with more than one affected member (Hardy, 1980) and the report of identical twins with the disease in the UK is unique (McConnochie et al., 1988).

Absorption and excretion of beryllium compounds

Information in human beings is incomplete but it appears that, after inhalation, the soluble compounds are cleared fairly readily from the lungs although a variable quantity may remain, whereas the relatively insoluble beryllium oxide is very slowly eliminated and is retained for long periods due, it is suggested, to its being bound to tissue proteins and only being released gradually (Reeves, 1968). Excretion occurs mainly via the kidneys and the amount depends upon the solubility of the compounds inhaled (Klemperer, Martin and Van Riper, 1951). A proportion that is not excreted, and is greater in acute than in chronic disease, is stored in the liver, spleen, lymph nodes and skeleton (Tepper, Hardy and Chamberlin, 1961). Mobilization and excretion of beryllium in the urine may continue for years so that urinary concentrations at any given time reflect only the amount released and not the total body burden (Preuss, 1975). There is no evident correlation between the presence or severity of disease and the quantity of beryllium excreted (Klemperer, Martin and Van Riper, 1951; Lieben, Dattoli and Vought, 1966).

Beryllium and its compounds are not absorbed through unbroken skin but readily enter cracks and abrasions; they are poorly absorbed from the gastrointestinal tract and no toxic effects from this route are on record (Preuss, 1975). Beryllium apparently crosses the placental 'barrier' but no disease in infants has been attributed to this (Tepper, Hardy and Chamberlin, 1961).

Tissue and urine analysis

The detection of beryllium in affected tissues plays an important role in diagnosis. However, the quantities detected show wide variation and only a poor correlation with extent and severity of disease (Tepper, Hardy and Chamberlin, 1961; Hardy, 1980). Small amounts of beryllium are sometimes found in the lungs of people with no known industrial exposure to beryllium compounds. This is usually attributed to the fact that urban air may contain small amounts of beryllium from the ash of some fossil fuels. Trace amounts of beryllium are present in Welsh coal (Chatterjee and Pooley, 1977) and are detectable in coal dust foci of coal workers' lungs (Jones Williams and Kelland, 1986). Although there is a potential source of exposure from naturally occurring beryllium in air, water, soils and even food stuffs (US Public Health Service, 1988), there are no known cases of disease from non-occupational sources.

Earlier results were based on fluorometric bulk analysis (Morrin method), but lack the sensitivity and ability to deal with small amounts of tissue that is available with modern atomic absorption spectrometry. However, an analytical study of beryllium disease, sarcoidosis and normal controls provided useful information (Sprince, Kazemi and Hardy, 1976).

1. In the control and sarcoid cases the lungs and lymph nodes contained only minute amounts of beryllium which were uniformly less than 0.02 µg/g dried tissue.
2. In 66 cases of beryllium disease the beryllium content of the lungs was in excess of 0.02 µg/g dried tissue in 82 per cent and the overall mean value was 1.19 µg/g (range = 0.004 to 45.7 µg/g). In mediastinal nodes the average level was 3.41 µg/g (range = 0.056 to 8.50 µg/g). Levels in peripheral lymph nodes were, however, lower than those in the lungs and mediastinal nodes.

In the UK series, using similar methods, lung beryllium content of chronic patients ranged from 0.02 to 15 µg/g dried tissue (Jones Williams, 1985).

More recent techniques are now available, not only to detect beryllium in parts per million, but to combine this with microscopic localization. There are two methods utilizing electron microscopy: *ion microprobe mass spectrometry* (IMMA) which has shown a good correlation with bulk analysis (Abraham, 1980), and a more experimental tool, *electron energy mass spectrometry* (EELS), where beryllium has been localized in phagolysosomes in the minutest quantity of 10^{-18} g (Dinsdale and Bourdillon, 1982).

In addition, there is now another qualitative, but not quantitative, technique of *laser microprobe mass spectrometry* (LAMMS), where beryllium can be localized using light microscopy (Jones Williams and Kelland, 1986). In a recent study (Jones Williams and Wallach, 1989), beryllium was detected within and confined to granulomas in all 31 cases of chronic disease examined (Figure 17.8) and was absent in the granulomas of 30 sarcoid patients. It was also detected in Schaumann bodies of beryllium disease and not in those of sarcoidosis. As beryllium is a natural constituent of coal (Chatterjee and Pooley, 1977), it is cautioned that sample areas should exclude coal dust foci as the authors' group found beryllium in such areas in 1 of 12 normal lungs and in 2 of 3 cases of coal pneumoconiosis. Beryllium was absent in other morphologically similar granulomas of Crohn's disease, isolated lymph node granulomas and, in another investigation, those of necrotizing sarcoidal granulomatosis (Gibbs, Jones Williams and Kelland, 1987). From the results of LAMMS analysis, and with bulk atomic absorption spectrometry with detection limits of around 1 part per million, it is most unlikely that disease can occur without detectable

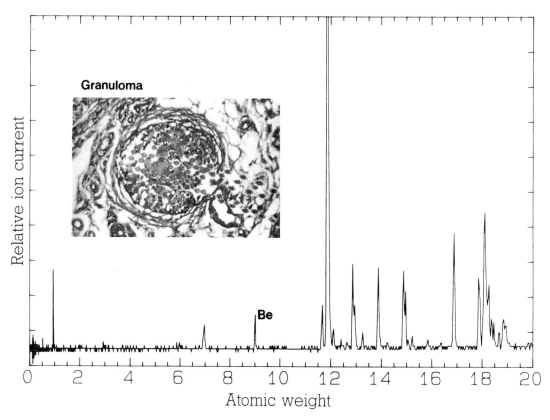

Figure 17.8 LAMMS spectrum showing beryllium peak (atomic weight = 9) found in the accompanying granuloma

beryllium which was inferred, using less sensitive methods, in earlier reports.

In conclusion, it is considered that finding beryllium within granulomas in a patient with a history of exposure and consistent clinical and radiographic features is diagnostic of beryllium disease.

The detection of beryllium in urine is probably of less value. Its presence certainly detects exposure but, as it may be found in the absence of clinical evidence of disease, it does not have the diagnostic significance of tissue assays (Tepper, Hardy and Chamberlin, 1961). As with tissue levels the amounts excreted in diseased patients show little correlation with extent of disease.

Biochemical abnormalities

An increase in circulating immunoglobulins has been repeatedly observed during exacerbations of chronic disease and this has prompted unfounded speculation that humoral antibodies may be involved. The concentrations of immunoglobulins are often raised but the Ig types affected have varied in different reports; in one the predominant increase was in IgA in 17 of 35 patients with chronic disease (Deodhar, Barna and Van Ordstrand, 1973); in another it was IgG in 5 of 6 patients with disease and 13 of 22 individuals with beryllium exposure but no evidence of disease (Resnick, Roche and Morgan, 1970). The significance of these findings is uncertain but, as IgG and IgA are often elevated in sarcoidosis especially in female and black patients (Goldstein, Israel and Rawnsley, 1969; Buckley and Dorsey, 1970), Ig levels are of little practical value in diagnosis.

There is often an increase in urinary calcium in patients with chronic beryllium disease and, if renal function is impaired, hypercalcaemia results. The underlying reason for the high urinary calcium is obscure but, as beryllium is known to be excreted by the tubules (Underwood, 1951), cellular intoxication at this level is a possible explanation. It is not attributed to immobilization of the patient but to the activity of the disease (Tepper, Hardy and

Chamberlin, 1961; Stoeckle, Hardy and Weber, 1969). However, renal failure is rare unless calculi develop, reported by the latter in 7 per cent of one series, and may contain beryllium (Stoeckle, Hardy and Weber, 1969). Steroid therapy results in return to normal of the urinary calcium levels. Both hypercalcaemia (11 per cent) and renal calculi (1 per cent) of course may also occur in sarcoidosis (James and Jones Williams, 1985).

Hyperuricaemia develops in some cases of chronic beryllium disease and also in a proportion of patients with sarcoidosis. This appears to be due to impaired renal clearance rather than to an increased production of uric acid, but its cause is not understood. There is no correlation between hyperuricaemia and the nature and duration of exposure to beryllium, severity of disease or the presence of beryllium in the urine. Serum alkaline phosphatase activity has usually been reported to be normal (Tepper, Hardy and Chamberlin, 1961) but is often raised (25 per cent) in sarcoidosis (James and Jones Williams, 1985).

Raised levels of serum angiotensin-converting enzyme (serum ACE) are frequent in sarcoidosis (87 per cent) and, although not specific, are a useful index of activity and extent of disease (James and Jones Williams, 1985). Raised serum ACE levels are also correlated with a rise in lysozyme levels (Selroos et al., 1980). It was earlier claimed that serum ACE levels are normal in chronic beryllium disease and, thus, useful in the differential diagnosis (Sprince, Kazemi and Fanburg, 1980). However, their cases were on steroid therapy, which is known to depress serum ACE levels. It was later shown that serum ACE levels may be moderately raised in chronic beryllium disease, as found in another US series (Lieberman, 1985) and in the UK (McConnochie et al., 1988) and Japan (Studdy and James, 1983). Raised serum ACE levels therefore do not differentiate between sarcoidosis and beryllium disease.

antigenicity by virtue of its known property of easily complexing with plasma proteins and, thus, acting as a hapten. There is no evidence of humoral antibody involvement and everything points to cellular (type IV) immunity.

Skin hypersensitivity to beryllium can be passively transferred to normal guinea-pigs by the injection of lymphocytes, but not serum, from beryllium-sensitized guinea-pigs (Cirla, Barbiano di Belgiojoso and Chiappino, 1968). It also appears that transient contact sensitivity to beryllium can be transmitted by transfer factor (TF) from lymphocytes of human donors with strong cellular immunity to beryllium to human recipients 'primed' with subsensitizing doses of beryllium fluoride. Fourteen of 38 recipients (37 per cent) developed a positive patch test to beryllium fluoride 24 hours or more after receiving the transfer factor but this reactivity lasted more than a week in only four cases (Epstein and Byers, 1979). Further investigation is needed to confirm these findings and their significance: whether, for example, non-specific transfer factor might not work equally well.

There is ample evidence for the development of granulomas following intratracheal injections in skin-sensitized guinea-pigs (Reeves, 1980; Barna et al. 1981). Also, more recently, Barton et al. (1985) have shown, in vitro, that a positive blood sensitization and a positive alveolar lymphocyte sensitization can occur in rats.

Rabbits in which delayed hypersensitivity to beryllium sulphate has been induced develop antigen-specific alveolar macrophage migration inhibition. Beryllium sulphate is highly toxic to isolated alveolar macrophages in vitro causing swelling of mitochondria and disruption of the cell membrane and cellular sap, but, in striking contrast to the situation so far observed in humans and guinea-pigs, it depresses lymphocyte transformation in sensitized rabbits which show delayed skin reactivity and macrophage inhibition (Kang et al., 1977). Species difference might explain the depressed lymphocyte response but this requires clarification.

Immunological aspects

It has long been suggested that beryllium disease is mediated by immunological factors as evidenced by the positive skin-patch test, together with a low attack rate, around 1 per cent, variable, up to 20 years' latent period between exposure and development of disease (Jones Williams, 1993) and an apparent lack of a dose relationship (Sterner and Eisenbud, 1951). As the beryllium ion is too small to act as a complete antigen, it probably achieves

Beryllium patch test

Hypersensitivity to beryllium may be detected by the development of an erythematous reaction in 48 to 72 hours after patch testing with a solution of beryllium sulphate or nitrate (Curtis, 1959). Skin granulomas may develop in the patch area after 3 to 4 weeks. However, a positive response may occur in beryllium-exposed individuals with acute dermatitis or granulomatous lesions but no systemic involvement in the lungs or elsewhere; a small proportion of patients with chronic disease do not react at all (Stoeckle, Hardy and Weber, 1969). Furthermore, as Curtis showed, the test itself can induce hypersensitivity because control individuals with no beryllium exposure who are negative on initial testing react positively when the test is repeated. For these reasons, and the further possibility that exacerbation of existing beryllium disease might be provoked (Sneddon, 1955), it is generally regarded as unsuitable in clinical and industrial medical practice. However, Jones Williams, Nosworthy and Williams (1980) found that there were no complications in 20 patch-tested cases of beryllium disease, 16 of which were positive. A positive reaction is reversed by corticosteroids (Norris and Peard, 1963; Ambrosi et al., 1968).

Kveim test

The Kveim test is usually negative (Stoeckle, Hardy and Weber, 1969; Jones Williams, Nosworthy and Williams, 1980) and, provided that the Kveim suspension exhibits little cross-reactivity (Siltzbach, 1976), it is a valuable adjunct to differential diagnosis. It is of interest, however, that beryllium was detected by LAMMS analysis, in two Kveim-negative (without granulomas) sites, of four beryllium patients and taken as evidence of widespread dissemination (Jones Williams and Wallach, 1989). However, the Kveim test is negative in 10 to 15 per cent of cases of subacute and in 30 to 35 per cent of cases of chronic sarcoidosis (Mitchell et al., 1977). Prospective study of the Kveim test in a large number of cases of beryllium disease does not appear to have been carried out, but was reported as negative in 15 cases of chronic beryllium disease in the *UK Case Registry* (Jones Williams, 1993).

Tuberculin test

Although the response to the tuberculin test has not been studied with the same epidemiological vigour in beryllium disease as in sarcoidosis, and available evidence indicates that it is generally negative in chronic disease (Stoeckle, Hardy and Weber, 1969; Izumi et al, 1976; Price et al., 1977; Jones Williams, Nosworthy and Williams, 1980), in a factory survey in Japan there appeared to be a tendency for more healthy beryllium workers to be non-reactors than comparable groups of non-exposed workers. This was thought to imply beryllium sensitization and, possibly, an increased risk of developing beryllium disease (Izumi et al., 1976). However, continuing study of these workers over a further 3 years has not supported this. Three new cases of beryllium disease were tuberculin positive before its onset and negative at the time of diagnosis (Nishikawa and Izumi, 1980).

The behaviour of the lepromin reaction in chronic disease is not known.

Lymphocyte function

Due to disadvantages of using the patch test, there have been considerable developments in 'in vitro' tests of cellular immunity using peripheral and, more recently, bronchoalveolar lavage (BAL) lymphocytes.

It has been shown that sensitized T lymphocytes, on challenge with the relevant antigen, release a variety of lymphokines whose detection is thus an index of cellular, type IV, immunity (Bloom and Bennett, 1966). Two main tests have been examined: *macrophage migration inhibition factor* (MIF) and *lymphocyte transformation* (LT). Both are dependent on the incubation of lymphocytes with soluble beryllium salts. MIF can be detected either directly, using peripheral blood leucocytes, or indirectly by adding supernatants to guinea-pig macrophages. LT is best assessed by detection of incorporated tritiated thymidine in the transformed blast cells.

Peripheral blood lymphocytes

Early MIF results were encouraging, showing high positivity in small numbers of chronic cases with negative results in control subjects (Henderson et al., 1972; Marx and Burrell, 1973). Later results (Price et al., 1977), even with technical improvements (Williams and Jones Williams, 1982), proved disappointing, reproducibility was poor and control experiments failed to show an expected incidence of tuberculin sensitization in a normal population. Positive tests are suppressed by steroids but may reverse following discontinuation for 3 weeks. The LT test has now been shown to be superior to the MIF test (Williams and Jones Williams, 1982) and is in common use. Based mainly on visual scoring to enumerate blast transformation, Preuss, Deodhar and Van Ordstrand (1980) found a positive rate of 57 per cent of 47 patients, with weak positives in 6 per cent of healthy, potentially exposed beryllium workers and negative results in control subjects.

In a later study (Jones Williams and Williams, 1985), all of 16 patients tested yielded positive results with a total of 29 out of 31 in the UK Beryllium Registry (Jones Williams, 1993). Similar high positive rates of 16 out of 17 have been reported from the USA (Mroz et al., 1991).

It is concluded that the beryllium lymphocyte transformation test identifies sensitivity to beryllium and correlates with the presence of disease. What of the positive tests in otherwise healthy beryllium workers? This demonstrates that sensitivity is not necessarily an indication of disease, although recent findings using both blood and BAL lymphocyte tests coupled with lung biopsies suggest the presence of latent disease.

BAL lymphocytes

As shown by LT testing, BAL lymphocytes appear to be more responsive to beryllium stimulation than those from peripheral blood. Rossman et al. (1988) investigated 14 beryllium patients with proven pulmonary granulomas and found positive BAL transformation in all compared to only 6 (42 per cent) using blood lymphocytes. In 16 sarcoid and 6 normal subjects, the BAL test was negative, although using blood lymphocytes the test was positive in 3 sarcoid and in 2 normal subjects. None was on steroid therapy. Saltini et al. (1989) also found that BAL lymphocytes are more sensitive to beryllium than those from the peripheral blood. They showed that the involved cells are T-helper lymphocytes and that beryllium acts as a class II restricted antigen stimulating local proliferation of beryllium-specific T-helper lung lymphocytes. In another comparative study (Newman et al., 1989), only 7 of 12 cases showed enhanced BAL responses compared to blood. Positive BAL lymphocyte transformation tests have also been reported from Japan (Chihara et al., 1983) and in one of twins from the UK who initially had a negative but later a much weaker positive blood test (McConnochie et al., 1988).

There is now additional evidence to support the suggestion (Jones Williams and Williams, 1983) that LT testing is of value in monitoring the health of workers in beryllium-using industries. In a German study, 3 of 23 apparently healthy beryllium workers showed a positive blood LT test compared to only 1 of 20 other unexposed workers from the same factory. Two of the three were later diagnosed as chronic cases, on clinical, physiological and radiological grounds; the third subject remains well (Bargon et al., 1986). This contrasts with the Cardiff experience when both positive subjects (2 of 117) remained well up to 6 years later.

There is some evidence that positive LT tests may indeed be a marker of latent, preclinical disease. Newman et al. (1989) found that transbronchial biopsies of four of five LT-positive beryllium workers with little or no symptoms and thus unsuspected disease showed granulomas and claims that

the test definitely identified 'preclinical disease'. Though flawed by lack of tissue analysis, as with other workers, the BAL transformation was higher than the blood test.

Thus, all the present evidence confirms that chronic beryllium disease is mediated by cellular immunity and that in vitro tests of lymphocyte reactivity are of value in diagnosis and have a role in worker health surveillance (see page 589).

Criteria for diagnosis

Diagnosis is often difficult in view of the protean manifestations of the disease and its resemblance to other granulomatous disorders – especially sarcoidosis; at times, diagnosis may be impossible. Prolonged observation of the patient is sometimes needed before the diagnosis can be made with any certainty.

The criteria upon which diagnosis is made are now generally agreed, although emphasis on individual features may differ (Tepper, Hardy and Chamberlin, 1961; Jones Williams, 1977; Kriebel et al., 1988). These are: (1) history of exposure; (2) presence of granulomas in affected tissues; (3) detection of beryllium in tissue, particularly in granulomas; (4) evidence of hypersensitivity; (5) consistent clinical, radiographic and physiological features; and (6) exclusion of other granulomatous diseases.

History of exposure
This is an essential requirement. It may demand a most comprehensive enquiry into occupational details over at least 20 years, and the possibility of unsuspected exposure in such work as scrap metal reclamation and welding operations that may involve beryllium alloys. Furthermore, the possibility of para-occupational exposure (such as work near an annealing furnace) must be borne in mind. In some instances the manufacturer may be able to supply a detailed analysis of processes involved and the concentrations of beryllium in the workplace air over a period of some years.

Presence of granulomas
Although the hallmark of disease, these are indistinguishable from those in other disease and are, thus, not diagnostic (see 'Pathology').

Beryllium in tissues
Without evidence of beryllium in tissues, the diagnosis is always in doubt. Bulk analysis should be

Table 17.2 Comparison of chronic beryllium disease (CBD), sarcoidosis (S) and extrinsic allergic alveolitis (EAA)*: clinical features

Features	CBD	S(%)	EAA
Occupational exposure	Yes	No	Yes
Respiratory symptoms	Marked	Often minimal	Marked
Weight loss	Common	Rare	Rare
Erythema nodosum	Rare	30	Rare
Skin lesions	Implantation	30	No
Uveitis	No	27	No
Peripheral lymphadenopathy	No	27	No
Splenomegaly	Rare	12	No
Salivary glands	No	4	No
Central nervous system	Very rare	4	No
Beryllium patch test	Positive	No	No
Negative tuberculin	? Increase	66	Normal
Positive Kveim test	No	80	No
Prognosis	Poor	Good	Good

* Incidence based on James and Jones Williams (1985).

Table 17.3 Comparison of chronic beryllium disease (CBD), sarcoidosis (S) and extrinsic allergic alveolitis (EAA)*: radiographic and laboratory features

Features	CBD (%)	S (%)	EAA (%)
BHL	Rare	65	No
Bone cysts	No	3	No
Serum precipitins	No	No	Yes
Lymphocyte transformation	Yes	No	No
Raised serum ACE	Occasional	60	Occasional
Granulomas	100	100	100 acute not chronic
Alveolitis	Prominent	Inconspicuous	Prominent
Schaumann bodies	62	70	5
Fibrosis	100	10	10
Presence of beryllium	Yes	No	No

*Incidence based on James and Jones Williams (1985).

coupled with microscopic detection within granulomas. The finding of beryllium within granulomas is diagnostic of disease. Results of urine analysis are of less value (see page 583).

Evidence of hypersensitivity
The majority of, if not all, cases show in vitro lymphocyte sensitization. The tests may, however, be positive without other evidence of disease and so it is not always diagnostic (see 'Immunology').

Clinical, radiographic and physiological features
It is required that all are consistent with the diagnosis but none is specific (see earlier).

Exclusion of other granulomatous diseases
The major source of confusion is sarcoidosis, although others must be considered. Confusion may be compounded in that beryllium patients are not

immune from developing sarcoidosis (see 'Differential diagnosis').

In conclusion, a history of exposure is mandatory and, with beryllium-containing granulomas, it is diagnostic. Positive beryllium LT tests are strongly supportive of the diagnosis and may indicate subclinical disease. In the absence of a definite history and with negative analysis, every effort must be made to exclude other granulomatous diseases (Jones Williams, 1993).

Differential diagnosis

(James and Jones Williams, 1985)

A major cause of confusion is the identical morphology of granulomas in a wide variety of diseases.

Having excluded infective agents, sarcoidosis poses the most common problem and, to a lesser extent, extrinsic allergic alveolitis.

Infective agents

It is vitally important to exclude *Mycobacterium tuberculosis*, in particular miliary tuberculosis, by special stains and culture. In endemic areas, e.g. Ohio, *Histoplasma capsulatum* may mimic tuberculosis and sarcoidosis as well as beryllium disease. Histoplasmin skin and complement fixation tests are useful. Special stains and culture may be required which will assist also in excluding other fungi such as *Coccidioides* sp., *Aspergillus* sp., and *Cryptococcus* sp. Propionibacteria and *Yersinia* sp. are other bacteria that cause similar granulomas.

Sarcoidosis (Tables 17.2 and 17.3)

The merging of clinical, radiographic, physiological and histological features of sarcoidosis with those of chronic beryllium disease often may be confusing (Hardy, 1956). It is not always possible to be certain of occupational exposure, tissue may not be available for histology and tissue analysis unavailable. The following features, in particular, favour a diagnosis of sarcoidosis, with clinical evidence of extrapulmonary disease: erythema nodosum, spontaneous skin lesions, uveitis, peripheral lymphadenopathy and splenomegaly and, radiologically, the presence of bilateral hilar lymphadenopathy (BHL), in the absence of parenchymal changes, with spontaneous resolution. The diagnosis of sarcoidosis is supported by a positive Kveim test in association with a negative tuberculin test and, in lung biopsies, a paucity of alveolitis compared to granulomas.

Extrinsic allergic alveolitis
(Tables 17.2 and 17.3)

With the increasing recognition of the large variety of usually organic antigens capable of producing very similar clinical and pathological changes, a history of possible exposure should always be obtained. The agents range from *Thermoactinomycetes* sp. (farmers' lung), to avian protein (pigeon fanciers' lung), and to amoebae and humidifier lung. The diagnosis is dependent on a history of exposure, direct response to antigenic challenge, presence of circulating precipitins (although these may be present without evidence of disease), the rarity of extra-pulmonary lesions and absence of bilateral hilar lymphadenopathy. On histology, alveolitis is prominent and granulomas are most conspicuous around small airways.

Other pneumoconioses

In general, these rarely cause any difficulty as granulomas are absent. However, there are two rare examples: aluminium (DeVuyst et al., 1987) and titanium (Redline et al., 1986) hypersensitivity granulomas (see Chapter 11, page 254). Both metals may not only be granulogenic but are also associated with positive in vitro lymphocyte transformation, indicating delayed hypersensitivity. The diagnosis can be confirmed by the finding of the metal within granulomas, but care is required in that both, particularly aluminium, are found in considerable amounts in normal lungs (Jones Williams and Wallach, 1989).

Medical surveillance

From the foregoing, general industrial hygiene must be of a high standard. In the UK, beryllium disease, in any of its forms, is notifiable under the terms of the Factories Act 1961 (Section 83) and similar legislation is enforced in the USA. Careful records need to be kept of atmospheric pollution and, in high-risk areas, both workplace and individual machine exhaust ventilation are advisable. It is good practice not to employ workers with known respiratory disease or allergies, although such a population is not proven to be at greater risk. Pre-employment and regular clinical examination, together with chest radiographs, are considered necessary and will help to identify early disease. Routine lung function tests are probably not of value and routine blood counts serve no purpose. There is a case for pre-employment and periodic lymphocyte transformation tests because sensitization, although not proven, may delineate workers at increased risk (see 'Immunology'). Due to often-recorded, long latent periods between exposure and development of disease, medical supervision of ex-workers should be continued for up to 20 years.

References

Abraham, J.L. (1980) Microanalysis of human granulomatous lesions. In *Eighth International Conference on Sarcoidosis and Other Granulomatous Diseases* (eds W. Jones Williams and B.H. Davies), Alpha Omega Publishing, Cardiff, pp. 767–768

Agate, J.N. (1948) Delayed pneumonitis in a beryllium worker. *Lancet* **2**, 530–533

Ambrosi, L., Sartorelli, E., Sbertoli, C. and Secchi, G.C (1968) Two cases of chronic pulmonary granulomatosis caused by beryllium. *Med. Lav.* **59**, 321–333

Andrews, J.L., Kazemi, H. and Hardy, H.L. (1969) Patterns of lung dysfunction in chronic beryllium disease. *Am. Rev. Respir. Dis.* **100**, 791–800

Balmes, J.R., Cullen, M.R. and Robins, J.M. (1984) Epidemic chronic beryllium disease among scrap metal refiners. In *Occupational Lung Diseases* (eds J.B. Gee, W.T.C. Morgan and S.M. Brooks), Raven Press, New York, pp. 225

Bargon, J., Kronenberger, H., Bergman, N.L., Buhl, R., Meier-Sydow, J. and Mitron, P. (1986) Lymphocyte transformation test in a group of foundry workers exposed to beryllium and non exposed controls. *Eur. J. Respir. Dis.* **69**, (Suppl 146), 211–215

Barna, B.P., Chiang, T., Phillarisetti, S.G. and Deodhar, S.D. (1981) Immunologic studies of experimental beryllium lung disease in the guinea-pig. *Clin. Immunol. Immunopathol.* **20**, 402–411

Barton, R.W., Votto, J.J., Thrall, R.S. and McCormick, J.R. (1985) Granulomatous lung disease induced by endotracheal administration of beryllium in rat. *Sarcoidosis* **2**, 53

Bloom, B.R. and Bennett, B. (1966) Mechanism of a reaction 'in vitro' associated with delayed type hypersensitivity. *Science* **153**, 80–82

Buckley, C.E. and Dorsey, F.C. (1970) A comparison of serum immunoglobulin concentrations in sarcoidosis and tuberculosis. *Ann. Intern. Med.* **72**, 37–42

Chatterjee, T.K. and Pooley, F.D. (1977) Examination of some trace elements in South Wales coals. *Proceedings of the Australian Institute of Mining and Metallurgy*, No. 263

Chihara, J., Nagai, S., Fujimura, N., Hirata, T and Izumi, T. (1983) BAL lymphocyte findings in chronic beryllium disease (abstract), *Am. Rev. Respir. Dis.* **127**(4), Part 2, 64

Cirla, A.M., Barbiano di Belgiojoso, G. and Chiappino, G. (1968) La iperensibilita ai composti di berillio; trasferimento passivo nella cavia mediante cellule linfoidi. *Boll. Ist. Sieroter. Milan* **47**, 663–668

Cullen, M.R., Kominsky, J.R., Rossman, M.D., Cherniack, M.G., Daniele, R.P., Palmer, L., Nagel, G.P., McManus, K and Cruz, R. (1987) Chronic beryllium disease in a precious metal refinery. *Am. Rev. Respir. Dis.* **135**, 201–208

Curtis, G.H. (1959) The diagnosis of beryllium disease, with special reference to the patch test. *Archs Ind. Health* **19**, 150–153

Doedhar, S.D., Barna, B. and Van Ordstrand, H.S. (1973) A study of the immunological aspects of chronic berylliosis. *Chest* **63**, 309–313

DeVuyst, P., DuMortimer, P., Schandene, L., Estenne, M., Verhest, A. and Yernault, J.C. (1987) Sarcoid like granulomatosis induced by aluminium. *Am. Rev. Respir. Dis.* **135**, 493–499

Dinsdale, D. and Bourdillon, A.J. (1982) The ultrastructural localisation of the presence of beryllium in pulmonary granulomas. *Expl Mol. Pathol.* **36**, 396–402

Eisenbud, M. and Lisson, J. (1983) Epidemiological aspects of beryllium induced non malignant lung disease: A 30 year up date. *J. Occup. Med.* **25**, 196–202

Epstein, W.L. and Byers, V. (1979) Transfer of contact sensitivity to beryllium using dialysable leukocyte extracts (transfer factor). *J. Allergy Clin. Immunol.* **63**, 11–115

Freiman, D.G. and Hardy, H.L. (1970) Beryllium disease. *Human. Pathol.* **1**, 25–44

Gibbs, A.R., Jones Willams, W. and Kelland, D. (1987) Necrotising Sarcoidal Granulomatosis. *Sarcoidosis* **4**, 94–100

Goldstein, R.A., Israel, H.L. and Rawnsley, H.M. (1969) Effect of race and stage of disease on the serum immunoglobulins in sarcoidosis. *J. Am. Med. Assoc.* **208**, 1153–1155

Griggs, K. (1973) Toxic metal fumes from mantle-type camp lanterns. *Science* **181**, 842–843

Hardy, H.L. (1955) Epidemiology, clinical character and treatment of beryllium poisoning. *Archs Ind. Health* **11**, 273–279

Hardy, H.L. (1956) Differential diagnosis between beryllium poisoning and sarcoidosis. *Am. Rev. Tuberc.* **74**, 885–896

Hardy, H.L. (1980) Beryllium disease: a clinical perspective. *Environ. Res.* **21**, 1–9

Hardy, H.L. and Chamberlin, R.I. (1972) Beryllium disease. In *Toxicology of Beryllium* (ed. Irving R. Tabershaw). US Department of Health, Education and Welfare, Public Health Service Publication No. 2173, pp. 9–16

Hardy, H.L. and Tabershaw, J.R. (1946) Delayed chemical pneumonitis occurring in workers to beryllium compounds. *J. Ind. Hyg. Toxicol.* **28**, 197–211

Hardy, H.L., Rabe, E.W. and Lorch, S. (1967) United States Beryllium Case Registry (1952–1966). *J. Occup. Med.* **9**, 271–276

Hart, B.A. and Pittman, D.G. (1980) the uptake of beryllium by the alveolar macrophage. *J. Reticuloendothel Soc.* **27**, 49–58

Hasan, F.M. and Kazemi, H. (1974) Chronic beryllium disease: a continuing epidemiological hazard. *Chest* **65**, 289–293

Hazard, J.B. (1959) Pathologic changes of beryllium disease. *Archs Ind. Health* **19**, 179–183

Henderson, W.R., Fukuyama, K., Epstein, W.L. and Spitler, L.E. (1972) *In vitro* demonstration of delayed hypersensitivity in patients with berylliosis. *J. Invest. Dermatol.* **58**, 5–8

Hooper, W.F. (1981) Acute beryllium lung disease. *NC Med. J.* **42**, 551–553

Infante, P.F., Wagoner, J.K. and Sprince, N.L. (1980) Mortality patterns from lung cancer and non-neoplastic respiratory disease among white males in the Beryllium Case Registry. *Environ. Res.* **21**, 35–43

Izumi, T., Kobara, Y., Inui, S., Tokunaga, R., Orita, Y., Kitano, M. and Jones Williams, W. (1976) The first seven cases of chronic beryllium disease in ceramic factory workers in Japan. *Ann. NY Acad. Sci.* **278**, 636–652

James, E.M.V. and Jones Williams, W. (1974) Fine structure and histochemistry of epithelioid cells in sarcoidosis. *Thorax* **29**, 115–120

James, D.G. and Jones Williams, W. (1985) *Sarcoidosis and Other Granulomatous Disorders*, Series No. 24, *Major Problems in Internal Medicine*. W.B. Saunders, Philadelphia.

Jones Williams, W. (1958) A histological study of lungs in 52 cases of chronic beryllium disease. *Br. J. Ind. Med.* **15**, 84–91

Jones Williams, W. (1960) The nature and origin of Schaumann Bodies. *J. Pathol. Bacteriol.* **79**, 193–201

Jones Williams, W. (1977) Beryllium disease – pathology and diagnosis. *J. Soc. Occup. Med.* **27**, 93–96

Jones Williams, W. (1985) UK Beryllium Case Registry 1945–1985. *J. Pathol.* **146**, 284A

Jones Williams, W. (1993) Diagnostic criteria for chronic beryllium disease (CBD) based on the UK Registry 1945–1991. *Sarcoidosis* **10**, 41–43

Jones Williams, W. and Kelland, D. (1986) A new aid for diagnosing chronic beryllium disease: Laser Ion Mass Analysis (LIMA). *J. Clin. Pathol.* **39**, 900–901

Jones Williams, W. and Kilpatrick, G.S. (1974) Cutaneous and pulmonary manifestations of chronic beryllium disease. In *Proceedings of the VI International Conference on Sarcoidosis, 1972* (eds. K. Iwai and Y. Hosoda), University of Tokyo, pp. 141–145

Jones Williams, W. and Wallach, R. (1989) Laser Microprobe Mass Spectrometry (LAMMS) analysis of beryllium, sarcoidosis and other granulomatous diseases. *Sarcoidosis* **16**, 111–117

Jones Williams, W. and Williams, D. (1967) 'Residual bodies' in sarcoid and sarcoid-like granulomas. *J. Clin. Pathol.* **20**, 574–577

Jones Williams, W. and Williams, W.R. (1983) Value of beryllium lymphocyte transformation tests in chronic beryllium disease and in potentially exposed workers. *Thorax* **38**, 41–44

Jones Williams, W., Nosworthy, S.E. and Williams, W.R. (1980) UK Beryllium Case Registry *Eighth International Conference on Sarcoidosis and Other Granulomatous Diseases* (eds. W. Jones Williams and B.H. Davies), Alpha Omega Press, Cardiff, p.771

Jones Williams, W., Williams, W.R., Kelland, D. and Holt, P.J.A. (1988) Beryllium skin disease. In *Sarcoidosis and Other Granulomatous Disorders* (eds. C. Grassi, G. Rizzato and E. Pozzi), Excerpta Medica, Amsterdam, International Congress Series 756, pp. 689–690

Kang, K., Bice, D., Hoffman, E., D'Amato, R. and Salvaggio, J. (1977) Experimental studies in sensitization to beryllium, zirconium and aluminium compounds in the rabbit. *J. Allergy Clin. Immun.* **59**, 425–436

Karkinen-Jaaskelainen, M., Matta, K., Pasila, M. and Saxen, L. (1982) Pulmonary berylliosis: Report on a fatal case. *Br. J. Dis. Chest* **76**, 290–297

Klemperer, F.W., Martin, A.P. and Van Riper, J. (1951) Beryllium excretion in humans. *Archs Ind. Hyg.* **4**, 251–256

Kriebel, D., Brain, J.D., Sprince, N.L. and Kazemi, H. (1988) The pulmonary toxicity of beryllium. *Am. Rev. Respir. Dis.* **137**, 464–473

Lieben, J. and Metzner, F. (1959) Epidemiological findings associated with beryllium excretion. *Am. Ind. Hyg. Assoc. J.* **20**, 494–499

Lieben, J., Dattoli, J.A. and Vought, V.M. (1966) The significance of beryllium concentrations in urine. *Archs Environ. Med.* **12**, 331–334

Lieberman, J. (1985) Angiotensin–converting enzyme (ACE) and serum lysozyme in sarcoidosis. In *Sarcoidosis* (ed. J. Lieberman), Grune and Stratton, Orlando, pp. 145–159

McCallum, R.I., Rannie, I. and Verity, C. (1961) Chronic pulmonary berylliosis in a female chemist. *Br. J. Ind Med.* **18**, 133–142

McCarthy, D.S. and Sigurdson, M. (1978) Lung function in pulmonary sarcoidosis. *Irish. J. Med. Sci.* **147**, 413–419

McConnochie, K., Williams, W.R., Kilpatrick, G.S. and Jones Williams, W. (1988) Chronic beryllium disease in identical twins. *Br. J. Dis. Chest* **82**, 431–435

Maceira, J.M.P., Fukyama, K. and Epstein, W.L. (1984) Appearance of T cell subpopulations during the time course of beryllium induced granulomas. *J. Invest. Dermatol.* **83**, 314–316

Mancuso, T.F. (1980) Mortality study of beryllium industry workers' occupational lung cancer. *Environ. Res.* **21**, 48–55

Marx, J.J. and Burrell, R. (1973) Delayed hypersensitivity to beryllium compounds. *J. Immunol.* **111**, 590–598

Mitchell, D.N., Scadding, J.G., Heard, B.E. and Hinson, K.F.W. (1977) Sarcoidosis: histopathological definition and clinical diagnosis. *J. Clin. Pathol.* **30**, 395–408

Mroz, M.M., Kreiss, K., Lezotte, D., Campbell, P.A. and Newman, L.S. (1991) Re-examination of the blood lymphocyte transformation test in the diagnosis of chronic beryllium disease. *J. Allergy Clin. Immunol.* **88**, 54–60

Munro, C.S., Campbell, D.A., Collins, L.A. and Poulter, L.W. (1987) Monoclonal antibodies distinguish macrophages and epithelioid cells in sarcoidosis and leprosy. *Clin. Expl Immunol.* **68**, 282–287

Newman, L.S. and Kreiss, K. (1992) Non-occupational beryllium disease masquerading as sarcoidosis: Identification by blood lymphocyte proliferative responses to beryllium. *Am. Rev. Respir. Dis.* **145**, 1212–1214

Newman, L.S., Kreiss, K., King, T.E., Seay, S. and Campbell, P.A. (1989) Pathologic and immunologic alterations in early stages of beryllium disease. *Am. Rev. Respir. Dis.* **139**, 1479–1486

NIOSH (National Institute of Occupational Safety and Health) (1985) *National Occupational Exposure Survey (NOES)*, Washington DC

Nishikawa, S. and Izumi, T. (1980) A three year prospective study on Mantoux reaction of factory workers exposed to beryllium oxide. *Eighth International Conference on Sarcoidosis and Other Granulomatous Diseases* (eds. W. Jones Williams and B.H. Davies), Alpha Omega Press, Cardiff, pp. 722–727

Norris G.F. and Peard, M.C. (1963) Berylliosis. Report of two cases with special reference to the patch test. *Br. Med. J.* **1**, 378–382

Peyton P.F. and Worcester, J. (1959) Exposure data and epidemiology of the Beryllium Case Registry – 1958. *Am. Archs Ind. Health* **19**, 94

Preuss, O.P. (1975) Beryllium and its compounds. In *Occupational Medicine: Principles and Practical Applications* (ed. C. Zenz) Year Book Medical, Chicago, pp. 619–636

Preuss, O.P., Deodhar, S.D. and Van Ordstrand, H.S. (1980) Lymphoblast transformation in beryllium workers. *Eighth International Conference on Sarcoidosis and Other Granulomatous Diseases* (eds. W. Jones Williams and B.H. Davies), Alpha Omega Press, Cardiff, pp.711–714

Price, C.D., Jones Williams, W. Pugh, A. and Joynson, D.H. (1977) Role of *in vitro* and *in vivo* tests of hypersensitivity in beryllium workers. *J. Clin. Pathol.* **30**, 24–28

Redline, S., Barna, B.P., Tomashefki, J. and Abraham, J.C. (1986) Granulomatous disease associated with pulmonary deposition of titanium. *Br. J. Ind. Med.* **43**, 652–656

Rees, P.J. (1979) Unusual course of beryllium lung disease. *Br. J. Dis. Chest* **73**, 192–194

Reeves, A.L. (1980) Delayed hypersensitivity in experimental pulmonary berylliosis. *Eighth International Conference on Sarcoidosis and Other Granulomatous Diseases* (eds. W. Jones Williams and B.H. Davies), Alpha Omega Press, Cardiff, pp. 715–721

Reeves, A.L., Deitch, D. and Vorwald, A.J. (1967) Beryllium carcinogenesis: Inhalation exposure of rats to beryllium sulphate aerosol. *Cancer Res.* **27**, 439–445

Resnick, H., Roche, M. and Morgan, W.K.C. (1970) Immunoglobulin concentration in berylliosis. *Am. Rev. Respir. Dis.* **101**, 504–510

Robinson, F.R., Brokeshoulder, S.F., Thomas, A.A. and Cholak, J. (1968) Microemission spectrochemical analysis of human lungs for beryllium. *Am. J. Clin. Pathol.* **49**, 821–825

Rossman, M.D., Kern, J.A., Elias, J. A., Cullen, M.R., Epstein, P., Preuss, O.P., Markham, T.N. and Daniele, R.P. (1988) Proliferative response of bronchoalveolar lymphocytes to beryllium. *Ann. Intern. Med.* **108**, 687–693

Saltini, C., Weinstock, K., Kirby, M., Pinkston, P. and Crystal, R.G. (1989) Maintenance of alveolitis in chronic beryllium disease by beryllium-specific helper T cells. *N. Engl. J. Med.* **320**, 1103–1109

Selroos, O. and Grönhagen-Riska, C. (1979) Angiotensin converting enzyme. III Changes in serum level as an indicator of disease activity in untreated sarcoidosis. *Scand. J. Respir. Dis.* **60**, 328–336

Selroos, O., Tiitinen, C., Grönhagen-Riska, C., Fyhrquist, F. and Klockars, M. (1980) Angiotensin-converting enzyme and lysozyme in sarcoidosis. In *Eighth International Conference on Sarcoidosis and Other Granulomatas Diseases* (eds. W. Jones Williams and B.H. Davies), Alpha Omega Press, Cardiff, pp. 303–310

Siltzbach, L.E. (1976) Qualities and behaviour of satisfactory Kveim suspensions. *Ann. NY Acad. Sci.* **278**, 665–668

Sneddon, I.B. (1955) Berylliosis: a case report *Br. Med. J.* **1**, 1448–1449

Sprince, N.L. and Kazemi, H. (1980) US Beryllium Case Registry through 1977. *Environ. Res.* **21**, 44–47

Sprince, N.L. and Kazemi, H. (1983) Beryllium disease. In *Environmental and Occupational Medicine*, 1st ed. (ed. E. Rom), Little Brown, Boston, pp. 481–490

Sprince. N.L. Kazemi, H. and Fanburg, B.L. (1980) Serum angiotensin I converting enzyme in chronic beryllium disease. *Eighth International Conference on Sarcoidosis and Other Granulomatous Diseases* (eds. W. Jones Williams and B.H. Davies), Alpha Omega Press, Cardiff, pp. 287–2890

Sprince, N.L., Kazemi, H. and Hardy, H.L. (1976) Current (1975) problem of differentiating between beryllium disease and sarcoidosis. *Ann. NY Acad. Sci.* **278**, 654–664

Sprince, N.L., Kanarek, D.J., Weber, A.L., Chamberlin, R.I. and Kazemi, H. (1978) Reversible respiratory disease in beryllium workers. *Am. Rev. Respir. Dis.* **117**, 1011–1017

Steenland, K. and Ward, E. (1991) Lung cancer incidence among patients with beryllium disease. A cohort study. *J. natl Cancer Inst.* **83**, 1380–1385

Sterner, J.H. and Eisenbud, M. (1951) Epidemiology of beryllium intoxication *Archs Ind. Hyg.* **4**, 123–151

Stoeckle, J.D., Hardy, H.L. and Weber, A.L. (1969) Chronic beryllium disease. *Am. J. Med.* **46**, 545–561

Studdy, P.R. and James, D.G. (1983) The specificity and sensitivity of serum angiotensin converting enzyme in sarcoidosis and other diseases. Experience in twelve centres in six different countries. In *Ninth International Conference on Sarcoidosis and Other Granulomatous Disorders* (eds. J. Chretien, J. Marsac and J.C. Saltiel), Pergamon, Paris, pp. 332–344

Sussman, V.H., Lieben, J. and Cleland, J.G. (1959) An air-pollution study of a community surrounding a beryllium plant. *Am. Ind. Hyg. Assoc. J.* **20**, 504–508

Tepper, L.B., Hardy, H.L. and Chamberlin, R.I. (1961) *The Toxicity of Beryllium Compounds.* Elsevier, Amsterdam.

Underwood, A.L. (1951) *Studies on the Renal Excretion of Beryllium.* (USAEC Report UR–171.) University of Rochester

US Public Health Service (1988) *Toxicological Profile for Beryllium.* A.T.S.D.R/T.P.–88/07, E.P.A. 5, 1987

Utidjian, H.M.D. (1973) Criteria for recommended standards: occupational exposure to beryllium and its compounds. *J. Occup. Med.* **15**, 659–665

Van Furth, R., Diesselhoff den Dulk, M.M.C., Raeburn, J.A., Van Zwet, T.L., Crofton, R. and Blusse Van Oud Alblas, A. (1980) Characteristics, origin and kinetics of human and murine mononuclear phagocytes. In *Mononuclear Phagocytes* (ed. R. Van Furth), Martinus Nijhoff, The Hague, pp. 279–298

Van Ordstrand, H.S., Hughes, R. and Carmody, M.G. (1943) Chemical pneumonia in workers extracting beryllium oxide. *Cleveland Clin. Q.* **10**, 10–18

Vorwald, A.J. (1966) Medical aspects of beryllium disease. In *Beryllium. Its Industrial Hygiene Aspects* (ed. H.E. Stokinger), Academic Press, London, pp. 167–200

Wagoner, J.K., Infante, P.F. and Bayliss, D.L. (1980) Beryllium and etiological agent in the induction of lung cancer, non-neoplastic respiratory disease and heart disease among industrially exposed workers. *Environ. Res.* **21**, 15–34

Weber, A.L., Stoeckle, J.D. and Hardy, H.L. (1965) Roentgenologic patterns in long-standing beryllium disease. *Am. J. Roentgenol.* **93**, 879–890

Weber H.H. and Engelhardt, WE. (1933) Über eine Apparatur zur Erzeugung niedriger Staubkonzentrationen von grosser Konstanz und eine Methode zur mikrogravinctrischen Staubbestimmung. Anwendung bei der Untersuchang con Stauben aus der Beryllium gewinnung. *Zentrabl. Gewerbehyg. Unfallerhüt.* **10**, 41–47

Williams, D., Jones Williams, W. and Williams, J.E. (1969) Enzyme histochemistry of epitheliod cells in sarcoidosis and sarcoid-like granulomas. *J. Pathol.* **97**, 705–709

Williams, W.R. and Jones Williams, W. (1982) Comparison of lymphocyte transformation and macrophage migration inhibition tests in the detection of beryllium hypersensitivity. *J. Clin. Pathol.* **35**, 684–687

18

Non-neoplastic disorders due to metallic, chemical and physical agents

H.A. Waldron

In this chapter the various topics are considered under the broad categories of metals and chemical agents; it ends with a consideration of the respiratory hazards associated with welding, fire-smoke and near-drowning.

Metals and metalloids

Metalloids are elements that have some but not all the properties of true metals; those to be considered here include antimony, boron and selenium.

Metal fume fever

This is a relatively common, non-specific and self-limiting acute illness which most closely resembles an attack of influenza. It goes under a variety of names in different trades, including *brass founders' ague*, *welders' ague*, *copper fever*, *Monday morning fever*, *smelters' chills*, *zinc chills* and the *smothers*. It is caused chiefly by exposure to the fumes of zinc, copper and magnesium but may be less frequently caused by aluminium, antimony, cadmium, iron, manganese, mercury, nickel and tin. It is due to the inhalation of particles of these metals ranging in size from 0.05 to 0.5 μm formed when the metals are heated to their melting points in an oxidizing atmosphere. The symptoms are most probably due to a direct toxic action possibly involving the chemotaxis of neutrophils; it is unlikely that there is an immunological basis to the condition.

It occurs in welding, galvanizing and smelting operations and in the arc-air gouging process involving these metals especially under enclosed or poorly ventilated conditions (Sanderson, 1968). Thus, it is most commonly encountered among shipyard and other metal workers, and foundry men. Sculptors working in metal may be affected. Copper *dust* from the polishing of copper plates and from other sources may produce an identical syndrome but the term 'metal fume fever' cannot properly be applied to it (Gleason, 1968).

The illness commences a few hours after exposure and consists of thirst, dry cough, dry throat, nausea, headache, rigors, profuse sweating, fatigue, pains in the limbs, aching in the chest and dyspnoea without wheezing. The temperature rises to 38.9°C (102°F) or higher, and there is polymorphonuclear leucocytosis.

Functionally, Sturgist et al. (1927) found a 50 per cent reduction in vital capacity during the acute phase of zinc fume fever after inhalation of zinc oxide fume by normal persons, and considerable reduction in FEV_1 and FVC occurred 4 to 6 hours after specific inhalation challenges of zinc oxide fume in the working environment in a worker who had previously experienced zinc fume fever (Malo et al., 1990). A clear decrease of peak flow was also observed by Nemery and Damedts (1991) during the melting of copper, zinc and aluminium, lasting well into the following day in a metallurgical engineer suspected of having had metal fume fever.

Complete recovery is usual in 24 to 48 hours and the man is able to return to work. No permanent pulmonary damage occurs.

An excess of neutrophils, but not lymphocytes, has been noted in bronchoalveolar lavage fluid of a welder with zinc fume fever (Vogelmeier et al., 1987). In guinea-pigs, inhalation of 5 mg/m³ ultra-fine zinc oxide particles for 3 hours a day for 6 days caused interstitial oedema with infiltration by inflammatory cells, which also involved the alveolar ducts and alveoli (Lam et al., 1985).

Radiographic abnormalities during the illness have rarely been recorded, and were not mentioned in the earlier editions of this book. However, Langham Brown (1988) has described a case of a zinc sprayer (using molten zinc) in a shipyard who, after 6 hours' exposure, developed typical symptoms with a few crackles at the lung bases and widespread, bilateral, multiple, discrete opacities 3 to 4 mm in diameter with a tendency to confluence in the posteroanterior radiograph. A film taken 4 days later was normal. Similar, though less prominent, opacities, which also cleared within a few days, were reported by Malo et al. (1990) in a man who sprayed heated zinc onto iron jointing rings for concrete pipes. It seems probable that these changes have not been recognized because chest radiographs have rarely been taken at the time of the acute illness. For this reason, the frequency of their occurrence and whether or not they are also associated with inhalation of other metal fumes is not known. Certainly, zinc fume fever should be considered in the differential diagnosis of bilateral, discrete opacities in an acute illness of obscure cause in an otherwise fit patient of working age (Langham Brown, 1988).

One curious feature of metal fume fever is that men who are continuously exposed to the metal fume, which can bring on the symptoms, develop a tolerance to them. This tolerance is lost, however, after a short period away from work so that it recurs on the first day back; this is the explanation for the name Monday morning fever. The underlying cause of this phenomenon is not clear. No specific IgG antibodies have been detected in zinc fume fever (Malo et al., 1990).

The illness is well understood by those at risk and they are able to make the diagnosis themselves. Some of those who are severely affected or find the symptoms unacceptable may seek other employment.

Diagnosis may require differentiation from a wide variety of quite febrile disorders. Polymer fume fever, the features of which are identical apart from the fact that tolerance of exposure does not develop, is referred to in Chapter 23.

Treatment is symptomatic, consisting usually of rest, fluids and analgesics but, in severe illness, supplemental oxygen and corticosteroids may be necessary.

Aluminium

Respiratory risks from aluminium arise during the refining of its principal ore, *bauxite*, during the smelting of aluminium oxide to the metal, following exposure to abrasives manufactured from aluminium oxide (*corundum*) and following exposure to aluminium dust.

Sources of exposure

Refining of bauxite

Bauxite is a mixture of aluminium oxide, hydroxide and oxyhydroxide and it also contains iron oxide, titanium dioxide and aluminosilicate minerals (see Appendix I). The ore contains from 37 to 59 per cent of aluminium oxide from which the various combinations of aluminium, oxygen and hydrogen, known as *aluminas*, are extracted. The three aluminas extracted – aluminium trihydroxide [$Al(OH)_3$], aluminium oxyhydroxide (AlOOH) and aluminium oxide (Al_2O_3) – are heated to different temperatures to obtain materials with the physicochemical properties desired for the commercial uses to which they are later put. During heating water is lost and transitional forms of alumina are produced. Those formed by heating between 250 and 500°C have a much increased surface area and increased catalytic activity; it has been suggested that some of these transitional aluminas may be biologically active (Dinman, 1988). In recent years there has been a trend towards the use of less highly heated aluminas for smelting.

It is generally accepted that aluminium oxide is inert and its occupational exposure standard is based on the assumption that it is a nuisance dust only. Early studies of workers exposed to aluminium oxide (Sutherland, Meiklejohn and Price, 1937; Meiklejohn, 1963) seemed to confirm that exposure to this material was without adverse effects. Later experiments, however, indicated that some transitional forms of alumina were able to induce pulmonary fibrosis in animals when administered by the intratracheal route (King, Harrison and Mohanty, 1955; Stacy et al., 1959). Studies in which rats were exposed to synthetic fibrous alumina (Pigott, Gaskell and Ishmael, 1981) failed to show that it was either fibrogenic or carcinogenic.

Two cross-sectional studies of workers exposed to aluminium oxide have shown some changes in lung function and in chest radiographs (Townsend et al., 1985, 1988). The first study was of 1109 workers in a smelter which prepared a number of different aluminas, including some of the more active transitional forms. A decrement in FEV_1 was noted, but the effect of the alumina dust was far less marked than that of smoking. In the second study, which included 788 subjects, scanty, small, irregular opacities were found in the radiographs in slightly under 8 per cent. The prevalence was greater in smokers than in non-smokers, although in non-smokers with high cumulative exposure there was a moderate increase in prevalence with increasing duration of exposure. There was no increase in rounded opacities. In their summary of these findings, Morgan and Dinman (1989) suggest that the reduction in pulmonary function was most probably the result of the development of industrial bronchitis which is a non-specific response to dust exposure, and they emphasize that smoking had a much more deleterious effect on the lungs than exposure to aluminium oxide (see Chapter 10).

Aluminium smelting

Aluminium is prepared from its oxide by an electrolytic reduction process in which the oxide is dissolved in synthetic *cryolite* (Na_3AlF_6) in a large pot in which carbon electrodes are placed. A considerable amount of fluoride-containing effluent is produced during the process.

There is evidence to show that those tending the pots (pot-room workers), but not others, develop an asthma-like state which is generally referred to as pot-room asthma. It was first described by Frostad in 1936 in workers in a Norwegian smelter. The prevalence of this disorder varies from country to country with the highest rates (up to 4.5 per cent of workers) reported in Norway (Bruusgaard, 1960). Some authors (Kaltreideer et al., 1972; Discher and Breitenstein, 1976; Chen-Yeung, Wong and McLean, 1982, 1983) have failed to identify it at all, although a higher prevalence of cough and sputum and a lower ventilatory capacity have been noted in the exposed workers as compared with non-exposed controls.

An obstructive pattern in the results of pulmonary function tests is a not infrequent finding in pot-room workers (Field, 1984; Larsson et al., 1989) and some authors have been able to demonstrate bronchial hyperreactivity to challenge with histamine (de Vries et al., 1974) and methacholine. A recent Swedish study has confirmed a modest decrement in FEV_1 (93 per cent of predicted) in pot-room workers but none of the exposed workers had symptoms of airways' obstruction and there was no dose–response relationship between lung function and dust exposure. No evidence of bronchial hyperreactivity was noted. It should be noted that only non-atopic subjects were selected in this study and that environmental conditions were considerably more favourable than in many of the earlier studies; for example, the concentration of air-borne fluorides in the study by de Vries et al. (1974) was 13 times greater.

Bronchoalveolar lavage (BAL) from workers in the Swedish smelter was examined for evidence of alveolar damage but was found to be not much different from non-exposed controls. The concentration of alveolar cells and the distribution of the various cell subpopulations did not differ significantly from non-exposed controls, but the concentrations of albumin and fibronectin were greater, reflecting an increased alveolar capillary permeability and an activation of alveolar macrophages (Eklund et al., 1989). The authors concluded that their results were consistent with a low-grade alveolitis and explained the rather minimal findings as being due to low levels of exposure and the frequent use of respiratory protective equipment.

Summarizing these data, it may be concluded that there is reasonable evidence to support the view that work in pot-rooms may be associated in some cases with the development of signs of obstructive lung disease. The pathogenesis, however, is far from clear and no specific allergen has been identified; it is also not known whether pot-room exposure initiates asthma or merely precipitates symptoms in predisposed individuals (Abramson et al., 1989).

An association between carcinoma of the lung and production of aluminium is discussed in Chapter 19 ('Aluminium production', page 655).

Pulmonary fibrosis
Gilks and Churg (1987) have described a case of pulmonary fibrosis occurring in a Hispanic male who had worked in two aluminium smelters, for a short time pouring molten metal into moulds to make ingots and for a longer period in the pot-room. He died 10 years after the onset of symptoms and the lungs showed 'honeycombing' and fibrosis, particularly in the upper zones. Both fibrous and non-fibrous particles of aluminium were present in vast quantity and it was suggested that the presence of the fibrous material gave rise to the fibrosis in this case.

Abrasives

Abrasives are made from natural emery (which contains 50 to 70 per cent alumina) or from corundum, which is itself formed from calcined bauxite that is mixed with coke and iron and fused in an electric arc furnace to about 2000°C. During this process fumes are given off which contain aluminium oxide and free silica.

Abrasive wheels or emery cloth are produced by compacting loose grains of emery or corundum with silicon carbide. Natural emery seems to have little or no effect on the lungs although there were some early reports of abnormalities in the chest radiograph of workers using abrasives (Clark, 1929; Smith and Perina, 1948). It seems likely that these radiographic changes were due to concomitant exposure to free silica and not to the aluminium oxide.

Shaver's disease

One condition which is at least of historical interest in this connection is Shaver's disease, which occurred in workers engaged in the manufacture of corundum. It was first described by Shaver and Riddell in 1947 and again by Shaver in 1948. The original paper was an account of 23 workers whose main symptoms were those of dsypnoea, wheeze and a productive cough. As the disease progressed the patient became fatigued, weak and emaciated and frequently developed spontaneous pneumothorax heralded by the onset of chest pain. Chest radiographs showed the presence of reticulonodular changes throughout the lung fields which conglomerated, especially in the upper lobes, as the disease progressed. Honeycombing of the lungs, bullae and pneumothoraces were other common abnormalities noted in this condition.

An acute form of the disease was also described which was characterized by cough, fever, tachypnoea and cyanosis; the close resemblance of these symptoms to acute silicosis was evident.

Histologically, the lungs in the acute disease showed alveolar septal thickening and alveolar proteinosis; diffuse interstitial fibrosis was also noted. In the chronic form there were collagenous conglomerate masses with obliterative endarteritis and perivascular fibrosis.

Although it is now clear that this disease was due to exposure to free silica, and in particular to cristobalite (as suggested in the second edition of this book), the lungs of affected individuals seldom showed classic silicotic nodules or evidence of complicated silicosis. Deaths from the disease were usually due to progressive respiratory failure, but there was no increase in the prevalence of respiratory tuberculosis. No new cases of the disease have been reported since 1950 (Morgan and Dinman, 1989), no doubt due to the decreased exposure to free silica.

Aluminium powder

Aluminium powder is prepared in two forms: flakes or granules. Particulate aluminium is produced by spraying molten metal through an atomizer with the generation of spherical or elliptical particles; these are aluminium granules. Flake aluminium is produced by putting granules through a ball mill giving rise to flattened particles that have a very large surface area. To prevent the flakes sticking or impacting together, stearine is added during the milling. The aluminium stearate formed thereby coats the flakes, prevents them adhering, and also

slows down the rate of oxygenation. In the preparation of powder for paint manufacture, the aluminium particles are large and mixed with considerable quantities of stearine.

Pyro

This is a form of aluminium powder of very small particle size (<1 μm diameter) to which only small amounts of stearine are added. It is used, mixed with carbon, in the manufacture of fireworks. In the past great quantities of dust were produced during the manufacture of fireworks and levels of almost 1 mg/m^3 have been recorded (McLaughlin et al., 1962).

'Aluminium lung'

Exposure to aluminium powder may give rise to a form of pulmonary fibrosis described first by Goralewski (1940, 1947, 1950) and referred to by him as *Aluminiumlunge* (aluminium lung). Goralewski's cases were among men who were engaged in the manufacture of pyro which was used for explosives. Early studies in the UK failed to confirm Goralewski's findings, probably because the workers were exposed to particles of non-respirable size. In the late 1950s and early 1960s, however, cases did come to light (Jordan, 1961; Mitchell et al., 1961; McLaughlin et al., 1962).

The first symptoms of aluminium lung are breathlessness on exertion and a dry, non-productive cough. Spontaneous pneumothorax is common, generally preceded by chest pain. As with Shaver's disease, which aluminium lung closely resembles, there is an acute form in which the predominant symptoms are cough, pyrexia and tightness of the chest. Pulmonary fibrosis is the end-point of both forms of the disease, only the speed of onset differentiating them.

The symptoms are accompanied by inspiratory (often coarse) crackles in the lung, sometimes by finger clubbing and, in advanced cases, by cyanosis. Lung function tests show a restrictive type of impairment with an abnormal diffusing capacity. Radiographs may show nodular or coalescent opacities predominantly in the upper and middle zones of the lung fields.

Pathology

Pathological examination of the lungs shows the presence of interstitial fibrosis first affecting the upper lobes. Damaged alveoli are epithelialized and giant cells may be present; there are no silicotic nodules. At the end-stage of the disease, 'honeycombing' may be present with obliterative endarteritis and perivascular fibrosis. The aluminium content of the lung tissue is greatly elevated.

Pathogenesis

It is now known that it is only the aluminium granules that are *not* covered with stearine which are pathogenic. This conclusion was first suggested by Corrin (1963a, b) who proposed that the appearance of cases in the UK might be consequent upon the substitution of mineral oil for stearine during the manufacturing process. He showed that flakes coated with mineral oil react violently with water, whereas those coated with stearine do not. Later animal experiments served to confirm Corrin's observations. Thus, Gross and his colleagues (Gross, Harley and de Treville, 1973) were able to produce focal fibrosis in rats by the intratracheal injection of aluminium dust. However, the chronic inhalation of high concentrations of aluminium fume produced pneumonitis and alveolar proteinosis, but not fibrosis.

It seems probable that aluminium granules that are not coated with stearine are chemically active in the lungs and may undergo exothermic reactions leading to their hydrolysis (Dinman, 1987). Aluminium powder is now produced only with a stearine coat (at least in western Europe and North America) and cases of aluminium lung in these parts of the world should no longer occur.

Aluminium silicate

The report that a worker engaged in handling artificial aluminium silicate (mullite) used for cat litter had developed pulmonary fibrosis (Musk, Greville and Tribe, 1980) led to the supposition that his disease was related to his exposure. A later study of workers exposed to this material and of animals exposed to the material by intratracheal instillation has, however, failed to confirm that aluminium silicate has a significant toxic effect on the lungs (Musk et al., 1988). For more detailed discussion, see Chapter 16 (page 554).

Antimony trichloride and pentachloride

Antimony trichloride is produced by the interaction of chlorine with antimony or by dissolving antimony trisulphide with hydrochloric acid. Antimony pentachloride is formed by reaction of molten antimony trichloride with chlorine. Both are used for 'blueing' steel and colouring aluminium, pewter and zinc and as catalysts in organic synthetic processes. They are highly toxic substances which may cause pulmonary oedema (Gudzovskii, 1971; Cordasco and Stone, 1973).

Metallic antimony is discussed in Chapter 11 (page 265).

Arsenic

The chief interest of this metal in occupational pulmonary disease is its potential to cause cancer (see Chapter 19, page 651, for detailed discussion).

Boranes

The boranes are hydrogen compounds – boron hydrides – of boron (B) and those usually encountered in industry, *diborane, pentaborane* and *decaborane,* are highly toxic. Diborane is the most important in relation to lung disease and its toxicity has been compared to that of phosgene (Krackow, 1953).

Diborane (B_2H_6), a gas under ordinary conditions, produces great heat on hydrolysis igniting spontaneously in moist air and, on this account, is used in high energy fuels for rockets and high-flying aircraft. It is also employed in some welding processes, in the manufacture of fungicides and bactericides, and for polymerizing catalysts. It may be capable of producing an exothermic reaction in the lungs.

Acute, subacute and chronic effects are described (Lowe and Freeman, 1957; Cordasco et al., 1962). *Acute illness* follows exposure to high concentrations and is a clinical syndrome similar to metal fume fever (see page 593) with breathlessness, chest tightness, non-productive cough and wheezing which occurs in about 1 to 24 hours and lasts in most cases for 3 to 5 days. However, unlike metal fume fever, radiographic signs of bilateral pneumonic consolidation may develop but resolve in a few days. In the *subacute phase* cough, chest tightness, headache and drowsiness are most prominent. *Chronic disease* which follows recurrent low level exposure consists of unproductive cough, wheeze – which may be increased by exercise – and dyspnoea on effort which may occasionally last as long as 2 to 3 years before finally ceasing. Where ventilatory function tests have been done they have indicated a fairly severe degree of airflow obstruction which ultimately recovers.

The effects of pentaborane and decaborane are predominantly neurological: they include headache, drowsiness, muscle spasms and fasciculation but cough, chest tightness and inspiratory crackles may be present in some patients.

Treatment of acute disease may require oxygen and corticosteroids, and bronchodilators will be necessary for more protracted airways' obstruction.

Preventive measures include special conditions of storage, handling and processing, the use of respiratory protective equipment and informing personnel about the nature of the hazard.

Metallic boron is non-toxic.

Cadmium

Cadmium metal or its compounds may be either inhaled or ingested, but only the results of inhalation that occur in industry are relevant here.

Freshly generated cadmium fumes (cadmium oxide) are so toxic that at one time they were considered as a possible weapon of chemical warfare. Fume, produced when the metal burns in air, is orange–brown in colour and tends to settle as a fine dust on cold surfaces. The metal melts at 32°C (610°F) and boils at 767°C (1800°F).

Uses and sources of exposure

Cadmium is highly resistant to corrosion and is used in antifriction metal alloys for engine bearings, for electroplating iron and steel, in the plates of nickel–cadmium storage batteries, in brazing and soldering alloys, wires and rods; in copper alloys for cables and trolley wires, in electrical capacitors, as cadmium sulphide and sulphoselenide in the preparations of pigments for paints, ceramics, glass, plastics and leather; in pesticides and veterinary medicines, and as a neutron absorber in atomic reactors. It is worth noting that both cadmium and beryllium are used in the manufacture of non-sparking tools.

Any of these processes is a potential source of exposure to dust or fume. Exposure to fume may also occur during the smelting and refining of zinc, lead and copper ores in which cadmium is present; during the recovery of scrap metal containing cadmium, and occasionally outside industry as in the use of cadmium alloys by sculptors in metal and by enthusiasts in metallist hobbies.

Oxyacetylene burning and welding of cadmium-plated metal and silver brazing have proved to be especially hazardous (Beton et al., 1966; Blejer and Caplan, 1971) because they are often carried out in enclosed or ill-ventilated places. The fume is freshly generated and the risk is frequently unsuspected. Silver brazing is a form of high-temperature welding in which metal is joined by the application of heat from 985 to 1650°C (1800 to 3000°F) with a silver alloy filler (commonly containing cadmium) which melts at about 428°C (800°F). Cadmium-plated metals may resemble galvanized (zinc-plated) metals and be mistaken for them. A simple test for the detection of cadmium is to heat gently a *small* spot of the metal with the welding rod when the film formed in the presence of cadmium is golden-yellow but is smoke-grey if zinc is present (Blejer and Caplan, 1971). High frequency and gas soldering of cadmium-containing metal produce cadmium smoke of minute particle size.

The danger is heightened by the fact that concentrations of cadmium fume or dust sufficient to cause severe illness or death do not give rise to any early warning symptoms. Therefore, any process that may evolve cadmium fume or dust in the vicinity of a worker's 'breathing zone' must be regarded as potentially dangerous, that is, any form of heating, brazing, welding, soldering or grinding of cadmium-containing metals (Blejer and Caplan, 1971).

Cadmium fume consists of minute particles up to about 0.1 µm diameter which form aggregates with overall diameters that may be as large as 2.5 µm. Cadmium oxide and chloride dusts are soluble in mildly acid conditions and body fluids, but cadmium sulphides and selenosulphides are relatively insoluble.

Smokers are exposed to low concentrations of cadmium because some of the cadmium content of tobacco passes into the smoke and, although many foods contain measurable amounts of cadmium that are poorly absorbed from the gastrointestinal tract, cigarette smoke appears to be the chief non-industrial source of cadmium accumulation in the body – especially in heavy smokers. However, the quantity of cadmium in the smoke is very small: on average a cigarette contains 1 µg cadmium about 15 per cent of which is absorbed by the smoker (Nandi et al., 1969; Lewis et al., 1972).

Absorption and excretion

Cadmium is relatively easily taken up from the lung and, in general, about 40 per cent of an inhaled dose will be absorbed, depending on the particle size and solubility of the species which is encountered. In the blood, cadmium is mainly bound to the red cell and it is stored predominantly in the liver and kidney, these two organs containing about 50 per cent of the total body burden. In the kidney, which is the major target organ for cadmium, the metal is concentrated in the renal cortex where it is bound to metallothionein (Lauwerys, 1983).

The half-life of cadmium in the body is between 10 and 30 years so that, although body burdens of cadmium are negligible at birth, they rise steadily and are between 20 and 30 mg at the age of 50 years in those with no occupational exposure; cadmium workers may have body burdens some 10 times higher than this. Smokers tend to have slightly higher body burdens than non-smokers (Lauwerys and Bernard, 1986).

Excretion takes place mainly through the kidney and also increases slightly with age. In those with no occupational exposure the urinary concentration is usually below 2 μg/g creatinine; excretion in those with occupational exposure is discussed below.

Blood cadmium levels

In unexposed non-smokers, blood cadmium levels are usually below 0.5 μg/dl and, in smokers, less than 1 μg/dl. Levels in cadmium workers are obviously higher and mainly reflect the last few months' exposure (Lauwerys, 1983). It has been suggested that a level of 1 μg/dl should be taken as the no-effect threshold for long-term exposure to cadmium (Bernard et al., 1979; Buchet et al., 1980).

Pathology and pathogenesis

Acute disease

This is caused chiefly by freshly generated fume and is a 'chemical pneumonia' with oedema. It is estimated that a cumulative total exposure of 2500 mg/m³ cadmium oxide fume over 5 hours or 5 mg/m³ over an 8-hour period could be lethal (British Occupational Hygiene Society Committee on Hygiene Standards, 1977).

Respiratory tract
The trachea and bronchi are congested and inflamed. Petechiae may be present in the pulmonary pleura. The lungs are voluminous and massively oedematous with blood-tinged fluid which is also found in the airways. Oedema is less pronounced if the patient has survived a week or more.

Microscopically, the alveoli and terminal airways are filled with proteinaceous fluid, and large areas of intra-alveolar haemorrhage may be seen. There may be partial hyaline membrane formation (Blejer and Caplan, 1971). The alveolar walls are thickened by oedema and may contain many lymphocytes and neutrophils and a number of fibroblasts. There is hyperplasia and metaplasia of alveolar epithelial cells with much desquamation but in some cases many alveolar spaces are completely filled by masses of cuboidal cells (Patterson, 1947; Christensen and Olsen, 1957; Beton et al., 1966). The type of appearance varies according to intensity of exposure and the time the patient survives. If he recovers, these lesions resolve completely.

Experimentally, cadmium has a similar effect to ozone (see page 626) in animals in that there is initial desquamation of type I pneumocytes followed by proliferation of type II pneumocytes, and a striking increase in vascular permeability (Steele and Wilhelm, 1967; Carrington and Greene, 1970; Palmer, Snider and Hayes, 1975).

Kidneys
Toxic nephrosis occurs in cases of heavy exposure. Microscopically there is widespread cortical necrosis, occlusion of the glomerular vessels by thrombi and tubular damage which may be extensive and severe (Beton et al., 1966).

Chronic disease

This may result from repeated short exposures to moderate or low concentrations of cadmium oxide fume or of cadmium oxide, sulphide and stearate dusts over a prolonged period of time (Smith, Smith and McCall, 1960; Bonnel, 1965; Fribeg, 1971).

Effects on the lungs
Emphysema of both panacinar and centriacinar type found *post mortem* in a small number of cadmium-exposed individuals has been attributed to cadmium (Baader, 1952; Lane and Campbell, 1954; Gough, 1960, 1968; Smith, Smith and McCall, 1960). Mild peribronchiolar fibrosis has also been described (Baader, 1952). However, no post-mortem studies with long exposures to cadmium compared with those of appropriate matched controls appear to have been done.

The question of so-called 'cadmium emphysema' is discussed later.

An excess mortality from cancer of the lung among workers in one cadmium smelter was reported by Lemen et al. (1976) but this result has not been confirmed by the much larger study of Armstrong and Kazantzis (1983). In this study a cohort of 6995 men born before 1940 and exposed for at least 1 year between 1942 and 1970 was followed up to the end of 1979. There were marginally more deaths than expected from lung cancer (199 observed as against 185.6 expected; SMR of 107). This SMR (standardized mortality ratio) was not statistically significant and, moreover, the excess of deaths from lung cancer was not related to exposure. In a later study of lung cancer mortality at a lead–zinc–cadmium smelter, Kazantzis and a colleague (Ades and Kazantzis, 1988) found that mortality from the disease was related to estimates of cumulative exposure to arsenic and to lead but not to cadmium. These data all suggest that cadmium is not aetiologically associated with lung cancer in human beings. For further discussion, see Chapter 19 (page 651).

Effects on the kidneys
The effects of cadmium on the kidney are rather complex and, for a full discussion, the reader is referred to the paper by Lauwerys and Bernard

(1986). It is now generally accepted that toxic effects are not noted if the concentration in the renal cortex is below 200 µg/g (200 parts per million, p.p.m.). When the concentration reaches 215 p.p.m., renal dysfunction is likely to develop in 10 per cent of those with occupational exposure.

The excretion of cadmium in the kidney depends upon the saturation of metallothionein binding sites in the cortex. At low levels of exposure, when the total amount of cadmium absorbed has not saturated the binding sites, the amount excreted in the urine will reflect mainly the amount in the kidney. As the binding sites become increasingly saturated, so the level in the urine will reflect current exposure more accurately. This means that in newly exposed cadmium workers there is a time lag – depending on the intensity of exposure – before the urinary concentration can be correlated with environmental conditions. Once kidney damage has been caused, the levels of cadmium in the urine increase considerably.

The earliest sign of renal dysfunction in cadmium workers is tubular proteinuria and this seems to require exposure to 20 to 50 µg/m³ respirable cadmium for about 20 years (Lauwerys et al., 1974; Falck, Fine and Smith, 1983; Elinder et al., 1985; Ellis, Cohn and Smith, 1985; Mason et al., 1988). The low-molecular-weight proteins that are found include β₂-microglobulin (BMG) and retinol-binding protein (RBP). The estimation of β₂-microglobulin levels in the urine is widely used to monitor exposure to cadmium but there are some analytical difficulties resulting from the instability of β₂-microglobulin in acid urine and, for this reason, some authorities advocate the measurement of RBP instead (Bernard, Moreau and Lauwerys, 1982; Beetham et al., 1985). Recently, it has been suggested that the activity of *N*-acetyl-β-D-glucosaminidase (NAG) in the urine is a more sensitive indicator of cadmium absorption than β₂-microglobulin even at urinary cadmium levels as low as 10 µg/g creatinine (Kawada, Koyama and Suzuki, 1989).

The appearance of β₂-microglobulin in the urine is, however, the most frequently used index of cadmium-induced renal damage, but it is important to understand that it is not specific to cadmium intoxication.

β₂-Microglobulin is synthesized by most cells of the body and it is present in the serum in a mean concentration of 1.8 mg/l. It undergoes almost complete resorption by the renal tubules and the amount present in the urine represents only about 0.1 per cent of the total filtered – some 350 mg/day. Elevation of serum β₂-microglobulin can result from reduced glomerular filtration rate, increased synthesis or both factors operating together. Increased synthesis may be associated with carcinomatosis, certain lymphomas, chronic lymphatic leukaemias, multiple myeloma, rheumatoid arthritis, systemic lupus erythematosus, sarcoidosis and alcoholic liver damage. Increased excretion occurs in chronic pyelonephritis, reflux nephropathy even in the absence of infection, and a variety of interstitial nephropathies including those caused by phenacetin and salicylates (Schardijn et al., 1979).

It is evident that the conclusion that the appearance of β₂-microglobulin in the urine is a reflection of cadmium intoxication requires at least that other causes are excluded. The most persuasive criterion is, of course, a history of prolonged and heavy exposure at work. If there is a positive occupational history, and the concentration of β₂-microglobulin is consistently high (say, in excess of 1000 µg/l) and there is an increase in protein excretion, then renal damage due to cadmium can be assumed (Kazantzis, 1980).

The long-term consequences of an increased excretion of β₂-microglobulin is the subject of some debate. Cadmium-induced proteinuria progresses slowly but once started it is rarely reversible (Roels et al., 1982; Elinder et al., 1985). Because it does not invariably herald the progression to renal insufficiency, some workers consider that isolated occurrences of β₂-microglobulin in the urine are of no significance; however, there is a significant excess of deaths from renal disease in cadmium workers with more than 15 years' exposure (Kjellström, Firberg and Rahnster, 1979), so there is little room for complacency.

The renal aspects of cadmium intoxication have been considered at length because they are the chief, and frequently the only, evidence for the disease.

Other effects

Yellow pigmentation of the teeth is seen in some cases and mild hypochromic anaemia, believed to be due to iron deficiency and increased red cell destruction, may occur (Cotter and Cotter, 1951; Friberg, 1957).

In spite of the accumulation of cadmium in the liver cirrhosis or other chronic hepatic disorders do not seem to have been reported, nor does liver function appear to be adversely affected (Piscator, 1976). This may be due to cadmium combining with the low-molecular-weight protein, metallothionein, which probably exerts a protective effect (Webb and Etienne, 1977). The underlying reason for the toxicity of cadmium is believed to be inhibition of certain tissue enzyme systems (in the kidney, those regulating tubular resorption) which depend upon the presence of copper, cobalt and zinc ions (Kendrey and Roe, 1969; Mustafa et al., 1971).

'Cadmium emphysema'

The question as to whether or not exposure to cadmium causes emphysema has been much discussed. From 1950 onwards there were reports of changes in lung function and in chest radiographs in cadmium workers that were consistent with emphysema, and centriacinar or panacinar emphysema was reported in a small number of cadmium workers at autopsy. These early studies had a number of deficiencies that were reviewed in a leading article in *The Lancet* in 1973 (Leading Article, 1973). The weight of opinion then tended to swing against cadmium as a cause of emphysema and this was the view taken in the last edition of this book.

More recently, however, a study of 101 of the 102 men who had worked at a copper–cadmium alloy plant for 1 year or more after 1926, when the plant opened, has provided strong evidence to support the earlier studies. The men exposed to cadmium were compared with 96 men from the same factory matched for age and occupational status. Smoking habits were similar in the two groups but the cadmium workers showed a reduction in FEV_1, FEV_1/FVC, $TLCO$ and KCO compared with expected values derived from regression equations for the controls. The workers employed before 1950 and with the highest cumulative exposure (as judged from company records and atmospheric measurements from 1951 onwards) showed the greatest decrement in lung function. Moreover, 18 per cent of the cadmium workers had radiographic emphysema on independent assessment compared with 7 per cent of the controls (Davison et al., 1986).

If cadmium does cause emphysema then the mechanism by which it does so is not understood. Experimental studies in animals have shown that intratracheal administraton of cadmium chloride or cadmium acetate, or repeated exposure to cadmium chloride aerosol, causes functional and morphological abnormalities that are characteristic of pulmonary fibrosis and airspace enlargement. It has been suggested that in cigarette smokers, at least, emphysema may result from a loss of elastic fibres in the lung. Recently, it has been shown that guinea-pigs instilled with a single dose of 0.5 ml 0.025 per cent cadmium chloride do not suffer a loss of pulmonary elastin, and it was considered that the airspace enlargement was a consequence of the fibrosis produced (Snider et al., 1988).

Clinical features

Acute disease

There are no symptoms during exposure. They are delayed for several hours, commonly starting when the man has returned home and retired to bed, and are identical to those of 'metal fume fever' (see page 593) with the addition, in some cases, of abdominal cramps and diarrhoea. He may feel well enough to return to work the following day. But some 12 to 36 hours later there is dyspnoea, severe chest pain with a sense of precordial constriction (which may be mistaken for myocardial infarction), persistent cough with frothy sputum which may be blood stained, wheeze, weakness and malaise (Beton et al., 1966).

On examination of severely ill patients there is fever, central cyanosis, restlessness and the signs of pneumonia or pulmonary oedema. There may be mild proteinuria and toxic liver damage may be suggested by increased serum glutamate–oxalo-acetate transaminase (SGOT – now known as aspartate transaminase or AST) and bilirubin levels (Blejer and Caplan, 1971). Pronounced loss of weight occurs in patients who survive some days.

The chest radiograph reveals the appearances of pulmonary oedema which usually resolve in a week or two but may not disappear completely for 2 or 3 months (Evans, 1960; Karlish, 1960; Townsend, 1968) (Figure 18.1).

Complete recovery is usually rapid with appropriate treatment, although a mortality rate of 15 to 20 per cent due to respiratory failure was reported by Bonnell (1965), and fatalities still occur due in most cases to failure to make the diagnosis (Patwardhan and Finckh, 1976). In some of these death is caused by acute renal failure. In those who recover there are no sequelae, and later deterioration of ventilatory function (FEV_1 and FVC) and gas transfer over a period of years does not seem to occur (Townsend, 1968).

Diagnosis

Acute disease

The two most important requirements are a detailed occupational history from the patient or a workmate, and an awareness by the physician of the existence of this disorder and the work conditions that may give rise to it.

It is imperative that the diagnosis is made promptly and that the illness is not mistaken for harmless 'metal fume fever'. If symptoms persist – especially fever and severe chest pain – after 24 hours (when those of 'metal fume fever' have ceased) in a man with an appropriate or suspicious work history, acute poisoning must be suspected. A worker who has previously experienced 'metal fume fever' and is unware of recent exposure to cadmium fume may wrongly attribute his symptoms to 'metal fume fever' and not seek medical advice until the delayed effects of cadmium are established. It should be noted that the other most commonly mistaken diagnoses are bronchopneumonia, virus pneumonia, influenza and, occasionally, myocardial infarction.

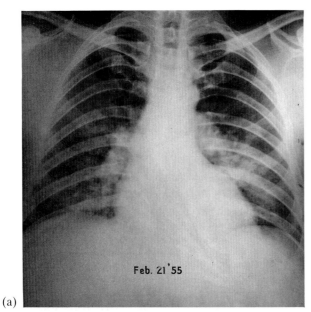

(a)

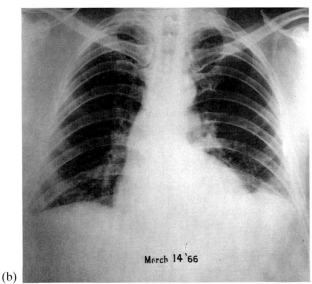

(b)

Figure 18.1 (a) Appearances of acute chemical pneumonia (pulmonary oedema) 1 week after heavy exposure to cadmium fume. Two months later, the radiograph was normal. (b) No evident abnormality (emphysema or hyperinflation) 11 years after the incident. This is the case of a welder and metal sheet worker in a small, ill-ventilated workshop who failed to remove the cadmium coating from the metal surface before welding. He developed intense burning pain in the chest, severe cough, vomiting and dyspnoea, but was symptom free in 3 weeks. There was no evidence of chronic respiratory disease during the rest of his life. He was a pinbowling enthusiast until shortly before his death from a non-respiratory illness. (Courtesy of Dr A.J. Karlish)

Chronic disease

There are no pathognomonic signs of chronic cadmium intoxication and diagnosis depends upon:

1. A positive history of prolonged, heavy exposure.
2. Increased excretion of cadmium in the urine (substantially above the normal of 2 μg/g creatinine).
3. Persistently and markedly elevated urinary concentrations of β_2-microglobulin or other tubular proteins in the absence of other known causes.
4. Other evidence of renal dysfunction.

Plasma and urinary calcium concentrations of calcium may be raised in some cases as a result of secondary hypoparathyroidism due to the chronic renal failure but these should not be considered as diagnostic features of cadmium intoxication.

Treatment

Acute chemical pneumonia and pulmonary oedema

First aid
1. Warmth and rest.
2. Administration of oxygen.
3. The patient must be warned against any exertion.

In hospital
1. Warmth and rest must be continued for several days over the period when delayed-onset pulmonary oedema may occur.
2. Oxygen administered by intermittent positive pressure ventilation.
3. Removal of bronchial exudates by suction tube. In many cases elective tracheotomy with a large cuff endobronchial tube is indicated.
4. Corticosteroids: early administration greatly improves the prognosis. In severely ill patients they should be given intravenously for a few days and thereafter in the form of prednisolone by mouth until recovery is established.
5. Chelating agents: calcium ethylenediamine tetra-acetic acid (EDTA) by the intravenous route has been recommended by some authorities but is regarded by Friberg (1971) as undesirable. If it is used the dose must be strictly controlled and renal function frequently checked. The reason for this is that it is nephrotoxic in combination with cadmium. The maximal recommended dose is 2.5 g/4.5 kg bodyweight, and for each 4.5 kg is 170 mg/hour, 330 mg/day or 1670 mg/week. No more than two such courses with a 1-week interval should be given (Blejer and Caplan, 1971). Dimercaprol (British anti-Lewisite) is contra-indicated.
6. Analgesics may be required for chest pain but morphine or other respiratory depressants should be avoided or given only in small doses.
7. A bronchodilator drug may give additional relief if wheezing is pronounced.

8. A broad-spectrum prophylactic antibiotic is probably desirable.

Chronic disease

The worker should be removed permanently from exposure to cadmium, and in most cases this is all that is necessary. But, occasionally, anaemia or renal malabsorption may require treatment. The use of EDTA should be avoided as it may worsen renal damage.

Prevention

General hygiene measures
1. The potential hazard of cadmium exposure and the processes and materials that can cause it should be made clear to all likely to be concerned. Brazers and welders should be familiarized with the orange–brown appearance of cadmium fume and warned of the danger of overheating cadmium–silver solders. A warning label should be firmly attached to all cadmium-containing materials and, whenever possible, cadmium-free silver-alloy fillers made available for silver brazing.
2. Efficient exhaust ventilation must be applied to alloying and refining furnaces, to all dusty operations and, whenever practicable, to welding and similar processes involving cadmium alloys. During oxyacetylene burning, welding or brazing in confined spaces where exhaust ventilation is impossible or when carried on outdoors (where dangerous concentrations of fume may still occur in workers' breathing zones) appropriate respirators must be worn. Men working in the vicinity of fume-producing processes should also have respirator protection.
3. The concentration of cadmium dust or fume in environmental and 'breathing zone' air should be monitored periodically and the results recorded.
4. Workers should not be allowed to eat, drink or smoke in workplaces where cadmium fume or dust may be present, and they should not take working clothes home.

Medical surveillance
In addition to routine clinical examination screening of urine at regular intervals for β_2-microglobulin is probably of value if the employee has been exposed for 10 years or more, but not otherwise (Adams, 1980). Urine is collected in metal-free polythene containers and part is refrigerated at -20°C for β_2-microglobulin analysis. Cadmium levels should also be determined. If proteinuria persists the work environment needs to be carefully surveyed. It would seem undesirable, however, to remove workers from exposure simply because a certain arbitrary limit of β_2-microglobulin is exceeded. This decision should rest on careful assessment of the features of each case (Kazantzis, 1980).

Regular assessment of ventilatory function – preferably at 6-monthly intervals – is recommended by the British Occupational Hygiene Society Committee on Hygiene Standards (1977).

Pre-employment examination of prospective entrants to processes in which there may be significant cadmium fume or dust should exclude those with a past history or current evidence of renal disease, and those with anaemia or chronic respiratory disease.

Occupational exposure limits
Occupational exposure to cadmium and its compounds is subject to a control limit which is the maximum concentration to which workers may be exposed for 40 hours a week. This level should never normally be exceeded. The control limit for all compounds, except cadmium sulphide, is 0.05 mg/m^3; for cadmium sulphide the limit is 0.04 mg/m^3.

Chromium

Metallic chromium is used extensively in the production of various alloys with nickel and molybdenum, cobalt, vanadium and niobium, and also in the chromate industry. Chromium plating is carried out by depositing chromium from a solution of chromic acid by electrolysis. Hexavalent sodium dichromate is employed in leather tanning, and other chromates are used for various purposes such as pigments for paints and ceramics, and mordants or fixatives in dyeing. Chromium may occasionally be present in arc welding fumes.

Chromite mining is referred to in Chapter 11.

Effects

Chromium is a powerful sensitizer and the metal, its chromates and dichromates, and chromic acid are all capable of causing asthma and dermatitis (Hicks, Hewitt and Lam, 1979) (see Table 21.7). Inhalation of high concentrations of chromic acid causes intense irritation of the upper and lower respiratory tracts with cough, dyspnoea, chest pain and radiographic changes (Meyers, 1950; Borghetti et al., 1977). Studies of workers in a ferrochromium and ferrosilicon producing plant showed some decrement in FVC and an increased prevalence of obstructive lung disease, but it was thought that these changes might have been due to the high total dust content in the atmosphere, rather than to the chromium itself (Langard, 1980).

Lung function studies among a cohort of chrome platers showed that both FVC and FEV_1 were reduced compared with non-exposed controls (Lindberg and Hedenstierna, 1983) and the authors concluded that a time-weighted 8-hour exposure in excess of $2 \mu g/m^3$ might cause a transient decrement in lung function.

A significant excess of carcinoma of the lung has been noted among chrome platers and chromate workers (see Chapter 19, page 653).

Cobalt

Cobalt is used for a variety of purposes and appears to be the cause of lung disease associated with the hard metal industry. Three types of disorder are attributed to it: *acute,* in the form of asthma; *sub-acute*, fibrosing alveolitis; and *chronic*, in the form of progressive DIPF – *hard metal disease.*

Cobalt (Co) is a silvery blue–white metal with magnetic properties which is obtained when copper is extracted from its ore. Various grades of cobalt powder are manufactured and the extra-fine grade is used in the manufacture of hard metal. The particles are rod shaped with a mean diameter of $1.4 \mu m$ and a length about 10 or 20 times greater but they break down during milling (L.R. Payne, 1979, personal communication).

It has a wide range of uses in industry, medicine and nuclear weapons, but its industrial applications only are considered here.

Industrial uses

1. *Metallic alloys*:
   (a) in combination with aluminium, nickel and other alloys to produce permanent magnets for the electrical and electronic industries;
   (b) in combination with nickel, chromium and molybdenum in the production of Vitallium for joint prostheses in orthopaedic surgery;
   (c) in the manufacture of high-speed steels.
2. *Tungsten carbide (hard-metal)*: this synthetic metal, which possesses exceptional properties of resistance to heat and wear and a hardness only slightly less than that of diamond, was first introduced in Germany in the 1920s and in the UK and the USA a decade later. Because its hardness increases with rising temperature the metal is used for high-speed cutting tools and drills which can operate at temperatures up to about 1090°C, and in armour plating, bullets and the nose cones of armour-piercing shells.

Tungsten carbide is produced by blending and heating tungsten (wolfram) and carbon in an electric furnace. It is then mixed and finely ground in a ball-mill with cobalt in quantities varying from 3 to 25 per cent in order to form a matrix for the tungsten carbide crystals. Other metals – such as chromium, nickel, titanium and tantulum – may be added according to the properties required in the final product. All these constituents are in a finely divided state having a mean diameter of about $1.5 \mu m$ (Coates and Watson, 1971). The powdered metal is next pressed into ingots or particular shapes. After pressing, it is fused (or sintered) in an electric furnace at approximately 1000°C, and the product finally heated to about 1500°C (cobalt melts at 1495°C). All these processes and dry grinding, drilling and finishing of hard-metal products, and cleaning equipment may be dusty if exhaust ventilation is inadequate. However, drilling and grinding operations usually require special coolant fluids in which varying amounts of cobalt dissolve and accumulate, and which form a fine aerosol spray. Lung disease appears to be more common in 'wet' (coolant-using) areas where cobalt occurs in ionized form but in lower concentrations than in 'dry' areas where it is non-ionized (Sjögren et al., 1980).

3. In the china, glass, paint and glaze industries as a clear blue pigment.
4. As a catalyst in the chemical and oil industries.

Respiratory effects

Acute

Pulmonary oedema
This occasionally follows exposure to high concentrations of cobalt fume, for example during melting and pouring the metal into moulds.

Asthma
Exposure to cobalt dust alone (as can occur during the milling of cobalt metal) may cause either asthma or dermatitis, or both. After a variable period in the hard-metal industry, a small but not insignificant proportion of workers may develop occupational asthma. One study found a prevalence of 5.6 per cent among workers who had been exposed for at least 5 years to a mean time-weighted average concentration of 0.05 mg cobalt/m^3 (Kusaka et al., 1986a). A much larger study of 1039 tungsten carbide production workers in the USA found a prevalence of work-related wheeze of 10.9 per cent; those with exposure greater than 0.05 mg/m^3 were more than twice as likely to develop wheeze than workers whose exposure was below 0.05 mg/m^3 (Sprince et al., 1988).

The symptoms of chest tightness and productive cough tend to occur at the end of the day or during the night. They remit during periods away from work but usually recur on the first day back. There is a beneficial response to bronchodilators and removal from exposure is curative in most, but not all, cases (Davison et al., 1983).

Bronchial provocation tests with cobalt are positive and may elicit an immediate, late or dual type of response (Davison et al., 1983; Kusaka et al., 1986a). Only a small proportion of those who respond to inhaled cobalt also have a positive patch test (Kusaka et al., 1986a).

The chest radiograph in most cases shows no abnormality but appearances similar to those of acute or subacute fibrosing alveolitis may develop in a small number (Bruckner, 1967; Tolot et al., 1970; Coates et al., 1973; Sjögren et al., 1980; Kusaka et al., 1986a).

A reduction in FEV_1 during the course of the working week with recovery when absent from work is apparently not uncommon in tungsten carbide workers following prolonged exposure (Alexandersson, 1979).

Although there is undoubtedly an immunological basis to cobalt asthma, there is also some evidence that hard-metal dust may cause bronchial irritation in previously unexposed subjects. Kusaka et al. (1986b) exposed 15 healthy young men to hard-metal dust at a concentration of 0.8 mg/m³ (mean cobalt concentration 38 μg/m³) for 6 hours and found a significant reduction in FVC but in no other indices of lung function. All the subjects developed a productive cough and a sore throat during the exposure but there were no abnormal signs in the chest.

Subacute

Fibrosing alveolitis

Cough which is usually non-productive, dyspnoea on exertion, loss of weight, inspiratory crackles at the lung bases and linear or ill-defined rounded opacities with prominent hilar shadows on the chest radiograph develop within a year or less and usually after only a few years in the hard-metal industry. Complete resolution occurs in some cases when exposure ceases but is incomplete in others. These changes may recur on re-exposure which, if repeated, might lead to progressive fibrosis.

The histological appearances are those of desquamating fibrosing alveolitis. Alveolar walls are thickened and infiltrated with lymphocytes, plasma cells and macrophages, and alveolar lining cells (type I pneumocytes) are swollen and many exfoliated. Granulomatous foci have also been reported (Joseph, 1968). Crystals identified as tungsten carbide by X-ray diffraction have been found in the macrophages (Miller et al., 1953; Lundgren and Öhman, 1954; Scherrer et al., 1970; Coates and Watson, 1973), and cobalt has been identified in the mediastinal lymph nodes of some workers (Sjögren et al., 1980).

Chronic

Hard-metal disease

This was first described as an abnormal radiographic appearance in Germany by Jobs and Ballhausen (1940). Occasional cases of progressive DIPF occur in susceptible workers after some years in the hard-metal industry: the time varies from 2 to 25 years but is usually in excess of 10. Cases have been described in most parts of the world, in Britain (Bech, Kipling and Heather, 1962), Europe (Reber and Burckhardt, 1970; Scherrer et al., 1970; Rüttner, Spycher and Stolkin, 1987; Meyer-Bisch et al., 1989), Sweden (Lundgren and Öhman, 1954; Ahlmark, Bruce and Nyström, 1960), Czechoslovakia and Russia (Bech, Kipling and Heather, 1962), Australia (Joseph, 1968) and the USA (Miller et al., 1953; Coates and Watson, 1971, 1973; Sprince et al., 1988). The probability of hard-metal workers developing fibrotic lung disease is substantially less than their prospect of developing asthma (Sprince et al., 1988).

The gross appearances of the lungs are those of widespread DIPF often with honeycomb cysts. The histological features are those of fibrosing alveolitis of the mural type. Collagen and elastic tissue are prominent in the alveolar walls and unusual giant cells are present (Figure 18.2). The giant cells comprise both type II alveolar epithelial cells and alveolar macrophages. The multinucleate macrophages are a distinctive feature of BAL from patients with hard-metal disease whereas the multinucleate alveolar cells are evident only in lung tissue (Davison et al., 1983). Electron microscopy reveals swelling of type I cells with the formation of numerous microvilli and groups of crystals identifiable as tungsten carbide within macrophages and their lysosomes and in alveolar walls (Coates and Watson, 1971, 1973). Elemental analysis of lung tissue from patients with hard-metal disease shows the presence of traces of tungsten, titanium, niobium, chromium and zirconium. Cobalt is not found in all cases, however; for example, in only four of nine examined by Rüttner, Spycher and Stolkin (1987). Iron and nickel are almost invariably present and there may be many other elements in the lungs, including silica. In view of the very mixed dust exposure to which hard-metal grinders are subjected, Rüttner and his colleagues proposed that the disease should be referred to as a 'mixed dust pneumoconiosis', rather than as hard-metal disease.

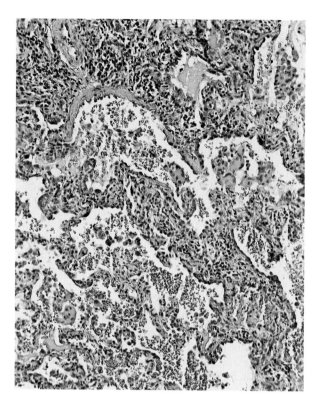

Figure 18.2 Microsection of the lung of a man who worked for 2 years in the final grinding process of tungsten carbide. There is pronounced interstitial cellular infiltration, fibrosis of alveolar walls and some metaplasia of alveolar lining cells. Large cells, many of which are multinucleated, lie free in the alveolar spaces (magnification × 120.) (Reproduced from Coates and Watson, 1971, with permission)

Effect on the myocardium

The possibility that prolonged exposure to high concentrations of cobalt dust in the hard-metal industry may occasionally result in fatal cardiomyopathy has been suggested (Barborik and Dusek, 1972; Kennedy, Dornan and King, 1981), and cobalt has been incriminated as the aetiological agent in an outbreak of cardiomyopathy in beer drinkers.

In a study of 30 hard-metal workers, Horowitz et al. (1988) found very little evidence for direct effects on the heart using radionuclide ventriculography although there was a weak but significant negative correlation ($r = -0.40$) between duration of exposure and resting left ventricular function. Workers with abnormal chest radiographs had relatively lower exercise right-ventricular ejection fractions and there was an inverse relationship between the severity of the radiographic changes and both rest and exercise right-ventricular ejection fractions. This was thought to be due to early pulmonary heart disease consequent upon pulmonary fibrosis.

Pathogenesis

The mechanism responsible for asthma is obscure but inhalation challenge with powdered cobalt or cobalt solution results in chest tightness and wheezing and decrements in lung function (Coates et al., 1973; Kusaka et al., 1986a); there is no response to powdered tungsten (Coates et al., 1973). In patients with allergic dermatitis due to metallic cobalt, skin patch tests with the powdered metal are positive but negative with other metals (Schwarz et al., 1945). This test has been found to be positive in hard-metal workers with both fibrosing alveolitis (DIPF) and skin sensitization (Sjögren et al., 1980), but in by no means all workers with hard-metal asthma (Kusaka et al., 1986a).

Particulate cobalt metal is strikingly toxic to the lungs of experimental animals when inhaled or injected by the intratracheal route. It results in haemorrhagic oedema, obliterative bronchiolitis and proliferation and desquamation of alveolar cells (Harding, 1950; Schepers, 1955a), whereas particulate tungsten metal, tantalum and titanium alone are relatively innocuous (Delahant, 1955; Schepers, 1955b,c; Kaplun and Mezencewa, 1960). Dust mixtures containing tungsten, titanium and cobalt cause a more pronounced effect than cobalt alone (Kaplun and Mezencewa, 1960). Finely divided cobalt, but not tungsten carbide, is toxic to normal human leucocytes in vivo, particularly in patients with fibrosing alveolitis (Coates and Watson, 1971).

There is no correlation between the quantity of cobalt in human lungs and severity of disease, however, although tungsten and titanium are almost always present (Bech, Kipling and Heather, 1962; Coates and Watson, 1971; Rüttner, Spycher and Stolkin, 1987). But there is a similar lack of correlation in beryllium disease (see Chapter 17). The high solubility of cobalt in biological fluids undoubtedly allows it to escape from the lungs. In ionized form it combines readily with proteins and amino acids and thus could conceivably act as a hapten capable of promoting immunological reactions both in the lungs and in the skin (Harding, 1950; Heath, Webb and Caffrey, 1969; Rae, 1975; Sjögren et al., 1980).

The failure of some metal-to-metal cobalt–chromium–molybdenum hip arthroplasties owing to necrosis of bone, muscle and joint capsule adjacent to the prosthesis has been attributed to the release of cobalt due to metal attrition; a similar observation has been made in bone fixed with such fracture plating (Halpin, 1975; Jones et al., 1975). The tissues adjacent to the prostheses often show a granulomatous reaction and tissue destruction (Rae, 1975). In these instances skin patch tests with cobalt were positive whereas those with nickel and chromium were negative, but a high incidence of allergy to chromium has also been found in some patients with metal-to-metal prostheses (Benson, Goodwin and

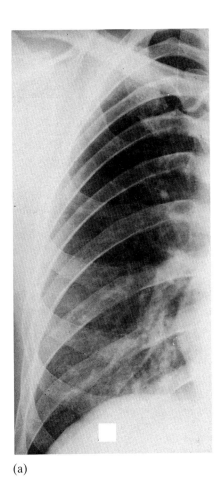
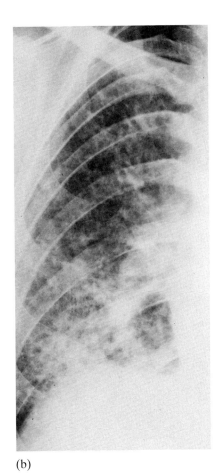

(a)   (b)

Figure 18.3 Radiographs of a man who worked with soft and hard tungsten carbide for 4 years. Fine linear opacities (ILO category s) are present in the lower half of the lung field in (a). (b) This radiograph was taken 10 years later and shows coarse linear and round opacities with some suggestion of 'honeycombing'. (Reproduced from Coates and Watson, 1971, with permission)

Brodyoff, 1975). Particulate cobalt and cobalt–chromium alloy have been shown to be cytotoxic to macrophages in vitro whereas chromium, molybdenum and titanium are not, and they are also strongly haemolytic to human erythrocytes, although chromium, molybdenum and titanium are only feebly so (Rae, 1975, 1978).

Thus, whereas tungsten is apparently inert, cobalt, whether free or in alloy form, is allergenic and cytotoxic and may be capable of provoking release of a fibrogenic agent from macrophages.

Although, unfortunately, few immunological studies appear to have been done in reported cases of hard-metal disease the following points are consistent with its being a specific entity – most probably due to cobalt – and not a coincidental fibrosing alveolitis:

1. Relationship of development of disease to exposure.

2. The average size range of the metallic particles is of the order of 1.2 to 1.9 μm (McDermott, 1971) so that a large proportion are capable of reaching the alveoli. Tungsten and associated metals are usually present in affected lungs although, of course, this does not establish proof of a causal relationship. The frequent absence of cobalt has been explained.

3. The reported association of subacute disease with positive cobalt patch tests.

4. Despite the fact that the number of recorded cases and apparent incidence of the disease are very small in relation to the numbers of workers exposed – in one American series, 9 out of 1500 (Coates and Watson, 1971) – the clinical features and pathology appear to be similar in all.

5. The allergenic potential and cytotoxicity of cobalt.

Although the exact mode of causation remains to be established with certainty, the features of reversible, or partly reversible, subacute disease and of progressive fibrosis are closely akin, respectively, to those of subacute and chronic extrinsic allergic alveolitis. It has, however, also been suggested that fine, tungsten oxide whiskers, 0.3 μm or less in diameter, formed during the reduction of tungsten trioxide with a gas phase to produce tungsten metal (Sahle and Berglund, 1981), have not been adequately considered as a possible cause of hard-metal disease (Sahle, 1992) [see Addendum, page 634].

Clinical features

The clinical, physiological and radiographic features are similar to those of DIPF from other causes, which is predominant in the lower halves of the lungs (Figure 18.3). In a few cases the disease has been fatal due to cardiorespiratory failure. As the atomic number of tungsten is 74 it might be expected that small dense radiographic opacities would be seen if sufficient dust is stored in the lungs but this seems rarely to have been described. However, computed tomography in workers exposed to hard metals is reported to show diffuse density of hilar and subcarinal lymph nodes, resembling that caused by calcification, yet not readily seen on standard radiographs. This might be an aid to identifying exposure (Mendelson et al., 1991). No investigations of circulating antibodies appear to have been reported but hyperglobulinaemia is recorded (Miller et al., 1953).

Diagnosis

A detailed occupational history is essential for identifying the cause of the asthma and in the diagnosis of the subacute and chronic forms of hard-metal disease. Identification of tungsten by lung biopsy confirms exposure and may imply the association of cobalt but does not prove the lung pathology to be that of hard-metal disease. Other possible causes must be excluded.

The value of cobalt patch tests in diagnosis of the subacute and progressive types of disease has still to be determined. Tests of lymphocyte transformation and leucocyte inhibition factor in response to cobalt might be of help (Christiansen, 1979; Mayor, Merritt and Brown, 1980).

Concentrations of cobalt in the blood and urine appear to correlate well with levels of exposure (Alexandersson, 1979).

Treatment

Hard-metal asthma responds to bronchodilators and removal from exposure may be curative in some but not all cases. The desquamative fibrosing alveolitis (cellular) stage of the disorder responds to treatment with corticosteroids. Prompt diagnosis is of the utmost importance and affected workers should not be permitted to return to exposure to hard-metal dust once they have recovered. The chronic form of the disease is not amenable to treatment.

Prevention

Dust from the various processes in the preparations of hard metal and the finishing of products should be reduced to a minimum by efficient exhaust ventilation of the high-velocity, low-volume type locally applied as in the machining of beryllium alloys (Chapter 17) (McDermott, 1971). Also the environmental air, both breathing-zone and general, should be monitored. As far as possible, coolant liquids with the lowest capacity for dissolving cobalt should be used.

Medical examination including chest radiographs and tests of ventilatory function should be carried out yearly, and atopic subjects should be excluded from work involving potential exposure. Workers who develop contact skin sensitivity and whose cobalt patch test is positive should probably be removed from exposure (Sjögren et al., 1980).

Copper

Copper as a potent cause of metal fume fever in workers exposed to finely divided oxide (for example, melting the metal in electric furnaces) is referred to earlier in this chapter.

Vineyard sprayers' lung

Lung disease which appears to be related to the use of copper sulphate as an anti-mildew spray has been described in Portuguese vineyard workers (Pimentel and Marques, 1969; Villar, 1974).

A solution of 1 to 2 per cent copper sulphate neutralized with hydrated lime and known as Bordeaux mixture is sprayed periodically on vines by manual or mechanical means. After prolonged exposure some workers develop dyspnoea on effort and bilateral, irregular and rounded opacities in their chest radiographs.

Examination of the lungs reveals green–blue patches on their surfaces and, on section, dark-blue, rounded and coalescent areas are found in all lobes. Microscopically, the appearances include lymphocytic infiltration and diffuse fibrosis of the alveolar walls, foreign body granulomas that stain for copper and, at a later stage, fibrohyaline nodular lesions that tend to coalesce; granulomas are also found in the liver. Lung changes, similar to those seen in sprayers, have been produced in guinea-pigs with Bordeaux mixture.

There is said to be an increased risk of lung cancer among the vine sprayers and, although this has been attributed to solutions containing arsenic, the excess has been noted among sprayers who only use copper solutions (Villar, 1974).

Lithium hydride (LiH)

This is a respiratory irritant gas that causes violent sneezing and coughing when microgram quantities are dispersed in air (Spiegl et al., 1956). It is used in the atomic energy industry, experimentally as a rocket fuel propellant due to its exothermic properties, as a reducing agent in the organic chemical industry and as a convenient means of transporting hydrogen.

It has been reported to have caused pulmonary oedema of rapid onset in a worker who entered a tank to investigate a gas leak. Intensive care treatment resulted in rapid recovery in about 48 hours. Other cases have occurred (Cordasco et al., 1965).

Manganese

Exposure to manganese dust may occur in the mining and crushing of *pyrolusite* ore and in some of the processes in which the dioxide is used. These include the manufacture of 'dry' electric batteries, extensive applications in the chemical industry, and for colouring glass. Metallic manganese is an important ingredient in a variety of alloys, in particular manganese steel.

Metal fume fever may follow exposure to nascent manganese dioxide fume, and this compound causes necrosis and haemorrhage in the lungs of experimental animals (Lloyd Davies, 1946; Lloyd Davies and Harding, 1949; Morichau-Beauchant, 1964). Exposure to manganese dioxide produced radiographic changes in a small number of monkeys exposed for 3 months or more and there is some evidence that animals exposed to a single dose have a decreased resistance to infection with *Klebsiella pneumoniae* and the influenza A virus (Maigretter et al., 1976). These last results may be related to observations that show that manganese dioxide can reduce the number and the viability of pulmonary macrophages, and their phagocytic ability in vitro (Graham et al., 1975; Walter et al., 1975).

In the light of these animal studies it is interesting that some authors in the early part of this century noted a high incidence of pneumonia in workers exposed to pyrolusite or to manganese dioxide (Baader, 1932; Lloyd Davies, 1946). In Lloyd Davies's study the mean annual incidence over 8 years was 26 per 1000 compared with a mean annual incidence of 0.73 per 1000 in a control group. Rather more recently Suzuki (1970) has shown that the incidence of pneumonia among workers in a ferromanganese plant was higher than in a control plant in the same area, and data from Yugoslavia have also revealed a higher prevalence of respiratory disorders in workers engaged in the production of manganese alloys (Saric et al., 1974; Saric and Lucic-Palaic, 1977). There was a relationship between smoking and the prevalence of respiratory disorders in the Yugoslavian workers, suggesting that smoking may act synergistically with manganese in the production of bronchitis.

The effects of manganese on the lung thus seem to be well established but they have, of course, been overshadowed by the effects that exposure to this metal and its compounds has on the central nervous system where it produces a parkinsonian-like syndrome.

Mercury

This silvery, metallic liquid has a boiling point of 357°C and vaporizes at room temperature. The smaller the globules the higher the vaporization rate becomes. The vapour is odourless.

Lung disease caused by mercury is uncommon but serious and sometimes fatal. In industry it is usually due to exposure in confined spaces.

Mercury is used in the electrical industry for the manufacture of mercury vapour lamps, transformers, rectifiers and dry cell batteries; in the chemical industry in electrolytic processes and in the manufacture of pharmaceuticals and fungicides; in metallurgy for the production of amalgams of silver, gold, tin and copper; and in the manufacture and repair of thermometers, barometers, manometers and vacuum pumps. Mercury-steam boilers and mercury-arc rectifiers are also used in power generation.

Accidental exposure in industry may result from spillage in the production of thermometers and manometers, and in laboratories and dental surgeries, although the use of mercury in the latter is declining. It may also result from rupture of mercury-vapour boilers and contamination by 'blown' manometers in generator plants, and from cleaning out tanks used for chemical electrolysis; recently a hazard from the repair of sphygmomanometers has been reported (Christensen, Krogh and Nielsen, 1937; King, 1954; Teng and Brennan, 1959; Tennant, Johnson and Wells, 1961; Milne, Christophers and de Silva, 1970; Merfield et al., 1976; Ide, 1986). Accidental exposure to mercury vapour has also been reported in the home from the heating of mercury or mercury-containing materials on stoves and this has caused fatalities in children (Campbell, 1948; Mathes et al., 1958; Hallee, 1969; Gore and Harding, 1987).

Pathology

The lungs of individuals who die within a day or two show severe tracheobronchitis with stratification of the epithelium of bronchioles, pulmonary oedema with proteinaceous exudate in the alveolar spaces and well-developed hyaline membranes. Small numbers of lymphocytes and large mononuclear cells are present in the alveolar walls and there are early proliferative changes of the lining and interstitial cells. At about 3 weeks, however, fairly extensive DIPF is present with early evidence of 'honeycombing', striking hyperplasia of alveolar lining cells many of which are atypical, and persistence of hyaline membrane (Liebow, 1975) (Figure 18.4). Mild DIPF has also been demonstrated some 5 months after exposure (Hallee, 1969).

Some of the inhaled mercury is exhaled and the rest apparently removed rapidly from the lungs. Experimental observations in monkeys and rabbits indicate that about 80 per cent of the mercury in the blood is in the erythrocytes leaving little free in the plasma (Berlin, Fazackerley and Nordberg, 1969). Urinary excretion of the metal correlates poorly with the quantity absorbed (Teisinger and Fiserova-Bergerova, 1965).

Clinical features

Symptoms do not usually develop until 1 to 4 hours after exposure. They include tightness in the chest, dyspnoea, persistent non-productive cough, fever and restlessness. Somewhat later, these symptoms may be followed by anorexia, nausea, vomiting, abdominal pain and arthralgia. The severity of the symptoms is dependent upon the severity of exposure.

Bilateral, diffuse inspiratory and expiratory crackles are present in the lung bases and the chest radiograph shows bilateral soft opacities similar to those of pulmonary oedema, most prominent in the lower halves of the lung fields. Pulmonary function tests may show a severe restrictive deficit with mild obstruction and impaired diffusion (Gore and Harding, 1987).

Among patients who survive – and recovery is the rule with prompt treatment – a proportion are found to have DIPF.

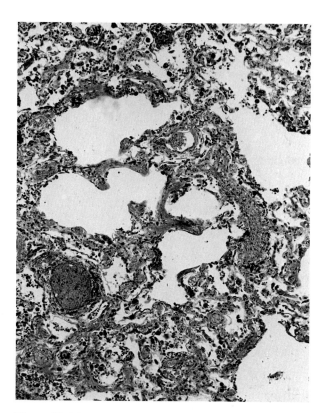

Figure 18.4 Interstitial and intra-alveolar fibrinous oedema caused by mercury vapour with cellular infiltration, desquamation of alveolar lining cells and some hyaline membrane formation. The radiograph was taken approximately 2 weeks after exposure. (magnification × 120). (Courtesy of Professor A.A. Liebow)

Diagnosis

In many cases in whom lung disease develops, exposure to mercury may not be part of their normal occupational pattern. Even those whose work regularly brings them into contact with the metal will not experience exposure sufficiently high to produce pulmonary symptoms. Therefore, the diagnosis of mercury-induced lung disease depends predominantly on obtaining a good history of accidental exposure. Blood mercury levels may be high (the normal value is <2 μg/dl) and the urinary concentration may also be high (normal is <5 μg/g creatinine). If mercury estimations are required, it is essential that they are carried out by a laboratory that has the necessary experience annd expertise; the results from routine biochemical laboratories should not be relied on.

Treatment

Corticosteroids should be started as soon as possible even in those who do not seem to be severely affected. Oxygen and other supportive measures will generally be required. Treatment with chelating agents is without effect and the use of BAL is considered to be potentially harmful because it increases the uptake of mercury by the brain.

Nickel

Nickel is used extensively in the production of nickel-based alloys including ferronickel, in the manufacture of steel, in nickel electroplating and in glass, enamels and ceramics. It may occur in some welding fumes. High-purity nickel is obtained from the decomposition of nickel carbonyl in the Mond process.

Acute effects

Asthma

Nickel, which is well known as a cause of allergic dermatitis, has been reported to cause late-type asthma which ceases at weekends and recurs on Mondays in the nickel plating industry and in the production of nickel carbonyl. In one case it was reproduced over a period of 5 hours by a single bronchial challenge with $NiSO_4$; gas transfer was not affected. Löffler's syndrome is also recorded in association with both asthma and dermatitis (Sunderman and Sunderman, 1961; McConnell et al., 1973) (see Table 21.7).

Chemical pneumonia and pulmonary oedema

These may follow exposure to nickel carbonyl. Nickel carbonyl [$Ni(CO)_4$] is a heavy, colourless, unstable liquid which is vaporized at 43°C. The vapour is highly toxic.

Acute disease caused by inhalation of the vapour has two phases: *immediate*, consisting of nausea, vomiting and severe headache which usually recovers fairly quickly; and *delayed*, the onset of which may vary from 10 to 36 hours – occasionally up to 8 days – after exposure, consisting of paroxysmal coughing, breathlessness, chest tightness, substernal pain and extreme weakness. The clinical and radiographic signs of pulmonary oedema and patchy bilateral consolidation develop.

Following heavy exposure death may occur in a few days when the lungs *post mortem* show haemorrhagic oedema with areas of consolidation, some of which may contain fibrinoid and be necrotic. Otherwise recovery, though slow, is complete (Sunderman and Kincaid, 1954).

Treatment requires the use of oxygen and corticosteroids. The value of chelating agents is doubtful.

Chronic effects

It is by no means certain that there are any chronic effects, although pulmonary fibrosis has been described in workers exposed to nickel carbonyl and both nickel and copper were present in the lungs of affected workers (Jones Williams, 1958). Pulmonary fibrosis has also been described in workers in a steel works in which there was exposure to nickel, but also to chromium and iron oxide (Jones and Warner, 1972). Epidemiological studies have failed to demonstrate any excess mortality from any respiratory diseases other than lung cancer (Doll, 1958; Morgan, 1958).

Carcinoma of lung

The possibility of nickel or nickel carbonyl being carcinogenic is referred to in Chapter 19 (page 654).

Osmium

Metallic osmium has a limited use in industry for certain alloys and in the chemical industry. It is innocuous but when heated, as in annealing, or at room temperature it evolves osmic acid or osmium tetroxide (OsO_4) which is used as a tissue fixative in electron microscopy. Osmium tetroxide is intensely irritant and toxic and, if inhaled even in small amounts, causes severe acute laryngotracheobronchitis with chest tightness and bronchospasm (McLaughlin, Milton and Perry, 1946), and may provoke pulmonary oedema in higher concentrations associated with accidental exposure. However, because the vapour is so irritant and nauseating, this is of rare occurrence. But accidental exposure to high concentrations would undoubtedly cause acute pulmonary oedema.

Prevention consists of good ventilation and storage of osmic acid in sealed containers.

Selenium compounds

Selenium is a semi-metal, or metalloid, with similar properties to sulphur. It is widely distributed in small quantities in igneous rocks, volcanic material and glacial drifts, chiefly in the form of metallic selenides or in combination with sulphur. It is obtained largely as a byproduct of processes involving selenium-containing sulphide minerals.

Selenium is most extensively used in the manufacture of metal plate rectifiers, photoelectric cells and other electronic devices. It is also employed as an additive to alloy steels, to decolorize poor grade green glass, in insecticides and with cadmium to produce orange and maroon pigments.

Elemental selenium is believed to be harmless to human beings but it burns readily in air producing dark-red selenium dioxide fume which is irritant and toxic. Hydrogen selenide gas, which may be evolved when the metal comes in contact with acid or water, is also dangerous.

Selenium dioxide (SeO$_2$)

Exposure to fume that smells of garlic may occur when selenium is added to furnaces or ladles and under other conditions of heating when it may also take the form of a light powder. Inhalation causes upper and lower respiratory tract irritation with cough and substernal pain and, in large amounts, may result in non-fatal pulmonary oedema. In addition, gastric irritation and epigastric pain after meals and, occasionally, haematuria may occur. But no chronic pulmonary effects appear to have been reported.

Hydrogen selenide (selenium anhydride, H$_2$Se)

Contact with this gas is less likely to arise in industry than exposure to selenium dioxide but it appears to be more toxic. Acute intoxication has occurred in laboratory workers and as a result of industrial accidents in processes where selenium is present, for example heating copper, zinc or lead; the production of glass; and roasting pyrites. Accidental leakage from cylinders of the gas has caused acute respiratory disease (Schecter et al., 1980).

The symptoms are similar to those caused by sulphur dioxide. Initially there is watering of the eyes and nose, sneezing, cough and chest tightness which recover fairly quickly. These are followed after about 6 to 8 hours by the symptoms and signs of pulmonary oedema often during the night. Severe dyspnoea with violent coughing, pneumomediastinum and subcutaneous emphysema have been reported 18 hours after exposure and were associated with severe obstructive and restrictive functional defects which slowly improved, although some impairment was still present 3 years later (Schecter et al., 1980). However, fatal cases have not been described and this may be attributable to hydrogen selenide being rapidly oxidized to elemental selenium on mucosal surfaces.

Treatment includes oxygen, diuretics and, probably, corticosteroids and antibiotics.

Prevention involves careful control of selenium-using processes, provision of goggles and respirators and storage of selenium away from acids and water (Clinton, 1947; Glover, 1970).

Dimethylselenide

Selenide is methylated in the liver to form dimethylselenide which is excreted through the lung and gives the breath a smell of garlic. Diskin and his colleagues (1979) reported the case of a man in whom numerous non-caseating perivascular granulomas were found as a coincidental finding at autopsy. The patient had worked for 50 years in a selenium refinery and died of myocardial infarction; he had no respiratory symptoms. It was suggested that the pathological changes in the lungs were consequent upon prolonged exposure to dimethylselenide and the authors concluded that this compound should be looked upon as a pulmonary toxin. They further suggested that their findings might require a revision of exposure standards in industry to avoid significant pathological changes in the lung. The fact that their patient survived to the age of 71 with no evidence of lung disease is not likely to lead to any rapid action on the part of the selenium industry or of those who promulgate hygiene standards.

Titanium tetrachloride

Titanium tetrachloride (an intermediary in the production of titanium metal) is used as a mordant for the dyeing industry, as a pigment and for military smokes and sky writing. It is highly corrosive and reacts violently with water to produce titanium particles, hydrochloric acid vapour and heat. Hydrochloric acid is probably released when unreacted titanium tetrachloride is inhaled due to hydrolysis in the humid conditions of the upper and lower respiratory airways. High concentrations of titanium tetrachloride may, therefore, cause acute rhinitis, tracheitis, bronchitis and pulmonary oedema.

Titanium tetrachloride is normally handled under inert conditions to avoid contact with oxygen and moisture in the air. In general, therefore, exposure of personnel is most unlikely to occur other than accidentally.

The clinical features that follow acute, severe exposure are those of pulmonary oedema with large amounts of proteinaceous fluid rich in fibrin, and swelling and hyperplasia of alveolar cells (Lawson, 1961). Diffuse endobronchial polyposis (similar to that which may occur in thermal and smoke injuries

– see page 631), in a chemical engineer some weeks after accidental inhalation of titanium tetrachloride, has also been described; recovery occurred in a year, although slight bronchial stenosis remained (Park et al., 1984). No respiratory symptoms appear to be caused by prolonged exposure to low concentrations.

Metallic titanium and titanium dioxide are discussed in Chapter 11.

Vanadium

Vanadium (atomic number 23) is found in combination with other elements in igneous and sedimentary rocks and in some petroleum deposits due to the fossilized remains of sea squirts of the tunicate family and sea cucumbers whose normal blood consists, in part, of vanadium.

Sources of exposure and uses

Vanadium ore is first crushed and dried ('inactive ore'), finely ground in a ball-mill ('active ore') and roasted; it is then mixed with sulphuric acid and the resulting precipitate, which is dried, is vanadium pentoxide. This is packed in bags. The roasting and bagging processes tend to produce most dust; grinding and crushing produce rather less.

Vanadium-bearing slags, produced on a large scale during the manufacture of steel from titaniferous magnetite, are becoming an increasingly important source of vanadium in some countries (for example, South Africa and the former USSR). Other important sources of vanadium-containing dusts are furnace residues from oil refineries, soot from oil-fired boilers and slags from the production of ferrovanadium (Williams, 1952). The soot is ground and treated with sodium hydroxide and slag is crushed, extracted with water, neutralized with sulphuric acid and filtered. In addition to vanadium, carbon dust is also produced by these processes. Deposit formed on heat-exchanger tubes of gas turbines contains some 11 to 20 per cent vanadium (Browne, 1955); its removal gives rise to a great deal of dust.

Carnotite ($K_2O \cdot 2UO_3 \cdot V_2O_5 \cdot 3H_2O$), a uranium-containing vanadium mineral found in South Australia and Colorado and Utah in the USA, forms the cementing material of sandstones and, being disseminated through them, must be mined with them. After mining it is milled and processed on a large scale as a uranium source. Mining and milling may thus carry a quartz risk, but the chief potential hazard to health lies in the production of radon decay products (Archer et al., 1962) (see Chapter 19, page 656).

Vanadium metal is used extensively for metal alloys: ferrovanadium and molybdenum–vanadium steels, and vanadium bronze and brass. Vanadium pentoxide and ammonium vanadate (NH_4VO_3) are used as catalysts in the manufacture of various chemicals and ammonium vanadate and other vanadium salts are also employed in inks, dyeing processes, paints, insecticides, photographic developer and glass production.

Pathology

Acute bronchitis and pneumonitis or bronchopneumonia may follow heavy exposure to vanadium pentoxide dust and fume. The pneumonic lesions are usually patchy but they may be widespread and confluent.

Wyers (1946) suggested, on the grounds of alleged abnormalities in chest radiographs of vanadium-exposed workers (but without the benefit of pathological examination of lungs), that permanent lung changes – interpreted as fibrosis – were caused by vanadium pentoxide, but Sjöberg (1950) and Williams (1952) did not confirm this. In fact, no pathological studies appear to be on record which demonstrate fibrosis in human lungs attributable to vanadium. However, mild cases of silicosis due to the presence of small quantities of quartz in the dust of dry sedimented dross seem to have occurred, although mining of the ore and exposure to metallic vanadium appear to be harmless.

Rabbits exposed to low concentrations of vanadium pentoxide for more than 8 months showed no evidence of pulmonary fibrosis and none resulted after its injection into the peritoneum of guinea-pigs (Sjöberg, 1950). Chronic exposure to this compound was found to produce inflammatory changes with haemorrhage, pneumonia and purulent bronchitis in rats (Roshchin 1967a,b).

Symptoms and physical signs

Exposure to fairly high concentrations of vanadium pentoxide dust (such as may result from the soot and bottom ash of oil-fired boilers in ships and electricity generating stations, from furnace residues of oil refineries and from slags in the production of ferrovanadium) causes intense irritation of the nose and eyes with lacrimation, sore throat and persistent, often violent, cough. The cough develops a few hours after exposure and persists for 7 to 10 days. It is often accompanied by a wheeze that may last 2 to 3 days (Lewis, 1959; Zenz and Berg, 1967; Lees, 1980). Wheezing is also more common in workers who have been exposed to low concentrations of vanadium pentoxide during its manufacture than in controls with no exposure (Kiviluoto, 1980).

On examination, wheezing is not always apparent, but transient, inspiratory crackles and wheezes may follow re-exposure. Sometimes wheezing is pronounced and associated with dyspnoea on exertion – in fact, it appears to be a late (non-immediate) asthmatic reaction (see Chapter 21). Bronchoscopy reveals diffuse hyperaemia of the mucosa of the trachea and bronchi with some viscid mucus. In the absence of pneumonic disease the patient is afebrile (Sjögren, 1950). Both symptoms and signs clear completely (Zenz and Berg, 1967). Signs of bronchopneumonic consolidation may, however, develop, following intense exposure.

Although chronic cough (Dutton, 1911) and dyspnoea (Wyers, 1946) have been attributed to vanadium exposure, there was no satisfactory evidence of a causal relationship. In Dutton's cases, pulmonary tuberculosis appears to have been responsible. Prospective studies of vanadium workers have not shown that the presence of chronic cough, breathlessness and abnormal physical signs can be ascribed to this cause, although 'bronchitis with bronchospasm' appears to be enhanced by repeated exposure to europium-activated yttrium orthovanadate (Sjöberg, 1950; Vintinner et al., 1955; Tebrock and Mackle, 1968). Based largely on the work of Roshchin (1968), it has been claimed (World Health Organization, 1988) that chronic vanadium intoxication produces 'profound changes in the respiratory organs' including diffuse pulmonary fibrosis, chronic bronchitis, chronic rhinitis and pharyngitis. Other published data (Sjöberg, 1950; Williams, 1952; Zenz and Berg, 1967) do not support this contention and, on balance, there seems little reason to change the opinion given in the previous edition that the association between vanadium exposure and the development of bronchitis and emphysema cannot be substantiated.

Lung function

No difference in vital capacity (VC) between exposed subjects and controls was found by Sjöberg (1950), and Vintinner et al. (1955) did not observe any significant impairment of other spirometric values. Kiviluoto (1980) found no significant difference in ventilatory function compared with matched controls in a group of vanadium pentoxide production workers exposed to concentrations ranging from 0.1 to 3.9 mg/m³ for an average of 11 years.

Zenz and Berg (1967) reported that, although volunteers exposed to 0.25 mg vanadium pentoxide/m³ for 8 hours complained of cough within 24 hours which ceased in 7 to 10 days, the values of their ventilatory function tests over a period of weeks did not fall below pre-exposure values even when exposure was repeated. However, men exposed to 523 µg/m³ time-weighted average of respirable dust (<10 µm) containing 15.3 per cent vanadium from the bottom ash of oil-fired boilers developed a pronounced fall in FEV_1 and FVC in 24 hours which did not fully return to normal in 8 days, although 4 weeks after exposure there were no residual defects (Lees, 1980). This author suggests that transient loss of function is not attributable simply to reflex bronchial reaction to irritation by an inert dust (Lees, 1980).

Radiographic appearances

Appearances of unilateral or bilateral pneumonic consolidation or, possibly, small areas of segmental collapse may be present after heavy exposure. Otherwise no abnormality is seen. Wyers (1946) reported fine linear markings ('X-ray reticulation') in three cases with low level exposure but the validity of this observation – which has never been confirmed (Williams, 1952; Tebrock and Mackle, 1968) – is most doubtful. Discrete opacities (pneumoconiosis) have not been described.

Diagnosis

Because the symptoms and signs are identical to those of an acute upper and lower respiratory infection it is necessary to identify recent exposure to vanadium pentoxide dust or fume, and to exclude viral or bacterial infection. In the absence of pneumonia, lack of fever supports the diagnosis. Detection of vanadium in the blood or urine significantly above the normal values (<0.1 µg/dl for blood; <1 µg/g creatinine for urine) is evidence of exposure.

The possibility of non-immediate vanadium-induced asthma should be borne in mind.

As vanadium does not cause any permanent radiographic abnormality there can be no confusion with pneumoconiosis or other forms of lung disease. If this is not understood abnormal radiographic shadows in a worker known to have been exposed to vanadium dust or fume in the past may be wrongly attributed to this cause and the responsible disease thus overlooked.

Prognosis

No permanent pulmonary damage appears to be attributable to exposure to vanadium pentoxide. Pneumonia usually recovers completely with appropriate treatment but, occasionally, after heavy exposure, it may be fatal.

Treatment

Apart from bronchopneumonia to which the standard principles apply, treatment is symptomatic.

Prevention

Efficient, well-fitting respirators for exposed personnel are essential. Routine annual spirometry and quantitative analysis of urinary vanadium as an index of the amount absorbed have been suggested (Lees, 1980).

Zinc

Zinc oxide fume has been referred to earlier as a potent cause of metal fume fever. In general, zinc salts are not harmful to the lungs but zinc chloride smoke is an important exception.

Zinc chloride is employed in galvanizing iron, oil refining, dry batteries and taxidermy, and has been used for smoke bombs in war time and for fire fighting exercises (Shenker, Speizer and Taylor, 1981). In smoke bombs zinc chloride is formed where zinc oxide and hexachloroethane are burnt together. Normally it is not hazardous, but if encountered in confined spaces the smoke can be lethal. At least 20 per cent of its small particles are deposited in the alveolar region, and larger particles cause thermal and hygroscopic injury to the mucosal surfaces of the airways (Pedersen, Hansen and Gronfeldt, 1984; Allen et al., 1992). Acute pulmonary oedema and chemical pneumonia occur and may progress to dense DIPF with fatal pulmonary heart disease within a few weeks. Ventilatory function may be greatly reduced (chiefly a restrictive defect) with severe hypoxaemia. The radiographic changes are those of pulmonary oedema or patchy irregular consolidation (Evans, 1945; Whitaker, 1945; Milliken, Waugh and Kadish, 1963), but with recovery appearances may return to normal (Allen et al., 1992).

The most appropriate treatment is not known. High-flow oxygen and corticosteroids are essential. The zinc-chelating agent acetylcysteine has been used without success but penicillamine, started early, appears to have been successful (Allen et al., 1992).

Prevention includes the wearing of respiratory protective equipment and protective clothing.

form. It is on record as causing severe pulmonary oedema (Cordasco and Stone, 1973).

Metallic zirconium and zircon are discussed in Chapter 11.

Non-metallic gases, vapours and mists

Many of these are irritant to mucous membranes and so are capable of causing inflammation of airways or pulmonary oedema if a sufficient concentration is inhaled. A highly soluble gas (ammonia, for example) gives rise to immediate and intense irritation of eyes, nose and upper respiratory tract which compels the exposed individual to make a prompt escape. In these circumstances only small amounts of the gas reach the lower respiratory tract, and the lungs are little, if at all, affected. But if escape is impossible or the concentration of the gas is high, sufficient quantities may reach the alveoli to provoke pulmonary oedema. An irritant gas of low solubility (such as nitrogen dioxide or phosgene), however, has no, or only a minor, irritant effect on the upper respiratory tract so that the worker may inhale considerable amounts before leaving the contaminated area, and its effects on the lungs may be delayed for a number of hours. Gases of intermediate solubility (such as chlorine) cause pulmonary oedema if exposure is fairly prolonged or concentration is high. In some instances – especially if the noxious gas is a respiratory depressant (for example, hydrogen sulphide and methyl bromide) – pulmonary oedema may be due to hypoxia of the lung rather than to direct assault by the gas on alveolar membranes.

In general, non-fatal cases of acute pulmonary damage from exposure to a noxious gas, vapour or mist appear to recover completely although secondary patchy pneumonia may occur during recovery resulting on occasion in small areas of permanent segmental fibrosis. However, few prolonged follow-up studies of substantial numbers of severe accidents seem to have been reported.

Zirconium tetrachloride ($ZrCl_4$)

This compound is produced during the reduction of its chloride in the preparation of the metal. It reacts violently with water and is usually found in gaseous

Acetaldehyde (ethanal, CH_3CHO)

This volatile, colourless liquid with a strong pungent odour is produced by oxidation of ethylene gas. Its main use is as an intermediary in the production of a large number of chemicals, but it is also used in the manufacture of synthetic resins, plastics, synthetic rubber and disinfectants. It is highly irritant to the respiratory tract and is narcotic.

Low concentrations cause irritation of the eyes and hypersecretion of the upper respiratory and bronchial mucus. High concentrations cause headache, stupor and acute pulmonary oedema which may not develop for some 24 hours.

Treatment, in most cases, consists simply of the relief of symptoms but, if there is suspicion of exposure to high concentrations, observation for development of pulmonary oedema should be maintained for at least 48 hours.

Prevention depends upon good ventilation, avoidance of spillages, and protective goggles and clothing.

Acetic acid

Acetic acid is used as a chemical feedstock for the production of plastics and a wide variety of chemicals and it is also to be found in the dye, rubber, pharmaceutical, food and textile industries. The vapour may produce immediate irritation to the eyes and upper respiratory tract and, if exposure is severe, pulmonary oedema. Rajan and Davies (1989) describe reversible airways' obstruction and interstitial pneumonitis in a maintenance fitter who was accidentally exposed to hot glacial acetic acid when he disconnected a pressurized pump for overhaul. He had first-degree burns which were immediately treated but, over the next 7 days, he developed exertional dyspnoea. On examination, he had inspiratory basal crackles with scattered wheezes. His chest radiograph showed the presence of patchy bilateral reticulonodular infiltration, especially at the lung bases. Lung function tests showed a marked decrement in FEV_1 and FVC and a reduced $TLCO$. Transbronchial biospy showed a diffuse, mainly mononuclear interstitial peumonitis; BAL contained excess numbers of macrophages and lymphocytes. The symptoms cleared promptly following treatment with corticosteroids and the authors speculated that the pneumonitis may have had an immunological basis.

Acrolein (acrylic aldehyde, CH_2CHCO)

This is an oily liquid produced by catalytic oxidation of propylene. In the liquid state it presents little hazard but, as it has a high vapour pressure, it may quickly form dangerous concentrations of a colourless, pungent, irritating gas.

It is used in the manufacture of plastics, textile finishes, acrylates, synthetic fibres and pharmaceuticals, and may be evolved when oils and fats containing glycerol are heated to high temperatures such as may occur in the production of soap, fatty acids and linseed oil, and during the reduction of animal fats.

Acrolein is intensely irritant at concentrations in excess of 5 p.p.m. Due to this, serious intoxication is rare because it is impossible to tolerate the effects for more than a brief period. However, accidental spillages or leakages from pipes or vessels may cause inhalation of high concentrations before the exposed workers can make their escape. Exposure is followed by productive cough, shortness of breath, chest tightness and the signs of pulmonary oedema. Fatalities have been reported following accidental exposure (Committee on Aldehydes, 1981).

Treatment with oxygen, corticosteroids and an antibiotic must be commenced as soon as possible because there is a risk of permanent lung damage.

Ammonia

Ammonia is a colourless, highly soluble, extremely irritant alkaline gas. It is used extensively in industry. Very large quantities are employed in the manufacture of soil fertilizers, and in the pharmaceutical and chemical industries. Its other important uses include: refrigeration, the manufacture of plastics and explosives, oil refining and as an additive to furnaces to inhibit oxidation.

In most instances exposure to the gas occurs as a result of rupture or leakage of tanks or other containers, fractured pipes or valve failures. The general public may also be affected if transporter tanks are involved in road or rail accidents (Caplin, 1941; Kass et al., 1972; Walton, 1973; Sobonya, 1977).

Due to its high solubility ammonia causes chemical burns of eyes, skin, oropharynx and upper respiratory tract. There is severe burning pain in the mouth and throat followed quickly by a feeling of suffocation with cough, copious watery sputum and difficulty in breathing. With exposure to high concentrations death occurs from asphyxia due to obstructive laryngeal oedema; with lower exposures the severity of symptoms varies.

In death shortly after exposure the post-mortem appearances are those of severe laryngeal and pulmonary oedema with haemorrhage (Walton, 1973). In patients who survive for some days bacterial infection supervenes, and terminal pneumonia due to *Nocardia asteroides* has been described

(Sobonya, 1977). Many who survive acute disease recover completely, though slowly, but others may be left with bronchiectasis (which may be severe and widespread) and fibrous obliteration of the small airways (Kass et al., 1972; Sobanya, 1977). Hence, long term, if not permanent, impairment of respiratory function (chiefly airflow obstruction) may sometimes result (Leduc et al., 1992).

Clinically, the heavily exposed individual is in respiratory distress with blood-stained sputum, cyanosis, stridor, loss of voice and fever; in addition to the signs of pulmonary oedema, there are chemical burns of varying degree. The chest radiograph may show the features of pulmonary oedema but correlation between the severity of clinical disease and radiographic appearances seems to be poor; often there is no evident abnormality. Patients with no abnormal physical signs in the chest tend to recover in 24 hours whereas those with abnormal signs have a more protracted and complicated course. Thus, the clinical signs are the best guide to prognosis (Montague and MacNeil, 1980).

Treatment is a matter of urgency in severely affected individuals and often requires an intensive care regimen. The complication of serious secondary pulmonary infection must be anticipated. Otherwise conservative medical treatment is usually sufficient.

Chlorine

Chlorine is a greenish-yellow gas, two and a half times heavier than air, the toxic qualities of which were exploited in the First World War. It is used in the manufacture of innumerable chemicals varying from pharmaceuticals to plastics, and for disinfecting water. It is usually transported commercially by road, sea or rail as a liquid under pressure. Exposure may occur during a manufacturing process, from leakage of pipes or tanks, from accidental spillage during transportation or as a result of mixing chlorine bleach with an acid cleaner (Chasis et al., 1947; Jones, 1952; Joyner and Durel, 1962; Kowitz et al., 1967; Weill et al., 1969). Swimming pool attendants may also be accidentally exposed when changing gas cylinders (Decker and Koch, 1978).

The injurious effects of the gas are thought to be due to its potent oxidative properties which liberate nascent oxygen – a protoplasmic poison – from water and to the fact that hydrochloric acid is formed (Kramer, 1967). The changes in the lungs may be those of oedema with some fibrin and the formation of hyaline membrane in alveoli, and early bronchiolar damage and obstruction of small blood vessels by thrombi. Brief concentrations of 3 to 5 p.p.m. of the gas appear to be tolerated without injury, but exposure to 5 to 8 p.p.m. for a signifi-cantly long period may cause mild acute illness. Levels of 14 to 21 p.p.m. are dangerous and when over 40 p.p.m. acute pulmonary oedema occurs. The effects of exposure, however, depend not only on the concentration of gas but also on duration of exposure, and the presence or absence of pre-existing disease. The very young and the aged suffer more severely than healthy adults (Kramer, 1967).

Clinical features

Symptoms of over-exposure consist of smarting of the eyes, lacrimation, rhinorrhoea, severe persistent cough, dyspnoea, retrosternal chest pain and a sense of constriction. Nausea, epigastric pain and vomiting may also occur. In spite of the severity of the symptoms, the patient usually recovers quickly when removed from the area of contamination. With higher concentrations of gas there is pink, frothy sputum, and restlessness, severe respiratory distress, central cyanois, widespread, coarse crackles – often with wheezing – and low-grade fever (Beach, Sherwood Jones and Scarrow, 1969). The patient is critically ill for some 48 hours and, even with appropriate treatment, it may be some weeks before dyspnoea on exertion finally ceases.

The chest radiograph of severely ill patients shortly after exposure shows the signs of pulmonary oedema that may occasionally be followed in a few days by bronchopneumonic consolidation. However, although both oedema and secondary infection are uncommon complications, death sometimes occurs (Flake, 1964; Beach, Sherwood Jones and Scarrow, 1969).

In fatal cases there is acute laryngotracheobronchitis and large quantities of frothy, bloody fluid in the lungs and airways. Microscopy shows massive pulmonary oedema, and some alveolar spaces filled with polymorphonuclear leucocytes and thrombosis in large proximal and central blood vessels. If death is delayed for 75 hours or so after exposure, hyaline membranes are present with fibrin in the capillary vessels (Weston et al., 1972).

After clinical recovery there are no residual respiratory symptoms and lung function returns to normal although this may take some months. For example, four or five chlorine plant workers who were accidentally exposed still had abnormal lung function tests 12 to 14 months after the accident (Kaufman and Burkons, 1971). However, Weill and his colleagues (Jones et al., 1986) followed up the victims of a severe gassing accident after a tanker train derailment in the USA and found that 3 weeks later there was no detectable difference in lung function relating to distance from the site of the spill or to the severity of the initial symptoms. Sixty of the victims were followed up over a 6-year period and the only changes in lung function that could be detected were those due to smoking.

Occasionally the develoment of pulmonary oedema is delayed for up to 2 days after exposure.

Long-term exposure of chlorine gas workers to concentrations of less than 1 p.p.m. is not associated with significant impairment of ventilatory function, but those who smoke have a lower maximum mid-expiratory flow rate than non-smokers (Chester, Gillespie and Krause, 1969).

Treatment

This is similar to that required for nitrogen dioxide poisoning with the exception of correction of methaemoglobulinaemia (see page 626). A broncho-dilator in nebulizer form is often recommended but may be unnecessary if corticosteroids are used. In healthy adults with mild poisoning, simple symptomatic treatment and oxygen at atmospheric pressure may be all that is needed. The case of intense exposure from which the individual cannot immediately escape is a medical emergency which demands prompt treatment of shock, coma and respiratory arrest.

Pre-employment medical examination of workers who may be exposed to a potential chlorine hazard should be done to exclude those with respiratory or cardiovascular disease.

Hydrogen chloride (hydrochloric acid, HCl)

This is evolved as a gas or vapour during the production of hydrochloric acid by various methods, in particular during decanting, the operation of pumps and the use of pouring frames. Accidental exposure may sometimes occur in the manufacture of dyes, fertilizers and textiles, in the rubber and ore refining industries, in fires and during welding in an atmosphere containing halogenated hydrocarbons. But serious exposures are rare because the highly irritant nature of the vapour quickly warns the worker of its presence.

Inhalation of a substantial quantity of vapour causes irritation of the upper respiratory tract, acute bronchitis, oedema of the glottis and pulmonary oedema.

Hydrogen fluoride (hydrofluoric acid, HF)

This is produced by the reaction of concentrated sulphuric acid and fluorspar (calcium fluoride). It is

a colourless gas which smells a little like chlorine, is readily soluble in water and forms a dense white vapour in moist air. It is used in the production of fluorocarbons and inorganic fluorides, in the refining of certain metals, as a constituent of some types of welding electrodes, as a catalyst for electrotinning of steel and in the chemical industry.

Hydrogen fluoride is highly irritant and toxic to the skin and mucous membranes, and inhalation causes burning of the nose, mouth and throat which may be followed by pulmonary oedema and pneumonia, the symptoms and signs of which, however, may not develop for 12 to 24 hours. The oedema may be severe enough to cause asphyxia requiring the full resources of an intensive care unit.

Preventative measures include special handling methods, exhaust ventilation and appropriate personal protection. Containers for transportation, duly labelled, are designed to prevent accidental spillage.

Other compounds of fluorine

Some other compounds of fluorine, including nitrogen fluoride and tetrafluorohydrazine, may also act as pulmonary irritants. Many of the compounds of fluorine, however, are physiologically inert, although some, such as sulphur hexafluoride, may produce extremely active breakdown products such as sulphur dioxide difluoride which may induce pulmonary oedema (Pilling and Jones, 1988). It is suggested elsewhere in this volume that some fluoro compounds such as sulphur hexafluoride and carbon tetrafluoride, which are extremely lipid soluble, may interfere with surfactants in the lung, thereby producing pulmonary oedema (see Chapter 2, page 26).

Hydrogen sulphide (sulphuretted hydrogen, H₂S)

This gas is classed as an asphyxiant because, following absorption from the lungs, it rapidly causes central respiratory paralysis. But it is also an irritant. It is encountered as a byproduct in the manufacture of some chemicals and dyes; in the rayon, tannery and rubber industries; in petroleum refining; in areas of volcanic activity; in mines with sulphide ores; in sewers; and in the fishing and fish meal industries – in which, incidentally, ammonia may also be a hazard (Dalgaard et al., 1972).

Exposure to concentrations greater than about 700 p.p.m. (which are, usually, accidental) causes death from respiratory failure due to depression of medullary centres before the irritant effects in the lungs have time to develop. More prolonged exposure to lower levels (for example, 300 to 600 p.p.m.) result in pain in the nose, throat and chest, cough, headache, and dizziness followed by pulmonary oedema which may be complicated by pneumonia.

Oedema is both inter- and intra-alveolar and haemorrhagic. There is widespread damage to type I pneumocytes and, to a lesser extent, to capillary endothelial cells (Biesold, Bachofen and Bachofen, 1974).

Respiratory failure can be reversed by prompt artifical respiration after removing the subject from exposure, otherwise intensive treatment for toxic pulmonary oedema is required.

Methyl bromide (bromethane)

This gas (CH_3Br) which has a low boiling point is used as a refrigerant, herbicide, fumigant insecticide, and in the manufacture of aniline dyes. It has also been employed as a fire extinguishing agent. Although one of the most toxic of the organic halides, it gives little warning of its presence to the senses and disperses slowly. It is thus highly dangerous especially if encountered in enclosed spaces.

Inhalation of high concentrations of the gas cause acute bronchitis with frothy, blood-stained sputum and signs of pulmonary oedema sometimes with haemorrhagic pleural effusions. In addition, there may be convulsions with other neurological abnormalities and subsequent coma. In such cases prognosis is poor. With exposure to lower concentrations pulmonary involvement is unusual but may occur in milder form, and the abnormalities (giddiness, convulsions, ataxia, pyramidal and extrapyramidal signs, EEG changes and anuria) are confined to the central nervous system and kidneys. Symptoms and signs generally develop some 2 to 4 hours after exposure but are often insidious and may be delayed for about 48 hours.

Diagnosis depends on history of exposure. The presence of convulsions and prominent neurological signs, however, may distract attention from involvement of the lungs.

Treatment of individuals with pulmonary symptoms and signs includes immediate removal from exposure, oxygen, corticosteroids and bed rest. Seizures require the use of anticonvulsive agents (Johnstone, 1945; Rathus and Landy, 1961).

Prevention involves mixing some pungent substances that can readily be smelled with the methyl bromide, the use of efficient halide detectors, effective ventilation and appropriate protective equipment. Methyl bromide can penetrate ordinary rubber gloves, and protective equipment should, therefore, be made of polyvinyl, neoprene or nitrile latex. If exposure to high concentrations is likely, respiratory protective equipment must be provided and workers should not work alone.

Oxides of nitrogen

The oxides of nitrogen include nitrous oxide (N_2O), nitric oxide (NO), nitrogen dioxide (NO_2), nitrogen trioxide (N_2O_3) and nitrogen tetroxide (N_2O_4). Nitrous oxide, of course, is a harmless anaesthetic gas. The other oxides which may occur in industry originate as NO. Nitric oxide is fairly stable having a half-life of about 10 p.p.m./hour and, therefore, converts slowly to NO_2 (the situation in the case of explosions may be different) (B.T. Commis, 1972, personal communication). Nitrogen dioxide may polymerize to N_2O_4 which is so unstable that it promptly dissociates to NO_2. These gases are often popularly, but incorrectly, referred to as 'nitrous fumes'. Nitrogen dioxide is a reddish-brown gas which is heavier than air, has an odour like domestic bleach and is the oxide of medical importance.

Nitrogen dioxide may be encountered in a wide variety of industrial situations: during the manufacture and use of nitric acid, and the manufacture of explosives; during welding, electroplating and engraving; in the exhaust from metal cleaning processes; in forage tower silos; during shot-firing in mines and other blasting operations; from slow burning of gun-cotton and cordite; and from the exhaust of diesel engines. Nitrogen dioxide is used as a constituent of jet engine and missile fuels. It has also occurred as an accidental contaminant of nitrous oxide for anaesthesia (Clutton-Brock, 1967).

The occurrence of nitrogen dioxide in metal welding and cutting is referred to in the section of welding (page 629).

The oxides of nitrogen and their effects on human and animal lungs are comprehensively reviewed by the World Health Organization (1977).

Forage tower silos

The need for a reliable supply of bulk fodder for cattle in winter months led to the adoption of ensilage of grass or other green crops. This began on the European continent in the mid-nineteenth century and spread to Britain (Jenkins, 1884). At first, lined pits or adapted barns were used but the method was a failure owing to lack of understanding of the biological processes involved. The tower silo was introduced to the eastern counties of England from the USA at the beginning of this century (Hall, 1923). However, it was not generally adopted because of the expense involved, and above-ground clamps, later with devices for self-feeding of cattle, were in common use until the 1950s (Turner, 1953). Then, a new type of American tower silo with mechanical loading and distributing equipment came to Britain in the late 1950s and has been installed increasingly since, its stark outline in the countryside being a mark of agricultural change (Figure 18.5).

Concentrations of nitrogen dioxide produced during the preparation of silage may be sufficiently high to cause death to a worker entering a silo (Delaney, Schmidt and Stroebel, 1956; Grayson, 1956; Lowry and Schuman, 1956; Desbaumes, 1968; Anonymous, 1970).

Evolution of carbon dioxide – which is detected first (Commins, Raveney and Jesson, 1971) – and NO_2 begins a few hours after silo filling commences, is maximal in 1 to 2 days and continues at a decreasing rate for a week or 10 days (Lowry and Schuman, 1956). At the same time, the concentration of oxygen falls. The processes that underlie the production of these gases are not wholly understood but appear broadly to be as follows.

Carbohydrates in the crops yield acetic and lactic acids and CO_2 due to degradation by bacteria. The nitrate content of plants is derived chiefly from inorganic nitrates which are converted into nitrites by enzymatic action; it is increased by soils highly nitrated by fertilizers, by drought and by immaturity of the plants. The potential concentration of NO_2 is said to be roughly proportional to the amount of nitrate in the silage crop by some authors (Lowry and Schuman, 1956) but not by others (Commins, Raveney and Jesson, 1971). The nitrites react with the acids to form nitrous acid (HNO_2) which decomposes to water, NO and NO_2 as the temperature of the silage rises due to fermentation (Grayson, 1956). Temperatures 3½ feet (105 cm) below the silage surface may range from 40.6 to 57°C (Delaney, Schmidt and Stroebel, 1956). Initially the concentration of NO is higher than that of NO_2 but later this situation is reversed and the ratio NO_2/NO rises (Commins, Raveney and Jesson, 1971). Some N_2O_4 is also evolved but breaks down rapidly to NO_2. According to the type of crop, its pH and moisture content, bacterial activity may, in addition, give rise to free ammonia, butyric acid and free amines.

The presence and concentrations of the gases vary widely in different towers but there is no evidence that those made of concrete slats are less likely to develop potentially dangerous concentrations, due to their porosity, than steel towers (Jesson, 1972).

Both CO_2 and NO_2, being about one and a half times heavier than air, are concentrated at or near the silage surface and in depressions. Dangerous amounts of gas may be present, not only for a few days after filling, but also some months later if the silo has remained unopened. The silage surface and silo wall may be stained yellow–red and a similar

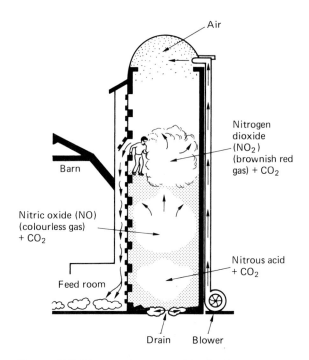

Figure 18.5 Diagram (not to scale) of a forage tower silo. (Adapted from Ramirez and Dowell, 1971, with permission)

coloured vapour may be seen above the surface. An open door in the discharge (or feed) chute permits the gases to flow down into an attached barn (Figure 18.5). A person entering the silo does so normally through a chute door above the silage surface. He climbs the vertical chute ladder, opens one of the chute doorways at the appropriate height, climbs through the narrow opening and jumps on to the surface which may be a few feet below. If he becomes unwell due to the effects of accumulated gases he may be physically incapable of the effort necessary to retrace his path through the door and down the ladder. When the surface is convex he is more likely to encounter higher gas concentrations immediately on entry than when it is concave, but a concavity may also contain high concentrations (Figure 18.6). Levelling the silage surface, therefore, may be a dangerous procedure if the difference between its highest and lowest levels exceeds the height of a man (Jesson, 1972). When the surface is concave the peripheral concentration of gas may be too low at breathing level to be detected by smell and so cause a false sense of security on entry, whilst the higher concentrations at the surface and in depressions may make descent into a depression and its disturbance during levelling, or an accidental fall, especially hazardous (Figure 18.7). Furthermore, the movement of men in a tower disturbs the gases and may release gas trapped in the silage.

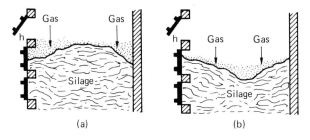

Figure 18.6 Diagram showing two different contours of the silage surface. Gas is likely to be encountered by the farm worker as he climbs on to a convex surface (a) from the hatch (h) or descends into a central concavity (b) disturbing pockets of NO_2 gas

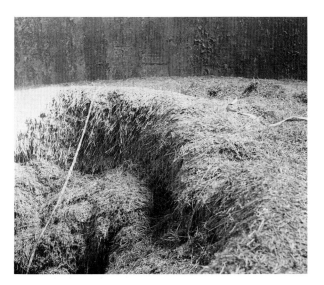

Figure 18.7 Photograph showing a concavity in the silage some 5 or 6 feet deep in the silage surface. The potential danger of the situation is evident. (Courtesy of Mr M.W. Jesson and the National Institute of Agricultural Engineering, Silsoe, Bedfordshire)

The presence of high CO_2 and low oxygen concentrations are important as they cause deep breathing which facilitates penetration of nitrogen dioxide to alveolar level and so enhances its effect (Commins, Raveney and Jesson, 1971). High concentrations of gas render a man helpless in two or three minutes (Anon, 1970).

Respiratory illness due to nitrogen dioxide in silos is known as *silo fillers' disease*. Its potential seriousness and the increasingly widespread use of tower silos indicate the necessity for a general awareness of the risks involved.

Groves and Ellwood (1989) recommend that some form of testing should be undertaken prior to entering silos. They found that a safe level of carbon dioxide was a good indicator of safe levels of oxygen but that the converse was not always the case. Thus, apparently safe levels of oxygen could be accompanied by levels of carbon dioxide and nitrogen dioxide that were in excess of the occupational exposure limits. If any form of testing is to be used, then measurements of both oxygen and carbon dioxide concentrations should be made, but it must be admitted that, in practice, few farmers would be likely to wish to invest in the necessary apparatus.

Mining

Nitrogen dioxide is produced in varying degree by the firing of nitro-explosive charges in mines and from the exhaust of diesel haulage locomotives.

The regular use of 'exhaust gas conditioners' on diesel engines in British coal mines greatly reduces the output of NO_2, and concentrations of the gas in the vicinity of these engines and in the driver's cab are usually well below the recommended TLV. The average concentration of NO_2 appears to be about 10 per cent of the nitrogen oxides in undiluted exhaust gases (Godbert and Leach, 1970). Recent studies have found no evidence that, as has sometimes been suggested, exhaust emissions cause chronic airways' obstruction in miners (Attfield, Trabant and Wheeler, 1982; Reger and Attfield, 1983; Robertson et al., 1984; Ames et al., 1988; Leigh and Wiles, 1988).

Concentrations of gas from shot-firing only reach dangerous levels under conditions of imperfect detonation of charges or poor ventilation which may exist, for example, in tunnelling operations. Ventilation in most areas of coal mines is good and serious pulmonary disease does not, therefore, occur. However, as there is some speculation that shot-firing in coal mines might constitute a hazard to underground workers the matter must be discussed in a little more detail. If an effect were produced it would be most likely to occur in men ('deputies' and shot-firers) working on headings and in tunnels, although in British coal mines it is the practice that they do not return to the working place for at least 10 minutes after firing more than six charges, or at least 5 minutes after firing six or less.

Both NO and NO_2 are produced by the explosion, the former being present in larger quantity, and the production of these gases varies little with the different explosives used but those with a negative or near-negative oxygen balance give rise to smaller quantities of gas. The gases are evolved in the form of a bolus and the rate at which this travels away from the explosion and is dispersed is determined by the velocity of the ventilating air. As the bolus passes a given point the concentration of the gases rises rapidly and then gradually falls, and the further it travels from source the more the gases are diluted. Hence, peak concentrations are very brief and the men are not likely to be exposed to them because they are outside the area. There is, moreover, no evidence that such transient peak concentrations have any medical significance.

Thus, in general, coal miners have not been exposed to the risk of developing acute disease (Kronenberger, 1959) though four possible cases of pulmonary oedema attributed to high exposure to shot-firing gases in 1960/1961 were reported by Kennedy (1972).

A variety of conditions influence the amount of oxides produced. They include the nature and quantity of explosive, the method of stemming and detonation, the area of the working place and the air volume. Therefore, although the concentrations vary from place to place those to which miners are subjected are uniformly low (Graham and Runnicles, 1943; Powell, 1961; Godbert and Leach, 1970). The average concentrations of mixed oxides for a whole working shift at the return end of the coalface has been found to be 4 p.p.m. (Graham and Runnicles, 1943), but may now be lower since the introduction of power loading in the 1960s. There is no satisfactory evidence to suggest that such concentrations are injurious to health.

Other occupational hazards

Burning furnishings or fires in chemical plants may evolve nitrogen oxides and firemen fighting the blaze may be exposed. Workers in burning buildings are also, of course, at risk. For example, in the 1929 Cleveland Clinic fire some 50 000 nitrocellulose X-ray films were destroyed with the evolution of NO, CO and HCN. Ninety-seven workers died immediately from the effects of the CO and the HCN and another 26 died within the next month, most probably from the effects of NO (Gregory, Malinoski and Sharp, 1969). Three American astronauts were exposed to NO_2 for 4 to 5 minutes due to the inadvertent firing of the Reaction Control System in the Apollo–Soyuz space craft and they developed pulmonary oedema the day after splashdown (Hatton et al., 1977).

Chemical effects

The severity of the effect of NO_2 depends mainly on its concentration and the duration of exposure to it, and is similar whatever its mode of origin. Unlike most water-soluble gases it is only feebly irritant to the upper respiratory tract. The reason for this is believed to be that, owing to its relatively low solubility, its conversion to HNO_2 and HNO_3 – which are the cause of its harmful effects in the lungs – occurs slowly in water or humid air and is not maximal, therefore, until it reaches the peripheral airways and alveoli resulting in pulmonary oedema and chemical pneumonia (Pattey, 1963).

Nitric acid apparently dissociates in the lungs into nitrates and nitrites resulting in local tissue damage and the formation of methaemoglobulin (Clutton-Brock, 1967); methaemoglobulinaemia is known to follow exposure to high concentrations of NO_2.

Experimental observations

In animals

Short-term exposure of animals to 7 to 16 p.p.m. NO_2 causes endothelial damage with transudation of fluid into alveolar spaces and airspaces, impairment of surfactant activity and airway's closure (Dowell, Kilburn and Pratt, 1971). Oedema, haemorrhage, hyperinflation, desquamation of the respiratory epithelium and bronchopneumonia are produced by the inhalation of the higher oxides of nitrogen (Shiel, 1967). Long-term exposure of animals to 12 to 26 p.p.m. NO_2 has been reported to cause bronchiolar hyperplasia and mild centriacinar dilatation of alveoli (Freeman and Haydon, 1964), and some partial closure of terminal bronchioles by fibrosis and occasional attenuation and fracture of alveolar walls has been described many weeks after prolonged exposure to an average of 15 p.p.m. NO_2 had ceased (Freeman, Crane and Furiosi, 1969).

Drozdz, Kucharz and Szyja (1977) reported that guinea-pigs exposed to 2 mg/m³ NO_2 for 180 days develop emphysema-like lesions and reduction in collagen content of the lungs. But Kleinerman (1979) found that, in hamsters exposed to approximately 30 p.p.m. NO_2 – a high concentration – for 22 hours daily for 3 weeks, total collagen content decreased within 4 days but returned to normal in about 14 days, and that both collagen and elastin content were normal 3 weeks after exposure had stopped. It has been suggested that alteration in collagen and elastin content and emphysema-like lesions in animals may be caused by enzyme activity but prolonged exposure of hamsters to 30 p.p.m. NO_2 revealed no evidence of proteolytic enzyme activity (Kleinerman and Rynbrandt, 1976; Rynbrandt and Kleinerman, 1977). Interestingly, Kleinerman and Wright (1961) observed reversal of the lung lesions caused by single or multiple treatments of animals with nitrates.

In a series of in vitro experiments with 'macrophage-like cells' and sheep erythrocytes, Davis et al. (1978) found no overall differences between the cytotoxic effects of pure coal dust and samples onto which high levels of NO_2 had been adsorbed.

In man

To what extent (if at all) these and similar observations are relevant to human beings is uncertain. But some evidence of degradation of lung collagen, deduced from changes in urinary hydroxylysine glycosides, was observed in the Apollo astronauts who developed pulmonary oedema after short exposure to high concentrations of NO_2 – average 250 p.p.m. (510 mg/m³) (Hatton et al., 1977).

Healthy young men challenged with 5 p.p.m. NO_2 for 2 days developed a significant increase in airways' resistance and a decrease in alveolar–arterial oxygen pressure differences (Hackney and Linn, 1979); no adverse effects were noted with exposure to levels up to 1 p.p.m. (Hackney et al., 1975; Folinsbee et al., 1978). Patients with asthma, however, may be rendered much more sensitive to the effects of bronchoconstrictors by concentrations of nitrogen dioxide as low as 0.1 p.p.m. (Orehek et al., 1976).

Pathology

The gross appearances of the lungs in rapidly fatal cases following exposure to large concentrations of NO_2 are those of haemorrhagic oedema with watery blood-tinged fluid in the airways and patches of pneumonia; in patients who survive for a few weeks before finally succumbing there are small palpable nodules and haemorrhagic areas.

Microscopy of rapidly fatal cases shows, in addition to oedema, extensive damage of the respiratory epithelium which may be completely shed in the small bronchi and bronchioles, and in the later cases, generalized infiltration of alveolar walls with lymphocytes, numerous macrophages in alveolar spaces and bronchiolitis obliterans in various stages of organization which is responsible for the palpable nodules (McAdams, 1955; Darke and Warrack, 1958; Moskowitz, Lyons and Cottle, 1964). If the patient recovers, these lesions usually resolve completely, especially if he has been treated with corticosteroids (Moskowitz, Lyons and Cottle, 1964).

Clinical features

The absence of immediate and pronounced irritation of the upper respiratory tract allows the worker to inhale gas for some time without distress. Irritation of the throat does not apparently occur until concentration of the oxides of nitrogen reaches 60 p.p.m. and cough not until it is 100 p.p.m. (Pieters and Creyghton, 1951). Severe headache and dizziness which have sometimes been complained of by magazine attendants, 'deputies' and shot-firers in coal mines have been caused more by absorption of the nitroglycerin of explosives cartridges through the skin or by ingestion, or to the inhalation of carbon monoxide from an exploded charge than by

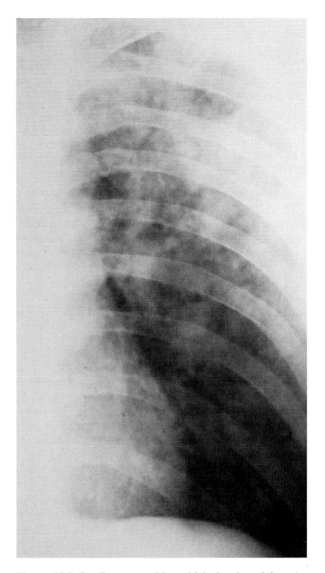

Figure 18.8 Confluent opacities which developed 3 to 4 weeks after exposure to high concentrations of nitrogen dioxide in a tower silo. The appearances in the right lung field were similar. Complete resolution and symptomatic recovery subsequently occurred. (Courtesy of Dr R.H.G. Greenspan, Connecticut, USA)

nitrogen dioxide (Powell and Lomax, 1960). But dizziness may occur early in some cases of NO_2 exposure due to the production of systemic hypotension.

The onset of respiratory symptoms is delayed for 3 to 30 hours after exposure (although some transient choking and tightness in the chest, and sometimes central chest pain with profuse sweating, may occur during exposure) so that, in some cases, a worker may return to work before becoming ill. However, in the mixed gas conditions which may be encountered in a tower silo a worker may rapidly be rendered senseless.

Table 18.1 Summary of extrinsic agents and injuries that can cause pulmonary oedema

Inorganic	Organic	Physical
Ammonia	Acetic acid	Fire smoke
Antimony oxide*	Acetaldehyde	Pulmonary barotrauma*
Antimony pentachloride	Acrolein	due to compression (see Chapter 25)
Antimony trichloride	Chlorinated camphene*	and decompression (see Chapter 24)
Bismuth pentachloride	Dioxane	Blast
Cadmium	Dimethyl sulphate*	Blunt trauma
Chlorine	Methyl bromide	Near-drowning
Cobalt	Nickel carbonyl	High altitude*
Hydrogen chloride	Organophosphates*	
Hydrogen fluoride	Phosgene	
Hydrogen selenide	Polytetrafluoroethylene*	
Lithium hydride	Toluene diisocyanate	
Mercury vapour	in high concentrations*	
Nitrogen dioxide	Trimellitic anhydride*	
Osmium tetroxide		
Ozone		
Phosphine		
Selenium dioxide		
Sulphur dioxide		
Sulphur hexafluoride (degraded)		
Titanium tetrachloride		
Zinc chloride		
Zirconium tetrachloride		

A worker known or suspected to have been exposed to any of these agents or conditions should be placed under close medical supervision for at least 72 hours *even if there are no significant symptoms immediately after exposure.*
*See appropriate chapters.

The patient becomes acutely ill with paroxysmal cough, wheeze, frothy blood-stained sputum, nausea, vomiting, increasing dyspnoea, restlessness and anxiety. He is feverish (38.3 to 38.9°C) with central cyanosis (which may be deep in the presence of methaemoglobinaemia) and there are widespread inspiratory crackles and polymorpholeucocytosis. There may be systemic hypotension and evidence of haemoconcentration due to intrapulmonary fluid loss; the chest radiograph reveals the ill-defined, woolly opacities characteristic of pulmonary oedema. Death from respiratory failure may occur at this stage.

Patients who recover may pass into a latent period lasting *2 to 6 weeks* during which time they continue to improve, and abnormal clinical and radiographic signs disappear, and then suddenly they relapse with a *second acute episode* similar to the first without having been re-exposed to the gas. The radiographic appearances consist either of small opacities (which have been mistaken for miliary tuberculosis) or confluent, ill-defined opacities (Becklake et al., 1957) (Figure 18.8). The reason for this 'rebound' episode (which does not occur in every case) is uncertain: it may be due to recurrence of oedema provoked by a minor infection in lungs in which repair of previously damaged alveolar epithelial cells is incomplete. If this is so, it is perhaps surprising that the phenomenon does not appear to be caused

by any other toxic gas. It is also possible that it corresponds to the development of bronchiolitis obliterans. However, recovery is usual with prompt treatment with corticosteroids, but irreversible bronchiolar fibrosis seems to have occurred in a few untreated cases (Moskowitz, Lyons and Cottle, 1964; Milne, 1969; Horvath et al., 1978).

Hence, there are three distinct clinical stages:

1. Acute oedema.
2. A period of apparent recovery.
3. Relapse in a second acute illness. This stage may develop even though the stage 1 illness may have been mild.

Lung function during stages 1 and 3 shows variable abnormal patterns but vital capacity is much reduced, airways' resistance increased, gas distribution uneven and gas transfer impaired. Serial tests during the delayed acute stage have shown normal elastic recoil and airflow resistance with reduction of dynamic compliance dependent on respiratory frequency, and hypoxaemia on exercise suggesting dysfunction of the small airways (Fleming, Chester and Montenegro, 1979). Although airways' obstruction and reduction of gas transfer may be present for weeks or months after the chest radiograph has cleared, it is rare to find any permanent abnormality of function (Becklake et al. 1957; Ramirez and Dowell, 1971; Jones, Proudfoot and Hall, 1973), but mild hyperinflation (Moskowitz, Lyons and Cottle, 1964) or airways' obstruction have occasionally been reported although, in most of these cases, lung function values have not been recorded prior to exposure.

The chest radiograph clears quickly with treatment without evidence of residual lung damage.

Does exposure to nitrogen dioxide cause irreversible pulmonary damage?

This, in fact, poses two questions which must be considered separately.

1. *Does acute disease with pulmonary oedema result in permanent lung damage?* As indicated in the previous section, complete recovery is the rule in those cases of pulmonary oedema or bronchiolitis obliterans which have been followed for a sufficient length of time and is hastened by treatment with corticosteroids. However, varying degrees of pulmonary dysfunction may persist in occasional cases due, possibly, to unresolved bronchiolitis, and some follow-up studies can be criticized for being too short and lacking smoking histories and adequate clinical and physiological assessment (Horvath et al., 1978).
2. *Does intermittent, long-term exposure to low concentrations cause emphysema?* From his clinical and physiological investigation of 100 cases of coalminers exposed to oxides of nitrogen during shot-firing underground, Kennedy (1972, 1974) contends that 'nitrous fumes' cause emphysema. However, there are some important deficiencies in this study which put the validity of the conclusion in doubt:
   (a) the men investigated were not randomly selected and appear to have been referred because they had respiratory symptoms (McLintock, 1972);
   (b) there was no matched control group;
   (c) smoking habits were not taken into account;
   (d) the presence or absence of other pulmonary disease was not mentioned;
   (e) NO – which converts slowly to NO_2 – and NO_2 were not monitored separately (Bergman, 1972).
   Similar criticisms apply to two other reports of workers exposed in non-mining occupations in which the same conjecture was advanced with the additional complication that the men had also been exposed to other toxic agents (Vigdortschik et al., 1937; Kosmider et al., 1972) (see also Chapter 10, page 249).

Because the open flames of gas cookers produce short-term peaks in NO_2 in cooking areas, studies have been carried out to determine the prevalence of respiratory disease and lung function in those living in households where gas cookers are used compared with those living where cooking is done with electricity. Keller and his colleagues (Keller et al., 1979a, b) found no adverse effects but Speizer, Ferris and Bishop (1980) found that children from homes with gas cookers did have a greater history of respiratory illness before the age of 2 years and had had significantly lower FEV_1 and FVC measurements when corrected for height, and when suitable adjustments were made for social class and smoking habits of their parents. Measurements of NO_2 in one home showed a level of 0.55 p.p.m. when the oven was in use and a level of 0.25 p.p.m. when a single gas burner was lit. This subject has been reviewed in more detail by Spengler and Sexton (1983) and by Fischer et al. (1985).

Despite these pointers to some adverse effects in young children by low levels of nitrogen dioxide, there are no comparable data that suggest that occupational exposures cause irreversible pulmonary damage and Horvath's statement that 'there is no conclusive evidence that long term exposure to low levels of NO_2 leads to emphysema or chronic bronchitis in humans' seems still to be the most reasonable summary of the evidence (Horvath et al., 1978). The results of the study on coal miners referred to in the previous edition do not yet appear to have seen the light of day.

Diagnosis

Awareness of the pattern of illness caused by NO_2 and a detailed occupational and medical history will usually point to the diagnosis but it may be necessary to exclude myocardial infarction. It is vital that diagnosis is made without delay and that a second acute episode is not mistaken for pneumonia because failure to use appropriate corticosteroid treatment at this stage may be fatal. Even with immediate appropriate treatment mortality from acute disease may be as high as 30 per cent (Ramirez and Dowell, 1971).

Acute farmers' lung may also occur as a result of disturbing mouldy material immediately below the silage surface while removing the top seal or unloading ('topping') of grass or grain (see Chapter 20, page 681). The history is all important for differentiation. The risk of silo fillers' disease is associated with freshly filled silos and is, therefore, present during the harvest season; the worker may have noticed both the smell and the yellow–red colour of the gas. Extrinsic allergic alveolitis is most likely to occur in winter or spring due to moulding of the previous summer's harvest, and the signs of NO_2 gas will have been absent. The presence of methaemoglobinaemia may help to identify silo fillers' disease.

It is possible that widespread pulmonary fibrosis which has occasionally been attributed to silage gases in the past was in reality chronic extrinsic allergic alveolitis.

Treatment

In all cases in which there has been a significant, or suspicion of significant, exposure to NO_2 admission to hospital for 48 to 72 hours is imperative. If signs of pulmonary oedema and respiratory distress develop, corticosteroids should be commenced immediately and, in some patients, oxygen, possibly with assisted ventilation, may be necessary. Steroid treatment should be continued for at least 8 weeks to prevent relapse and the development of bronchiolitis obliterans (Horvath et al., 1978). Other measures which may be needed are as follows:

1. Antibiotics: their use is indicated only if evidence of infection supervenes.
2. Reconversion of methaemoglobulinaemia by an initial dose of methylene blue 2 mg/kg intravenously and subsequent doses titrated against the methaemoglobulin concentration in the blood (Prys-Roberts, 1967).
3. Correction of haemoconcentration in some cases.
4. The use of a vasopressor drug in the event of severe systemic hypotension.

The patient should be kept under observation for at least 3 months from the date of exposure.

Prevention

Good ventilation is the most important measure in any potential NO_2 hazard. Some welding processes can be subjected to exhaust ventilation techniques. Respirators used in enclosed spaces must be of approved type as some models are ineffective against NO_2.

Special measures apply to forage tower silos. These include:

1. Thorough ventilation of the tower by use of the blower (see Figure 18.5) for at least half an hour before entry (Jesson, 1972).
2. A safety harness to which a rope can be attached should be worn and two workmates should be in attendance outside the tower.
3. If it is necessary to enter a silo during filling (for example, to level the silage by hand), this should be done immediately after the last load and not left until the following day when gas may already have been evolved.

It has also been recommended that, after opening a chute door, the worker should immediately climb above it in order to be higher than any remaining gas that might escape. However, Jesson (1972) has shown that this manoeuvre cannot be relied upon and may be hazardous as the direction of airflow after the chute door is opened varies with wind direction.

Workers must be educated about the risks involved in their industry. The 8-hour time-weighted average (TWA) exposure limits for nitrogen dioxide and nitric oxide are 3 and 25 p.p.m. respectively; the 10-minute short-term TWA exposure limits are 5 and 35 p.p.m.

Ozone

Ozone is a highly toxic gas and one of the most powerful oxidizing substances known. It is normally present in the atmosphere in minute quantities without any harmful effect but it occurs in increased concentrations at high altitudes. Significant amounts may enter the cabins of aircraft at altitudes greater than 30 000 feet (9000 m) (Bennett, 1962; Young, Shaw and Bates, 1962) (see Chapter 24, page 795). It is produced in lightning and high-tension, non-sparking, electrical discharges in air or oxygen. It is used in industry for sterilizing water, bleaching paper, flour and oils and deodorizing organic factory effluents by masking, but not destroying, the odour (Pattey, 1963).

The evolution of potentially dangerous levels of ozone from atmospheric oxygen by ultraviolet radiation produced by gas-shielded, welding and arc-air gouging is referred to in the section on 'Welding and similar processes'. Ultraviolet radiation from air-conditioning equipment and office photocopying machines may give rise to low levels but, in ordinary ventilated areas, these are unlikely to be harmful.

The effects of ozone on the lungs of experimental animals have been extensively studied especially in the USA where they have been prompted in part by the anxiety of the high levels generated during the production of photochemical smog. Alveolar type I cells are most susceptible to the effects of ozone and undergo necrosis whereas type II cells are remarkably resistant and proliferate to replace them even during continuous exposure to the gas (Stephens et al., 1974; Mustafa and Tierney, 1978; Castleman et al., 1980). Clara cells and alveolar macrophages are also stimulated, although the function of pulmonary macrophages may be inhibited (Huber et al., 1971).

The death of cells in the lung results in a decrease in enzyme activity which is followed by a reparative phase in which enzyme activity is elevated. These metabolic changes can be demonstrated following continuous exposure for 7 days to concentrations of 0.8 p.p.m. or lower (Mustafa et al., 1983). Ozone also increases the susceptibility of experimental animals to bacterial pneumonia. This is probably because the membrane damage to the macrophage impairs their ability to produce the superoxide anion radical which reduces bactericidal activity (Witz, Amuroso and Goldstein, 1983; Ryder-Powder et al., 1988).

The intracellular effects of ozone are similar to those of ionizing radiation and both produce reactive free-radical intermediates. Antioxides and radical-trapping agents such as quinones, ascorbic acid and α-tocopherol protect against the toxic effects of ozone as does the intracellular enzyme superoxide dismutase; it has been suggested that elaboration of the latter may protect the lungs of those chronically exposed to polluted air (Hackney et al., 1975).

Clinical features

Ozone is 10 to 15 times more toxic than NO_2 (Stokinger, 1965).

Acute illness following heavy exposure (in excess of 2 p.p.m.) is either rapid in onset consisting of severe headache, substernal pain and dyspnoea (suggesting myocardial infarction) or develops more slowly with irritation of the nose and eyes which may last for a day or so, with severe cough, blood-stained sputum, dyspnoea and fever. Symptoms, physical signs and radiographic appearances are those of pulmonary oedema. Exposures of from 5 to 20 p.p.m. from 1 hour or more may be fatal (Kleinfeld, Giel and Tabershaw, 1957; Stokinger, 1965; EMAS, 1972).

Concentrations of 0.4 to 0.5 p.p.m. inhaled for 3 hours a day for 5 days caused reduction in FVC and specific airways' conductance in healthy volunteers, but subsequently there were no significant differences and respiratory symptoms ceased after the second day (Farrell et al., 1979). This phenomenon is known as 'adaptation' and takes place even in sensitive subjects, although the process takes longer (Horvath, Gliner and Folinsbee, 1981). Adaptation can also be induced in rats (Tepper et al., 1989), but apparently not dogs (Kleeberger et al., 1988). The effect on the airways seems to be mediated by histamine and some metabolites of arachidonic acid and it can be prevented by the administration of cromolyn sodium (Fouke, Delemos and McFadden, 1988; Kleeberger et al., 1988).

It has been reported that with concentrations of 0.5 p.p.m. there is no significant increase in gas transfer or in static compliance (Kerr et al., 1975). More recent studies, however, have shown that there is an increase in the permeability of the respir-

atory epithelium. Volunteers were exposed to 0.4 p.p.m. ozone for 2 hours while performing exercise on a treadmill. The rate of pulmonary clearance of ^{99m}Tc-DTPA (^{99m}Tc-labelled diethylenetriamine pentaacetic acid) was measured by sequential posterior lung imaging with a gamma camera and the mean clearance increased from 0.59 to 1.75 per cent minute (Kehrl et al., 1987).

Although levels of less than 0.5 p.p.m. have an inhibitory effect on acetylcholinesterase, this is not apparently related to the presence of bronchoconstriction (as revealed by FEV_1 and maximal expiratory flow rates) which, at these concentrations, occurs only in smokers (Fabbri et al., 1979). A study of 1330 flight attendants showed that those who worked for airlines flying at high altitudes, where ozone levels of up to 0.5 p.p.m. may be found, were much more likely to complain of chest pain, chest tightness, difficulties in breathing and persistent cough than those flying on low-altitude commuter airlines (Reed, Glaser and Kaldor, 1980). More recently, however, Harding (1988) has found that concentrations of 1.0 p.p.m. have been recorded in subsonic commercial aircraft flying at 40 000 feet without any evidence of distress in passengers and crew. The reason for this discrepancy is not immediately obvious, but it does suggest that the effects of exposure to low levels of ozone in healthy individualso require more thorough examination (see Chapter 24, page 795).

Treatment

In cases of acute illness this is similar to that required for the effects of nitrogen dioxide, but methaemoglobulinaemia does not occur.

Prevention

Local exhaust ventilation is necessary where significant concentrations of the gas may occur but is unlikely to be adequate unless measures to screen off the ozone-producing source are taken (Frant, 1963).

Phosgene (carbonyl chloride, $COCl_2$)

This gas – used as a poison gas in the First World War – is many times more toxic than chlorine, is about three and a half times heavier than air and has a sweet, pungent smell resemblng new mown hay which, however, may not be detected at low concentrations.

Situations in which phosgene may cause poisoning are as follows: the chemical industry in which it is used as a chlorinating agent in the synthesis of organic compounds such as dyes; in the metallurgical industry for separation of certain metals by chlorination; during welding of metals cleaned with chlorinated hydrocarbons such as carbon tetrachloride and trichlorethylene which yield the gas when heated; the use of chlorinated hydrocarbons for fire fighting; and the use of paint removers such as methylene chloride in heated enclosed spaces (Gerritsen and Buschmann, 1960; Seidelin, 1961; Doig and Challen, 1964; English, 1964; Everett and Overholt, 1968). Although phosgene occurs in fires in which there is burning polyvinyl chloride (PVC) its quantity is very small and makes little or no contribution to the overall toxicity of the decomposition products (Wooley, 1971).

Because phosgene is less soluble than ammonia or chlorine its effects are directed predominantly at the deeper parts of the lung. In the lung, phosgene undergoes hydrolysis producing nascent hydrochloric acid which destroys the permeability of the alveolar epithelium. Significant quantities of the gas can be inhaled before any symptoms develop. At first there may be cough with some breathlessness and tightness in the chest but, with low concentrations, these initial symptoms may be mild or absent. The symptoms and signs of pulmonary oedema and respiratory distress follow, but often not until 24 or 48 hours after first exposure. Collapse in hypovolaemic shock may then occur with coma and death. The pathological changes include inter- and intra-alveolar oedema with sloughing of the bronchiolar mucosa.

Patients who survive recover completely over a period of 1 to 2 weeks and, as far as is known, have no permanent lung damage (Seidelin, 1961; English, 1964).

Prolonged exposure to minute concentrations of phosgene does not appear to have any adverse effects.

Phosphine (hydrogen phosphide, PH_3)

Exposure to this colourless gas which has the foul odour of rotten fish is uncommon and usually accidental and unexpected. It may occur under the following conditions: handling of hot phosphoric acid; processing of wet ferrosilicon metals due to the presence of metallic phosphides as impurities; production of acetylene; from aluminium phosphate stored under unsatisfactory moist conditions; welding of steel coated with phosphate rust-proofing; during the manufacture of phosphide agricultural insecticides and the striking surfaces of matchboxes with phosphorus sesquisulphide; and the use of calcium phosphide in the pyrotechnics industry. As a rule the offensive smell warns workers of its

presence but the odour threshold is sufficiently high for dangerous concentrations to be unrecognized.

Aluminium phosphide, which releases phosphine, may be used as a grain fumigant in preference to methyl chloride because, although it is more toxic than methyl chloride, it is said to be safer under actual conditions of work (Hayes, 1971). Accidental poisoning with fatalities has been reported in some of the crew and their families of a grain freighter when phosphine leaked from the hold (Wilson et al., 1980).

Inhalation of phosphine causes weakness, faintness, cough, dyspnoea and, in concentrations over about 300 p.p.m., pulmonary oedema which usually occurs within 24 hours but is occasionally delayed for a few days after exposure. Concentrations above 400 to 600 p.p.m. are rapidly fatal with convulsions and coma (Pattey, 1963).

Treatment is similar to that for pulmonary oedema due to other toxic gases but absolute rest is necessary in seriously ill patients, and exposed individuals who do not appear to be seriously affected must be kept under close medical supervision for at least a week.

Sulphur dioxide (SO_2)

This gas, which is more than twice as heavy as air, is an intense respiratory irritant because it is first hydrated and then oxidized to sulphuric acid on mucosal surfaces. The most commonly encountered toxic gas, it is used extensively in the chemical and paper industries, and in bleaching, fumigation, refrigeration and preserving. It also occurs as a byproduct of smelting sulphide ores and during the action of sulphuric acid on reducing agents. In the USA some 500 000 workers are believed to be at risk of exposure to acute sulphur dioxide inhalation (Charan et al., 1979).

An accident involving five previously healthy men in the paper industry working inside or near a digester tank partly filled with wooden chips, and who were exposed to varying concentrations of the gas, exemplifies the range of effects it can have. Two men inside the tank were able to climb out but died within 5 minutes in respiratory arrest and shock with pink frothy fluid around their mouths. The pharyngeal and laryngeal mucosa had a coagulated appearance and, microscopically, the superficial columnar epithelium was widely denuded. The lungs and airways were filled with pink proteinaceous oedema fluid but there was no inflammation, cell infiltration and no disruption of alveolar walls. The three survivors outside the tank experienced tightness in the chest with intense dyspnoea, and soreness of eyes, nose and throat. Crackles and rhonchi were heard in their lungs but chest radiographs were normal. One of these men subsequently developed irreversible airways' obstruction with air trapping, hyperinflation and dyspnoea on slight exertion; and another (who was a smoker) had a mild degree of airflow obstruction 4 months after exposure. The third (a non-smoker), had no lung function abnormalities shortly after exposure or subsequently (Charan et al., 1979).

As a rule most individuals who survive acute exposure recover completely.

Exposure to low concentrations of sulphur dioxide has been extensively investigated largely because it was formerly the most important environmental contaminant in industrial and domestic air pollution. The principal physiological response is a mild degree of bronchial constriction which can be found in human subjects (Lawther et al., 1975; Linn et al., 1987). The effect is particularly apparent in asthmatic individuals but does not seem to be related to atopy (Koenig et al., 1981; Sheppard et al., 1981; Linn et al., 1987). Similar alterations in lung function are noted in experimental animals; however, recent evidence suggests that the response is not due to an altered state in the contractile elements in the lung but probably represents the expression of an inhibitory influence of the muco-epithelial barrier (Shore et al., 1987).

Studies of workers chronically exposed to SO_2 show very little, if any, alteration in lung function (Ferris, Puleo and Chen, 1979; Federspiel et al., 1980), perhaps because those who remain in occupations in which exposure occurs become adapted. Mortality studies of workers exposed to SO_2 in pulp and paper mills have not shown any excess of deaths from respiratory disease (Jäppinen, 1987; Hennenberger, Ferris and Monson, 1989).

Welding and similar processes

As a variety of potential respiratory hazards may exist in these processes it may be helpful to group them together in one section but, as the subject is large and complex, only a brief outline is attempted.

Welding

Welding is the process whereby metal or other thermoplastic materials are joined together by the application of heat or pressure, or a combination of both, with or without the use of a filler metal. Many different types of welding are used in industry and welders constitute one of the largest occupational groups; for example, there are well over 100 000 welders in the UK and 500 000 in the USA (HMSO, 1979; Stern, 1981). There are several potential respiratory hazards associated with welding arising from the use of materials employed in the process; from fumes arising from the metals or plastics being welded together; from the evolution of pollutant gases; and some environmental hazards from working in the same proximity as those using potentially toxic materials. The specific effects of these materials in the lungs have been described earlier in this chapter, or elsewhere in the book.

Types of welding

Heat is applied to the materials to be welded by a gas flame or with an electric current.

Gas welding

Gas welding is used for welding thin materials and where low temperature gradients are required in order to avoid cracking. The most common gases used are acetylene, natural gas and propane mixed with oxygen in order to achieve higher temperatures than would be possible if the gas were used on its own. It is important to remember that oxyacetylene torches may also be used to cut through metal and hazards may arise when painted metal structures are demolished in this way if the paint contains lead or other heavy metals.

Arc welding

In this process, heat is generated by striking an arc between an electrode and the base metal. Some molten metal is usually added to the join either from the electrode itself which consists of a core wire with an electrode coating (*consumable electrode process*) or from a separate filler rod (*non-consumable electrode process*). The metal to be welded is protected from oxidization by the use of an inert gas shield. Many arc welding processes are automatic or semi-automatic, but if it is carried out manually the process is known as *manual metal arc* (MMA) or *open arc welding*.

Non-consumable electrode processes
Here the electrode is carbon or tungsten. In the latter case shielding is provided by the use of helium or argon or a mixture of the two; the process is referred to as tungsten–inert gas (TIG) welding.

Consumable electrode processes

The electrodes used here are either uncoated and provided with a gas shield or they are covered with a flux coat that vaporizes in the arc to form a shielding gas and a slag which reacts with the molten metal to protect the cooling weld. If an inert gas is used as the shield, the process is referred to as metal–inert gas (MIG) welding. In some cases small amounts of an active gas (usually carbon dioxide) which reacts with the base metal are added to the helium and argon; this is known as *metal–active gas (MAG) welding*.

The electrodes used in arc welding may contain fluoride (basic electrodes) or titanium dioxide (rutile electrodes), and a wide variety of coatings may be used, for example, cellulose, metallic oxides and salts, silica and various silicates including asbestos, feldspar and mica.

Plasma arc welding

This uses a mixture of hydrogen, helium, argon or nitrogen (or a mixture of these gases). The arc is formed at a small orifice through which the gas flows. The plasma consists of ionized gas at a temperature of about 24 000°C which forms into a jet under the gas pressure and becomes an intense flame beyond the nozzle. Shielding is provided by inert gases either singly or in combination.

Resistance welding

This involves the application of a powerful compressive force to the components being welded while a strong low voltage electric current flows through them generating heat at the interface. *Spot welding, flash welding* and *electroslag welding* are types of resistance welding.

Welding on coated surfaces

Welding or cutting painted surfaces is well known to give rise occasionally to cadmium or lead poisoning. Metal surfaces may be covered with a variety of other coatings, however, such as rust-proofing material or plastic or synthetic resins as insulating layers. The result is that many organic and inorganic compounds can be liberated when they are vaporized at the welding temperatures (see Chapter 21).

Soldering and brazing

Soldering and brazing are processes whereby the parts to be joined form an alloy with a metal derived from a solder. The processes differ in the type of solder that is used; soldering (or soft-soldering) uses a solder that melts below 450°C and that frequently contains lead and tin. Brazing employs a hard solder that melts at higher temperatures. Hard solders usually contain zinc and copper, and silver and cadmium are added to lower the melting temperature.

Fluxes are used to protect the metal surface and to dissolve any oxides that form with atmospheric oxygen. Corrosive fluxes contain zinc and ammonium chlorides whereas non-corrosive fluxes contain colophony resin (see Chapter 21).

Health hazards associated with welding

Welding involves a potential exposure to a wide variety of gases, fumes and dusts and the health effects of this type of work have been intensively studied (for a review see Stern and Berlin, 1986). In addition to the effects on the respiratory tract there is the danger of 'arc-eye' resulting from the ultraviolet radiation generated during arc welding; there is also the risk of explosion or electrocution, and the ever-present risk of burns.

The most common acute effect on the lungs is metal fume fever which is described earlier in the chapter. Effects, including pulmonary oedema, may also be noted from exposure to ozone which is formed during gas-shielded welding of aluminium or, to a lesser extent, stainless steel (Ulfvarson, 1981; Sjögren and Ulfvarson, 1985). Respiratory symptoms in aluminium welders have been connected with their exposure to ozone (Sjögren and Ulfvarson, 1985). Carbon monoxide can be formed when carbon dioxide is used as a shielding gas and carboxyhaemoglobin levels may be elevated if the work is carried out with inadequate ventilation (de Kretser, Evans and Waldron, 1964). Nitrogen dioxide may be produced in substantial concentrations during gas or arc welding when no shielding is used. In practice, however, the risk from nitrogen dioxide is not great if ventilation is adequate or if the process is carried out in an open shop, although pulmonary oedema has been reported in welders working under less than ideal conditions (Norwood et al., 1966). Basic electrodes coated with calcium fluoride emit fluoride in the fume, but post-shift urinary concentrations of fluorides are not unacceptably high (Sjögren, Hedström and Lindstedt, 1984).

If welding is carried out in an atmosphere that contains halogenated hydrocarbons there is a risk that the ultraviolet radiation produced will cause them to decompose to phosgene in the case of perchloroethylene or 1,1,1-trichloroethane, or to dichloroacetyl chloride in the case of trichloroethylene. These solvents are commonly used as degreasing agents in the engineering industry and so welders will not uncommonly come into contact with them. As with nitrogen dioxide, the hazard may be more theoretical than actual.

Other gases that might give rise to acute effects include phosphine from metal coated with phosphate rust-proofing material, acrolein and formaldehyde from alkyl and epoxy resin coatings, and isocyanates from polyurethane resin coatings.

Among the chronic respiratory effects, the most common is siderosis from the inhalation of iron oxide which can be found in considerable quantities in the lungs (Kaponen and Gustafson, 1980; Kalliomaki and Rahkonen, 1981; Kalliomaki and Kalliomaki, 1983; Funahashi et al., 1988), and the most serious, the development of asthma from the use of colophony resins (this is discussed in detail in Chapter 21) and the possible risk of cancer.

Siderosis is symptomless but fibrotic changes have been reported in welders that were not considered to be due to the concomitant presence of silica with iron in the lung (Funahashi et al., 1988). However, the occasional presence of lesions of 'mixed dust fibrosis' (rarely conglomerate masses) or irregular fibrosis in arc welders is certainly not caused by iron dust. Possible explanations are discussed in Chapter 11 (page 257). The most likely seems to be exposure to one of the polymorphs of silica from an unrecognized source. Irregular fibrosis may be due to asbestos from nearby insulation work.

Some studies have shown an increased prevalence of chronic bronchitis (Mur and Teculescu, 1985; Sjögren and Ulfvarson, 1985) but others have not been able to find major differences between welders and control subjects except in an increased rate of sickness absence from respiratory disorders (McMillan, 1978; Hayden et al., 1984). Some mortality studies have shown an increased risk from lung cancer which appears to be related to asbestos (Newhouse, Oakes and Wooley, 1985) or hexavalent chromium during stainless steel welding (Sjögren, 1980; Becker and Claude, 1985; Sjögren and Gustavsson, 1987), or to both chromium and nickel (Stern, 1987); these results have not always been replicated by others (McMillan and Pethybridge, 1983) (see Chapter 19).

Considering the great variety of work and exposure conditions subsumed by the term 'welding', it is no surprise that the results of lung function studies in welders have yielded both positive (Oxhøj and Bake, 1979; Kalliomaki and Kalliomaki, 1982; Mur and Teculescu, 1985) and negative (McMillan, 1979; Hayden et al., 1984; Sjögren and Ulfvarsson, 1985) results.

Summary

Welders work under such different conditions and may be exposed to such different materials that the wisdom of considering them all together may be questioned. What is important when trying to determine whether or not symptoms in an individual may be due to his or her work is to obtain as precise an account as possible of the type of welding because from this a better knowledge of the range of possible exposures will be gained.

Prevention

1. Education of welders in the potential risks and their avoidance.
2. Good general and local exhaust ventilation.
3. Wearing of respiratory protective equipment in confined spaces if these are not efficiently ventilated.
4. Monitoring of welders' breathing zone for toxic fumes and gases.
5. The value of periodic medical examination of welders in ordinary welding shops has been doubted on the grounds that they do not appear more likely to develop serious pulmonary disease than other workers (Antti-Poika, Hassi and Pyy, 1977). However, routine examinations are clearly desirable in processes in which there is a risk of asthma (see Chapter 21). Individuals with established chronic pulmonary disease should probably be excluded from welding.

Fire smoke

Acute respiratory injury either with or without external burns has long been known to occur in victims of fires but chronic sequelae are unusual. Workers and other personnel may be caught in major conflagrations in factories, offices, mines, ships and aircraft; and firemen, unless protected by appropriate breathing apparatus, are at risk.

It is important to stress that respiratory injury may occur in the absence of cutaneous burns. Immediately following exposure there is cough and soreness of the throat which recover quickly but, after an asymptomatic interval varying from 8 to 24 hours, cough with thick tenacious sputum and sometimes slight haemoptysis, hoarseness of voice and central chest pain occur. In badly affected individuals, there is severe breathlessness with bilateral, basal, fine inspiratory crackles and widespread rhonchi. The clinical and radiographic features of pulmonary oedema are present at this stage in some, but not all, cases (Hampton, 1971). Secondary respiratory infection is particularly apt to develop and has been shown to occur after 24 hours in dogs exposed to high concentrations of wood smoke (Stephenson et al., 1975).

A wide variety of materials may be involved in fires including wood, wool, leather, cork and synthetic polymer foams – in particular PVC and polyurethane. The resulting products differ according to what extent they undergo combustion or pyrolysis. *Combustion* consists of thermal decomposition of organic material in an oxygen atmosphere: *pyrolysis* is thermal decomposition in an oxygen-depleted atmosphere. Both occur to a varying degree in fires and, in general, the products of complete combustion are less harmful than those of incomplete combustion (Kimmerle, 1976). Thus, toxic gases that may occur in fires include carbon monoxide, the oxides of nitrogen, hydrogen chloride (from PVC), aldehydes and toluene diisocyanate 'smoke' which, at high temperatures, yields hydrogen cyanide. Release of phosgene from burning PVC, however, is negligible (Wooley, 1971; Stark, 1972; Wooley and Palmer, 1976). Hydrogen chloride gas, which is rarely encountered in industry under normal conditions, is highly irritant and may cause severe pulmonary oedema.

Pathology

The trachea and major airways are intensely hyperaemic with oedema in the submucosal layers, variable mucosal necrosis and fibrinous exudate with pronounced cellular infiltrations. The progression of upper airways' oedema may lead to the obliteration of the aryepiglottic folds, the arytenoid eminences and the interarytenoid areas and occlusion of the airway (Haponik et al., 1987). Pulmonary oedema is present in severe cases of exposure. These effects are said to be due to the smoke and its various components rather than to thermal burns (Hampton, 1971), although the severity of changes does correlate with the size of cutaneous burns or their presence on the face and neck (Haponik et al., 1987). However, diffuse endobronchial polyposis, which sometimes occurs a few weeks after the accident, appears to be a sequel of thermal injury, and to resolve spontaneously after some months (Adams et al., 1979; Williams, Vanecko and Glassroth, 1983). Bronchiectasis, bronchiolitis obliterans and tracheobronchial stenosis have also been reported as chronic complications of severe thermal burns (Di Vincenti, Pruitt and Reckler, 1971; Arora and Aldrich, 1980).

Pulmonary function

Firemen have been found to have no impairment of respiratory function 1 month after exposure to dense smoke, and a 3-year study of firemen showed no increased annual loss of ventilatory function (Musk, Peters and Wegman, 1977; Tashkin et al., 1977). The major, and apparently independent, factor in airways' obstruction in firemen, in fact, is cigarette smoking but a few non-smokers may have symptomless dysfunction of the small airways, the significance of which is uncertain (Loke et al., 1980). However, a study of 30 firemen examined immediately after and up to 18 months following severe smoke exposure showed 'a significant decrement' in FEV_1 and FVC which did not improve, accompanied by a high prevalence of non-specific respiratory symptoms throughout the follow-up period by comparison with matched controls. The authors suggest that impaired lung function may result more from repeated exposures than from a sudden decrease due to a specific exposure (Unger et al., 1980). As this fire was in a warehouse where complex chlorinated hydrocarbons were stored it is likely that the men had substantial exposure to phosgene. Significant quantities of sulphur dioxide, benzene and dichlorofluoromethane have also been reported in the breathing zones of firemen (Brandt-Rauf et al., 1988).

Firemen have been found to have increased alveolar permeability as measured by the rate of disappearance of ^{99m}Tc-DTPA (Minty and Royston, 1985) but, generally, no other short- or long-term impairment in lung function has been reported (Musk, Peters and Wegman; 1977; Tashkin et al., 1977; Douglas et al., 1985; Horsfield et al., 1988; Brandt-Rauf et al., 1989), although, if respiratory protection is not worn, some significant obstructive changes are present (Brandt-Rauf et al., 1989). In the study of West Sussex firemen by Horsfield and his colleagues (Horsfield et al., 1988), firemen had a lower rate of annual deterioration in lung function than their controls which was thought to be a reflection of selection procedures, continued physical training and the regular use of breathing apparatus. The major, and apparently independent, factor in airways' obstruction in firemen is, in fact, cigarette smoking (Loke et al., 1980; Douglas et al., 1985).

In a study which did show a significant decrement in FEV_1 and FVC following severe smoke exposure, the authors (Unger et al., 1980) suggested that the impairment in lung function may have resulted from repeated exposure. However, as the fire that the men attended was in a warehouse in which chlorinated hydrocarbons were kept it is possible that they experienced a substantial exposure to phosgene.

Evidence suggestive of sustained airflow obstruction of the small airways has been reported in a small number of the survivors of the King's Cross underground station fire in 1987 after 2 years. However, a varnish on the escalators and advertising panels contained a polyurethane base which could have generated toxic products including cyanide gas (Fogarty et al., 1991) – especially if combustion was incomplete due to an oxygen-depleted atmosphere (Kimmerle, 1976).

Mortality

Mortality studies of firemen have shown them to have a death rate which is lower than the general population (Musk et al., 1978; Eliopulos et al., 1984; Vena and Fielder, 1987) and this has been attributed to the so-called healthy worker effect. The most recent study of firemen in Seattle, Tacoma and Portland has confirmed the overall favourable death rate (SMR = 82), but found an increased risk of dying from non-malignant respiratory disease (SMR = 142) (Rosenstock et al., 1988).

Treatment

As smoke inhalation is potentially life threatening immediate action is required. Substantial doses of corticosteroids for a few days only with appropriate antibiotics are recommended in individuals with respiratory distress and also in those without if there has been heavy exposure. Oxygen may be required. Even if initially relatively symptomless, all persons who have had significant exposure to smoke should be kept under medical surveillance for at least 48 hours (Hampton, 1971).

The combination of extensive surface burns and smoke inhalation is especially menacing and requires attention to colloid and crystalloid adjustment as well as cardiorespiratory resuscitation. In cases of smoke inhalation alone normal spirometry shortly after the accident excludes significant exposure (Whitener et al., 1980).

Prognosis

Most patients who survive have no permanent lung damage although full recovery may not occur for some months. However, bronchial stenosis or bronchiectasis with airflow obstruction and, possibly, small airways' obstruction may occasionally follow (Kirkpatrick and Bass, 1979; Whitener et al., 1980; Fogarty et al., 1991).

Blast wave and blunt trauma effects

These include blast injuries in air from explosions in factories, ships and mines and other confined spaces; and in water where divers, seamen and armed forces personnel may be affected. Blunt trauma may be caused by falls into water from a height or blows on the chest wall. Alveolar rupture often occurs due, probably, to a shearing injury of the lungs and not to overinflation as is the case in 'burst lung' caused by decompression pulmonary barotrauma (see Chapter 25). In many cases, especially those of blast in water or blunt trauma, there may be no fracture of ribs or penetrating injury of the chest although ecchymosis over the area of impact is usual.

The effects of blast under water are more pronounced than in air owing to the greatly increased pressure wave generated in underwater explosions caused by the relative incompressibility of water and the higher velocity of sound in water than in air. In addition to individuals who are immersed at the time of an explosion, pilots who fire their ejection seats to escape from submerged aircraft may be injured in this way.

Clinical features are cough, frothy blood-stained sputum or frank haemoptysis and crackles in the lungs. As a rule multiple small opacities of so-called acinar-filling type appear within a few hours and are usually most prominent adjacent to the area of maximum impact. Subcutaneous emphysema, mediastinal emphysema, pneumothorax (often bilateral) and haemothorax may subsequently develop. Pulmonary oedema, delayed for some 24 to 48 hours is a common complication of blast injury (Fallon, 1940; Williams, 1942; Watt, 1977; Robertson, Lakshminarayan and Hudson, 1978).

Pathologically, the surface of the lungs is contused and large quantities of blood are present in the alveoli and airways.

Treatment includes bronchial aspiration, oxygen, corticosteroids as anti-inflammatory agents and prophylactic antibiotics. There is some controversy concerning the use of positive pressure ventilation (as is also the case in pulmonary barotrauma) because of the risk of inducing air embolism and surgical emphysema. But volume-cycled mechanical ventilation with positive end-expiratory pressure sufficient to maintain arterial oxygen pressure above 60 mmHg in a group of attempted suicide cases who had fallen 50 m into water did not provoke any incidents of air embolism (Robertson, Lakshminarayan and Hudson, 1978). Treatment of pneumothorax may be necessary.

Patients who recover usually do so without sequelae but some may have permanent, diffuse unilateral or bilateral pleural fibrosis. Occasionally empyema occurs.

Near-drowning

Near-drowning is survival – usually as the result of successful resuscitation – after immersion in salt or fresh water. In spite of an apparently good recovery, however, death may follow some hours later from 'secondary drowning' which is generally considered to be the result of pulmonary oedema, aspiration pneumonia, airflow obstruction, anoxaemia and acidosis (Rivers, Orr and Lee, 1970; Modell, Graves and Ketover, 1976). It has also been shown that victims of near-drowning may develop interstitial fibrosis (Grauser and Smith, 1975) and foreign body granulomatosis (Noguchi, Kimula and Ogata, 1985). The case of Noguchi and his colleagues was that of a racing driver who aspirated muddy water when his car overturned in a puddle. He was rescued after about 10 minutes and developed dyspnoea and a cough which produced muddy sputum. He died 17 days after the accident and autopsy showed the presence of massive fibrosis, more severe in the lower lobes where the alveolar structure was mostly destroyed and replaced with fibrous tissue. Numerous epithelioid cell granulomas with crystalline foreign bodies were found in the middle and upper lobes; elemental analysis of the crystals showed that they contained silicon and lesser amounts of aluminium, calcium, titanium, iron and potassium. There seems little doubt that the changes in what the authors called 'muddy lung' were caused by the irritant effects of silica-containing mud. Gravel and larger stones may also be aspirated into the lungs from the hypopharynx, but these can be removed by repeated bronchoscopy using both rigid and fibreoptic instruments. Complete recovery is, then, possible (Hal Cragun, Grover and Dunn, 1992).

Thus, aspiration of mud, sand or gravel in near-drowning accidents is sometimes encountered as an unusual and rare form of occupational lung disease.

Addendum

Cobalt

Swennen et al. (1993) have now supplied evidence that suggests that exposure to cobalt alone – as metal, oxides or salts – does not cause parenchymal changes in the lungs, and that interaction with other air-borne matter (in particular, tungsten carbide which increases the bioavailability of cobalt) appears to be necessary for pulmonary fibrosis to occur.

References

Abramson, M.J. (1989) Does aluminium smelting cause lung diseases? *Am. Rev. Respir. Dis.* **139**, 1042–1057

Adams, C., Moisan, T., Chandrasekhar, A.J. and Warpeha, R. (1979) Endobronchial polyposis secondary to thermal inhalation injury. *Chest* **75**, 643–645

Adams, R. (1980) β2-Microglobulin levels in nickel–cadmium battery workers. In: *Occupational Exposure to Cadmium.* Report on seminar: London, 20 March 1980. Cadmium Association, London, pp. 41–42

Ades, A.E. and Kazantzis, G. (1988) Lung cancer in a non-ferrous foundry: the role of cadmium. *Br. J. Ind. Med.* **45**, 435–442

Ahlmark, A., Bruce, T. and Nyström, A. (1960) *Silicosis and Other Pneumoconiosis in Sweden.* Heinemann, London, pp. 361–365, 371–373

Alexandersson, R. (1979) Investigations of the effects of exposure to cobalt. VI. Exposure, assimilation and pulmonary effects of cobalt in the tungsten carbide industry. *Arbete och Hälsa (Vetenskaplig skriftserie)*, Arbetars-kyddsverket, Stockholm

Allen, M.B., Crisp, A., Snook, N. and Page, R.L. (1992) 'Smoke-bomb' pneumonitis. *Respir. Med.* **86**, 165–166

Ames, R.G., Piacitelli, G.M., Reger, R.B. and Gamble, J.F. (1988) Effects of exposure to diesel emissions among coal miners: a prospective evaluation. *Ann. Occup. Hyg.* **32** (suppl. 1), 635–643

Anon (1970) Check on poison gas in tower silos. *Farmer and Stockbreeder* **84**, 11

Antti-Poika, M., Hassi, J. and Pyy, L. (1977) Respiratory disease in arc welders. *Int. Archs Occup. Environ. Health* **40**, 225–330

Archer, V.E., Magnuson, H.H., Holaday, D.A. and Lawrence, P.A. (1962) Hazards to health in uranium mining and milling. *J. Occup. Med.* **4**, 55–60

Armstrong, B. and Kazantzis, G. (1983) The mortality of cadmium workers. *Lancet* **1**, 1425–1427

Arora, N. and Aldrich, T.K. (1980) Bronchiolitis obliterans from a burning automobile. *S. Med. J.* **73**, 507–510

Attfield, M.D., Trabant, G.D. and Wheeler, R.W. (1982) Exposure to diesel fumes and dust in six potash mines. *Ann. Occup. Hyg.* **26** (nos 1–4), 817–831

Baader, E.W. (1951) Die chronische Kadmiumvergiftung. *Dtsch. Med. Wschr.* **76**, 484–487

Baader, E.W. (1952) Chronic cadmium poisoning. *Ind. Med. Surg.* **21**, 427–430

Barborik, M. and Dusek, J. (1972) Cardiomyopathy accompanying industrial cobalt exposure. *Br. Heart J.* **34**, 113–116

Beach, F.X.M., Sherwood Jones, E. and Scarrow, G.D. (1969) Respiratory effects of chlorine gas. *Br. J. Ind. Med.* **26**, 231–236

Bech, A.O., Kipling, M.D. and Heather, J.C. (1962) Hard metal disease. *Br. J. Ind. Med.* **19**, 239–252

Becker, N. and Claude, J. (1985) Cancer risk of arc welders exposed to fumes containing chromium and nickel. *Scand. J. Work Environ. Health* **11**, 75–82

Becklake, M.R., Goldman, H.I., Boxman, A.R. and Freed, C.C. (1957) The long-term effects of exposure to nitrous fumes. *Am. Rev. Tuberc.* **76**, 398–409

Beetham, D., Dawnay, A., London, J. and Cattwell, C.C. (1985) A radio-immunoassay for retinol-binding protein in serum and urine. *Clin. Chim. Acta* **31**, 1364–1367

Behnke, A.R. (1945) Decompression sickness incident to deep sea diving and high altitude ascent. *Medicine* **24**, 381–402

Bennett, G. (1962) Ozone contamination of high altitude aircraft cabins. *Aerospace Med.* **33**, 969–973

Benson, M.K.D., Goodwin, P.G. and Brodyoff, J. (1975) Metal sensitivity in patients with joint replacement arthroplastics. *Br. Med. J.* **4**, 374–375

Bergman, I. (1972) Nitrous fumes and coal miners with emphysema. Discussion. *Ann. Occup. Hyg.* **15**, 301

Berlin, M., Fazackerley, J. and Nordberg, G. (1969) The uptake of mercury in the brains of mammals exposed to mercury vapor and to mercuric salts. *Archs Environ. Health* **18**, 719–729

Bernard, A.M., Moreau, D. and Lauwerys, R.R. (1982) Comparison of retinol-binding protein and β_2-microglobulin determination in urine for the early detection of tubular proteinuria. *Clin. Chim. Acta* **126**, 1–7

Bernard, A., Roels, H.A., Buchet, J.P., Mason, P.L. and Lauwerys, R. (1977) α_1-Antitrypsin level in workers exposed to cadmium. In: *Clinical Chemistry and Chemical Toxicology of Metals* (ed. S.A. Brown), Elsevier, Amsterdam, pp. 161–164

Bernard, A., Goret, A., Buchet, J.P., Roels, H. and Lauwerys, R. (1979) Comparison of sodium dodecyl sulfate-polyacrylamide gel electrophoresis with quantitative methods for the analysis of cadmium-induced proteinuria. *Int. Archs Occup. Environ. Health* **44**, 139–148

Beton, D.C., Andrews, G.S., Davies, H.J., Howells, L. and Smith, G.F. (1966) Acute cadmium fume poisoning. *Br. J. Ind. Med.* **23**, 292–301

Biesold, J., Bachofen, M. and Bachofen, H. (1974) Pulmonary oedema due to hydrogen sulfide. *Swiss National Science Foundation* (3. 394–0. 74)

Blejer, H.P. and Caplan, P.E. (1971) *Occupational Health Aspects of Cadmium Fume Poisoning*, 2nd ed. Bureau of Occupational Health and Environmental Epidemiology, California

Bonnell, J.A. (1965) Cadmium poisoning. *Ann. Occup. Hyg.* **8**, 45–50

Borghetti, A., Mutti, A., Cavatorta, A., Falzoi, M., Cigala, F. and Franchini, I. (1977) Indices renaux d'exposition aigue et d'impregnation chronique par le chrome. *Med. Lav.* **68**, 355–363

Brandt-Rauf, P.W., Fallon, L.F., Tarantini, T., Idema, C. and Andrews, L. (1988) Health hazards of fire fighters: exposure assessment. *Br. J. Ind. Med.* **45**, 606–612

Brandt-Rauf, P.W., Cosman, B., Fleming Fallon, L., Tarantini, T. and Idema, C. (1989) Health hazards of fire fighters: acute pulmonary effects after toxic exposures. *Br. J. Ind. Med.* **46**, 209–211

British Occupational Hygiene Society Committee on Hygiene Standards: Subcommittee on Cadmium (1977) Hygiene standards for cadmium. *Ann. Occup. Hyg* **20**, 215–228

Browne, R.C. (1955) Vanadium poisoning from gas turbine. *Br. J. Ind. Med.* **12**, 57–59

Bruckner, H.C. (1967) Extrinsic asthma in a tungsten carbide worker. *J. Occup. Med.* **9**, 518–519

Bruusgaard, A.A. (1960) Asthma-like disease among Norwegian aluminium plant workers. *Tidskr. Nor. Laegefor.* **80**, 796–797

Buchet, J.P., Roels, H., Bernard, A. and Lauwerys, R.R. (1980) Assessment of renal function of workers exposed to inorganic lead, cadmium or mercury vapour. *J. Occup. Med.* **22**, 741–747

Campbell, N.S. (1948) Acute mercurial poisoning by inhalation of metallic vapour in an infant. *Can. Med. Assoc. J.* **58**, 72–75

Caplin, M. (1941) Ammonia-gas poisoning. *Lancet* **2**, 95–96

Carrington, C.B. and Green, T.J. (1970) Granular pneumocytes in early repair of diffuse alveolar injury. *Archs Intern. Med.* **126**, 464–465

Castleman, W.L., Dungworth, D.L., Schwarz, L.W. and Tyler, W.S. (1980) Acute respiratory bronchiolotis. *Am. J. Pathol.* **98**, 811–827

Charan, N.B., Myers, C.G., Lakshminarayan, S. and Spencer, T.M. (1979) Pulmonary injuries associated with acute sulphur dioxide inhalation. *Am. Rev. Respir. Dis.* **119**, 555–560

Chasis, H., Zapp, J.A., Bannon, J.H., Whittenberger, J.L., Helm, J., Doheny, J.L. and MacLeod, C.D. (1947) Chlorine accident in Brooklyn. *Occup. Med.* **4**, 152–176

Chen-Yeung, M.R., Wong, R. and McLean, L. (1982) Health of workers in an aluminium smelter at Kitimat, B.C. In: *Respiratory System. Health Protection in Primary Aluminium Production*, Vol. II, New Zealand House, London, pp. 45–46

Chen-Yeung, M., Wong, R. and McLean, L. (1983) Epidemiologic health study of workers in an aluminium smelter in British Columbia. *Am. Rev. Respir. Dis.* **127**, 465–469

Christensen, H., Krogh, M. and Nielsen, M. (1937) Acute mercury poisoning in a respiration chamber. *Nature* **139**, 626

Christensen, F.C. and Olsen, E.C. (1957) Cadmium poisoning. *Archs Ind. Health* **16**, 8–13

Christiansen, K.J. (1979) The correlation between prosthesis failure and metal sensitivity as determined by a new immunological technique. *J. Bone Jt Surg.* **61B**, 240

Clark, W.I. (1929) The dust hazard in the abrasive industry. *J. Ind. Hyg.* **11**, 92

Clinton, M. (1947) Selenium fume exposure. *J. Ind. Hyg. Toxicol.* **29**, 225–227

Clutton-Brock, J. (1967) Two cases of poisoning by contamination of nitrous oxide with higher oxides of nitrogen during anaesthesia. *Br. J. Anaesth.* **39**, 388–392

Coates, E.O. and Watson, J.H.L. (1971) Diffuse interstitial lung disease in tungsten carbide workers. *Ann. Intern. Med.* **75**, 709–716

Coates, E.O., Jr, and Watson, J.H.L. (1973) Pathology of the lung in tungsten carbide workers using light and electron microscopy. *J. Occup. Med.* **15**, 280–286

Coates, E.O., Jr, Sawyer, H.J., Rebusk, J.W., Kvale, P.H. and Sweet, L.W. (1973) Hypersensitivity bronchitis in tungsten carbide workers. *Chest* **64**, 390

Commins, B.T., Raveney, F.J. and Jesson, M.W. (1971) Toxic gases in tower silos. *Ann. Occup. Hyg.* **14**, 275–283

Committee on Aldehydes (1981) *Formaldehyde and Other Aldehydes*. National Academy Press, Washington

Cordasco, E.M. and Stone, F.D. (1973) Pulmonary oedema of environmental origin. *Chest* **64**, 182–185

Cordasco, E.M., Cooper, R.W., Murphy, J.V. and Anderson, C. (1962) Pulmonary aspects of some toxic experimental space fuels. *Dis. Chest* **41**, 68–74

Cordasco, E.M., Kosti, H., Vance, J.W. and Golden, L.N. (1965) Pulmonary edema of non-cardiac origin. *Archs Environ. Health* **11**, 588–596

Corrin, B. (1963a) Aluminium pneumoconiosis. I. in vitro comparison of stamped aluminium powders containing different lubricating agents and granular aluminium powder. *Br. J. Ind. Med.* **20**, 264–267

Corrin, B. (1963b) Aluminium pneumoconiosis. II. Effect on the rat lung of intratracheal injections of stamped aluminium powders containing different lubricating agents and of a granular aluminium powder. *Br. J. Ind. Med.* **20**, 268–276

Cotter, L.H. and Cotter, B.H. (1951) Cadmium poisoning. *Archs Ind. Hyg.* **3**, 495–504

Dalgaard, J.B., Dencker, F., Fallentin, B., Hansen, P., Kaempe, B., Steensberg, J. and Wilhardt, P. (1972) Fatal poisoning and other health hazards connected with industrial fishing. *Br. J. Ind. Med.* **29**, 307–316

Darke, C.S. and Warrack, A.J.N. (1958) Bronchiolitis from nitrous fumes. *Thorax* **13**, 327–333

Daum, S., Anderson, H.A., Lilis, R., Lorimer, W.V., Fischbein, S.A., Miller A. and Selikoff, I.J. (1977) Pulmonary changes among titanium workers. *Proc. R. Soc. Med.* **70**, 31–32

Davis, J.M.G., Gormley, I.P., Collings, P., Ottery, J. and Robertson, A. (1978) Studies on the cytotoxicity of coal dust samples, including the effects of adsorbed nitrous fumes. *Institute of Occupational Medicine, Edinburgh, Final Report* 6244–00/8/105

Davison, A.G., Fayers, P.M., Newman Taylor, A.J., Venables, K.M., Darbyshire, J.H., Pickering, C.A.C., Holden, H., Smith, N.J., Mason, H. and Scott, M. (1986) Cadmium inhalation and emphysema. *Thorax* **41**, 714

Davison, A.G., Haslam, P.L., Corrin, B., Coutts, I.I., Dewar, A., Riding, W.D., Studdy, P.R. and Newman-Taylor, A.J. (1983) Interstitial lung disease and asthma in hard-metal workers: bronchiolar lavage, ultrastructural, and analytical findings and results of bronchial provocation tests. *Thorax* **38**, 119–128

de Kretser, A.J., Evans, W.D. and Waldron, H.A. (1964) Carbon monoxide hazard in the CO_2 arc-welding process. *Ann. Occup. Hyg.* **7**, 253–259

de Vries, K., Lowenberg, A., Coster van Voorhuout, H.E.V. and Ebels, J.H. (1974) Langzeit beobachtungen bei Fluorwasserstoffexposition. *Pneumologie* **150**, 149–154

Decker, W.J. and Koch, H.F. (1978) Chlorine poisoning at the swimming pool: an overlooked hazard. *Clin. Toxicol.* **13**, 377–381

Delahant, A.B. (1955) An experimental study of the effects of rare metals on animals lungs. *Archs Ind. Health* **12**, 116–120

Delaney, L.T., Schmidt, H.W. and Stroebel, C.F. (1956) Silofillers' disease. *Proc. Staff Meet. Mayo Clin.* **31**, 189–198

Desbaumes, P. (1968) Intoxications mortelles par les gaz de fermentation de silos agricoles (oxyde de carbone et oxydes d'azote). *Arch. Tox.* **23**, 160–164

Di Vincenti, F.C., Pruitt, B.A. and Reekler, J.M. (1971) Inhalation injuries. *J. Trama* **11**, 109–117

Dinman, B.D. (1987) Aluminium in the lungs. II. The pyro conundrum. *J. Occup. Med.* **29**, 869–876

Dinman, D.B. (1988) Alumina-related pulmonary disease. *J. Occup. Med.* **30**, 328–335

Discher, D.P. and Breitenstein, B.D. (1976) Prevalence of chronic pulmonary disease in aluminium potroom workers. *J. Occup. Med.* **18**, 379–386

Diskin, C.J., Tomasso, C.L., Alper, J.C., Glaser, M.L. and Fliegel, S.E. (1979) Long-term selenium exposure. *Archs Intern. Med.* **139**, 624–626

Doig, A.I. and Challen, P.J.R. (1964) Respiratory hazards of welding. *Ann. Occup. Hyg.* **7**, 223–229

Doig, A.T. and Duguid, L.N. (1951) *The Health of Welders.* HMSO, London

Doll, R. (1958) Cancer of the lung and nose in nickel workers. *Br. J. Ind. Med.* **15**, 217–223

Douglas, D.B., Douglas, R.B., Oakes, D. and Scott, G. (1985) Pulmonary function of London firemen. *Br. J. Ind. Med.* **42**, 51–54

Dowell, A.R., Kilburn, K.H. and Pratt, P.C. (1971) Short-term exposure to nitrogen dioxide. *Archs Intern. Med.* **128**, 74–80

Drozdz, M., Kucharz, E. and Szyja, J. (1977) Effect of chronic exposure to nitrogen dioxide on collagen content in lung and skin of guinea pigs. *Environ. Res.* **13**, 369–377

Dutton, W.F. (1911) Vanadiumism. *J. Am. Med. Assoc.* **56**, 1648

Edmonds, C. (1976) Barotrauma. In: *Diving Medicine* (ed. R.H. Strauss), Grune and Stratton, New York, San Francisco and London, pp. 49–61

Eklund, A., Arns, R., Blaschke, E., Hed, J., Hjertquist, S-O., Larsson, K., Lowgren, H., Nyström, J., Skold, C.M. and

Tornling, G. (1989) Characteristics of alveolar cells and soluble compounds in bronchiolar lavage fluid from nonsmoking aluminium potroom workers. *Br. J. Ind. Med.* **46**, 782–786

Elinder, C-G., Edling, C., Lindberg, E., Kagedal, B. and Vesterberg, O. (1985) β2-Microglobulinuria among workers previously exposed to Cd: follow-up and dose–response analysis. *Am. J. Ind. Med.* **8**, 553–564

Eliopulos, E., Armstrong, B.K., Spickett, J.T. and Heyworth, F. (1984) Mortality of fire fighters in Western Australia. *Br. J. Ind. Med.* **41**, 183–187

Ellis, K.J., Cohn, S.H. and Smith, T.J. (1985) Cadmium inhalation exposure estimates: their significance with respect to kidney and liver cadmium burdens. *J. Toxic. Environ. Health* **15**, 173–187

EMAS (1972) *Ozone Notes of Guidance.* Chief Employment Medical Adviser, Health and Safety Executive, London

English, J.M. (1964) A case of probable phosgene poisoning. *Br. Med. J.* **1**, 38

Evans, D.M. (1960) Cadmium poisoning. *Br. Med. J.* **1**, 173–174

Evans, E.H. (1945) Casualties following exposure to zinc chloride smoke. *Lancet* **2**, 368–369

Everett, E.D. and Overholt, E.L. (1968) Phosgene poisoning. *J. Am. Med. Assoc.* **205**, 243–245

Fabbri, L., Mapp, C., Rossi, A., Sarto, F., Trevisan, A. and De Rosa, E. (1979) Pulmonary changes due to low level occupational exposure to ozone. *Med. Lav.* **4**, 307–312

Falck, F.J., Fine, L.J. and Smith, R.G. (1983) Occupational Cd exposure and renal status. *Am. J. Ind. Med.* **4**, 541–549

Farrell, B.P., Kerr, H.D., Kulle, T.J., Sauder, L.R. and Young, J.L. (1979) Adaption in human subjects to the effects of inhaled ozone after repeated exposure. *Am. Rev. Respir. Dis.* **119**, 725–730

Federspiel, C.F., Layne, J.T., Auer, C. and Bruce, J. (1980) Lung function among employees of a copper mine smelter: lack of effect of chronic sulfur dioxide exposure. *J. Occup. Med.* **22**, 438–444

Ferris, B.G., Jr, Puleo, S. and Chen, H.Y. (1979) Mortality and morbidity in a pulp and paper mill in the United States: a ten year follow-up. *Br. J. Ind. Med.* **36**, 127–134

Field, G.B. (1984) Pulmonary function in aluminium smelters. *Thorax* **39**, 743–751

Fischer, P., Remijn, B., Brunekreef, B., van der Lende, R., Schouten, J. and Quanjer, P. (1985) Indoor air pollution and its effect on pulmonary function of adult and non-smoking women. *Int. J. Epidemiol.* **14**, 221–226

Flake, R.E. (1964) Chlorine inhalation. *N. Engl. J. Med.* **271**, 1373

Fleming, G.M., Chester, E.H. and Montenegro, H.D. (1979) Dysfunction of small airways following pulmonary injury due to nitrogen dioxide. *Chest* **75**, 720–721

Fogarty, P.W., George, P.M.J., Solomon, M., Spiro, S.G. and Armstrong, R.F. (1991) Long term effects of smoke inhalation in survivors of the King's Cross underground station fire. *Thorax* **46**, 914–918

Folinsbee, L.J., Horvath, S.M., Bedi, J.F. and Delehunt, J.C. (1978) Effect of 0.62 p.p.m. NO_2 on cardiopulmonary function in young male non-smokers. *Environ. Res.* **15**, 199–205

Fouke, J.M., Delemos, R.A. and McFadden, E.R. (1988) Airway response to ultra short-term exposure to coma. *Am. Rev. Respir. Dis.* **137**, 326–330

Frant, R. (1963) Formation of ozone in gas-shielded welding. *Ann. Occup. Hyg.* **6**, 113–125

Freeman, G. and Haydon, G.B. (1964) Emphysema after low-level exposure to NO_2. *Archs Environ. Health* **8**, 125–128

Freeman, G., Crane, S.C. and Furiosi, N.J. (1969) Healing in rat lung after subacute exposure to nitrogen dioxide. *Am. Rev. Respir. Dis.* **100**, 622–676

Friberg, L. (1957) Deposition and distribution of cadmium in man in chronic poisoning. *Archs Ind. Health* **16**, 27–29

Friberg, L. (1971) Cadmium, alloys, compounds. In: *Encyclopedia of Occupational Health and Safety*, International Labour Office, Geneva, pp. 233–234

Frostad, E.W. (1936) Fluoride intoxication in Norwegian aluminium plant workers. *Tidsskr. Nor. Laegef.* **56**, 179–182

Funahashi, A., Schlueter, D.P., Pintar, K., Bemis, E.L. and Siegesmund, K.A. (1988) Welders' pnemoconiosis: tissue elemental microanalysis by energy dispersive X-ray analysis. *Br. J. Ind. Med.* **45**, 14–18

Gerritsen, W.B. and Bushmann, C.H. (1960) Phosgene poisoning caused by the use of chemical paint removers containing methylene chloride in ill-ventilated rooms heated by kerosene stoves. *Br. J. Ind. Med.* **17**, 187–189

Gilks, B. and Churg, A. (1987) Aluminium-induced pulmonary fibrosis: do fibers play a part? *Am. Rev. Respir. Dis.* **136**, 176–179

Gleason, R.P. (1968) Exposure to copper dust. *Am. Ind. Hyg. Assoc. J.* **29**, 461–462

Glover, J.R. (1970) Selenium and its industrial toxicology. *Ind. Med. Surg.* **39**, 50–54

Godbert, A.L. and Leach, E. (1970) *Research Report 265*. A preliminary survey of the pollution of mine air by nitrogen oxides from diesel exhaust gases. Safety in Mines Research Establishment, Sheffield

Goralewski, G. (1940) Zur Symptomatologie der Aluminium-Staublunge. *Arch. Gewerbepath. Gewerbehyg.* **10**, 384–408

Goralewski, G. (1947) Die Aluminiumlunge: eine neue Gewerbeerkrankung. *Z. ges. inn. Med.* **2**, 665–673

Goralewski, G. (1950) Die Aluminiumlunge. Eine klinische Studie. *Arbeitsmedizin* **26**

Gore, I. and Harding, S.M. (1987) Sinker lung: acute metallic mercury poisoning associated with the making of fishing weights. *Alabama J. Med. Sci.* **24**, 267–269

Gough, J. (1960) Emphysema in relation to occupation. *Ind. Med. Surg.* **29**, 283–285

Gough, J. (1968) The pathogenesis of emphysema. In: *The Lung*, (eds. A.A. Liebow and D.E. Smith), Williams and Wilkins, Baltimore, pp. 124–126

Graham, J.A., Gardner, D.E., Walters, M.D. and Coffin, D.L. (1975) Effect of trace metals on phagocytosis by alveolar macrophages. *Infect. Immunol.* **11**, 1278–1283

Graham, J.I. and Runnicles, D.F. (1943) Nitrous fumes from shot-firing in relation to pulmonary disease. In: *Chronic Disease in South Wales Coal Miners*. Medical Research Council Special Report Series No. 244, pp. 187–213

Grauser, F.L. and Smith, W.R. (1975) Pulmonary interstitial fibrosis following near-drowning and exposure to short-term high oxygen concentrations. *Chest* **68**, 373–375

Grayson, R.R. (1956) Silage gas poisoning: nitrogen dioxide pneumonia, a new disease in agricultural workers. *Ann. Intern. Med.* **45**, 393–408

Gregory, K.L., Malinoski, V.F. and Sharp, C.R. (1969) Cleveland clinic fire survivorship study, 1929–1965. *Archs Environ. Health* **18**, 508–512

Groves, J.A. and Ellwood, P.A. (1989) Gases in forage tower silos. *Ann. Occup. Hyg.* **33**, 519–535

Gudzovskii, G.A. (1971) Antimony: alloys and compounds. *Encyclopedia of Occupational Health and Safety,* Vol. 1, ILO, Geneva, pp. 112–114

Hackney, J.D. and Linn, W.S. (1979) Koch's postulates updated: a potentially useful application to laboratory research and policy analysis in environmental technology. *Am. Rev. Respir. Dis.* **119**, 849–852

Hackney, J.D., Linn, W.S., Mohler, J.G., Pedersen, E.E., Breisacher, P. and Russo, A. (1975). Experimental studies on human health effects of air pollutants. II. Four-hour exposure to ozone alone and in combination with other pollutant gases. *Archs Environ. Health* **30**, 379–384

Hal Cragun, W., Grover, B. and Dunn, T. (1992) Acute respiratory failure associated with a motor vehicle accident. *Chest* **102**, 1581

Hall, A.D. (1923) Can silage be substituted for roots? *J. Farmers Club*, March 20–21

Hallee, T.J. (1969) Diffuse lung disease caused by inhalation of mercury vapor. *Am. Rev. Respir. Dis.* **99**, 430–436

Halpin, D.S. (1975) An unusual reaction in muscle in association with a Vitallium plate: a report of possible metal hypersensitivity. *J. Bone Jt Surg.* **57B**, 451–453

Haponik, E.F., Meyers, D.A., Munster, A.M., Smith, P.L., Britt, E.J., Wise, R.A. and Bleecker, E.R. (1987) Acute upper airway injury in burn patients. *Am. Rev. Respir. Dis.* **135**, 360–366

Hampton, T.R.W. (1971) Acute inhalation injury. *J. R. Naval Med. Service* **57**, 4–9

Harding, H.E. (1950) Notes on the toxicology of cobalt metal. *Br. J. Ind. Med.* **7**, 76–78

Harding, R.M. (1988) Medical aspects of special types of flight. In: *Aviation Medicine*, 2nd ed. (eds. J. Einsting and P. King), Butterworths, London, pp. 478–479

Hatton, D.V., Leach, C.S., Nicogossian, A.E. and Di Ferrante, N. (1977) Collagen breakdown and nitrogen dioxide inhalation. *Archs Environ. Health* **32**, 33–36

Hayden, S.P., Pincock, A.C., Hayden, J., Tyler, L.E., Cross, K.W. and Bishop, J.M. (1984) Respiratory symptoms and pulmonary function of welders in the engineering industry. *Thorax* **39**, 442–447

Hayes, W.J. (1971) Insecticides, rodenticides and other economic poisons. In: *Drull's Pharmacology in Medicine*, 4th edn (ed. J.R. di Palma), McGraw Hill, New York, pp. 1256–1276

Heath, J.C., Webb, M. and Caffrey, M. (1969) The interaction of carcinogenic metals with tissues and body fluids. Cobalt and horse serum. *Br. J. Cancer* **23**, 153–166

Hennenberger, P.K., Ferris, B.G. and Monson, R.R. (1989) Mortality among pulp and paper workers in Berlin, New Hampshire. *Br. J. Ind. Med.* **46**, 658–664

Hicks, R., Hewitt, P.J. and Lam, H.F. (1979) An investigation of the experimental induction of hypersensitivity in the guinea pig on material containing chromium, nickel and cobalt from arc welding fumes. *Int. Archs Allergy Appl. Immunol.* **59**, 265–272

HMSO (1979) *Occupational Mortality Tables*, HMSO, London

Horowitz, S.F., Fischbein, A., Matza, D., Rizzo, J.N., Stern, A., Machac, J. and Solomon, S.J. (1988) Evaluation of right and left ventricular function in hard metal workers. *Br. J. Ind. Med.* **45**, 742–746

Horsfield, K., Guyatt, A.R., Cooper, F.M., Buckman, M.P. and Cumming G. (1988) Lung function in West Sussex firemen: a four year study. *Br. J. Ind. Med.* **45**, 116–121

Horvath, E.P., doPico, G.A., Barbee, R.A. and Dickie, H.A. (1978) Nitrogen dioxide-induced pulmonary disease. *J. Occup. Med.* **20**, 103–110

Horvath, S.M., Gliner, J.A. and Folinsbee, L.J. (1981) Adaptation to ozone: duration of effect. *Am. Rev. Respir. Dis.* **123**, 496–501

Huber, G.L., Mason, R.J., La Force, M., Spencer, N.J., Gardner, D.E. and Coffin, D.L. (1971) Alteration in the lung following the administration of ozone. *Archs Intern. Med.* **128**, 81–93

Ide, C.W. (1986) Mercury hazards arising from the repair of sphygmomanometers. *Br. Med. J.* **292**, 1409–1410

Jäppinen, P. (1987) A mortality study of Finnish pulp and paper workers. *Br. J. Ind. Med.* **44**, 580–587

Jesson, M.W. (1972) *Removal of Gases from a Forage Tower Prior to Entry*. Report No. 3. National Institute of Agricultural Engineering, Silsoe, Beds

Jobs, H. and Ballhausen, C. (1940) Quoted by Bech, A.O., Kipling, M.D. and Heather, J.C. (1962)

Johnstone, R.T. (1945) Methyl bromide intoxication in a large group of workers. *Ind. Med. Surg.* **14**, 495–497

Jones, A.T. (1952) Noxious gases and fumes. *Proc. R. Soc. Med.* **45**, 609–610

Jones, D.A., Lucas, H.K., O'Driscoll, M., Price, C.H.G. and Wibberley, B. (1975) Cobalt toxicity after McKee hip arthroplasty. *J. Bone Jt Surg.* **57B**, 289–296

Jones, G.R., Proudfoot, A.T. and Hall, J.T. (1973) Pulmonary effects of acute exposure to nitrous fumes. *Thorax* **28**, 61–65

Jones, J.G. and Warner, C.G. (1972) Chronic exposure to iron oxide, chromium oxide and nickel oxide fumes in metal dressers in a steelworks. *Br. J. Ind. Med.* **29**, 168–177

Jones, R.N., Hughes, J.M., Glinmeyer, H. and Weill, H. (1986) Lung function after acute chlorine exposure. *Am. Rev. Respir. Dis.* **134**, 1190–1195

Jones Williams, W. (1958) The pathology of the lungs in five nickel workers. *Br. J. Ind. Med.* **15**, 235–242

Jordan, J.W. (1961) Pulmonary fibrosis in a worker using an aluminium powder. *Br. J. Ind. Med.* **18**, 21–23

Joseph, M. (1968) Hard metal pneumoconiosis. *Australas. Radiol.* **12**, 92–95

Joyner, R.E. and Durel, E.G. (1962) Accidental liquid chlorine spill in a rural community. *J. Occup. Med.* **4**, 152–154

Kalliomaki, P.L. and Kalliomaki, K. (1982) Respiratory status of stainless steel and mild steel welders. *Scand. J. Work Environ. Health* **8** (suppl. 1), 117–121

Kalliomaki, P.L. and Kalliomaki, K.K. (1983) Lung measurements of particles retained in the lungs. *Scand. J. Work Environ. Health* **9**, 219–222

Kalliomaki, P.L. and Rahkonen, E. (1981) Lung retained contaminants, urinary chromium and nickel among stainless steel welders. *Int. Archs Occup. Environ. Health* **49**, 67–75

Kaltreider, N.L., Elder, M.J., Cralley, L.V. and Colwell, M.O. (1972) Health survey of aluminium workers with special reference to fluoride exposure. *J. Occup. Med.* **14**, 531–541

Kaplun, Z.S. and Mezencewa, N.W. (1960) Experimentellstudie uber die toxische Wirkung von Staub bei der Erzengung von Sintermettallen. *J. Hyg. Epidemiol. Microbiol. Immunol.* **4**, 390–399

Kaponen, M. and Gustafson, T. (1980) Dusts in steel-making plants: lung contamination among iron workers. *Int. Archs Occup. Environ. Health* **47**, 35–45

Karlish, A.J. (1960) Cadmium poisoning. *Br. Med. J.* **1**, 173–174

Karstens, A.I. and Welch, B.E. (1971) Spacecraft atmospheres. In: *Aerospace Medicine*, 2nd edn (ed. H.W. Randel), Williams and Wilkins, Baltimore, pp. 668–669

Kass, I., Zamel, N., Dobry, C.A. and Holzer, M. (1972) Bronchiectasis following ammonia burns of the respiratory tract. *Chest* **62**, 282–285

Kaufman, J. and Burkons, D. (1971) Clinical, roentgenologic and physiologic effects of acute chlorine exposure. *Archs Environ. Health* **23**, 29–33

Kawada, T., Koyama, H. and Suzuki, S. (1989) Cadmium NAG activity and β2-microglobulin in the urine of cadmium pigment workers. *Br. J. Ind. Med.* **46**, 52–55

Kazantzis, G. (1980) *Occupational Exposure to Cadmium*, Report

on Seminar: London, 20 March, 1980. Cadmium Association, London, pp. 55–56, 58–61

Kehrl, H.R., Vincent, L.M., Kowalski, R.J., Horstman, D.H. O'Neill, J.J., McCartney, W.H. and Bromberg, P.A. (1987) Ozone exposure increases respiratory epithelium permeability in humans. *Am. Rev. Respir. Dis.* **135**, 1124–1128

Keller, M.D., Lanese, R.R., Mitchell, R.I. and Cote, R.W. (1979a) Respiratory illness in households using gas and electricity for cooking. 1. Survey and incidence. *Environ. Res.* **19**, 495–503

Keller, M.D., Lanese, R.R., Mitchell, R.I. and Cote, R.W. (1979b) Respiratory illness in households using gas and electricity for cooking. 11. Symptoms and objective findings. *Environ. Res.* **19**, 504–515

Kendrey, G. and Roe, F.J.C. (1969) Cadmium toxicology. *Lancet* **1**, 1206–1207

Kennedy, A., Dornan, J.D. and King, R. (1981) Fatal myocardial disease associated with industrial exposure to cobalt. *Lancet* **1**, 412–414

Kennedy, M.C.S. (1956) Aluminium powder inhalations in the treatment of silicosis of pottery workers and pneumoconiosis of coal-miners. *Br. J. Ind. Med.* **13**, 85–99

Kennedy, M.C.S. (1972) Nitrous fumes and coal-miners with emphysema. *Ann. Occup. Hyg.* **15**, 285–300

Kennedy, M.C.S. (1974) Nitrous fume poisoning in coal-miners. *Rev. Inst. Hyg. Mines* **29**, 167–174

Kerr, H.D., Kulle, T.J., McIlhany, M.L. and Swidersky, P. (1975) Effects of ozone on pulmonary function in normal subjects. *Am. Rev. Respir. Dis.* **111**, 763–773

Kimmerle, G. (1976) Toxicity of combustion products with particular reference to polyurethane. *Ann. Occup. Hyg.* **19**, 269–273

King, E.J., Harrison, C.V. and Mohanty, G.P. (1955) The effect of various forms of alumina on the lungs of rats. *J. Pathol. Bacteriol.* **69**, 81–93

King, G.W. (1954) Acute pneumonitis due to accidental exposure to mercury vapor. *Ariz. Med.* **11**, 335

Kirkpatrick, M.B. and Bass, J.B. (1979) Severe obstructive lung disease and smoke inhalation. *Chest* **76**, 108–110

Kiviluoto, M. (1980) Observations on the lungs of vanadium workers. *Br. J. Ind. Med.* **37**, 363–366

Kjellstrom, T., Firberg, L. and Rahnster, D. (1979) Mortality and cancer morbidity among cadmium-exposed workers. *Environ. Health Persp.* **28**, 199–204

Kleeberger, S.R., Kolbe, J., Adkinson, N.F., Peters, S.P. and Spannhake, E.W. (1988) The role of mediators in the response of the canine peripheral lung to 1 p.p.m. ozone. *Am. Rev. Respir. Dis.* **137**, 321–325

Kleinerman, J. (1979) Effects of nitrogen dioxide on elastin and collagen contents of lung. *Archs Environ. Health* **34**, 228–232

Kleinerman, J. and Rynbrandt, D. (1976) Lung proteolytic activity and serum protease inhibition after NO2 exposure. *Archs Environ. Health* **31**, 37–41

Kleinerman, J. and Wright, G.W. (1961) The reparative capacity of animal lungs after exposure to various single and multiple doses of nitrite. *Am. Rev. Respir. Dis.* **83**, 423–424

Kleinfeld, M., Giel, C. and Tabershaw, I.R. (1957) Health hazards associated with inert-gas-shielded metal arc welding. *Archs Ind. Health* **15**, 27–31

Koenig, J.Q., Pierson, W.E., Hirke, M. and Frank, R. (1981) Effects of SO2 plus NaCl aerosol combined with moderate exercise on pulmonary function in asthmatic adolescents. *Environ. Res.* **25**, 340–348

Kosmider, S., Ludyga, K., Misiewicz, A., Drozdz, M. and Sagan, J. (1972) Experimentalle and klinische Untersuchungen über emphysembildende Wirkung der Stickstoffoxyde. *Zentrabl. Arbeitsmed.* **22**, 362–368

Kowitz, T.A., Reba, R.C., Parker, R.T. and Spicer, W.S. (1967) Effects of chlorine gas upon respiratory function. *Archs Environ. Health* **14**, 545–558

Krackow, E.H. (1953) Toxicity and health hazards of boron hydrides. *Archs Ind. Hyg. Occup. Med.* **8**, 335–339

Kramer, C.G. (1967) Chlorine. *J. Occup. Med.* **9**, 193–196

Kronenberger, F.L. (1959) Bronchiolitis after shot-firing in a colliery. *Br. J. Dis. Chest* **53**, 308–313

Kusaka, Y., Yokoyama, E., Sera, Y., Yamamoto, S., Kyono, H., Skirakawa, T. and Gotto, S. (1986a) Respiratory diseases in hard metal workers: an occupational hygiene study in a factory. *Br. J. Ind. Med.* **43**, 474–485

Kusaka, Y., Ichikawa, Y., Shirakawa, T. and Goto, S. (1986b) Effect of hard metal dust on ventilatory function. *Br. J. Ind. Med.* **43**, 486–489

Lam, H.F., Conner, M.W., Roger, A.E., Fitzgerald, S. and Amdur, M.O. (1985) Functional and morphological changes in the lungs of guinea pigs exposed to freshly generated ultrafine zinc oxides particles. *Toxic. Appl. Pharmacol.* **78**, 29–38

Lane, R.E. and Campbell, A.C.P. (1954) Fatal emphysema in two men making a copper cadmium alloy. *Br. J. Ind. Med.* **11**, 118–122

Langard, S. (1980) A survey of respiratory symptoms and lung function in ferrochromium and ferrosilicon workers. *Int. Archs Occup. Environ. Health* **46**, 1–9

Langham Brown, J.J. (1988) Zinc fume fever. *Br. J. Radiol.* **61**, 327–329

Larsson, K., Edlund, A., Arns, R., Lowgren, H., Nystrom, J., Sunderstrom, G. and Tornling, G. (1989) Lung function and bronchial reactivity in aluminium potroom workers. *Scand. J. Work Environ. Health* **15**, 296–301

Lauwerys, R.R. (1983) *Industrial Chemical Exposure: Guidelines for Biological Monitoring*. Biomedical Publications, Davis

Lauwerys, R.R. and Bernard, A.M. (1986) Cadmium and the kidney. *Br. J. Ind. Med.* **43**, 433–435

Lawson, J.J. (1961) The toxicity of titanium tetrachloride. *J. Occup. Med.* **3**, 7–12

Lawther, P.J., McFarlane, A.J., Waller, R.E. and Brooks, A.G.F. (1975) Pulmonary function and sulphur dioxide, some preliminary findings. *Environ. Res.* **10**, 355–367

Leading article (1973) Cadmium and the lung. *Lancet* **2**, 1134–1135

Leduc, D., Bris, P., Lheureux, P., Gevenois, P.A., De Vuyst, P. and Yernault, J.C. (1992) Acute and long term respiratory damage following inhalation of ammonia. *Thorax* **47**, 755–757

Lees, R.E.M. (1980) Changes in lung function after exposure to vanadium compounds in fuel oil ash. *Br. J. Ind. Med.* **37**, 253–256

Leigh, J. and Wiles, A.N. (1988) Effects of diesel equipment usage on prevalence of chronic bronchitis, lung carcinoma and ischaemic heart disease in coal workers. *Ann. Occup. Hyg.* **32** (suppl. 1), 1196–1198

Lemen, R.A., Lee, J.S., Wagoner, J.K. and Blejer, H.P. (1976) Cancer mortality among cadmium production workers. *Ann. NY Acad. Sci.* **27**, 273–279

Lewis, C.E. (1959) The biological effects of vanadium exposure. II The signs and symptoms of occupational vanadium exposure. *Archs Ind. Hyg.* **19**, 497–503

Lewis, G.P., Jusko, W.J., Coughlin, L.L. and Hartz, S. (1972). Contribution of cigarette smoking to cadmium accumulation in man. *Lancet* **1**, 291–292

Liebow, A.A. (1975) Definition and classification of interstitial pneumonias in human pathology. *Prog. Respir. Res.* **8**, 1–33

Lindberg, E. and Hedenstierna, G. (1983) Chrome plating. Symptoms, findings in the upper airways, and effects on lung function. *Archs Environ. Health* **38**, 367–374

Linn, W.S., Avol, E.L., Peng, R-C., Shamoo, D.A. and Hackney, J.D. (1987) Replicated dose–response study of sulfur dioxide effects in normal, atopic and asthmatic volunteers. *Am. Rev. Respir. Dis.* **136**, 1127–1134

Lloyd-Davies, T.A. (1946) Manganese pneumonitis. *Br. J. Ind. Med.* **3**, 111–135

Lloyd-Davies, T.A. and Harding, H.E. (1949) Manganese pneumonitis. *Br. J. Ind. Med.* **6**, 82–90

Loke, J., Farmer, W., Matthay, R.A., Putman, C.E. and Walker Smith, G.J. (1980) Acute and chronic effects of fire fighting on pulmonary function. *Chest* **77**, 369–373

Lowe, H.J. and Freeman, G. (1957) Boron hydride (Borane) intoxication in man. *Archs Ind. Health* **16**, 523–533

Lowry, T. and Schuman, L.M. (1956). 'Silo-filler's disease' – a syndrome caused by nitrogen dioxide. *J. Am. Med. Assoc.* **162**, 153–160

Lundgren, K.D. and Öhman, J. (1954) Pneumokoniose in der Hartmetall-industrie. *Virchows Arch. [A] Pathol. Anat. Physiol.* **325**, 259–284

McAdams, A.J. (1955) Bronchiolitis obliterans. *Am. J. Med.* **19**, 314–322

McAllum, R.I. and Leathart, G.L. (1975) Pneumoconiosis in zirconium workers. *Proceedings of the Eighteenth International Congress on Occupational Health*, ICOH, Brighton

McConnell, L.H., Fink, J.N., Schlueter, D.P. and Schmidt, M. G. Jr (1973) Asthma caused by nickel sensitivity. *Ann. Intern. Med.* **78**, 888–890

McDermott, F.T. (1971) Dust in the cemented carbide industry. *Am. Ind. Hyg. Assoc. J.* **32**, 188–193

McLaughlin, A.I.G., Kazantzis, G., King, E., Teare, R.J. and Owen, R. (1962) Pulmonary fibrosis and encephalopathy associated with inhalation of aluminium dust. *Br. J. Ind. Med.* **19**, 253–263

McLaughlin, A.I.G., Milton, R. and Perry, K.M.A. (1946) Toxic manifestations of osmium tetroxide. *Br. J. Ind. Med.* **3**, 183–186

McLintock, R.S. (1972) Discussion. *Ann. Occup. Hyg.* **15**, 301

McMillan, G.H.G. (1978) Studies of the health of welders in naval dockyards. *Ann. Occup. Hyg.* **21**, 377–392

McMillan, G.H.G. (1979) The health of welders in naval dockyards: acute changes in respiratory function during standardized welding. *Ann. Occup. Hyg.* **22**, 19–32

McMillan, G.H.G. (1983) The health of welders in naval dockyards: the risk of asbestos-related diseases occurring in welders. *J. Occup. Med.* **25**, 727–730

McMillan, G.H.G. and Heath, J. (1979) The health of welders in naval dockyards: acute changes in respiratory function during standardized welding. *Ann. Occup. Hyg.* **22**, 19–32

McMillan, G.H.G. and Pethybridge, R.J. (1983) The health of welders in naval dockyards: proportional mortality study of welders and two control groups. *J. Occup. Med.* **33**, 75–84

Maigretter, R.Z., Erhlich, R., Fenters, J.D. and Gardner, D.E. (1976) Potentiating effects of manganese dioxide on experimental respiratory infections. *Environ. Res.* **11**, 386–391

Malo, J-L., Malo, J., Cartier, A. and Dolovich, J. (1990) Acute lung reaction due to zinc inhalation. *Eur. Respir. J.* **3**, 111–114

Mason, H.J., Davison, A.J., Wright, A.L., Guthrie, C.J.G., Fayers, P.M., Venables, K.M., Smith, N.J., Chettle, D.R., Franklin, D.M., Scott, M.C., Holden, H.C., Gompertz, D. and Newman-Taylor, A.J. (1988) Relations between liver cadmium, cumulative exposure, and renal function in cadmium alloy workers. *Br. J. Ind. Med.* **45**, 793–802

Mathes, F.T., Kirschner, R., Yow, M.D. and Brennan, J.C. (1958) Acute poisoning associated with inhalation of mercury vapor. *Pediatrics* **22**, 675–688

Mayor, M.B., Merritt, K. and Brown, S.A. (1980) Metal allergy and the surgical patient. *Am. J. Surg.* **139**, 477–479

Meiklejohn, A. (1963) The successful prevention of silicosis among china biscuit workers in the North Staffordshire potteries. *Br. J. Ind. Med.* **20**, 255–263

Mendelson, D.S., Gendal, E.S., Janus, C.L. and Fischbein, A. (1991) Computed tomography of the thorax in workers exposed to hard metals. *Br. J. Ind. Med.* **48**, 208–210

Merfield, D.P., Taylor, A., Gemell, D.M. and Parish, J.A. (1976) Mercury intoxication in a dental surgery following unreported spillage. *Br. Dent. J.* **141**, 179–186

Meyer-Bisch, C., Pham, Q.T., Mur, J-M., Massin, N., Moulin, J-J., Teculescu, D., Carton, B., Pierre, F. and Baruthio, F. (1989) Respiratory hazards in hard metal workers: a cross sectional study. *Br. J. Ind. Med.* **46**, 302–309

Meyers, J.B. (1950) Acute pulmonary complications following inhalation of chromic acid mist. *Archs Ind. Hyg.* **2**, 742–747

Miller, C.W., Davies, M.W., Goldman, A. and Wyatt, J.P. (1953) Pneumoconiosis in the tungsten carbide tool industry. *Archs Ind. Hyg.* **8**, 453–465

Milliken, J.A., Waugh, D. and Kadish, M.E. (1963) Acute interstitial pulmonary fibrosis caused by smoke bomb. *Can. Med. Assoc. J.* **88**, 36–39

Milne, J.E.H. (1969) Nitrogen dioxide inhalation and bronchiolitis obliterans. *J. Occup. Med.* **11**, 538–547

Milne, J., Christophers, A. and de Silva, P. (1970) Acute mercurial pneumonitis. *Br. J. Ind. Med.* **27**, 334–338

Minty, B.D. and Toyston, D. (1985) Changes in permeability of the alveolar-capillary barrier in fire-fighters. *Br. J. Ind. Med.* **42**, 631–634

Mitchell, J., Manning, G.B., Molyneux, M. and Lane, R.E. (1961) Pulmonary fibrosis in workers exposed to finely powdered aluminium. *Br. J. Ind. Med.* **18**, 10–20

Modell, J.H., Graves, S.A. and Ketover, A. (1976) Clinical course of 91 consecutive near-drowning victims. *Chest* **70**, 231–238

Montague, T.J. and MacNeil, A.R. (1980) Mass ammonia inhalation. *Chest* **77**, 496–498

Morgan, J.G. (1958) Some observations on the incidence of respiratory cancer in nickel workers. *Br. J. Ind. Med.* **15**, 224–234

Morgan, W.K.C. (1962) Arc welders' lung complicated by conglomeration. *Am. Rev. Respir. Dis.* **85**, 570–575

Morgan, W.K.C. and Dinman, B.D. (1989) Pulmonary effects of aluminium. In: *Aluminium and Health. A Critical Review* (ed. H.J. Gitelman), Marcell Dekker, New York, pp. 203–234

Morichau-Beauchant, G. (1964) Pneumonies manganiques. *J. fr. Méd. Chir. thorac.* **18**, 300–312

Morley, R. and Silk, S.J. (1970) The industrial hazard of nitrous fumes. *Ann. Occup. Hyg.* **13**, 101–107

Moskowitz, R.L., Lyons, H.A. and Cottle, H.R. (1964) Silofiller's disease. *Am. J. Med.* **36**, 457–462

Mur, J-M. and Teculescu, D. (1985) Lung function and clinical findings in a cross sectional study of arc welders: an epidemiological study. *Int. J. Occup. Environ. Health* **57**, 1–17

Musk, A.W., Greville, H.W. and Tribe, A.E. (1980) Pulmonary disease from occupational exposure to an artificial aluminium silicate used for cat litter. *Br. J. Ind. Med.* **37**, 367–372

Musk, A.W., Peters, J.M. and Wegman, D.H. (1977) Lung function in firefighters: 1. A three-year follow-up of active subjects. *Am. J. Publ. Health* **67**, 626–629

Musk, A.W., Manson, R.R., Peters, J.M. and Peters, R.K. (1978) Mortality among Boston firefighters. *Br. J. Ind. Med.* **35**, 104–108

Musk, A.W., Beck, B.D., Greville, H.W., Brain, J.D. and Bohannon, D.E. (1988) Pulmonary disease from exposure to an artificial aluminium silicate: further observations. *Br. J. Ind. Med.* **45**, 246–250

Mustafa, M.G. and Tierney, D.F. (1978) Biochemical and metabolic changes in the lung with oxygen, ozone and nitrogen dioxide toxicity. *Am. Rev. Respir. Dis.* **118**, 1061–1066

Mustafa, M.G., Cross, C.E., Munn, R.J. and Hardie, J.A. (1971) Effects of divalent metal ions on alveolar macrophage membrane adenosine triphosphatase activity. *J. Lab. Clin. Med.* **77**, 563–571

Mustafa, M.G., Elsayed, N.M., Graham, H.A. and Gardner, D.E. (1983) Effects of ozone exposure on lung metabolism. *Adv. Modern Environ. Toxicol.* **5**, 57–73

Nandi, M., Jick, H., Slone, D., Shapiro, S. and Lewis, G.P. (1969) Cadmium content of cigarettes. *Lancet* **2**, 1329–1330

Nemery, B. and Damedts, M. (1991) Respiratory involvement in metal fume fever. *Eur. Respir. J.* **4**, 764–765

Newhouse, M.L., Oakes, D. and Wooley, A.J. (1985) Mortality of welders and other craftsmen at a shipyard in NE England. *Br. J. Ind. Med.* **42**, 406–410

Nishiyama, K., Suzuki, Y., Fujii, N., Yano, H., Miyai, T. and Onishi, K. (1975) Effect of long-term exposure to manganese particles. II. Periodical observation of respiratory organs in monkeys and mice. *Jap. J. Hyg.* **30**, 117–123

Noguchi, M., Kimula, Y. and Ogata, T. (1985) Muddy lung. *Am. J. Clin. Pathol.* **83**, 240–244

Norwood, W.D., Wisehart, D.E., Earl, C.A., Adley, F.E. and Anderson, D.E. (1966) Nitrogen dioxide poisoning due to metal cutting with oxyacetylene torch. *J. Occup. Med.* **8**, 301–306

Orehek, J., Massari, J.P., Gayrard, P., Grimaud, C. and Charpin, J. (1976) Effect of short-term low-level nitrogen dioxide exposure on bronchial sensitivity of asthmatic subjects. *J. Clin. Invest.* **57**, 301–307

Oxhøj, H. and Bake, B. (1979) Effects of electric arc welding on ventilatory lung function. *Archs Environ. Health* **34**, 211–221

Palmer, K.C., Snider, G.L. and Hayes, J.A. (1975) Cellular proliferation induced in the lung by cadmium aerosol. *Am. Rev. Respir. Dis.* **112**, 173–179

Park, T., Di Benedetto, R., Morgan, K., Colmers, R. and Sherman, E. (1984) Diffuse endobronchial polyposis following a titanium tetrachloride inhalation injury. *Am. Rev. Respir. Dis.* **130**, 315–317

Patterson, J.C. (1947) Studies on the toxicity of inhaled cadmium. *J. Ind. Hyg.* **29**, 294–301

Pattey, F.A. (1963) In: *Industrial Hygiene and Toxicology*, Vol. II (eds. D.W. Fassett and D.D. Irish), Interscience Publishers, John Wiley and Sons, New York and London, pp. 883–884

Pedersen, C., Hansen, C.P. and Gronfeldt, W. (1984) Zinc chloride smoke poisoning following employment of smoke ammunition. *J. Dan. Med. Assoc.* **146**, 2397

Pieters, H.A.J. and Creyghton, J.W (1951) *Safety in the Chemical Laboratory*. Butterworths, London

Pigott, G.H., Gaskell, B.A. and Ishmael, J. (1981) Effects of long term inhalation of alumina fibres. *Br. J. Expl Pathol.* **62**, 323–331

Pilling, K.J. and Jones, H.W. (1988) Inhalation of degraded sulphur hexafluoride resulting in pulmonary oedema. *J. Soc. Occup. Med.* **38**, 82–84

Pimentel, J.C. and Marques, F. (1969) Vineyard sprayer's lung: a new occupational disease. *Thorax* **24**, 678–688

Piscator, M. (1976) Health hazards from inhalation of metal fumes. *Environ. Res.* **11**, 268–270

Powell, M. (1961) Toxic fumes from shotfiring in coal mines. *Ann. Occup. Hyg.* **3**, 162–183

Powell, M. and Lomax, A. (1960) The toxic effects of handling and firing explosives in coal mines. *Ann. Occup. Hyg.* **2**, 141–151

Princi, F. (1947) A study of industrial exposures to cadmium. *J. Ind. Hyg.* **29**, 315–320

Prys-Roberts, C. (1967) Principles of treatment of poisoning by higher oxides of nitrogen. *Br. J. Anaesth.* **39**, 432–438

Rae, T. (1975) A study of the effects of particulate metals of orthopaedic interest on murine macrophages in vitro. *J. Bone Jt Surg.* **57B**, 444–450

Rae, T. (1978) The haemolytic action of particulate metals. *J. Pathol.* **125**, 81–89

Rajan, K.G. and Davies, B.H. (1989) Reversible airways obstruction and interstitial pneumonitis due to acetic acid. *B. J. Ind. Med.* **46**, 67–68

Ramirez, R.J. and Dowell, A.R. (1971) Silo-filler's disease: nitrogen dioxide-induced lung injury. *Ann. Intern. Med.* **74**, 569–576

Rathus, E.M. and Landy, P.J. (1961) Methylbromide poisoning. *Br. J. Ind. Med.* **18**, 53–57

Reber, E. and Burckhardt, P. (1970) Uber Hartmetallstaublungen in des Schweiz. *Respiration* **27**, 120–153

Redline, S., Barna, B.P., Tomashefski, J.F. and Abraham, J.L. (1986) Granulomatous disease associated with pulmonary deposition of titanium. *Br. J. Ind. Med.* **43**, 652–656

Reed, D., Glaser, S. and Kaldor, J. (1980) Ozone toxicity symptoms among flight attendants. *Am. J. Ind. Med.* **1**, 43–48

Reger, R.B. and Attfield, M.D. (1983) Diesel emissions and associated respiratory health effects in mining. In: *Health Issues Related to Metal and Non-metallic Mining* (eds W.L. Wagner, W.N. Rom and J.A. Merchant), Butterworths, London and Sydney, pp. 393–412

Rivers, J.F., Orr, G. and Lee, H.A. (1970) Drowning. Its clinical sequelae and management. *Br. Med. J.* **1**, 157–161

Robertson, H.T., Lakshminarayan, S. and Hudson, L.D. (1978) Lung injury following a 50-metre fall into water. *Thorax* **33**, 175–180

Robertson, A., Dodgson, J., Collings, P. and Seaton, A. (1984) Exposure to oxides of nitrogen: respiratory symptoms and lung function in British coalminers. *Br. J. Ind. Med.* **41**, 214–219

Roels, H., Bernard, A., Buchet, J.P., Goret, A., Lauwerys, R., Chettle, D.R., Harvey, T.C. and Al Haddad, I. (1979) Critical concentration of cadmium in renal cortex and urine. *Lancet* **1**, 221

Roels, H., Djubgang, J., Buchet, J.P. and Lauwerys, R. (1982) Evolution of cadmium-induced renal dysfunction in workers removed from exposure. *Scand. J. Work Environ. Health* **8**, 191–200

Roshchin, A.V. (1967a) Toxicology of vanadium compounds used in modern industry. *Hyg. Sanit.* **32**, 345–352

Roshchin, A.V. (1967b) Vanadium. In: *Toxicology of the Rare Metals* (ed. Z.I. Israelson), Israel Program for Scientific Translations, Jerusalem, pp. 52–59

Rosenstock, L., Demers., P., Heyer, N.J. and Barnhart, S. (1988) Firefighting is associated with an increased risk for mortality from non-malignant respiratory disease. *Am. Rev. Respir. Dis.* **137**, Suppl. 251

Rüttner, J.R., Spycher, M.A. and Stolkin, I. (1987) Inorganic particulates in pneumoconiotic lungs of hard metal grinders. *Br. J. Ind. Med.* **44**, 657–660

Ryder-Powell, J.E., Amoruso, M.A., Czerniecki, B., Witz, G. and Goldstein, B.D. (1988) Inhalation of ozone produces a decrease in superoxide anion radical production in mouse alveolar macrophages. *Am. Rev. Respir. Dis.* **138**, 1129–1133

Rynbrandt, D. and Kleinerman, J. (1977) Nitrogen dioxide and pulmonary proteolytic enzymes. *Archs Environ. Health* **32**, 165–172

Sahle, W. (1992) Possible role of tungsten oxide whiskers in hardmetal pneumoconiosis. *Chest* **102**, 1310

Sahle, W. and Berglund, S. (1981) The morphology of slightly reduced tungsten trioxide equilibrated with CO–CO_2 gaseous buffers with and without addition of water. *J. Less Common Metals* **79**, 271–280

Sanderson, J.T. (1968) Hazards of the arc-air gouging process. *Ann. Occup. Hyg.* **11**, 123–133

Saric, M. and Lucic-Paliac, S. (1977) Possible synergism of exposure to airborne manganese and smoking habit in occurrence of respiratory symptoms. In: *Inhaled Particles IV*, Pergamon Press, Oxford, pp. 773–779

Saric, M., Lucic-Palaic, S., Paukovic, R. and Holetic, A. (1974) Respiratory effects of manganese. *Archs High Rad.* **25**, 15–26

Scanlon, P.D., Seltzer, J., Ingram, R.H., Reid, L. and Drazen, J.M. (1987) Chronic exposure to sulfur dioxide. *Am. Rev. Respir. Dis.* **135**, 831–839

Schardijn, G., van Eps, L.W.S., Swaak, A.J.G., Kager, J.C.G.M., and Persijn, J.P. (1979) Urinary β_2-microglobulin in upper and lower urinary-tract infections. *Lancet* **1**, 805–807

Schecter, A., Shanske, W., Stenzler, A., Quintilian, H. and Steinberg, H. (1980) Acute hydrogen selenide inhalation. *Chest* **77**, 554–555

Schepers, G.W.H. (1955a) The biological action of particulate cobalt metal. *Archs Ind. Health* **12**, 127–133

Schepers, G.W.H. (1955b) The biological action of particulate tungsten metal. *Archs Ind. Health* **12**, 134–136

Schepers, G.W.H. (1955c) The biological action of tantalum oxide. *Archs Ind. Health* **12**, 121–123

Scherrer, M., Parambadathumalail, A., Burki, H., Senn, A. and Zürcher, R. (1970) Drei Falle von Hartmetallstaublunge. *Schweiz. Med. Wschr.* **100**, 2251–2255

Schwarz, L., Peck, S.M., Blair, K.E. and Markuson, K.E. (1945) Allergic dermatitis due to metallic cobalt. *J. Allergy* **16**, 51–53

Seidelin, R. (1961) The inhalation of phosgene in a fire extinguisher accident. *Thorax* **16**, 91–93

Shaver, C.G. (1948) Further observations of lung changes associated with the manufacture of alumina abrasives. *Radiology* **50**, 760–769

Shaver, C.G. and Riddell, A.R. (1947) Lung changes associated with the manufacture of alumina abrasives. *J. Ind. Hyg. Toxic.* **29**, 145–157

Shenker, M.B., Speizer, F.E. and Taylor, S.O. (1981) Acute upper respiratory symptoms resulting from exposure to zinc chloride aerosol. *Environ. Res.* **25**, 317–324

Sheppard, D.A., Saisho, A., Nadel, J.A. and Boushey, H.A. (1981) Exercise increases sulfur dioxide induced bronchoconstriction in asthmatic subjects. *Am. Rev. Respir. Dis.* **123**, 486–491

Shiel, O.M.F. (1967) Morbid anatomical changes in the lungs of dogs after inhalation of higher oxides of nitrogen during anaesthesia. *Br. J. Anaesth.* **39**, 413–424

Shore, S.A., Kariya, S.T., Andeerson, K., Skornik, W., Feldman, H.A., Pennington, J., Godleski, J. and Drazen, J.M. (1987) Sulfur-dioxide-induced bronchitis in dogs. *Am. Rev. Respir. Dis.* **135**, 640–647

Simonsson, B.G., Sjöberg, A., Rolf, C. and Haeger-Aronsen, B. (1985) Acute and long-term airway hyperreactivity in aluminium-salt exposed workers with nocturnal asthma. *Eur. J. Respir. Dis.* **66**, 105–118

Sjöberg, S. (1950) Vanadium pentoxide dust. *Acta Med. Scand. Suppl.* **238**

Sjögren, B. (1980) A retrospective cohort study of mortality among stainless steel welders. *Scand. J. Work Environ. Health* **6**, 197–200

Sjögren, B. and Gustavsson, L.H. (1987) Mortality in two cohorts of welders exposed to high and low levels of hexavalent chromium. *Scand. J. Work Environ. Health* **13**, 247–251

Sjögren, B. and Ulfvarson, V. (1985) Respiratory symptoms and pulmonary function among welders working with aluminium, stainless steel and railway tracks. *Scand. J. Work Environ. Health* **11**, 27–32

Sjögren, B., Hedstrom, L. and Lindstedt, G. (1984) Urinary fluoride concentration as an estimate of welding fume exposure from basic electrodes. *Br. J. Ind. Med.* **41**, 192–196

Sjögren, I., Hillerdal, G., Anders, A. and Zetterström, O. (1980) Hard metal lung disease: importance of cobalt in coolants. *Thorax* **35**, 653–659

Smith, A.R. and Perina, A.E. (1948) Pneumoconiosis from synthetic abrasive minerals. *Occup. Med.* **5**, 396–402

Smith, J.P., Smith, J.C. and McCall, A.J. (1960) Chronic poisoning from cadmium fume. *J. Pathol.* **80**, 287–296

Snider, G.L., Lucey, E.C., Faris, B., Jung-Legg, Y., Stone, P.J. and Franzblau, C. (1988) Cadmium-chloride-induced air-space enlargement with interstitial pulmonary fibrosis is not associated with destruction of lung elastin. *Am. Rev. Respir. Dis.* **137**, 918–923

Sobonya, R. (1977) Fatal anhydrous ammonia inhalation. *Human Pathol.* **8**, 293–299

Spiegl, C.J., Scott, J.K., Steinhardt, H., Leach, L.J. and Hodge, H.C. (1956) Acute inhalation toxicity of lithium anhydride. *Archs Ind. Health* **14**, 468–470

Speizer, F.E., Ferris, B. and Bishop, Y.M.M. (1980) Respiratory disease rates and pulmonary function in children associated with NO₂ exposure. *Am. Rev. Respir. Dis.* **121**, 3–8

Spengler, J.D. and Sexton, K. (1983) Indoor air pollution: a public health perspective. *Science* **221**, 9–17

Sprince, N.L., Oliver, L.C., Eisen, E.A., Greene, R.E. and Chamberlin, R.I. (1988) Cobalt exposure and lung disease in tungsten carbide production. *Am. Rev. Respir. Dis.* **138**, 1220–1226

Stacy, B.D., King, E.J., Harrison, C.V., Nagelschmidt, G. and Nelson, S. (1959) Tissue changes in rats' lungs caused by hydroxides, oxides and phosphates of aluminium and iron. *J. Pathol. Bacteriol.* **77**, 417–426

Stark, G.W.V. (1972) Smoke and toxic gases from burning plastics. *Trans. I. Mar. Eng.* **84**, 25–34

Steele, R.H. and Wilhelm, D.L. (1967) The inflammatory reaction in chemical injury II. *Br. J. Expl Pathol.* **48**, 592–607

Stephens, R.J., Sloan, M.A., Evans, M.J. and Freeman, G. (1974) Early response of lungs to low levels of ozone. *Am. J. Pathol.* **74**, 31–58

Stephenson, S.F., Esrig, B.C., Polk, H.C. Jr and Fulton, R.L. (1975) The pathophysiology of smoke inhalation injury. *Ann. Surg.* **182**, 652–660

Stern, R.M. (1981) Process-dependent risk of delayed health effects for welders. *Environ. Health Persp.* **41**, 235–253

Stern, R.M. (1983) Assessment of risk of lung cancer for welders. *Archs Environ. Med.* **38**, 148–155

Stern, R.M. (1987) Cancer incidence among welders: possible effects of exposure to extremely low frequency electromagnetic radiation (ELF) and to welding fumes. *Environ. Health Persp.* **76**, 221–229

Stern, R.M. and Berlin, A. (1986) *Health Hazards and Biological Effects of Welding Fumes and Gases.* Elsevier, Amsterdam

Stokinger, H.E. (1965) Ozone toxicology: a review of research and industrial experience, 1954–1964. *Archs Environ. Health* **10**, 719–731

Sturgis, C.C., Drinker, P. and Thomson, R.M. (1927) Clinical observations on the effect of experimental inhalation of zinc oxide by apparently normal persons. *J. Ind. Hyg.* **9**, 88–97

Sunderman, F.W. and Kincaid, J.F. (1954) Nickel poisoning. II. Studies on patients suffering from acute exposure to vapors of nickel carbonyl. *J. Am. Med. Assoc.* **155**, 889–894

Sunderman, F.W. and Sunderman, F.W. Jr (1961) Löffler's syndrome associated with nickel sensitivity. *Archs Intern. Med.* **107**, 405–408

Sutherland, C.L., Meiklejohn, A. and Price, F.N.R. (1937) An inquiry into the health hazard of a group of workers exposed to alumina dust. *J. Ind. Hyg. Toxic.* **19**, 312–319

Suzuki, Y. (1970) Environmental contamination by manganese. *Jap. J. Ind. Health* **12**, 529–533

Swennen, B., Buchet, J-P., Stánescu, D., Lison, D. and Lauwerys, R. (1993) Epidemiological survey of workers exposed to cobalt oxides, cobalt salts, and cobalt metal. *Br. J. Ind. Med.* **50**, 835–842

Tashkin, D.P., Genovesi, M.G., Chopra, S., Coulson, A. and Simmons, M. (1977) Respiratory status of Los Angeles fireman: one-month follow-up after inhalation of dense smoke. *Chest* **71**, 445–449

Tebrock, H.E. and Mackle, W. (1968) Exposure to europium-activated yttrium orthovanadate. *J. Occup. Med.* **10** 692–696

Teisinger, J. and Fiserova-Bergerova, V. (1965) Pulmonary retention and excretion of mercury vapors in man. *Ind. Med. Surg.* **34**, 580–584

Teng, C.T. and Brennan, J.C. (1959) Acute mercury vapour poisoning. A report of four cases with radiographic and pathologic correlation. *Radiology* **73**, 354–361

Tennant, R., Johnson, H.J. and Wells, J.B. (1961) Acute bilateral pneumonitis associated with the inhalation of mercury vapour. *Conn. Med.* **25**, 106–109

Tolot, F., Girard, R., Dortit, G., Tabourin, G., Galy, P. and Bourret, J. (1970) Manifestations pulmonaires des 'métaux durs': troubles irritatifs et fibrose (Enquête et observations cliniques). *Archs mal. prof. Méd. trav.* **31**, 453–470

Townsend, M.C., Enterline, P.E., Sussman, N.B., Morgan, W.K.C., Belk, H.D. and Dinman, B.D. (1985) Pulmonary function in relation to total dust exposure at a bauxite refinery and alumina-based chemical products plant. *Am. Rev. Respir. Dis.* **132**, 1174–1180

Townsend, M.C., Sussman, N.B., Enterline, P.E., Morgan, W.K.C., Belk, H.D. and Dinman, B.D. (1988) Radiographic abnormalities in relation to total dust exposure at a bauxite refinery and alumina-based chemical products plant. *Am. Rev. Respir. Dis.* **138**, 90–95

Townshend, R.H. (1968) A case of acute cadmium pneumonitis: lung function tests during a four-year follow-up. *Br. J. Ind. Med.* **25**, 68–71

Turner, C. (1953) Self-feeding of silage. *Agriculture* **60**, 358–359

Ulvarson, S. (1981) Survey of air contaminants from welding. *Scand. J. Work Environ. Health* **11**, 27–32

Unger, K.M., Snow, R.M., Mestas, J.M. and Miller, W.C. (1980) Smoke inhalation in firemen. *Thorax* **35**, 838–842

Vena, J.E. and Fiedler, R.C. (1987) Mortality of a municipal worker cohorts: IV fire fighters. *Am. J. Ind. Med.* **11**, 671–684

Vigdortschik, N.A., Andreeva, E.C., Matussevitsch, I.Z., Nikulina, M.M., Frumina, L.M. and Stritor, V.A. (1937) The symptomatology of chronic poisoning with oxides of nitrogen. *J. Ind. Hyg. Toxicol.* **19**, 469–473

Vilar, T.G. (1974) Vineyard sprayers' lung. *Am. Rev. Respir. Dis.* **110**, 545–555

Vintinner, F.J., Vallenas, R., Carlin, C.E., Weiss, R., Macher, C. and Ochoa, R. (1955) Study of health of workers employed in mining and processing vanadium ore. *Archs Ind. Health* **12**, 635–642

Vogelmeier, C., Konig, G., Bencze, K. and Frhumann, G. (1987) Pulmonary involvement in zinc fume fever. *Chest* **92**, 946–48

Walters, M.D., Gardner, D.E., Aranyi, C. and Coffin, D.L. (1975) Metal toxicity for rabbit alveolar macrophages in vitro. *Environ. Res.* **9**, 32–47

Walton, M. (1973) Industrial ammonia gassing. *Br. J. Ind. Med.* **30**, 78–86

Watt, J. (1977) The role of the services in accident and disaster. *J. R. Naval Med. Serv.* **63**, 117–125

Webb, M. (1975) Cadmium. *Br. Med. Bull* **31**, 246–250

Webb, M. and Etienne, A.T. (1977) Studies on the toxicity and metabolism of cadmium-thionein. *Biochem. Pharmacol.* **26**, 15–30

Weill, H., George, R., Schwarz, M. and Ziskind, M. (1969) Late evaluation of pulmonary function after acute exposure to chlorine gas. *Am. Rev. Respir. Dis.* **99**, 374–379

Weston, J.T., Liebow, A.A., Dixon, M.G. and Rich, T.H. (1972) Untoward effects of exogenous inhalants on the lung. *J. Forensic Sci.* **17**, 199–279

Whitaker, P.H. (1945) Radiological appearances of the chest following partial asphyxia by a smoke screen. *Br. J. Radiol.* **18**, 396–397

Whitener, D.R., Whitener, K.M., Robertson, K.J., Baxter, C.R. and Pierce, A.K. (1980) Pulmonary function measurements in patients with thermal injury and smoke inhalation. *Am. Rev. Respir. Dis.* **122**, 731–739

Williams, D.O., Vanecko, R.M. and Glassroth, J. (1983) Endobronchial polyposis following smoke inhalation. *Chest* **84**, 754–776

Williams, E.R.P. (1942) Blast effects in warfare. *Br. J. Surg.* **30**, 38–49

Williams, N. (1952) Vanadium poisoning from cleaning oil fired boilers. *Br. J. Ind. Med.* **9**, 50–55

Wilson, R., Lovejoy, F.H., Jaeger, R.J. and Landrigan, P.L. (1980) Acute phosphine poisoning aboard a grain freighter: epidemiologic, clinical and pathological findings. *J. Am. Med. Assoc.* **244**, 148–150

Wirz, G., Amuroso, M.A. and Goldstein, B. (1983) Effect of ozone on alveolar macrophage function. *International Symposium on the Biomedical Aspects of Ozone and Related Photochemical Oxidants,* Vol. V of *Advances in Modern Environmental Toxicology* (eds S.D. Lee, M.G. Mustafa and M.A. Mehlman), Princeton Scientific, Princeton, pp. 263–272

Wooley, W.D. (1971) Decomposition products of PVC for studies of fires. *Br. Polymer J.* **3**, 186–193

Wooley, W.D. and Palmer, K.N. (1976) Plastics in fires and toxic hazards. *Building Res. Estb. News* **37**, HMSO, London

World Health Organization (1977) Oxides of nitrogen. *Environmental Health Criteria 4.* WHO, Geneva

World Health Organization (1988) Vanadium. *Environmental Health Criteria 81.* WHO, Geneva

Wyers, H. (1946) Some toxic effects on vanadium pentoxide. *Br. J. Ind. Med.* **3**, 177–182

Young, W.A., Shaw, D.B. and Bates, D.V. (1964) Effect of low concentrations of ozone on pulmonary function in man. *J. Appl. Physiol.* **19**, 765–768

Zenz, C. and Berg, B.A. (1967) Human responses to controlled vanadium pentoxide exposure. *Archs Environ. Health* **14**, 709–712

19

Lung cancer

J.M. Harrington and L.S. Levy

Introduction

As a target organ for cancer, the lung is important in a number of ways. The two prime features are the poor prognosis that follows such disordered cell division in the lung and the frequency with which lung tumours occur in the populations of industrialized countries. The prognosis question relates to the fact that organs such as the lung and large intestine produce symptoms late, so many such tumours are incurable at the time of diagnosis. Such a poor prognosis is compounded in public health terms by the sheer numbers of cases of lung cancer currently occurring in developed countries. Various estimates exist for different countries but in the USA over 100 000 people die each year from the disease (Doll and Peto, 1981; Lemen, 1986; Frank, 1987). Most of the cases are in men and, until recently, the number of new cases has been rising rapidly. In females, the rate has only recently shown a dramatic rise as the rises in male rate have begun to show signs of slowing down. By 1985, lung cancer had overtaken breast cancer as the leading cause of death in females and lung cancer accounts for about a third of all cancer deaths in the USA in males and about a sixth in females. Similar figures exist for other Western countries, so that the toll in disease and death is of major public health importance.

The common fatal cancers occur in large measure as a result of so-called lifestyle factors. In the case of lung cancer, smoking cigarettes is the undisputed leading cause of the disease. Indeed tobacco has been estimated to cause between 25 and 40 per cent of all cancers (Doll and Peto, 1981). To the authors' knowledge, only two reviews have attempted to assess the impact of occupational factors on lung cancer: Simonato, Vineis and Fletcher (1988) and Vineis and Simonato (1991) estimate that, depending on the agent and the type of exposure assessment adopted, between 0.6 and 40 per cent of lung cancers in employed populations are attributed to occupation.

Other causes of the disease are, however, worth mentioning although the purpose of this chapter is to review the occupational factors that can lead to lung cancer. Thus for completeness, it is important to note the other aetiological factors or agents that have been cited. Familial clustering has been reported, vitamin A deficiency has been mooted as a risk factor and atmospheric pollution (undefined) is statistically associated with the disease which demonstrates a clear urban/rural gradient (Alderson, 1986).

In this chapter, however, the focus will be on occupational factors with the exception of asbestos and asbestiform fibres as well as synthetic mineral fibres, the carcinogenic properties of which are dealt with in Chapters 14 and 16. Recent reviews of occupationally related lung cancer include those by Alderson (1986), Simonato and Lavalle-Hawkin (1983), NCI Oncology Reviews (1986), Blot (1985), Lemen (1986), Cotes and Steel (1987), and Frank (1987), and the literature on the subject is extensive. Particularly useful accounts by agent or process are contained in the *IARC Monograph Series* which currently runs to 58 volumes. Supplement 7, published in 1987, reviews and updates the first 42 volumes. This series is perhaps the most thorough and independent analysis of the epidemiological evidence linking agents and processes to cancer and the reader is advised to consult these volumes for detailed critiques of the evidence for carcinogenicity. Thus, with some exceptions, the bulk of the references cited in this chapter relate to work published in the last 5 years.

However, the story of occupationally induced lung cancer starts in the Middle Ages when Agricola (1494–1555) described the health and working conditions of underground silver miners in the Carpathian Mountains of Central Europe. He noted the 'galloping consumption' that afflicted these men and also drew attention to the atrocious working conditions in the mines. His treatise *De Re Metallica*, published at the time of his death, emphasized the need to ventilate the mines and thereby diminish the concentrations of noxious agents which he felt caused the fatal lung diseases seen in the miners. These mines no longer produce silver, but are still a source of radioactive ores such as uranium. Thus it seems highly likely that the bronchial tissues of mediaeval miners were exposed to leakage of radon gas from the rock surfaces, and that the 'galloping consumption' was, in fact, lung cancer.

Nevertheless, lung cancer was a relatively rare disease until this century. Its incidence was noted to rise in the third decade of the twentieth century and, at the same time, reports appeared linking this rise with exposure to the coal carbonization process. By the 1940s arsenic and chromium were suspected of causing lung cancer and the first reports linking the disease to asbestos had also begun to appear (Blot, 1985).

The veritable epidemic that followed in the succeeding three decades has been linked (correctly) with cigarette smoking but has also meant that it is vitally important to separate out the occupational factors from the smoking factors, and indeed to analyse these data for interaction. Such procedures require the use of in vitro and in vivo experimental studies as well as epidemiological techniques. Whereas cell cultures and animal studies can and do point the finger of suspicion at certain agents or processes that may be found in the workplace, it is the epidemiological method that has emerged as the most relevant procedure for identifying and quantifying human risk factors for various occupationally related diseases especially cancer.

The search for aetiological agents

The role of in vitro and in vivo experimental studies

Since the first reported experimental induction of cancer of the skin in rabbits, by the repeated application of coal tar (Yamagiwa and Ichikawa, 1918), a huge range of animal and other biological models has been developed and used to try both to identify and to explain the mode of action of substances that may give rise to human cancer. Initially, whole animal models were used simply to try to identify the substances capable of causing cancer, but, in the 1950s and 1960s, it became apparent through biochemical research that many of the carcinogens that were being studied were capable of reacting

with or damaging nuclear DNA. It was thus considered an important step when the scientific community accepted the paradigm that all, or at least most, carcinogens acted through a mutational mechanism in which the carcinogen caused a fundamental change to the controlling DNA of a target cell, causing mutation and leading to uncontrolled proliferation, and hence to cancer. This reasoning led to the somatic mutation theory of cancer and a proliferation of research activity which showed that many organic carcinogens operated, usually with some metabolic activation at least in part, through such a mechanism. Thus, the next logical step to take was the development of a whole range of in vivo and in vitro biological models which looked at DNA damage or some measurable expression of such damage as a surrogate for expensive and time-consuming, large-scale whole animal lifetime testing of rodents. Many of these toxicological tools utilize bacteria or cell cultures of mammalian cells and have advanced our knowledge of the carcinogenic mechanism as well as having identified many potentially hazardous substances. An excellent review and critical appraisal of both long- and short-term tests was published by the IARC (1986).

However, life is not quite so simple that we can use these models as biological litmus tests for the detection of human carcinogens. First, not all carcinogens are genotoxic and thus would not demonstrate a positive response in such bioassays and, secondly, it is now known that carcinogenesis is a multistage process, the first stage of which (initiation) is probably a genotoxic event, but that a carcinogen may influence this initial stage or any of the later stages. Hence a carcinogen could well be a non-genotoxic substance which may cause a pool of already altered (initiated) cells to move, or progress, from one stage to the next. Such a carcinogen would not be picked up by any conventional bioassay based solely on genetic damage or an expression thereof. The implication for testing is that all such steps in human cancer need to be identified and then related to an appropriate biological model, be it an initiation or a progressional step. Clearly, this cannot always be the case. Even using whole animal models presupposes that all the stages leading to human lung cancer can be or are mimicked, or at least have some kind of corresponding counterpart in an animal model in which a frank neoplasm is the end-point.

Moving on to consider the role of whole animal studies in lung cancer aetiology, it is necessary to explore the way in which the animal model has been used and to fit the study type into one of the following possible purposes:

1. Models in which the lung was simply used as one of the three routes of entry to the body to mimic human occupational exposure to investigate some 'systemic' carcinogen.

2. Models in which the lung was primarily exposed as the target tissue to investigate a putative lung carcinogen.

3. Models in which the development of lung tumours was used as a bioassay model for a carcinogen per se but not specifically for lung carcinogens, for example, the mouse strain A model (Shimkin and Stoner, 1975) in which the incidence of the rapid induction of pulmonary adenomas is measured. In this case, test substances are given by the intraperitoneal route and the increase in these tumours is used to signify the action of a carcinogen, not just a lung carcinogen. Here the lesion has no clear human counterpart nor is the route of exposure important, so it would be difficult to use this model to specify a lung carcinogen.

In the case of (1) and (2), lung cancers can be induced in experimental species, usually rats, by the use of a variety of methods, including intratracheal instillation and intrabronchial implantation as well as inhalational exposure. The major problems of evaluation with any such investigation relates to the histogenesis of the induced lesion; the dose extrapolation to humans if the histogenesis is thought comparable to human lung cancer; and the possibility that the experimental dose used has overloaded the normal defence mechanism, in some form of unrealistic way, and thus, although the induced neoplasm appears genuine, the means of obtaining it are unrealistic and cannot be extrapolated to human exposure – hence the probable human risk. This latter case is exemplified where the lungs are overloaded to the extent that other major pathological changes occur in the lung such as severe scarring – in such cases it is not unusual to see the development of metaplastic squamous lesions with extensive keratinization. These, in isolation, appear remarkably similar to squamous carcinomas. The standard cancer protocol for carcinogens proposed and commonly used (US National Toxicology Program, 1984) suggest that the dose used in cancer tests is set at the maximum tolerated dose (MTD), that is, the dose that produces a sublethal toxic effect in, say, about 10 per cent of the highest dosed group. Such an effect would be one such as a loss of body weight. The assumption is that cancer may occur at dose levels below that producing other toxic effects. Also the relatively small number of animals, 100, compared to the potentially exposed human population is such that the dose is increased to maximize the chances of producing a positive result with even a weak carcinogen. This raises the possibility of eliciting a seemingly positive response by a mechanism not normally encountered even by a heavily exposed human population. As an example, in a inhalation study rats were exposed 8 hours/day for 2 years to a dust of chromium (IV) dioxide. Apart from a dose-related inflammatory response, a number of rats developed lesions within the lung described as keratin cysts and others described as cystic keratinized squamous-cell carcinomas. A cautionary note by the authors (Lee et al., 1988) pointed out that, although the study appeared to point to a carcinogenic response caused by the chromium dioxide, a form of chromium not previously noted for its genotoxicity, the lesions were not 'true' malignancies, but related to an overload or 'nuisance' dust reaction and did not represent a true carcinogenic response. Thus, even when a bronchial lesion with an apparently human counterpart is described in a rodent study, much care is needed in interpretation for human risk assessment purposes.

The other side of the coin is the production of false-negative results from animal studies. Here, a useful example to bear in mind is arsenic which, although appearing to be a well-documented human lung carcinogen, has generally failed to produce convincing evidence of lung tumours in animal models.

The overall impression that is reached when examining the multiplicity of data produced from animal and other submammalian studies in the identification of human carcinogens is that vast amounts of information and clues for human cancer caused by carcinogens have been produced, particularly in the specification of particular substances as an adjunct to epidemiology. However, much care needs to be taken when trying to identify lung carcinogens specifically. This must be questioned particularly when examining the results of rodent studies and here a number of key questions must be asked.

1. Were there sufficient numbers in each group? (Usually 100 – this minimum number is required for acceptable evidence of a negative result.)

2. Was the dosing schedule of sufficiently high concentration and duration? Usually 8 hours/day for the major part of the animal's life in the case of inhalation studies and at near the maximum tolerated dose in the case of the highest dosed group.

3. Did the experimental technique expose the target tissue sufficiently?, that is, the bronchial epithelium of both major and minor airways.

4. Did the substance produce tumours with a comparative human counterpart? There is an expectation of squamous carcinomas, adenocarcinomas or other carcinomas arising from the bronchial epithelium, such as small cell and large cell carcinomas.

5. Were the tumours produced in a dose-related fashion? Normally in toxicology investigations, a dose–response relationship would be expected as evidence of a true effect. This may not always be the case but the lack of such a relationship certainly requires detailed scrutiny of the results.

6. Were there other pathological changes in the lung that could be related to any concomitant tumours? – as, for example, the appearance of microscopic tumours in the parenchyma of the lung which is severely scarred or fibrosed by the administered substance. This phenomenon should certainly make us question the significance of such lesions.

Some of these difficulties will be discussed further under 'The mechanism of lung carcinogenesis'.

The conclusion is, therefore, that, although experimental studies can be useful in the identification of human carcinogens, including lung carcinogens, rodent studies that expose the lung can be particularly invaluable in specifying chemicals and substances. Nevertheless, great care must be taken in the interpretation of the results of such studies.

The role of epidemiology

Although the uses and abuses of epidemiology are dealt with in Chapter 8, it is important to emphasize here that the bulk of the human evidence suggesting a definite, probable or possible role in carcinogenesis for a given agent or process has been evaluated in a particular way. The approach used in this chapter mirrors the IARC stance and the reader is urged to adopt a similar stance – as outlined in the preamble to each monograph – whenever faced with conclusions based on epidemiological evidence.

Epidemiology is not an exact science but it is the best available means of coming to some consensus when faced with a growing body of literature in which different studies may come to different conclusions. The epidemiologist, in contrast to the experimental scientist, cannot control or, sometimes, even measure the exposures of the population he or she wishes to investigate. Thus, in many cases, epidemiologists have to make the best use of the data sources available to them, warts and all. Nevertheless, as Hogstedt once said, paraphrasing a popular advertising slogan, epidemiology is the real thing. It is the stuff of human exposures; so, just because it may be difficult, is no excuse to ignore it.

Doll (1984), in a masterly review of the problems in interpreting occupational cancer studies, cites certain criteria as necessary prerequisites for concluding that a causal relationship exists between an agent and a cancer. These are the following:

1. The strength of the association between the agent and the cancer.
2. A satisfactory exclusion of bias, confounding and chance.
3. The evidence of corroborative data from repeated studies.

4. A relationship between incidence and intensity of dose.
5. A relationship between incidence and the duration of exposure and time since first exposure.

In general, only two types of epidemiological study warrant serious consideration: the longitudinal (or cohort) study and the case-referent (or case-control) study – the analytical studies. Correlation studies where a population may be viewed with no a priori hypothesis, can raise interesting leads but these are, by definition, no more than hypothesis-generating exercises. Case reports are rarely of sufficient merit to be included in the final evaluation of an agent's carcinogenic potential. IARC, in its evaluations, rightly places great weight on large, well-designed, analytical studies with accurate exposure data, a long and thorough follow-up and good diagnostic techniques. The final placing of the agent or process on the scale – 1, 2A, 2B, 3 and 4 – takes the animal and in vitro data into account, but animal data alone, however convincing, cannot classify an agent as a grade 1 carcinogen. One of the tantalizing, and challenging, features of the current state of knowledge is that there is a large number of compounds known to be animal carcinogens but for which little, or no, human data are available.

Epidemiology is a useful study method because it should lead to prevention. This aspect is discussed in a later section but suffice it to say here that, although studies vary, there are over one and a half million people in the USA who are occupationally exposed to each of the following known or suspected agents: formaldehyde, fibres, cadmium and arsenic (Spiezer, 1986). This number is more than doubled for 'organic particles' and one estimate suggests that there have been 100 000 excess cases of lung cancer due to cadmium and a similar number due to arsenic in the USA (Peters et al., 1986). The lung is the most commonly known site for excess cancer incidence in one review of 37 occupations and in 60 occupations reporting any cancer excess (Simonato and Levalle-Hawkin, 1983).

Thus, there is considerable scientific and public health concern to improve the epidemiological method and to evaluate agents and processes for their carcinogenic potential. What follows in the remainder of this chapter could, perhaps, be summarized in a table. Here, only those agents or processes for which good quality studies are available have been included. Nevertheless, the inexactitude of our knowledge on even some of the most clear-cut associations is unsatisfactory. This is particularly true for processes where listing 'nickel refining' or 'iron/steel founding' does little to suggest what would be the definitive steps that need to be taken in order to diminish worker exposure. For chromium, there is an urgent need to distinguish compounds that are carcinogenic from those that are not. A recent IARC evaluation suggesting that the occupation of painting carries a carcinogenic risk does little to help the preventive medicine specialist in diminishing the risk in such an ubiquitous trade when the agent or agents remain obscure.

There is a continuing need for epidemiological studies (Doll, 1984) for three main reasons:

1. To demonstrate risks overlooked or tentatively suggested by laboratory tests.
2. To estimate the level of exposure that is deemed to be socially acceptable.
3. To check the correctness of the conclusions about a cancer hazard by monitoring the effect of its removal.

The mechanism of lung carcinogenesis

The use of experimental observations

Much of this chapter deals with evidence of occupational cancers coming from epidemiological studies. This is not accidental because such studies provide the most convincing evidence. However, as noted earlier, convincing as it might be, such studies do not always point to a specific causative agent, especially if the working group in which the increased lung cancer risk has been shown to exist are exposed to a pot-pourri of air-borne substances. This makes effective practical control of the situation difficult. In such cases the use of experimental tools or models is invaluable. The role of in vivo and in vitro models is discussed under 'The search for aetiological agents'. A vast amount of literature is available on the biology of cancer, mainly owing to the efforts, in the 1960s and 1970s, related to tobacco smoke as an aetiological agent. Much of this information is thus useful in understanding lung cancer caused by other extrinsic, including occupational, factors. Most of our knowledge on the mechanism of cancer is based on observational changes rather than on a detailed understanding of the molecular changes that must surely take place. Thus, such terms as 'early' and 'late' factors in carcinogenesis and co-carcinogens are observational terms used to describe events rather than to explain them. Fuller understanding comes from a combination of epidemiological observation, a clear pathological understanding of the changes from normal to neoplastic cells and an acceptable understanding of molecular events that accompany such changes. Nowhere can the need be

greater than in the development of lung cancer. The key considerations that need to be put together from available theoretical knowledge and experimental investigations to help explain epidemiological clues are the following:

1. An understanding of the basic classification of carcinogens.
2. Metabolism and molecular events leading to cancer.
3. Histopathological changes leading to induced lung cancer.
4. Histopathological changes shown in animal studies related by specific substance exposure.

A basic classification of carcinogens

Earlier, it was briefly noted that cancer was generally considered to be a multistage process and that, in theory, a carcinogen could effect any of these stages. Early investigations on mouse skin (Berenblum and Schoental, 1947) indicated a two-stage process involving stages known as *initiation* (thought to be a fundamental change in nuclear DNA), followed by *promotion* (some non-genotoxic stimulus that caused the initiated cells to progress on to cancer). Each of these two stages was mediated by the sequential application of two separate chemicals (3,4-benzopyrene followed by croton oil). These stages are the equivalent of 'early' and 'late' factors involved in human cancer. This is not just of theoretical importance: a substance such as arsenic, which is thought to affect the late stages of cancer (see 'The role of in vitro and in vivo experimental studies'), if removed from the working environment can have a marked reducing effect on lung cancer incidence in a relatively short space of time. However, experimental observations have shown that carcinogens cannot be classified into initiators and promoters alone, and that the classification in Table 19.1, modified from Weisburger and Williams (1980), is probably the best classification available at present based on possible mechanisms of action.

Clearly, the bronchial epithelium will be a target tissue for a carcinogenic agent that can act through any of the classes, especially if it is inhaled in air.

Metabolism of carcinogens and molecular events leading to cancer

Genotoxic carcinogens ultimately must react with DNA with some kind of resultant cell transformation. Substances that can penetrate cell membranes

Table 19.1 Classes of carcinogenicity

A *Genotoxic*
  Direct-acting
  Bioactivated
  Indirect-acting
  Chronic tissue toxin

B *Non-genotoxic (possibly epigenetic)*
  Solid state
  Hormonal
  Immunosuppressive
  Co-carcinogen
  Promoter
  Chronic tissue toxin
    Toxic
    Traumatic
    Inflammatory

Modified from Weisburger and Williams (1980).

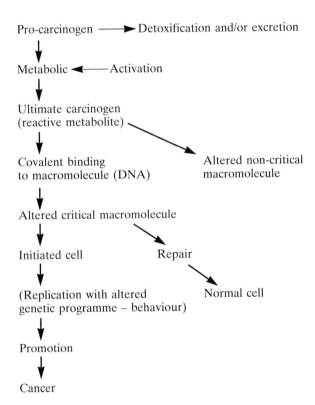

Figure 19.1 The process of carcinogenesis

and organelles prior to reacting with DNA are called direct-acting carcinogens (Figure 19.1). Many carcinogens, however, require some kind of enzymatic metabolic activation before they become active. The metabolites thus formed are able to react with DNA. Examples of such reactive metabolites are electrophilic species such as epoxides and carbonium ions. Figure 19.1 outlines the general framework within which genotoxic and non-genetic materials mediate cancerous changes.

Initially, it was thought that most human and animal carcinogens, with a few exceptions, were genotoxic, either with or without metabolic activation. These could thus be picked up readily in one or other of the in vitro tests outlined earlier. Unfortunately, it may well be that many carcinogens act as promoters at later stages in the carcinogenic process. These will be much harder to pick up in bioassays.

Histopathological aspects of occupationally induced cancer

A major difficulty in attributing lung cancer causation to a specific substance is that there does not appear to be any clear distinguishing histopathological type that is uniquely associated with specific substances or industrial exposures as such. This can be contrasted to the case of pleural mesothelioma, where the strong association with asbestos exposure presents overwhelming evidence of a causal link. Bronchial carcinomas that have been associated with occupational exposures cover the span of the histopathological types seen in the 'unexposed' population. Presumably this is because the target bronchial cells have a limited range of neoplastic expression when presented with a carcinogenic insult, be it tobacco smoke, other environmental carcinogens or an occupational carcinogen. Nevertheless, investigators have attempted to see if there were any differences in patterns or links which would assist in our understanding of both specific material and lung cancer types reported in epidemiological investigations, and the histogenesis of such lesions as pointers to causation.

There has been, over the last 60 years, various attempts to provide a unifying framework for the classification of lung cancer based on both location and histopathology, and the revised World Health Organization classification (WHO, 1982) into 13 histological types of carcinoma, although generally recognized, coexists with at least five other currently used classification systems. In spite of differences in detail, it is generally accepted that 90 per cent of all lung carcinomas are covered by four main histopathological categories: *squamous carcinoma*, *small cell carcinoma*, *large cell carcinoma* and *adenocarcinoma*. Terms such as 'anaplastic' or 'undifferentiated', although previously and, to some extent, still used, are generally subsumed in the four categories. The proportion of the four categories varies from study to study and occupational epidemiology, where histological classification is available, has attempted to look for predominance

Table 19.2 Histology of lung cancer

Cell type	Male		Female	
	Range (%)	*Median (%)*	*Range (%)*	*Median (%)*
Squamous carcinoma	17.9–68.9	41.3	2.9–43.1	18.6
Adenocarcinoma	3.2–34.1	17.9	10.2–66.7	45.1
Small cell carcinoma	0.0–63.6	19.4	0.0–44.6	11.0
Large cell carcinoma	0.0–25.0	0.3	0.0–19.0	0

Adapted from Modan (1978).

The percentages in many studies do not add up to 100 because not all categories are included or appear in the original text.

of one type or a change from the expected incidence of each type. As an example, Modan (1978), in an investigation of histological types of lung cancer in Israel, looked at the available literature on reported histological types in 43 world-wide studies (24 in males and 19 in females) including the USA, Norway, Israel, Singapore and Uganda. The proportions of each type, expressed as a percentage, are shown in Table 19.2.

The wide range observed is not surprising considering that it takes into account diagnoses based on biopsy procedures, although the median frequencies are around those that are most generally accepted. In an authoritative review of types of lung cancer from epidemiological studies, Ives, Buffler and Greenberg (1983) have tried to tease out the relationship between histopathological type and putative lung carcinogen. Their conclusions suggest the following relationships:

Arsenic exposure	Different lung cancer cell types predominate in different studies
Beryllium	Adenocarcinoma or small cell carcinoma predominates in a single study
Chromates	Squamous carcinoma
Nickel	Squamous carcinoma
Bis(chloromethyl) ether	Small cell carcinoma
Uranium miners	Small cell carcinoma (particularly high proportion)
Asbestos	Three out of four studies showed predominance of adenocarcinoma
PVC dust	Greater proportion of large cell and adenocarcinoma found

The general conclusion was that, although there was evidence of predominance in some areas, not

enough was known of the distribution of types of lung cancer in the general population, let alone in exposed populations and that this must be a priority for researchers and investigators.

Histogenesis of lung cancer related to occupational factors

There is a range of views on the development of lung cancer. As an example, Yesner (1980) has proposed the transition from small cell to large cell carcinoma and from large cell carcinoma to squamous cell carcinoma and adenocarcinoma. Clearly, this maturation transition from small cell carcinoma to squamous and adenocarcinoma is at variance with the hypothesis that small cell carcinomas arise from the neuroectoderm. Other theories relate to a single cell derivation from squamous and small cell carcinomas (Bereton et al., 1978), a continuum within the general group of small cell anaplastic carcinomas (Burdon, Sinclair and Henderson, 1979), or a transition between the small cell carcinomas (Abeloff et al., 1974). Probably the most conceptually satisfying of views which is not inconsistent with others, is that of Seydel, Chait and Gmelich (1975), who proposed, as a theory to explain the development of lung cancers, a gradual transition from normal, bronchial, respiratory, ciliated epithelium to squamous metaplasia to carcinoma-in-situ and, finally, to locally invasive carcinoma. This transition in human beings occurs over a 5- to 10-year period and the stages (fitting in with the multistage theory of carcinogenesis) are referred to as 'pre-neoplasia'. This concept has been accepted by Auerbach and his colleagues (Auerbach, Hammond and Garfinkel, 1979; Auerbach, 1980), to help explain the pathogenesis of bronchial carcinoma. They add an important rider that, from the point of view of prevention, each intermediate stage in the continuum of development of bronchial carcinoma is potentially reversible.

The term 'pre-neoplasia', used by many investigators to describe an atypical respiratory epithelial change that is not yet a neoplasm, is an area of much pathological controversy (Ives, Buffler and Greenberg, 1983). However, early work of Stanton (1974), and more recent studies by Levy and Venitt (1986), illustrate that the development of squamous metaplasia in the respiratory epithelium, in response to polycyclic hydrocarbon carcinogens or chromate-containing compounds, is not simply a non-specific response to injury, but rather a response to specific carcinogens. Stanton's work further showed that metaplasia preceded carcinoma by many months and only progressed to neoplasia in the presence of high concentrations of the carcinogen. Other investigators have found profound dysplastic changes in lung epithelia that had been exposed to carcinogens and already exhibited hyperplasia and metaplasia (Pour et al., 1976). Here, dysplasia was considered to be the true harbinger of neoplasia.

Relationship between animal lung cancer types and human lung cancer

Ideally, an animal investigation that would be of most use as a predictive model of human cancer would give a comparative histopathology to human lung cancer as well as giving an increase in lung tumour incidence in a dose-related fashion following exposure to a lung carcinogen. This of course presupposes a similar molecular mechanism and a similar histogenesis for cancer induction in animal and human lungs. This is not an unreasonable request given our knowledge of the histology of bronchial and parenchymal tissue in rodent models and human subjects. However, there are real differences in response between the two which may not just reflect an artefact due to experimental technique, but a true histogenic difference in response in pathogenesis leading to different forms of lung tumours. An example is the mouse where almost all malignant tumours caused by carcinogens are adenocarcinomas, often arising in parenchymal tissue. These are often difficult to distinguish from adenomas which are often found in many strains of mice. However, it is rare to find a squamous carcinoma in mouse lung. Moreover, although squamous cell carcinoma and adenocarcinoma can be experimentally induced in the rat, neither small cell carcinoma nor large cell carcinoma has been reported. These latter lesions also do not occur in the mouse. An interesting review by Adachi and Takemoto (1987) has compared lung tumour types found in human epidemiological studies with those from animal investigations using the same carcinogens. The authors generally agree with the observations of Ives, Buffler and Greenberg (1983). The correlation with animal data was not good, however, and although there was some agreement, such as squamous carcinoma in rats with chromates, the species response and the experimental technique (inhalation, intratracheal instillation or intrabronchial implantation) may have had more to do with the tumour response than any other factor.

In spite of these shortcomings, animal models still provide the best scientific test available to us to investigate putative human lung carcinogens or to help provide an explanation of occupational lung cancers arising from an air-borne 'cocktail' of substances in which a carcinogen may reside.

Review of agents and processes linked to human lung cancer

This section describes in more detail some of the justification for the evaluations given in Table 19.3 and, in addition, mentions some other agents or processes for which the evidence of lung carcinogenicity is either more tentative or involves relatively few exposed workers.

In 1986 the National Cancer Institute and the International Cancer Research Data Bank published a selection of nearly 500 papers on the subject of occupational lung cancer gleaned from the journals between 1982 and 1985. Apart from asbestos and ionizing radiation, this review concluded that there were six accepted carcinogenic agents (arsenic, chloromethyl ethers, chromium, mustard gas, nickel and polyaromatic hydrocarbons) and three accepted carcinogenic processes (welding, foundry work and rubber manufacture). The review notes the widespread interest in chloromethyl ethers, which is probably due to their high potency as carcinogens rather than to any widespread exposures. By contrast, mustard gas, a well-known carcinogen, has a surprisingly limited literature. For the future, the review highlights the need for more work to be done on differentiating risks by the type of lung cancer cell as well as reiterating the known difficulties of undertaking and reporting on good quality epidemiological studies. The histological problems are discussed under 'Histopathological aspects of occupationally induced cancer'.

Known carcinogens

Arsenic

Inorganic arsenic had been suspected as a skin carcinogen since the early 1800s but the first scientific evidence of a link with lung cancer came with a report on the mortality experience of a population of sheep dip manufacturers in England (Hill and Faning, 1948). This study, which is a model for any budding epidemiologist on how to produce a first-class study out of limited available data, noted a

Table 19.3 Occupationally related agents and/or processes associated with lung cancer (excluding asbestos, asbesti-form-like materials and synthetic mineral fibres)

Agent/Process	Definitive	Probable	Possible	Notes
Acrylonitrile		√		
Aluminium production	√			Probably pitch volatiles
Arsenic and/or compounds	√			
Beryllium and/or compounds	√			No individual compounds of beryllium specially identified
Bis(chloromethyl) ether and chloromethyl methyl ether	√			
Cadmium and/or compounds	√			No individual compounds of cadmium specially identified
Chlorinated toluenes			√	
Chromium and/or compounds	√			Mainly 'sparingly soluble' hexavalent compounds
Coal gasification	√			Probably coal-tar pitches
Coke production	√			Probably coal-tar pitches
1,2-Dibromochloropropane			√	
Dimethyl sulphate			√	
Epichlorhydrin			√	
Formaldehyde		√		
Underground mining with radon exposure	√			Including mining for uranium, iron, fluorspar, tin, niobium and mixtures of metals (zinc/silver/lead)
Iron and steel founding	√			Probably polyaromatic hydrocarbons
Mineral oils	√			Untreated or mildly refined varieties
Mustard gas	√			
Nickel refining	√			Compounds not identified ?Nickel subsulphide and nickel oxide
Pesticide application			√	Various agents implicated including chlordane, chlorophenoxy herbicides and hexachlorocyclohexane
Rubber manufacture		√		No agent(s) specifically identified
Silica			√	Crystalline variety ?Silicosis a risk factor (see Chapter 12, page 315)
Soots	√			
Vinyl chloride		√		Probably the monomer only
Welding		√		No agent(s) specifically identified

proportional mortality for lung cancer in the sheep dip workers of 31.8 per cent compared with only 15.9 per cent in a population of workers from three other factories (the skin cancer percentage difference was over tenfold). Other studies of vine growers and pesticide applicators, who both used arsenical sprays, followed. The bulk of modern epidemiological evidence resides with studies of metalliferous ore miners and smelters from several countries, where consistently high excesses of lung cancer have been described (IARC, 1987). A tenfold increase in the incidence of lung cancer has been found in smelter workers most heavily exposed to arsenic and dose–response relationships have been shown with regard to cumulative exposures. A re-analysis of one smelter in the USA which specialized in smelting metal ores with a high arsenic content has shown a trend in cancer mortality that follows arsenic levels in air and arsenic concentrations in urine (Enterline, Henderson and Marsh, 1987). Indeed, this paper re-evaluated previous exposure data estimates and found a much closer relationship than had been previously noted between excess cancer deaths and arsenic in urine (straight line) and arsenic levels in air (concave downward).

The value of biological monitoring, as opposed to environmental measures, is clearly demonstrated and is important – particularly for an element such as arsenic which has complex metabolic pathways. The Enterline study showed an eightfold excess in the highest exposure group whereas an update of an animal pesticide manufacturing plant found excesses no higher than twofold (Sobel et al., 1988). Further difficulty in evaluating exposure indices is seen in the latest study of the Ronnskar copper smelter population in Sweden (Jarup, Pershagen and Wall, 1989). In this report a clear dose–response relationship exists for average intensity of exposure to arsenic but not for length of exposure.

At these elevated cancer risks, confounding factors such as smoking and sulphur dioxide clearly play little part in explaining the effect, and yet it is interesting that a decrease in lung cancer risk after cessation of exposure to arsenic has been mentioned in some studies, possibly indicating a carcinogenic effect of arsenic at a late stage. This is consistent with the general view that arsenic is not a genotoxic carcinogen, but plays a part in cancer induction at a late stage. Although various types of lung cancer cell exist in the populations studied, a significant relative excess of adenocarcinomas has been observed in smelter workers (IARC, 1987).

In contrast to virtually all other human carcinogens, inorganic arsenic has failed to produce consistent and clear-cut cancers in experimental animals. The explanation for this fascinating scientific snippet remains elusive but, if discovered, might shed important light on the mechanism of carcinogenesis itself.

Bis(chloromethyl) ether (BCME) and chloromethyl methyl ether (CMME) (technical grade)

The alkylating agent CMME has been produced since the mid-1940s as a cross-linking agent for ion exchange resins and as an intermediate in the production of organic chemicals. Twenty years later it was noted that CMME was a mouse skin carcinogen and that BCME, which is a 2.8 per cent impurity in CMME, was an even more potent carcinogen. Its marked potency as an animal lung carcinogen was then demonstrated and epidemiological studies of workers in Germany, Japan and the USA followed. In their preliminary report from the USA in 1975, Albert et al. noted a 2.5-fold excess risk in exposed workers, but commented that in the most heavily exposed group the excess risk of lung cancer exceeded twentyfold with a particularly early age of onset. Maximal relative risks for BCME exposure appear to occur at 15 to 20 years after first exposure but this latency can be shortened with particularly heavy exposure (IARC, 1987). Another interesting feature is the apparent association between exposure and the development of small (oat) cell tumours.

The relationship of BCME exposure to smoking is conflicting but the tumours do develop in non-smokers. Indeed there is every indication that this agent is one of the most potent of all lung carcinogens.

Chromium and chromium compounds

The first indication that chromium compounds might be a cause of lung cancer came from reports in the 1940s of the chromate-producing industries in

Germany and the USA. The initial study from Machle and Gregorius in the USA suggested a relative risk for lung cancer of 25 (Blot, 1985). Other reports followed so that by the 1970s, dichromate production, chromate pigment manufacture and chrome plating had been implicated in the carcinogenic risk. Excess cancer risks in chrome alloy workers, welders and chrome pigment users are also suggested as being caused by chromium compounds (IARC, 1987).

A more recent British study of nickel chromium platers (Sorahan, Burges and Waterhouse, 1987) reported a lung cancer excess of 58 per cent which on further analysis suggested that a twofold excess existed for chrome bath operators versus other chrome workers. It was concluded that nickel exposure was not a confounding factor. Nine lung cancer cases in a population of Icelandic masons showed a 3.1-fold excess compared with national rates (Rafnsson and Johannesdottir, 1986) with a rising risk for 20-year exposure (3.7-fold) and 30-year exposure (6.3-fold). Cement dust was considered to cause the risk exposure, although the role of nickel and cobalt was deemed minor compared with that of chromium.

Despite the clear association between chromium compound exposure and lung cancer, difficulties remain in elucidating the carcinogenic potential of chromium and its salts. The metal in itself cannot be classified as carcinogenic because there is no evidence for this. The evidence for some compounds implies that they have different potencies (Norseth, 1986). This is exemplified particularly when considering the studies of chrome pigment makers. Chrome pigments and corrosion inhibitors are usually hexavalent and commonly include zinc, lead or strontium chromate. A small Norwegian study identified 24 workers previously exposed to zinc chromate out of a total chromium pigment worker population of 133. All six lung cancers occurred in the zinc chromate subgroup with 0.14 expected (Langård and Vigandar, 1983). In the UK, a group of 'pure' lead chromate workers was identified from a population of chrome pigment manufacturers at three plants. In the lead chromate group no lung cancer excess was found whereas, in the other two plants with mixed lead and zinc chromate exposure, the observed : expected ratios for high/medium exposure ranged from 13 : 5.9 to 5 : 0.9 (Davies, 1984).

In the UK, only one of the three plants manufacturing chromates and reported in the literature is still operating. In 1981, the results of following workers entering the industry after 1949 showed a fall in lung cancer excess from threefold to less than twofold when compared with workers whose employment started earlier. The latest update to 1988 shows an SMR for these workers of 102. However, an excess of nasal cancer (4 observed,

0.26 expected) has now appeared in the group with over 20 years' employment (Davies, Easton and Bidstrup, 1991). Major improvements in plant operation and safety precautions were instituted in the early 1950s, suggesting that such procedures have had an important influence on lung cancer risk in the plant population (DHSS, 1986).

By contrast with the difficulties of specifying which compounds are carcinogenic from epidemiological studies, the animal carcinogenicity tests clearly show a difference in carcinogenic potency between different chromium compounds (Levy, Martin and Bidstrup, 1986) and it was this evidence that finally swayed the Industrial Injuries Advisory Council in the UK to specify that, for chromium compounds, lung cancer could be a prescribed disease for workers exposed to the dust of zinc, cadmium and strontium chromate (DHSS, 1986).

Major difficulties still remain in evaluating the health risks of chromium and its compounds. It appears that sparingly soluble hexavalent chromium compounds carry the greatest risks of producing human lung cancer, and yet, the importance of particle size, crystal modification, surface charge, solubility or the ability of the compound to be phagocytosed still needs to be clarified (Norseth, 1986). The complex issue of bioavailability is clearly crucial to the understanding of how some chromium compounds, but definitely not all, can cause human cancer. The need to differentiate the guilty from the innocent is essential if preventive measures are to be targeted effectively where they are most needed (Levy, Martin and Venitt, 1987).

Mustard gas

Although the victims of mustard gas exposure in the First World War did not provide incontrovertible evidence of a risk of lung cancer, data from the manufacturers of this chemical weapon were much more clear-cut. A threefold excess of lung cancer, but a fortyfold excess of respiratory tract cancer, was noted in the Japanese proportional mortality study of mustard gas producers during the Second World War (Wada et al., 1988). A British study of similar workers at a similar time has recently been updated (Easton, Peto and Doll, 1988). Large and significant excesses were observed in a cohort of nearly 2500 men and 1000 women. The lung cancer excess was of the order of 50 per cent but excesses were much higher for larynx (2.7-fold), lip, tongue and salivary gland (threefold) and pharynx (5.5-fold). An analysis to determine the influence of cigarette smoking on these figures suggested that exposure to mustard gas adds to rather than multiplies the risk due to smoking. Similar additive effects can be construed from the Japanese studies.

Nickel and nickel compounds

The 1932 report of the Chief Inspector of Factories in the UK first drew attention to the possibility that nickel or its compounds might be human carcinogens. The plant in question was a nickel refinery in South Wales and epidemiological studies published later demonstrated a five- to tenfold excess risk of lung cancer and a 100- to 900-fold excess for nasal cancer. Changes to the plant operation and the level of personal worker protection in the mid-1920s were clearly demonstrated to have removed the major risk, because the increased risk was shown to be confined to those who started employment in the plant before 1930. The cancer hazard was thus focused on the early stages of nickel refining. Nickel carbonyl was considered unlikely to be involved whilst nickel subsulphide and nickel oxide emerged as the strongest candidates for suspicion (IARC, 1987).

Later reports from Canada and the USA confirmed the increased risks for lung and sinonasal cancers caused by exposure during nickel refining. In Norway, the roasting, smelting and electrolysis departments at the refinery carried the highest risk of respiratory organ cancer. Studies of nickel alloy workers have been inconclusive.

A recent evaluation of the epidemiological evidence for nickel carcinogenicity (Grandjean, Anderson and Neilson, 1988) reviewed data from studies of populations of refinery workers in Canada, the USA, South Wales and New Caledonia, a well as nickel mining industry workers. The authors concluded that nickel compounds from the calcining and sintering operations at refineries are strongly implicated. Nickel-using industries provide no clear-cut evidence of a carcinogenic risk. This conclusion is, in essence, confirmed by the 1990 Report of the International Committee on Nickel Carcinogenesis in Man.

In short, the finger of suspicion points most clearly to nickel oxide and other crystalline compounds such as nickel subsulphide. By contrast, exposure to amorphous nickel compounds, nickel ore, nickel metal and its alloys appear much less hazardous, although it would be imprudent in the current state of knowledge to assume that these compounds are without hazard.

Polycyclic aromatic hydrocarbons

There are a number of epidemiological studies in the literature which have assessed the lung cancer risks associated with a variety of industries such as gas retort, coke oven and steel industry workers, aluminium refiners, iron and steel founders, as well as populations of workers exposed to soot, pitch, tars and petroleum product exhaust fumes. What each of these studies appears to have in common is exposure to polycylic aromatic hydrocarbons (PAHs). Some of these industries will be dealt with later in the chapter – particularly if other confounding exposures might have contributed to the perceived lung cancer risk. Nevertheless, for many of these industries cited above, and from some case-control studies of lung cancer, the grouping by exposure to PAHs has emerged as a convenient, if somewhat vague, label for exposure characterization.

Polycyclic aromatic hydrocarbons constitute a large and complex group of compounds which are, in the main, generated during the incomplete combustion of carbonaceous products of which coal and oil usage are the most important occupational exposures. Cigarette smoke, of course, also contains a number of these compounds and so it is often difficult to distinguish lifestyle from occupational factors in such employed populations. Furthermore, the carcinogenic potency of individual compounds has been poorly defined and, thus, reviewers are left to describe as best they can the probable influence of an infinite variety of mixtures.

Coal carbonization

Excluding for a moment the well-known story of Percivall Pott and the chimney sweeps' scrotal cancer, suspicions of an increased lung cancer risk from PAHs first arose in the earlier part of this century with studies of workers in the coal carbonization processes (gas retort houses, coke ovens and gas generators). The largest investigation of this type was that conducted by Lloyd, Redmond and co-workers of the Pittsburgh steel mills in the USA. They established a cohort of 59 000 coke oven workers in 1953 and subsequently published a series of follow-up mortality studies (Lloyd, 1971; Redmond, 1983; Dong et al., 1988). Dose–response analyses have been produced for exposure to coal-tar pitch volatiles and these exposures have been reviewed in relation to lung cancer. Coke oven workers exhibited a large, statistically significant increase in lung cancer which was strongly associated with duration of exposure to coke oven fumes as well as to intensity of exposure, as shown by the fifteenfold differential risk of lung cancer between oven top-side workers and others who worked in less vulnerable jobs. Redmond (1983) calculated that even at the extant OSHA (Occupational Safety and Health Administration) standard for total particulate matter of $150 \, \mu g/m^3$ benzene-soluble fraction, an excess lung cancer risk of between 7 per cent and 50 per cent would still exist. Further work by Dong and his colleagues, using the Lloyd cohort and some Canadian coke oven populations, suggested that coke oven emissions are lung cancer

initiators with, in addition, some evidence of a multistage influence on tumour generation.

The destructive distillation of coal to produce gas has been known, for a number of years, to lead to increased incidences of scrotal, skin, bladder and respiratory tract tumours (IARC, 1987). Although most of these gas-retort house processes are now defunct, the possibility that such processes could be resurrected in countries lacking cheap and available gas supplies raises the possibility that this occupational cancer risk could reappear.

Aluminium production

An excess of lung cancer exists in the aluminium industry which, on reflection, mirrors the experience of the gas and coke oven workers, that is, a review of death certificates shows that persons employed in the industry are at a high risk of developing cancer. Furthermore, men employed in certain work areas with exposures related to those found at the coke plants appear to be at the greatest risk.

Although studies supporting this hypothesis have emanated from a number of countries, the best documented group is the Canadian aluminium production workers (Gibbs, 1985) who worked in the Soderberg process. This process of electrolytic reduction of aluminium generates a number of toxic substances into the atmosphere of the pot rooms, including coal-tar pitch volatiles. Lung cancer excesses of 40 to 50 per cent were found (as well as other cancer excesses such as cancer of the oesophagus and bladder). Analysis of lung cancer mortality by increasing years of exposure, tar-years of exposure and years since first exposure to tar revealed a steady, statistically significant, increasing trend. Whilst a similar trend existed for bladder cancer, no such clear-cut pattern was found for oesophagus or stomach cancers. The influence of smoking on these figures was assessed.

There is sufficient evidence, therefore, to suggest that the lung cancer excess associated with aluminium production is linked to exposure to pitch volatiles.

Chimney sweeps

The carcinogenicity of soot has been demonstrated by numerous studies over the past 200 yeas for skin cancer – particularly the skin of the scrotum. More recently, cohorts of chimney sweeps in Sweden and Denmark have shown a significantly increased risk of lung cancer (IARC, 1987). A more recent mortality study of nearly 5500 Swedish chimney sweeps revealed a 2.5-fold excess of lung cancer with a clear-cut increasing trend with years of exposure (Gustavsson, Gustavsson and Hogstedt, 1987).

Although smoking histories were not available, cigarette smoking is not likely to have seriously biased these estimates.

Printing industry

Epidemiological studies on the risks of cancer associated with work in the printing industry have shown excesses at several sites including the lung. The excesses were usually modest (10 to 60 per cent) but were consistent (Malker and Gemme, 1987). Little or no specific exposure information is usually available in these studies and, assuming that smoking has a confounding effect, the major alternative hypothesis is occupational exposure to the mists in printing and typography rooms, which includes a wide range of materials such as mineral oils, carbon black, ink pigments, dyes and solvents.

Diesel exhaust fumes

Diesel engines emit a complex mixture of aromatic hydrocarbons including the nitropolycyclic group (Matanoski et al., 1986). Excess lung cancer risks have been reported in professional drivers (Balarajan and McDowall, 1988), railroad workers (Garshick et al., 1988) and from studies of cancer patients in an hypothesis generating exercise (Siemiatyki et al., 1988a). Cigarette smoke also contains these nitrated hydrocarbons and could act as a major confounding factor given the relatively modest lung excesses noted in the studies.

Radon and radon daughters

Everyone is continuously exposed to radon and its radioactive daughters. All rocks and soils contain the primordial series headed by uranium-238 and the fifth member of the series, radium, which decays to gaseous radon (Harley et al., 1986), although most of the radon remains in the uranium-bearing rocks and only a proportion escapes into the air (see Appendix I, page 865). Occupational exposures to radon and its decay products are largely confined to underground miners – particularly those mining uranium, hematite, tin and fluorspar.

The Carpathian silver miners of the Middle Ages seem to be first group of workers identified as dying of radon-induced lung cancer, and further studies this century of the Czechoslovak uranium mines confirm this view (Lemen, 1986). Underground iron ore mines in England, Sweden, Czechoslovakia, Italy and France have consistently shown a higher incidence of lung cancer in the presence of exposure to radon daughters than surface workers (Battista et al., 1988; IARC, 1988). A recent follow-up of the English miners has shown that the excess risk was largely confined to workers employed before 1967, although the diminished risk thereafter seems more to do with workers leaving the industry than to improved mine ventilation (Kinlen and Willows, 1988). In Italy, pyrites miners were shown to have (depending on years of exposure) an excess of 13 to 21 cases of lung cancer per million person years and working level month (a *working level month* – WLM – is 1.3×10^5 MeV of α activity in 1 litre of respired air for 170 hours of exposure).

Excess lung cancer has also been described following exposure to radon and thoron daughters in a Swedish niobium mine (Solli et al., 1985), in residents near the phosphate mines of central Florida (Stockwell et al., 1988), where the phosphate ore is known to contain uranium-238, in underground fluorspar miners in Newfoundland (Morrison et al., 1988), and Cornish tin miners (Hodgson and Jones, 1990).

Suspect agents

Acrylonitrite

Acrylonitrite is used in the production of plastics, textile fibres and synthetic rubber. Four studies of these workers have been published – two from the USA, and one each from the UK and Germany (IARC, 1987). Lung cancer excesses have been noted in all four studies, although they are modest (less than twofold) and could have been subject to confounding factors such as smoking as well as other occupational exposures, given that the factories produced textile fibres, rubber or polymerized products of acrylonitrite.

Beryllium

Much of the evidence concerning the carcinogenic potential of beryllium comes from studies of workers in plants in Pennsylvania and Ohio and from a register of beryllium disease cases in the USA. The studies and their interpretation have, however, been the source of much heated debate (Saracci, 1985). Lung cancer excesses of 40 per cent were found in the US cohorts of workers compared with the general population and non-exposed factory populations. For cases of beryllium disease, a threefold excess was noted for subjects with acute beryllium disease but not among those with chronic beryllium disease. As the lung cancer excess for the beryllium workers tended to be concentrated in those workers employed for less than 5 years, this finding would fit with the hypothesis that heavy exposure to beryllium, possibly resulting in the worker leaving the industry prematurely, is the causative agent in the subsequent development of lung cancer. The dispute revolves around the interpretation of an excess risk mainly noted in workers with a relatively short exposure, but not in those who worked longest in the industry. Short-term workers may be different in many ways from the long-term employees, and evidence of an excess lung cancer risk in short-term talc workers supports this view (Lamm et al., 1988). Nevertheless, if beryllium exposure is heavy enough to cause acute beryllium disease, the length of exposure may be less relevant here than the dose (see Chapter 17, page 581).

Cadmium

The first indication that a cadmium compound might have a carcinogenic effect appeared in 1961 after subcutaneous injection into rats. Whilst it has been known that cadmium could play a role in causing acute and chronic non-malignant respiratory disease, it is only recently that evidence has been gathered that cadmium or its compounds might cause respiratory cancer (Oberdorster, 1986).

Four populations of cadmium-exposed workers form the bulk of the epidemiological evidence. In the UK, the workers in a variety of cadmium-exposed industries were found to have an increased risk of lung cancer (Kazantzis, Lamm and Sullivan, 1988) with a trend in excess from 12 per cent in the 'always low' category of exposure to 21 per cent in 'ever medium' to 94 per cent in 'ever high'. It appears, however, that the majority of lung cancer deaths were from one large non-ferrous smelter where exposures were in the medium/low category with a relationship to length of employment in the smelter but not to cumulative exposure to cadmium. A 30 per cent excess of lung cancer was also found in the population of nickel–cadmium battery workers in the UK (Sorahan, 1987), but no trend with years of exposure was found. The US study by Thun et al. (1985) of 602 cadmium smelter workers is the only study to show a clear association between cadmium exposure and lung cancer. Although, even here, smoking data were inadequate (and cigarette smoke contains cadmium), arsenic exposure was another possible confounder in the early years of plant operations. The authors, however, contend that these compounds do not account for their findings.

The question of whether cadmium or its compounds are pulmonary carcinogens in human beings remains debatable. Certainly cadmium compounds are carcinogens to a number of organs in animal, including the lung following inhalation. The chemical form of the inhaled cadmium may well be important. Cadmium oxide and cadmium chloride seem to be equally toxic to the lung, but cadmium sulphide exhibits a lower acute pulmonary toxicity. Whether these non-malignant effects of different salts mirror their carcinogenic potential remains to be seen.

This topic is also referred to in Chapter 18 (page 599).

Formaldehyde

Formaldehyde is present in the environment from natural and industrial sources. In industry, formaldehyde is produced in large quantities and used in many applications. Therefore, the discovery that formaldehyde was a respiratory tract carcinogen in rats (and perhaps in mice) produced a flurry of activity to review human exposures. A number of epidemiological studies have now been published using different designs and investigating a variety of occupational exposures with conflicting results. Cancers have been noted in excess for a number of sites in more than one study, but some of the study populations overlap (IARC, 1987). Slight excesses in the occurrence of lung cancer have been noted in several studies but these excesses have shown no consistent pattern with increasing level or duration of exposure to formaldehyde. The evidence for human lung carcinogenicity (or indeed for nasal cancer) must be concluded as being limited on present evidence (Nelson et al., 1986). Many problems of interpretation compound the issue. The doses in the rodent experiments were high enough to cause acute nasal mucosal damage – an environment inimicable to continued occupational exposure. Furthermore the rapidity with which exogenous formaldehyde enters the endogenous pool raises questions concerning its ability to affect DNA cross-linkages, particularly at the site of first contact – mainly the upper respiratory tract. But epidemiological studies have not confirmed such a risk of malignancy in human subjects. The role of smoking also remains unanswered so that the low incidence of lung cancer in formaldehyde-exposed populations of physicians, for example, is difficult to interpret. Hence, the present evidence suggests that formaldehyde does not have a high carcinogenic potential. Given the widespread past occupational exposures to formaldehyde, it can, thus, be concluded that formaldehyde is, at most, a weak human carcinogen.

Silica

Although the causal connection between occupational quartz exposure and silicosis is well established, the question of whether silica can cause lung tumours remains debatable. The matter was first raised 50 years ago but recently a number of papers have addressed the issue anew. The finding of an increased risk of lung cancer in foundry workers started the process and since then a number of papers have appeared which link silicosis with lung cancer (IARC, 1987). Three recent studies illustrate the issues involved: Steenland and Beaumont (1986), in a mortality study of 1905 granite cutters in the USA, found 97 cases of lung cancer – a 19 per cent excess. When these cases were compared with 137 other cases and evidence of silicosis as a contributory cause of death was analysed, it was found that there was a threefold excess of lung cancer in subjects suffering from silicosis. In Sweden, a population of 280 ceramic workers who contracted silicosis were followed up (Tornling, Hogstedt and Westerholm, 1988) and an 88 per cent increase in lung cancer was observed. In Italy, a relative risk of two for lung cancer was noted in a case-control study of ceramic workers – 3.9 for those with silicosis but 1.4 (not significant) for those without (Forastiere et al., 1986).

Epidemiological studies of both exposed populations and subjects with silicosis give indications of the carcinogenicity of a working environment containing crystalline silica with or without other exposures to PAHs or radon daughters. Few studies provide smoking data. If the carcinogenic effect is real, it seems to be greatest in workers with silicosis which raises the possibility that the carcinogenic effect requires the fibrotic process to initiate the malignant change (Simonto and Saracci, 1990).

This matter is discussed in more detail in Chapter 12 (page 315).

Vinyl chloride monomer

Although vinyl chloride monomer is known to cause angiosarcoma of the liver, attention has focused in recent years on its ability to induce tumours at other sites such as the brain, lung and the lympho-haemopoietic system. Doll (1988) reviewed the epidemiological studies concerning the effects of exposure to vinyl chloride and found that only four studies were of sufficient power and design to warrant serious consideration. For lung cancer the US and UK studies show 'small' excesses for lung cancer in the longest exposed workers, whilst for four countries combined, comprising 14 plants, the observed : expected fibres for lung cancer were 31.5 : 30.72. However, the expected figures may be an overstatement. Doll concludes that the evidence for vinyl chloride being a human lung carcinogen is weak but, in view of the positive animal studies, a small risk to human beings could well exist. The case is not proven.

Synthetic (man-made) mineral fibres

The question as to whether these are carcinogenic in human beings is discussed in Chapter 16 (page 563).

Suspect processes

Foundries

Work in iron and steel foundries had been suspected of carrying a risk of lung cancer for the last 50 years, but until recently, such a suspicion was largely based on national occupational mortality statistics such as the UK Decennial Supplements (Blot, 1985). In the last few years several cohort studies of foundry workers have been published which, in general, show moderately elevated risks for lung cancer of between 1.5- and 2.5-fold (IARC, 1987) with some also showing elevation for gastrointestinal tract tumours. All these studies suffered from problems of inadequate definition of confounding factors and, not infrequently, from difficulties of ensuring that the smaller – and arguably the dirtier – workplaces provided adequate employment data to trace the individual numbers of the cohort (Fletcher and Ades, 1984). A recent update of this study (Sorahan and Cooke, 1989) confirms the previous elevated SMR for lung cancer – now 147 based on 441 deaths.

The difficulties of delineating the exposure characteristics of the cohort members are much greater. Certainly there are a number of known or suspect carcinogens in the working environment. These include polycylic aromatic hydrocarbons, aromatic amines, silica, metal fumes of one sort or another and formaldehyde. Smoking data are also frequently lacking although, at measured risks of this magnitude, smoking cannot account for all the excess. Indeed, a recent Polish study (Becher et al., 1989) suggests that an excess (up to twofold) is present after allowing for smoking. But the agent or agents in foundry work that cause this excess of lung cancer remain as yet unidentified. The possibility of acid mists as an aetiological factor is now under serious consideration (Steenland and Beaumont, 1989).

Rubber industries

Observations of bladder tumours among workers in the rubber industry in the UK in the 1950s led to the establishment of large-scale cohort studies of rubber workers both in the UK and the USA. These study populations have been followed since then and they continue to provide a valuable source of epidemiological data on the hazards of the industry.

As the incidence of bladder tumours has waned following the control or prohibition of the most potent carcinogens in the aromatic amine group, attention in these cohorts has switched to a review of other tumour sites. The literature on rubber workers' mortality is vast and so this review will concentrate on a few recent reports. Sorahan et al. (1986) re-analysed the mortality experience of 36 000 British rubber workers first employed at 1 of 13 plants during the period 1946–1960 and now followed to 1980. Statistically significant excesses were noted for stomach, liver and lung cancer. For lung cancer the excess was 33 per cent based on 1191 deaths and, in a recent update (Sorahan et al., 1989), the excess remains at 31 per cent. Analysis by regression models was used to compare exposure characteristics for these cases. An association was found between duration of employment in jobs principally associated with fume or solvent exposure, or both, for cancer of the lung in workers in the tyre sector. These authors do not feel that this association with tyres is meaningful alone but could imply a more widespread risk. Smoking data were not available but were not considered likely to provide an explanation of the excess. They postulate a causal link between 'occupational exposures' in the rubber industry and lung cancer but cannot identify specific carcinogens.

A similar, although smaller, cohort of Swedish rubber workers has also recently been updated (Gustavasson, Hogstedt and Holmberg, 1986). Here the cohort of nearly 9000 workers revealed an excess for lung cancer but only in those followed for more than 40 years since first employment. An analysis by country of origin suggested that the excess was particularly marked in immigrant Finns and Danes rather than the indigenous Swedes.

In the USA, studies by Monson and co-workers had revealed a lung cancer excess in the tyre-curing sections of rubber manufacturing plants and a case-control study of 40 such deaths in one plant has revealed that occupational exposures are related to the incidence of cases in terms of duration of exposure in reclaim, chemicals and special products manufacture (Andjelkovich et al., 1988). The excess risk in workers in these areas with more than 5 years' exposure ranged from 2.2- to 4.9-fold, with the excess noted in both smokers and non-smokers but with the greatest excess in smokers. Similar results were found in a cohort of rubber factory workers in Shanghai (Zhang et al., 1989). They found an excess risk of 8.3 in workers who did not smoke but 28.2 in workers who smoked.

Again, unfortunately, the likely causal agents for these consistent excesses of lung cancer have not been identified.

Welding

A number of studies of cohorts of welders has noted lung cancer excesses of 30 to 50 per cent (Blot, 1985), although the possible confounding effects of smoking, and asbestos exposure, remain important but ill-defined. Two recent studies have looked at shipyard workers and both found an elevation in lung cancer. In the US study (Rinsky et al., 1988), the object of the study was to evaluate a previously reported excess of leukaemia. Lung cancer excesses found were reviewed by primary exposure groupings with modest excesses of 23 per cent, 24 per cent and 46 per cent for radiation, asbestos and welding respectively. The authors conclude that the probable cause of the lung cancer excess was a combination of welding and asbestos exposure. Similarly in Finland, Tola et al. (1988) found a 20 per cent lung cancer excess in shipyard workers. The highest excess (53 per cent) was in pipe fitters and this they attributed to asbestos exposure.

There is no doubt that welders as a group do experience excess respiratory disease, both malignant and non-malignant, but these excesses are not particularly large and frequently less than twofold. The possible causative factors are legion and include smoking, metal fume, asbestos and a variety of other gaseous irritants. As in previous industries listed in this section, no clear evidence has emerged implicating specific carcinogens. Only a few animal studies have been reported and these have been negative, although collected foundry fume has been shown to be mutagenic in short-term bacterial mutation tests (see also Chapter 18, page 629).

Possible agents or processes

In this section, the epidemiological evidence for an association between agent or process and lung cancer is rather more tenuous. Although some specific points will be outlined, many of the data can be described as little more than hypothesis generation. Typical of this sort of study are ones that begin by noting a geographical clustering of cases. Many such studies could be listed but (biased) preference is given to a case-control study by Harrington et al. (1978) which reviewed the occupational and residential histories of 858 cases of lung cancer in the coastal counties of Georgia, USA where excess lung cancer rates were noted in a previous national cancer mapping exercise. Construction workers were found to have a twofold excess – and a later study linked this to asbestos exposure. The industrial concentrations in this part of Georgia were wood and paper industries where a threefold excess was found for lung cancer in the rural counties of the region. Other recent case-control studies of lung cancer have found statistically significant associations with construction, leather, wood, gas and coke industries, and in bakers and cooks in young to middle-aged men (Coggon et al., 1986), and with wood dust (Siemiatyki et al., 1986). However, Damber and Larsson (1987), as well as noting known associations with underground miners, found a 70 per cent excess for woodpulp workers and a twofold excess for asphalt and concrete workers in Sweden. A decreased risk for lung cancer was found for farmers and foresters which is in contrast to a case-control study from Shanghai (Levin et al., 1988) where farmers had a 60 per cent excess risk. Exposure to wood dusts revealed an elevated risk although the textile industry had a significantly low risk. In France, Benhamou, Benhamou and Flamant (1988) noted a 24 per cent excess in farmers, 80 per cent in plumbers and pipe fitters and 40 per cent in motor vehicle drivers. In two northern Italian industrial areas the wood workers showed nearly a threefold excess (Ronco et al., 1988) with non-significant excesses of 57 per cent to fivefold in workers in the chemical and metal industries.

The value of such studies is limited. They are only the first stage in the epidemiological process. Analytical (hypothesis-testing) studies must follow. What follows here is a 'pot-pourri' of publications which no more than suggests that certain agents and processes are worthy of further scrutiny as a possible cause of occupationally induced lung cancer.

Chlorinated toluenes

Two small studies from Japan and the UK had previously noted lung cancer excesses in workers exposed to chlorinated toluenes, including benzotrichloride, benzyl chloride, benzoyl chloride and related chemicals (IARC, 1987). A further cohort of 697 similarly exposed US workers has been studied (Wong, 1988) with seven cases of respiratory cancer. Attempts at closer scrutiny of chemical exposures suggest an increasing trend with years since first employment and years of exposure. The lung cancer excess arising in laboratory employees (based on only two cases) was 1200-fold. An update of the UK study to 1984 confirms the excess lung cancer risk but fails to implicate specific chlorinated toluenes (Sorahan and Cathcart, 1989).

Cobalt

Cobalt exposure has been associated with hard-metal disease. A recent study of 1876 hard-metal workers in Sweden (Hogstedt, 1988) was reported to have a twofold excess of lung cancer in the subcohort of workers exposed long term (based on seven deaths), whilst in France, four lung cancer deaths noted in a cohort study of cobalt and sodium workers at an electrochemical plant produced at 4.6-fold excess risk. A nested case-control study of nine lung cancer deaths noted that four (44 per cent) had worked with cobalt (Mur et al., 1987).

Dimethyl sulphate

Dimethyl sulphate is an alkylating agent and case reports of bronchial carcinoma in association with occupational exposure are supported by clear-cut evidence of in vitro and in vivo carcinogenicity and mutagenicity (IARC, 1987).

Epichlorhydrin

This chemical is an alkylating agent used in the production of synthetic glycerin and epoxy resins and is known to be a lung carcinogen in mice. One study of a human population at two plants in the southern states of America found an excess risk of lung cancer (6 observed cases, 4.2 expected), although previous work in the manufacture of isopropyl alcohol is a possible confounder (Enterline, 1982).

Butchers and meat industry workers

Correspondence in the pages of *The Lancet* in 1982 and 1983 suggested that reviews of national occupational mortality statistics in the UK and Denmark had revealed an excess of lung cancer among butchers and meat cutters with evidence from Denmark that smoking might not explain the excess. The exposures that were mooted as possible causative factors included nitrosamines, butylated hydroxyanisole (BHA), butylated hydroxytoluene (BHT), as well as smoke and fumes emitted from the thermal decomposition of plastic films used to wrap meat. A cohort study of 13 844 US meat cutters revealed 90 per cent excess of lung cancer which decreased to 20 per cent after allowance for geographical variation, (Johnson et al., 1986), although 34 per cent of the cases occurred in the under 50-year-old age group. Excesses for bone cancer (tenfold) and Hodgkin's disease (twofold) also raised the possibility of a role for oncogenic viruses in the cancers observed. Further studies of meat industry employees from New Zealand (Reif, Pearce and Fraser, 1989) and the UK (Coggon et al., 1989) support the hypothesis that exposure to freshly slaughtered meat may lead to a modest excess of lung cancer in exposed workers, but the data from these studies do not suggest any specific aetiological agents.

Painters

Painters (and paint makers) are potentially exposed to a wide range of chemicals including petroleum solvents, toluene, xylene, ketones, alcohols, ethers and glycol ethers. Painters are also exposed to chlorinated hydrocarbons used as paint strippers. Chromates and, in the past, asbestos have been used in paint formulations. Furthermore, painters working on construction sites and in shipyards could be exposed to asbestos in the working environment.

IARC have recently evaluated painters as an occupational group and found a modest (20 to 50 per cent), but consistent, excess of lung cancer in studies ranging from national mortality statistics to analytical epidemiological studies of painting populations (IARC, 1989). Smoking, where allowed for, still left an unexplained excess of the order of 30 per cent. Other tumour sites such as the gastrointestinal and urinary tracts and the lymphohaemopoietic system also showed excesses. Whilst data on paint manufacture were deemed inadequate for evaluation, the studies on painters were considered consistent and valid enough to warrant a 'sufficient cause' rating.

There is no doubt that paints have contained – or do contain – some known or suspect carcinogens, but it is difficult to take specific preventive health measures following such an evaluation. Many of the studies evaluated were of the type described earlier or were the findings in cohort studies of many occupational groups analysed for multiple-cause risk factors. Thus, the usefulness of such a classification, involving as it does hundreds of thousands of paint makers and millions of painters world wide, is limited without further specific data.

Pesticide applicators

Pesticides contain a variety of chemical formulations – some of which in the past certainly contained arsenicals. Recent studies of pesticide applicators in East Germany (Barthel, 1981) and the USA (Blair et al., 1983; MacMahon et al., 1988) provided somewhat conflicting results. Superficially each shows an excess of lung cancer (89 per cent, 35 per cent and 58 per cent respectively). In the Barthel and Blair studies, the excess was greater with longer periods of exposure, whereas the MacMahon study excess was limited to persons employed for less than 5 years. The MacMahon study found no excess in termite exterminators, thus suggesting that chlordane and heptochlor would not be the likely carcinogens. Blair, by contrast, found a non-significant excess in a similar group of applicators. In East Germany, apparently, chlordane and heptochlor are not available. Thus, the question remains as to whether the excess is real and, if it is, what might the carcinogen(s) be.

Wood industries

IARC have reviewed several subsections of this industrial grouping: carpentry and joining, furniture and cabinet making, and lumber and saw mill industries (IARC, 1987). Whilst there is no doubt that sinonasal cancer is causally linked to furniture and cabinet making, the evidence in any of the industries for a lung cancer risk is limited, with the US study suggesting a 20 per cent excess in carpenters and joiners, whereas a Finnish case-control study of wood industry workers with lung cancer found a 3 per cent excess associated with wood dust but a five- to thirteenfold excess for exposure to unspecified pesticides or phenol when a 10-year latency was applied (Kauppinen et al., 1986). These elevated risk ratios were, however, based on less than 10 cases in each group.

Prevention

The major preventive measure available to reduce the huge toll of disease and death from lung cancer remains the elimination of tobacco smoking. It is estimated that more than 90 per cent of the lung cancer cases in one Norwegian case-control study would have been prevented if smoking had not been a factor (Kjuus, Langård and Skjaerven, 1986). The so-called aetiological fraction related to occupational exposure varied from 22 to 47 per cent but interaction between smoking and the workplace carcinogen may also play a part. Saracci (1987) attempted to assess interaction in a wide-ranging review of available epidemiological evidence. In a thoughtful and thorough analysis, he concludes that certain agents do interact with tobacco smoking with differing results. In summary his findings are:

Arsenic	Additive to multiplicative
Asbestos	Multiplicative
Chlorinated methyl ethers	Possibly less than additive
Nickel	Additive
Radon	Additive to multiplicative

By contrast, even less has been done to determine if any workplace exposures have a *subtractive* effect on lung cancer. There is some evidence, for example, that selenium might be protective (Gerhardsson et al., 1985).

In short, the elimination of one or other (smoking or workplace factors) could have a disproportionately large effect on the incidence of lung cancer in cases where interaction seems to exist. Given the difficulty in persuading people to change their lifestyles, there is much to be said for applying measures beyond their control or will – namely lowering the workplace exposures.

From the epidemiological point of view, too few studies have good smoking data to allow such inter-actions to be assessed and retrospective collection of smoking histories – particularly from the relatives of decedents – is frequently inaccurate. Nevertheless all is not as bleak as it appears. Steenland and Schnorr (1988) estimated that a reliance on current smoking data is a fair estimate although as smoking prevalence is changing in industrialized countries, this might underestimate the role of smoking. However, it is too facile – and incorrect – to dismiss even moderate excesses of lung cancer on the basis that smoking data are unavailable. Several studies have looked at the possible effect of different smoking patterns on lung cancer excesses. The estimates all agree quite closely:

Axelson (1978) <50 per cent
Asp (1987) <30 per cent
Blair, Hoar and Walrath (1985) <30 per cent
Siemiatycki et al. (1988a,b) <40 per cent

Thus, any lung cancer excess noted to be greater than 50 per cent cannot be readily dismissed even if smoking histories are unavailable. Indeed, in the review by Simonto, Vineis and Fletcher (1988), which only included studies that assessed smoking as a confounder, they concluded that smoking had a limited effect which was unlikely to alter estimates by more than 20 to 25 per cent. A doubling effect should give serious cause for considering an exposure factor in the workplace.

Future considerations

The epidemiological method upon which this chapter has so heavily depended is flawed. Not only are the health outcome and exposure indices often incompletely ascertained but human beings are exposed to a variety of possible harmful agents with differing doses and durations in a lifetime's experi-ence. Thus, the task of delineating specific work-place carcinogens from epidemiological studies will always be problematic. Nevertheless, many agents and processes have been declared carcinogenic. Therefore, a major concern for the future is the energetic pursuit of improving the working environ-ment to ensure even lower concentrations of these known carcinogens. If possible, substitution of the

harmful agent with a less dangerous material should be implemented.

Further work is clearly needed on the possible interaction of different agents with each other and with smoking. Indeed, few studies attempt to look for histological differences in lung tumours which might be a pointer in the direction of evaluating how important workplace, as opposed to lifestyle, exposures might be (Brownson et al., 1987).

It is also important to improve the clarification of specific agent exposures in order to diminish the number of vague processes as compared with specific agents that appear in Table 19.3.*

So far as the search for aetiological agents is concerned, the time has come for epidemiologists to move away from further studies of lung carcinogens, where even the dose–response effect has been described, and move on to look at agents for which positive animal data exist in an attempt to find human exposed populations. In other words the asbestos story is now one of control or elimination, with a redirected effort towards the hundreds of known animal carcinogens. There will always be a place for the hypothesis-generating study but epidemiology has never discovered any carcinogen (with the possible exception of the serendipitous finding of nasal cancer in boot and shoe manufac-turers). The first clue to new hazards in the workplace commonly comes from those closest to it: the occupational health specialist and, particularly important, the workers themselves. It is foolish and arrogant to ignore concerns about health that emanate from the shop floor.

Conclusions

Although lung cancer is a public health issue of enormous proportions, the role of the workplace in its initiation is an important factor in diagnosis and prevention. Workplace exposure in lung cancer cases probably accounts for at least 5 per cent of the total and contributes to the disease in at least a further 5 per cent of cases. Thus, occupational factors contribute to a significant minority of cases and, in attributable risk terms, the numbers of cases of lung cancer that could be prevented make atten-tion to the workplace an important public health issue.

*After this chapter was completed the IARC (Monograph Series 54, 1991) reported that it had identified sulphuric acid and other strong acid mists as proven human carcinogens (group 1), and it reclassified beryllium and cadmium compounds to this same group as well (not yet published) (see Table 19.3).

Further carcinogens will be discovered with time but it is important to remember that occupational diseases are rarely, if ever, eliminated, as smallpox seems to have been. Many agents or processes have not been – or cannot be – removed from the working environment. The diseases they are capable of producing are thus kept at bay by vigilant and rigorous adherence to the best work practices and such practices should invariably become more stringent as technology allows. Occupational factors in the genesis of lung cancer will, therefore, remain important for the foreseeable future.

References

Abeloff, M.D., Eggleston, J.C., Mendelsohn, G., Ettinger, D.S. and Baylin, S.B. (1974) Changes in morphologic and biochemical characteristics of small cell carcinoma of the lung. A clinicopathologic study. *Am. J. Med.* **66**, 757–764

Adachi, S. and Takemoto, K. (1987) Occupational lung cancer: a comparison between humans and experimental animals. *Jap. J. Ind. Health* **29**, 345–357

Albert, R.E., Pasternak, B.S., Shore, R.E., Lippmann, M., Nelson, N. and Ferris, B. (1975). Mortality patterns among workers exposed to chloromethyl ethers – A preliminary report. *Environ. Health Perspect.* **11**, 209–214

Alderson, M.R. (1986) *Occupational Cancer*. Butterworths, London

Andjelkovich, D.A., Abdelghany, N., Matthew, R.M. and Blum, S. (1988) Lung cancer case control study in a Rubber manufacturing plant. *Am. J. Ind. Med.* **14**, 559–574

Asp, A. (1982) Confounding by variable smoking habits in different occupational groups. *Scand. J. Work Environ. Health* **10**, 325–326

Auberbach, O. (1980) Natural history of carcinoma of the lung. In: *Pulmonary Diseases and Disorders* (ed. A.P. Fishman). McGraw-Hill, New York, pp. 1388–1396

Auerbach, O., Hammond, E.C. and Garfinkel, L. (1979) Changes in bronchial epithelium in relation to cigarette smoking, 1955–60 vs 1970–77. *N. Engl. J. Med.* **300**, 381–386

Axelson, O. (1978) Aspects of confounding in occupational health epidemiology. *Scand. J. Work Environ. Health* **4**, 98–102

Balarajan, R. and McDowall, M.E. (1988) Professional drivers in London: A mortality study. *B. J. Ind. Med.* **45**, 483–486

Battista, G., Belli, S., Carboncini, F., Comsa, P., Levante, G., Sartorelli, P., Strambi, F., Valentini, F. and Axelson, O. (1988) Mortality among pyrites miners with low level exposure to radon daughters. *Scand. J. Work Environ. Health* **14**, 280–285

Barthel, E. (1981) Increased risk of lung cancer in pesticide-exposed male agricultural workers. *J. Toxicol. Environ. Health* **8**, 1027–1040

Becher, H., Jedrychowski, Flak E., Gomola, K. and Wahrendorf, J. (1989) Lung cancer, smoking and employment in foundries. *Scand. J. Work Environ. Health* **15**, 38–42

Benhamou, S., Behamou, E. and Flamant, R. (1988) Occupational risk factors of lung cancer in a French case control study. *Br. J. Ind. Med.* **45**, 231–233

Berenblum, I. and Schoental, R,C, (1947) Carcinogenic constituents of coal-tar. *Br. J. Cancer* **1**, 157

Bereton, H.D., Matthews, M.M., Costa, J., Kent, C.H. and Johnson, R.E. (1978) Mixed anaplastic small-cell and squamous-cell carcinoma of the lung. *Ann. Intern. Med.* **88**, 805–806

Blair, A., Hoar, S. and Walrath, J. (1985) Comparison of crude and smoking adjusted standardised mortality ratios. *J. Occup. Med.* **27**, 881–884

Blair, A., Grauman, D.J., Lubin, L.H. and Fraumeni, J.E. (1983) Lung cancer and other causes of death among licensed pesticide applicators. *J. Natl Cancer Instit.* **71**, 31–37

Blot, W.J. (1985) Lung cancer and occupational exposures. In: *Lung Cancer – Causes and Prevention* (eds M. Mixell and P. Correa), Verlag Chemical International, Deerfield, FL, pp. 47–64

Brownson, R.C., Reif, J.S., Keefe, T.J., Ferguson, S.W. and Pritzel, J.A. (1987) Risk factors for adenocarcinoma of the lung. *Am. J. Epidemiol.* **125**, 26–34

Burdon, J.C.W., Sinclair, R.A. and Henderson, M.M. (1979) Small cell carcinoma of the lung. Prognosis in relation to histologic subtype. *Chest* **76**, 302–304

Coggon, D., Pannett, B., Osmond, C. and Acheson, E.D. (1986) A survey of cancer and occupation in young and middle aged men: Cancer of the respiratory tract. *Br. J. Ind. Med.* **43**, 332–338

Coggon, D., Pannett, B., Pippard, E.C. and Winter, P.D. (1989) Lung cancer in the meat industry. *Br. J. Ind. Med.* **46**, 188–191

Cotes, J.A. and Steel, J. (1987) Occupational lung cancer. In: *Work-related Lung Disorders*, Blackwell Scientific, Oxford, pp. 42–263

Damber, L.A. and Larsson, L.G. (1987) Occupational and male lung cancer: a case control study in North Sweden. *Br. J. Ind. Med.* **44**, 446–453

Davies, J.M. (1984) Lung cancer mortality among workers making lead chromate and zinc chromate pigment at three English factories. *Br. J. Ind. Med.* **41**, 158–169

Davies, J.M., Easton, D.F. and Bidstrup, P.L. (1991) Mortality from respiratory cancer and other causes in United Kingdom chrome production workers. *Br. J. Ind. Med.* **48**, 299–313

Department of Health and Social Security (1986) *Occupational Lung Cancer – A Report of the Industrial Injuries Advisory Council.* Cm37, HMSO, London

Doll, R. (1984) Occupational cancer: problems of interpreting human evidence. *Ann. Occup. Hyg.* **28**, 291–305

Doll, R. (1988) Effects of exposure to vinyl chloride. *Scand. J. Work Environ. Health* **14**, 61–78

Doll, R. and Peto, J. (1981) *The Causes of Cancer.* Oxford University Press, Oxford

Dong, M.H., Redmond, C.K., Mazumdar, S. and Costantino, J.P. (1988) A multistage approach to the cohort analysis of lifetime lung cancer risk among steel workers exposed to coke oven emissions. *Am. J. Epidemiol.* **128**, 860–873

Easton, D.R., Peto, J. and Doll, R. (1988) Cancers of the respiratory tract in mustard gas workers. *Br. J. Ind. Med.* **45**, 652–659

Enterline, P.E. (1982) Importance of sequential exposure in the production of epichlorhydrin and isopropanol. *Ann. NY Acad. Sci.* **381**, 344–349

Enterline, P.E., Henderson, V.L. and Marsh, G.M. (1987) Exposure to arsenic and respiratory cancer. *Am. J. Epidemiol.* **125**, 929–938

Fletcher, A.C. and Ades, A. (1984) Lung cancer mortality in a cohort of English foundry workers. *Scand. J. Work Environ. Health* **10**, 7–16

Forastiere, F., Lagorio, S., Michelozzi, P., Cavariani, F., Arca, M., Borgia, P., Perucci, C. and Axelson, O. (1986) Silica, silicosis and lung cancer among ceramic workers: a case referent study. *Am. J. Ind. Med.* **10**, 363–370

Frank, A.L. (1987) Occupational cancer of respiratory tract. In: *Occupational Cancer and Carcinogens – Occupational Medicine State of the Art Reviews*, vol. 2, no. 1. Hanley & Balfor Inc., Philadelphia, pp. 71–83

Garshick, E., Schenker, M.B., Munoz, A., Segal, M., Smith, T.J., Woskie, S.R., Hammond, K. and Spiezer, F.E. (1988) A retrospective cohort study of lung cancer and diesel exhaust exposure in rail road workers. *Am. Rev. Respir. Dis.* **137**, 820–825

Gerhardsson, L., Brune, D., Nordberg, I.G.F. and Wester, P.O. (1985) Protective effect of selenium on lung cancer in smelter workers. *Br. J. Ind. Med.* **42**, 617–626

Gibbs, G.W. (1985) Morbidity of alumium reduction plant workers, 1950 through 1977. *J. Occup. Med.* **27**, 761–770

Grandjean, P., Anderson, O. and Neilson, G.D. (1988) Carcinogenicity of occupational nickel exposure: an evaluation of the epidemiological evidence. *Am. J. Ind. Med.* **13**, 193–209

Gustavsson, P., Gustavsson, A. and Hogstedt, C. (1987) Excess mortality among Swedish chimney sweeps. *Br. J. Ind. Med.* **44**, 738–743

Gustavsson, P., Hogstedt, C. and Holmberg, B. (1986) Mortality and incidence of cancer among Swedish rubber workers 1952–1981. *Scand. Work Environ. Health* **2**, 538–544

Harley, N., Samet, J.M., Cross, F.T., Hess, T., Muller, J. and Thomas, D. (1986) Contribution of radon and radon daughters to respiratory cancer. *Environ. Health Perspect.* **70**, 17–21

Harrington, J.M., Blot, W.J., Hoover, R.N., Housworth, W.J., Heath, C.W. and Fraumeni, J.F. (1978) Lung cancer in coastal Georgia. A death certificate analysis of occupation *J. Natl Cancer Instit.* **60**, 295–298

Hill, A.B. and Faning E.L. (1948) Studies in the incidence of cancer in a factory handling inorganic compounds of arsenic. *Br. J. Ind. Med.* **5**, 1–15

Hodgson, J.J. and Jones, R.D. (1990) Mortality of a cohort of tin miners 1941–1986. *Br. J. Ind. Med.* **47**, 665–676

Hogstedt, C. (1988) Identification of cancer risks from chemical exposures – an epidemiologic programme at the Swedish National Institute of Occupational Health. *Scand. J. Work Environ. Health* **14**, suppl. 1, 17–20

International Agency for Research on Cancer (1986) *Long-term and Short-term Assays for Carcinogens: a Critical Appraisal.* IARC Scientific Publication No. 83, Lyon

International Agency for Research on Cancer (1987) Monographs. An evaluation of carcinogenic risk to humans. *Overall Evaluation of Carcinogenicity: An Updating of IARC Monographs Vols 1–42*, Suppl. 7, IARC, Lyon

International Agency for Research on Cancer (1988) *Man Made Mineral Fibre and Radon, Vol. 43*, IARC, Lyon.

International Agency for Research on Cancer (1989) Some organic solvents, resin monomers and related compounds, pigments and occupational exposures in paint manufacture and painting. *Vol. 47.* IARC, Lyon

Ives, J.C., Buffler, P.A. and Greenberg, S.D. (1983) Environmental associations and histopathologic patterns of carcinoma of the lung: The challenge and dilemma in epidemiologic studies. *Am. Rev. Respir. Dis.* **128**, 195–209

Jarup, L., Pershagen, G. and Wall, S. (1989) Cumulative arsenic exposure and lung cancer in Smelter workers: A dose response study. *Am. J. Ind. Med.* **15**, 31–41

Johnson, E.S., Fischman, H.R., Matanoski, P.M. and Diamond, E. (1986) Cancer mortality among white males in the meat industry. *J. Occup. Med.* **28**, 23–32

Kauppinen, T.P., Partanen, T.J., Nurminen, M.M., Nickels, J.I., Hernberg, S., Hakulinen, T.R., Pukkala, E. and Savonen, E.T. (1986) Respiratory cancers and and chemical exposure in the wood industry: a nested case/control study. *B. J. Ind. Med.* **43**, 84–90

Kazantzis, G., Lam, T-H. and Sullivan, K.R. (1988) Morbidity of cadmium exposed workers. *Scand. J. Work Environ. Health* **14**, 220–223

Kinlen, L.J. and Willows, A.N. (1988) Decline in lung cancer hazard: a prospective study of the morbidity of iron ore miners in Cumbria. *Br. J. Ind. Med.* **45**, 219–224

Kjuus, H., Langård, S. and Skjaerven, R. (1986) A case referent study of lung cancer, occupational exposure and smokers. Etiological fraction of occupational exposures. *Scand. J. Work Environ. Health* **12**, 210–215

Lamm, S.H., Levine, M.S., Starr, J.A. and Tirey, S.L. (1988) Analysis of excess lung cancer risk in short term employees. *Am. J. Epidemiol.* **127**, 1202–1209

Langård, S. and Vigander, T. (1983) Occurrence of lung cancer in workers producing chromium pigments. *Br. J. Ind. Med.* **40**, 71–74

Lee, K.P., Ulrich, C.E., Geil, R.G. and Trochimowicz, H.J. (1988) Effect of inhaled chromium oxide dust on rats exposed for two years. *Fund. Appl. Toxic.* **10**, 125–145

Lemen, R.A. (1986) Occupationally induced lung cancer epidemiology. In: *Occupational Diseases* (ed. J.A. Merchant), National Institute of Occupational Safety and Health, Washington DC, US Department, Health and Health Services, pp. 629–656

Levin, L.I., Zheng, W., Blot, W.J., Gao, Y-T. and Fraumeni, J.R. (1988) Occupation and lung cancer in Shanghai: a case control study. *Br. J. Ind. Med.* **45**, 450–458

Levy, L.S., Martin, P.A. and Bidstrup, P.L. (1986) An investigation of the potential carcinogenicity of a range of chromium-containing compounds. *Br. J. Ind. Med.* **43**, 243–256

Levy, L.S., Martin, P.A. and Venitt, S. (1987) Carcinogenicity of chromium and its salts. *Br. J. Ind. Med.* **44**, 355–357

Levy, L.S. and Venitt, S. (1986) Carcinogenicity of chromium compounds: the association between bronchial metaplasia and neoplasia. *Carcinogenesis* **7**, 831–836

Lloyd, J.W. (1971) Long term mortality study of steel workers: V: respiratory cancer in coke plant workers. *J. Occup. Med.* **13**, 53–68

MacMahon, S., Monson, R.R., Wang H.H. and Zheng, T. (1988) A second follow up of mortality in a cohort of pesticide applicators. *J. Occup. Med.* **30**, 429–432

Malker, H.S.R. and Gemne, G. (1987) A register – epidemiology study on cancer among Swedish printing industry workers. *Archs. Environ. Health* **42**, 73–82

Matanoski, M., Fishbein, L., Redmond, C., Rosenkranz, H. and Wallace, L. (1986) Contribution of organic particulates to respiratory cancer. *Environ. Health Perspect.* **70**, 37–49

Modan, B. (1978) Population distribution of histological types of lung cancer. Epidemiological aspects in Israel and review of the literature. *Israel J. Med. Sci.* **14**, 772–784

Morrison, H.I., Semeciw, R., Mao, Y. and Wigle, D.T. (1988) Cancer mortality among a group of fluorspar miners exposed to radon progeny. *Am. J. Epidemiol.* **128**, 1266–1275

Mur, J.M., Moulin, S.J., Charruyer-Seinerra, M.P. and Lafitte, J. (1987) A cohort mortality study among cobalt and sodium workers in an electrochemical plant. *Am. J. Ind. Med.* **11**, 75–81

National Cancer Institute/International Cancer Research Data Bank (1986) *Oncology Review: Selected Abstracts on Potential Occupational Causes of Cancer. 1. Respiratory Tract,* US Health and Hygiene Service, Washington DC

Nelson, N., Levine, R., Albert, R.E., Blair, A.E., Griesemer, A., Landrigan, P.J., Stayner, L.T. and Swenberg, J.A. (1986) Contribution of formaldehyde to respiratory cancer. *Environ. Health Perspect.* **70**, 23–35

Norseth, T. (1986) The carcinogenicity of chromium and its salts. *Br. J. Ind. Med.* **43**, 649–651

Oberdorster, G. (1986) Airborne cadmium and the carcinogenesis of the respiratory tract. *Scand. J. Work Environ. Health* **12**, 523–537

Peters, J.M., Thomas, D., Falk, H., Oberdorster, G. and Smith, T.J. (1986) Contribution of metals to respiratory cancer. *Environ. Health Perspect.* **70**, 71–83

Pour, P., Stanton, M.F., Kuscher, M., Laskin, S. and Shabad, L.M. (1976) Tumours of the respiratory tract. In: *Pathology of Tumours in Laboratory Animals*, Vol. 1, *Tumours of the Rat*, Part 2, IARC, Lyon, pp. 1–44

Rafnsson, V. and Johannesdottir, S.G. (1986) Mortality among masons in Iceland. *Br. J. Ind. Med.* **43**, 522–525

Redmond, C.K. (1983) Cancer mortality among coke oven workers. *Environ. Health Perspect.* **52**, 67–73

Reij, J.S., Pearce, N.E. and Fraser, J. (1989) Cancer risks among New Zealand meat workers. *Scand. J. Work Environ. Health* **15**, 24–29

Report of International Committee on Nickel Carcinogenesis in Man (1990) *Scand. J. Work Environ. Health* **16**, 1–82

Rinsky, R.A., Melius, J.M., Hornung, R.W., Zumwalde, R.D., Waxweiler, R.J., Landrigan, P.J., Bierbaum, P.J. and Murray, W.E. (1988) Case control study of lung cancer in civilian employees at the Portsmouth Naval Shipyard, Kittery, Maine. *Am. J. Epidemiol.* **127**, 55–64

Ronco, G., Ciccone, G., Mirabelli, D., Troia, B. and Vineis, P. (1988) Occupation and lung cancer in two industrial areas of Northern Italy. *Int. J. Cancer* **41**, 354–358

Saracci, R. (1985) Beryllium: epidemiological evidence. In: *Interpretation for Negative Epidemiological Evidence for Carcinogenicity* (eds N.J. Wald and R. Doll), IARC Scientific Publication No. 65, Lyon, pp. 203–219

Saracci, R. (1987) The interactions of tobacco smoking and other agents in cancer aetiology. *Epidem. Rev.* **9**, 175–193

Seydel, H.G., Chait, A. and Gmelich, J.T. (1975) The natural history of cancer of the lung. In: *Cancer of the Lung* (eds H.G. Seydel, A. Chait and J.T. Gmelich), John Wiley, New York, pp. 52–63

Shimkin, M.B. and Stoner, G.D. (1975) Lung tumours in mice: application to carcinogenesis bioassay. *Adv. Cancer Res.* **21**, 1–58

Siemiatycki, J., Richardson, L., Gerin, M., Goldberg, M., Dewar, R., Desy, M., Campbell, S. and Wacholder, S. (1986) Associations between several sites of cancer and nine organic dusts: results from a hypothesis generating case/control study in Montreal 1979–1983. *Am. J. Epidemiol.* **123**, 235–249

Siemiatycki, J., Gerin, M., Stewart, P., Nadon, L., Dewar, R. and Richardson, L. (1988a) Associations between several sites of cancer and ten types of exhaust and combustion products. *Scand. J. Work Environ. Health* **14**, 79–90

Siemiatycki, J., Wacholder, S., Dewar, R., Cardis, E., Greenwood, C. and Richardson, L. (1988b) Degree of confounding bias related to smoking, ethnic groups, and socio-economic status in estimates of the association between occupation and cancer. *J. Occup. Med.* **30**, 617–625

Simonato, L. and Lavallee-Hawkin, J. (1983) Evidenza epidemiologica di rischio cancerogeno a carico del polmone connesso con l'ambiente lavaratino. *International Congress Proceedings: Il carcinoma del polmone epidemiologa with prevenzione*, Padova 6–8 October 1983, pp. 87–97

Simonato, L. and Saracci, R. (1990) Epidemiological aspects of the relationship between exposure to silica dust and lung cancer. In: *Occupational Exposure to Silica and Cancer Risk* (eds. L. Simonato, A.C. Fletcher R. Saracci and T.L. Thomas), IARC, Lyon, pp. 1–5

Simonato, L., Vineis, P. and Fletcher, A.C. (1988) Estimates of the proportion of lung cancer attributable to occupational exposure. *Carcinogenesis* **9**, 1159–1165

Sobel, W., Bond, G.G., Baldwin, C.L. and Du Commun, D.J. (1988) An update of respiratory cancer and occupational exposure to arsenicals. *Am. J. Ind. Med.* **13**, 263–270

Solli, H.M., Anderson, A., Strawden, E. and Langard, S. (1985) Cancer incidence among workers exposed to radon and thoron daughters at a niobium mine. *Scand. J. Work Environ. Health* **11**, 7–13

Sorahan, T. (1987) Mortality of lung cancer among a cohort of nickel– cadmium battery workers: (1946–84) *Br. J. Ind. Med.* **44**, 803–809

Sorahan, T. and Cathcart, M. (1989) Lung cancer mortality among workers in a factory manufacturing chlorinated toluenes: 1961–84. *Br. J. Ind. Med* **46**, 425–427

Sorahan, T. and Cooke, M.A. (1989) Cancer mortality in a cohort of United Kingdom steel foundry workers: 1946–85. *Br. J. Ind. Med.* **46**, 74–81

Sorahan, T., Burges, D.C.L. and Waterhouse, J.A.H. (1987) A mortality study of nickel/chromium platers. *Br. J. Ind. Med.* **44**, 250–258

Sorahan, T., Parkes, H.G., Veys, C.A. and Waterhouse, J.A.H. (1986) Cancer mortality in the British rubber industry. 1946–1980. *Br. J. Ind. Med.* **43**, 363–373

Sorahan, T., Parkes, H.G., Veys, C.A., Waterhouse, J.A.H., Straughan, J.K. and Nutt, A. (1989) Mortality in the British rubber industry 1946–85. *Br. J. Ind. Med.* **46**, 1–11

Speizer, F.E. (1986) A review of the risks of respiratory cancer from airborne contaminants. *Environ. Health Perspect.* **70**, 9–15

Stanton, M.F. (1974) Fibre carcinogenesis: Is asbestos the only hazard? *J. Natl Cancer Instit.* **52**, 633

Steenland, K. and Beaumont, J. (1986) A proportionate mortality study of granite cutters. *Am. J. Ind. Med.* **9**, 189–201

Steenland, K. and Beaumont, J. (1989) Further follow up and adjustment for smoking in a study of lung cancer and acid mists. *Am. J. Ind. Med.* **16**, 347–354

Steenland, K. and Schnorr, T. (1988) Availability and accuracy of cancer and smoking data obtained from next of kin for decedants in a retrospective cohort study. *J. Occup. Med.* **30**, 348–353

Stockwell, H.G., Lymann, G.H., Waltz, J. and Peters, J.T. (1988) Lung cancer in Florida: Risks associated with residence in the central Florida phosphate mining region. *Am. J. Epidemiol.* **128**, 78–84

Thun, M.J., Schnorr, T.M., Smith, A.B., Halperin, W.E. and Lemen, R.A. (1985) Mortality among a cohort of US cadmium production workers – an update. *J. Natl Cancer Instit.* **74**, 325–333

Tola, S., Kalliomaki, P-L., Pukkala, E., Asp, S. and Korkala, M-L. (1988) Incidence of cancer among welders, platers, machinists and pipe fitters in shipyards and machine shops. *Br. J. Ind. Med.* **45**, 209–218

Tornling, G., Hogstedt, C. and Westerholm, P. (1988) Lung cancer incidence among Swedish ceramic workers with silicosis. In: *Progress in Occupational Epidemiology* (eds C. Hogstedt and C. Reuterwall), Excerpta Medica, Amsterdam, pp. 167–170

US National Toxicology Program (1984) Report of the NTP ad hoc Panel on chemical carcinogenesis testing and evaluation,

Washington DC. US Department of Health and Human Services

Vineis, P. and Simonato, L. (1991) Proportion of lung and bladder cancer in males resulting from occupation: a systematic approach. *Archs Environ. Health* **46**, 6–15

Wada, S., Nisihmoto, Y., Miyanishi, M., Kambe, S. and Miller R.W. (1968) Mustard gas as a cause of respiratory neoplasia in man. *Lancet* **1**, 1161–1163

Weisburger, J.H. and Williams, G.M. (1980) Chemical carcinogens. In: *Toxicology* (eds J. Doull, C.D. Klaassen and M.O. Admur), MacMillan, London, pp. 84–138

World Health Organization (1982) The World Health Organization histological typing of lung tumours. *Am. J. Clin. Pathol.* **77**, 123–136

Wong, O. (1988) A cohort mortality study of employees exposed to chlorinated chemicals. *Am. J. Ind. Med.* **14**, 417–431

Yamagiwa, K. and Ichikawa, K. (1918) Experimental study of the pathogenesis of carcinoma. *J. Cancer Res.* **3**, 1

Yesner, R.C. (1980) The spectrum of lung cancer histopathology. In: *Prevention and Detection of Cancer*, Part II, Vol. 2 (ed. H.E. Neiburgs), Marcel Dekker, New York, pp. 1403–1407

Zhang, Z-F., Yu, S-Z., Li, W-X. and Choi, B.K. (1989) Smoking, occupational exposure to rubber and lung cancer. *Br. J. Ind. Med.* **46**, 12–15

20

Extrinsic allergic bronchioloalveolitis (hypersensitivity pneumonia)

C.A.C. Pickering and Anthony J. Newman Taylor

Introduction

The range of extrinsic organic agents that can be inhaled as fine particulate matter or aerosols in occupational or other circumstances and give rise to lung disease is large. It includes vegetable dusts (notably fungal spores), proteins of animal and piscine origin, various pathognomonic micro-organisms (such as bacteria, *Rickettsia* and *Chlamydia*), vegetable and mineral oils, and certain organic chemicals.

This chapter is concerned with hypersensitivity lung disease due to antigenic proteins or other matter.

Hypersensitivity lung disease, in general, is the result of different types of allergic reaction and takes two distinct forms – *asthma* and *extrinsic allergic bronchioloalveolitis* (hypersensitivity pneumonia in the USA). Occasionally both types of disorder occur in the same individual. Occupational asthma is discussed in Chapter 21 and other disorders caused by organic agents in Chapters 22 and 23.

Extrinsic allergic bronchioloalveolitis (hypersensitivity pneumonia)

This is a generic term for a common manifestation of a variety of causes. It can be defined as a clinical disorder due to the inhalation of particulate antigenic, organic material and is characterized in its *acute phase* by constitutional symptoms, the presence of specific precipitating antibodies (precipitins) in many cases and by lymphocytic infiltration and sarcoid-type granulomas in the walls of alveoli and small airways; in its *chronic phase* it is characterized by an irreversible and often progressive diffuse intrapulmonary fibrosis. It must be emphasized, however, that the 'acute' phase is often clinically subacute and not an illness of abrupt onset. The majority of affected individuals are non-atopic.

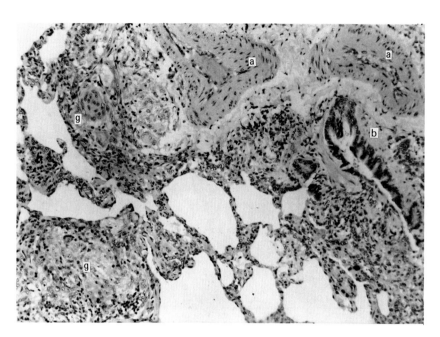

Figure 20.1 Acute extrinsic alveolitis in a farmer. Sarcoid-type granulomas (g) and infiltration of alveolar walls by lymphocytes and plasma cells; arteries (a) and involvement of the wall of a bronchiole (b) with narrowing of its lumen. Magnification × 120. (Courtesy of Dr R.M.E. Seal)

Due to the fact that the disease process involves respiratory bronchioles as well as alveoli, the term 'alveolitis' falls short and 'bronchioloalveolitis' is preferable (Seal, 1975). However, this being understood, allergic alveolitis will be used throughout for convenience.

A large group of allergens is now known or believed to cause extrinsic allergic alveolitis (Table 20.1) and there appears to be no limit to the potential sources. Recent additions include *wine growers' lung* (Popp et al., 1987), *fertilizer workers' lung* (Kagen et al., 1981), *potato riddlers' lung* (Greene and Bannan, 1985) and *woodmen's disease* (Dykewicz et al., 1988). In general, they fall into two major groups: microbial spores arising from moulding vegetable matter and animal proteins, principally avian in origin. One important characteristic of these various allergens is that the particles are sufficiently small for a high proportion of them to penetrate to and deposit in the gas-exchanging region of the lungs. The spores of thermophilic actinomycetes associated with farmers' lung, for example, range from 0.7 to 2.0 μm in diameter. The spores of *Aspergillus clavatus,* the cause of malt workers' lung, are slightly larger in diameter, being about 3.5 μm. Avian protein aggregates are considerably smaller. The disease is usually associated with an occupation or hobby, because a high level of exposure to the allergen is required to induce sensitization.

It should be realized that the specific causal agent has only been identified in a small number of the disease types listed and evidence of an immunological mechanism (if, in fact, one is involved) is not always complete. The presence of precipitins in some cases is, of course, evidence of an immunological reaction but not necessarily of its involvement in pathogenesis. Furthermore, they are often present in the absence of disease, but the development of the clinical features of disease in association with repeated exposure to a particular material is a reasonably good indication of a causal relationship.

The pathology, pathogenesis and clinical characteristics will be considered first in general terms followed by an outline of features peculiar to each type of the disease.

Pathology

Acute disease

Details of the pathology of acute disease have been obtained almost entirely from biopsy material taken at varying intervals from the onset of symptoms. Bronchoscopically the large bronchi are usually intensely congested (Fuller, 1953).

Microscopic appearances

Initially there is oedema of the lungs with a predominantly lymphocytic infiltration and thickening of

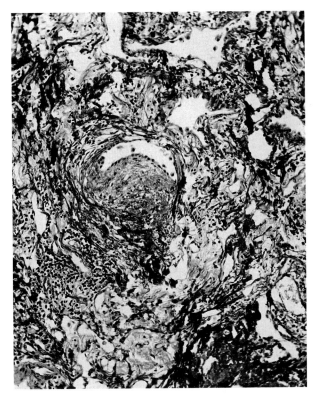

Figure 20.2 Subacute extrinsic allergic alveolitis in a bird fancier showing a large granulomatous lesion in the wall of a bronchiole almost obstructing its lumen, round cell infiltration and early changes of DIPF. Magnification × 120. (Reproduced with permission from Hinson, 1970)

alveolar walls and plasma cells are usually – but not always – prominent. Within the first 2 weeks, as oedema subsides, numerous non-caseating, sarcoid-type epithelioid granulomas with Langhans' giant cells develop (Figure 20.1). These changes were referred to as 'acute granulomatous pneumonitis' by Dickie and Rankin (1958).

The granulomas, many of which are surrounded by a narrow band of collagen fibres, are similar in appearance to those seen in sarcoidosis, chronic beryllium disease, tuberculosis without caseation, brucellosis, and various fungal and protozoal infections (Jones Williams, 1967). But they sometimes contain birefringent bodies which are thought to be of vegetable origin (Molina, 1976). They occur in alveolar walls and in the walls of terminal and respiratory bronchioles which they may almost obliterate (Figures 20.1 and 20.2) and they tend to favour the centre of the lobule. Bronchiolitis is fairly common and the walls of related pulmonary arteries and arterioles are occasionally thickened by swelling of their muscle fibres and endothelial cells (Seal, 1975). Necrosing vasculitis is, however, not seen.

In contrast to sarcoidosis granulomas are not found in the hilar lymph nodes (Seal et al., 1968).

An exceptional case of extremely acute disease in a young farmer showed numerous discrete, grey-coloured, miliary nodules throughout the lungs to the naked eye. The nodules consisted of large numbers of lymphocytes, epithelial cells and early reticulin formation, but relatively few plasma cells and neutrophils, and no granulomas. Acute necrosing alveolitis was also present (Barrowcliff and Arblaster, 1968). It is possible, however, that this may have been a case of acute mycoplasma pneumonia which can produce *Faenia rectivirgula (Micropolyspora faeni)*-like precipitins.

The granulomas resolve in about 3 or 4 months and are replaced by a substantial lymphocytic infiltration of alveolar walls and scattered lymphoid follicles with germinal centres. The inflammatory thickening of the walls is more pronounced than that seen in sarcoidosis. Some reticulin or fine collagen fibrosis may also be present. Hyalinized granulomas, similar to those seen in some cases of sarcoidosis and chronic beryllium disease, do not occur. This may reflect different rates of 'turnover' of macrophages and their derivative epithelial cells (Spector, 1971).

Thermophilic actinomycetes have been isolated from lung biopsy specimens (Wenzel et al., 1964) and fungal spores can sometimes be identified with special stains.

Little is known of the pathology during the transition period from acute to chronic disease.

Chronic disease

Macroscopic appearances

There may be some thickening of the pulmonary pleura although this is not often prominent. However, in advanced disease multiple, thick-walled, 'hob-nail' cysts ('air blebs') are common.

The cut surface of the lungs displays the appearances of a fine DIPF which is confluent in places forming large, irregular, solid masses. Smooth-walled 'honeycomb' cysts up to 2 or 3 cm in diameter are often associated with the fibrosis. Characteristically these changes are distributed predominantly in the upper halves of the lungs but occasionally this is reversed, and advanced diseases may be generalized (Figure 20.3). In some cases the fibrosis is so delicate and the cysts so small that they are not readily identified if the lungs are not prepared by formalin perfusion or barium sulphate impregnation (see Appendix III). Such fine fibrosis and dilated airspaces may be mistaken for emphysema.

Microscopic appearances

There is diffuse collagenous fibrosis of alveolar walls, around terminal and respiratory bronchioles

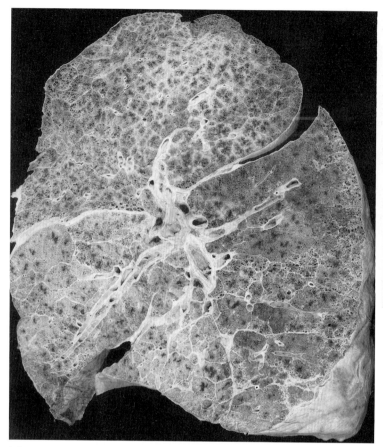

(a)

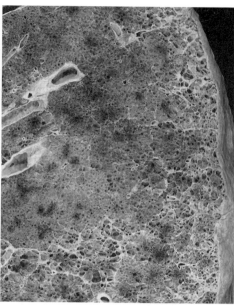

(b)

Figure 20.3 Naked eye appearances of chronic extrinsic alveolitis in a farmworker. (a) Whole lung slice; (b) widespread, sharply demarcated DIPF with numerous small honeycomb cysts in lower lobe. Note diffuse thickening of pulmonary pleura. (Courtesy of Dr R.M.E. Seal)

and perivascular zones. Large tracts of collagen are often a feature of the fibrotic areas which may extend to the periphery of the lobule. Scattered bronchiolitis, which is said to occur in about one-third of cases, may be seen and is sometimes associated with centrilobular emphysema (Seal, 1975). Granulomas are absent but a few may still be found if the latent period since the episode of acute disease is not longer than about 12 months. Foreign body giant cells containing birefringement material of uncertain identity may be present but plasma cells are usually absent, although substantial numbers may be found in the medulla of hilar lymph nodes (Seal et al., 1968). Medial thickening of pulmonary arteries indicative of pulmonary hypertension will usually be seen in the more advanced cases.

Pathogenesis

The pathogenesis of extrinsic allergic alveolitis involves immunological mechanisms and, in all probability, other non-immunological factors, but,

owing to conflicting experimental results and controversy over the significance of the serological findings, it is not readily explained.

The features of farmers' lung and bird fanciers' lung which are the most common types of extrinsic allergic alveolitis and, thus, the most extensively studied probably apply to all the other types (Table 20.1).

Immunological mechanisms

Humoral immunity

Evidence for disease being a consequence of complement-fixing immune complex deposition in alveoli includes the following:

1. High concentrations of IgG antibody are present in the serum of individuals with acute disease.
2. Reactions in the skin to intradermal injection of antigen have the time characteristics of an Arthus reaction, and perivascular IgG and complement are demonstrable by immunofluorescence on biopsy.

Table 20.1 Types of extrinsic allergic alveolitis

Type	Nature of responsible aerosol	Nature of antigen
Farmers' lung	Mouldy hay, straw or grain	*Faenia rectivirgula, Thermoactinomyces vulgaris, T. thalpophilus*
Bird fanciers' lung	Bloom, droppings	Avian proteins
Bagassosis	Mouldy sugar cane	*T. sacchari*
Mushroom workers' lung	Compost dust	Thermophilic actinomycetes, mushroom spores
Malt workers' lung	Mouldy barley	*Aspergillus clavatus*
Suberosis	Mouldy corkbark dust	*Penicillium frequentans*
Maple bark strippers' lung	Mouldy bark dust	*Cryptostroma corticale*
Wood pulp workers' disease	Mouldy bark dust	*Alternaria* sp.
Air-conditioner disease	Dust or mist	*F. rectivirgula, A. pullulans, T. vulgaris, Cephalosporium* sp.
Humidifer fever	Contaminated water	Endotoxin?
Sewage sludge disease	Dust of heat-treated sludge	Gram-negative bacteria
Sauna-takers' disease	Contaminated steam	*Aureobasidium pullulans*
Sequoiosis	Mouldy sawdust – redwood	*Aureobasidium pullulans, Graphium* sp.?
Cheese washers' lung	Mould dust	*Penicillium casei*, acarids?
Dry rot lung	Mould dust	*Merulius lacrymans*
Wheat weevil lung	Mouldy grain and flour dust	*Sitophilus granarius*
Animal handlers' lung	Dust or dander, hair particles and dried urine of rats	Serum and urine proteins
Fish meal workers' lung	Fish meal dust	Fish proteins
Diisocyanate alveolitis	Vapour	TDI and MDI
Pyrethrum alveolitis	Insecticide aerosol	Pyrethrum
Pituitary snuff takers' lung	Therapeutic snuff	Pig or ox protein
Winegrowers' lung	Mould dust	*Botrytis cinerea*
Potato riddlers' lung	Straw dust	*F. rectivirgula*
Fertilizer workers' lung	Air-borne bacteria	*Streptomyces albus*
Woodmen's disease	Mouldy bark dust	*Penicillium* sp.
Laboratory workers' lung	Pauli's reagent	Sodium diazobenzenesulphate

TDI = toluene diisocyanate.
MDI = methylene diphenyl diisocyanate.

3. Natural exposure to and inhalation tests with antigen provoke reaction in gas-exchanging parts of the lung with similar time characteristics to reactions in the skin.

This does not explain the characteristic feature of acute extrinsic allergic alveolitis: sarcoid-type granulomas which are not associated with type III Arthus reactions. However, granulomas have been induced experimentally by injection of antigen–antibody complexes that are not complement fixing (Spector and Heesom, 1969). The pathological features of the case of Barrowcliff and Arblaster (1968), referred to earlier, are consistent with an Arthus reaction.

Precipitins against particular antigenic components may mediate reactions in one individual but not in another. Thus, they are often found in healthy (asymptomatic) persons who have had similar exposure as well as in those with disease. Precipitins to thermophilic actinomycetes are present in a proportion (about 18 per cent) of healthy farmers (Pepys, 1969) and to avian antigens in up to 40 per cent of asymptomatic pigeon fanciers (Fink et al., 1968), but rarely in budgerigar and parrot fanciers

(Pepys, 1977). This may reflect different levels of exposure to the antigen or sensitivity of the test – IgA ELISA – being more frequently found (ELISA = enzyme-linked immunosorbent assay).

There is some evidence that type I allergy, which is mediated by reaginic IgE or by short-term sensitizing IgG antibodies (see Chapter 4) may be required for the development of the type III reaction (Pepys, 1969; Cochrane, 1971). This has been invoked to explain why precipitins are more often present in affected than in non-affected individuals (Pepys, 1978). However, specific precipitins are absent in some persons with proven extrinsic allergic alveolitis. This may reflect the sensitivity of the precipitin test or failure to identify the correct causative antigen. In spite of the uncertainty of the part played by precipitins and their relevance in diagnosis, they provide evidence of exposure and are the chief means by which most types of extrinsic allergic alveolitis have been, and are, first identified.

Although the complexity of antigens in farmers' lung makes quantification of the related antibodies difficult, IgG, IgM and IgA antibodies are demonstrable by immunofluorescent and radio-immunoassay techniques (Parratt et al., 1975; Patterson et al., 1976). Similarly IgG antibodies capable of fixing complement and small quantities of IgM and IgA antibodies have been demonstrated in pigeon fanciers' disease and also in healthy individuals with similar exposures to birds (Fink, Tebo and Barboriak, 1969; Moore and Fink, 1975; Boren et al., 1977). Deposits of IgG and complement have occasionally been found in lesions of pulmonary vasculitis (Ghose et al., 1974), but evidence of pulmonary vasculitis is rarely found in lung biopsy material and then only in the face of recent acute disease (Sutinen et al., 1983). A consistent finding in extrinsic allergic alveolitis, but not in sarcoidosis, is the presence of IgM in the bronchoalveolar fluid; the IgG albumin ratio is greater than 1 in extrinsic allergic alveolitis but less than 1 in sarcoidosis (Weinberger et al., 1978). Indeed, IgG and IgA levels in bronchial lavage fluid of individuals with bird (pigeon) fanciers' lung are significantly higher than in exposed but healthy persons (Calvanico et al., 1980). The IgG subclass, IgG3, is increased in farmers' lung patients compared with 'control' farmers, suggesting that they have a tendency to produce this antibody type (Stokes, Turton and Turner-Warwick, 1981).

Precipitin tests in routine use (usually agar gel diffusion techniques) are relatively insensitive and may fail to demonstrate antibodies in all cases, whereas radio-immunoassay will detect them in most (Parratt and Boyd, 1976). This probably explains some, but not all, cases of precipitin-negative disease and may make the interpretation of some earlier investigations difficult.

Hay dust, *Faenia rectivirgula* (*M.faeni*) and pigeon serum antigens are capable of activating the C3 component of complement in vitro directly with intervention of antibody – that is, by the alternative pathway (Berrens, Guikders and Van Dijk, 1974; Edwards, Baker and Davies, 1974; Edwards, 1976; Marx and Flaherty, 1976; Bice et al., 1977) (see Chapter 4, page 54). It is suggested that after inhalation the antigens are rapidly ingested by macrophages causing them to secrete C3-cleaving enzymes. The resultant activated C3 (C3b) then stimulates macrophages to release other factors (which include fibrogenic factor) and leucocytes to produce tissue-damaging enzymes (Schorlemmer et al., 1977) (Figure 20.4). However, it is not clear either whether the same antigens can activate both classic and alternative pathways or whether the activation of one or other pathway is determined by the *nature* of the antigen or by the *amount* inhaled. Whilst this hypothesis explains some cases of precipitin-negative acute extrinsic allergic alveolitis, it does not readily account for the characteristic granulomas. However, transient granulomas with Langhans' giant cells have been shown to develop 8 days after intratracheal deposition of mouldy hay dust in unsensitized rats and rabbits, apparently

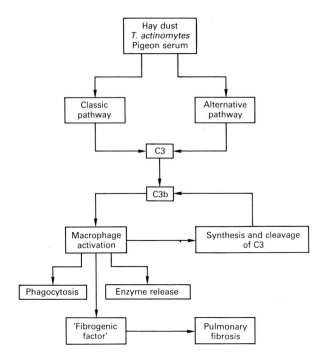

Figure 20.4 Schema of suggested interaction between the complement system and macrophages in extrinsic allergic alveolitis

without the involvement of a specific immunological response (Edwards, Wagner and Seal, 1976, 1980). Other antigens that cause extrinsic allergic alveolitis have not yet been shown to activate the alternative pathway of complement.

Massive exposure of farmworkers to a variety of saprophytic fungi when unsealing silos has been reported to cause disease similar to extrinsic allergic alveolitis (see 'Organic dust toxic syndrome') which has been suggested as being caused by this mechanism.

T-lymphocyte-dependent response

The granulomatous nature of extrinsic allergic alveolitis is more characteristic of a T lymphocyte than an immune complex inflammatory response. Until the advent of the technique of bronchoalveolar lavage (BAL), evidence for T-cell involvement in the human disease was largely lacking.

There is evidence, in experimental animals, that thermophilic actinomycetes, a major source of antigen in extrinsic allergic alveolitis, have an adjuvant effect on both antibody production and type IV cell-mediated immunity (Bice et al., 1977). It has been suggested that, in human beings, both immune complex and T-lymphocyte-dependent responses are involved in the pathogenesis of extrinsic allergic alveolitis (Pepys, 1978). Such a concept is supported by recent bronchoalveolar lavage studies (see Chapter 4).

The initial event following antigen challenge is the migration of polymorphonuclear leucocytes into the alveoli (Costabel et al., 1984; Fournier et al., 1985) which may be the outcome of an immune complex-mediated reaction. This neutrophil migration occurs in response to the release of neutrophil chemotactic factors which can be demonstrated in bronchoalveolar lavage fluid (Yoshizawa et al., 1986). The degree of chemotactic activity is related to the activity of the disease, being highest in the acute stages. The neutrophil recovery in BAL is transient and by 8 days after antigen challenge the numbers of neutrophils have returned to pre-challenge levels (Fournier et al., 1985). This is succeeded by an increase in the number of T lymphocytes recovered at BAL which is the characteristic finding of both subacute and chronic allergic alveolitis (Bernardo et al., 1979; Cormier et al., 1986). It is also found in cases of active pulmonary sarcoidosis – a disease from which allergic alveolitis must be differentiated. The absolute number of T lymphocytes in active sarcoidosis is usually less than in allergic alveolitis. There is also a difference in the proportions of T-cell subset populations in these two diseases. In allergic alveolitis there is a predominance of CD_8 (cytotoxic-suppressor) T lymphocytes and a decrease in the $CD_4:CD_8$ ratio of T lymphocytes in BAL (see Chapter 4, page 66). This contrasts with sarcoidosis (and beryllium disease) where there is a predominance of CD_4 (inducer) T lymphocytes (Leatherman et al., 1984; Rossman et al., 1988). The presence of increased numbers of CD_8 T lymphocytes, however, does not necessarily reflect the presence of disease. In both asymptomatic dairy farmers and pigeon breeders, increased numbers of T lymphocytes with a predominance of CD_8 phenotype have been reported in the BAL fluid (Solal-Celigny et al., 1982; Leatherman et al., 1984). T lymphocytes have been reported from cases of disease to show functional differences from those of asymptomatic exposed workers. Whereas T lymphocytes from asymptomatic individuals inhibit the blood lymphocytic response to stimulation by pigeon serum, BAL lymphocytes from cases of disease do not inhibit and may stimulate this response (Keller et al., 1984). Follow-up studies of asymptomatic farmers with BAL lymphocytosis over 2 to 3 years have not demonstrated the development of disease in any individual (Cormier et al., 1986). It remains to be seen whether evidence of disease will develop on longer follow-up.

Recent observations have identified an additional cell, the *mast cell*, which may be involved in the cell-mediated immune process. BAL samples from patients with extrinsic allergic alveolitis have revealed the presence of increased numbers of mast cells compared to samples from controls, sarcoidosis or cryptogenic fibrosing alveolitis (Haslam et al., 1987). After removal of patients from exposure to the antigen, the mast cell counts initially rise (Soler et al., 1987) and later fall to normal (Haslam et al., 1987). The mast cells are thought to be of 'mucosal' type and ultrastructurally have a greater similarity to bronchial subepithelial mast cells than to pulmonary interstitial or dermal connective tissue mast cells. The role of the mast cell in the inflammatory process of extrinsic allergic alveolitis still needs to be clarified.

Host factors

Only a very small proportion of people exposed regularly to the known causes of extrinsic allergic alveolitis ever develop disease. This suggests that individual susceptibility is important in its development. Initially reports suggested that there was an association between certain HLA antigens (notably B8) and the occurrence of farmers' lung and pigeon fanciers' lung (Allen et al., 1975; Flaherty et al., 1975; Berrill and Van Rood, 1977; Sennekamp, Rittner and Vogel, 1977; Terho et al., 1981) and also that individuals with P_2 positive blood group were less likely than other groups to develop pigeon fanciers' lung (Effler, Roland and Redding, 1976). However, Rodey et al. (1979) and Terho et al. (1981) found no association between any HLA phenotypes that they examined. Similarly, Flaherty et al. (1980) found no significant correlations between any of the serologically detectable HLA-A, -B and -C loci antigens and farmers' lung.

A host factor of importance in the development of disease is the smoking habit of the exposed individuals. A survey of Devon farmers showed that precipitins to *F. rectivirgula* (*M. faeni*) were significantly more prevalent among non-smokers and ex-smokers than among smokers (Morgan et al., 1973). This increased prevalence of precipitins has subsequently been confirmed for both avian and farmers' lung antigens in non-smokers both with and without disease; the intensity of the antibody response, however, does not appear to be affected by smoking habits (Morgan et al., 1975; Boyd et al., 1977; Warren, 1977; Cormier et al., 1986). The explanation may well lie in changes in the local immunological system in the lungs of smokers (Holt and Keast, 1977; Andersen et al., 1982) or in antigen presentation by macrophages (Editorial, 1985).

Summary

It seems likely that some or all of the pathogenic mechanisms described may be involved in the development of extrinsic allergic alveolitis in varying degree at different stages and that the immunoregulation of T-lymphocyte activity in the lungs is particularly important in the translation of the immunological to the inflammatory response in the alveoli.

Clinical features

There is considerable variability in the initial presentation and subsequent course of extrinsic allergic alveolitis. In 1953, Fuller suggested that farmers' lung occurred in three phases: an acute, subacute and chronic phase. A similar classification has been suggested for pigeon fanciers' (breeders') lung (Fink et al., 1968). Boyd et al. (1982) introduced a time factor into the patterns of disease seen in pigeon fanciers. They described symptom complexes which included acute progressive, acute intermittent non-progressive and recurrent non-acute disease. It is likely that similar symptom patterns occur in farmers' lung.

Acute and subacute disease

Symptoms

Characteristically these occur about 4 to 8 hours following heavy exposure to the offending antigen, although they may take several days to develop fully. They include cough, rigors, sweating, fever, marked anorexia, muscle and joint pains, and occasionally nausea and vomiting. Breathlessness on effort is invariable and sometimes severe. Haemoptysis is rare. Pain in the chest does not occur other than from cough–fracture of ribs.

The pattern of symptoms, however, varies from patient to patient. In some they are predominantly systemic, in others, respiratory. They may be mild or very severe. Due to the similarity of the symptoms to those of a variety of bacterial and viral diseases, it is essential to obtain a detailed history of relevant exposure. This is especially true of subacute disease in which increasing breathlessness, fever and ill-health may take some days to develop making its origin difficult to recognize.

Providing there is no further exposure to the cause, symptoms usually subside after about 48 hours, but they may not cease completely for 7 to 10 days. Profound loss of weight may be associated with acute episodes of disease and in some cases dyspnoea on effort may persist for a few months.

Physical signs

There is tachycardia and fever which may be as high as 46°C (106°F) and, in patients with predominantly respiratory symptoms, there may be dyspnoea at rest. The severity of the dyspnoea may be sufficiently severe to require hospital treatment. Central cyanosis is sometimes present, and restlessness and apprehension may be prominent. These signs may take several days to become established.

Fine- to medium-pitched, often patchy, crackles may be heard towards the end of full inspiration over the lower halves of the lung fields. They disappear completely with recovery. In addition, inspiratory 'squawks' may also be heard (see Chapter 6). Wheezes are not a feature of the disease but may occur in a small number of patients (Pepys, 1969). There are no signs of consolidation or pleural effusion.

Chronic disease

Symptoms

After repeated acute episodes, a variable amount of sputum and dyspnoea on effort develops, in most cases, increasing progressively after each separate illness although, sometimes, these symptoms occur after a single episode of acute disease. By contrast, in those cases in which there has been recurrent exposure to low concentrations of mould dust, symptoms develop insidiously without any antecedent acute episode; this is particularly apt to occur in bird fanciers' lung associated with long contact with only one or two birds. Dyspnoea tends gradually to worsen in most cases without further exposure to antigen, but the degree of change is variable. There are no constitutional symptoms.

Physical signs

There are no characteristic signs. Central cyanosis is not evident at rest until disease is advanced but may be observed after effort when it is less advanced. Clubbing of the fingers is rarely seen. Signs of widespread fibrosis with deviation of the trachea and impairment of chest expansion of the more affected side are sometimes present. Adventitious sounds are heard in only a minority of cases but, when they are, they consist of inspiratory crackles, either in the latter part of inspiration or pan-inspiratory, of medium to coarse quality. Persistent, late, inspiratory 'squawks' often audible at the mouth, are a feature of some cases (see Chapter 6, page 150). Wheeze is absent. The rarity of clubbing and infrequency of adventitious sounds contrast with the findings in idiopathic DIPF.

The signs of pulmonary heart disease and congestive heart failure may occur in advanced disease.

Investigations

Acute and subacute disease

Lung function

The earliest abnormality to occur is widening of the alveolar–arterial P_{O_2} gradient on exertion. This is followed by a reduction in vital capacity (VC), total lung capacity (TLC) and compliance, and a decrease in gas transfer that tends to be proportional to the reduction in VC. In some cases the decrement in gas transfer is due to inequality of ventilation–perfusion ratios as is shown by a normal gas transfer coefficient (K_{CO}) and a significant increase in arterial oxygen tension on breathing pure oxygen. In others there is an alveolar membrane component indicated by a low K_{CO}. Evidence of airflow obstruction as determined by FEV_1 (forced expiratory volume in 1 second) and FVC (forced vital capacity) is absent but flow–volume curves reveal increased up-stream airflow resistance which is probably situated in the small airways due to their involvement in the disease process (Warren, Tse and Cherniak, 1978). In certain instances the inflammatory process may predominantly involve the bronchioles with only a patchy alveolitis being present (Harries, Heard and Geddes, 1984) causing reduced flow rates at low lung volumes, a raised residual volume, normal total lung capacity and impaired gas transfer. The degree of impairment of these functional parameters varies from mild to severe according to the severity of the disease.

Bronchial hyperreactivity is demonstrable in a proportion of cases (Freedman and Ault, 1981; Monkare et al., 1981) and may persist for months following an acute episode. Most lung function abnormalities resolve within 6 weeks in most patients treated with corticosteroids (Hapke et al., 1968) and in 12 months in the majority who are not treated. However, some individuals continue to demonstrate abnormalities in gas transfer and compliance after becoming asymptomatic and after the chest radiograph has returned to normal (Williams, 1963; Allen, Williams and Woolcock, 1976).

Radiographic appearances

In mild attacks the chest film may remain normal. Rarely, it may be normal associated with severe physiological abnormalities (Arshad, Braun and Sunderrajan, 1987). Otherwise abnormalities vary from barely detectable changes to widespread coarse opacities similar to the appearance of acute beryllium disease (see Figure 17.1) or acute pulmonary oedema.

The earliest changes consist of very fine, pinpoint opacities (a 'ground glass' or miliary appearance) in the central two-thirds or lower zones of the lung fields and may be so subtle as to be overlooked

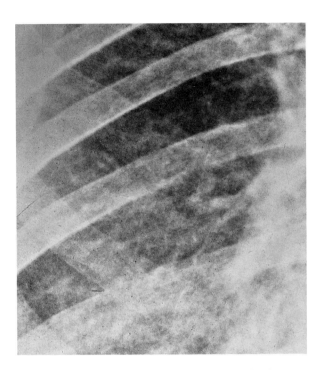

Figure 20.5 Small opacities due to extrinsic allergic alveolitis in a farmer's wife. The appearances were uniformly distributed throughout both lung fields. Complete resolution occurred

(Figure 20.5). They are often only detected in retrospect by comparison with films taken after the patient has recovered. The use of an anteroposterior (AP) in addition to a standard posteroanterior (PA) film viewed with a hand lens increases the likelihood of their detection.

More definite abnormalities consist of discrete, well-defined opacities ranging from pinpoint size to about 3 mm in diameter in the middle and lower zones of the lung fields, but frequently sparing the costophrenic angles (see Figure 20.7a). In severe attacks larger, blotchy opacities are seen. However, the degree of radiographic abnormality correlates poorly with the severity of the symptoms.

Larger opacities usually disappear within 2 or 3 weeks after avoidance of exposure, but the fine type may last up to 6 months before clearing. If fine opacities fail to resolve in 6 to 12 months they are unlikely to do so and will ultimately be replaced by the changes of chronic fibrotic disease (Hapke et al., 1968).

Evidence of bilateral hilar node enlargement or of pleural effusion is not seen.

Serology

Precipitins specific to the antigen responsible for the disease are present in the majority of cases – about 90 per cent – if sufficiently sensitive tests are used.

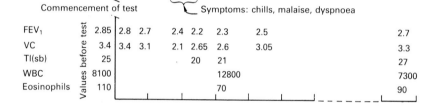

Figure 20.6 Systemic and pulmonary reactions to inhalation challenge with avian antigens in a patient with 'bird breeders' lung'. (Courtesy of Professor J. Pepys)

Bronchoscopy

The advent of fibreoptic bronchoscopy and the ability to lavage and biopsy the lung provides additional important assistance in diagnosing allergic alveolitis. Bronchoalveolar lavage in both acute and chronic disease reveals the presence of a lymphocytic alveolitis. The absence of a lymphocytic alveolitis in an individual still in contact with the antigen thought to be causing his or her disease would exclude the diagnosis (Voisin et al., 1981; Cormier et al., 1986).

Transbronchial biopsies may yield tissue containing non-caseating granulomas (Arshad, Braun and Sunderrajan, 1987).

Bronchial (inhalation) provocation tests

Some years ago it was shown that controlled inhalation of the relevant antigen is followed by a systemic reaction in 4 to 8 hours after challenge accompanied by a transient rise in temperature, mild leucocytosis, restriction of ventilation and fall in FEV_1 and, in some instances, gas transfer (Figure 20.6). In a small proportion of cases this is preceded by an immediate asthmatic reaction with airflow obstruction (Pepys, 1969). More recently it has been confirmed that there are six practical measurements which indicate a positive late response to challenge: increase of body temperature (>37.2°C), circulating

neutrophils $\geq$ +2500/mm²), exercise minute ventilation ($\geq$ +15 per cent) and exercise respiratory frequency ($\geq$ +25 per cent); and decrease of circulating lymphocytes ($\geq$ –500/mm³ with lymphopenia) and FVC ($\geq$ –15 per cent). These confirmatory tests have specificities of approximately 95 per cent and sensitivities of 85 to 48 per cent. Auscultation and chest radiography and measurement of T_L and lung volume subdivisions are too insensitive to be useful. However, challenge doses sufficient to provoke significant changes in these tests may be potentially dangerous and are, if possible, better avoided (Hendrick et al., 1980). But, in general, provocation tests are only indicated in suspect cases of extrinsic allergic alveolitis in which precipitin tests are negative and chest radiographs normal (Harries, Burge and O'Brien, 1980) (see also Chapter 21, page 727).

Skin reactions

In general these are of little value due mainly to the fact that there are few suitable extracts available which do not cause non-specific reactions. An exception to this is an intracutaneous test with avian extract but it is unlikely to provide more information than specific precipitins (see 'Bird fanciers' lung'). The Kveim test appears to be negative in many cases (Molina, 1976).

Haematology

There are no specific abnormalities. The sedimentation rate is raised and there is a mild polymorphonuclear leucocytosis but no eosinophilia. These changes are short-lived.

Sputum

There are no unusual features on naked eye or microscopic examination. But different strains of the *Thermoactinomyces* sp. can be cultured from specimens expectorated by patients who have been exposed to mouldy hay (see 'Farmers' lung'), and the percentage of T lymphocytes among the total number of cells in bronchoalveolar lavage fluid is significantly increased (see 'Pathogenesis').

Lung biopsy

This is rarely necessary or justifiable. It is discussed briefly under 'Diagnosis'.

Chronic disease

Lung function

Patterns of impaired function are variable. The most common pattern is a restrictive ventilatory defect, increased RV/TLC ratio and impaired gas transfer (RV = residual volume). However, in some patients there is reduction of gas transfer and compliance with or without decrease in lung volume, but no evidence of airflow obstruction. In others – about a third – there is slight to moderate, irreversible airflow obstruction (reduced $FEV_1/FVC\%$ and increased RV) which may be due to bronchiolitis obliterans of terminal and respiratory bronchioles as a sequela of granulomatous infiltration (see 'Pathology'). In yet other patients both types of functional impairment are combined (Dickie and Rankin, 1958; Hapke et al., 1968). Compliance is usually reduced (increased elastic recoil), often considerably, but in some cases it is increased together with reduction of airflow indicating associated emphysematous changes (Warren, Tse and Cherniack, 1978).

There is sometimes a discrepancy between the symptoms complained of and the values of lung function tests at rest which may be near normal. This is analogous to the situation in early asbestosis and chronic beryllium disease.

Cardiac catheterization reveals the presence of pulmonary hypertension in some cases which appears to be caused by obliterative reduction of the vascular bed as pulmonary scintigraphy with ^{131}I has shown (Bishop, Melnick and Raine, 1963; Molina, 1976).

Radiographic appearances

These vary according to the severity of the disease. They range from fine, linear or rounded, ill-defined opacities to coarse linear opacities that tend to radiate from the hilar regions and, in advanced disease, are accompanied by tracheal deviation and distortion, lobar contraction, and by small translucent areas caused by cyst formation (Figures 20.7 and 20.8). By contrast with acute disease these appearances predominate in the upper and middle zones, and are often more pronounced on one side. They are indistinguishable from fibrocavernous tuberculosis, chronic sarcoidosis and, in some cases, allergic bronchopulmonary aspergillosis. Undue translucency of the lower zones may be present. Occasionally fibrotic appearances are more predominant in the middle or lower zones than in the upper zones.

Chronic disease may also be represented by small discrete opacities when these remain unchanged for about a year. They do not necessarily progress to the 'fibrotic' appearances just described. If serial chest films are not available these opacities could, in the presence of an acute respiratory illness, be interpreted as evidence of acute extrinsic allergic alveolitis or of some unrelated disease.

Serology

In the case of chronic disease the chance of demonstrating precipitins becomes less as the time since the last acute episode increases. Precipitins are still present in about 80 per cent of cases up to 3 years after an attack of acute farmers' lung disease, but in only about 20 per cent when the interval is longer than 3 years (Hapke et al., 1968).

Lung biopsy

This is discussed in the next section.

Diagnosis

Extrinsic allergic alveolitis in its acute form must be distinguished at times from a variety of other respiratory diseases which occur fortuitously or originate from the same occupational environment. The chronic form may need to be differentiated from widespread fibrosis due to other causes.

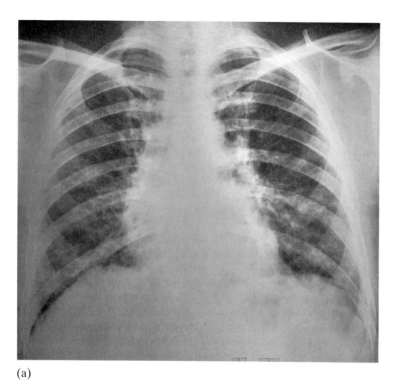

(a)

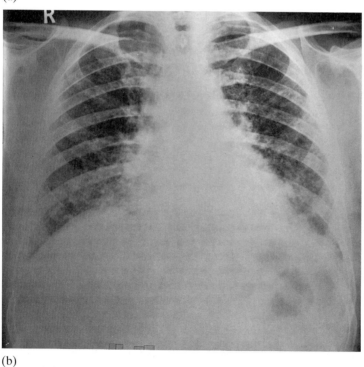

(b)

Figure 20.7 Chronic extrinsic allergic alveolitis in a cattleman handling straw, hay, grain and cattle bedding for 16 years. No definite episodes of acute disease but a heavy 'cold' and lassitude reported in the autumn of 1972. Productive cough, dyspnoea on effort and loss of weight 3 years later. (a) 1975: widespread irregular opacities with no evident cystic appearances; disease of moderate severity. Clinically: pronounced finger clubbing and localized inspiratory crackles. Precipitins: *F. rectivirgula* positive in moderately high titre; *A. fumigatus* weakly positive; *T. vulgaris* negative. (b) 1978: progression of small round and irregular opacities and increase in heart size due to pulmonary heart disease. Coarse inspiratory and expiratory crackles in all lobar regions.

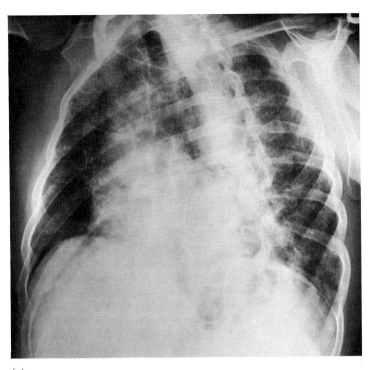

(a)

Figure 20.7 (c) Left 45 degree anterior oblique view on the same day shows particulate involvement of the upper zone of the right lung. *Post mortem*: by naked eye shows multiple 'hobnail' air blebs of the pulmonary pleura; widespread, fairly coarse DIPF with 'honeycomb' cysts up to 1.5 cm in diameter involving all lobes and sharply demarcated from adjacent normal lung. Microscopically: features of chronic extrinsic allergic alveolitis; no granulomas. Death from cardiorespiratory failure

The history is extremely important. It should include precise details of the occupational exposure. Careful enquiry into hobbies (such as pigeon racing and budgerigar breeding) and the keeping of domestic pets (for example, budgerigars or parrots) is also necessary in many cases of acute or chronic lung disease presenting for diagnosis. Of equal importance is the history of the development and nature of the symptoms. The historical details, together with the associated clinical, radiographic and bronchoalveolar lavage features (and, in acute disease and a proportion of cases of chronic disease, the presence of specific precipitins), establish the diagnosis in the majority of cases.

Bronchial provocation tests are rarely necessary except in cases in which proof of one of the rarer causes of extrinsic allergic alveolitis is required.

'Open' lung biopsy, as a rule, is not indicated but may be needed to exclude other causes of fibrosing alveolitis in some cases of precipitin-negative acute disease and other causes of diffuse interstitial pulmonary fibrosis (DIPF) in chronic disease.

Granulomas are readily found in most cases of acute and subacute disease (Reyes et al., 1976).

Acute and subacute disease

The difference between the sudden onset of fever, rigors and dyspnoea of acute disease and the gradual development of ill-health, fever, loss of weight, increasing breathlessness and widespread shadowing in the chest radiograph of subacute disease must be borne in mind. Of the two modes of presentation the subacute is probably more common and is more difficult to recognize promptly.

Diagnosis rests on a detailed history of occupation and the mode of onset of disease, characteristic constitutional and respiratory symptoms and signs, the presence of relevant precipitating antibodies and consistent radiographic appearances. Lung function tests are of no diagnostic help. It must be remembered that, in taking the history, the patient may not be aware that he has been in contact with

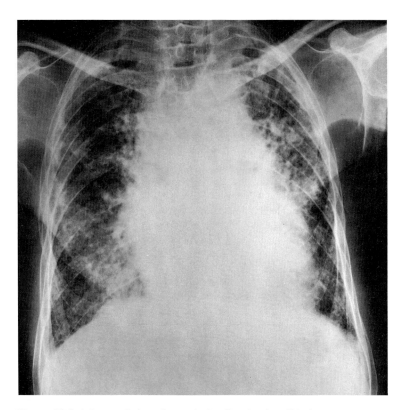

Figure 20.8 Advanced chronic extrinsic allergic alveolitis in a farmworker with no history of initial episodes of acute disease. Coarse rounded and irregular opacities in all zones which tend to be predominant in the upper and middle zones. Large heart shadow due to severe pulmonary heart disease

the relevant antigenic source (for example, mouldy hay). In mild cases there are no dramatic symptoms.

The following diseases may need to be distinguished.

Influenza

Acute extrinsic allergic 'alveolitis' is most frequently confused with an influenzal illness, but the history of exposure and delayed onset of symptoms should lead to the correct diagnosis.

Acute bronchitis

Extrinsic allergic alveolitis is differentiated by unproductive or slightly productive cough; by rapidly developing breathlessness; by the presence of inspiratory crackles in the lower halves of the lung fields in the absence of rhonchi; and by a lack of response to treatment with antibiotics and bronchodilators.

Late asthma

The time of onset may be identical. Differentiation may be difficult initially if, as is often the case, wheeze is absent and if mouldy hay or avian precipitins are present, which is likely in farm workers and bird fanciers respectively. This applies especially to asthma due to storage mites ('barn allergy') which is referred to on page 686 and in Chapter 21 (page 719).

Atypical viral or mycoplasmal pneumonia

These are similar but the physical signs and radiographic signs of consolidation are distinct from extrinsic allergic alveolitis. Serological tests may be required.

Miliary tuberculosis

Differentiation here rests mainly upon the occupational and clinical history, and upon the presence of precipitins. Resolution of radiographic abnormalities after treatment with antituberculous drugs is of no diagnostic assistance because most cases of acute extrinsic allergic alveolitis recover spontaneously. In both diseases the tuberculin test is often negative.

Allergic bronchopulmonary aspergillosis

This may occur in atopic farm workers (who usually have a history of extrinsic asthma) after exposure to mouldy hay with a high content of aspergillus spores but the features of the disease are entirely different from those of farmers' lung. They consist of a more rapid onset after exposure, an asthmatic attack with evident wheeze, expectoration of solid brown plugs of sputum which contain fungal mycelia, eosinophilia of sputum and peripheral blood, immediate (type I) and late (type III) skin responses to extracts of *Aspergillus fumigatus* which do not occur in farmers' lung, and radiographic evidence of lung consolidation or collapse.

Psittacosis – ornithosis

This disease, which affects birds of the parrot family, pigeons and turkeys, may be acquired by farmers and people keeping or handling birds, or coming into contact with their droppings. It is distinguished by high titres of antibodies to *Chlamydia* group B and the fact that the radiographic appearances are usually those of patchy consolidation or collapse which is often unilateral. The presence of precipitins to thermoactinomycetes or avian proteins does not help differentiation (see Chapter 22).

Silo-fillers' disease

Although the onset of symptoms may resemble that of acute extrinsic allergic alveolitis it is usually more rapid, but in some cases it may be delayed for 2 or 3 weeks. As a rule the clinical and radiographic features are those of pulmonary oedema but occasionally they may be identical to those of acute extrinsic allergic alveolitis. However, the nature of the exposure should point to the diagnosis, although it should be remembered that moulding of silo contents may ultimately occur and cause acute extrinsic allergic alveolitis when they are disturbed after the silo is re-opened (see Chapter 18).

Sarcoidosis

In extrinsic allergic alveolitis the work history, mode of onset of the illness, basal inspiratory crackles, absence of radiographic evidence of hilar lymph-adenopathy and rapid recovery with resolution of radiographic abnormalities make confusion with sarcoidosis unlikely. Furthermore, the Kveim test is usually negative.

Acute fibrosing alveolitis

The progressive nature of most cases of cryptogenic disease, rapid deterioration of the patient's condition especially in Hamman–Rich-type disease, and the absence of precipitins to a specific antigen distinguish this from extrinsic allergic alveolitis. However, in some cases the possibility of previous administration of drugs capable of causing allergic alveolitis may need to be excluded, for example, hydrochlorothiazide, nitrofurantoin and sodium cromoglycate (Beaudry and Laplante, 1973; Goldstein and Janicki, 1974; Sheffer, Rocklin and Goetzl, 1975).

Chronic disease

If chronic disease does not follow single or repeated episodes of acute disease, or if these have passed unrecognized, diagnosis can be very difficult. The difficulty is emphasized by the fact that there are no characteristic physiological or radiographic features, and that relevant precipitins are unlikely to be present more than 3 years after the last exposure; furthermore, precipitins may be found in farmers who have lung fibrosis due to another cause. Unlike acute and subacute disease, there are no constitutional symptoms.

Diagnosis depends upon a careful and detailed history of work, hobbies, domestic pets and past respiratory illnesses, and upon exclusion of other causes of lung fibrosis. Biopsy may be necessary in disease of insidious onset but can be indecisive when it has been present for more than 12 months as by then epithelioid granulomas have disappeared.

As stated previously the radiographic changes may take two forms:

1. A widespread fibrotic pattern usually in the upper halves of the lung fields but sometimes in the lower halves.
2. Widespread round opacities.

Differentiation may have to be made from the following diseases.

Fibrocavernous tuberculosis

Past clinical, bacteriological and therapeutic history indicate the diagnosis in most cases and, in some, *Mycobacterium tuberculosis* can be cultured from the sputum. Occasionally, the organism isolated is *M. avium* which may originate from exposure to birds.

Chronic fungal disease

Certain pathogenic fungi are occasionally encountered in the same environmental conditions as some of the causal agents of extrinsic allergic alveolitis and may cause disease with similar clinical and radiographic features. These include (but not in the UK) histoplasmosis, coccidioidomycosis and sporotrichosis. Differentiation in some cases might be difficult because only limited help can be expected from skin and serological tests in these diseases, although the relevant organisms may be recovered from the sputum (see later in this chapter).

Chronic sarcoidosis

Although this is irreversible, the absence of hilar lymphadenopathy and extrathoracic stigmata of sarcoidosis together with a negative Kveim test in chronic extrinsic allergic alveolitis should distinguish the two disorders. However, the reactivity of the tuberculin test may also be reduced in extrinsic allergic alveolitis (Scadding, 1967). The clinical history is crucial.

Pathologically, the presence of plasma cells and the absence of sarcoid-type granulomas in hilar lymph nodes and other organs exclude sarcoidosis; Schaumann bodies, common in sarcoidosis, are rare in extrinsic allergic alveolitis (Seal et al., 1968).

Other forms of DIPF

The lack of relevant occupational history and the fact that, in most cases, they favour the lower parts of the lungs differentiate them from chronic extrinsic alveolitis. The histological features of both disease groups are often sufficiently similar to make microscopic differentiation difficult or impossible. The possibility of fibrosis due to certain drugs has to be borne in mind (see Chapter 15).

Asbestosis

Difficulty may sometimes arise when exposure to asbestos and exposure to a known cause of extrinsic allergic alveolitis have both occurred, although the two diseases should rarely be confused. However, both may occasionally be seen in the same patient. This question is discussed in more detail in Chapters 14 and 15.

Chronic beryllium disease

The occupational history is usually sufficient for differentiation. Otherwise beryllium and epithelioid granulomas are not found in chronic extrinsic allergic alveolitis (see Chapter 17).

'Mixed dust fibrosis'

The occupational history is usually sufficient. However, coincident chronic bird fanciers' lung may also be present on occasion (see Chapter 12).

Prognosis and complications

Acute and chronic disease

After a single attack, complete recovery is the rule in 2 to 12 weeks if the patient ceases to be exposed to the offending antigen. However, cessation of antigen exposure is frequently not possible for economic reasons in farmers and among pigeon breeders usually for psychosocial reasons. It was originally suggested (Dickie and Rankin, 1958) that continuous re-exposure or numerous subacute episodes could lead to progressive fibrosis. Recent longitudinal studies among both farmers and pigeon breeders (Cormier and Belanger, 1985; Monkäre and Haahtela, 1987; Bourke et al., 1989) suggest that progressive lung damage is unusual. In a series of 86 patients with farmers' lung followed over 5 years, minor abnormalities in diffusing capacity only were observed in 40 per cent of farmers (Monkäre and Haahtela, 1987). Among a group of 21 pigeon breeders followed over 10 years, symptoms had improved in the majority despite continued antigen exposure (Bourke et al., 1989). There is some evidence that symptomatic recurrences may be an important determining factor in those who do develop progressive disease (Braun et al., 1979; Schmidt et al., 1988).

Spontaneous pneumothorax is a rare complication.

Treatment

Acute disease

As soon as the diagnosis is made, the patient must be removed from exposure. This alone results in improvement. If the attack is severe he should be reassured and corticosteroids – the only treatment of any value – administered in the form of prednisolone in adequate dosage (about 40 mg/day) for 2 weeks, followed by 20 mg daily until resolution of clinical and radiographic signs is complete. Although corticosteroids are effective in improving clinical status and shortening acute episodes of disease they do not appear to influence the long-term recovery rate (Monkäre and Haahtela, 1987; de Gracia et al., 1989).

Chronic disease

There is, of course, no treatment for fibrotic disease, but in some cases of moderately advanced disease acute lesions may also be present as a result of the most recent exposure to mouldy material and, in these, trial of corticosteroids is worth while.

Farmers' lung

There is an old country tradition that mouldy hay has a baneful effect on the lungs. Over 150 years ago an illness with similar symptoms to farmers' lung and associated with handling mouldy hay was described in an Icelandic journal. The disease was called 'heysott' or 'haysickness' (Björnsson, 1960; Eliasson, 1982). However, it was not until 1932 that it was first recorded in the English medical literature by Campbell at Carlisle in the UK. He accurately described the characteristic features of acute disease in a group of farmworkers exposed to mouldy hay, but Pickles (1944) appears to have coined the term 'farmers' lung'. Other descriptions followed in England from Lancashire (Fawcitt, 1938), Yorkshire (Pickles, 1944), Devon (Fuller, 1953), in Wales (Staines and Forman, 1961), in Scotland and in Eire (Joyce and Kneafsey, 1955). Detailed study has also been done in the USA (for example, Dickie and Rankin, 1958; Emanuel et al., 1964; Rankin et al., 1967), Scandinavia (Tornell, 1946), Switzerland (Hoffman, 1946), Australia (Cooper and Greenaway, 1961) and Finland (Terho, Lammi and Heinonen, 1980). The literature on the subject is now extensive. Extrinsic allergic alveolitis due to exposure to mouldy hay and straw also occurs in cattle and horses (Pirie et al., 1971; Pauli, Gerber and Schatzmann, 1972).

Organisms associated with farmers' lung

Farmers' lung is characteristically associated with inhalation of the spores of thermophile actinomycetes, a group of Gram-positive filamentous

bacteria growing at temperatures between 30 and 65°C. The species include *Faenia rectivirgula (Micropolyspora faeni,* previously identified erroneously with *Thermopolyspora polyspora), Thermoactinomycetes (Micropolyspora) vulgaris* and *Saccharomonospora (Thermomonospora) viridis.* They occur in hay and other substrates that have heated spontaneously and may be accompanied by such mesophilic actinomycetes as *Streptomyces griseus* and *S. albus. Thermoactinomyces vulgaris* was previously regarded as a very variable species (Kuster and Locci, 1964) but it now seems probable that it should be divided into at least two species: *T. vulgaris* and *T. thalpophilus* (Cross and Unsworth, 1977). Confusion has been caused by the proposal of the name *T. candidus* for strains corresponding most closely to the original description of *T. vulgaris* while retaining the latter name of strains corresponding to *T. thalpophilus* (Kurup, Barboriak and Fink, 1975). Thus, *T. candidus* should be considered a synonym of *T. vulgaris* whilst another species, *T. antibioticus,* is probably synonymous with *T. thalpophilus. T. vulgaris* colonies appear to be more numerous in hay than *T. thalpophilus,* but *T. thalpophilus* colonies are stronger growing and produce an antibiotic inhibitory to *T. vulgaris.*

Antigenic preparations of isolates identified as *F. rectivirgula* and *T. vulgaris* have been widely used to determine the presence of antibodies in exposed farm workers and in the diagnosis and epidemiological study of farmers' lung. However, most of the antigens 'T. vulgaris' have originated from isolates of *T. thalpophilus* as a consequence of the stronger growth of this species. *T. vulgaris* differs antigenically from *T. thalpophilus* and may induce precipitins in exposed subjects more readily (Greatorex and Pether, 1975; Terho and Lacey, 1979). This may explain many precipitin-negative cases of farmers' lung and suggests that earlier work was probably incomplete (Cross and Unsworth, 1976, 1977). More recently, three specific *F. rectivirgula* antigens have been identified which correspond to precipitins that occur only in individuals with disease, but not in those exposed but lacking disease symptoms (Treuhaft et al., 1979).

The relative abundance of micro-organisms colonizing hay may vary between countries and with the method of haymaking used. Thus, hays associated with farmers' lung in Finland show less evidence of spontaneous heating and contain fewer actinomycete spores than British hays. Only *T. vulgaris* is sometimes abundant whilst precipitins to *T. vulgaris* are more frequent than those to *T. thalpophilus.* Precipitins to fungi of the *Aspergillus glaucus* group are also found (Terho and Lacy, 1979).

Aspergillus fumigatus antibodies sometimes occur but their significance in pathogenesis is uncertain (Pepys and Jenkins, 1965; Roberts, Wenzel and Emanuel, 1976; Katila and Mäntyjärvi, 1978).

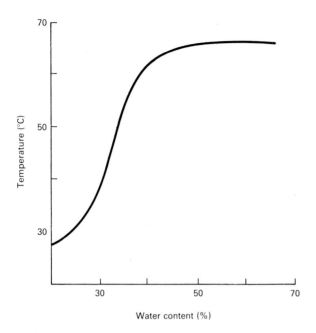

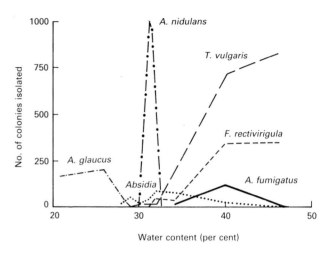

Figure 20.10 The effect of water content on the growth trends of some relevant fungi and actinomycetes in stored hay. (Reproduced with permission from Dr J. Lacey and the Editor of *World Crops*)

Figure 20.9 The relationship of the temperature generated in stored hay to its water content. (Reproduced with permission from Dr J. Lacey and the Editor of *World Crops*)

Conditions for growth

Water is essential for the growth of fungi. Few can grow if the equilibrium relative humidity is less than 65 per cent (Figure 20.9). Microbial heating is limited to a maximum of 65 to 70°C, but chemical processes may sometimes be initiated leading to further heating, and eventually to spontaneous ignition. Heating is ultimately limited by loss of water from the material, so that it cools to ambient temperature.

Successive stages in the heating process are caused by a sequence of different micro-organisms, of which fungi and actinomycetes are probably the most important. When water content is low, the *Aspergillus glaucus* group of fungi predominates and, due to respiration, increases the water content of the fodder. This permits other fungi to become established leading, in turn, to the proliferation of a succession of fungus and actinomycete species which favour increasing water content and temperature. Self-heating of fodder in this fashion encourages exuberant growth of such thermotolerant and thermophilic species as *T. thalpophilus*, *T. vulgaris*, *F. rectivirgula* and *A. fumigatus* when the water content exceeds 35 per cent and the temperature rises to 50°C or more (Festenstein et al., 1965) (Figure 20.10). The characteristics of hay types are exemplified in Table 20.2.

For storage with little or no moulding, the water content of hay must be less than 20 per cent, and of grain about 14 per cent. The spore content of good hay will usually be less than 5 million spores/g dry weight, compared with over 100 million spores/g in mouldy hay, and sometimes in excess of 1000 million spores/g in a farmers' lung type hay (Gregory et al., 1963).

When rainfall is high it is more difficult to make good hay without artificial drying, and the chances of moulding are therefore greater. This results in geographical and seasonal variations in the incidence of farmers' lung and other diseases related to hay moulding, for example, mycotic abortion in cattle due to aspergillus or mucor infections (Hugh-Jones and Austwick, 1967).

The same principles relating water content and heating to fungal growth apply, in general, to grain, bagasse, mushroom compost and other substrates (see appropriate sections in this chapter).

Thus, farmers' lung is a disorder associated with cold and humid weather conditions often in mountainous and semimountainous regions.

Sources of exposure

Turning and stacking hay in the field and removing it to storage present little hazard. Exposure most often occurs when stored mouldy hay crops are handled during such operations as opening bales of hay and straw for animal feeding and bedding and poultry bedding, and when moving and threshing

Table 20.2 Characteristics of different hay types

| *Hay type* | *Water content at baling (%)* | *Maximum temperature reached (%)* | *Spore content* (millions/g) | |
			Fungi	*Actinomycetes and bacteria*
Very mouldy	35–50	50–65	10–100	350–1200
Mouldy	20–30	35–45	2–60	3–250
Good	15–20	22–26	0.1–7	0.5–8

Reproduced with permission from Dr J. Lacey and Editor of *World Crops*.

mouldy grain. Many of these activities may be carried out in poorly ventilated barns, sheds, shippens or partly open buildings so that the spore cloud – which may consist of up to 1600 million spores/m³ air (most of which are actinomycetes) (Lacey and Lacey, 1964) – is not diluted by clean air, and exposure is intense. The risk of exposure to mouldy material in these enclosed surroundings may occur at any time of the year, but is likely to be highest in the late winter and early spring months (Terho, Lammi and Heinonen, 1980). Exposure may also occur during unloading of grass or grain silos.

However, in addition to farmworkers, others who may be exposed to mouldy straw, hay and grain include stable hands (including, until recent years, pit pony ostlers underground in coal mines), poultry workers, attendants of zoo and circus animals, petshop workers, and packers of glass and crockery who use straw.

Incidence and prevalence

In the British Isles, and also elsewhere in Europe, acute disease may occur sporadically throughout the year, but the incidence increases from September, reaches a peak from February to April and then declines rapidly. Sporadic cases may occur at any time. In general more cases have been reported in men than in women, probably a reflection of farming habits. In contrast, in Finland women are more frequently affected than men (Monkäre and Haahtela, 1987); children may also acquire the disease (Staines and Forman, 1961; Bureau et al., 1979). The highest 'attack rate' is between the ages of 41 and 60 years. Staines and Forman (1961) found a varying regional prevalence of 11.5/100 000 of the farming population in East Anglia, 73.1 in south-west England and 193.1/100 000 in Wales; they computed that a conservative estimate of the annual incidence might be about 1000. In Caithness (Scotland) the incidence of acute and chronic farmers' lung grouped

together is 110/100 000 of the farming population (Boyd, 1971). In Orkney, Ayrshire and East Lothian the prevalence of precipitin-positive cases has been reported as 43, 36 and 0 per 1000 respectively (Grant et al., 1972).

On the basis of disease associated with moderate to strong serological results, the prevalence rate for men ranged from 87/1000 in Devon to 302/1000 in mid-Wales (Morgan et al., 1975); in the farming population of Somerset the prevalences of both serologically positive and negative cases have been reported to be 23/1000 (Pether and Greatorex, 1976). Among 343 farm workers in north-west Ireland (Counties Sligo, Leitrim and Donegal) nine, of whom two had precipitins to *F. rectivirgula (M. faeni)*, were considered to have farmers' lung – a prevalence of 2.6 per cent (Shelley et al., 1979). In Wisconsin (USA) a prevalence of 9 to 12 per cent has been recorded in adult males exposed to mouldy hay (Madsen et al., 1976). A postal survey of 12 056 farmers in Finland (Heinonen et al., 1982) demonstrated a prevalence of farmers' lung symptoms of 1.6 per cent. In Italy, Saia et al. (1984) reported a prevalence of farmers' lung symptoms in 1.4 per cent of farmers.

Obviously, prevalence rates are influenced by farming standards and vary according to whether diagnosis rests solely on symptomatology or on the acceptance of only precipitin-positive cases, and also upon the precipitin tests employed.

Other considerations

Sputum

Thermophilic actinomycetes have apparently been isolated from the sputum of patients who have not been in contact with mouldy hay for 3 years, but not from other individuals without such exposure (Greatorex and Pether, 1976). This suggests that spores may, perhaps, germinate and form vegetative cells in the lungs.

Persistence of precipitins

When there is no further exposure, precipitins may disappear in 3 to 5 years after an acute episode (Rankin et al., 1967; Hapke et al., 1968), although, in about a third of cases, they are still present some 10 years later (Braun et al., 1979).

Additional factors in causation

There is some evidence that farmers' lung may not be due solely to *Thermoactinomycetes* sp. (see page 683). When *F. rectivirgula (M. faeni)* alone is administered by intratracheal injection to guinea-pigs, they do not develop any lesions of allergic alveolitis, whereas with mouldy hay dust they do and the reaction is still more severe with a mixture of both (Zaidi et al., 1971). Furthermore, it appears that farmers with extrinsic allergic alveolitis have also had significant exposure to many other respiratory pathogens (Marx et al., 1977). In Finland mesophilic fungi are more abundant in hay than in Britain and fungi of the *A. glaucus* group, particularly *A. umbrosus,* may be implicated in the development of farmers' lung in this country (Terho and Lacey, 1979).

'Barn allergy'

This consists of rhinitis and allergic asthma in farmworkers caused by hypersensitivity to storage mites resident in hay, straw and grain (see next section). Before a firm diagnosis of acute or subacute 'farmers' lung' is made, whether or not specific 'farmers' lung' precipitins are present, storage mite allergy should always be considered and trial treatment with sodium cromoglycate may help to prove it. In some cases, however, the diagnosis may only be reached by bronchial provocation tests and assessment of gas transfer (Cuthbert et al., 1979).

Prevention

The chief aim is to dry hay or grain sufficiently by natural or artificial means (such as barn drying) and to prevent re-wetting during storage so that no moulding or heating can take place. Good ventilation of barns and storage buildings is required. Dust respirators of special design effectively prevent the inhalation of spores (Gourley and Braidwood, 1971), and should be worn by farmworkers known to have had a previous attack of farmers' lung and who are likely to be exposed to mouldy material. However, many find masks difficult to tolerate and refuse to wear them during heavy work (Smyth et al., 1975).

One per cent of concentrated propionic acid, well mixed with grain before it is loaded into the silo for storage, prevents the growth of fungi and bacteria and, thus, a rise in temperature favouring the growth of thermophilic organisms. A practical method of treating hay in this manner, however, has not yet been developed.

Substitution of silage for hay has been advocated as a preventive measure and is employed by some farmers.

Ideally, a farmworker who has had more than one acute attack should change his occupation, but usually he has no inclination or little aptitude for other work and, if self-employed, change may be impossible.

Grain dusts

This is an appropriate point for brief general discussion of the composition and possible harmful effects of grain dusts, although they are also considered under 'Organic dust toxic syndrome'.

Grain dust is a heterogeneous material consisting of particles from various cereals such as wheat, barley, oats, rye and maize. It may contain a large number of contaminants including seeds, pollens, bacteria and their endotoxins, fungi and their metabolites, insects such as the grain weevil, mites, mammalian debris, quartz, and chemical pesticides and herbicides. However, composition varies according to the geographical areas and climatic conditions in which the grain is grown, transported and stored. On the whole, little is known about the effects of pure grain dusts or their various contaminants on health. Certainly some of them are of 'respirable size' and they may constitute about 40 per cent of the total suspended dust although qualitative and quantitative details are lacking (Yoshida and Maybank, 1978). There is some evidence that exposure to grain dusts is associated with excessive loss of lung function (Chan-Yeung et al., 1980). In regard to allergic lung disease – extrinsic allergic alveolitis and asthma – the debris and excreta of mites and insects and the microflora are important. 'Barn allergy' has just been referred to, but see also Chapter 21 (page 719).

The presence of free silica due to contamination by soil containing quartz and from opaline 'silica cells' in wheat and other cereals is unlikely to present a silicosis risk because, in general, its amount is very small, although in one analysis it was reported to range from 1.2 to 6.5 per cent (Blackman, 1969; Farant and Moore, 1978). No radiographic evidence of silicosis was found in a survey of 3000 grain workers (Cotton and Dosman, 1978).

Microflora of grain dusts (Lacey, 1980)

Grain dusts can be broadly grouped into two types according to whether they are produced during harvesting or storage. The microflora evolve continuously from harvest, through the early stage of storage of dry grain to the later stages of storage of moist grain and in accumulated grain deposits in silos and grain elevators. As cereal plants grow they may be infected by phytopathogenic fungi with airborne spores and, as they ripen, both grain and straw are colonized by a variety of saprophytic fungi. Hence, combined harvester dust contains enormous numbers of spores and fungal hyphae as well as bacteria. Spores of *Cladosporium* spp. appear to be most abundant but those of *Verticillium, Paecilomyces, Alternaria, Epicoccum, Ustilago* and *Puccinia* species are common.

Although cladosporium and alternaria spores are known to be allergenic (Hyde, 1972), a survey of British farmworkers showed that 35 per cent had positive skin-prick tests to *Aphanocladium album, Verticillium lecanii* and *Paecilomyces farinosus* extracts and that over 50 per cent had precipitins to these species, whereas only 18 per cent were skin test positive to *Cladosporium* and *Alternaria* spp. (Darke et al., 1976).

The composition of air-borne dust from stored grain varies greatly according to the conditions of storage, because the microflora change in relation to the aeration of the grain bulk, its water content and degree of spontaneous heating. As in the case of hay (see page 683 and Figures 20.9 and 20.10), the more the rising water content and heating increase the microflora the more prolific thermophilic and thermotolerant organisms – which are potential pathogens – become. The nature of air-borne spores, therefore, is determined by storage conditions and varies accordingly. As the water content and temperature increase respectively to about 30 per cent and 50 to 65°C, the greater will be the number of organisms such as *Absydia corymbifera, Mucor pusillus, T. vulgaris, F. rectivirgula (M. faeni), A. fumigatus* and possibly others that may present a risk of extrinsic allergic alveolitis or lung infection. Near-anaerobic conditions, such as may occur in sealed silos, limit heating and microbial growth, whereas aerated maltings favour the growth of *A. clavatus* and *A. fumigatus* (see malt-workers' lung). A study in grain elevators in Canada (Manitoba) has shown that the microflora were similar in all and consisted almost entirely of bacteria, *Penicillium*, yeasts, *Aspergillus flavus, A. fumigatus, T. vulgaris* and *Streptomyces albus*.

Barley grain for cattle fodder stored in concrete silos in different parts of Britain has also been studied. The grain, which contained 23 to 40 per cent water, was covered by straw or chopped wilted grass with or without a polyethylene or butyl rubber sheeting. Heating and moulding of the uppermost layer of grain was found to depend on the rate at which the grain was removed from the silo and on the efficiency of the top seal. Thus, the nature and number of organisms and air-borne spores associated with grain stored by this method show very considerable variation. Species known to be potentially pathogenic to humans and animals were most abundant in and immediately below the top seal, unless this formed silage, and when the temperature during unloading was in excess of 35°C. Removing the top seal or unloading grain causes a rapid and large increase in the spore content of the air in silos.

It is not known if fungal enzymes and metabolites are harmful to the lungs, but they may have a role in the pathogenesis of 'organic dust toxic syndrome' which is discussed in the next section.

Bacteria are universally present in grain and this raises the possibility that endotoxins of some species may be responsible for lung disease. Endotoxin of *Erwinia herbicola* is reported to be common in grain in Poland and has been suggested as a cause of respiratory disease in farmworkers (Dutkiewicz, 1978). However, this organism is uncommon in Canadian grain elevators and British grain silos, although it frequently colonizes plant surfaces before harvest.

The development of new techniques in harvesting and storing grain has, to some extent, increased the risks of microbial growth and the quantities of air-borne dust produced. Preventive measures include: air-filtered driving cabs on combine harvesters; drying grain to a safe water content and maintaining this during storage until used; good ventilation of grain handling areas; treatment of grain for cattle fodder with propionic acid to prevent moulding; and ensuring rapid emptying of most grain silos to prevent the production of large concentrations of spores of potentially pathogenic fungi. The recognition and prevention of respiratory disease from grain dust requires the co-operation of doctors, microbiologists and engineers.

Organic dust toxic syndrome

An acute febrile illness following the inhalation of massive amounts of fungi was first described in 1975 by Emanuel, Wenzel and Lawton in a group of farmworkers. They named the condition pulmonary mycotoxicosis because they regarded a toxin from the fungus as the likely cause. Febrile episodes in the absence of other signs of alveolitis have been well described in farmers (Malmberg et al., 1988). These have, in the past, been referred to as precipitin-negative farmers' lung (Edwards, Baker and Davies, 1974) and atypical farmers' lung (Jones, 1982). Similar episodes have been reported in a number of different environments including grain elevators (doPico et al., 1982), sewage treatment plants (Rylander et al., 1976) and grain silos (Pratt and May, 1984). In 1986, it was proposed that these principally febrile responses to different types of usually agricultural dusts should be called the 'organic dust toxic syndrome' (doPico, 1986). The evidence that has now accumulated would appear to justify regarding this syndrome as a distinct entity.

The clinical features of organic dust toxic syndrome have now been well described (May et al., 1986; Rask-Anderson, 1989). Characteristically, the farmer experiences shivering episodes associated with a cough, breathing difficulties, muscle aches, headaches, chest tightness and nausea. The episodes last for 24 to 72 hours and are sufficiently severe to require a period of bedrest in the majority of affected individuals. On physical examination, the patient is febrile and tachypnoeic with tachycardia, and inspiratory crackles may be present at the lung bases (May et al., 1986; Rask-Anderson, 1989). A leucocytosis is present with a relative increase in neutrophils. Precipitating antibodies to extracts of the organic dust to which the individual has been exposed are absent (Emanuel, Wenzel and Lawton, 1975; Lecours, Laviolette and Cormier, 1986; May et al., 1986). Pulmonary function tests in the majority of patients are normal, although arterial blood gas tensions may show a widening of the alveolar–arterial oxygen gradient. Significant arterial desaturation is rare (May et al., 1986). The chest radiograph is characteristically normal. Occasionally minor interstitial infiltration is present. Bronchoalveolar lavage during the early acute stage reveals a neutrophil alveolitis. At 1 month this resolves to become a mild to moderate lymphocytic alveolitis (Lecours, Laviolette and Cormier, 1986).

The febrile episodes of organic dust toxic syndrome in an individual may occur infrequently, specifically following an unusually high exposure to organic dust. An important feature of the syndrome is the complete recovery of the person and his or her subsequent ability to work exposed to the organic dust at lower levels without a recurrence of symptoms. The differentiation of this condition from extrinsic allergic alveolitis is, therefore, important because the employment advice given in these two situations is quite different. Extrinsic allergic alveolitis in a farmer has important long-term consequences with the possible development of permanent lung damage and disability if exposure does not

cease. In organic dust toxic syndrome, the recovery is full and future episodes can be prevented by avoiding massive exposures to organic dusts.

Bird fanciers' (breeders') lung

This was first recorded in workers handling goose and duck feathers (Plessner, 1960) and in a budgerigar breeder (Pearsall et al., 1960), but 'pneumonitis' of unknown cause in people exposed to pigeon excreta had, in fact, been reported by Feldman and Sabin in 1948. The disease is thought to be related to exposure to avian proteins in dry dust of the droppings, and sometimes of the feathers of a variety of birds: pigeons, budgerigars (parakeets), parrots, turtle doves, turkeys and chickens (Reed, Sosman and Barbee, 1965; Hargreave et al., 1966; Elman et al., 1968; Hinson, 1970; Boyer et al., 1974; Warren and Tse, 1974; Molina, 1976; Schatz et al., 1976). Pigeon droppings have been considered to be the major environmental source of antigen (Fredericks, 1978). However, as Boyd et al. (1982) point out, pigeon droppings are hygroscopic, bulky and do not desiccate easily and a more likely source of antigen is pigeon bloom. This waxy powder coats the feathers of racing pigeons, is readily dispersed in pigeon lofts and is produced in abundance, particularly when birds are in peak racing condition. The bloom is derived from feathers and consists of keratin granules of average size of the order of 1 μm coated with a soluble antigenic material, probably pigeon IgA (Boyd et al., 1982).

The *prevalence* of bird fanciers' lung is difficult to determine; the majority of surveys have been of volunteer populations, thus introducing unknown biases. It probably depends upon types of birds and modes of exposure to them. Among pigeon fanciers it is variously reported as 1/1000 (Molina, 1976), 1.4/1000 (Maesen, 1972), 6 per cent (Moore et al., 1974), 21 per cent (Christensen, Schmidt and Robbins, 1975) and 10.4 per cent (Banham et al., 1986); and among budgerigar fanciers in Britain it is calculated to lie between 0.5 and 7.5 per cent (Hendrick et al., 1987a). There is far less information available on the rates of respiratory disease among poultry and turkey farmers. Elman et al. (1968) in a study of 58 poultry farmers found no evidence of allergic alveolitis. In a study of turkey raisers (Boyer et al., 1974), 6 per cent had symptoms consistent with an allergic alveolitis. It has been speculated (Boyd et al., 1982) that the apparent lack of clinical disease in the poultry and turkey industries relates to the poorly developed feathers and much lower bloom content of these non-flying birds.

Features of exposure

Exposure occurs during cleaning out pigeon lofts, bird cages and poultry houses. People likely to be exposed include those who breed budgerigars or pigeons professionally or as a hobby, pet shop workers, aviary attendants, poultry farmers, and budgerigar and parrot fanciers who keep one bird. Those who look after many birds (such as pigeon fanciers) experience intermittent exposure to high concentrations of antigen at 1- to 2-weekly intervals during cleaning of lofts or cages, and typical acute disease may develop, whereas those who keep one or two pet birds at home are exposed more or less continuously to low concentrations of antigen and in them the development of disease is gradual and insidious. This insidious onset is marked only by progressive dyspnoea on effort. Severe fibrosis is likely to be established by the time the patient is first seen. Occasionally it is fatal within 2 to 3 years of the first complaint of symptoms (Edwards and Luntz, 1974).

Acute exposure to antigen is associated with three types of response (Boyd et al., 1982). The *first* is that of acute progressive disease with severe, debilitating symptoms requiring total removal from the source of antigen. The *second,* and most common, response is that of acute intermittent, non-progressive disease. The individual experiences classic symptoms, but only after a heavier than normal avian exposure. The symptoms rapidly resolve over 24 to 48 hours. The *third* response is that of recurrent non-acute disease which is characterized by the presence of low-grade, non-specific symptoms including cough, sputum, lassitude and malaise, improving rapidly following withdrawal of antigen. When all contact with the birds is stopped, complete clinical recovery is the rule, although in some patients irreversible chronic disease may persist. But, as in the case of farmers' lung, not all people exposed to avian antigens develop evidence of disease. The disease may occur in the children of pigeon and budgerigar enthusiasts and appears to be of more insidious onset than in adults (Stiehm, Reed and Tooley, 1967; Chandra and Jones, 1972).

Among poultry farmers typical acute disease appears to be rare, although it has been reported: tightness in chest and cough are complained of by a minority after prolonged exposure (Elman et al., 1968). Horses in contact with chickens have developed similar disease (Mansmann and Osborn, 1971).

Pathology and immunology

The pathology has already been described. Lung biopsy in acute disease reveals infiltration of lymphocytes and plasma cells, reticulin proliferation and sarcoid-type granulomas in alveolar walls and spaces (Nash, Vogelpoela and Becker, 1967; Hensley et al., 1969). Unlike allergic alveolitis due to other causes large macrophages with pale vacuolated cytoplasm ('foam cells') are often seen in the granulomas. Honeycomb cysts are common in chronic disease.

That avian antigens are causally responsible is demonstrated by the fact that acute respiratory and constitutional symptoms, basal inspiratory crackles and impaired gas transfer result about 6 hours after inhalation of a dilute aerosol of pigeon or budgerigar serum by patients who have previously had acute disease (Reed, Sosman and Barbee, 1965; Hargreave et al., 1966). Precipitins and typical lesions of allergic alveolitis with foam cells and granuloma formation occur in rats after prolonged inhalation of dust containing pigeon droppings (Fink, Hensley and Barboriak, 1969). If inhalation tests are used in diagnosis the initial extracts must be weak in order to avoid prolonged respiratory symptoms which may require treatment with corticosteroids.

Precipitins against avian antigens are found in the serum of the majority of patients with acute pigeon breeders' disease and in some 16 per cent of pigeon fanciers with no evidence of disease (Barboriak, Sosman and Reed, 1965), but they are absent in unexposed people. Important factors influencing antibody response are the duration of exposure and the number of birds kept (Banham, Lynch and Boyd, 1978). However, there does not appear to be a correlation between the intensity of exposure and the response. The intensity of antibody response is closely associated with the presence of symptoms: 86.6 per cent of those with serum antibody concentrations greater than 60 μg/ml experience classic symptoms of pigeon fanciers' lung (Banham et al., 1986). Precipitating antibodies to pigeon bloom extract are also detectable in pigeon fanciers with significantly higher antibody levels in those with most severe symptoms and a higher incidence of precipitins to bloom compared to pigeon serum (Banham et al., 1982). This may prove clinically relevant in those individuals experiencing classic symptoms of pigeon fanciers' lung but whose conventional precipitin tests are negative.

Precipitating antibodies to chick antigen are also present in a majority of unaffected poultry farmers (Elman et al., 1968) and there is a significantly higher prevalence of precipitins among symptomatic workers in the turkey raising and processing industry than among asymptomatic workers (Boyer et al., 1974). In budgerigar fanciers, the situation is remarkably different because precipitins are not found in exposed healthy subjects, although they are present in almost all those with allergic alveolitis confirmed by inhalation tests (Faux et al., 1971). These differences in correlation with disease are poorly understood, but may be due to differing potency of the various antigens, as well as to a variable intensity of individual exposures.

The precipitating antibodies in pigeon breeders' disease are directed against pigeon IgG and IgM (Diment and Pepys, 1977) and an antigen (not present in the serum) that cross-reacts with pigeon γ-globulin and appears to be IgA derived either from the intestinal tract (Tebo, Fredericks and Roberts, 1977) or from pigeon bloom. To detect specific antibodies to pigeon antigens, a purified fraction of pigeon dropping extract is required as the whole extract causes a variety of non-specific reactions (Tebo, Moore and Fink, 1977).

Cross-reaction between different antigens is sometimes observed. Precipitins against *F. rectivirgula (M. faeni)* and *Aspergillus fumigatus* have been found in some cases of bird fanciers' lung and precipitins against pigeon excreta are occasionally present in patients with farmers' lung.

Intradermal tests with purified pigeon antigen give positive immediate responses in the skin suggesting the presence of reaginic IgE in some sensitized individuals. This is followed later by an Arthus-type reaction (Pepys, 1969). In contrast to farmers' lung, the Arthus-type skin reaction to avian antigens is closely associated with the presence of precipitins and may, therefore, be a useful pointer to diagnosis.

Clinical features

Lung function returns to normal in most patients when they cease their contact with birds. Although lung function may continue to deteriorate if they remain exposed, a major group of patients with 'acute recurring non-progressive' disease experience no deterioration in lung function over many years despite continued exposure to antigen and a persistent antibody response (Bourke et al., 1989). As in farmers' lung, irreversible airways' obstruction is sometimes present but can later recover completely (Nash, Vogelpoel and Becker, 1967; Dinda, Chatterjee and Riding, 1969).

There is evidence that the duration of symptomatic exposure influences the degree of recovery (de Gracia et al., 1989). In a series of 22 patients with bird fanciers' lung, those with less than 2 years' avian contact made a full recovery; a significant proportion of those exposed for longer than 2 years were left with respiratory impairment.

It is particularly important to identify the disorder in a child – often manifested as a failure to thrive – because permanent lung damage may develop unless contact with the birds is stopped.

Acute disease should not be confused with psittacosis; although the symptoms can be somewhat similar, in psittacosis they develop after an incubation period of 7 to 14, occasionally up to 30, days, and lung consolidation may occur (see Chapter 22, page 763). However, the possibility that both diseases can occur in the same patient must be borne in mind (Molina, 1976).

Chronic disease of insidious development due to continuous contact with birds in the home (chiefly budgerigars) is probably sufficiently prevalent, although uncommon, to cause possible diagnostic confusion in individuals who have worked in a known occupational dust hazard – for example, the asbestos industry, coal mining, foundry – particularly because the keeping of budgerigars by the families of workers in these and other industries is fairly common.

In Britain, about 0.3 per cent of the population keep pigeons whereas budgerigars are apparently kept in 5 to 6 million homes. On these estimates, if 12 per cent of the general population is exposed to budgerigars, then between 65 and 90/100 000 are likely to have bird fanciers' lung, although mildly in most cases. Hence, bird fanciers' lung is believed to be about ten times more common than farmers' lung owing to the much larger population at risk – only about 1.1 per cent of the general population work in farming (Hendrick et al., 1978a). Therefore, *when taking the occupational history of a patient with suspected lung disease the question of birds in the home or in hobby activity should never be omitted.*

False-positive complement fixation titres to egg-grown respiratory virus preparations have been found in some patients with acute pigeon fanciers' lung and regarded as antibodies directed against antigens from hens' eggs in which the test viruses were grown. Such antigens were, in fact, demonstrated in the virus preparations. Therefore, due to the clinical similarities between influenza, psittacosis and acute bird fanciers' lung, it is essential that a diagnosis of influenza or psittacosis should not be made in bird fanciers on the grounds of a single raised titre or a fourfold rise of complement fixation titre without appropriate control tests with avian antigens being made (Newman Taylor et al., 1977).

Prevention

The most important precept in the management of patients with acute (or subacute) disease is permanent avoidance of contact with offending birds.

However, most individuals who develop symptoms will modify their exposure to antigen by reducing contact and by wearing respiratory protection and may successfully control their symptoms in this way. There is now a greater awareness among the pigeon fancying community of the dangers of pulmonary sensitization to their pigeons and many wear respiratory protection during periods of high antigen exposure to prevent the development of disease.

It should be remembered that antigen may persist in the birds' environment after they have been removed.

Bird fanciers' lung, farmers' lung, coeliac disease and 'egg eaters' lung'

An association between adult coeliac disease (gluten-sensitive enteropathy) and diffuse interstitial pulmonary disease was reported by Hood and Mason (1970), Lancaster-Smith, Benson and Strickland (1971) and later by Berrill et al. (1975), and it was thought likely that the lung disease might be an autoimmune fibrosing alveolitis. But it was soon observed that avian precipitins were present in many of these patients (Lancaster-Smith et al., 1974) and all of those studied by Berrill et al. (1975) proved to have had contact with birds. Thus, it was suggested that the lung pathology was bird fanciers' lung and that intestinal absorption of avian antigens might be a factor in its pathogenesis or persistence.

However, precipitins against avian antigens common to the pigeon, budgerigar and hen, but distinct from the antigens usually associated with bird fanciers' lung, have been found in patients with coeliac disease who were not exposed to birds (Morris et al., 1971; Faux, Hendrick and Anand, 1978). This antigen is a component of hen egg yolk but not of bird droppings, and is present in the birds' serum. It has been referred to as 'coeliac-associated' antigen to distinguish it from 'bird fanciers' lung-associated' antigen (Faux, Hendrick and Anand, 1978). Hence, the precipitins are unlikely to result from bird dust inhalation. There is, in addition, an association between the degree of intestinal mucosal damage and the presence of precipitins to 'coeliac-associated' antigen in coeliac patients (Hendrick et al., 1978b). The source of antigen is probably partly cooked or uncooked eggs in various foods.

It is not known whether the precipitins in the cases with lung disease reported by Berrill et al. (1975) were directed against 'bird fanciers' lung-associated' or 'coeliac-associated' antigen, but, as villous atrophy was present in all, it seems likely that they were of the latter category. However, important evidence that the lung disease is not bird fanciers' lung is provided by the fact that bronchial challenge tests with avian protein had no ill-effects on lung function of affected patients (Benson et al., 1972).

It is possible, as Faux, Hendrick and Anand (1978) suggest, that because 'bird fanciers' lung-associated' antigens were found in eggs in addition to 'coeliac-associated' antigens, some patients with bird fanciers' lung may respond unfavourably to eating eggs. Indeed, some of the patients studied by Hendrick et al. (1978b) disliked or avoided eggs which they thought caused gastrointestinal discomfort, malaise and even dyspnoea on effort. Established bird fanciers' lung could be followed by 'egg eaters' lung', which might become particularly severe if the patient had coincident coeliac disease owing to defective mucosal processing of ingested avian antigens, even if there is no causal association between the two diseases. This might apply equally to farmers' lung because cases with coeliac disease have been reported (Robinson, 1976; Robinson et al., 1981). Similarly, diffuse lung disease in patients with coeliac disease who do not keep birds might arise primarily as a result of ingested egg or other food antigens.

Another hypothesis, which needs investigation, has been suggested, namely, that antibodies to bird gut mucosa cross-react with the patients' gut mucosa and this provokes simultaneous coeliac disease (Purtilo, Bonica and Yang, 1978).

Both coeliac disease and some types of 'fibrosing alveolitis' are more common in individuals with the HLA-8 antigen (Stokes et al., 1972; Turton et al., 1978) and it may be that the concurrence of the two disorders is the result of a common immunological dysfunction.

Summary

When considering diagnosis it is important to bear in mind that patients with active coeliac disease are likely to have precipitins to avian serum, even in the absence of exposure to birds or of lung disease, so that, in patients with suspected bird fanciers' lung, the presence of antibodies requires careful interpretation. However, although the two precipitin groups are distinguished, 'bird fanciers' lung-associated' precipitins are not pathognomonic of bird fanciers' lung, nor does their absence exclude it (Hendrick et

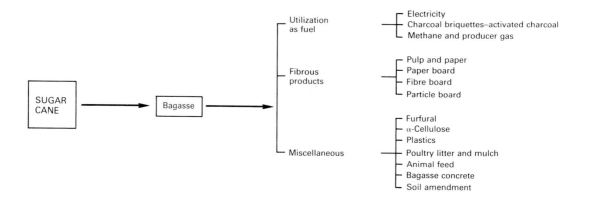

Figure 20.11 Uses of bagasse. (Adapted with permission from Paturau, 1969)

al., 1978b). For this reason it may be necessary to perform bronchial challenge tests to establish the diagnosis of bird fanciers' lung, and certainly contact with the birds under suspicion should be discontinued. In view of the apparent lack of a strong association between bird fanciers' lung and coeliac disease, routine jejunal biopsy is probably not desirable (Hendrick et al., 1978b).

Bagassosis

Bagasse is the fibrous cellulose residue of sugarcane stalk after it has been crushed and the juice extracted. It consists of tough 'true fibre' and soft 'pith' tissue from the inner stalk. Pith absorbs water readily and, if present in any quantity, hinders drying. It is fibrous, tough and has good insulating qualities for heat and sound.

Sugar-cane is grown in the West Indies, India, Pakistan, Brazil, Cuba, Argentina, the southern USA, South Africa, Australia and Mexico. After the extraction of sugar, bagasse may be baled for storage.

Baling is done in a press similar to a hay baler. The bales are bound by steel wire and stacked in the open in such a fashion as to allow ventilation. Stacks may be protected against rain by a covering of asbestos or plastic sheeting. The bagasse is stored for about 12 months, when it may be transferred to another plant for compression into smaller compact bales for transportation. The baling plant operates during the few months in the year when the crop is gathered.

Fresh bagasse stored in bales heats spontaneously to 54°C in 5 days then cools to 40°C before rising again after about 33 days to 49°C. However, bagasse with a water content of 27 per cent heats to 49°C in 3 days (Lacey, 1969). Hence, the growth of many different species of fungi and thermophilic and mesophilic actinomycetes is favoured in bagasse with this degree of moisture. Fermentation of residual sugar by yeasts probably assists the initial heating.

Since the late 1950s, the Ritter system of bulk storing unpithed or partly depithed bagasse has been used in some industrial plants. It consists of keeping large mounds of loose, unbaled bagasse wet with a 'biological' liquor containing molasses and lactic acid-producing bacteria until required for use. Continuous moistening with automatic sprinklers keeps the water content to a minimum of 50 to 60 per cent. The importance of this system is that it effectively eliminates the production of actinomycete-bearing dust during the mechanical processing of bagasse (Paturau, 1969; Lehrer et al., 1978). Mouldy bagasse contains enormous numbers of fungal spores – probably as many as 500 000 000/g dry weight (Buechner, 1968) – and, although these were earlier identified as *T. vulgaris* (Seabury et al., 1968), it is now known that they consist in fact chiefly of a much more abundant, but closely related, species of thermoactinomytes, *T. sacchari*.

Bagassosis has the same acute and chronic forms as farmers' lung, but is more often found in the acute form. It follows exposure to the dust of dry, mouldy bagasse but not of fresh or autoclaved bagasse. It was described in New Orleans (Jamison and Hopkins, 1941) and, although most of the reported cases have occurred in the southern states of the USA (Sodeman and Pullen, 1944; Buechner et al., 1958, 1964), there have been many others in

Britain (Castleden and Hamilton-Paterson, 1942; Hunter and Perry, 1946; Hargreave, Pepys and Holford-Strevens, 1968), Italy (Cangini, 1951), India (Ganguly and Pal, 1955; Viswanathan et al., 1963), the Philippines (Dizon, Almonte and Anselmo, 1962), Spain (González de Vega et al., 1966) and the West Indies (Hearn, 1968). It is apt to occur in sporadic outbreaks when workers are exposed to mouldy material.

Uses of bagasse

Bagasse has many possible uses and these are summarized in Figure 20.11. Bagasse in briquettes is employed as a fuel to generate electricity in cane-producing areas, although it is now largely replaced by oil. Charcoal is produced by carbonization (see Chapter 13, 'Activated carbons'), and methane by anaerobic fermentation of the cellulose fraction. Manufacture of different types of paper and board has become increasingly important in recent years. Particle board can be moulded to any shape for the furniture container, motor car and ship-building industries, and fibre board is used for acoustic and thermal insulation. Furfural, which is also known as furfuraldehyde and is produced by acid hydrolysis of the xylan in bagasse, is employed in the refining of lubricating oils and the manufacture of resins. Bagasse is also used in the production of viscose rayon and as a filler and extender in the reinforced thermosetting plastics. For details of the many uses of bagasse see Paturau (1969).

Sources of exposure

A potential risk of bagassosis exists in the following processes if bagasse is dry and mouldy: removing bales from stacks to the compressing plant, the compressing operation, opening or shredding of bales in the factory, hammer-milling bagasse to desired particle size, during various manufacturing operations (including the grinding of hardboard), and moving and turning bagasse for ·cattle and poultry bedding. In a British factory before the Second World War, bales were opened using a wet process, but when, in the altered circumstances of the war, they were opened dry, cases of bagassosis occurred (Hunter and Perry, 1946).

The growth of bacteria and fungi in bagasse can now be prevented, however, by treating it when fresh with 1 per cent propionic acid before or after milling. This has greatly increased the potential of bagasse in manufacturing.

Pathology and immunology

The pathology of acute disease has the same features as acute farmers' lung, including granulomas (Sodeman and Pullen, 1943; Bradford, Blalock and Wascom, 1961; Buechner, 1962), but some cases are remarkable for the presence of large numbers of plasma cells both in the alveolar walls and spaces. Chronic disease consists of diffuse interstitial fibrosis with bronchiolectasis – mainly in the upper parts of the lungs – and pleural thickening (Buechner, 1962).

Precipitins are present in some two-thirds of patients during or shortly after an acute attack of bagassosis, but disappear within 1 to 3 years (Salvaggio et al., 1969). *Thermoactinomyces vulgaris* was thought to be the chief, if not only, antigenic source (Seabury et al., 1968), and inhalation of extract of *T. vulgaris,* but not of *F. rectivirgula* by men suffering from bagassosis appeared to reproduce the symptoms of the disease. However, Lacey (1971) subsequently identified the organism as *T. sacchari.* This explains why precipitins to genuine *T. vulgaris* extracts have not been demonstrated (Hargreave, Pepys and Holford-Strevens, 1968; Holford-Strevens, 1971). But when extracts of *T. sacchari* were tested by immunoelectrophoresis and agar-gel double diffusion against sera from patients with bagassosis in the USA and from exposed workers in Trinidad, characteristic precipitin reactions occurred (J. Lacey, 1971, personal communication). These reactions could not be altered by absorption of the sera with *T. vulgaris* extracts (Holford-Strevens, 1971). However, one of the subjects who reacted to extracts of *T. vulgaris* reacted similarly to extracts of *T. sacchari* (Lacey, 1971) and immunoelectrophoresis suggests that the two species may contain some antigens in common.

Thus, *T. sacchari* appears to be the major source of antigen in mouldy bagasse which is responsible for bagassosis. However, it is possible, as may be the case in farmers' lung, that other components (in particular, bagasse dust itself) may be involved in pathogenesis. Experimental work lends some support to this possibility (Kawai et al., 1972; Bhattacharjee, Saxena and Zaidi, 1980).

Allergic bronchopulmonary aspergillosis may occasionally occur in bagasse-exposed workers (see Chapter 22, page 766).

Serum IgG and IgA, but not IgM, levels are raised in acute bagassosis (Salvaggio et al., 1969).

Bagasse contains a small amount of quartz (about 0–1 to 0–2 per cent) derived from the soil and, because of this, some authorities have suggested that bagassosis is a form of silicosis. There is no foundation for this belief and it is evident that the pathogenesis and pathology of the disease do not resemble silicosis in any way.

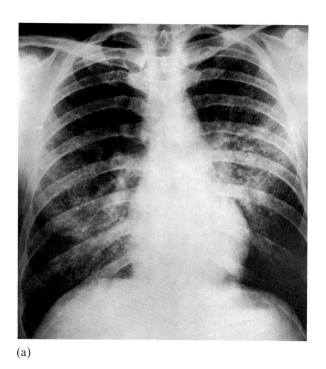

(a)

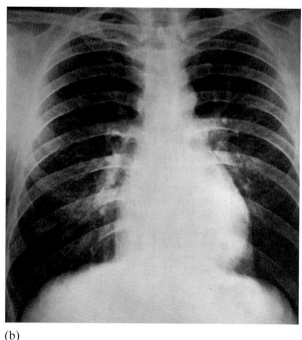

(b)

Figure 20.12 Subacute bagassosis in a worker in the UK handling mouldy bagasse for manufacture of laminated boards. Precipitins to the relevant organism are present. (a) Multiple round mid-zone opacities preceded by a few months of lassitude, breathlessness and loss of weight. Note clearer lower zones. (b) Resolution almost complete 6 weeks later. Ultimately complete recovery

Clinical features

The symptoms, physical signs and radiographic appearances of both acute and chronic disease are similar to those of farmers' lung (Figure 20.12), but in a number of acute cases there is no evident abnormality of the chest film.

Lung function tests during acute disease reveal some reduction of TLC, VC and gas transfer which subsequently return to normal in most cases (Weill et al., 1966). Vital capacity in exposed workers without disease may be significantly lower than in unexposed workers, but the reason for this has not been ascertained (Hearn, 1968). However, a single episode of bagassosis can produce dyspnoea on effort, permanent reduction of lung volume and gas transfer, and hyperventilation on exercise (Miller, Hearn and Edwards, 1971).

Treatment

As in the case of farmers' lung, the majority of patients with acute disease recover spontaneously in 4 to 12 weeks after being removed from exposure. Corticosteroids in adequate dose may hasten clini-

cal recovery, but do not appear to influence the rate at which lung function returns to normal (Pierce et al., 1968).

Prevention

The application of 1 per cent propionic acid to milled fresh bagasse before baling effectively prevents moulding even after bales are stored in the open for more than 12 months. However, the Ritter system and continuous moistening of large, loose mounds of bagasse have been used increasingly. This and carrying out grinding and shredding operations in the open, the use of exhaust ventilation and enclosure of machinery (where possible) have greatly reduced both the incidence of the disease and the prevalence of *T. sacchari* precipitins in the workers (Lehrer et al., 1978). High-efficiency respirators may be worn under some circumstances but are intolerable in hot and humid climates.

If more than one acute attack has occurred, the worker should be removed from further exposure to bagasse and should not transfer to agricultural work in which there could be contact with mouldy hay or fodder.

Mushroom workers' lung

Mushroom workers' lung was first reported in the USA among Puerto Rican mushroom farmworkers in 1959 (Bringhurst, Byrne and Gershon-Cohen, 1959) and is characterized by the same acute constitutional and respiratory symptoms and signs as farmers' lung; however, only two cases of doubtful chronic disease appear to have been observed (Sakula, 1967; Jackson and Welch, 1970; Chan-Yeung, Grzybowski and Schonell, 1972). It appears to be remarkably uncommon considering that mushroom cultivation is carried out on a large scale in Britain, the USA and European countries. However, there have been no epidemiological studies in Britain studying either the prevalence or incidence of this disease and it is probable that the illness is more common than reports suggest and often goes unrecognized.

The production process of mushroom cultivation involves the preparation of a compost consisting of horse manure, pig manure or chicken litter mixed with wheat straw and allowed to ferment in piles over a period of 7 days in the open air (*phase 1*). In recent years compost for mushroom cultivation has been produced commercially and supplied to mushroom farms. It is then transferred to open trays and pasteurized by heating to 49 to 60°C usually using steam for 5 to 7 days and then allowed to cool (*phase 2*). The pasteurization process promotes a heavy growth of thermophilic and thermotolerant actinomycetes, including *F. rectivirgula (M. faeni)* and *T. vulgaris* and various fungi (Fergus, 1964; Craveri, Guicciardi and Pacini, 1966). The mushroom spawn is then added to the freshly pasteurized compost. This process in the past has been carried out manually with the worker spawning the mushrooms standing over the trays of compost which were being mechanically agitated. This mechanical agitation leads to high concentrations of air-borne micro-organisms. Random sampling of air in a spawning shed has yielded counts of the order of 700×10^6 spores/m³ (Lacey, 1973). The mushroom spawn is adherent to cereal grains and does not itself become air-borne. After spawning the compost is moved to growing sheds where it is maintained at a temperature of 20°C and a humidity of about 90 per cent. When the mushroom crop has been picked the mushroom compost is steam heated to 60°C, after which the compost is taken out and disposed of.

The commercial production of mushroom compost, the spawning process and the disposal of compost are the chief sources of exposure to the spores of thermophilic actinomycetes and are phases at which outbreaks of disease may occur. Exposure to mushroom spores themselves may occur in the growing sheds, depending on the strain of mushroom being cultivated. In Britain, *Agaricus bisporus* is usually cultivated. This mushroom only liberates its spores when fully mature and is usually picked when immature. Outbreaks of disease have not been described during this production phase in Britain, whereas *Pleurotus ostreatus (P. florida)*, cultivated in other countries, releases spores in large numbers from a very early stage of growth and is another cause of allergic alveolitis in mushroom workers (Berruchon and Oury, 1981).

Clinical and immunological features

Mushroom workers may develop respiratory disease at any of the phases of mushroom production: mushroom compost preparation (Phillips et al., 1987), most frequently during the spawning process (Bringhurst, Byrne and Gershon-Cohen, 1959; Sakula, 1967; Chan-Yeung, Grzybowski and Schonell, 1972), mushroom growth (Hou, 1985), picking and sorting (Von Betz, 1985) and during the disposal of spent compost (Lockey, 1974).

There is considerable variation in the duration of exposure in relation to the development of symptoms. These usually first occur after some weeks or months of symptom-free work in the industry, although occasionally they develop within hours of first exposure (Stewart, 1974). In general, in affected workers the time between starting work and awareness of symptoms is from 4 to 6 hours (Chan-Yeung, Grzybowski and Schonell, 1972; Stewart, 1974).

The symptoms are those of acute extrinsic allergic alveolitis described already. Cough and sputum are frequent presenting symptoms and the sputum may be blood stained. The respiratory physiological abnormalities are those of a restrictive defect with impaired gas transfer. Occasionally, a predominantly obstructive defect occurs (Johnson and Kleyn, 1981). Radiographic changes, which range from bilateral miliary opacities in the middle and lower zones to confluent, ill-defined opacities in the same regions, are usually present (Stewart, 1974).

Precipitins to *F. rectivirgula* and *T. vulgaris* are found in very few cases even after concentration of the serum, but precipitins to a variety of other thermophilic actinomycetes may be present, although none is common to all workers (Stewart and Pickering, 1974). Hence, with so rich a microflora as provided by mushroom compost it is possible that other organisms are involved. It is Lacey's experience that *Thermomonospora*-like organisms are more abundant than *F. rectivirgula* and *T. vulgaris* (J. Lacey, 1971, personal communication). Precipitating antibodies against mushroom compost may be demonstrated in affected workers but they may occur in unaffected workers and unexposed controls (Chan-Yeung, Grzybowski and Schonell, 1972).

Although the clinical features of mushroom workers' lung are usually consistent with an immunological basis, the development of symptoms on first exposure (Stewart, 1974) suggests that non-immunological or para-immunological mechanisms may also be involved.

The spores of the mushrooms (*P. florida*) are highly allergenic. Acute symptoms of extrinsic allergic alveolitis may be associated with the inhalation of spores and a large proportion of exposed workers may be affected (von Betz, 1985). Prick and intradermal skin tests with spore extract give dual skin reactions, and serum precipitins against the spore extract are present in the serum of affected workers (Schulz, Felten and Hausen, 1974).

The causal allergens of mushroom workers' lung, therefore, arise from two sources: the mushroom compost itself which is rich in thermophilic actinomycetes and from which no specific causal allergen has been identified, and from the mushroom spores, particularly those of *P. florida*.

It has been suggested that nitrogen dioxide might be evolved by the compost (see 'silo-fillers' disease', Chapter 18) and cause the disease (Bringhurst, Byrne and Gershon-Cohen, 1959), but there is no evidence that significant concentrations of the gas occur and no reason whatsoever to believe that it plays any part in the pathogenesis of mushroom workers' lung.

Diagnosis and prevention

It is important to bear this form of extrinsic allergic alveolitis in mind when a mushroom farmworker has an acute febrile respiratory disease, especially if the illness is not necessarily severe. All the acutely ill patients in Stewart's (1974) group were first considered to have bronchopneumonia and were treated for such without effect. In other instances (Jackson and Welch, 1970), a lung biopsy has been required to establish the diagnosis. A worker who has more than one attack should be advised to leave the industry and, probably, avoid any other work carrying a known risk of extrinsic allergic alveolitis.

Further outbreaks of mushroom workers' lung should be rare. The spawning of mushroom compost is now fully automated in most mushroom farms and appropriate respiratory protection has controlled respiratory disease among the mushroom pickers and sorters (Schulz, Felten and Hausen, 1974; von Betz, 1985).

Malt workers' lung

Although the features of acute extrinsic allergic alveolitis in malt workers were first recorded in 1928 (Vallery-Radot and Giroud), the significance of this observation has only recently been recognized (Riddle et al., 1968; Channel et al., 1969). The disease occurs in distillery maltsmen and brewery workers. The prevalence of symptomatic disease with lung function changes in a few but without abnormal physical signs of radiographic changes is reported to be 5.2 per cent among workers in the Scottish malting industry (Grant et al., 1976), but in the industry as a whole some cases may have been unrecognized. A chronic form of the disease does not seem to have been described, although chronic respiratory symptoms appear to be more common among malt workers than controls (Riddle, 1974).

In the malting process barley from the farms is dried in hot-air kilns, stored in silos for at least 8 weeks, and dehydrated in steeping tanks with hypochlorite as a mild fungicide. It is then treated by traditional or mechanized processes. In the traditional process the barley is spread out on open concrete floors (open-floor malting) and allowed to germinate. The temperature of the grain is maintained at 18°C by turning and raking the grain periodically (which also releases carbon dioxide and water) or by varying the thickness of the layer. The heat is produced by the respiration of the barley during germination. When the process has reached the desired stage of germination, it is stopped by drying the malt at 82°C in a hot air kiln in which it is turned periodically to facilitate drying. It is then ready for the distillery. In modern maltings the process is partly or wholly mechanized (drum-method) so that dust exposure is either much reduced or eliminated and, correspondingly, so is the prevalence of disease. However, open-floor malting is believed to be essential for the characteristic flavour of high quality Highland malt whisky but, in this case, due, probably, to the fact that only high quality local, and not imported, barley is used, the prevalence of extrinsic allergic alveolitis is low (Grant et al., 1975).

The disease is apparently caused by *Aspergillus clavatus* (Riddle et al., 1968; Channel et al., 1969). *A. clavatus* is a recognized contaminant of grain (Panasenko, 1967). Small amounts of inoculum may be present on grain or barley in the field, but there are also many opportunities of infection in the malting process and the suitable conditions on the malt floor lead to rapid proliferation. The spores are present in husks and malt grist, which implies that they can withstand the temperatures reached in the kilns (Channel et al., 1969). Riddle et al. (1968) have suggested that the growth of fungi is encouraged by the presence of a large percentage of split corns, by maintenance of a higher floor temperature (24°C) assisted by spraying the grain with water to shorten the germination time; and that the hypochlorite treatment encourages the growth of *A. clavatus* by suppression of other organisms. Malt workers may be exposed to spore dust, therefore, when turning barley on the malt floor and malt in the malt kilns, and also when cleaning the kilns (Channel et al., 1969).

The sputum of all exposed workers, irrespective of whether or not they have evidence of disease, contains spores of *A. clavatus*. Precipitins against *A. clavatus* are present in the serum of men with symptoms in increasing prevalence according to their severity and also in a proportion of healthy employees, but not in normal unexposed employees nor in patients with suspected farmers' lung (Channel et al., 1969). Skin-prick tests suggest that symptoms are usually associated with a type III reaction to *A. clavatus* (Grant et al., 1976), and bronchial challenge tests with *A. clavatus* spores reproduce the disease in men who have previously suffered from it.

Some workers also have precipitins to *Aspergillus fumigatus, Penicillium granulatum, Penicillium citrinium* and *Rhizopus stolonifer,* which are common contaminants of malt floors, but without evidence of respiratory disease (Riddle, 1974).

When contamination of the malting process with *A. clavatus* is discovered clinical, radiographic and serological tests should be carried out on all exposed employees, and the possibility of allergic alveolitis considered in the event of acute respiratory disease.

The application of mechanical methods in some distilleries and breweries has greatly decreased or eliminated the chance of workers inhaling spores and of developing allergic alveolitis.

Suberosis

Cork workers in Portugal – who number more than 20 000 – are prone to lung disease which has been attributed to work dust (Cancella, 1959). In atopic workers it has the features of bronchial asthma with transient opacities in the chest radiograph, but in non-atopic workers it is an extrinsic allergic alveolitis with the same clinical, physiological and radiographic features as farmers' lung (Ávila and Villar, 1968; Pimentel and Ávila, 1973). Persons with acute or subacute alveolitis appear to recover completely when removed from the working environment.

Cork is the bark of *Quercus suber* L, a species of oak growing in Spain and Portugal. A wide variety of jobs are involved in its processing: sorting, grading and boiling cork bark in the open air; work in cork storage warehouses; cutting and preparing discs, stoppers ('corks') and other materials; and finishing, for example standing, grading and packing the products. Machine and other maintenance workers not directly involved with the process also work in the factor (Ávila and Lacey, 1974). Cork bark is burnt to produce a black pigment, Spanish black.

Cork bark may become mouldy after being boiled and stacked wet for straightening purposes in hot, damp warehouses. Dust which consists of cork and the spores of numerous different fungi, including *Penicillium frequentans* (Westling), is encountered in high concentrations during destacking and the preparatory manufacturing stages of discs and stoppers ('corks') (Ávila and Lacey, 1974).

The pathology of acute disease consists of infiltration of alveolar walls with lymphocytes, histiocytes and, later, fibroblasts, and by the appearance of sarcoid-type granulomas with peripheral lymphocytic infiltration. In chronic disease there is dust pigmentation and DIPF with honeycombing and obliterative changes in small vessels (Ávila and Villar, 1968). The size of the spores of *P. frequentans* and some of the other air-borne fungi will allow them to penetrate to alveolar level whereas cork particles tend to be larger (Ávila and Lacey, 1974), although they are consistently present in lung lesions (Pimentel and Ávila, 1973).

That *P. frequentans* is probably the chief cause of this form of extrinsic allergic alveolitis is indicated by the facts that:

1. Precipitins against *P. frequentans* are present in the sera of almost all (98 per cent) of affected workers but in only very few (7 per cent) unaffected workers.
2. Extracts of the fungus give a type III skin reaction in patients with disease.
3. Bronchial challenge tests with the extract reproduce the symptoms.
4. Radiographic changes are significantly correlated with the concentration of air-borne fungus spores (Ávila and Lacey, 1974).

Although air-borne cork particles are fewer and larger than the fungal spores, it has been suggested that they may play some part in pathogenesis on the grounds that the incidence of precipitins correlates with the numbers of air-borne cork particles and that cork particles are commonly present in the granulomatous lesions (Ávila and Lacey, 1974). However, the presence of cork particles in the lesions is not necessarily proof of cause. It is possible, nonetheless, that particulate cork might facilitate the production of disease by the fungus (see Bagassosis, page 692).

There is no evidence that the dust of clean, non-mouldy cork causes lung disease. This point is important because exposure to cork dust in such activities as the cutting and buffing of corn-containing products (for example, floor tiles) is fairly common.

Maple bark strippers' disease (coniosporosis)

Acute respiratory disease in men who stripped the bark off maple trees was first reported by Towey, Sweany and Huron in 1932 since when a number of cases of allergic granulomatous alveolitis have been reported (Emanuel, Lawton and Wenzel, 1962; Emanuel, Wenzel and Lawton, 1966; Wenzel and Emanuel, 1967). Although Towey, Sweany and Huron referred to the disorder as 'bronchial asthma' the clinical and radiographic features they described were typical of acute extrinsic allergic alveolitis. The cause of the disease is inhalation of spores of *Cryptostroma (Coniosporum) corticale* which are ovoid and measure 4 to 5 μm in their greater axis. This fungus causes disease under the bark of maples, hickories, bass woods and sycamores (Gregory and Waller, 1951). Wenzel and Emanuel (1967) found that *C. corticale* was not present in maples before they were felled but developed during prolonged storage afterwards. Exposure to the spores occurred mainly in paper mills during stripping of logs by hand or mechanical means, sawing, and shaking small log chippings through screens to remove bark fragments. A chronic form of the disease does not seem to have been observed.

Precipitins specific for the spore extract are present in affected workers and also in exposed, but seemingly unaffected, workers some of whom, however, have had subclinical disease (Emanuel, Wenzel and Lawton, 1966). Experimental work with *C. corticale* in rats supports the conclusion that delayed hypersensitivity plays an important role in maple bark disease (Tewksbury, Wenzel and Emanuel, 1968).

Biopsy of lung tissue during the illness reveals sarcoid-type granulomas and some degree of diffuse interstitial fibrosis, and the presence of spores. The fungus can be grown from the tissue on Sabouraud's agar supplemented with an aqueous extract of maple wood (Emanuel, Wenzel and Lawton, 1966). The spores in the lungs closely resemble *Histoplasma capsulatum* but are distinguished by being stained black with Gomori's methenamine

silver nitrate technique (Emanuel, Wenzel and Lawton, 1966). Histoplasmin skin and complement fixation tests are negative.

Preventive measures consist of spraying logs during debarking with water containing detergent, remote control of some operations, the wearing of special respirators, monitoring of spore concentrations in the mill, and regular clinical, serological and radiographic examinations. The disease can be controlled by these means, but continual vigilance is necessary.

Similar type, prolonged exposure to the fungus *Alternaria* in logs during the preparation of wood pulp for the manufacture of paper may also cause allergic alveolitis (*wood-pulp workers' disease*). Characteristic symptoms and radiographic changes occur and lung biopsy has shown features consistent with allergic alveolitis. Bronchial challenge with alternaria extract has reproduced symptoms of the disease (Schlueter, Fink and Henley, 1972).

Air conditioner lung disease

'Humidifier fever' or '*Befeuchterfieber*' was first described in 1959 by Pestalozzi in a group of workers in a carpentry shop who had been exposed to air from a humidifier contaminated by bacteria and fungi. Respiratory and constitutional symptoms consistent with extrinsic allergic alveolitis have also been reported in relation to air-conditioning systems contaminated with micro-organisms. The disorder was originally attributed to *F. rectivirgula (M. faeni)* spores released into the atmosphere of an office from a contaminated air-conditioning system in the USA (Banaszak, Thiede and Fink, 1970). Subsequently, episodes of disease have been associated with air-conditioning systems in homes, offices, operating rooms and factories – especially in industries requiring carefully controlled humidity, such as printing, stationery and the manufacture of textiles (Fink et al., 1971; Sweet et al., 1971; Weiss and Soleymani, 1971; Hodges, Fink and Schlueter, 1974; Friend et al., 1977; Medical Research Council Symposium, 1977; Campbell et al., 1979). However, although in some respects humidifier fever may be similar to extrinsic allergic alveolitis there are significant differences which suggest the existence of two distinct syndromes:

1. Extrinsic allergic alveolitis which is predominant in the descriptions of disease in the USA and Switzerland (Scherrer et al., 1978).
2. 'Humidifier fever' proper.

Extrinsic allergic alveolitis

Symptoms, physical signs, lung function and radiographic changes are identical to those of acute, subacute or chronic extrinsic allergic alveolitis due to other causes. Chronic disease appears to consist of the gradual onset of dyspnoea on exertion without previous acute disease. Only two outbreaks of this disease, caused by contamination of an air-conditioning system or a central heating system, have been described in Britain (Fergusson, Milne and Crompton, 1984; Robertson et al., 1987). The illness has been attributed to thermophilic actinomycetes (*T. vulgaris* and *T. thalpophilus* – see page 683) growing in water of air-conditioning systems and to spores of *Aureobasidium pullulans* (*Pullularia*) – the organism associated putatively with sequoiosis (see page 700) – in steam from stagnant water poured over a heating element in a home sauna bath (*sauna-takers' disease*) (Metzger et al., 1976); to steam from contaminated water in a hot tub room (*Cladosporium cladosporoides*) (Jacobs et al., 1986); to growth of micro-organisms in carpet felt made damp by a leaking central heating system (*Penicillium chrysogenum* and *P. cyclopium*) (Fergusson, Milne and Crompton, 1984); and to contamination of the evaporative core of a car air conditioner by *T. candidus* (Kumar, Marier and Leech, 1981). Serum precipitins to actinomycetes or other implicated allergens are present in most cases and, in a few, the antigen has been demonstrated in lung tissue by immunofluorescence. Inhalation challenge with cultured organisms has reproduced the illness (Fink et al., 1976).

'Humidifier fever'

This illness varies between one of mild 'flu-like symptoms with myalgia associated with a low grade fever to an acute illness consisting of malaise, myalgia, fever, headache and breathlessness. These symptoms usually resolve in 24 hours. One of the differentiating features between 'humidifier fever' and extrinsic allergic alveolitis is their symptom periodicity. In 'humidifier fever' symptoms are most severe on the first day of the working week, improving rapidly over the remainder of the week. They recur on re-exposure after an absence from work. In extrinsic allergic alveolitis, symptoms tend to increase in severity with continued exposure to the allergen. Investigations of outbreaks of 'humidifier fever' in Britain, including factories such as printing, stationery and textile manufacture and an operating room, have shown that usually only a minority of workers are affected, prevalence rates varying between 2.5 and 40 per cent (Edwards, Griffiths and

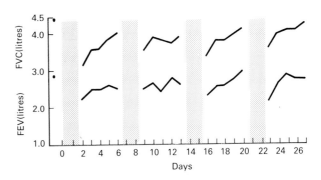

Figure 20.13 Spirometry during 1 month in a worker with intermittent malaise, cough and fever in a factory where air-conditioning units were contaminated with a variety of organisms. The stippled columns indicate weekends. Measurements taken at 16:00 each day: indicates daily FVC and FEV$_1$ measured at 16:00 when he was asymptomatic and working in an uncontaminated part of the factory. (Reproduced with permission from Pickering et al., 1976)

Mullins, 1976; Pickering et al., 1976; Friend et al., 1977; Parrott and Blyth, 1980; Cockcroft et al., 1981). No radiographic changes were observed in any of these outbreaks, although a single case of 'humidifier fever' has been described with radiographic changes (Anderson, McSharry and Boyd, 1985). The periodicity of symptoms in this individual with intermittent symptoms through the working week and the associated profound weight loss is more in keeping with extrinsic allergic alveolitis than with 'humidifier fever'. The incidence of the illness is highest in the winter months due to the greater use of humidifiers during this period.

Symptoms and changes in pulmonary function are most pronounced on return to work on a Monday and improve progressively over the remainder of the working week similar to grades C1 and C2 byssinosis (Figure 20.13) (see Chapter 21, page 732). The physical findings are the same as those of extrinsic allergic alveolitis.

The specific responsible organism(s) has not been identified but serum precipitins against crude humidifier extracts are present in both affected, and unaffected but exposed, workers. In workers exposed to heavily contaminated humidifiers, the presence and amount of antibody present are determined by the individual's length of exposure and smoking habits (Finnegan et al., 1985). There is a strong inverse relationship between current smoking and precipitins. This effect of smoking reversed 3 years after stopping smoking. The duration of exposure also has a major effect with a clear dose–response relationship demonstrable between length of employment and the presence and amount of antibody. In general, no consistent relationships between precipitins and individual fungi or bacteria have been evident. Several causes of 'humidifier fever' have been proposed on the basis of serological testing including bacterial endotoxins (Rylander et al., 1978; Flaherty et al., 1984), *Bacillus subtilis* (Parrott and Blyth, 1980) and amoebae (Medical Research Council Symposium, 1977; Edwards, 1980). Air-borne endotoxin was also implicated in an outbreak among printers exposed to humidifier water contaminated with *Pseudomonas* sp. (Rylander and Haglind, 1984). However, a study of four outbreaks of humidifier fever (Finnegan et al., 1987) found no correlation between the presence of antibodies to amoebae and the presence of 'humidifier fever' symptoms. Bronchial provocation studies with extracts of individual organisms isolated from a contaminated humidifier have failed to reproduce the disease in affected individuals (Pickering et al., 1976). Nonetheless, provocation studies with an extract of contaminated water itself induces the typical symptoms of 'humidifier fever' in affected subjects but not in unexposed controls (Friend et al., 1977). The pattern of the challenge reaction is similar in nature, rate of onset and duration to the 'late alveolar reaction' provoked by appropriate antigens in extrinsic allergic alveolitis (Newman Taylor et al., 1978).

Conclusions

The clinical features of 'humidifier fever' are very variable and the causal agents are yet to be clearly defined. Unlike typical acute (or subacute) extrinsic allergic alveolitis, where the source of exposure is usually well defined and dust concentrations high, the level of air-borne material sufficient to cause an episode of 'humidifier fever' in susceptible individuals appears to be extremely low. It has been suggested that the febrile illness might be caused by bacterial endotoxins. This would be consistent with the apparent tachyphylaxis which affected individuals demonstrate. However, the clinical features of this disease, with a minority of exposed individuals affected and the often prolonged periods of exposure before developing disease, would suggest an immunological aetiology. The two important differences between 'humidifier fever' and extrinsic allergic alveolitis are the absence of both radiographic changes and persisting disability in the former disease. This may be related to antigen presentation. In 'humidifier fever', soluble antigen might produce soluble aggregates and resultant complement consumption, whereas in extrinsic allergic alveolitis the antigen tends to be particulate and relatively insoluble, persisting in the lung and leading to granuloma formation. Whatever the causes and mechanisms of this disorder prove to be, two points are important:

1. The clinician must be aware of its existence and of the different forms it may take. If only a few individuals in the workforce are affected and the humidifier is used only intermittently, the diagnosis may be difficult to make (Newman Taylor et al., 1978). A history of a recurrent febrile illness, often with respiratory symptoms but normal chest radiograph, may call for investigation of the conditions in which the patient works including systematic observations at work. Inhalational challenge testing may be necessary for a definitive diagnosis.

2. Prevention of the growth of organisms in the humidifier system will avoid the development of disease. A rich flora grows readily in recirculated water reservoirs, particularly when the humidifier has a washing in addition to a humidifying function. Droplet nuclei containing antigen are released into the working environment by these contaminated humidification systems. At the present time the growth of organisms is frequently controlled by the regular introduction of biocides into the humidifier water. This method should be discouraged because we have no knowledge of the effects of long-term exposure of working populations to low levels of this group of chemicals. Regular cleaning, which may be made difficult by poor design, and regular dumping of humidifier water at night or over weekends will reduce microbial growth. Steam injection systems in place of cold water sprays will also prevent microbial growth.

At present air-conditioner disease is not a notifiable disease in Britain; its true prevalence is, therefore, unknown.

Rare causes of extrinsic allergic alveolitis

Sequoiosis

A granulomatous alveolitis has been reported in a man exposed to mouldy sawdust of the giant redwood (*Sequoia sempervirens*) in whose serum precipitins against extracts of saw-mill dust were found (Cohen et al., 1967). The responsible organisms have not been positively identified, but may be *Graphium* or *Aureobasidium pullulans*.

Cheese workers' lung

The clinical features of extrinsic allergic alveolitis have been observed both in Swiss cheesemakers engaged in washing moulds off the surface of cheeses (De Week, Gutersohn and Bütikofer, 1969; Molina, 1976) and in a worker packaging blue cheese (Campbell et al., 1983). Among the cheese washers 10 to 15 per cent workers are affected and precipitins of IgG class against *Penicillium casei* were present in their sera. In the blue cheese worker, specific IgG to *Penicillium roqueforti* was detected both in the serum and in the bronchoalveolar lavage fluid.

Asthmatic symptoms also occur in cheese washers and may be difficult to differentiate from acute extrinsic allergic alveolitis; indeed, both may occur together (Wüthrich and Keiser, 1970). Molina (1976) has found acarids of *Dermatophagoides* spp. on the surface of cheese and preliminary investigation of Cantal cheese workers has shown specific serum precipitins against acarid extracts. The cheese mites *Aleurobius farinae* and *Tyrolichus casei* may be implicated (Renaud et al., 1979).

It is clear that cheese manufacture involves exposure of workers to moulds on the surface of cheeses and as an integral part of the cheese itself, and also to mites, all of which are potentially allergenic.

Dry rot lung

Acute allergic alveolitis with typical radiographic changes has been observed in association with asthma and shown to be due to the fungus *Merulius lacrymans* from extensive dry rot in the patient's home. Skin testing showed a dual reaction to the fungus extract and specific IgE and IgG precipitins were present. Complete recovery followed removal from exposure (O'Brien et al., 1978). Asthma caused by the spores of this fungus is well recognized (see Chapter 21).

Wheat weevil lung

For many years it has been known that asthma may occur in sensitive granary or farmworkers exposed to grain and flour dust (Frankland and Lunn, 1965; Lunn, 1966). This may be caused by a variety of mites and fungi, but the wheat weevil (*Sitophilus granarius*) can give rise, not only to a pronounced immediate (type I) allergy, but also to precipitating antibodies (Jimenez-Diag, Lahoz and Canto, 1947). Delayed (type III) sensitivity with constitutional symptoms, basal inspiratory crackles and impairment of gas transfer have been produced in an atopic worker by inhalation challenge 3 hours after

an immediate asthmatic reaction. Precipitins against weevil extract were found in his serum after concentration, and intradermal injection of weevil extract caused a delayed, Arthus-type reaction (Lunn and Hughes, 1967). The source of the antigen is weevil protein.

Animal handlers' lung

Recurrent episodes of acute extrinsic allergic alveolitis have been described in a research assistant handling rats for experimental purposes. Skin-prick tests to rat serum were positive and precipitins against rat serum, urine and pelt, but not fur, were present. Rat urine contains large amounts of serum protein and was probably the chief source of antigen. The patient's symptoms recurred with radiographic changes on deliberate or inadvertent re-exposure to rats or mice. Thus, air-borne proteins of the urine, dander and hair particles of rats and, possibly, other experimental animals are a source of antigen capable of provoking extrinsic allergic alveolitis in laboratory workers (Carroll et al., 1975).

Close contact with gerbils (small rodents also known as jerboas) is also reported to cause acute disease, presumably for similar reasons (Korenblat et al., 1977).

Fish meal workers' lung

Features of acute disease have been reported in an employee of a factory manufacturing animal foods in which fish meal was incorporated. Intracutaneous tests gave a dual response to fish meal extracts, and bronchial challenge was followed by basal inspiratory crackles and fall in T_L after 5 hours. Multiple serum precipitins against fish meal antigens were present (Ávila, 1971).

Diisocyanate alveolitis

Organic isocyanates are extensively used in the manufacture of synthetic rubbers, adhesives and paints, and as a catalyst in porcelain finishing and moulding sands; they are known to be a potent cause of asthma and are discussed in Chapter 21. However, occasionally acute extrinsic allergic alveolitis may occur in individuals exposed to toluene diisocyanate (Charles et al., 1976), methylene diphenyl diisocyanate (Malo and Zeiss, 1982) and hexamethylene diisocyanate (Malo et al., 1983). A mixed picture of allergic alveolitis and bronchial asthma has also been described (Malo et al., 1983; Vergnon et al., 1985). The clinical, radiographic bronchoalveolar lavage and bronchial biopsy findings are characteristic of an extrinsic allergic alveolitis (Vergnon et al., 1985; Takazakura et al., 1987). Immunologically, specific IgG antibodies to isocyanate bound to human serum albumin have been identified both in the serum (Malo and Zeiss, 1982) and in bronchoalveolar lavage fluid (Bascom et al., 1985) of sensitized individuals. The prognosis in diisocyanate alveolitis is not well documented. No cases of progressive lung fibrosis have been described. However, in order to prevent irreversible lung damage, immediate removal from exposure to antigen is essential.

Pyrethrum alveolitis

Pyrethrum consists of powdered flower heads of the plant *Anacyclus pyrethrum*, and has insecticidal properties.

Repeated heavy exposure to a pyrethrum-based insecticide in the home is reported to have caused subacute extrinsic allergic alveolitis with radiographic changes and granuloma-like lesions and DIPF on lung biopsy. Skin tests with pyrethrum produced a dual response (Carlson and Villaveces, 1977).

Bacillus subtilis alveolitis

A minor epidemic of 'hypersensitivity pneumonitis' in six members of a family apparently caused by *B. subtilis* released from wood dust in the flooring of an old bathroom during its restoration has been described by Johnson et al. (1980). They suggest that this organism should be considered as a potential cause of irreversible lung damage in susceptible people.

Pauli's reagent alveolitis

Acute extrinsic alveolitis caused by sodium diazobenzene sulphate (Pauli's reagent) used in chromatography has been reported in an atopic medical laboratory technician by Evans and Seaton (1979). Bronchial challenge resulted in immediate and late airflow obstruction, and clinical, physiological, radiographic and histological evidence of

allergic alveolitis. Complete recovery followed withdrawal from exposure. The fact that other workers in the laboratory were unaffected and that this appears to be the first case on record suggests that the reaction was related to increased susceptibility due to the atopic status of the subject.

Pituitary snuff takers' lung

Cases of extrinsic allergic alveolitis apparently caused by therapeutic snuffs containing powdered extracts of pig or ox pituitary glands in patients with diabetes insipidus were reported in the past (Mahon et al., 1967; Harper et al., 1970). As this method of treatment has now ceased, they no longer count.

References

Allen, D.H., Williams, G.V. and Woolcock, A.J. (1976) Bird breeders' hypersensitivity pneumonitis: progress studies of lung function after cessation of exposure to the provoking antigen. *Am. Rev. Respir. Dis.* **114**, 555–566

Allen, D.H., Basten, A., Williams, G.V. and Woolcock, A.J. (1975) Familial hypersensitivity pneumonitis. *Am. J. Med.* **59**, 505–514

Andersen, P., Pedersen, O.F., Bach, B. and Bonde, G.J. (1982) A current view of pigeon fanciers' lung. *Clin. Allergy* **12**, 53–59

Anderson, K., McSharry, C.P. and Boyd, G. (1985) Radiographic changes in humidifier fever. *Thorax* **40**, 312–313

Arshad, M., Braun, S.R. and Sunderrajan, E.V. (1987) Severe hypoxaemia in farmers' lung disease with normal findings on chest roentgenogram. *Chest* **91**, 274–275

Ávila, R. (1971) Extrinsic allergic alveolitis in workers exposed to fish meal and poultry. *Clin. Allergy* **1**, 343–346

Ávila, R. and Lacey, J. (1974) The role of *Penicillium frequentans* in suberosis (respiratory disease in workers in the cork industry). *Clin. Allergy* **4**, 109–117

Ávila, R. and Villar, T.G. (1968) Suberosis. Respiratory disease in cork workers. *Lancet* **1**, 620–621

Banaszak, E.F., Thiede, W.H. and Fink, J.N. (1970) Hypersensitivity pneumonitis due to contamination of air conditioners. *N. Engl. J. Med.* **183**, 271–276

Banham, S.W., Lynch, P. and Boyd, G. (1978) Environmental and constitutional factors determining hypersensitivity to avian antigens in pigeon fanciers. *Thorax* **33**, 674

Banham, S.W., McKenzie, H., McSharry, C., Lynch, P.P. and Boyd, G. (1982) Antibody against a pigeon bloom-extract: a further antigen in pigeon fanciers' lung. *Clin. Allergy* **12**, 173–178

Banham, S.W., McSharry, C., Lynch, P.P. and Boyd, G. (1986) Relationships between avian exposure, humoral immune response and pigeon breeders' disease among Scottish pigeon fanciers. *Thorax* **41**, 274–278

Barboriak, J.J., Sosman, A.J. and Reed, C.E. (1965) Serological studies in pigeon breeder's disease. *J. Lab. Clin. Med.* **65**, 600–604

Barrowcliff, D.F. and Arblaster, P.G. (1968) Farmer's lung: a study of an early acute fatal case. *Thorax* 23, 490–500

Bascom, R., Kennedy, T.P., Levitz, D. and Zeiss, C.R. (1985) Specific broncho-alveolar lavage IgG antibody in hypersensitivity pneumonitis from diphenylmethane diisocyanate. *Am. Rev. Respir. Dis.* 131, 463–465

Beaudry, C. and Laplante, L. (1973) Severe allergic pneumonitis from hydrochlorothiazide. *Ann. Intern. Med.* 78, 251–253

Benson, M.K., Lancaster-Smith, M.J., Perrin, J., Holborrow, E.J. and Pepys, J. (1972) Serum immunoglobulins, autoantibodies and avian precipitins in adult coeliac disease. *Ninth International Congress of Gastroenterology,* 1972, Paris, Abstract, p.398

Bernardo, J., Hunninghake, G.W., Gadek, J.E., Ferrans, V.J. and Crystal, R.G. (1979) Acute hypersensitivity pneumonitis: serial changes in lung lymphocyte subpopulations after exposure to antigen. *Am. Rev. Respir. Dis.* 120, 985– 994

Berrens, L., Guikers, C.L.H. and van Dijk, A. (1974) The antigens of pigeon breeder's disease and their interaction with human complement. *Ann. NY Acad. Sci.* 221, 153– 162

Berrill, W.T. and Van Rood, J.J. (1977) HLA-DW6 and avian hypersensitivity. *Lancet* 2, 248–249

Berrill, W.T., Eade, O.E., Fitzpatrick, P.F., Hyde, I., McLeod, W.M. and Wright, R. (1975) Bird fancier's lung and jejunal villous atrophy. *Lancet* 2, 1006–1008

Berruchon, J. and Oury, M. (1981) Le poumon de champignononniiste. *Med. Intern.* 16, 162–171

Bhattacharjee, J.W., Saxena, R.P. and Zaidi, S.H. (1980) Experimental studies on the toxicity of bagasse. *Environ. Res.* 23, 68–76

Bice, D.E., McCarron, K., Hoffman, E.O. and Salvaggio, J.E. (1977) Adjuvant properties of *Micropolyspora faeni. Int. Archs. Allergy Appl. Immunol.* 55, 267–274

Bishop, J.M., Melnick, S.C. and Raine, J. (1963) Farmer's lung: studies of pulmonary function and aetiology. *Q. J. Med.* 32, 257–258

Björnsson, O. (1960) Quoted by Staines, F.H. and Forman, J.A.S. (1961) A survey of 'farmer's lung'. *J. Coll. Gen. Practnrs Res. Newsl.* 4, 351–382

Blackman, E. (1969) Observations on the development of silica cells of the leaf sheaf of wheat (*Triticum aistium*). *Can. J. Bot.* 47, 827–848

Boren, M.N., Moore, V.L., Abramoff, P. and Fink, J.N. (1977) Pigeon breeder's disease. Antibody response of man against a purified component of pigeon dropping extract. *Clin. Immunol. Immunopathol.* 8, 108–115

Bourke, S.J., Banham, S.W., Certer, R., Lynch, P. and Boyd, G. (1989) Longitudinal course of extrinsic allergic alveolitis in pigeon breeders. *Thorax* 44, 415–418

Boyd, D.H.A. (1971) The incidence of farmer's lung in Caithness. *Scott. Med. J.* 16, 261–262

Boyd, G., Madkour, M., Middleton, S. and Lynch, P. (1977) Effect of smoking on circulating antibody levels to avian protein in pigeon breeder's disease. *Thorax* 32, 651

Boyd, G., McSharry, C.P., Banham, S.W. and Lynch, P.P. (1982) A current view of pigeon fancier's lung. A model for pulmonary extrinsic allergic alveolitis. *Clin. Allergy* 12(suppl.), 53–59

Boyer, R.S., Klock, L.E., Schmidt, C.D., Hyland, L., Maxwell, K., Gardner, R.M. and Renzetti, Jr, A.D. (1974) Hypersensitivity lung disease in the turkey raising industry. *Am. Rev. Respir. Dis.* 109, 630–635

Bradford, J.K., Blalock, J.B. and Wascom, C.M. (1961) Bagasse disease of the lungs. *Am. Rev. Respir. Dis.* 84, 582– 585

Braun, S.R., doPico, G.A., Tsiatis, A., Horvath, E., Dickie, H.A.

and Rankin, J. (1979) Farmer's lung disease: Long term clinical and physiological outcome. *Am. Rev. Respir. Dis.* 119, 185–191

Bringhurst, L.S., Byrne, R.N. and Gershon-Cohen, J. (1959) Respiratory disease of mushroom workers. *J. Am. Med. Assoc.* 171, 15–18

Buechner, H.A. (1962) Bagassosis: a true pneumoconiosis. *Ind. Med. Surg.* 31, 311–314

Buechner, H.A. (1968) Quoted by Seabury et al. (1968)

Buechner, H.A., Prevatt, A., Thompson, J. and Blitz, O. (1958) Bagassosis – a review, with further historical data, studies of pulmonary function and results of adrenal steroid therapy. *Am. J. Med.* 25, 234–247

Buechner, H.A., Aucoin, E., Vignes, A.J. and Weill, H. (1964) The resurgence of bagassosis in Louisiana. *J. Occup. Med.* 6, 437–442

Calvanico, N.J., Ambegaonkar, S.P., Schlueter, D.P. and Fink, J.N. (1980) Immunoglobulin levels in bronchoalveolar lavage fluid from pigeon breeders. *J. Lab. Clin. Med.* 96, 129–140

Campbell, I.A., Cockcroft, A.E., Edwards, J.H. and Jones, M. (1979) Humidifier fever in an operating theatre. *Br. Med. J.* 2, 1036–1037

Campbell, J.A., Kryda, M.J., Treuhaft, M.W., Marx, J.J. and Roberts, R.C. (1983) Cheese workers' hypersensitivity pneumonitis. *Am. Rev. Respir. Dis.* 127, 495–496

Cancella, de Carvalho (1959) Suberose. Alteraçoes pulmonares relacionadas com a inalação de poeiras de cortiça. Dissertaçao de Dontoramento, Lisboa

Cangini, G. (1951) Casidi bagassosi in Italia. *Lotta c. tuberc.* 21, 300

Carlson, J.E. and Villaveces, J.W. (1977) Hypersensitivity pneumonitis due to pyrethrum. *J. Am. Med. Assoc.* 237, 1718–1719

Carroll, K.B., Pepys, J., Longbottom, J.L., Hughes, D.T.D. and Benson, H.G. (1975) Extrinsic allergic alveolitis due to rat serum proteins. *Clin. Allergy* 5, 443–456

Castleden, L.I.M. and Hamilton-Paterson, J.L. (1942) Bagassosis. An industrial lung disease. *Br. Med. J.* 2, 478–480

Chan-Yeung, M., Grzybowski, S. and Schonell, M.E. (1972) Mushroom worker's lung. *Am. Rev. Respir. Dis.* 105, 819–822

Chan-Yeung, M., Schulzer, M., Maclean, L., Dorken, E. and Gryzbowski, S. (1980) Epidemiologic health survey of grain elevator workers in British Columbia. *Am. Rev. Respir. Dis.* 121, 329–338

Chandra, S. and Jones, H.E. (1972) Pigeon fanciers' lung in children. *Archs Dis. Child.* 47, 716–718

Channel, S., Blyth, W., Lloyd, M., Weir, D.M., Amos, W.M.G., Littlewood, A.P., Riddle, H.F.V. and Grant, I.W.B. (1969) Allergic alveolitis in maltworkers. *Q. J. Med.* 38, 351–376

Charles, J., Bernstein, A., Jones, B., Jones, D.J., Edwards, J.H., Seal, R.M.E. and Seaton, A. (1976) Hypersensitivity pneumonitis after exposure to isocyanates. *Thorax* 31, 127–136

Christensen, L.T., Schmidt, C.D. and Robbins, L. (1975) Pigeon breeder's disease – a prevalence study and review. *Clin. Allergy* 5, 417–430

Cockcroft, A., Edwards, J., Bevan, C., Campbell, I., Collins, G., Houston, K., Jenkins, D., Latham, S., Saunders, M. and Trotman, D. (1981) An investigation of operating theatre staff exposed to humidifier fever antigens. *Br. J. Ind. Med.* 38, 144–151

Cohen, H.I., Merigan, T.C., Kosek, J.C. and Eldridge, F. (1967) Sequoiosis. *Am. J. Med.* 43, 785–794

Cormier, Y. and Belanger, J. (1985) Long-term physiologic outcome after acute farmers' lung. *Chest* 87, 796–800

Cormier, Y., Belanger, J., Leblanc, P. and Laviolette, M. (1986)

Bronchoalveolar lavage in farmers' lung disease: diagnostic and physiological significance. *Br. J. Ind. Med.* **43**, 401–405

Cooper, I.A. and Greenaway, T.M. (1961) Farmer's lung: a case report. *Med. J. Aust.* **2**, 980–981

Costabel, U., Bross, K.J., Marxen, J. and Matthys, H. (1984) T-lymphacytosis in bronchoalveolar lavage fluid of hypersensitivity pneumonitis. *Chest* **85**, 514–518

Cotton, D.J. and Dosman, J.A. (1978) Grain dust and health. III. Environmental factors. *Ann. Intern. Med.* **89**, 420–421

Craveri, R., Guicciardi, A. and Pacini, N. (1966) Distribution of thermophilic actinomycetes in compost for mushroom production. *Ann. di Microbiol.* **16**, 111–113

Cross, T. and Unsworth, B.A. (1976) Farmer's lung: a neglected antigen. *Lancet* **1**, 958–959

Cross, T. and Unsworth, B.A. (1977) List of actinomycete names: alternative proposals for the genus *Thermoactinomyces*. *Actinomycetes and Related Organisms* **12**, 6–11

Cuthbert, O.D., Brostoff, J., Wraith, D.G. and Brighton, Q.D. (1979) 'Barn allergy': asthma and rhinitis due to storage mites. *Clin. Allergy* **9**, 229–236

Darke, C.S., Knowelden, J., Lacey, J. and Ward, A.M. (1976) Respiratory disease of workers harvesting grain. *Thorax* **31**, 293–302

de Gracia, J., Morell, F., Bofill, J.M., Curull, V. and Orriols, R. (1989) Time of exposure as a prognostic factor in avian hypersensitivity pneumonitis. *Respir. Med.* **83**, 139–143

de Week, A.L., Gutersohn, J. and Bütikofer, E. (1969) La maladie des laveurs de fromage ('Käsenwascherkrankheit'): une forme particulière du syndrome du poumon du fermir. *Schweiz. Med. Wochenschr.* **99**, 872–876

Dickie, H.A. and Rankin, J. (1958) Farmer's lung: an acute granulomatous interstitial pneumonitis occurring in agricultural workers. *J. Am. Med. Assoc.* **167**, 1069–1076

Diment, J.A. and Pepys, J. (1977) Avian erythrocyte agglutination tests with the sera of bird fanciers. *J. Clin. Pathol.* **30**, 29–34

Dinda, P., Chatterjee, S.S. and Riding, W.D. (1969) Pulmonary function studies in bird breeder's lung. *Thorax* **24**, 374–378

Dizon, G.D., Almonte, J.B. and Anselmo, J.E. (1962) Bagassosis and silicosis in the Philippines. *J. Philipp. Med. Assoc.* **38**, 865–872

doPico, G.A. (1986) Report on diseases. *Am. J. Ind. Med.* **10**, 261–265

doPico, G.A., Flaherty, D., Bhansali, P. and Chavaje, N. (1982) Grain fever syndrome induced by inhalation of airborne grain dust. *J. Allergy Clin. Immunol.* **69**, 435–443

Dutkiewicz, J. (1978) Exposure to dust-borne bacteria in agriculture. I. Environmental studies. *Archs Environ. Health* 250–259

Dykewicz, M.S., Laufer, P., Patterson, R., Roberts, M. and Sommers, H.M. (1988) Woodman's disease: Hypersensitivity pneumonitis from cutting live trees. *J. Allergy Clin. Immunol.* **81**, 455–460

Editorial (1985) Smoking, occupation, and allergic lung disease. *Lancet* **1**, 965

Edwards, J.H. (1976) A quantitative study on the activation of the alternative pathway of complement by mouldy hay dust and thermophilic actinomycetes. *Clin. Allergy* **6**, 19–25

Edwards, J.H. (1980) Microbial and immunological investigations and remedial action after an outbreak of humidifier fever. *Br. J. Ind. Med.* **37**, 55–62

Edwards, J.H., Baker, J.T. and Davies, B.H. (1974) Precipitin test negative farmer's lung – activation of the alternative pathway of complement by mouldy hay dust. *Clin. Allergy* **4**, 379–388

Edwards, J.H., Griffiths, A.J. and Mullins, J. (1976) Protozoa as sources of antigen in 'humidifier fever'. *Nature* **264**, 438–439

Edwards, C. and Luntz, G. (1974) Budgerigar-fancier's lung: a

report of a fatal case. *Br. J. Dis. Chest* **68**, 57–64

Edwards, J.H., Wagner, J.C. and Seal, R.M.E. (1976) Pulmonary responses to particulate materials capable of activating alternative pathway of complement. *Clin. Allergy* **6**, 155–164

Edwards, J.H., Wagner, J.C. and Seal, R.M.E. (1980) Production of granulomas by organic dusts deposited endotracheally. *Eighth International Conference on Sarcoidosis and Granulomatous Disease* (eds W. Jones Williams and B.H. Davies), Alpha Omega Publishing, Cardiff, pp. 99–103

Effler, D., Roland, F. and Redding, R.A. (1976) The P blood group system in pigeon breeder's disease. *Chest* **70**, 719–725

Eliasson, O. (1982) Farmers' lung disease: a new historical perspective from Iceland. *J. Hist. Med. Allied Sci.* **37**, 440–445

Elman, A.J., Tebo, T., Fink, J.N. and Barboriak, J.J. (1968) Reactions of poultry against chicken antigens. *Archs Environ. Health.* **17**, 98–100

Emanuel, D.A., Lawton, B.R. and Wenzel, F.J. (1962) Maple bark disease. Pneumonitis due to *Coniosporium corticale*. *N. Engl. J. Med.* **266**, 333–337

Emanuel, D.A., Wenzel, F.J. and Lawton, B.R. (1966) Pneumonitis due to *Cryptostroma corticale* (Maple bark disease). *N. Engl. J. Med.* **274**, 1413–1418

Emanuel, D.A., Wenzel, F.J. and Lawton, B.R. (1975) Pulmonary mycotoxicosis. *Chest* **67**, 293–297

Emanuel, D.A., Wenzel, F.J., Bowerman, C.I. and Lawton, B.R. (1964) Farmer's lung. Clinical pathologic and immunologic study of twenty four patients. *Am. J. Med.* **37**, 392–401

Evans, W.V. and Seaton, A. (1979) Hypersensitivity pneumonitis in a technician using Pauli's reagent. *Thorax* **34**, 767–770

Farant, J.P. and Moore, C.F. (1978) Dust exposure in the Canadian grain industry. *Am. Ind. Hyg. Assoc. J.* **39**, 177–194

Faux, J.A., Hendrick, D.J. and Anand, B.S. (1978) Precipitins to different avian serum antigens in bird fancier's lung and coeliac disease. *Clin. Allergy* **8**, 101–108

Faux, J.A., Wide, L., Hargreave, F.E., Longbottom, J.L. and Pepys, J. (1971) Immunological aspects of respiratory allergy in budgerigar (*Melopsittacus undulatus*) fanciers. *Clin. Allergy* **1**, 149–158

Fawcitt, R. (1938) Occupational diseases of the lungs in agricultural workers. *Br. J. Radiol.* **11**, 378–392

Feldman, H.A. and Sabin, A.B. (1948) Pneumonitis of unknown aetiology in a group of men exposed to pigeon excreta. *J. Clin. Invest.* **27**, 533

Fergus, C.L. (1964) Thermophilic and thermotolerant moulds and actinomycetes of mushroom compost during peak heating. *Mycologia* **56**, 267–284

Fergusson, R.J., Milne, L.J.R. and Crompton, G.K. (1984) Penicillium allergic alveolitis: faulty installation of central heating. *Thorax* **39**, 294–298

Festenstein, G.N., Lacey, J., Skinner, F.A., Jenkins, P.A. and Pepys, J. (1965) Self heating hay and grain in Dewar flasks, and the development of farmer's lung antigens. *J. Gen. Microbiol.* **41**, 389–407

Fink, J.N. and Schlueter, D.P. (1978) Bathtub refinisher's lung: An unusual response to toluene diisocyanate. *Am. Rev. Respir. Dis.* **118**, 955–959

Fink, J.N., Hensley, G.T. and Barboriak, J.J. (1969) An animal model of a hypersensitivity pneumonitis. *J. Allergy* **46**, 156–161

Fink, J., Tebo, T. and Barboriak, J.J. (1969) Characterization of human precipitating antibody to inhaled antigens. *J. Immunol.* **103**, 244–251

Fink, J.N., Sosman, A.J., Barboriak, J.J., Schlueter, D.P. and Holmes, R.A. (1968) Pigeon breeders' disease. A clinical study of a hypersensitivity pneumonitis. *Ann. Intern. Med.* **68**, 1205–1219

Fink, J.N., Banaszak, E.A., Thiede, W.H. and Barboriak, J.J.

(1971) Interstitial pneumonitis due to hypersensitivity to an organism contaminating a heating system. *Ann. Intern. Med.* **74**, 80–83

Fink, J.N., Banaszak, E.F., Barboriak, J.J., Hensley, G.T., Kurup, V.P., Scanlon, G.T., Schlueter, D.P., Sosman, A.J., Thiede, W.H. and Unger, G.F. (1976) Interstitial lung disease due to contamination of forced air systems. *Ann. Intern. Med.* **84**, 406–413

Finnegan, M.J., Pickering, C.A.C., Davies, P.S. and Austwick, P.K.C. (1985) Factors affecting the development of precipitating antibodies in workers exposed to contaminated humidifiers. *Clin. Allergy* **15**, 281–292

Finnegan, M.J., Pickering, C.A.C., Davies, P.S., Austwick, P.K.C. and Warhurst, D.C. (1987) Amoebae and humidifier fever. *Clin. Allergy* **17**, 235–242

Flaherty, D.K., Iha, T., Chmelik, F., Dickie, H. and Reed, C.E. (1975) HLA-8 in farmer's lung. *Lancet* **2**, 507

Flaherty, D.K., Braun, S.R., Marx, J.J., Blank, J.L., Emanuel, D.A. and Rankin, J. (1980) Serologically detectable HLA – A, B and C loci antigens in farmers' lung disease. *Am. Rev. Respir. Dis.* **122**, 437–443

Flaherty, D.K., Deck, F.H., Cooper, J., Bishop, K., Winzenburger, P.A., Smith, L.R., Bynum, L. and Witmer, W.B. (1984) Bacterial endotoxin isolated from a water spray air humidification system as a putative agent of occupation-related lung disease. *Infect. Immunol.* **43**, 206–212

Fournier, E., Tonnel, A.B., Gosset, P.H., Wallaert, B., Ameisen, J.C. and Voisin, C. (1985) Early neutrophil alveolitis after antigen inhalation in hypersensitivity pneumonitis. *Chest* **88**, 563–566

Frankland, A.W. and Lunn, J.A. (1965) Asthma caused by the grain weevil. *Br. J. Ind. Med.* **22**, 157–159

Fredericks, W. (1978) Antigens in pigeon dropping extracts. *J. Allergy Clin. Immunol.* **61**, 221–223

Freedman, P.M. and Ault, B. (1981) Bronchial hyperreactivity to methacholine in farmers' lung disease. *J. Allergy Clin. Immunol.* **67**, 59–63

Friend, J.A.R., Gaddie, J., Palmer, K.N.V., Pickering, C.A.C. and Pepys, J. (1977) Extrinsic allergic alveolitis and contaminated cooling-water in a factory machine. *Lancet* **1**, 297–300

Fuller, C.J. (1953) Farmer's lung: a review of present knowledge. *Thorax* **8**, 59–64

Ganguly, S.K. and Pal, S.C. (1955) Early bagassosis. *J. Indian Med. Assoc.* **34**, 253–254

Ghose, T., Landrigan, P., Killeen, R. and Dill, J. (1974) Immunopathological studies in patients with farmer's lung. *Clin. Allergy* **4**, 119–129

Goldstein, R.A. and Janicki, B.W. (1974) Immunologic studies in nitrofurantoin induced pulmonary disease. *Med. Ann. Distr. Columbia* **43**, 115–119

González de Vega, N., Zamora, A., Cano, M. and Fernández Castany, A. (1966) Nuestra experiencia personal sobre la bagazosis en Espana Enferm. *Tórax* **15**, 215–237

Gourley, C.A. and Braidwood, G.D. (1971) The use of dust respirators in the prevention of recurrence of farmer's lung. *Trans. Soc. Occup. Med.* **21**, 93–95

Grant, I.W.B., Blackadder, E.S., Greenberg, M. and Blyth, W. (1976) Extrinsic allergic alveolitis in Scottish maltworkers. *Br. Med. J.* **1**, 490–493

Grant, I.W.B., Blyth, W., Wardrop, V.E., Gordon, R.M., Pearson, J.C.G. and Mair, A. (1972) Prevalence of farmer's lung in Scotland. A pilot survey. *Br. Med. J.* **1**, 530–534

Greatorex, F.B. and Pether, J.V.S. (1975) Use of serologically distinct strain of *Thermoactinomyces vulgaris* in the diagnosis of farmer's lung disease. *J. Clin. Pathol.* **28**, 1000–1002

Greene, J.J. and Bannan, L.T. (1985) Potato riddler's lung. *Irish Med. J.* **78**, 282–284

Gregory, P.H. and Waller, S. (1951) *Cryptostroma corticale* and sooty bark disease of sycamore. (Acerpseudoplantanus:) *Trans. Br. Mycol. Soc.* **34**, 579–597

Gregory, P.H., Lacey, J., Festenstein, G.N. and Skinner, F.A. (1963) Microbial and biochemical changes during moulding of hay. *J. Gen. Microbiol.* **33**, 147–174

Hapke, E.J., Seal, R.M.E., Thomas, G.D., Hayes, M. and Meek, J.C. (1968) Farmer's lung. *Thorax* **23**, 451–468

Hargreave, F.E., Pepys, J. and Holford-Strevens, V. (1968) Bagassosis. *Lancet* **1**, 619–620

Hargreave, F.E., Pepys, J., Longbottom, J.L. and Wraith, D.G. (1966) Bird breeder's (fancier's) lung. *Lancet* **1**, 445–449

Harper, L.O., Burrell, R.G., Lapp, J.L. and Morgan, W.K.C. (1970) Allergic alveolitis due to pituitary snuff. *Ann. Intern. Med.* **73**, 581–584

Harries, M.G., Burge, P.S. and O'Brien, I.M. (1980) Occupational type bronchial provocation tests: testing with soluble antigens by inhalation. *Br. J. Ind. Med.* **37**, 248–252

Harries, M.G., Heard, B. and Geddes, D. (1984) Extrinsic allergic bronchiolitis in a bird fancier. *Br. J. Ind. Med.* **41**, 220–223

Haslam, P.L., Dewar, A., Butchers, P., Primett, Z.S., Newman-Taylor, A. and Turner-Warwick, M. (1987) Mast cells, atypical lymphocytes, and neutrophils in bronchoalveolar lavage in extrinsic allergic alveolitis. *Am. Rev. Respir. Dis.* **135**, 35–47

Hearn, C.E.D. (1968) Bagassosis: An epidemiological, environmental and clinical survey. *Br. J. Ind. Med.* **25**, 267–282

Heinonen, O.P., Husman, K., Terho, E.O. and Vohlonen (1982) Farmers' lung, asthma and chronic bronchitis in the Finnish farming population with respect to atopy, smoking and precipitin antibodies. *Eur. J. Respir. Dis.* **63**, 124s, 38

Hendrick, D.J., Faux, J.A. and Marshall, R. (1978) Budgerigar-fancier's lung: the commonest variety of allergic alveolitis in Britain. *Br. Med. J.* **2**, 81–84

Hendrick, D.J., Faux, J.A., Anand, B., Piris, J. and Marshall, R. (1978) Is bird fancier's lung associated with coeliac disease? *Thorax* **33**, 425–428

Hendrick, D.J., Marshall, R., Faux, J.A. and Krall, J.M. (1980) Positive 'alveolar' responses to antigen inhalation provocation tests: their validity and recognition. *Thorax* **35**, 415–427

Hensley, G.T., Garancis, J.C., Cherayil, G.D. and Fink, J.N. (1969) Lung biopsies in pigeon breeder's disease. *Archs Pathol.* **87**, 572–579

Hinson, K.F. (1970) Diffuse pulmonary fibrosis. *Human Pathol.* **1**, 275–288

Hodges, G.R., Fink, T.N. and Schlueter, D.P. (1974) Hypersensitivity pneumonitis caused by a contaminated cool-mist vapouriser. *Ann. Intern. Med.* **85**, 501–504

Hoffman, W. (1946) Die Dreschkrankheit. *Schweiz. Med. Wochenschr.* **76**, 988–990

Holford-Strevens, V. (1971) Quoted by J. Lacey (1971)

Holt, P.G. and Keast, D. (1977) Environmentally induced changes in immunological function: acute and chronic effects of inhalation of tobacco smoke and other atmospheric contaminants in man and experimental animals. *Bacteriol. Rev.* **41**, 205–216

Hood, J. and Mason, A.M.S. (1970) Diffuse pulmonary disease with transfer defect occurring with coeliac disease. *Lancet* **1**, 445–448

Hou, J. (1985) Clinical and X-ray features of lung disease in 43 cases in mushroom workers. *Chung Hua Chieh Ho Ho Hu Hsi Hsi Chi Ping Tsa Chih* **8**, 44–46

Hugh-Jones, M.E. and Austwick, P.K.C. (1967) Epidemiological studies of bovine mycotic abortion. *Vet. Rec.* **81**, 273–276

Hunter, D. and Perry, K.M.A. (1946) Bronchiolitis resulting from the handling of bagasse. *Br. J. Ind. Med.* **3**, 64–74

Hyde, H.A. (1972) Atmospheric pollen and spores in relation to allergy. *Clin. Allergy* **2**, 153–179

Jackson, E. and Welch, K.M.A. (1970) Mushroom worker's lung. *Thorax* **25**, 25–30

Jacobs, R.L., Thorner, R.E., Holcomb, J.R., Schwietz, L.A. and Jacobs, F.O. (1986) Hypersensitivity pneumonitis caused by *Cladosporium* in an enclosed hot-tub area. *Ann. Intern. Med.* **105**, 204–206

Jamison, C.S. and Hopkins, J. (1941) Bagassosis – a fungus disease of the lung. *New Orleans Med. Surg. J.* **93**, 580–582

Jimenez-Diaz, C., Lahoz, C. and Canto, G. (1947) The allergens of mill dust. Asthma in millers, farmers and others. *Ann. Allergy* **5**, 519–525

Johnson, C.L., Bernstein, I.L. Gallagher, J.S., Bonventre, P.F. and Brooks, S.M. (1980) Familial hypersensitivity pneumonitis induced by *Bacillus subtilis*. *Am. Rev. Respir. Dis.* **122**, 339–348

Johnson, W.M. and Kleyn, J.G. (1981) Respiratory disease in a mushroom worker. *J. Occup. Med.* **23**, 49–51

Jones, A. (1982) Farmers' lung: an overview and prospectus. *Ann. Am. Conf. Gov. Ind. Hyg.* **2**, 171–181

Jones Williams, W. (1967) The pathology of sarcoidosis. *Hosp. Med.* **2**, 21–27

Joyce, J.C. and Kneafsey, D. (1955) Farmer's lung. *J. Irish Med. Assoc.* **37**, 313–315

Kagan, S.L., Fink, J.N., Schleuter, D.P., Kurup, V.P. and Fruchtman, R.B. (1981) *Streptomyces albus*: a new cause of hypersensitivity pneumonitis. *J. Allergy Clin. Immunol.* **68**, 295–299

Katila, M-L. and Mäntyjärvi, R.A. (1978) The diagnostic value of antibodies to the traditional antigens of farmer's lung in Finland. *Clin. Allergy* **8**, 581–587

Kawai, T., Salvaggio, J., Lake, W. and Harris, J.O. (1972) Experimental production of hypersensitivity pneumonitis with bagasse and thermophilic actinomycete antigen. *J. Allergy Clin. Immunol.* **50**, 276–288

Keller, R.H., Swartz, S., Schlueter, D.P., Bar-Sela, S. and Fink, J.N. (1984) Immunoregulation in hypersensitivity pneumonitis: phenotypic and functional studies of bronchoalveolar lavage lymphocytes. *Am. Rev. Respir. Dis.* **130**, 766–771

Korenblat, P., Slavin, R., Winzenburger, P., Marks, E. and Wenneker, M.D. (1977) Gerbil keeper's lung – a new form of hypersensitivity pneumonitis (Abstract). *Ann. Allergy* **38**, 437

Kumar, P., Marier, R. and Leech, S.H. (1981) Hypersensitivity pneumonitis due to contamination of a car air conditioner. *N. Engl. J. Med.* **305**, 1531–1532

Kurup, V.P., Barboriak, J.J. and Fink, J.N. (1975) *Thermoactinomyces candidus*, a new species of thermophilic actinomycetes. *Int. J. Syst. Bacteriol.* **25**, 150–154

Kuster, E. and Locci, R. (1964) Taxonomic studies of the genus *Thermoactinomyces*. *Int. Bull. Bact. Nomencl. Taxon.* **14**, 109–114

Lacey, J. (1969) Bagassosis. *Rothamsted Experimental Station Report for 1968*. Part 1, p. 133

Lacey, J. (1971) *Thermoactinomyces sacchari* sp. nov., a thermophilic actinomycete causing bagassosis. *J. Gen. Microbiol.* **66**, 327–338

Lacey, J. (1973) Actinomycetes in soils, composts and fodders. In: *The Actinomycetates* (eds G. Sykes and F.A. Skinner), London: Academic Press, p. 231

Lacey, J. (1980) The microflora of grain dusts. In *Occupational Lung Disease – Focus on Grain Dust and Health* (eds J.A. Dosman and D.J. Cotton), Academic Press, London, pp. 417–440

Lacey, J. and Lacey, M.E. (1964) Spore concentrations in the air of farm buildings. *Trans. Br. Mycol. Soc.* **47**, 547–552

Lancaster-Smith, M.J., Benson, M.K. and Strickland, I.D. (1971) Coeliac disease and diffuse interstitial lung disease. *Lancet* **1**, 473–476

Leatherman, J.W., Micheal, A.F., Schwartz, B.A. and Hoidal, J.R. (1984) Lung T cells in hypersensitivity pneumonitis. *Ann. Intern. Med.* **100**, 390–392

Lecours, R., Laviolette, M. and Cormier, Y. (1986) Bronchoalveolar lavage in pulmonary mycotoxicosis (organic dust toxic syndrome). *Thorax* **41**, 924–926

Lehrer, S.B., Turner, E., Weill, H. and Salvaggio, J.E. (1978) Elimination of bagassosis in Louisiana paper manufacturing plant workers. *Clin. Allergy* **8**, 15–20

Lockey, S.D. (1974) Mushroom workers' pneumonitis. *Ann. Allergy* **33**, 282–288

Lunn, J.A. (1966) Millworker's asthma. Allergic responses to the grain weevil (*Sitophilus granarius*). *Br. J. Ind. Med.* **23**, 149–152

Lunn, J.A. and Hughes, D.T.D. (1967) Pulmonary hypersensitivity to the grain weevil. *Br. J. Ind. Med.* **24**, 158–161

Madsen, D., Klock, L.E., Wenzel, F.J., Robbins, J.L. and Schmidt, C.D. (1976) The prevalence of farmer's lung in an agricultural population. *Am. Rev. Respir. Dis.* **13**, 171–174

Maesen, F.P.V. (1972) *Pigeon Breeder's Lung*. N. Vuitgeverij Winants, Heerlen, Hasselt

Mahon, W.E., Scott, D.J., Ansell, G., Manson, G.L. and Fraser, R. (1967) Hypersensitivity to pituitary snuff with miliary shadowing in the lungs. *Thorax* **22**, 13–20

Malmberg, P., Rask-Andersen, A., Hoglund, S., Kolmodin-Hedman, B. and Guernsey, J.R. (1988) Incidence of organic dust toxic syndrome and allergic alveolitis in Swedish farmers. *Int. Arch. Allergy Appl. Immunol.* **87**, 47–54

Malo, J-L. and Zeiss, C.R. (1982) Occupational hypersensitivity pneumonitis after exposure to diphenylmethane diisocyanate. *Am. Rev. Respir. Dis.* **125**, 113–116

Malo, J-L., Ouimet, G., Cartier, A., Levitz, D. and Zeiss, C.R. (1983) Combined alveolitis and asthma due to hexamethylene diisocyanate (HDI), with demonstration of cross respiratory and immunologic reactivities to diphenylmethane diisocyanate (MDI). *J. Allergy Clin. Immunol.* **72**, 413–419

Mansmann, R.A. and Osborn, B.I. (1971) Hypersensitivity pneumonitis to chickens in horses. *J. Allergy Clin. Immunol.* **51**, 103

Marx, J.J. and Flaherty, D.K. (1976) Activation of the complement sequence by extracts of bacteria and fungi associated with hypersensitivity pneumonitis. *J. Allergy Clin. Immunol.* **57**, 328–334

Marx, Jr. J.J., Kettrick-Marx, M.A., Mitchell, P.D. and Flaherty, D.K. (1977) Correlation of exposure to various respiratory pathogens with farmer's lung disease. *J. Allergy Clin. Immunol.* **60**, 169–173

May, J.J., Stallones, L., Darrow, D. and Pratt, D.S. (1986) Organic dust toxicity (pulmonary mycotoxicosis) associated with silo unloading. *Thorax* **41**, 919–923

Medical Research Council Symposium (1977) Humidifier fever. *Thorax* **32**, 653–663

Metzger, W.J., Patterson, R., Fink, J., Semerdjam, R. and Roberts, M. (1976) Sauna-takers disease. *J. Am. Med. Assoc.* **236**, 2209–2211

Miller, G.J., Hearn, C.E.D. and Edwards, R.H.T. (1971) Pulmonary function at rest and during exercise following bagassosis. *Br. J. Ind. Med.* **28**, 152–158

Molina, C. (1976) *Broncho-pulmonary Immunopathology.* Churchill Livingstone, Edinburgh, London and New York (translated by J. Pepys)

Monkäre, S. (1988) Influence of corticosteroid treatment on the course of farmers' lung. *Eur. J. Respir. Dis.* **64**, 283–293

Monkäre, S. and Haahtela, T. (1987) Farmers' lung: a 5-year follow-up of eighty-six patients. *Clin. Allergy* **17**, 143–151

Monkäre, S., Haahtela, T., Ikonen, M. and Laitinen, L.A. (1981) Bronchial hyperreactivity to inhaled histamine in patients with farmers' lung. *Lung* **159**, 145–151

Moore, V.L., Fink, J.N., Barboriak, J.J., Ruff, L.L. and Schlueter, D.P. (1974) Immunologic events in pigeon breeder's disease. *J. Allergy Clin. Immunol.* **53**, 319–328

Morgan, D.C., Smyth, J.T., Lister, R.W. and Pethybridge, R.J. (1973) Chest symptoms and farmer's lung: a community survey. *Br. J. Ind. Med.* **30**, 259–265

Morgan, D.C., Smyth, J.T., Lister, R.W., Pethybridge, R.J., Gilson, J.C., Callaghan, P. and Thomas, G.O. (1975) Chest symptoms in farming communities with special reference to farmer's lung. *Br. J. Ind. Med.* **32**, 228–234

Morris, J.S., Read, A.E., Jones, B., Cotes, J.E. and Edwards, J.H. (1971) Coeliac disease and lung disease. *Lancet* **1**, 754

Nash, E.S., Vogelpoel, L. and Becker, W.B. (1967) Pigeon breeder's lung – a case report. *S. Afr. Med. J.* **41**, 191–193

Newman Taylor, A., Pickering, C.A.C., Turner-Warwick, M. and Pepys, J. (1978) Respiratory allergy to a factory humidifier contaminant present as pyrexia of undetermined origin. *Br. Med. J.* **2**, 94–95

Newman Taylor, A.J., Taylor, P., Bryant, D.H., Longbottom, J.L. and Pepys, J. (1977) False positive complement fixation tests with respiratory virus preparations in bird fanciers with allergic alveolitis. *Thorax* **32**, 563–566

O'Brien, I.M., Bull, J., Creamer, B., Sepulveda, R., Harries, M., Bunge, P.S. and Pepys, J. (1978) Asthma and extrinsic allergic alveolitis due to *Merulius lacrymans*. *Clin. Allergy* **8**, 535–542

Panasenko, V.T. (1967) Ecology of microfungi. *Bot. Rev.* **33**, 189–215

Parratt, D. and Boyd, G. (1976) Farmer's lung: a neglected antigen. *Lancet* **1**, 1294

Parratt, D., Nielsen, K.H., Boyd, G. and White, R.G. (1975) The quantitation of antibody in farmer's lung syndrome using a radioimmunoassay. *Clin. Expl Immunol.* **20**, 217–225

Parrott, W.F. and Blyth, W. (1980) Another causal factor in the production of humidifier fever. *J. Soc. Occup. Med.* **30**, 63–65

Patterson, R., Roberts, M., Roberts, R.C., Emanuel, D.A. and Fink, J.N. (1976) Antibodies of different immunoglobulin classes against antigens causing farmer's lung. *Am. Rev. Respir. Dis.* **114**, 315–324

Paturau, J.M. (1969) *By-products of the Cane Sugar Industry.* Elsevier, Amsterdam

Pauli, B., Gerber, H. and Schatzmann, U. (1972) Farmer's Lung beim pferd. *Pathol. Microbiol.* **38**, 200–214

Pearsall, H.R., Morgan, E.H., Tesluk, H. and Beggs, D. (1960) Parakeet dander pneumonitis. Acute psittaco-kerato-pneumoconiosis. *Bull. Mason Clin.* **14**, 127–137

Pepys, J. (1969) *Hypersensitivity Diseases of the Lungs due to Fungi and Organic Dusts.* Karger, Basel

Pepys, J. (1977) Clinical and therapeutic significance of patterns of allergic reactions of the lungs to extrinsic agents. *Am. Rev. Respir. Dis.* **116**, 573–588

Pepys, J. (1978) Antigens and hypersensitivity pneumonitis. *J. Allergy Clin. Immunol.* **61**, 201–203

Pepys, J. and Jenkins, P.A. (1965) Precipitin (FLH) test in farmer's lung. *Thorax* **20**, 21–35

Pestalozzi, C. (1959) Febrile Gruppener Krankungen in einer Modellschreinerei durch Inhalation von mit Schimelpilzen Kontaminiertem Befeuchterwasser ('Befeuchterfieber'). *Schweiz. Med. Wochenschr.* **89**, 710–713

Pether, J.V.S. and Greatorex, F.B. (1976) Farmer's lung disease in Somerset. *Br. J. Ind. Med.* **33**, 265–268

Phillips, M.S., Robinson, A.A., Higenbottam, T.W. and Calder, I.M. (1987) Mushroom compost workers' lung. *J. R. Soc. Med.* **80**, 674–677

Pickering, C.A.C., Moore, W.K.S., Lacey, J., Holford-Strevens, V.C. and Pepys, J. (1976) Investigation of a respiratory disease associated with an air-conditioning system. *Clin. Allergy* **6**, 109–118

Pickles, W.N. (1944) The country doctor and public health. *Publ. Health* **58**, 2–5

Pierce, A.K., Nicholson, D.P., Miller, J.M. and Johnson, R.L. (1968) Pulmonary function in bagasse worker's lung disease. *Am. Rev. Respir. Dis.* **97**, 561–570

Pimentel, J.C. and Ávila, R. (1973) Respiratory disease in cork workers ('suberosis']. *Thorax* **28**, 409–423

Pirie, H.M., Dawson, C.O., Breeze, R.G., Wiseman, A. and Hamilton, J. (1971) A bovine disease similar to farmer's lung: extrinsic allergic alveolitis. *Vet. Rec.* **88**, 346–350

Plessner, M.M. (1960) Une maladie des trieurs de plumes: la fièvre de canard. *Archs Mal. prof. Méd. trav.* **21**, 67–69

Popp, W., Ritschka, L., Zwick, H. and Rauscher, H. (1987) 'Beerenausleselunge' oder Winzerlunge – eine exogen-allergische Alveolitis ausgelost durch Botrytis cinerea-sporen. *Prax. Klin. Pneumonol.* **41**, 165–169

Pratt, D.S. and May, J.J. (1984) Feed-associated respiratory illness in farmers. *Archs Environ. Health* **39**, 43–48

Purtilo, D.T., Bonica, A. and Yang, J.P.S. (1978) Bird fancier's lung and coeliac disease. *Lancet* **1**, 1357–1358

Rankin, J., Kobayashi, M., Barbee, R.A. and Dickie, H.A. (1967) Pulmonary granulomatoses due to inhaled organic antigens. *Med. Clin. N. Am.* **51**, 459–482

Rask-Anderson, A. (1989) Organic dust toxic syndrome among farmers. *Br. J. Ind. Med.* **46**, 233–238

Reed, C.E., Sosman, A. and Barbee, R.A. (1965) Pigeon breeder's lung. *J. Am. Med. Assoc.* **193**, 261–266

Renaud, J., Pétavy, A.F., Duriez-Vauchelle, T., Guillot, J. and Coulet, M. (1979) Analyse antigénique des acariens du fromage et vue d'une étude de la maladie des fromagers. *Rev. fr. Mal. Respir.* **7**, 441–447

Reyes, C.N., Emanuel, D.A., Roberts, R.C., Marx, Jr, J.J. and Wenzel, F.J. (1976) The histopathology of farmer's lung (60 consecutive cases) [abstract]. *Am. J. Clin. Pathol.* **66**, 460–461

Riddle, H.F.V. (1974) Prevalence of respiratory and sensitization by mould antigens among a group of malt workers. *Br. J. Ind. Med.* **31**, 31–35

Riddle, H.F.V., Channell, S., Blyth, W., Weir, D.M., Lloyd, M., Amos, W.M.G. and Grant, I.W.B. (1968) Allergic alveolitis in a maltworker. *Thorax* **23**, 271–280

Roberts, R.C., Wenzel, F.J. and Emanuel, D.A. (1976) Precipitating antibodies in a midwest dairy farming population toward the antigens associated with farmer's lung disease. *J. Allergy Clin. Immunol.* **57**, 518–524

Robertson, A.S., Burge, P.S., Wieland, G.A. and Carmalt, M.H.B. (1987) Extrinsic allergic alveolitis caused by a coldwater humidifier. *Thorax* **42**, 32–37

Robinson, T.J. (1976) Coeliac disease with farmer's lung. *Br. Med. J.* **1**, 745–746

Robinson, T.J., Nelson, S.D., Haire, M., Middleton, D., McMillan, S.A. and Evans, J.P. (1981) Jejunal villous changes associated with farmers' lung. *Postgrad. Med. J.* **57**, 697–701

Rodey, G.E., Fink, J., Koethe, S., Schlueter, D., Witkowski, J., Bettonville, P., Rimm, A. and Moore, V. (1979) A study of HLA-A, B, C and DR specificities in pigeon breeder's disease. *Am. Rev. Respir. Dis.* **119**, 755–759

Rossman, M.D., Kern, J.A., Elias, J.A., Cullen, M.R., Epstein, P.E., Preuss, O.P., Markham, T.N. and Daniele, P. (1988). Proliferative response of broncho-alveolar lymphocytes to beryllium: a test for chronic beryllium disease. *Ann. Intern. Med.* **108,** 687–693

Rylander, R. and Haglind, P. (1984) Airborne endotoxins and humidifier disease. *Clin. Allergy* **14,** 109–112

Rylander, R., Anderrson, K., Belin, L., Berglund, G., Bergstrum, R., Hanson, L-A., Lundholm, M. and Mattsby, I. (1976) Sewage workers' syndrome. *Lancet* **2,** 478–479

Rylander, R., Haglind, P., Lundholm, M., Mattsby, I. and Stenqvist, K. (1978) Humidifier fever and endotoxin exposure. *Clin. Allergy* **8,** 511–516

Saia, B., Mastrangelo, G., Marcer, G. and Reggio, O. (1984) Prevalence and risk factors of chronic respiratory disease in a farming population. *Med. Lav.* **75**(2), 101–109

Sakula, A. (1967) Mushroom worker's lung. *Br. Med. J.* **3,** 708–710

Salvaggio, J., Arquembourg, P., Seabury, J. and Buechner, H. (1969) Bagassosis IV. Precipitins against extracts of thermophilic actinomycetes in patients with bagassosis. *Am. J. Med.* **46,** 538–544

Scadding, J.G. (1967) *Sarcoidosis.* Eyre and Spottiswoode, London, p. 160

Schatz, N., Patterson, R., Fink, J., Momore, V., Rodey, G., Cunningham, A., Roberts, M. and Harris, K. (1976) Pigeon breeder's disease. III. A study of a family exposed to doves. *Clin. Expl. Immunol.* **24,** 33–41

Scherrer, M., Imhof, K., Weickhardt, W. and Lebek, G. (1978) Befeuchterfieber in einer Giesserei. *Rev. Suisse Med. (Praxis)* **67,** 1855–1861

Schlueter, D.P., Fink, J.N. and Henley, G.T. (1972) Wood pulp worker's disease: a hypersensitivity pneumonitis caused by *Alternaria. Ann. Intern. Med.* **77,** 907–914

Schmidt, C.D., Jensen, R.L., Christensen, L.T., Crapo, R.O. and Davis, J.J. (1988) Longitudinal pulmonary function changes in pigeon breeders. *Chest* **93,** 359–363

Schorlemmer, H.W., Edwards, J.H., Davies, P. and Allison, A.C. (1977) Macrophage responses to mouldy hay dust. *Micropolyspora faeni* and zymosan by the alternative pathway. *Clin. Expl. Immunol.* **27,** 198–207

Schulz, K.H., Felton, G. and Hausen, B.M. (1974) Allergy to the spores of *Pleurotus florida. Lancet* **1,** 29

Seabury, J., Salvaggio, J., Buechner, H. and Kunder, V.G. (1968) The pathology of the acute and chronic stages of farmer's lung. *Thorax* **23,** 469–489

Seabury, J., Salvaggio, J., Buechner, H. and Kunder, V.G. (1968) Bagassosis III. Isolation of thermophilic and mesophilic actinomycetes and fungi from mouldy bagasse. *Proc. Soc. Expl. Biol. Med.* **129,** 351–360

Seal, R.M.E. (1975) Pathology of extrinsic allergic bronchiolo-alveolitis. In *Alveolar Interstitium of the Lung. Progress in Respiratory Research,* pp. 66–73 (eds H. Herzog, F. Basset and R. Georges)

Seal, R.M.E., Hapke, E.J., Thomas, G.O., Meek, J.C. and Hayes, M. (1968) The pathology of the acute and chronic stages of farmer's lung. *Thorax* **23,** 469–489

Sennekamp, J., Rittner, C. and Vogel, F. (1977) HLA-B8 in pigeon fancier's lung. *Lung* **154,** 148–149

Sheffer, A.L., Rocklin, R.E. and Goetzl, E.J. (1975) Immunologic components of hypersensitivity reactions to cromolyn sodium. *N. Engl. J. Med.* **293,** 1220–1224

Shelley, E., Dean, G., Collins, D., Dinah, R., Evans, J. and McHardy, J. (1979) Farmer's lung: a study in North-West Ireland. *J. Irish Med. Assoc.* **72,** 261–264

Smyth, J.T., Adkins, G.E., Lloyd, M., Moore, B. and McWhite, E. (1975) Farmer's lung in Devon. *Thorax* **30,** 197–203

Sodeman, W.A. and Pullen, R.L. (1943) Bagasse disease of the lungs. *New Orleans Med. Surg.* **95,** 558–560

Sodeman, W.A. and Pullen, R.L. (1944) Bagasse disease of the lungs. *Archs Intern. Med.* **73,** 365–374

Solal-Celigny, P.H., Laviolette, M., Hebert, J. and Cormier, Y. (1982) Immune reactions in the lungs of asymptomatic dairy farmers. *Am. Rev. Respir. Dis.* **126,** 964–967

Soler, P., Nioche, S., Valeyre, D., Basset, F., Benveniste, J., Burtin, C., Battesti, J.P., Georges, R. and Hance, A.J. (1987) Role of mast cells in the pathogenesis of hypersensitivity pneumonitis. *Thorax* **42,** 565–572

Spector, W.G. (1971) The cellular dynamics of granulomas. *Proc. R. Soc. Med.* **64,** 941–942

Spector, W.G. and Heesom, N. (1969) The production of granu-lomas by antigen–antibody complexes. *J. Pathol.* **98,** 31–39

Staines, F.H. and Forman, J.A.S. (1961) A survey of 'farmer's lung'. *J. Coll. Gen. Practnrs Newsl.* **4,** 351–382

Stewart, C.J. (1974) Mushroom worker's lung – two outbreaks. *Thorax* **29,** 252–257

Stewart, C.J. and Pickering, C.A.C. (1974) Mushroom worker's lung. *Lancet* **1,** 317

Stiehm, E.R., Reed, C.E. and Tooley, W.H. (1967) Pigeon breeder's lung in children. *Pediatrics* **39,** 904–915

Stokes, P.L., Asquith, P., Holmes, G.K.T., Mackintosh, P. and Cooke, W.T. (1972) Histocompatibility antigens associated with adult coeliac disease. *Lancet* **2,** 162–164

Stokes, T.C., Turton, C.W.G. and Turner-Warwick, M.T. (1981) A study of immunoglobulin G subclasses in patients with farmer's lung. *Clin. Allergy* **11,** 201–207

Sutinen, S., Reijula, K., Huhti, E. and Karkola, P. (1983) Extrinsic allergic bronchiolo-alveolitis: serology and biopsy findings. *Eur. J. Respir. Dis.* **64,** 271–282

Sweet, L.C., Anderson, J.A., Callies, Q.C. and Coates, E.O. Jr (1971) Hypersensitivity pneumonitis related to a home furnace humidifier. *J. Allergy Clin. Immunol.* **48,** 171–178

Takazakura, E., Tsuji, H., Makino, H., Terada, Y., Sugiusa, H. and Kitagawa, S. (1987) Two cases of hypersensitivity pneumonitis due to isocyanate in foundry cast workers. *Nippon Kyobu Shikkar Gakkai Zasshi* **25,** 924–928

Tebo, T.H., Fredericks, W.W. and Roberts, R.C. (1977) The antigens of pigeon breeder's disease. II. Isolation and charac-terisation of antigen PDE. *Int. Archs Allergy Appl. Immunol.* **54,** 553–559

Tebo, T.H., Moore, V.L. and Fink, J.N. (1977) Antigens in pigeon breeder's disease. *Clin. Allergy* **7,** 103–108

Terho, E.O. and Lacey, J. (1979) Microbiological and serological studies of farmer's lung in Finland. *Clin. Allergy* **9,** 43–52

Terho, E.O., Lammi, S. and Heinonen, O.P. (1980) Seasonal variation in the incidence of farmer's lung. *Int. J. Epidemiol.* **9,** 219–223

Terho, E.O., Koskimies, S., Heinonen, O.P. and Mantyjarvi, R. (1981) HLA and farmer's lung. *Eur. J. Respir. Dis.* **63,** 361–362

Tewksbury, D.A., Wenzel, F.J. and Emanuel, D.A. (1968) An immunologic study of maple bark disease. *Clin. Expl. Immunol.* **3,** 857–863

Törnell, E. (1946) Thresher's lung. *Acta Med. Scand.* **125,** 191–219

Towey, J.W., Sweany, H.C. and Huron, W.H. (1932) Severe bronchial asthma apparently due to fungus spores found in maple bark. *J. Am. Med. Assoc.* **99,** 453–459

Treuhaft, M.W., Roberts, R.C., Hackbarth, C., Emanuel, D.A. and Marx, J.J. Jr (1979) Characterization of precipitin response to *Micropolyspora faeni* in farmer's lung disease by quantitative immunoelectrophoresis. *Am. Rev. Respir. Dis.* **119,** 571–578

Turton, C.W.G., Morris, L.M., Lawler, S.D. and Turner-Warwick, M. (1978) HL-A in cryptogenic fibrosing alveolitis. *Lancet* **1,** 507–508

Vallery-Radot, P. and Giroud, P. (1928) Sporomycose des pelleteurs de grains. *Bull. Soc. méd. Hop. Paris* **52,** 1632–1645

Vergnon, J.M., Riffat, J., Boncheron, S., Fournet, P. and Emonot, A. (1985) Extrinsic allergic broncho-alveolitis to isocyanates: a new observation. *Arch. mal. Prof.* **46,** 321–325

Viswanathan, R., de Monte, A.J.H., Shivpuri, D.N., Venkitasubramanian, T.A., Tandon, H.D., Chandrusekhars, S., Jaion, S.K., Gupta, I.M., Singh, P., Gambhie, K.K., Randhawa, H.S. and Singh, V.N. (1963) Bagassosis. *Indian J. Med. Res.* **51,** 563–633

Voisin, C., Tonnel, A.B., Lahoute, C., Robin, H., Lebas, J. and Aerts, C. (1981) Bird fanciers' lung: studies of broncho-alveolar lavage and correlations with inhalation provocation tests. *Lung* **159,** 17–22

von Betz, B. (1985) Austernpilzzuchterlunge. Klinik und pravention einer form der exogen allergischen alveolitis. *Arbeitzmed. Sozialmed. Praventivmed.* **20,** 241–244

Warren, C.P.W. (1977) Extrinsic allergic alveolitis: a disease commoner in non-smokers. *Thorax* **32,** 567–569

Warren, C.P.W. and Tse, K.S. (1974) Extrinsic allergic alveolitis owing to hypersensitivity to chickens – significance of sputum precipitins. *Am. Rev. Respir. Dis.* **109,** 672–677

Warren, C.P.W., Tse, K.S. and Cherniack, R.M. (1978) Mechanical properties of the lung in extrinsic allergic alveolitis. *Thorax* **33,** 315–321

Weill, H., Buechner, H.A., Gonzales, E., Herbert, S.J., Aucoin, E. and Ziskind, M.M. (1966) Bagassosis: A study of pulmonary function in 20 cases. *Ann. Intern. Med.* **64,** 737–747

Weinberger, S.E., Kelman, J.A., Elson, N.A., Young, R.C. Jr., Reynolds, H.Y., Fulmer, J.D. and Crystal, R.G. (1978) Bronchoalveolar lavage in interstitial lung disease. *Ann. Intern. Med.* **89,** 459–466

Weiss, N.S. and Soleymani, D.A. (1971) Hypersensitivity lung disease caused by contamination of an air conditioning system. *Ann. Allergy* **29,** 154–156

Wenzel, F.J. and Emanuel, D.A. (1967) The epidemiology of maple bark disease. *Archs Environ. Health* **14,** 385–389

Wenzel, F.J., Emanuel, D.A., Lawton, B.R. and Magnin, G.E. (1964) Isolation of the causative agent of farmer's lung. *Ann. Allergy* **22,** 533

Williams, J.V. (1963) Inhalation and skin tests with extracts of hay and fungi in patients with farmer's lung. *Thorax* **18,** 182–196

Wüthrich, B. and Keiser, G. (1970) Das Käsewascherasthma Abgrenzung gegenuber die Käsewascherdrankei. *Schweiz. Med. Wochenschr.* **100,** 1108–1111

Yoshida, K. and Maybank, J. (1978) Physical and environmental characteristic of grain dusts. *Ann. Intern. Med.* **89,** 420–421

Yoshizawa, Y., Ohdama, S., Tanoue, M., Tanaka, M., Ohtsuka, M., Uetake, K. and Hasegawa, S. (1986) Analysis of bronchoalveolar lavage cells and fluids in patients with hypersensitivity pneumonitis: possible role of chemotactic factors in the pathogenesis of the disease. *Int. Archs Allergy Appl. Immunol.* **80,** 376–382

Zaidi, S.H., Dogra, R.K.S., Shanker, R. and Chaudra, S.V. (1971) Experimental farmer's lung in guinea pigs. *J. Pathol.* **105,** 41–48

21

Occupational asthma and byssinosis

Anthony J. Newman Taylor and C.A.C. Pickering

Occupational asthma

Anthony J. Newman Taylor

Introduction

Asthma is usually defined as *narrowing of the airways that is reversible over short periods of time, either spontaneously or as a result of treatment*. This definition focuses on the characteristic variability of airways' calibre which distinguishes asthma from other less reversible causes of airflow limitation, in particular obstructive bronchiolitis and alveolar wall destruction caused by inhaled tobacco smoke. Another important characteristic of asthma is *airways' hyperresponsiveness*. Airways' responsiveness describes the ease with which a variety of non-specific provocative stimuli, such as exercise and inhaled histamine and methacholine, provoke acute transient airways' narrowing. Patients with asthma whose airways are hyperresponsive require smaller than normal doses of such stimuli to provoke narrowing of the airways. These physiological abnormalities – which have been used to define asthma – are probably manifestations of a characteristic pattern of *airways' inflammation* with bronchial epithelial cell desquamation and infiltration with eosinophils and lymphocytes. Indeed, asthma might be defined pathologically as *desquamative eosinophilic bronchitis*.

Inducers of asthma are agents that cause airways' inflammation and hyperresponsiveness. *Inciters* of asthma are agents that provoke acute airways' narrowing in individuals with hyperresponsive airways but which do not cause airways' inflammation or increase airways' responsiveness. *Inducers* may initiate asthma and cause airways' inflammation, as the outcome of either toxic damage to the airways or an acquired specific hypersensitivity response. 'Toxic' inducers

include viral respiratory tract infections and reactive chemicals; 'hypersensitivity' inducers include high-molecular-weight proteins, other complex biological molecules and low-molecular-weight chemicals that may form haptens with body proteins. 'Inciters' of acute airways' narrowing may be physical, such as exercise and the inhalation of cold dry air, chemical, such as inhaled sulphur dioxide, or pharmacological, such as histamine and methacholine. Inducers initiate and increase the severity of asthma; inciters increase the frequency of attacks of acute airways' narrowing. Avoidance of exposure to an inducer will reduce airways' hyperresponsiveness and the severity of asthma, which may resolve; avoidance of exposure to an inciter, whilst reducing the frequency of provoked attacks, will not reduce airways' hyperresponsiveness or the severity of the disease.

Both inciters and inducers may be encountered in the workplace. Irritant chemicals, inhaled as gas, vapour or fume, and cold air in cold storage areas and outdoors, may incite acute airways' narrowing in individuals with asthma. Inhalation of reactive chemicals in toxic concentrations can initiate asthma which, although usually transient, may be prolonged. Asthma caused by inhalation of toxic chemicals has been entitled RADS (*reactive airways' dysfunction syndrome*) by Brooks, Weiss and Bernstein (1985). Most cases of asthma initiated by agents inhaled at work fulfil the criteria of an acquired hypersensitivity response, and the term 'occupational asthma' is usually reserved to describe *asthma induced by sensitization to an agent inhaled at work*. Although less common, the other circumstances in which asthma may be initiated or provoked at work should be appreciated.

Importance of occupational asthma

The contribution of occupational asthma to the prevalence of asthma in both the UK and elsewhere is not known. Different authors have suggested that occupational causes in their countries account for between 2 per cent (Introna, 1966) and 15 per cent (Kobayashi, 1974) but the basis of none of these estimates is secure. At present we are limited to information about the numbers receiving compensation and to reports given to surveillance schemes, both of which are likely to provide underestimates of the true frequency of disease. In the UK, occupational asthma is currently prescribed for statutory compensation for 14 groups of agents. The number of 'awards' made in 1989 was 214.

The most promising potential source of information about the incidence of occupational causes of asthma in the UK is the voluntary surveillance scheme of work-related disease, started in January 1989, to which respiratory and occupational physicians report. In 1989, 2101 new cases were notified. Asthma (554 cases: 26 per cent) was the most frequent cause; other causes included mesothelioma (16 per cent), pneumoconiosis (15 per cent), benign pleural disease (11 per cent) and allergic alveolitis (6 per cent) (Meredith, Taylor and McDonald, 1991). The annual incidence rate for occupational asthma, calculated per million working population was 22 per million. The rate in men was approximately twice that of women and increased in both men and women with age. The rates varied from less than 10 per million in professional management, clerical and selling occupational groups to 114 per million in industries processing non-metal and electrical materials and those engaged in painting, assembly and packing. The estimated incidence of occupational asthma in high-risk occupational groups is shown in Table 21.1. The most important agents reported as causes of occupational asthma were isocyanates which accounted for 22 per cent of cases; also grain, wood dusts and laboratory animals together were responsible for 17 per cent. The reported rates in the UK are lower than in Finland, one of the few countries where new cases of occupational lung disease are still registered. In 1981, 156 new cases of asthma were registered in a working population of some 2.2 million, an incidence of 71 per million (Keskinen, 1983) (as compared to the estimated UK national rate of 22 per million). However, within the UK, considerable differences in regional rates were reported, the lowest rate being in West Yorkshire (8 per million) and the highest in West Midlands Metropolitan County (63 per million) – similar to the reported incidence in Finland. Meredith, Taylor and McDonald (1991) suggest that the differences in

regions may be, at least in part, attributable to differences in ascertainment and reporting, and that the true incidence of occupational asthma may be some three times the reported national rate.

Most epidemiological studies of occupational asthma reported to date have estimated its prevalence in working populations exposed to a particular agent, that is, the proportion of the current workforce who have occupational asthma (variously defined). Because many who develop asthma will leave an occupation that exposes them to the cause of their symptoms, estimates of disease prevalence are also likely to underestimate (probably seriously) the true frequency of disease. Nevertheless, owing to the difficulties and expense of longitudinal studies of working populations, the majority of information currently available about the frequency of asthma caused by specific agents is derived from cross-sectional studies.

Causes of occupational asthma

The number of reported causes of occupational asthma is already enormous and, with the development of biotechnology and the constant introduction of newly synthesized chemicals, the number is likely to grow. The recognized causes at present include proteins of animal, vegetable and microbial origin, naturally occurring organic chemicals,

Table 21.1 Incidence of occupational asthma in high-risk occupational groups as reported to SWORD project

Occupational group	Cases	Population	Rate/million per year
Welders/solderers electronic assemblers	35	220 068	159
Laboratory technicians and assistants	26	127 478	204
Metal-making and treating	14	56 270	249
Plastics-making and processing	27	66 005	409
Bakers	29	70 839	409
Chemical processors	31	73 189	424
Coach and spray painters	35	54 737	639
Other painters	21	201 225	104

After Meredith et al. (1991)

Table 21.2 Causes of occupational asthma: animals, their excreta and secreta

Cause	Occupation	Selected references
Laboratory animals: rats, mice, guinea-pigs etc.	Laboratory workers	Newman Taylor, Longbottom and Pepys (1977); Gross (1980); Slovak and Hill (1981); Cockroft et al. (1981); Swanson et al. (1984); Venables et al. (1988)
Pig urine		Harries and Cromwell (1982)
Birds:		
Pigeons, budgerigars	Bird breeders	Hargreave and Pepys (1972)
Bats	Office workers	El-Ansary et al. (1987)
Arthropods (arachnids and insects):		
Storage mites	Farmers	Ingram et al. (1979); Blainey et al. (1986); van Hage-Hamsten et al. (1985)
Locusts	Research workers	Tee et al. (1988); Frankland (1953)
Housefly (*Musca domestica*)	Laboratory workers	Tee et al. (1985)
Grain weevil (*Sitophilus granarius*)	Laboratory workers	Frankland and Lunn (1965)
Northern fowl mite (*Ornithonyssus sylvarium*)	Poultry workers	Lutsky, Teichtahl and Bar-Sela (1984)
Cockroach	Laboratory workers	Bernton, McMahon and Brown (1972)
Cricket	Field contact	Harfi (1980)
Carmine (from *Coccus cactis*)	Cosmetic dye manufacture	Burge et al. (1979a)
Silkworm larvae	Silkworm sericulture	Kobayashi (1974)
Chironomid larvae (*Chironomus thummi thummi*)	Pet fish food	Baur et al. (1982)
Cockroach (*Blatella germanica* and *Blatella americana*)	Laboratory workers	Steinberg et al. (1987)
Gypsy moth (*Lymantria dispar* caterpillar)	Laboratory workers	Etkind et al. (1982)
Fruit fly (*Drosophila melanogaster*)	Laboratory workers	Spieksma et al. (1986)
Meal worm (*Tenibrio molitor* larvae)	Warehouse fishbait handlers	Bernstein, Gallagher and Bernstein (1983)
Shellfish:		
Crab	Crab processing	Cartier et al. (1984)
Prawn	Prawn processing	Gaddie et al. (1980)
Hoya	Oyster farm	Iyo et al. (1980)
Fish:		
Trout	Fish preparation	Sherson, Hansen and Sigsgaard (1989)
Eggs	Bakery workers	Edwards et al. (1983)

synthetic organic chemicals and inorganic chemicals, in particular metal salts. Tables 21.2 to 21.7 identify some of the more important of these causes, but do not aim to be comprehensive.

Disease mechanisms

Inciters

Agents that provoke acute transient airways' narrowing in individuals act through several different mechanisms.

Exercise and hyperventilation of cold dry air probably stimulate mast cell mediator release. Sulphur dioxide stimulates sensory nerve endings in the bronchial epithelium. Histamine acts directly on bronchial blood vessels and smooth muscle, and methacholine on muscarinic receptors in the airways. Acute asthma has been described in those spraying crops with organophosphorous insecticides which, as cholinesterase inhibitors, probably also act by stimulating muscarinic receptors in the airways (Weiner, 1961).

Toxic inducers

The original report of RADS by Brooks and Lockey (1981) described 13 workers with no previous

Table 21.3 Causes of occupational asthma: plants and vegetable products

Causes	Occupation	Selected references
Grain dust	Grain handlers	Warren, Chermick and Tse (1974); Davies, Green and Schofield (1976); Chan-Yeung, Wong and MacLean (1979)
Wheat/rye flour	Bakers and millers	Hendrick, Davies and Pepys (1976); Björksten et al. (1977); Block et al. (1983); Prichard et al. (1985); Walsh et al. (1985); Musk et al. (1989)
Green coffee bean	Food process workers	Lehrer, Kerr and Salvaggio (1978)
Castor beans	Coffee bean baggers and handlers	Figley and Rawling (1950)
	Seamen and laboratory workers	Davison et al. (1983a)
Psyllium	Laxative manufacture	Busse and Schoenwetter (1975)
Tea fluff	Teaworkers	Uragoda (1970)
Tobacco leaf	Tobacco manufacture	Gleich et al. (1980)
Baby's breath (*Gypsophila*)	Florist	Twiggs et al. (1982a)
Weeping fig	Plant keeper	Axelsson, Skedinger and Zetterstöm (1985)
Gums:		
Gum acacia	Printers	Fowler (1952)
Gum tragacanth	Gum manufacture	Gelfand (1943)

Table 21.4 Causes of occupational asthma: wood dusts

Cause	Occupation	Selected references
Western Red Cedar (*Thuja plicata*)	Woodworkers	Chan-Yeung et al. (1973)
	Woodworkers	Chan-Yeung et al. (1984)
	Timber millers, joiners and carpenters	Gandevia and Milne (1970)
	Carpenters	Pickering, Batten and Pepys (1972)
Tanganyika aningre	Woodworkers	Paggiaro et al. (1981)
African maple (*Seferoxylon triplochiton*)	Woodworkers	Hinojosa et al. (1984)
Eastern white cedar (*Thuja occidentalis*)	Woodworkers	Cartier et al. (1986)
Cedar of Lebanon (*Cedrus libani*)	Carpenters	Greenberg (1972); Sosman et al. (1969)
Iroko (*Chloro-hora exelcsa*)	Carpenters	Pickering, Batten and Pepys (1972)
South African boxwood		Harvey Gibson (1905)
	Shuttlemakers	Hay (1907)
Mansonia		Bridge (1935)
Oak	Sawmiller	Sosman et al. (1969)
Mahogany	Patterns' maker	Sosman et al. (1969)
Abiruana		Booth, LeFoldt and Moffitt (1976)
Cocabolla (*Dalbergia retusa*)	Wood finishers	Eaton (1973)
Kejaat (*Pterocarbus angblensis*)	Wood machinist	Ordman, (1949)
California Redwood (*Sequoia sempervirens*)	Carpenter	Chan-Yeung and Abboud (1976)
	Woodworkers	doPico (1978)
Ramin (*Gonystylus bancanus*)	Woodworkers	Howie, Boyd and Moran (1976)
African zebrawood (*Microberlinia*)	Woodworkers	Bush, Yunginger and Reed (1978)
Ebony (*Diospyros crassiflora*)	Carpenters	Maestrelli, Marcer and Dal Vecchio (1987)
Obeche		Hinojosa et al. (1986)
Ash (*Fraxinus americana*)	Woodworkers	Malo and Cartier (1989)
Palisander	Woodworkers	Godnic-Cvar and Gomzi (1990)

respiratory symptoms who developed symptomatic and functional evidence of bronchial asthma within hours of exposure to toxic air-borne concentrations of respiratory irritants such as chlorine and ammonia. Increased airways' responsiveness to methacholine was present in five of six tested. In the majority of cases, symptoms resolved within weeks. In a later report, Brooks, Weiss and Bernstein (1985) reported the findings in bronchial biopsies in two patients with RADS. These showed evidence of

Table 21.5 Causes of occupational asthma: enzymes and drugs

Causes	Occupations	Selected references
Enzymes		
Alcalase from *B. subtilis*	Detergent manufacture	Flindt, (1969); Pepys et al. (1969); Newhouse et al. (1970); Greenberg, Milne and Watt (1970); Mitchell and Gandevia, (1971); Weill, Naddell and Ziskind (1971); Juniper et al. (1977)
Papain		Milne and Brandt (1975); Flindt (1979); Baur et al. (1982)
Bromelain	Pharmaceutical worker	Baur and Fruhmann (1979a)
	Blood group laboratory workers	Gailhoffer et al. (1988)
α-Amylase		Flindt (1979)
Pancreatic extract	Bread manufacture	Baur et al. (1986)
	Pharmaceutical worker	Pilat, Popa and Tecoulescou (1967)
	Parents of cystic fibrosis (CF) children	Dolan and Myers (1974)
	Paediatric nurse	Hayes and Newman Taylor (1991)
Hog trypsin		Colten et al. (1975)
Drugs		
Psyllium	Laxative manufacture	Busse and Schoenwetter (1975); Bardy (1987)
Methyldopa	Manufacture	Harries et al. (1979)
Salbutamol intermediate	Manufacture	Fawcett, Pepys and Erooga (1976)
Amprolium	Poultry feed mixer	Greene and Freedman (1976)
Dichloramine	Manufacture	Popa et al. (1969)
Piperazine	Process worker and chemist	Pepys, Pickering and Loudon (1972)
Spiramycin	Manufacturing engineering	Davies and Pepys (1975)
Penicillins	Manufacture	Davies, Hendrick and Pepys (1974)
Phenylglycine acid chloride	Ampicillin manufacture	Kammermeyer and Mathews (1973)
Ipecacuanha	Manufacture	Luczynska et al. (1984)
Cimetidine	Manufacture	Coutts et al. (1984)
Isoniazid	Hospital pharmacist	Asai et al. (1987)
Tetracycline	Manufacture	Menon and Das (1977); Fawcett and Pepys (1976)
Sulphathiazole	Manufacture	Popa et al. (1969)
Gentian powder	Pharmacists	Kobayashi (1974)
Phosdrin (organophosphate insecticide)	Manufacture	Weiner (1961)
Cephalosporins	Manufacture	Coutts et al. (1981)

airways' inflammation with some, but not all, of the changes regarded as characteristic of asthma. They reported bronchial epithelial desquamation with mucous cell hyperplasia and bronchial wall infiltration with plasma cells and lymphocytes, but no eosinophils and no evidence of smooth muscle hyperplasia or basement membrane thickening.

More recently three cases of persistent asthma in policemen initiated by inhalation of chemical vapour from a single roadside truck accident have been reported. Symptoms and abnormal lung function (including airways' responsiveness measured in two of the three) persisted for 5 years in two and for the 2 years of follow-up in the third (Promisloff et al., 1990).

Whether asthma and airways' hyperresponsiveness in these cases are the direct consequence of persistent airways' inflammation or the outcome of other effects, such as neural damage consequent upon epithelial cell injury, is unknown. There is also, not surprisingly, no evidence for normal airways' function and responsiveness prior to the respiratory irritant exposure, and the validity of RADS depends upon the assumption that the absence of previously reported respiratory symptoms implies normal lung function, including airways' responsiveness.

Hypersensitivity inducers

In the great majority of cases, asthma caused by both complex biological molecules (both proteins and others) and low-molecular-weight chemicals

Table 21.6 Causes of occupational asthma: low-molecular-weight chemicals (including soldering fluxes and dyes)

Cause	Occupation	Selected references
Diisocyanates:		
Toluene (TDI)	TDI use:	
	Varnishes	Pepys et al. (1972)
	TDI manufacture	Butcher et al. (1977)
	Workers in adjacent offices	Carroll, Secombe and Pepys (1976)
	Foam manufacture	Gandevia (1964)
	Various uses/print ink and laminating adhesive	O'Brien et al. (1979a,b); Durham et al. (1987)
Diphenylmethane (MDI)	Foam manufacture	Tanser et al. (1973)
	Foundry workers	Zammitt-Tabbona et al. (1983); Johnson et al. (1985)
Hexamethylene (HDI)	Spray painters	O'Brien et al. (1979a)
Acid anhydrides:		
Naphthalene (NDI)	Rubber manufacture	Harries et al. (1979)
Phthalic (PA)	Paint manufacture	Kern (1939); Maccia et al. (1976); Fawcett et al. (1977); Durham et al. (1987)
Trimellitic (TMA)	Paint	Fawcett, Newman Taylor and Pepys (1977)
	Chemical workers	Zeiss et al. (1977); Zeiss et al. (1983)
Tetrachlorophthalic (TCPA)	Electronics factory	Shlueter et al. (1978); Howe et al. (1983) Venables et al. (1987)
Maleic (MA)		Topping et al. (1986); Durham et al. (1987)
Hexahydrophthalic		Moller et al. (1985)
Himic		Berstein et al. (1984)
Fluxes		
Aminoethylethanolamine	Aluminium soldering	Sterling (1967); Pepys et al. (1972)
Colophony	Electronics and hot melt glue	Fawcett, Newman Taylor and Pepys (1976)
	Electronics soldering	Burge et al. (1979b, 1980)
	Solder wire manufacture	Burge et al. (1981)
Other chemicals		
Ethylenediamine	Photography	Lam and Chan-Yeung (1980)
Triethylenetetramine	Aircraft fitter	Fawcett, Newman Taylor and Pepys (1977)
Dimethylethanolamine	Spray painting	Vallieres et al. (1977)
Azodicarbonamide	Manufacture	Slovak (1981)
Chloramine T	Brewery	Bourne, Flindt and Walker (1979)
Formaldehyde	Dialysis nurses	Hendrick and Lane (1977); Nordman et al. (1985)
Glutaraldehyde	Bronchoscopy nurses	Corrado (1986)
Cyanoacrylates	Cyanoacrylate glues	Locewicz et al. (1987)
Methyl methacrylate		Locewicz et al. (1987)
Furfuryl alcohol	Foundry workers	Cockroft et al. (1980)
p-Phenylenediamine	Fur stripers	Silbermann and Sorrell (1959)
Persulphates and henna	Hairdressers	Pepys, Hutchcroft and Breslin (1976)
Freon		Malo, Gagnon and Cartier (1984)
Tannic acid		Johnston et al. (1951)
Hexachlorophene (sterilizing agent)	Hospital staff	Nagy and Orosz (1984)
Reactive dyes	Fabric dye workers	Alanko et al. (1978); Docker et al. (1987)

(organic and inorganic) fulfil the classic criteria for an allergic response which von Pirquet defined as a state of 'specific acquired altered reactivity', however mediated or expressed, which follows initial exposure to a foreign protein:

1. Asthma occurs in a proportion, usually a minority, of those exposed to the particular agent. For example, only about 5 to 10 per cent of isocyanate or laboratory animal workers develop asthma.

2. Asthma develops only after an initial symptom-free period of exposure. This commonly has a duration of weeks or months, but it can be years. The majority of cases of asthma in laboratory animal workers (Gross, 1980), isocyanate

Table 21.7 Causes of occupational asthma: metals and metal salts

Cause	Occupation	Selected references
Platinum salts	Precious metal refining	Hunter, Milton and Perry (1945); Roberts (1951); Pepys, Pickering and Hughes (1972); Dally et al. (1980); Venables et al. (1989a,b)
Nickel	Metal plating	McConnell et al. (1973); Block et al. (1983); Malo et al. (1982)
Chromium	Chrome plating	Joules (1952); Novey, Habib and Wells (1983)
Stainless steel	Welding	Keskinen, Kalliomaki and Alanko (1980)
Cobalt	Hard metal manufacture and grinding	Bruckner (1967); Davison et al. (1983b)
Vanadium	Gas turbine cleaner	Browne (1955)
	Boiler cleaner	Williams (1952)

workers (Butcher et al., 1977) and platinum refinery workers (Venables et al., 1989a) occur in the first 1 to 2 years of exposure. The risk of developing asthma for those who survive this initial period is considerably less.

3. Asthmatic responses (both reduced airways' calibre and increased airways' responsiveness) are provoked by the inhalation of the specific cause of asthma in concentrations that do not cause such changes in others similarly exposed and of which the individual him- or herself was previously tolerant. In TDI-sensitive individuals, asthma may be provoked by inhalations of toluene diisocyanate (TDI) in atmospheric concentrations of 0.001 part per million (p.p.m.) – about one-twentieth of the concentration to mucosal surfaces of 0.5 p.p.m. (Henschler, Assman and Meyer, 1962).

These characteristics have stimulated research into evidence for a specific immunological response, and in particular for evidence of IgE to the specific causes of occupational asthma. A specific IgE response to a particular agent is usually inferred from the ability of a water-soluble extract of either the responsible substance or a hapten–protein conjugate to elicit an immediate 'weal and flare' response in the skin. Alternatively, specific IgE can be identified directly in serum by tests such as the radioallergosorbent test (RAST). Using one or other of these methods, specific IgE has been identified in most cases of occupational asthma caused by proteins of animal, vegetable or microbial origin. These include the excreta and secreta of animals such as rats and mice (Newman Taylor, Longbottom and Pepys, 1977) and locusts (Tee et al., 1988), wheat and rye flour (Björksten et al., 1977) and the enzyme alcalase from *Bacillus subtilis* (Pepys et al., 1973).

Specific IgE has also been reported in cases of asthma caused by several low-molecular-weight chemicals. These include acid anhydrides (Newman Taylor et al., 1987), platinum salts (Cleare et al., 1976), reactive dyes (Docker et al., 1987),

isocyanates (Butcher et al., 1980) and plicatic acid (Tse, Chan and Chan-Yeung, 1982).

A specific immunological response to a particular agent may simply be the outcome of exposure to it. The implication of the involvement of a particular agent in the pathogenesis of occupational asthma requires evidence that demonstrates a clear relationship to cases of asthma in exposed populations. This has been investigated in relatively few situations, but a clear relationship between specific IgE antibody and asthma has been found in workforces exposed to laboratory animals (Venables et al., 1988), locusts (Tee et al., 1988) and tetrachlorophthalic anhydride (Howe et al., 1983). No consistent relationship between specific IgE and asthma has been reported for either isocyanates or plicatic acid and there is no evidence of a specific immunological response in cases of colophony-induced asthma. Although specific IgE antibody to isocyanates and plicatic acid has been reported, specific IgE is only present in some 15 per cent of those with occupational asthma caused by TDI (Butcher et al., 1980) and in 40 per cent of Western Red Cedar (*Thuja plicata*) workers with asthma caused by plicatic acid (Tse, Chan and Chan-Yeung, 1982). This may be due to the involvement of other patterns of immunological response (B-cell or T-cell mediated), although to date no convincing evidence for this has been provided. It may also reflect either the difficulties of working with highly reactive chemicals, such as isocyanates, in in vitro systems or the failure to prepare the relevant in vivo hapten–protein conjugate for the in vitro test. Reactants of the isocyanate–water reaction may form in the respiratory tract and these, rather than the parent isocyanate, bind to body proteins. Similarly, colophony is a mixture of pinewood resin acids and aldehydes and it remains unclear which is (or are) the biologically relevant molecule(s).

The lack of evidence for a specific immunological response, in many cases of asthma caused by non-protein molecules in particular isocyanates and plicatic acid, has stimulated studies that have examined the role of non-immunological mechanisms. Plicatic acid has been shown to release histamine from non-sensitized human and pig lung (Evans et al., 1974) and to activate the classical pathway of complement (Chan-Yeung, Gicas and Henson, 1980). TDI has been found to inhibit the in vitro stimulation of lymphocyte adenylate cyclase by isoprenaline in a dose-dependent fashion (Davies et al., 1977), possibly by covalent binding of the isocyanate group to the membrane receptor. Hypothetically, TDI could therefore cause asthma by β-adrenoreceptor inhibition. TDI did not, however, inhibit isoprenaline-induced tracheal smooth muscle relaxation (Mackay and Brooks, 1983). A hypothesis in which asthma is caused by non-immunological and pharmacological activities of these chemicals fails to explain both the well-documented latent interval between initial exposure to TDI or plicatic acid and the development of asthma, and the observation that in sensitized individuals inhalation of the specific chemical cause, such as TDI or acid anhydrides, induces an increase in non-specific airways' responsiveness (Durham et al., 1987).

Coutts et al. (1984) found that the prevalence of work-related nasal and lower respiratory symptoms in a workforce manufacturing the drug cimetidine increased with increasing duration of exposure during the working week. In a cohort study of enzyme detergent workers, Juniper et al. (1977) found that the incidence of developing an immediate skin test response to an extract of the *Bacillis subtilis* enzyme alcalase was increased in the higher intensity categories of exposure.

Very little evidence has been reported in support of suggestions that the risk of sensitization to inhaled chemicals, such as isocyanates, is increased among those exposed to high atmospheric concentrations during 'spills' or other accidents. Weill et al. (1981) reported that 7 of 13 cases of asthma caused by TDI in a TDI manufacturing plant followed a brief period of high-intensity exposure. The frequency of such an occurrence in members of the workforce not developing occupational asthma was not reported.

Contributory factors to the development of occupational asthma

Three major factors have been reported as contributing to the development of occupational asthma in exposed populations: exposure, atopy and tobacco smoking. Of these, exposure, even though it is the most directly amenable to control, has to date received the least attention.

Exposure

No studies so far reported have examined the incidence of occupational asthma in relation to measured exposure. A study of bakery workers, which examined the prevalence of work-related respiratory symptoms and airways' responsiveness in relation to estimated and measured total dust exposure, found an increased prevalence of both symptoms and airways' hyperresponsiveness among those who had worked at any time in dustier conditions (Musk et al., 1989). Burge et al. (1981), in a cross-sectional study of colophony workers, found a gradient of work-related respiratory symptoms in relation to measured levels of colophony.

Atopy

Atopy is usually defined in immunological terms as occurring in those who produce IgE antibodies readily on contact with common environmental allergens (Pepys, 1973). Atopy is commonly identified by the ability of extracts of one or more common inhalant allergens (which in the UK would usually include grass pollens, the house-dust mite *Dermatophagoides pteronyssinus* and cat fur) to elicit an immediate 'weal and flare' response in the skin. Studies of workforces have consistently shown that, by this definition, between about one-quarter and one-third have one or more immediate skin test responses to these extracts, that is, between about one-quarter and one-third are 'atopic'.

IgE antibody production and asthma caused by several agents inhaled at work have been reported to occur more commonly among atopics. This association is probably best described for asthma caused by laboratory animal excreta (Venables et al., 1988), *B. subtilis* enzymes (Juniper et al., 1977) and the complex platinum salt, ammonium hexachloroplatinate. There is no evidence that atopics are at increased risk of developing asthma caused by isocyanates (Butcher et al., 1977) or plicatic acid (Chan-Yeung, 1982). Several studies have reported an association between asthma caused by laboratory animals and atopy (Cockroft et al., 1981; Slovak and Hill, 1981; Venables et al., 1988). In these studies, work-related chest symptoms occurred some four to five times more frequently in atopic than in non-atopic laboratory animal workers, and the prevalence of skin test responses to laboratory animal urine extracts was greater in atopics. However, no significant association of atopy with other manifestations of laboratory animal allergy – rhinitis, conjunctivitis or urticaria – was found. Juniper et al. (1977) found, in their cohort study of enzyme detergent workers, that at each level of exposure the presence of an immediate skin test response to alcalase was greater among atopics than among non-atopics. Dalley et al. (1980) found an increased incidence of skin-prick reactions to ammonium hexachloroplatinate, and respiratory symptoms in atopics employed in a platinum refinery. This study did not examine the effect of smoking, and a later study (Venables et al., 1989a) found that the increased risk associated with atopy was smaller than with tobacco smoking and was not significant when smoking was taken into account.

The relationship between atopy and occupational asthma has assumed considerable importance in some industries where atopy is used as a tool for pre-employment selection. Although, as mentioned earlier, the risk of sensitization and asthma may be greater in atopics than in non-atopics, several arguments weigh against the use of identification of atopics for this purpose. Atopy discriminates poorly: about one-quarter to one-third of the adult workforce have been found to have one or more immediate skin-test responses to common environmental allergens; even among laboratory animal workers, where the risk of developing asthma is some four to five times greater among atopics, asthma only occurs in a minority of exposed atopics and the cost of excluding the minority of the atopics who may develop asthma is to exclude up to one-third of a potential workforce. Furthermore, the prevention of asthma caused by agents inhaled at work is better based upon environmental control rather than upon seeking out 'susceptible' individuals.

Tobacco smoking

Tobacco smoking has been reported to increase the risk of developing specific IgE antibody and asthma to several different agents inhaled at work. Specific IgE antibody has been found to occur some four to five times more frequently in smokers than in non-smokers exposed at work to tetrachlorophthalic anhydride (TCPA) (Venables et al., 1985a) and ispaghula (Zetterström et al., 1981); also a positive skin-prick test is likewise more frequent among smokers exposed at work to the green coffee bean (Zetterström et al., 1981) and to ammonium hexachloroplatinate (Venables et al., 1989a). The

risk of developing occupational asthma is also increased although usually less than for the specific IgE. All seven cases of TCPA-induced asthma in one factory were smokers (Howe et al., 1983) and the risk of smokers developing asthma was some twofold greater among smokers who worked in a platinum refinery (Venables et al., 1989a) and among those who processed snow crabs (Cartier et al., 1984).

The 'adjuvant' effect of smoking on IgE production has also been observed in animal experiments. Inhaled tobacco smoke potentiated the IgE response to inhaled but not to subcutaneous ovalbumin (Zetterström et al., 1985), suggesting a local effect on the airways. Other respiratory irritants have been shown to cause a similar enhancing effect: ozone inhaled concurrently with platinum salts increased the frequency of IgE antibody production and asthma in monkeys (Biagini et al., 1986) and sulphur dioxide inhaled concurrently with ovalbumin by guinea-pigs increased the rate of immunological and airways' responses in a dose-dependent fashion (Riedel et al., 1988). The local effect of tobacco smoke and other respiratory irritants, inhaled concurrently with novel antigen, suggest the existence of a mechanism such as increased mucosal permeability of the airways caused by local airways' injury that increases antigen access to submucosal immunocompetent cells.

Examples of occupational asthma

It is not practical to discuss all the known causes of occupational asthma. Many are listed in Tables 21.2 to 21.7; some important examples of these will be described in more detail.

Laboratory animals
(in particular rats and mice)

Laboratory animal allergy is one of the most important causes of occupational allergy and asthma. Some 32 000 persons (scientific, technical and administrative staff) have been estimated to work with laboratory animals (Cockroft et al., 1981). Cross-sectional surveys of laboratory animal workers have consistently found prevalence rates of laboratory animal allergy (LAA) of between 15 and 30 per cent (Gross, 1980; Cockroft et al., 1981; Davies and McArdle, 1981; Schumacher, Tait and Holmes, 1981; Slovak and Hill, 1981; Beeson et al., 1983; Agrup et al., 1986). A more recent survey found a 44 per cent prevalence of symptoms consistent with LAA and a 11 per cent prevalence of LAA chest symptoms in 138 pharmaceutical employees exposed at work to laboratory animals (Venables et al., 1989a) and a prospective study estimated the incidence of laboratory animal allergy to be 15 per cent and of asthma 2 per cent, in the first year of work with animals (Davies et al., 1983).

Extracts of urine proteins of rats and mice elicit immediate skin test responses and, when inhaled, provoke asthmatic reactions in sensitized workers (Newman Taylor, Longbottom and Pepys, 1977). The important urinary proteins seem to be an α_2-globulin in the rat and a prealbumin in the mouse – proteins excreted particularly by postpubertal male animals (Newman Taylor, Longbottom and Pepys, 1977). The mouse prealbumin is probably also secreted by sebaceous glands (Price and Longbottom, 1987).

The steady-state concentration of animal urine proteins in air is determined by the ratio of the rates of generation and removal. The major factors that determine generation of urine proteins are animal density (the relationship of animal numbers to the volume of the room) and working activities (for example, cage cleaning and sweeping). The major factors that influence the reduction of air-borne allergen concentration are ventilation, air filtration and humidity. Twiggs et al. (1982a) found the concentration of mouse urine protein in the air of an animal laboratory to vary between 1.8 and 825 µg/m³ and it was influenced by both animal density and level of work activity. Similarly, Price and Longbottom (1988) found that the concentration of mouse, rat and rabbit allergens was increased by greater animal density and increased work activity, such as cleaning an animal room or animal handling. Edwards, Beeson and Dewdney (1983) found that the concentration of rat urine protein in air was appreciably reduced by increased ventilation rates and by increased humidity.

Grain dust

Grain dust is a complex mixture of grain, its disintegration products and organic constituents, whose composition depends upon whether the grain is encountered during harvesting or in storage. For the purposes of considering contaminants that may cause occupational asthma, it is convenient to distinguish harvest from storage dust.

Harvest dust

Growing and ripening grains are important sources of the saprophytic grain spores of several different fungi. These include *Alternaria tenuis* and *Cladosporium herbarum* whose spores are released into the air by day and *Didymella exitialis* whose spores are released into the air at night and after rainfall. In the UK, spores of *A. tenuis* and *C. herbarum* are present in the air throughout the year, rising from a few hundred per m³ in the winter months to 10 000 and 1 000 000 per m³, respectively, in the late summer and autumn months. During harvesting, total air-borne spore counts can reach 10^8 per m³ of which some 75 per cent are *C. herbarum* and 25 per cent *A. tenuis*. The spores are blown free by the wind with air-borne concentrations maximal in dry windy weather. In contrast, the spores of *D. exitialis* are expelled into the air after absorption of water and their air-borne concentration is maximal in conditions of high humidity (and therefore during the night) and after rainfall (Harries et al., 1985).

Inhalation of spores of *A. tenuis*, *C. herbarum* and *D. exitialis* can stimulate IgE antibody production and cause asthma. The three fungi share several allergens (Tee, Gordon and Newman Taylor, 1987). In their study of Lincolnshire farmers, Darke et al. (1976) found that nearly one-quarter reported acute respiratory symptoms during the harvesting period. Their symptoms had usually developed after several years of farm work and occurred particularly in those most heavily exposed to grain dust, drivers of combine harvesters and those working in grain bins or near grain driers and elevators.

Storage dust

The capacity of stored grain to support the growth of moulds and mites is determined primarily by its water content. Moulding can occur at water contents of between 10 per cent and 15 per cent and mites that feed on the moulds also grow at this water content. Grain stored with this content of water may become infested with storage mites of which the most important in the UK are *Leptidoglycus destructor*, *Acaris siro* and *Glycyphagus domesticus*. Inhalation of mites and their excreta can stimulate IgE antibody production and cause asthma (Ingram et al., 1979). In a study of Essex farmers, Blainey et al. (1986) found that nearly one-fifth had asthma that they considered to be caused by storage mites. In a survey of Swedish farmers in Gotland (an island in the Baltic sea), van Hage-Hamsten et al. (1985) estimated the prevalence of respiratory symptoms caused by storage mite allergy to be 6.2 per cent.

Inhalation tests with grain dust and grain dust extract have been reported to provoke an asthmatic response (Warren, Chermick and Tse, 1974; Davies, Green and Schofield, 1976; Chan-Yeung, Wong and MacLean, 1979). However, it is not clear from these reports whether the asthma was provoked by constituents of the grain or by its contaminants.

Enzymes

Enzymes are widely and increasingly used commercially for a variety of purposes. The incorporation of proteolytic enzymes into detergent powders is probably the most widely appreciated but other uses include fungal α-amylase in the manufacture of bread, papain as a meat tenderizer and bromelin used as tenderizer and reaction booster in blood grouping laboratories. Enzymes are proteins and when inhaled can cause asthma. The risks of asthma occur primarily among the enzyme producers and the manufacturers of products that incorporate them. Allergy to enzymes was reported in a small number of consumers using enzyme-containing detergents in Sweden and the USA during the early period of manufacture when powdered non-granulated enzyme products were marketed (Belin et al., 1970; Zetterström and Wide, 1974). However, any important risk to consumers seems to have been markedly reduced with the introduction of granulated enzymes (Zetterström, 1977; Pepys et al., 1985).

The introduction of recombinant DNA technology has increased the potential for producing enzymes and other proteins of commercial value and the risk to those exposed to them in production and manufacture remains unless measures are taken to minimize the risk of their becoming air-borne.

The respiratory hazard of inhalation of proteolytic enzymes during detergent manufacture was initially identified by Flindt (1969) and Pepys et al. (1969). Subsequent epidemiological studies in the UK (Greenberg, Milne and Watt, 1970; Newhouse et al., 1970), the USA (Weill, Waddell and Ziskind, 1971) and Australia (Mitchell and Gandevia, 1971) demonstrated high rates of skin-prick test responses and respiratory symptoms consistent with asthma. In a 7-year follow-up study of a detergent enzyme workforce exposed to the *B. subtilis* enzyme, alcalase, Juniper et al. (1977) showed a clear relationship between the development of a positive skin test reaction to alcalase and exposure category and atopy (Table 21.8).

The influence of atopy was reported in other studies and a further analysis of these data (Editorial, 1985) has also shown an effect of smoking.

Considerable reductions in the levels of air-borne enzyme dust have been achieved by encapsulation

Table 21.8 Percentage of exposed workforce who develop positive skin-prick test to alcalase

Exposure	Percentage workforce with atopic status	
	Positive	*Negative*
'High'	40	25
'Intermittent'	20	4.5

of the enzyme powder to form granules of aerodynamic diameters in excess of 150 μm. Subsequent reports would suggest that reduction in the risk of sensitization and asthma occurred in parallel with these changes (Juniper et al., 1977), but other measures, such as the exclusion of atopics, occurred concurrently.

Flindt (1979) and Milne and Brandt (1975) also drew attention to the hazards of papain and α-amylase to those exposed to it in production and use. Subsequently, Baur et al. (1986) reported cases of asthma in bakers caused by α-amylase used in bread manufacture.

Bromelin is a purified protease of pineapple. Baur and Fruhmann (1979a) described occupational rhinitis and asthma in a pharmaceutical worker which had been provoked by inhaled and ingested bromelin and which was associated with an immediate skin-prick test response to bromelin. They also demonstrated cross-reactivity between IgE binding to bromelin and papain. Gailhoffer et al. (1988) reported four cases of occupational allergy (with asthma) provoked by handling bromelin among blood group laboratory workers. All four had specific IgE to bromelin.

Occupational asthma caused by inhaled papain has been reported in those exposed to it occupationally. Baur and Fruhmann (1979b) reported asthma and rhinitis associated with evidence of specific IgE to papain in seven of eleven people exposed to papain at work, nine of whom worked in a kitchen where papain was used to tenderize meat; the other two worked in a pharmaceutical factory that produced papain-containing digestives.

Wood dusts

Asthma has been reported in workers exposed to wood dust as being caused by the dusts of many different woods (see Table 21.4). The wood that has been most studied is the Western Red Cedar (*Thuja plicata*). It is the most important cause of occupational asthma in British Columbia (Chan-Yeung,

Lam and Koener, 1982). Asthma caused by Western Red Cedar has been found in 4.1 per cent of cedar mill workers (Chan-Yeung et al., 1984) and 13.5 per cent of those studied by Brooks et al. (1981).

Western Red Cedar-induced asthma was first described by Gandevia and Milne (1970) who reported six cases of asthma and four of rhinitis in patients exposed to the wood dust in their work. Inhalation testing in four with a water-soluble extract of Western Red Cedar provoked late and nocturnal asthmatic responses. In a later study of 22 cases, Chan-Yeung et al. (1973) found that asthmatic responses provoked by inhalation of water-soluble extracts of Western Red Cedar could be reproduced by inhaling plicatic acid – a water-soluble constituent unique to Western Red Cedar which is the major fraction (40 per cent) of the non-volatile components of the wood.

Tse, Chan and Chan-Yeung (1982) identified IgE specific to crude cedar extract coupled to Sepharose and specific to plicatic acid conjugated to human serum albumin in the sera of 8 out of 18 cases of Western Red Cedar asthma diagnosed by inhalation testing. Specific IgE was not found in the sera of 16 control subjects or in 10 individuals in whom inhalation of plicatic acid did not provoke an asthmatic response.

Chan-Yeung, Lam and Koener (1982) reported their findings in 125 wood workers with occupational asthma diagnosed by inhalation testing with either crude cedar extract or plicatic acid. Symptoms had developed on average some 3 to 4 years from initial exposure. At follow-up between 1 to 9 years (average 3½ years), 50 remained employed and 75 had left the industry. All 50 who remained exposed had continuing symptoms and so too did 50 per cent (37 of 75) of those who had left. The time since leaving did not differ between those with and those without symptoms (average of 40 months). Whereas the concentration of methacholine that provoked a 20% fall in FEV_1 (PC_{20}) had increased since diagnosis in those whose symptoms had improved (on average from 2.98 to 10.68), those with continuing symptoms showed no change (on average 0.47 at diagnosis and 0.32 at follow-up), similar to those who had remained exposed (1.81 at diagnosis and 0.89 at follow-up). The factors associated with continuing symptoms and hyperresponsiveness of the airways at follow-up were longer duration of exposure (87.6 vs 33.9 months), longer duration of symptomatic exposure before diagnosis (49 vs 17.2 months), greater abnormality of lung function and methacholine PC_{20} at diagnosis, and a greater likelihood of a dual than a lone late asthmatic response provoked by specific inhalation testing. This study provided the clearest evidence that chronic asthma is caused by prolonged symptomatic exposure to an occupational cause and the most persuasive argument for early identification and avoidance of further exposure.

Flour

The estimated incidence of occupational asthma in bakery workers is one of the four highest of the occupational groups reported to the UK surveillance scheme (see Table 21.3). Although grain contaminants such as mites and moulds have been suggested as causes, current evidence would implicate cereal flour proteins as the most important cause. Hendrick, Davies and Pepys (1976) studied two bakers with occupational asthma in whom inhalation of wheat and rye flour in one and wheat flour in the other provoked dual asthmatic responses. Skin testing with the same flours elicited immediate responses in both. Interestingly, ingestion of uncooked flour provoked no adverse reactions. Block et al. (1983) studied eight patients in whom inhalation testing provoked an immediate asthmatic response with rye flour in four and with wheat in the two of these four tested. Specific IgE to rye and wheat flour extract was present in the sera of six of the eight including all those in whom inhalation tests provoked asthma.

Björksten et al. (1977) identified specific IgE to wheat extract by RAST in the sera of 9 of 21 bakers with asthma. Five of these nine, but none of those without IgE to wheat, had specific IgE to rye extract suggesting common cross-reacting antigens. Blands et al. (1976) identified 40 proteins in wheat flour, 20 of which cross-reacted with rye flour. IgE present in the sera of 13 allergic bakers bound to 18 of these 40 wheat proteins. Walsh et al. (1985) found that IgE binding was greatest to the water-soluble albumins in flour; binding also occurred to the water-insoluble gliadins and glutenins. Baur et al. (1986) reported asthma, rhinitis and conjunctivitis associated with flour contact in 35 of 118 bakery and confectionery workers. All 35 had specific IgE to wheat flour and, of these, 33 had specific IgE to rye flour. In addition, 12 had specific IgE to fungal α-amylase (from *Aspergillus oryzae*) – an important flour additive. Inhalation testing with the enzyme in four of these subjects provoked immediate rhinitis or asthma.

Prichard et al. (1985) studied 176 male bakers who represented 90 per cent of all bakers in Perth, Western Australia. Of these, 15 per cent had immediate skin test responses and specific IgE to water-soluble wheat proteins. The presence of antibodies was associated with an increased prevalence of work-related respiratory symptoms and measurable airways' hyperresponsiveness. In a companion paper, Prichard, Ryan and Musk (1984) reported that 20 of the 176 fulfilled their definition of work-related asthma. Increased airways' responsiveness to inhaled methacholine and immediate skin test responses to both wheat flour proteins and to common inhalant allergens were more prevalent in these 20. However, whilst the prevalence of skin test reactions to wheat flour increased with increasing duration of exposure, that of common inhalant allergens declined, suggesting that atopics were selected out of this employment. In a cross-sectional study of a bakery in the UK, Musk et al. (1989) found that of 318 employees 19 per cent had work-related nasal symptoms and 13 per cent work-related chest symptoms. Both were associated with current exposure to higher dust concentrations in the factory. Measurable airways' responsiveness to inhaled histamine was associated with higher exposure to dust concentrations at any time during employment.

Acid anhydrides

Acid anhydrides are low-molecular-weight chemicals used industrially as curing agents in the production of epoxy and alkyd resins and in the manufacture of the plasticizer dioctyl phthalate. Epoxy and alkyd resins have widespread applications as paints, plastics and adhesives. Six acid anhydrides – phthalic (PA) (Maccia et al., 1976), trimellitic (TMA) (Fawcett, Newman Taylor and Pepys, 1977; Zeiss et al., 1977), tetrachlorophthalic (TCPA) (Howe et al., 1983), maleic (MA) (Topping et al., 1986; Durham et al., 1987), hexahydrophthalic (Moller et al., 1985) and himic (Bernstein et al., 1984) – have been reported to cause occupational asthma; inhalation tests with the causal acid anhydride provoked asthmatic responses, and specific IgE or IgG antibodies (or both) to the specific anhydride conjugated to human serum albumin have been identified in the sera of the great majority of cases, although this is less frequent with maleic than with the other anhydrides. Zeiss et al. (1977) identified four separate clinical syndromes caused by TMA for which they have proposed separate mechanisms: toxic airways' irritation; immediate IgE-mediated rhinitis and asthma; IgG-mediated late asthma with systemic symptoms ('TMA 'flu'); and pulmonary haemorrhage–haemolytic anaemia syndrome as the outcome of antibody binding to circulating red blood cells and to pulmonary vascular cells. The distinction between 'immediate' and late 'asthmatic' reactions with 'influenza' and their different pattern of immunological response have not been consistently observed by others and it seems likely that asthma caused by acid anhydrides (including TMA) may be associated with IgE or IgG or both, although (specific) IgE and IgG4 seem to be associated more with asthma and IgG with exposure. The pulmonary haemorrhage–haemolytic anaemia syndrome is real but rare. Studies of the specificity of the IgE binding to acid anhydrides and to their conjugates with human and bovine serum albumin suggest that the anhydride is involved in the IgE binding site (Topping et al., 1986), findings consistent with the results of Landsteiner and van der Scheer (1936) who demonstrated that hapten configuration profoundly affects antibody binding.

Seven patients with TCPA-induced asthma were followed up for 4 years from avoidance of exposure (Venables et al., 1987). One of the seven died 1 year after leaving work. All the others had continuing symptoms consistent with persistent airways' hyperresponsiveness and the five in whom it was undertaken had measurable PC_{20} to inhaled histamine. During the period of follow-up, IgE antibody fell exponentially and in parallel in all six with a half-life $(t_{1/2})$ of 1 year suggesting that they were not further exposed to TCPA during this period and that IgE continues to be secreted for years after the last exposure.

Complex platinum salts

The complex platinum salt ammonium hexachloroplatinate is an essential intermediate in the refining of platinum – a corrosion-resistant metal used as a catalyst and in jewellery. Allergy to platinum salts in refinery workers was first reported by Hunter, Milton and Perry (1945). Subsequently, Pepys, Pickering and Hughes (1972) showed that inhalation of the salt provoked an asthmatic response and that the salt without protein conjugation provoked an immediate skin test response. The presence of specific IgE antibodies has been inferred from passive-transfer studies in human subjects and monkeys using sera from sensitized patients (Pepys et al., 1979).

The incidence of occupational allergy in the platinum refining industry was high in the UK in the mid-1970s. In a cohort study of 91 workers who entered employment in a platinum refinery in the 2 years, 1973 and 1974 (Venables et al., 1989a), 22 developed respiratory symptoms and an immediate skin test response to ammonium hexachloroplatinate. The risk was greatest in the first year of employment and smoking was the single most important predictor of developing a positive skin test reaction.

Colophony

Colophony is pine wood resin, the major use of which is as a soft solder flux in the electronics industry. Colophony fume which is generated during soldering is a complex mixture of resin acids and aldehydes of which the most important is abietic acid. Asthma caused by inhaled colophony fume was first reported by Fawcett, Newman Taylor and Pepys (1976) and subsequently further investigated by Burge and his colleagues.

Inhalation of colophony fume during soldering has been shown to provoke an asthmatic response in sensitized individuals (Fawcett, Newman Taylor and Pepys, 1976; Burge et al., 1980). Burge et al. (1979a) found, in a cross-sectional survey of an electronics factory where colophony was used as a soft solder flux, that 22 per cent of 446 shop-floor employees had work-related respiratory symptoms as compared with 16 per cent of those working in other parts of the factory. Some of those sensitized were not solderers but worked in the vicinity of those who soldered. Of the employees of this factory who had left during 3½ years before the survey, a significantly greater proportion had worked on the factory floor than in other parts of the factory and this excess could largely be accounted for by those leaving with work-related respiratory symptoms (Perks et al., 1979). In a survey of a factory that manufactured colophony flux-cored solder, Burge et al. (1981) found the prevalence of work-related respiratory symptoms to be related to measured atmospheric concentrations of colophony. Whereas 21 per cent of those in the high exposure group had symptoms, only 4 per cent of the low exposure group had symptoms.

To date, no studies have reported any convincing evidence for a specific immunological response to colophony or its constituents.

Burge (1982b) followed up 39 electronics workers with asthma 1 to 4 years after initial investigation by inhalation testing with colophony. Inhalation testing with colophony had provoked an asthmatic response in 28, but not in 11, who were considered not to have occupational asthma. Twenty of the 28 had left work, of whom 18 had continuing respiratory symptoms; 8 had been relocated at work all of whom had continuing symptoms, worse during the working week than during absences from work. Airways' response to inhaled histamine, measured at the time of diagnosis and at follow-up, had returned to normal in half of those who had left work but in only one of the eight relocated.

Asthma caused by inhaled colophony has been reported, although considerably less frequently, in occupations not associated with electronics soldering. These include a tool setter for whom colophony was a constituent of an emulsified oil mist generated when it was used as a coolant (Hendy, Beattie and Burge, 1985), a man exposed to unheated solid colophony while making a bitumen mixture (Burge et al., 1986) and a Hong Kong chicken plucker who dipped his chickens into heated liquid colophony prior to plucking.

Diisocyanates

Diisocyanates are bifunctional molecules used commercially to polymerize polyhydroxyl and polyglycol compounds to form polyurethanes. Diisocyanates also react with water to evolve carbon dioxide, a reaction exploited in the manufacture of flexible polyurethane foam. The urethane reaction is exothermic and the heat generated is sufficient to evaporate diisocyanates with high vapour pressures such as toluene diisocyanate (TDI) and hexamethylene diisocyanate (HDI). Significant evaporation of diisocyanates with low vapour pressures such as diphenyl methane diisocyanate (MDI) and naphthalene diisocyanate (NDI) occurs when heated. In order to reduce the amount of diisocyanate available for evaporation during polyurethane formation, adducts of diisocyanate with other organic compounds such as glycerol have been manufactured. However, although less diisocyanate evaporates when the compounds are sprayed, as in spray painting, high concentrations of aerosolized isocyanates are generated which can be inhaled.

Polyurethanes have widespread applications and exposure to diisocyanates or isocyanate adducts occurs in many different occupational circumstances: these include the manufacture of flexible and rigid polyurethane foam, the application of two-part polyurethane paints by brush and by spray painting, and in flexible packaging production where diisocyanates are used in inks and as laminating adhesives. It has been estimated that in the USA the use of polyurethanes will reach 2.2 million tonnes by 1990 and that between 50 000 and 1 000 000 workers there are exposed to isocyanates at work.

Inhaled diisocyanates probably cause four different respiratory reactions.

1. Toxic bronchitis and asthma caused by isocyanate inhalation in toxic concentrations. Exposure to TDI in an atmospheric concentration of 0.5 p.p.m. causes irritation of mucosal surfaces – eyes, nose and throat (Henschler, Asmann and Meyer, 1962). Persistent asthma and airways' hyperresponsiveness (RADS) following a single inhalation of TDI in toxic concentrations has also been reported (Luo, Nelson and Fischbein, 1990).
2. Bronchial asthma caused by sensitization to diisocyanates.
3. Accelerated decline of FEV_1: the rate of decline of FEV_1 in non-smokers exposed in a manufacturing plant with high cumulative exposures was similar to the rate of decline in both the low and high exposure groups of smokers. No additive effect of TDI with smoking was reported (Diem et al., 1982).
4. Extrinsic allergic alveolitis which has been reported particularly in workers exposed to MDI

(Zeiss et al., 1980; Malo and Zeiss, 1982) but also to HDI (Malo et al., 1983).

Of these, bronchial asthma caused by hypersensitivity to isocyanates has been the most frequently reported and seems to be the most important. Asthma has been reported to be caused by each of the diisocyanates: TDI (Pepys et al., 1972; Butcher et al., 1979), MDI (Tanser, Bourke and Blandford, 1973; Zammitt-Tabbona et al., 1983), HDI (O'Brien et al., 1979a) and NDI (Harries et al., 1979). TDI and MDI have been the most widely used and are the major causes of asthma. Weill et al. (1981), in a study of workers employed at a new TDI manufacturing plant, identified 12 workers (some 4 per cent of the total workforce) who had developed asthma during a 5-year period, of whom 9 developed asthma in the first year of employment. The average exposure to TDI monitored by paper tapes was 0.002 p.p.m. One-half had been exposed to spills, six were maintenance workers, one a laboratory worker and only five process workers. A cross-sectional study of a steel coating plant, where TDI had been introduced into the process some years before, identified 21 cases of asthma out of a total of 221 (Venables et al., 1985b) which was probably an underestimate of the true number of cases. Johnson et al. (1985) reported 12 cases of asthma in 78 iron and steel foundry workers exposed to MDI, which was considered as the most probable cause of the asthma.

Inhalation tests with TDI have shown that, in sensitized workers, asthmatic response may be provoked by exposure to very low atmospheric concentrations – in one report by 0.001 p.p.m. (O'Brien et al., 1979b). Late asthmatic responses provoked by isocyanates are associated with the development of an increase in non-specific airways' responsiveness (Durham et al., 1987) and cells recovered from bronchoalveolar lavage during a late asthmatic reaction provoked by TDI have an increased proportion of neutrophils (Fabbri et al., 1987). The characteristics of TDI-induced asthma suggest that it has an allergic basis, which has stimulated a considerable research effort into the identification of a specific immunological response that is consistently related to the development of asthma in exposed individuals. To date, although evidence for a specific immunological response has been found (see page 716), it has only been detected in a small minority of cases (some 15 per cent).

Studies of the outcome of isocyanate-induced asthma have consistently found that about half of the cases continue to have asthma several years after avoidance of exposure. Paggiaro et al. (1984) reported that 8 of 12 patients with TDI-induced asthma, confirmed by inhalation testing, continued to have episodic respiratory symptoms after 2 years' avoidance of exposure. Airways' responsiveness to

inhaled bethanechol remained increased in 7 of the 11 tested. All 15 patients with TDI-induced asthma, who had remained exposed during this 2-year period, continued to have respiratory symptoms and increased airways' hyperresponsiveness. Lozewicz et al. (1987) studied 50 patients with diisocyanate-induced asthma at least 4 years after avoidance of exposure. Forty-one (82 per cent) continued to have respiratory symptoms of whom about a half required treatment at least once a week. Airways' responsiveness was increased in 14 of the 21 tested at follow-up (Paggiaro et al., 1984).

Diagnosis of occupational asthma

Early recognition of occupational asthma and accurate identification of the specific cause are important. Remission of symptoms and restoration of lung function (including the loss of airways' hyperresponsiveness) can follow avoidance of exposure to the specific cause. The limited evidence available from follow-up studies suggests that continuing exposure to its cause after the onset of asthma adversely affects prognosis. More than half of 75 patients with Western Red Cedar-induced asthma were found at follow-up to have chronic asthma 1 to 9 years after avoidance of exposure (Chan-Yeung, Lam and Koener, 1982). A major determinant of continuing asthma in this population was longer duration of exposure after the onset of asthmatic symptoms. Accurate diagnosis is also important to avoid advising those whose asthma is not occupationally caused to change or leave their jobs unnecessarily. Misdiagnosis can be as harmful as missing the diagnosis.

The diagnosis of occupational asthma is usually suggested by the history. It usually (but of course not always) occurs in an individual exposed at work to a recognized sensitizing agent. The onset of symptoms occurs after an initial symptom-free period of exposure (of weeks, months or years) to the specific cause in concentrations which now provoke asthma. Symptoms are worse during periods at work, often progressing in severity during the working week, and improve during absences from work, such as weekends or holidays. Symptoms may be most severe or are on occasions only present after leaving work at the end of the working day or in the night. They may also persist for several days after the last exposure so that improvement does not occur during a 2-day weekend absence and is only appreciated during a longer (1- or 2-week) holiday absence from work. The patient may also be aware of others at his place of work who have developed similar respiratory symptoms.

Occupational asthma needs to be distinguished from asthma not occupationally caused and from chronic airflow limitation, both of which may be aggravated by respiratory irritants inhaled at work such as cold air or sulphur dioxide. It should also be distinguished from other causes of episodic respiratory symptoms, such as hyperventilation, which may be associated with periods at work.

Investigations

The most direct method of demonstrating a cause and effect relationship between exposure to a specific agent and the development of asthma is through provocation of both acute airways' narrowing and increased non-specific airways' responsiveness by the agent. Inhalation testing in all cases of occupational asthma is neither justifiable nor feasible and in the majority of cases the diagnosis can be made with sufficient confidence from the history, supported by serial measurements of lung function or immunological tests or both. Inhalation tests with the specific agent should be reserved for those in whom the results from other investigations do not provide sufficient evidence on which to base advice about future employment.

Lung function measurements

The most commonly used method for diagnosis of asthma – measurement of lung function on a single occasion before and after inhalation of bronchodilator to demonstrate reversible airflow limitation – has not proved to be a sensitive diagnostic test of occupational asthma and is clearly not specific for an occupational cause. Chan-Yeung, Lam and Koener (1982) found that 80 per cent of cases with asthma caused by Western Red Cedar had a normal FEV_1 at the time of diagnosis. Similarly, Burge, in a study of isocyanate workers, found a single FEV_1

measurement made at work, in those in whom inhalation tests with TDI provoked an asthmatic response, was no different from that in non-asthmatic workers in the factory (Burge, 1982a). Lung function tests to support the diagnosis of occupational asthma need to demonstrate asthma (variable airways' narrowing) and its relationship to work. Measurement of lung function before and after a working shift has been examined for this purpose. Burge (1982a) compared the change in FEV_1 before and after a working shift in 49 asthmatic electronic workers exposed to colophony with 46 symptomless workers from the same factory. FEV_1 fell by 20 per cent in only 22 per cent of those with asthma and in 11 per cent of the comparison group. The change in lung function was greatest during the first day back at work following an absence and diminished (primarily because of progressive waking reduction in lung function) during the working week.

These results suggest that a 20 per cent fall in FEV_1 across a working shift is neither a sensitive nor a specific test of occupational asthma.

The ideal test should demonstrate that exposure at work reproducibly provokes asthma (airways' narrowing or airways' hyperresponsiveness) of increasing severity during periods at work with improvement during absences from work. To date, the most acceptable (to patients) and reliable test for this purpose has been serial self-recorded measurements of peak flow. These are made on a sufficient number of occasions during the day and for a sufficient length of time to allow the demonstration of consistent changes in relation to periods at and away from work. This can only be done by the individual making and recording his or her own results and self-recorded peak flow measurements are now widely used in the UK for this purpose. Patients are lent a mini-peak flowmeter, instructed in its use and asked to record the best of three results (of which the best two should be within 20 l/min of each other) at 2-hourly intervals from waking to sleeping for a period of 1 month. It is essential for the period of recording to include periods of exposure to the suspected cause of asthma and desirable to include a period away from work longer than a 2-day weekend, preferably a 1- to 2-week holiday.

The diagnostic value of self-recorded peak flow measurements depends upon the reproducibility of the forced expiratory manoeuvres as well as the compliance and honesty of the individual tested. Concurrent drug treatment can seriously interfere with the results, particularly when treatment is increased during periods at work and reduced during absences from work. Where possible, treatment should not be altered during the period of recordings; at a minimum all treatment taken should be recorded.

The results can be conveniently summarized as the maximum, minimum and average value for each day. No generally agreed criteria for a positive or negative test have been established, but Burge et al. validated the results of peak flow measurements by comparison with the results of inhalation tests in colophony (Burge, O'Brien and Harries, 1979a) and isocyanate (Burge, O'Brien and Harries, 1979b) workers with suspected occupational asthma and found them to be both sensitive and specific for occupational asthma. Graneek (1988) examined the results of serial peak flow records in patients who had also undergone inhalation tests. They found that those whose peak flow results did not show asthma did not react on inhalation testing, unless they had not been exposed to the particular cause during the period of the measurements. Those with peak flow measurements which showed evidence of work-related asthma reacted on inhalation testing, provided the appropriate agent was used in the inhalation test. The major problem lay in the group whose peak flow records showed evidence of asthma without work relationship of whom half reacted in inhalation testing. The most usual reason for this false negative response was insufficient time away from work to allow recovery to occur.

An interesting case of a 'false-positive' peak flow record was reported by Venables et al. (1989b). A woman with asthma made her first peak flow recording of the non-working days 2 hours later than on working days, by when her daily 'morning dip' had recovered and her record therefore appeared to show weekend improvement.

Cartier et al. (1986) have reported a modified method of self-recorded peak flow measurements with fewer recordings made each day to improve compliance, supplemented by serial measurements of airways' responsiveness to increase 'objectivity'.

Immunological investigations

The application of immunological tests (both skin and serological tests) in the investigation of occupational asthma has increased due to:

1. Identification of the nature and source of the responsible proteins (and therefore more relevant extracts for testing), for example, identification of laboratory animal urine as a major source of allergenic protein and the recognition of added fungal amylase as an allergenic constituent of some flours.
2. Preparation of hapten–protein conjugates suitable for immunological testing, for example, human serum albumin in conjugates with acid anhydrides and reactive dyes.

3. Development of reliable methods for identification of specific immunoglobulins – particularly a specific IgE in serum.

Specific IgE antibody – most commonly identified by the radioallergosorbent test (RAST) – has been found in the sera of cases of occupational asthma caused by many allergens of animal, vegetable and microbial origin. These include the *B. subtilis* proteolytic enzyme, alcalase (Pepys et al., 1973), grain storage mites (Ingram et al., 1979), rat and mouse urine proteins (Newman Taylor, Longbottom and Pepys, 1977) and locusts (Tee et al., 1988). In addition, specific IgE antibody that binds to hapten–protein conjugates has been identified in the sera of cases of asthma caused by acid anhydrides, including phthalic (Maccia et al., 1976), trimellitic (Zeiss et al., 1977) and tetrachlorophthalic (Howe et al., 1983) anhydrides and to several reactive dyes (Luczynska and Topping, 1986).

The identification of specific IgE in serum is only diagnostically valuable if its presence is closely associated with cases of occupational asthma in exposed populations. It is important that the test is not positive in any but a small number of unexposed or exposed without asthma. This has been demonstrated for relatively few of the causes of occupational asthma, but has been shown for locusts (Tee et al., 1988) (Figure 21.1) and for one of the acid anhydrides (Howe et al., 1983) (Figure 21.2).

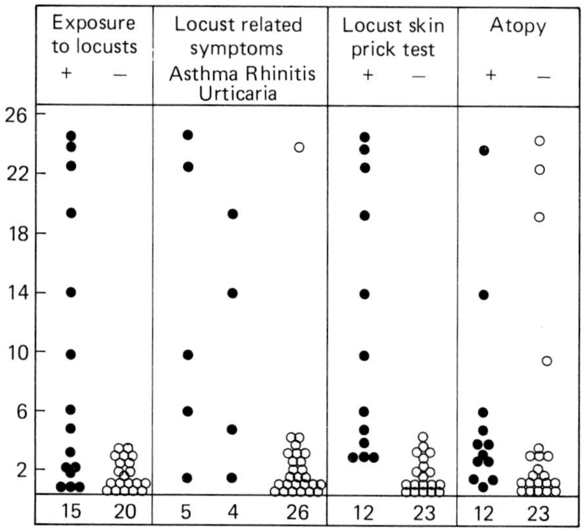

Figure 21.1 Specific IgE antibody expressed as RAST binding percentage to locust extract in 35 individuals working in a research centre in relation to locust exposure, allergic symptoms, immediate skin test reaction to locus extract and atopic status. Specific IgE is only present in those exposed to locusts who have a skin test response and, with only one exception, is limited to those with allergic symptoms. There is no apparent relationship with atopy

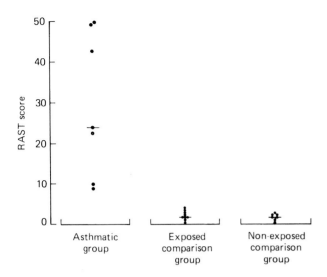

Figure 21.2 Specific IgE antibody expressed as RAST score in serum to tetrachlorophthalic anhydride – human serum albumin conjugate in group of seven patients from one factory with occupational asthma, eight comparably exposed individuals from the same factory and eight unexposed individuals. There is no overlap in this study group between the cases of asthma and their controls

For several of the low-molecular-weight causes of occupational asthma (including isocyanates and colophony), either no evidence of a specific immunological response has been found or, if found, no consistent relationship has been demonstrated between the immunological response and asthma. Several studies (for example, Butcher et al., 1980) have found specific IgE antibody to isocyanates in only 15 per cent of cases of isocyanate-induced asthma. It still remains unclear whether this reflects the difficulties of working with highly reactive chemicals in vitro and a failure to prepare the relevant in vivo conjugate or asthma caused by non-immunological mechanisms.

Inhalation testing

Inhalation testing with occupational materials is a potentially hazardous investigation which should only be undertaken, where indicated, in specialized centres by staff experienced in the techniques. It should be used to obtain specific information on which to base decisions about the future management of an individual patient. Physicians will vary in the extent to which they will require such information to come to a decision in any individual case. Nevertheless, four major indications for inhalation

testing for diagnostic purposes in occupational asthma can be identified:

1. Where the agent thought to be a cause of asthma has not previously or reliably been shown to induce asthma.
2. Where an individual with evidence of work-related asthma (for example, from history of serial peak expiratory flow records) is exposed at his or her place of work to more than one recognized cause of asthma and recognition of the specific agent is relevant to decisions about future employment (for example, in relation to a proposed relocation at work).
3. Where asthma is of such severity (for example, sufficient to have necessitated hospital inpatient or casualty care or to require treatment with oral corticosteroids) that it is considered unjustifiable for the individual to continue to be exposed to the possible cause of asthma in the uncontrolled conditions of work.
4. Where the diagnosis of occupational asthma remains in doubt after other appropriate investigations have been completed.

Inhalation testing whose sole purpose is in support of a legal claim would seem hard to justify.

The objective in an occupational inhalation test is to expose the individual to the putative cause of the asthma in circumstances that resemble as closely as possible the conditions of exposure at work. The tests should be made single blind. Wherever possible, concentrations of exposure should be based on knowledge of the exposures experienced at work and the physical conditions of exposure (for example, size of dust particles, temperatures to which materials are heated) should be similar to those at work.

The different methods used in inhalation testing depend primarily on the physical state of the test material. Soluble proteins (for example, laboratory animal urine and serum proteins) are inhaled as nebulized extracts in solution. Volatile organic liquids (for example, toluene diisocyanate) may be painted onto a flat surface in increasing concentrations or generated by passing a stream of warm air over the surface of the liquid. The atmospheric concentration generated can be measured with an appropriate monitor and the appropriate exposure dose estimated from previous experience. Exposure to dusts (for example, antibiotics and ammonium hexachloroplatinate) is achieved by tipping the test material, usually diluted in dried lactose, between two trays. Personal samplers can be worn to measure exposure concentrations during the test.

Changes in lung function provoked by inhalation tests are simply and reliably identified by regular measurements of forced expiratory volume in one second (FEV$_1$), forced vital capacity (FVC) and peak expiratory flow rate (PEFR) made before and for at least 24 hours after each test. Changes are compared with the results following an appropriate control exposure, each test being made on a separate day.

Different patterns of asthmatic response provoked by inhalation tests have been distinguished by their time of onset and duration. *Immediate* reactions develop within minutes of the test exposure and resolve spontaneously within 1 to 2 hours. These are not associated with an increase in non-specific airways' responsiveness. This pattern of asthmatic reaction may be provoked by specific sensitizing agents – both proteins and low-molecular-weight-chemicals – and by non-specific provocative stimuli such as exercise. *Non-immediate* or *late reactions* develop one or more hours after the test inhalation – most commonly after some 3 to 4 hours and can persist for 24 to 36 hours. 'Non-immediate' reactions are usually associated with an increase in non-specific airways' responsiveness which can be identified at 3 hours after the test inhalation prior to the onset of the late reaction (Durham et al., 1987) and may persist for several days after measurements of airways' calibre have returned to pre-test values.

A *dual reaction* is an immediate reaction followed by a late reaction. *Recurrent nocturnal* reactions are occasionally provoked by a single test exposure (Newman Taylor et al., 1979): asthmatic reactions occur at night with complete or partial recovery in the intervening days and are probably a manifestation of an induced increase in non-specific airways' responsiveness (see also Chapter 6, pages 140 and 143).

Ideally, to be confident that the results of inhalation testing show a cause-and-effect relationship, changes in lung function on test days and control days should be shown to be reproducible and, where appropriate, dose dependent. However, such strict criteria – particularly the second – usually cannot be fulfilled, often due to time constraints.

It is important to appreciate that inhalation tests, although often considered as the gold standard for the diagnosis of occupational asthma, can give 'false' negative results. This may result from testing with the wrong material, when exposure to more than one sensitizing agent is encountered in the place of work (particularly where there is no previously recognized cause of asthma). Another more interesting and potentially less remediable problem is the temporary loss of reactivity to the specific agent that can occur after a period of avoidance of exposure. That this is not a true loss of sensitivity is demonstrated by the recurrence of asthma that follows after a few days' return to exposure at work.

The methods of inhalation testing and the interpretation of provoked reactions have been reviewed by Newman Taylor and Davies (1981).

Summary of diagnostic investigations

In the majority of cases, the diagnosis of occupational asthma can be made, without the need for hospital inpatient investigation, from:

1. Exposure at work to an agent recognized to cause occupational asthma.
2. A history of work-related respiratory symptoms that have developed after an initial symptom-free period of exposure.
3. Reliable self-recorded serial peak flow records that show consistent deterioration during periods at work and improvement during absences from work.
4. Where applicable and relevant, evidence of a specific immunological response (usually immediate skin test response or specific IgE in serum) to the inhaled agent.

However, circumstances remain where the diagnosis cannot be made with sufficient confidence to justify recommendations about future employment, and inhalation testing with the putative cause is indicated.

Outcome of occupational asthma

Until relatively recently, it had been generally believed that asthma caused by an agent inhaled at work invariably resolved when exposure to the initiating cause was avoided. Several recent reports particularly, but not exclusively, of cases of asthma initiated by low-molecular-weight chemicals have found that asthma persists in a significant proportion (frequently in excess of 50 per cent) for several years after avoidance of exposure, and possibly indefinitely. Occupational causes of asthma may therefore initiate chronic symptomatic asthma.

Follow-up studies have been reported the most for cases of asthma caused by Western Red Cedar, isocyanates, colophony, acid anhydrides and in snow crab process workers.

Chan-Yeung, MacLean and Paggiaro (1987) reported their findings in 232 cases of occupational asthma caused by Western Red Cedar and diagnosed by inhalation testing seen, on average, 4 years from initial diagnosis. Of the 136 who had avoided exposure, 40 per cent had recovered and 60 per cent had continuing asthma. Those with persistent symptoms had continuing airways' hyperresponsiveness with histamine PC$_{20}$ measurements not significantly different from their value at diagnosis and similar to those with continuing exposure.

In a study of TDI-induced asthma, Paggiaro et al. (1984) found that after 2 years' avoidance of exposure, 8 of 12 cases had continuing respiratory symptoms and 7 of 11 had increased airways' responsiveness to inhaled bethanechol. In another study of 50 cases of isocyanate-induced asthma (all diagnosed by inhalation testing), Lozewicz et al. (1987) found that 82 per cent had continuing respiratory symptoms four or more years after avoidance of exposure. Airways' responsiveness was increased in 14 of the 21 tested at follow-up. Paggiaro et al. (1990) have reported the findings in bronchial biopsies and at bronchoalveolar lavage (BAL) in 10 patients suffering from TDI-induced asthma with persistent symptoms 4 to 40 months after avoidance of exposure to TDI. Bronchial biopsy showed eosinophil, neutrophil and lymphocyte infiltration of the submucosa with epithelial damage and thickening of basement membranes – pathological changes characteristic of chronic bronchial asthma. Eosinophil numbers in BAL were increased in four of five with persistent airways' hyperresponsiveness, but in only one of five in whom airways' hyperresponsiveness had improved.

Burge (1982b) followed up 28 electronics workers with asthma caused by colophony 1 to 4 years from diagnosis by inhalation testing. Of the 20 who had left work, 18 continued to have respiratory symptoms. Airways' responsiveness to inhaled histamine, measured at diagnosis and follow-up, had returned to normal in half of those who had left work, but in only one of eight who had been relocated and remained at work. In another follow-up study of electronics workers, Venables et al. (1987) reported their findings in seven women whose asthma had been caused by tetrachlorophthalic anhydride (TCPA) seen 4½ years after avoidance of exposure. One had died; the remaining six reported improvement in their symptoms, but five continued to need treatment and to be awakened on occasions by respiratory symptoms. Airways' responsiveness to inhaled histamine was measurable in the five tested. Specific IgE to TCPA–HSA (HSA = human serum albumin) was measured in serial blood samples taken during the 4-year period and it was found to decline exponentially with a half-life of 1 year. The consistent and parallel falls in specific IgE in these patients make it very improbable that their continuing asthma could be attributed to continuing, albeit indirect or unrecognized, exposure to TCPA. Malo et al. (1988) studied 31 snow crab workers with occupational asthma, diagnosed by inhalation tests, after 5 years from their last exposure. All denied exposure to crab meat by inhalation or ingestion. Respiratory symptoms persisted in all 31, of whom 26 had a measurable metacholine PC_{20}. Although FEV_1, FEV_1/FVC and PC_{20} improved during the initial period of avoidance of exposure, FEV_1/FVC plateaued by 1 year and PC_{20} by 2 years.

Byssinosis

C.A.C. Pickering

The term 'byssinosis' ($\beta\acute{v}\sigma\sigma\sigma\zeta$ = flax and the linen made from it) introduced by Proust in 1877 and first employed in the UK by Oliver (1902), embraces a gradation of respiratory symptoms due to the exposure to the dust of cotton, flax, soft hemp and, to a limited degree, sisal which range from acute dyspnoea with cough and reversible breathlessness and chest tightness on one or more days of a working week to (it is believed) permanent respiratory disability due to irreversible airflow obstruction.

Although cotton and flax have been used in the manufacture of textiles since times of antiquity, byssinosis does not seem to have been recognized or, possibly, to have existed until the introduction of mechanized processes in the early nineteenth century (Patissier, 1822). In 1831, Kay described a respiratory disease, cotton spinners' phthisis, characterized by a work-related cough associated with a sensation of uneasiness under the sternum. The first clear description of the symptom pattern now usually associated with byssinosis was given by Mareska and Heyman in 1845:

> All the workers have told us that the dust bothered them much less on the last days of the week than on the Monday and Tuesday. The masters find the cause of this increased sensitivity to be in the excesses of the Sunday, but the workers never fail to attribute it to the interruption of work which they say makes them lose, in part, their habituation to the dust.

To this description would now be added an increased severity of symptoms on the first day at work after a period of absence longer than a weekend.

Byssinosis was generally overlooked in the UK until surveys of the cotton industry were started about 30 years ago. The disorder was then thought to be mostly confined to Lancashire cotton workers (Schilling, 1956) and flax workers in Northern Ireland (Smiley, 1951) where it is commonly known as 'poucey chest' ('poucey' is a dialect word meaning dirty or nasty). But it was subsequently reported to occur in Scotland (Smith et al., 1962), the Netherlands, Germany, Sweden, the USA, Egypt, Greece, India and Taiwan (Bouhuys et al., 1967a), Spain (Bouhuys et al., 1976b), Belgium (Tuypens, 1961), Australia (Gandevia and Milne, 1965a), Israel (Chwat and Mordish, 1963), Tanzania (Mustafa et al., 1978), Hong Kong (Morgan and Ong, 1981), China (Lu et al., 1987) and The Cameroons (Takam and Nemery, 1988).

At this point it is important to note that other symptoms have been described and may still occur following exposure to cotton, flax or hemp because they are distinct from byssinosis. They are referred to respectively as mill fever, weavers' cough and mattress makers' fever.

Mill fever (factory fever)

This is characterized by slight fever, cough, malaise, rigors and rhinitis which occur in some workers on *first contact* with cotton, flax, soft hemp or kapok dust. The symptoms, which are mild, usually last a few hours or, sometimes, days but cease as exposure continues (Greenhow, 1860; Arlidge, 1892; Gill, 1947; Uragoda, 1977). Its prevalence among new workers is not accurately known but assessments varying from 10 to 80 per cent have been made (Doig, 1949; Harris et al., 1972; Uragoda, 1977). The cause is uncertain but may be due to endotoxins of contaminating Gram-negative bacteria in the vegetable dusts and in mill air (Rylander and Lundholm, 1978) (see page 739).

Whether or not mill fever predisposes to the subsequent development of byssinosis is not known but, according to Gill (1947), byssinosis does not occur in the absence of a preceding history of mill fever.

Weavers' cough

This was an acute respiratory illness identical with late asthma, but accompanied by fever and malaise, in workers machining cotton yarns treated with flour paste or tamarind seed extract and was believed to be due to contaminating fungi (Collis,

1915). However, tamarind extract appears to have been responsible in some of these cases. Acclimatization does not occur and both new and old workers are equally affected. The asthma may last for months (Vigliani, Parmeggiani and Sassi, 1954).

Mattress makers' fever

Acute symptoms occurred from 1 to 6 hours after starting work and consisted of fever, rigors, malaise, nausea and vomiting but none of the features of asthma. The cause was attributed to contamination of cotton by the Gram-negative bacillus *Aerobacter cloacae*, and the disease may well have been a form of extrinsic allergic alveolitis (Neal, Schneiter and Caminita, 1942).

Sources of exposure

Cotton (*Gossypium* spp.)

The chief sources of dust production occur: in the ginnery where seeds are removed from the cotton after picking in a special machine, the 'gin'; in the 'mixing room' during opening of bales of cotton; in the 'blow room' where the cotton is beaten and blown to eliminate dust and short fibres; and in the 'cardroom' where carding engines comb the fibres and remove dirt and defective material. The fibres are then gathered and twisted into fine strands for spinning. Other dusty operations are 'stripping', which consists of removing dust and cotton fibre adherent to the wire teeth of the carding engine, and 'grinding' (sharpening) the teeth.

Air-borne dust consists of broken cotton fibres, bracts (thin, brittle leaves surrounding the stem of the cotton boll which cannot be separated from the cotton), pericarps, bacteria, fungi and minerals. Particles vary from 3.8 cm (1½ inches) in length to less than 2 μm diameter. The larger air-borne particles visible to the naked eye consist mainly of broken cotton fibres up to 2.5 cm in length – which are apparently innocuous – and fragments of plant debris too large to enter the lungs which are known as *fly*. 'Coarse' grade cotton produces more dust than the 'fine' grade when the fibres are long. Although, in general, there has been less dust in spinning than in carding rooms, there may be a risk of increased concentrations in spinning and winding rooms equipped with high-speed machines.

Flax (*Linum usitatissimum*)

Although the industry has contracted owing to substitution of synthetic fibres, flax is still used (often with hemp) to manufacture linen (an Old English word for flax) and yarn for rope, twine, thread, hosepipes, tarpaulins, fishing nets and clothing. In Britain this industry is confined to Northern Ireland and Scotland.

Until the early 1960s flax fibre was separated from the woody parts of the plant (that is, 'retting') by a putrefative process but this has subsequently been replaced by a chemical method.

Bales of flax are first opened and small bundles separated out by hand, mixed, and then passed into a machine which combs out and straightens the fibres and eliminates dirt ('hackling'). Tow produced during 'hackling' or received in bales is passed through a carding machine to be opened and agitated. All these processes are dusty but carding particularly so.

Fibres are next further straightened on 'drawing frames' and then formed into slivers of uniform thickness, twisted and wound on to bobbins. Much fine dust is produced. The yarn is then spun dry, half-dry or wet; only dry spinning gives off substantial amounts of dust. Winding, twisting and cabling of rope causes significantly smaller dust concentration than opening, hackling, carding and spinning (Smith et al., 1969).

Hemp

(Soft hemp, *Cannabis sativa*; also known as English or Irish hemp; hard hemp or Manilla hemp, *Musa textiles*; Mauritius hemp, *Furcraea gigantea*)

It appears that only soft hemp, which is a stem fibre unlike the others which are leaf fibres, is associated with the development of byssinosis. It is used in the manufacture of rope and yarn.

After the hemp plant has been 'retted' it is dried, beaten (batted) to removed wood particles, 'hackled' and baled (Bouhuys et al., 1967b). Until recently this was a flourishing industry in Calosa de Segura in Spain, but is now in rapid decline due to the increased use of synthetic fibres.

Batting and hackling are very dusty activities, but dust concentration during cabling, twisting and polishing rope are low (Smith et al., 1969).

Jute

(Fibre from bark of *Corchorus capsularis* and *C. oliterius*)

This is grown mainly in India and Pakistan and is used in the manufacture of carpets, felt, wadding and, in combination with flax, in various types of cloth. Retted jute is received by the mill in bales, the opening of which is dusty; mixing grades of fibres, carding and drawing fibre are also dusty processes.

Sisal

(Fibre from the leaves of *Agave sisalana*)

Sisal is employed chiefly in rope manufacture. The leaves are decorticated and brushed – a very dusty process – and the resulting fibre baled. Opening the bales and carding fibre also produce much dust.

Kapok

(A cotton-like fibre from the fruits of the tropical tree, *Ceiba pentandra*)

The tree grows in the Philippines, Indonesia, Thailand, India, Sri Lanka and East and West Africa. Its pods are husked by hand and then ginned manually or mechanically. Machinery, collecting and bagging are dusty processes (Uragoda, 1977).

Coir

(This is a fibre obtained from husks of the coconut, *Cocos nucifera*)

It is used in the manufacture of brushes, rope, twine, nets, sacks and matting. Sri Lanka is the chief producer and it is imported by many countries but especially the United Kingdom, Eire, Germany and Japan. The husks are retted in brackish water, milled and then mechanically teased, twisted and hackled according to the purpose for which it is required (Uragoda, 1975).

Rayon

(Generic term for synthetic fibre produced from cellulose)

No untoward effects have been observed among workers in rayon spinning mills (Tiller and Schilling, 1958; Berry et al., 1973).

Natural history of byssinosis

As stated earlier byssinosis is a particular form of extrinsic asthma caused in some exposed workers by cotton, flax, hemp or, to a lesser extent, sisal dust with resultant breathlessness, tightness or oppression in the chest and objective evidence of airways' obstruction over progressively longer periods of the working week and which may be prevented or reduced by certain drugs (see page 740). Thirty years ago, Gill (1947) stated that established byssinosis is characterized by 'asthma-like nocturnal attacks'. Byssinotic symptoms do not apparently result from exposure to coir, kapok and jute (Uragoda, 1975, 1977; Žuškin, Valić and Bouhuys, 1976).

In most cases byssinosis does not develop until there has been 10 or more years' exposure to cotton flax or hemp and it is unusual under 5 years. There is some evidence that atopic status may influence the development of respiratory disease in cotton workers (page 734). However, asthmatic individuals who frequently react severely and immediately to cotton dust and others who develop symptoms shortly after starting work almost certainly leave the industry at an early stage (Harris et al., 1972).

The stages of byssinosis are sufficiently well defined to allow subdivision on clinical grounds and the scheme of clinical grades suggested by Schilling et al. (1963) has been widely used.

Clinical grades

For clarity these are prefixed by 'C' to distinguish them from the functional ('F') grades referred to in the next section.

Grade C½   Occasional chest tightness of the chest on the first day of the working week.

Grade C1   Tightness of the chest or difficulty in breathing or both on each first day only of the working week.

Grade C2   Tightness of the chest or difficulty in breathing or both on the first day and other days of the working week.

Grade C3   Grade C2 symptoms accompanied by evidence of permanent respiratory disability from reduced ventilatory capacity.

The early symptoms cease completely when the worker is removed from exposure to the relevant vegetable fibre. Progression to more severe symptoms appears to be very variable. Some workers do not seem to progress beyond the early stages and never develop permanent respiratory disability, whereas others reach this stage within a few years. These differences may be influenced by smoking habits. Symptomatology is discussed further on page 741.

Functional grades

Theroretically, the immediate, or acute, effect of exposure to dust can be determined by measuring FEV$_1$ before and at the end of a working shift on the first working day after a period (usually a weekend) away from work. The difference between these values is the basis of the grading system suggested by Bouhuys, Gilson and Schilling (1970). An FEV$_1$ value below 80 per cent of predicted normal is taken as abnormal. When an abnormal value is recorded the test should be repeated after administration of a bronchodilator. It is, of course, necessary that the prediction data are valid for the populations examined. The grades are as follows:

Grade F0   No demonstrable acute effect of the dust on ventilatory capacity; no evidence of chronic ventilatory impairment.

Grade F½   Slight acute effect of dust on ventilatory capacity; no evidence of chronic ventilatory impairment.

Grade F1   Moderate acute reduction of ventilatory impairment.

Grade F2   Evidence of slight-to-moderate irreversible impairment of ventilatory capacity.

Grade 3   Evidence of moderate-to-severe irreversible impairment of ventilatory capacity.

These clinical and functional grading systems have limitations. The clinical grades do not take into account the irritant effects of dust exposure or the acute lung function changes which may occur in the absence of symptoms. The functional grading system relies on usually very small absolute changes in FEV$_1$ which are subject to error that may be both significant and misleading. These important shortcomings have led to a new proposed system of classification combining both clinical and function grades (WHO, 1983).

Classification	*Symptoms*
Grade 0	No symptoms
Byssinosis	
Grade B1	Chest tightness and/or shortness of breath on most of first days back at work
Grade B2	Chest tightness and/or shortness of breath on the first and other days of the working week
Respiratory tract irritation (RTI)	
Grade RTI1	Cough associated with dust exposure
Grade RTI2	Persistent phlegm (that is, on most days during 3 months of the year) initiated or exacerbated by dust exposure
Grade RTI3	Persistent phlegm initiated or made worse by dust exposure either with exacerbations of chest illness or persisting for 2 years or more
Lung function	
1. Acute changes:	
No effect	A consistent* decline in FEV$_1$ of less than 5 per cent or an increase in FEV$_1$ during the working shift

Mild effect	A consistent* decline of between 5 and 10 per cent in FEV_1 during the working shift
Moderate effect	A consistent* decline of between 10 and 20 per cent in FEV_1 during the working shift
Severe effect	A decline of 20 per cent or more in FEV_1 during the working shift

2. Chronic changes:

No effect	FEV_1† – per cent of predicted values‡
Mild-to-moderate effect	FEV_1† – 60 to 79 per cent of predicted values‡
Severe effect	FEV_1† less than 60 per cent of predicted values‡

*A decline occurring in at least three consecutive tests made after an absence from dust exposure of 2 days or more.
†Predicted values should be based on data obtained from local populations or similar ethnic and social class groups.
‡By a pre-shift test after an absence from dust exposure of 2 days or more.

This new classification system has now been applied in a recent epidemiological study (Parikh et al., 1986).

In all epidemiological studies data for each worker must include his or her age, the nature and duration of his or her work, smoking habits and the presence of other respiratory disease. It should be pointed out, however, that all functional grading systems are, on the whole, limited to specially controlled investigations. There are a number of reasons for this. For the purposes of routine medical examination in the clinic and factory, there are a number of factors influencing lung function measurement, including the level of dust exposure, variation in dust exposure, variation in dust exposure, recent cigarette smoking and concurrent respiratory infections. The measurements must be made using standardized techniques and appropriately calibrated instruments (American Thoracic Society, 1979).

A similar gradation of symptoms and impairment of ventilatory capacity also occurs among flax and soft hemp workers (Mair et al., 1960; Elwood et al., 1965) and in sisal workers (Mustafa et al., 1978; Thomas, Elwood and Elwood, 1988). In sisal workers, the effects may be absent or mild and transient (Velvart, 1971, 1972).

Incidence and prevalence

Byssinosis occurs throughout the world where cotton, flax and soft hemp fibres are processed, but cotton dust is most commonly responsible. Jute does

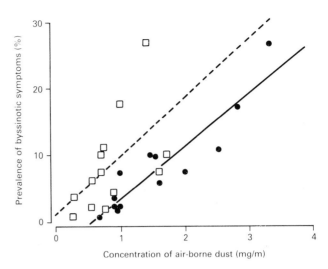

Figure 21.3 The concentration of air-borne dust-less 'fly' (C_{TWA}) measured in the personal breathing zone (□) and in the work zone (●) versus the prevalence of byssinotic symptoms (PBS) in workrooms grouped according to the work process (opening and blowing, carding, spinning, and winding and beaming), and the quality of the fibre spun (synthetic + cotton, fine-to-medium cotton, medium-to-coarse cotton, and waste synthetic + waste cotton). ----- PBS = 0.85 + (8.9 × C_{TWA}); —— PBS = –4.5 + (7.9 × C_{TWA}). (Reproduced, with the permission of the British Occupational Hygiene Society, from Cinkota, 1988b)

not cause the symptoms associated with byssinosis although mild changes in ventilatory function have been described in workers milling the fibre (Gandevia and Milne, 1965b; Valić and Žuškin, 1971).

The prevalence of disease in cotton workers varies according to the duration of employment in the industry, the quantity and quality of air-borne dust in the workroom, and the smoking habit of the individual (Cinkotai et al., 1988a). Plant debris and other foreign matter (that is, 'cotton trash') associated with cotton fibre appear to be the source of the agent or agents that cause byssinosis and 'medium' to 'coarse' dust from this source may be encountered in the separation of cotton from lint (the ginning process), opening of the stripping and grinding of carding machines. The prevalence of all grades of byssinosis is proportional to the total concentration of dust of 'medium' and 'coarse' cotton less 'fly' (that is, coarse waste cotton), and to duration of exposure (Žuškin and Valić, 1972). The correlation of the prevalence of byssinosis and the concentration of air-borne dust is significantly better when dust concentrations are measured in the personal breathing zone compared to area dust sampling (Figure 21.3) (Cinkotai et al., 1988a).

In countries where dust exposure levels have been reduced, there has been a progressive fall in the prevalence of byssinosis. In England between 1963 and 1966, the total prevalence of byssinosis grades C½ and C2 was 26.9 per cent and was higher in 'coarse' rather than in 'medium' cotton mills (Molyneux and Tombleson, 1970). In the mid-1970s, the prevalence had fallen to 17.4 per cent (Cinkotai and Whitaker, 1978) and by the mid-1980s to 3.9 per cent (Cinkotai et al., 1988a).

There is considerable variation in the reported prevalence of byssinosis around the world. In the Sudan, a prevalence of 37 per cent has been reported in a coarse spinning mill (Elkarim and Onsa, 1987), in the USA a prevalence of 5.7 per cent (Jones et al., 1979), in The Cameroons a prevalence of 18 per cent (Takam and Nemery, 1988), in China a prevalence of 5.6 per cent (Lu et al., 1987) and in Australia a prevalence of 1.1 per cent (Gun et al., 1983). These variations are influenced by dissimilar working conditions, and dust composition and concentration.

Byssinosis is associated with dust concentration and years of exposure. The highest prevalence occurs among cardroom workers and the lowest among ring spinners (Berry, Molyneux and Tombleson, 1974; Cinkotai et al., 1988a). Expressing dust exposure in terms of a time-weighted dust measurement (that is, dust concentration = length of exposure or mg years/m³) it has been reckoned that approximately 10 per cent of workers exposed to 0.5 mg/m³ cotton dust for 40 years will have byssinosis (Fox et al., 1973). A recent study (Cinkotai et al., 1988b), using current dust exposure levels measured in the personal breathing zone, suggests that at an exposure level of 1 to 2 mg/m³, less than 5 per cent of cotton spinners contract byssinosis and at 0.7 mg/m³ less than 1 per cent.

The prevalence of byssinosis is higher in men than in women. This would appear to be due to factors other than a true sex difference (Cinkotai et al., 1988a). Among spinners in England and Sweden, prevalence has been reported to be 2.7 per cent and 17 per cent respectively (Haglind, Lundholm and Rylander, 1981; Cinkotai et al., 1988a). In cotton seed (non-textile) mills in which levels of respiratory and total dust were high, prevalence has been found to be low, although there was a mean decline in ventilatory function over a working shift, but not on Fridays (Jones et al., 1977).

In flax workers, byssinosis was apparently equally prevalent in all parts of the mill and lower grade symptoms were common in those over 35 years of age (Mair et al., 1960; Carey et al., 1965). A prevalence of 22.9 per cent has been reported in Egyptian flax workers (Noweir, Amine and Osman, 1975), 11 per cent in flax workers in Russia (Zaritskala, 1979) and 1.7 per cent in flax workers in Poland (Szulc, 1971). The method of flax processing influences the

prevalence of byssinosis. The introduction of chemical in place of biological retting appears to eliminate the disease (Bouhuys et al., 1963).

Effects of smoking

Smokers have a greater incidence of byssinosis and loss of ventilatory function at all levels of dust exposure and also show a greater tendency to develop byssinosis with increasing dust exposure than non-smokers. Among cotton workers, smokers have significantly more byssinosis of each grade than non-smokers after allowing for dust concentration and length of exposure (Elwood et al., 1965; Bouhuys et al., 1967b; Fox et al., 1973; Merchant et al., 1973a; Berry, Molyneux and Tombleson, 1974). A similar effect has been observed in flax and Tanzanian sisal workers (Smith et al., 1962; Carey et al., 1965; Noweir Amine and Osman, 1975; Mustafa et al., 1978). However, in two more recent studies in Egypt (Noweir et al., 1984) and in Sweden (Haglind, Lundholm and Rylander, 1981) no association was observed between current smoking and byssinosis, although in the latter study there was a significant excess of byssinosis among ex-smokers. These studies suggest that smoking habits are becoming less important in relationship to the development of byssinosis. Fox et al. (1973) and Berry, Molyneux and Tombleson (1974) found that the prevalence of 'chronic bronchitis' (MRC Definition, see Chapter 9) is unrelated to dust concentrations, but Merchant et al. (1972) and Cinkotai et al. (1988a) concluded that byssinosis and 'chronic bronchitis' (hypersecretion of mucus) are both influenced by cotton and dust exposure and cigarette smoking. Evidence of bronchitis is not, however, always present (Imbus and Suh, 1973). In Australian cotton mill workers, the prevalence of productive cough and of impairment of respiratory function was not found to be specifically attributable to exposure to cotton dust and was less that that observed in current cigarette smokers (Field and Owen, 1979).

Effects of atopic status

Cotton dust is frequently contaminated by Gram-negative bacteria, endotoxin and a variety of different fungi. It may be anticipated that atopic cotton workers would develop airways' responses of both a specific (allergic) and non-specific nature as a consequence of this type of dust exposure. In a study in cotton workers of the effect of atopy on cross-shift ventilatory decline on a Monday, Jones et al. (1980) demonstrated, in one of the three exposure groups studied, a significant association between mean declines in FEV_1 and FEF_{25-75} across the workshift and atopic status. In a study of healthy, non-asthmatic adults (previously unexposed to cotton) (Sepulveda et al., 1984) exposed to cotton dust in an artificial cardroom, the mean decline in FEV_1 was significantly greater in atopic compared to non-atopic subjects. This response is probably determined by the presence of increased airways' reactivity which is frequently present in atopic individuals. Because this airways' response occurs on first exposure to cotton dust, it may lead to this group of susceptible workers leaving the cotton industry early. In two studies in which the atopic status of cotton workers and of individuals was examined, the prevalence of atopy was found to be significantly lower than that found in the general population, suggesting that atopic subjects select themselves out of the industry prematurely to prevent recurrent symptoms (Jones et al., 1980; Honeybourne, Finnegan and Pickering, 1985).

There is evidence of an early high labour turnover in Finnish cotton-spinning mills (Koskela et al., 1990), where one in ten employees left within 2 weeks and one in four within 3 weeks of taking up employment.

Pathology

No specific abnormalities have been identified. Grey–black, macular pigmentation may be present in the lungs but there is no fibrosis. In cotton workers, cotton fibres, which are highly birefringent when viewed by polarized light, are occasionally seen. Round or oval bodies up to 10 μm diameter with a central black core surrounded by a yellowish coating which stains positively for iron may also be present (so-called 'byssinosis bodies'), but they have no diagnostic significance (Gough, 1959).

A post-mortem study (without control cases) of 43 British cotton workers diagnosed as having byssinosis during life revealed the following: no significant emphysema in 27 (63 per cent) but a varying amount of centriacinar emphysema in 10 (23 per cent) and panacinar type in 6 (14 per cent) (Edwards et al., 1975). Smoking habits were known in all but 9 of the 43 cases: 'significant' emphysema was present in 4 of 17 life-long non-smokers, and in 9 of 17 smokers (Rooke, 1981). Microscopy showed occasional minimal fibrosis but no granulomas or any other evidence of extrinsic allergic alveolitis, and the pulmonary blood vessels were unremarkable. But mucous gland hyperplasia and hypertrophy of smooth muscle (expressed as the airways' wall formed by muscle) were observed in lobar but not in segmental bronchi: findings that are consistent with asthma. Takizawa and Thurlbeck (1971)

found that the amount of bronchial smooth muscle in chronic bronchitic subjects with no history of wheezing was the same as that in non-bronchitic subjects, but that in chronic bronchitic subjects who had suffered bouts of wheezing the muscle was increased in amounts comparable to those seen in known asthmatic subjects. However, it is likely that varying degrees of muscle hyperplasia will be present in chronic bronchitic subjects according to the varying intensities of bronchospasm these patients may have; and, before valid specific inferences can be drawn from the presence of muscle hyperplasia, a frequency distribution curve of muscle proportions in bronchi obtained from random autopsies and from patients with chronic bronchitis is required (Thurlbeck, 1976). To these could be added patients with byssinosis but, unfortunately, the accuracy of this diagnosis in individual subjects during life is by no means certain depending, as it so often does, on subjective criteria.

A more recent retrospective study of the lungs of 49 cotton textile workers in the USA with smoking habits and appropriate control cases revealed a significant association between cotton dust exposure and mucous gland hyperplasia and goblet cell metaplasia, but none with emphysema; also there was no significant or consistent difference in pigmentation between cotton and non-cotton workers. It was concluded that irreversible airflow obstruction and morphological emphysema in textile workers are most probably related to smoking and not to the occupational exposure (Pratt, Vollmer and Miller, 1980).

The quantitative and qualitative features of mast cells in the tracheobronchial tree do not seem to be known, but in other asthmatic patients their numbers are apparently decreased and the prevalence of degranulated and disrupted cells increased (Salvator, 1961).

In view of an early report of an excess of systemic hypertension in heavily exposed cotton operatives (Schilling, Goodman and O'Sullivan, 1952), it is of interest that left ventricular weights in the subjects described by Edwards et al. (1975) did not substantiate this.

Rüttner, Spycher and Engeler (1968) described widespread pulmonary fibrosis in a cotton mill worker but this appears to have been the end-result of sarcoidosis, and the incidental finding of cotton fibre by electron microscopy and of 'byssinosis bodies' does not, in fact, imply a causal relationship.

Pathogenesis

The potential of vegetable textile fibres to produce byssinosis ranges from potent to negligible in this order: cotton, flax, soft hemp and sisal. There is

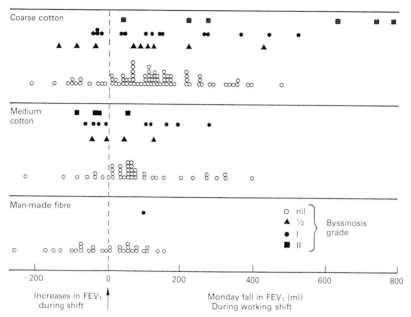

Figure 21.4 This figure shows the effect the type of mill dust has in determining the difference in Monday fall in FEV_1 among workers without byssinosis, the negligible mean fall in FEV_1 in synthetic fibre mills and that the Monday fall of FEV_1 was related to symptoms of byssinosis only in the coarse cotton mills. The relationship between Monday fall in FEV_1 and byssinosis is weak. (Reproduced, with permission, from Berry et al., 1973)

controversy in regard to the effect of sisal which, in general, appears to be minimal. Slight reduction in ventilatory capacity in sisal rope workers has been attributed to lubricant additives used as fibre softeners and not to sisal dust (Baker et al., 1979).

Cotton and other vegetable dusts have been conveniently classified by Gilson et al. (1962) into size grades: 'coarse' – greater than 2 mm; 'medium' – 2 mm down to 7 μm; and 'respirable' – less than 7 μm.

Cotton plant parts consist of bract, leaf, vein material, petiole, capsule, cotyledon and pericarp (which includes exocarp, mesocarp and endocarp). The potential for cotton trash to produce fine particulate material is determined by the friability of its components. Bract – the leaf-like structure that enfolds the cotton boll – and wood fragments are the most friable and thus the most abundant 'respirable' (less than 10 μm) components of raw cotton; lint and seed coat are the least friable (Morey, 1979). However, cotton dust and trash contain bacteria, fungi, fragments of other plants (such as weeds and grasses) and inorganic material from the soil. The range of organic chemical contents is, therefore, enormous; it includes carbohydrates, proteins, lipids, amines, lignins, tannins, phenolic pigments, terpenes, terpinoid alcohols, carbonyl compounds and epoxides. However, bract is believed to contain the active agent, or agents, that cause the airways' obstruction of byssinosis,

although the bioactivity of bark and stem dusts that account for 25 per cent of the 'respirable' dust is not known (Wakelyn et al., 1976; Morey, 1979).

The bioactivity of cotton is greatly reduced by washing and steaming before processing (Merchant et al., 1973b, 1974; Imbus and Suh, 1974); the compounds in cotton dust causing byssinosis are, therefore, likely to be water soluble. It is interesting to note that, in the early days of the cotton industry in Lancashire, cotton was washed and dried before being carded and carding engines were designed for washed cotton (Aitken, 1795; Chapman, 1904).

The ventilatory capacity of workers with symptoms of byssinosis falls when they are exposed to cotton dust during a working day, but is also falls – although to a lesser degree – under similar conditions in workers who do not have byssinosis (Figure 21.4) (Berry et al., 1973). However, this study does not document the presence or absence of symptoms in the non-byssinotic worker. In a recent study of cotton workers, airways' reactivity was found to be increased in both symptomatic non-byssinotic and byssinotic workers when compared to asymptomatic cotton workers matched for work area and dust exposure (Fishwick et al., 1992). The factor determining the presence and degree of shift changes in lung function may be the degree of airways' reactivity that is present. It was originally believed that byssinosis is closely related to overall dustiness

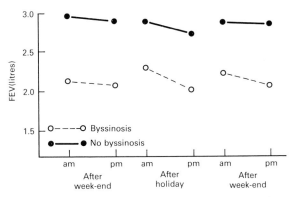

Figure 21.5 Change in $FEV_{0.75}$ on Mondays in male cardroom workers before the holiday, immediately after the holiday and 1 week later. (Reproduced with permission of the President from the International Conference on Respiratory Diseases in Textile workers, Alicante, 1968)

(Roach and Schilling, 1960). Later a good correlation between byssinosis and the measurement of total dust-less fly was demonstrated (Fox et al., 1973). The most recent study, relating the prevalence of byssinotic symptoms to current air-borne dust levels, continues to show a good correlation between dust level and byssinotic symptoms (Cinkotai et al., 1988b). The correlation was significantly better for personal breathing-zone measurements compared to area dust measurements. The 'respirable' and 'medium' components of the total dust have also been shown to correlate significantly with the prevalence of respiratory symptoms (Molyneux and Berry, 1971).

An interesting feature of the production of the disorder is revealed by an observation in cotton workers. Those who have been away from dust exposure for longer than a weekend (that is, for 2 weeks) show a significantly higher first FEV_1 reading and a significantly lower final FEV_1 reading than is usual on the day of return to work, whereas in workers without byssinosis, the first reading is barely different from usual, although the final reading is significantly lower (McKerrow and Molyneux, 1971) (Figure 21.5).

The mechanism by which cotton and other vegetable fibre dusts cause narrowing of airways is not understood. A number of hypotheses have been suggested, the most important of which are as follows:

1. Non-immunological local release of histamine in the lungs.
2. An antigen–antibody reaction.
3. Bacterial endotoxins.
4. Fungal enzymes.
5. Non-specific pharmacological mediator release.

Local histamine release

Symptoms identical to the 'Monday feeling' may occur with similar changes in lung function in healthy volunteers by inhalation challenge in the laboratory with cotton dusts or aerosols of aqueous cotton extracts. The response begins after 10 to 15 minutes and lasts some hours, although repeat challenge after 24 hours has no effect (McKerrow and Molyneux, 1971; Bouhuys, 1976). Changes in function include decreased FEV_1 and vital capacity (VC), increased airways' resistance, impaired maximum expiratory flow–volume curves, without any fall of gas transfer (see page 742). Washed cotton dust, with similar physical properties, produces neither symptoms nor physiological changes on inhalation, suggesting that washing removes the causal agent (McDermott, Skidmore and Edwards, 1971). It was postulated that the agent might be a histamine-liberating substance in the cotton dust because histamine is a well-known powerful bronchoconstrictor and, although the amount of histamine in cotton is minute, extracts of cotton, flax and hemp dusts have been shown to release histamine from human lung tissue in vitro (Bouhuys, Lindell and Lundin, 1960; Nicholls, Nicholls and Bouhuys, 1966; Hitchcock, Piscitelli and Bouhuys, 1973). Histamine-releasing activity of various extracts is measured by adding them to guinea-pig, rat, pig or human lung tissue or to smooth muscle preparations or porcine platelets (Ainsworth, Newman and Harley, 1979). However, until the agent that causes byssinosis is established, these techniques are of limited value for the assessment of the byssinosis-producing potential of cotton and other vegetable dusts (Nicholls and Skidmore, 1975).

Aqueous extracts of Western Red Cedar wood, fungal spores and dimethylhydantoin formaldehyde resin also cause direct histamine release in vitro (Evans and Nicholls, 1974; Battigelli et al., 1976; Nicholls, 1976).

Just as the bronchoconstrictor effect of histamine aerosol inhaled by human volunteers is potentiated by the β-adrenergic receptor blocking agent, propranolol, and prevented by atropine. The effect of challenge inhalations of hemp dust is similarly potentiated and inhibited by these drugs (Bouhuys, 1971).

Blood histamine levels have been shown to be elevated in both flax and cotton workers. This elevation occurs within 2 hours of starting work and is seen in all workers (Norweir, Abdel-Kader and Omran, 1984). Histamine levels had fallen to baseline measurements by the second morning in all workers except those with grade 2 byssinotic symptoms.

The histamine metabolite – 1-methyl-4-imidazole acetic acid – is also found to be elevated in the 24-hour urinary specimens of control subjects following

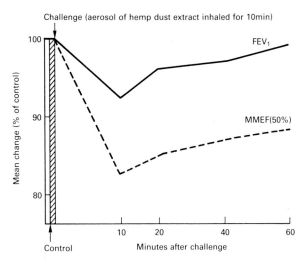

Figure 21.6 Mean acute changes in FEV$_1$ and MMEF (50 per cent) following challenge with hemp dust extract in healthy volunteers. (Adapted, with permission, from Zuskin et al., 1975)

inhalation of cotton dust, but there is no increase after the inhalation of washed cotton.

These various observations have led to the suggestion that acute changes of lung function provoked in normal people might be due to histamine release from the lungs, and the unusually low final FEV$_1$ values on the first day back at work after a holiday in workers without byssinosis are consistent with the possibility of an increase in histamine reserves during the holiday (McKerrow and Molyneux, 1971). The successive decrease in the asthmatic response during the working week has been attributed to tachyphylaxis due to depletion of endogenous histamine (Nicholls, Nicholls and Bouhuys, 1966). A variety of the many chemical compounds in cotton and hemp dust has been suggested as the cause of byssinosis by stimulating the release of histamine, but none has yet been positively identified as the responsible agent (Textile Research Institute, 1978).

The weaknesses in this hypothesis are that direct histamine release alone does not satisfactorily explain the time relationships of byssinosis, and also the immediate response provoked by bronchial challenge in healthy volunteers (Figure 21.6) does not usually occur in 'natural byssinosis'. However, it may be important in the pathogenesis of other work-related symptom complexes experienced by cotton workers.

Antigen–antibody reaction

The proposition that a specific hypersensitivity response is involved in the pathogenesis of byssinosis is suggested by the time interval between first exposure and the development of symptoms, and by the fact that only a minority of workers are now affected. However, skin tests using cotton dust extracts have failed to differentiate between normal, atopic and byssinotic subjects (Cayton, Furness and Maitland, 1952). Total IgE measurements (Petronio and Bovenzi, 1983) in textile cotton workers, both with and without byssinosis, showed no significant differences between groups and there was no relationship between the level of total IgE and the clinical grade of byssinosis. More recently, Mundie et al. (1985), using a radioallergosorbent test and skin test to cotton dust extract, demonstrated negative results in all byssinotic workers and positive results in some non-byssinotic workers. Intradermal skin tests with a cotton bract extract in naïve subjects induced both immediate and late skin responses (Schachter et al., 1985). Biopsies of each phase were obtained. These revealed oedema in the early phase followed by a mixed cellular perivascular infiltration. Degranulation of mast cells was noted throughout the reaction. This may have important implications in terms of responses of airways in subjects exposed to cotton dust.

Precipitating IgG antibody against an antigen in cotton is present in cotton workers and unexposed persons. Its titre is highest in workers with byssinosis, lower in those without byssinosis and lowest in the unexposed subjects. It has been suggested that the symptoms of byssinosis are caused either directly by a late Arthus-type reaction in the walls of airways or indirectly by the reaction liberating a pharmacologically active substance (see Chapter 4, 'Immunopathology – type IV hypersensivity'). The fact that symptoms of grades B1 and B2 byssinosis disappear while the worker is still exposed to the dust is explained on the grounds that, as long as exposure continues, antibody is progressively removed from the circulation leaving insufficient to produce a reaction, whereas after a period away from the dust, during which antibody is not removed, its titre is increased by the time the worker is re-exposed (Massoud and Taylor, 1964). The presence of precipitins in control subjects may have been due to antibodies to other antigens cross-reacting with cotton antigens.

Subsequently, Taylor Massoud and Lucas (1971) demonstrated that the precipitin titre is greater at the beginning of the working week than at the end, and is increased after returning from a week's holiday. Titration of precipitins before and after challenge inhalation of cotton antigen, by byssinotic and non-byssinotic cardroom workers, revealed smaller titres 6 hours after inhalation than before. Although 'Monday' symptoms were reproduced by inhalation of antigen, reduction in FEV$_1$ did not occur (Massoud, Taylor and Lucas, 1971). However, evidence of antibody production in normal subjects and increases of Ig levels after 10 days were not confirmed (Popa et al., 1969; Edwards et al., 1970) and subsequently Edwards and Jones (1974) found the reaction of the so-called byssinosis antigen to be remarkably non-specific. Although Kamat et al. (1979) have reported a significant increase in serum IgG and a fall in IgD and IgM in workers with byssinosis, this has not been confirmed by other workers who found normal levels of immunoglobulins and complement in byssinotic workers (Mundie, Pilia and Ainsworth, 1985). The current evidence suggests that it is unlikely that either immediate hypersensitivity or immune complex formation is playing a direct causative role in the pathogenesis of byssinosis (Mundie, Pilia and Ainsworth, 1985).

Bacterial endotoxins

There is good evidence that 'mill fever' (see page 730), which may occur in workers in cotton, flax, hemp and grain mills, is caused by the inhalation of the endotoxins of bacteria or other organisms growing in these materials (Pernis et al., 1961; Rylander and Lundholm, 1978). This has raised the question that byssinosis might also be caused by endotoxins, especially as it was reported to occur in workers in factories where flax and hemp were biologically retted (during which bacteria and fungi might be expected to flourish) but not in those where these fibres were chemically retted with alkali (Bouhuys, Hartogensis and Korfage, 1963; Bouhuys et al., 1967b).

Both bacteria and fungi are present in baled cotton and thus in the mill atmosphere. Gram-negative chromogenic bacteria (mainly of the genus *Enterobacter*) are much more prevalent than fungi and, although among the many species of fungi that have been isolated *Thermoactinomyces vulgaris* and *Faenia rectivirgula* (*Micropolyspora faeni*) may be widespread, they are seldom as abundant as other species, in particular *Penicillium* spp., *Cladosporium* spp. and *Aspergillus* spp. Endotoxin is derived from lipopolysaccharide cell wall material from Gram-negative bacteria. The concentrations of endotoxin in cotton mill dust range from 0.2 mg/m^3 to 1.5 mg/m^3 dust (Cinkotai, Lockwood and Rylander, 1977).

Cumulative exposures to air-borne bacteria, protease content of air-borne dust and concentration of 2- to 4-mm particles in cotton cardroom air correlate significantly with byssinotic symptoms (Cinkotai and Whitaker, 1978). Cavagna, Foa and Vigliana (1969) found a better correlation between byssinosis prevalence and concentration of air-borne endotoxins than with the total amount of dust. In a study of naïve subjects (that is, healthy subjects with no previous exposure to cotton dust) Castellan et al. (1984) found, similarly, that the acute bronchoconstrictor response to cotton dust correlated best with endotoxin levels and least well with gravimetric dust levels. However, in a study in cotton textile mills, although air-borne endotoxin levels were significantly correlated with the prevalence of chronic bronchitis, no similar relationship was demonstrated to the prevalence of byssinosis or to acute FEV_1 decline across the working shift (Kennedy et al., 1987).

Recent studies have also cast doubt on the role of endotoxin in the acute airways' constrictor response in 'naïve' subjects. Volunteers challenged with aqueous extracts of cotton bracts demonstrated no correlation between the degree of airways' constriction and the concentration of endotoxin, and continued to demonstrate airways' responses after the almost complete elimination of endotoxin from the bract extracts (Buck, Wall and Schachter, 1986). Provocation tests in normal subjects using flax dust containing a known concentration of endotoxin, and using pure endotoxin at the same concentration, produced an airways' constrictor response to flax dust, but no similar response to endotoxin (Jamison and Lowry, 1986).

The role of endotoxin in the pathogenesis of byssinosis remains unclear. It may not be the primary offending agent.

Fungal enzymes

Cotton mill dust contains proteolytic enzymes (Braun et al., 1973; Chinn, Cinkotai and Lockwood, 1976). Significant correlations have been shown between dust enzyme levels and acute FEV_1 decline across the working shift (Braun et al., 1973). There is, however, strong evidence against the involvement of enzymes in that in woollen mills (Cinkotai, 1976) and cotton willowing mills (Chinn, Cinkotai and Lockwood, 1976), both of which have high enzyme levels, byssinosis is either absent or relatively rare.

Non-specific pharmacological mediator release

It is clear from research in both human beings and animals that cotton dust is biologically highly active and able directly to release a variety of inflammatory mediators and to recruit into the airways' cells further promoting inflammation.

Cotton dust extract in in vitro experiments (Rylander and Snella, 1976; Wilson et al., 1980; Mundie, Boackle and Ainsworth, 1983), has been shown to activate complement by both the alternative and classical pathways (Mundie, Boackle and Ainsworth, 1983). However, the complement activating component of cotton dust extract has not been identified. Endotoxin concentrations did not correlate with complement activation and the removal of polyphenolic tannins did not abolish the complement-activating capacity of the cotton dust extract (Mundie, Boackle and Ainsworth, 1983). The complement fragment C5a is chemotactic for polymorphonuclear leucocytes and can cause release of leukotrienes (Stimler et al., 1982). Leukotrienes C_4 and D_4 are themselves potent bronchoconstrictors (Bisgaard, Groth and Dirksen, 1983) (see Chapter 4, 'Specific (acquired) immune defences').

In vivo experiments in animals have demonstrated the release of arachidonic acid metabolites, $PGF_{2\alpha}$ and thromboxane A_2, the release of 5-hydroxytryptamine occurring maximally 4 hours after challenge (Mundie, Whitener and Ainsworth, 1985). The major source of thromboxane A_2 release in vivo in animals is platelets. Cotton dust contains known platelet aggregators including polyphenolic tannins (Rohrbach et al., 1984) and 5-hydroxytryptamine (De Clerk and Herman, 1983). In addition, *Enterobacter agglomerans*, a major bacterial contaminant of cotton dust, is thought to induce the release of platelet-activating factor from polymorphonuclear leucocytes (Holt et al., 1983). Support for this pathway of mediator release in human subjects is derived from the observation by Bomski, Otawski and Bomska (1971) that a peripheral thrombocytopenia occurred in byssinotic workers during the working shift. This would be consistent with the aggregation of platelets occurring in the lung following cotton dust inhalation. There are, therefore, a variety of different mechanisms that may be operating singly or in combination with each other and leading to airways' inflammation in cotton-exposed individuals.

The effect of drugs

The effects on respiratory responses to cotton dust following the administration of a variety of different drugs have been evaluated. An antihistamine (Bouhuys, 1963) and a bronchodilator (Valić and Žuškin, 1972) will reduce or prevent the observed fall in FEV_1 across a working shift. In a study comparing the effects of disodium cromoglycate, beclomethasone dipropionate and salbutamol (Fawcett et al., 1978), salbutamol was found to be most effective and disodium cromoglycate least effective in preventing changes in FEV_1 in a group of cotton workers. Žuškin and Bouhuys (1967) examined the effect of disodium cromoglycate on the bronchoconstriction caused by hemp dust in a group of healthy subjects. They found considerable protection from a single dose of disodium cromoglycate, but this protection was short-lived and was lost 9 hours after the last dose of the drug.

Susceptibility to byssinosis

Flax workers whose fathers had been exposed occupationally to flax dust (especially if they had had byssinosis) are apparently less likely to develop byssinotic symptoms than fellow workers whose fathers had no such history (Noweir, Amine and Osman, 1975). Although the histocompatibility antigen, HLA-B27, is significantly more common in individuals with flax byssinosis, it is not necessary for the development of byssinosis in these workers and its presence may be associated with other genes (Middleton et al., 1979). It has been suggested that cotton workers who have had mill fever are more prone to develop byssinosis than those who have not (Gill, 1947). It is now very rare for byssinotic subjects to give a history of mill fever.

Is byssinosis distinct from other forms of bronchial asthma?

Byssinosis has been regarded as a separate entity on the following grounds (Schilling, 1956; Bouhuys, 1976):

1. Most asthmatics are hypersensitive to histamine, but this is 'not a regular finding in byssinosis' (Bouhuys, 1967).
2. A large proportion of textile workers may be affected by byssinosis, but in other forms of asthma the number of workers affected is usually very small.
3. The symptoms of byssinosis are delayed (that is, are not immediate) and improve during the working week.
4. Skin tests with dust extracts correlate poorly with byssinosis by comparison with skin tests in atopic asthma.

However, the prevalence of both byssinosis and occupational asthma varies greatly. The prevalence of byssinosis may be extremely low in comparable processes (Field and Owen, 1979) and the prevalence of occupational asthma may be very high (complex platinum salts) (Hunter, Milton and Perry, 1945). Although Bouhuys (1976) stated that histamine reactivity was not a regular finding in byssinosis, a recent study has found a good correlation between the presence of both respiratory symptoms and byssinosis in cotton workers, and evidence of increased bronchial reactivity (Fishwick et al., 1992). The pattern of grades B1 and B2 byssinosis is consistent with late-onset asthma, and recovery on subsequent days of the working week also occurs in some other forms of occupational lung disease (for example, 'humidifier fever', see Chapter

20). The improvement in airways' function over the working week in byssinosis may be more apparent than real. Merchant et al. (1974), studying grade 2 byssinotic subjects, found that the largest shift decline in FEV_1 occurred on Monday, but the mean daily FEV_1 tended to fall over the week, with the lowest FEV_1 occurring at the end of the working week. Lack of correlation with skin test reactions in other forms of occupational asthma is also fairly common due to the difficulty in making appropriate preparations of some industrial agents. In addition byssinosis may not be antibody mediated. Hence, although the underlying mechanism of byssinosis is not fully understood, its general features are those of occupational asthma. The clinical history of improvement of symptoms over the working week differentiates byssinosis from other forms of occupational asthma.

Symptoms

The symptoms of byssinosis, which are distinct from those of 'mill fever' have already been summarized under 'Clinical grades' (page 732). Acute symptoms consist of chest tightness and breathlessness (grades B1 and B2) which develop during the afternoon of the work day, although in severe cases they occur a few hours after starting work in the morning. Cough, sputum and wheezing are also experienced by byssinotic subjects. The frequency is related to the grade of byssinosis – the higher the grade the more frequent the prevalence of these symptoms. Smoking does not influence the prevalence of additional respiratory symptoms in byssinotic subjects, except among ex-smokers who have a higher prevalence of cough and sputum (Pickering, 1989). The expression 'tightness', incidentally, is commonly used to refer to the sensation of breathlessness experienced by patients with lower airways' disease, especially asthma, which has a vague but more 'internal' localization than the 'inability to get in enough air' associated with cardiac, neurological and other lung diseases (Widdicombe, 1979) (see Chapter 6).

The 'Monday feeling' of grade C½, consisting of chest tightness alone, occurring only on some Mondays (or first day back at work) has now been abandoned (see 'Clinical grading'). Chest tightness sometimes associated with cough, breathlessness, wheezing and fatigue experienced on the first day of most working weeks but ceasing completely on the second day of the working week is grade B1. Grade B1 symptoms are best exemplified in the words of a cotton stripper and grinder who had been exposed to cotton dust for 10 years (Schilling, 1950):

Monday is a different day to me. Getting to 11 o'clock I feel tight in the chest and short of wind, but I have no cough. Towards 5.30 I feel done and struggle for breath and I can't walk at my ordinary speed. I am a dead horse on Mondays, but could fell a bull on Tuesdays.

In many workers there may be no further progression of symptoms during their work in the textile industry and when they leave symptoms cease completely leaving no residual disability.

Grade B2 is characterized by a gradual progression of symptoms. Chest tightness and breathlessness increase in severity and, although usually worse by Mondays, are present on other days of the week. Days on which cleaning takes place (Fridays) have also been associated with particularly severe symptoms.

The functional grading has now been separated from these clinical grades into two categories: *acute changes* – the measurement of decline in FEV_1 across the working shift; and *chronic changes* – the measurement of FEV_1 when away from contact with cotton dust. Each grading is classified from 'no effect' up to a 'severe effect'.

Morbidity and mortality

Initial epidemiological studies in England demonstrated evidence of morbidity and excess mortality in cotton workers. Hill (1930) found high death rates from respiratory disease among strippers and grinders compared to workers in the ring room and warehouse. Earlier, Collis (1909) described a high prevalence (74 to 91 per cent) of an asthma-like condition in strippers and grinders, and observed that it was unusual for these men to remain in the cardroom over the age of 45. Over recent years there has been a progressive reduction in dust levels within cotton mills. This has been associated with a decrease in the prevalence of byssinosis. The effect of these environmental changes on the outcome of byssinosis remains poorly documented. Several mortality studies have failed to demonstrate an increased mortality among cotton textile workers (Berry and Molyneux, 1981; Merchant and Ortmeyer, 1981) or among flax workers (Elwood et al., 1982). In view of the findings of a recent study of a normal population, where a strong correlation between impaired lung function and increased mortality was found, it could be concluded that, in the absence of an excess of respiratory deaths in cotton workers, exposure to cotton dust is not associated with permanent respiratory disability (Peto et al., 1983). However, a recent mortality study (Hodgson and Jones, 1990) of 3458 cotton workers, whilst demonstrating a lower than expected total mortality and mortality for respiratory disease, showed an increased mortality from respiratory disease in those reporting symptoms of byssinosis.

The available evidence suggests that cotton dust exposure does not cause an accelerated loss of lung function in cotton workers as a whole, but that byssinosis itself is associated with an excess morbidity and mortality due to respiratory disease.

Physical signs

As a rule there are no abnormal signs in grades B1 and B2, although expiratory wheeze is sometimes present. Breath sounds may be impaired in some individuals with chronic changes of moderate-to-severe degree.

Investigations

Lung function

There is a progressive reduction of ventilatory capacity (as indicated by FEV_1) and an increase in airways' resistance throughout the working day in grades B1 and B2 byssinosis, and also some unevenness of distribution of inspired gas (McKerrow et al., 1958; Cotes, 1979). Decline in FEV_1 may occur during the working day without respiratory symptoms (Berry et al., 1973; Imbus and Suh, 1973). Maximum mid-expiratory flow (MMF) is also reduced and may be more sensitive in detecting airflow obstruction than FEV_1. Closing volume is a less sensitive, unreliable and more time-consuming test (Fairman et al., 1975; Žuškin et al., 1975). Observations by Field and Owen (1979) in Australia indicate that a fall in MMF occurs early in a shift and is consistent with constriction of distal airways, whereas reduction in FEV_1 and PEFR (peak expiratory flow rate), which is indicative of involvement of larger airways, occurs later and more gradually. These authors also found that the Monday morning fall in MMF was rarely accompanied by chest symptoms, in contrast to the reported findings in Europe and North America, which they suggest are due to extraneous factors.

There is little published work on the level of airways' reactivity in byssinotic subjects. The initial studies gave differing results. In a group of cardroom workers increased airways' reactivity was demonstrated in the highest grades of byssinosis (9 out of 12 workers) (Massoud et al., 1967), whereas Bouhuys (1967) demonstrated increased airways'

reactivity in only 2 of 11 byssinotic subjects. In a study measuring the pre- and post-shift levels of airways' reactivity (Haglind, Bake and Belin, 1983) of a group of byssinotic and non-byssinotic subjects, the baseline level of airways' reactivity was found to be increased in the byssinotic subjects and increased further over the shift in 11 of the 16 byssinotic subjects. In a recent study byssinotic workers had significantly increased airways' reactivity compared to asymptomatic controls (Fishwick et al., 1992).

Gas transfer remains within normal limits (Žuškin et al., 1975), the presence of an impaired gas transfer being related to the individual's past smoking habits rather than to his or her cotton dust exposure (Honeybourne and Pickering, 1986).

The most practical lung function tests for routine use in industry are, however, FEV_1 or PEFR.

Radiographic appearances

Byssinosis is not characterized by any abnormality of the chest radiograph.

Intradermal tests

Intradermal skin tests with cotton extracts have given varying results. However, positive results have not differentiated between byssinotic and non-byssinotic workers.

Diagnosis

Ideally the diagnosis of grades B1 and B2 rests on:

1. A history of industrial exposure to cotton, flax or soft hemp dust.
2. A typical history of these clinical grades.
3. Fall in FEV_1 or MMF across the first working shift of the working week.

In clinical practice, the objective evidence of ventilatory function at the time of the symptoms is not always available and the diagnosis then depends entirely on the reliability of the patient's history. Hence, the technique of eliciting the history either directly from the patient or via a questionnaire is all important. It is essential to avoid leading questions, such as 'Is your chest tight on Mondays?'. The history or questionnaire should elicit the presence of relevant symptoms and their periodicity in a stepwise fashion, initially establishing the presence or absence of chest tightness or breathing difficulty, then the days of the week when this symptom is present and finally the day or days when it is most severe. Every effort should be made to measure

FEV$_1$ or PEFR before, during and after a working shift and, if possible, at regular intervals during a weekend or holiday period. The influence of diurnal variation on ventilatory capacity, both in healthy and chronic bronchitic individuals, must be taken into account.

Summary

1. The acute respiratory and constitutional symptoms of variable intensity of 'mill fever' and 'mattress makers' fever' are separate from byssinosis and the distinction has to be borne in mind. The occasional use of the term 'Monday fever' for grade B1 byssinosis is both incorrect and confusing.
2. Byssinosis grades B1 and B2 behave as 'late' asthma.
3. The immediate asthmatic response in healthy persons on bronchial challenge with textile dust extracts or visiting a mill may not be relevant to 'natural' byssinosis in susceptible workers.
4. The functional chronic airways' changes in byssinosis are an uncertain entity. Because life-long non-smoking byssinotic subjects may demonstrate these changes, they are not solely related to past smoking habits.
5. The features of extrinsic allergic alveolitis are absent.

Treatment

Workers with grades B1 and B2 byssinosis should be removed from areas of dust exposure.

The prophylactic effects of antihistamines, salbutamol, beclomethasone and disodium cromoglycate have already been referred to. However, their use as a therapeutic measure is no substitute for prevention.

Prevention

Prevention depends upon the co-operation of engineering and medical disciplines.

Dust control

The most effective preventive measure is the replacement of natural by synthetic fibres. Although this has been achieved to some extent in Europe and the USA, it is small by comparison with the world increase in cotton production; and, while the production of flax has declined that of hemp has not changed significantly.

Plant already in existence in established factories should be enclosed as far as is practicable and subjected to local exhaust ventilation, that is, cotton gins and opening and mixing and carding machines. But removal of dust is often inefficient due to unsatisfactory design, application and maintenance of equipment. The difficulty has been accentuated in recent years by rising production demands requiring a great increase in the speed of carding machines and, consequently, of the dust output. A proportionally greater demand, therefore, has been placed upon ventilation systems. Effective methods of water washing and steam treatment of raw cotton before processing are under active investigation.

General ventilation is also necessary and recirculated air must be efficiently filtered. Dust should be removed from machines, mill floors, ventilation equipment and other surfaces by vacuum cleaners.

Where sporadically large concentrations of dust occur (for example, stripping and grinding of carding machines) the operatives should wear efficient respirators.

Dust control measures and sampling techniques are related to current TLVs which are under review because the composition and biological activity of textile dusts can vary significantly in different processing operations so that a series of dust levels may be needed.

Suggested methods of control

1. Spraying of ripening cotton with bactericides and fungicides.
2. Treatment of raw cotton with gaseous hydrogen chloride or acetic acid because acids have been found to inactivate the active component in cotton bracts and dust.

Medical surveillance of workers

Pre-employment examination

All prospective employees in vegetable textile industries should be examined. Examinations should include a questionnaire similar to that of the Medical Research Council with additional details of atopic family history, personal history of allergy and asthma, physical examinations, FEV$_1$, PEFR or MMF and a chest radiograph. Investigation of atopic status by skin-prick tests to common allergens should be done in each case, and atopic subjects probably excluded.

It is advisable that moderate-to-heavy cigarette smokers and persons with chronic or recurrent respiratory disease should be placed in low- or no-risk areas; but in practice, in the case of the smokers, there is probably little chance of achieving this. Individuals with a FEV_1 less than 60 per cent of the predicted normal value should not be exposed to dust.

There is at present no practical immunological method of detecting individual susceptibility.

Periodic medical examinations

These serve two purposes: to identify workers who develop a pronounced reaction to the dust; and to provide a biological assessment of the efficiency of dust control and sampling in specific processes.

During the first month of his employment the worker's FEV_1 should be recorded before and after 6 hours of commencing his shift on the first day of a working week. If a significant decrease occurs he should be transferred to a less dusty area.

Systematic clinical examinations and recording of FEV_1, PEFR or MMF should be done annually in all exposed workers. Those who are prone to develop substantial disability can be identified by comparing the annual fall of their FEV_1 with the predicted normal value after the effects of diurnal variation and cigarette smoking are allowed for. They should be moved to a no-risk area as soon as this is recognized.

References

Agrup, G., Beilin, L., Sjostedt, L. and Skerfving, S. (1986) Allergy to laboratory animals and laboratory technicians and animal keepers. *Br. J. Ind. Med.* **43**, 128–129

Ainsworth, S.K., Neuman, R.E. and Harley, R.A. (1979) Histamine release from platelets for assay of byssinogenic substances in cotton mill dust and related materials. *Br. J. Ind. Med.* **36**, 35–42

Aitken, J. (1795) *A Description of the Country from Thirty to Forty miles around Manchester.* Republished 1968. David and Charles, Newton Abbott

Alanko, K., Keskinen, H., Bjorksten, F. and Ojjanen, S. (1978) Immediate-type-hypersensitity to reactive dyes. *Clin. Allergy* **8**, 25–31

American Thoracic Society (1979) ATS statement – Snowbird workshop on standardisation of spirometry. *Am. Rev. Respir. Dis.* **119**, 831–838

Arlidge, J.J. (1892) *The Hygiene Disease and Mortality of Occupations.* Percival, London, pp. 354–358

Asai, A., Shimoda, T., Hara, K. and Fujiwara, K. (1987) Occupational asthma caused by isonicotinic acid hydrazide (INH) inhalation. *J. Allergy Clin. Immunol.* **80**, 578–582

Axelsson, G., Skedinger, M. and Zetterström, O. (1985) Allergy to weeping fig – a new occupational disease. *Allergy* **40**, 461–464

Baker, M.D., Irwig, L.M., Johnston, J.R., Turner, D.M. and Bezuidenhout, B.N. (1979) Lung function in sisal ropemakers. *Br. J. Ind. Med.* **36**, 216–219

Baldo, B.A., Krilis, S. and Taylor, K.M. (1982) IgE-mediated acute asthma following inhalation of a powdered marine sponge. *Clin. Allergy* **12**, 179–186

Bardy, J.D., Malo, J.L., Seguin, P., Ghezzo, H., Desjardins, J., Dolovich, J. and Cartier, A. (1987) Occupational asthma and IgE sensitization in a pharmaceutical company processing psyllium. *Am. Rev. Respir. Dis.* **135**, 1033–1036

Battigelli, M.C. Fischer, J.J., Craven, P.L. and Foarde, K.K. (1976) The etiology of byssinosis. *Am. Rev. Respir. Dis.* **113**, 100 (Abstract)

Baur, X. and Fruhmann, G. (1979a) Allergic reactions including asthma to the pineapple protease bromelain following occupational exposure. *Clin. Allergy* **9**, 443–450

Baur, X. and Fruhmann, G. (1979b) Papain induced asthma: diagnosis by skin test, RAST and bronchial provocation test. *Clin. Allergy* **9**, 75–81

Baur, X., Dewair, M., Fruhmann, G., Aschauer, H., Pfletschinger, J. and Braunitzer, G. (1982) Hypersensitivity to chironomides (non-biting midges): localization of the antigenic determinants within certain polypeptide sequences of hemoglobins (erythrocruorins) of *Chironomus thummi thummi* (Diptera). *J. Allergy Clin. Immunol.* **69**, 66–76

Baur, X., Fruhmann, G., Haug, B., Rasche, B., Reiher, W. and Weiss, W. (1986) Role of aspergillus amylase in bakers' asthma. *Lancet* **1**, 43

Beeson, M.F., Dewdney, J.M., Edwards, R.G., Lee, D. and Orr, R.G. (1983) Prevalence and diagnosis of laboratory animal allergy. *Clin. Allergy* **13**, 433–442

Belin, L., Hoborn, J., Falsen, E. and Andre, J. (1970) Enzyme sensitisation in consumers of enzyme containing washing powders. *Lancet* **2**, 1153–1157

Bernstein, D.I., Gallagher, J.S. and Bernstein, I.L. (1983) Mealworm asthma: clinical and immunologic studies. *J. Allergy Clin. Immunol.* **72**, 475–480

Bernstein, D.I., Gallagher, J.S., D'Souza, L. and Bernstein, I.L. (1984) Heterogeneity of specific IgE responses in workers sensitised to acid anhydride compounds. *J. Allergy Clin. Immunol.* **74**, 794–801

Bernton, H.S., McMahon, R.F. and Brown H. (1972) Cockroach asthma. *Br. J. Dis. Chest* **66**, 61–66

Berry, G. and Molyneux, M.K.B. (1981) A mortality study of workers in Lancashire cotton mills. *Chest* **79S**, 11S–15S

Berry, G., Molyneux, M.K.B. and Tombleson, J.B.L. (1974) Relationship between dust level and byssinosis and bronchitis in Lancashire cotton mills. *Br. J. Ind. Med.* **31**, 18–27

Berry, G., McKerrow, C.B., Molyneux, M.K.B., Rossiter, C.E. and Tombleson, J.B.L. (1973) A study of the acute and chronic changes in ventilatory capacity of workers in Lancashire cotton mills. *Br. J. Ind. Med.* **30**, 25–36

Biagini, R.E., Moorman, W.J., Lewis, T.R. and Bernstein, I.L. (1986) Ozone enhancement of platinum asthma in a primate model. *Am. Rev. Respir. Dis.* **134**, 719–725

Bisgaard, H., Groth, S. and Dirksen, H. (1983) Leukotriene D4 induced bronchoconstriction in man. *Allergy* **38**, 441–443

Björksten, F., Backman, A., Jarvinen, K., Lehti, A.J., Savilahti, H., Syvanen, P. and Karkkeinen, T. (1977) Immunoglobulin E specific to white wheat and rye flour proteins. *Clin. Allergy* **7**, 473–483

Blainey, A.D., Topping, M.D., Ollier, S. and Davies, R.J. (1986) Specific IgE to storage mites in Essex farmers. *Thorax* **41**, 251–252

Blair Smith, A. Bernstein, D.I., Aw, T.C., Gallagher, J.S., London, M., Kopp, S and Carson, G.A. (1987) Occupational asthma from inhaled egg protein. *Am. J. Ind. Med.* **12**, 205–218

Blands, J., Diamant, B., Kailos, P., Kallosdefner, L. and Lowenstein, H. (1976) Flour allergy in bakers. *Int. Archs Allergy Appl. Immunol.* **52**, 392

Block, G. and Chan-Yeung, M. (1982) Asthma induced by nickel. *J. Am. Med. Assoc.* **247**, 1600–1602

Block, G., Tse, K.S., Kajjek, K., Chan, H. and Chan-Yeung, M. (1983) Bakers asthma. Clinical and immunological studies. *Clin. Allergy* **13**, 359–370

Bomski, H., Otawski, J. and Bomska, H. (1971) Hamatologische und serologische untersuchungen bei byssinosegefahrdeten arbeitern. *Int. Arch. Arbeitsmed.* **27**, 309–323

Booth, B.H., LeFoldt, R.H. and Moffitt, E.M. (1976) Wood dust hypersensitivity. *J. Allergy Clin. Immunol.* **57**, 352–357

Bouhuys, A. (1963) Prevention of Monday dyspnoea in byssinosis: a controlled trial with an antihistamine drug. *Clin. Pharmacol. Ther.* **4**, 311–314

Bouhuys, A. (1967) Response to inhaled histamine in bronchial asthma and in byssinosis. *Am. Rev. Respir. Dis.* **95**, 89–93

Bouhuys, A. (1971) Byssinosis. *Archs Environ. Health* **23**, 405–407

Bouhuys, A. (1976) Byssinosis: scheduled asthma in the textile industry. *Lung* **154**, 3–16

Bouhuys, A., Gilson, J.C. and Schilling, R.S.F. (1970) Byssinosis in the textile industry. *Archs Environ. Health.* **21**, 475–478

Bouhuys, A., Hartogensis, F. and Korfage, H.J.H. (1963) Byssinosis prevalence and flax processing. *Br. J. Ind. Med.* **20**, 320–323

Bouhuys, A., Lindell, S.E. and Lundin, G. (1960) Experimental studies in byssinosis. *Br. Med. J.* **1**, 324–326

Bouhuys, A., Heaphy, L.J. Jr., Schilling, R.S.F. and Welborn, J.W. (1967a) Byssinosis in the United States. *N. Engl. J. Med.* **277**, 170–175

Bouhuys, A., Lindell, S.E., Roach, S.A. and Schilling, R.S.F. (1967b) Byssinosis in hemp workers. *Archs Environ. Health* **14**, 533–544

Bourne, M.S., Flindt, M.L.H. and Walker, J.M. (1979) Asthma due to industrial use of chloramine. *Br. Med. J.* **2**, 10–12

Bousquet, J., Dhivert, H., Clauzel, A-M., Hewitt, B. and Michel, F-B. (1985) Occupational allergy to sunflower pollen. *J. Allergy Clin. Immunol.* **75**, 70–74

Braun, D.C., Scheel, L.D., Tuma, J. and Parker, L. (1973) Physiological response to enzymes in cotton dust. *J. Occup. Med.* **15** 241–244

Bridge, J.C. (1935) *Annual Report of the Chief Inspector of Factories and Workshops*, 60. HMSO, London

Brooks, S.M. and Lockey, J. (1981) Reactive airways dysfunction syndrome (RADS). A newly defined occupational disease. *Am. Rev. Respir. Dis.* 1–3 (suppl. 133)

Brooks, S.M., Weiss, M.A. and Bernstein, K. (1985) Reactive airways dysfunction syndrome (RADS): persistent asthma syndrome after high level irritant exposures. *Chest* **88**, 376–384

Brooks, S.M., Edwards, J.J., Apol, A. and Edwards, F.H. (1981) An epidemiologic study of workers exposed to Western Red Cedar and other wood dusts. *Chest* **80** (suppl.), 30–32

Browne, R.C. (1955) Vanadium poisoning from gas turbines. *Br. J. Ind. Med.* **12**, 57–59

Bruckner, H.C. (1967) Extrinsic asthma in a tungsten carbide worker. *J. Occup. Med.* **9**, 518–519

Bryant, D.H. (1985) Asthma due to insecticide sensitivity. *Aust. NZ J. Med.* **15**, 66–68

Buck, M.G., Wall, J.H. and Schachter, E.N. (1986) Airway constrictor response to cotton bract extracts in the absence of endotoxin. *Br. J. Ind. Med.* **43**, 220–226

Burge (1982a) Single and serial measurement of lung function in the diagnosis of occupational asthma. *Eur. J. Respir. Dis.* **63** (suppl. 123), 147–159

Burge, P.S. (1982b) Occupational asthma in electronics workers caused by colophony fumes: follow-up of affected workers. *Thorax* **37**, 348–353

Burge, P.S., Hendy, M. and Hodgson, E.S. (1984). Occupational asthma, rhinitis and dermatitis due to tetrazene in a detonator manufacturer. *Thorax* **39**, 470–471

Burge, P.S., O'Brien, I.M. and Harries, M.G. (1979a) Peak flow rate records in the diagnosis of occupational asthma due to colophony. *Thorax* **34**, 308–316

Burge, P.S., O'Brien, I.M. and Harries, M.G. (1979b) Peak flow records in the diagnosis of occupational asthma due to isocyanates. *Thorax* **34**, 317–323

Burge, P.S., O'Brien, I.M., Harries, M.G. and Pepys, J. (1979a) Occupational asthma due to inhaled carmine. *Clin. Allergy* **9**, 185–189

Burge, P.S., Parks, W., O'Brien, I.M., Hawkins, R. and Green, M. (1979b) Occupational asthma in an electronics factory. *Thorax* **34**, 13–18

Burge, P.S., Harries, M.G., O'Brien, I. and Pepys, J. (1980) Bronchial provocation studies in workers exposed to fumes of electronic soldering flux. *Clin. Allergy* **10**, 137–149

Burge, P.S., Edge, G., Hawkins, E.R., White, V. and Newman Taylor, A.J. (1981) Occupational asthma in a factory making flux cord solder containing colophony. *Thorax* **36**, 828–834

Burge, P.S., Finnegan, M., Horsfield, N., Emery, D. Austwick, P., Davies, P.S. and Pickering, C.A.C. (1985) Occupational asthma in a factory with a contaminated humidifier. *Thorax* **40**, 248–254

Burge, P.S., Wieland, A., Robertson, A.S. and Weir, D. (1986) Occupational asthma due to unheated colophony. *Br. J. Ind. Med.* **43**, 559–560

Bush, R.K., Yuninger, J.W. and Reed, C.E. (1978) Asthma due to African zebrawood (*Microberlinia*). *Am. Rev. Respir. Dis.* **117**, 601–603

Busse, W.W. and Schoenwetter, W.F. (1975) Asthma from psyllium in laxative manufacture. *Ann. Intern. Med.* **83**, 361–362

Butcher, B.T., Jones, R.N., O'Neil, E. et al. (1977) Longitudinal study of workers employed in the manufacture of toluene diisocyanate. *Am. Rev. Respir. Dis.* **116**, 411

Butcher, B.T., Karr, R.M., O'Neil, C.E. et al. (1979b) Inhalation challenge and pharmacologic studies of toluene diisocyanate (TDI) sensitive workers. *J. Allergy Clin. Immunol.* **64**, 146–152

Butcher, B.T., O'Neill, C.E., Reed, M.A. and Salvaggio, J.E. (1980) Radioallergosorbent testing of toluene di-isocyanate reactive individuals using *p*-tolyl isocyanate antigen. *J. Allergy Clin. Immunol.* **66**, 213–216

Carey, G.C.R., Elwood, P.C., McAulay, I.R., Merrett, J.D. and Pemberton, J. (1965) Byssinosis in flax workers in Northern Ireland: A report to the Minister of Labour and National Insurance, The Government of Northern Ireland, HM Stationery Office, Belfast

Carino, M., Elia, G., Molinini, R., Nuzzaco, A. and Ambrosi, L. (1985) Shrimpmeal asthma in the aquaculture industry. *Med. Lav.* **76**, 471–475

Carroll, K.B., Secombe, C.J.P. and Pepys, J. (1976) Asthma due to non-occupational exposure to toluene di-isocyanate. *Clin. Allergy* **6**, 99–104

Cartier, A., Malo, J.L., Forest, F., Lafranc, M., Pineau, L., St-Aubin, J.J. and Dubois, J.Y. (1984) Occupational asthma in snow crab processing workers. *J. Allergy Clin. Immunol.* **74**, 261–269

Cartier, A., Chan, H., Malo, J-L., Pinou, L., Tse, K.S. and Chan-Yeung, M. (1986) Occupational asthma caused by eastern white cedar (*Thuja occidentalis*) with demonstration that plicatic acid is present in this wood dust and is the caused agent. *J. Allergy Clin. Immunol.* **77**, 639–645

Castellan, R.M., Olenchock, S.A., Hankinson, J.L., Millner, P.D., Cocke, J.B., Bragg, C.K., Perkins, H.H. and Jacobs, R.R. (1984) Acute bronchostriction induced by cotton dust: dose related response to endotoxin and other dust factors. *Ann Intern. Med.* **101**, 157–163

Cavagna, G., Foa, V. and Vigliani, E.C. (1969) Effects in man and rabbits of inhalation of cotton dust or extracts and purified endotoxins. *Br. J. Ind. Med.* **26**, 314–321

Cayton, H.R., Furness, G. and Maitland, H.B. (1952) Studies in cotton dust in relation to byssinosis. Part II. Skin tests for allergy with extracts of cotton dusts. *Br. J. Ind. Med.* **9**, 186–196

Chan-Yeung, M. (1982) Immunologic and non-immunologic mechanisms in asthma due to W. red cedar (*Thuja plicata*). *J. Allergy Clin. Immunol.* **70**, 32–37

Chan-Yeung M. and Abboud, R. (1976) Occupational asthma due to California redwood (*Sequoia sempervirens*) dust. *Am. Rev. Respir. Dis.* **114**, 1027–1031

Chan-Yeung, M., Lam, S. and Koener, S. (1982) Clinical features and natural history of occupational asthma due to Western red cedar. *Am. J. Med.* **72**, 411–415

Chan-Yeung, M., Gicas, P.C. and Henson, P.M. (1980) Activation of complement by plicatic acid, the chemical compound responsible for asthma due to Western Red Cedar (*Thuja plicata*). *J. Allergy Clin. Immunol.* **65**, 333–337

Chan-Yeung, M., MacLean, L. and Paggiaro, P.L. (1987) Follow up study of 232 patients with occupational asthma caused by Western red cedar (*Thuja plicata*). *J. Allergy Clin. Immunol.* **79**, 792–796

Chan-Yeung, M., Wong, R. and MacLean, L. (1979) Respiratory abnormalities among grain elevator workers. *Chest* **72**, 461–467

Chan-Yeung, M., Barton, G.M., MacLean, L. and Grzybowski, S. (1973) Occupational asthma and rhinitis due to Western red cedar (*Thuja plicata*) *Am. Rev. Respir. Dis.* **108**, 1094–1102

Chan-Yeung, M., Vedal, S., Cuss, J., MacLean, L., Ennarson, D. and Tse, K.S. (1984) Symptoms, pulmonary function and bronchial hyper-reactivity in Western red cedar workers compared with those in office workers. *Am. Rev. Respir. Dis.* **130**, 1038–1041

Chapman, S.J. (1904) *The Lancashire Cotton Industry*. Manchester University Press, Manchester

Chwat, M. and Mordish, R. (1963) Byssinosis investigations into cotton plants in Israel. 14th International Conference in Occupational Health, Madrid, 1963. *International Congress Series No. 62*, Excerpta Medica, Amsterdam, pp. 572–573

Chinn, D.J., Cinkotai, F.F. and Lockwood, M.G. (1976) Airborne dust; its protease content and byssinosis in willowing mills. *Ann. Occup. Hyg.* **19**(2), 101–108

Cinkotai, F.F. (1976) The size-distribution and protease content of airborne particles in textile mill card rooms. *Am. Ind. Hyg. Assoc. J.* **37**, 234–238

Cinkotai, F.F. and Whitaker, C.J. (1978) Airborne bacteria and the prevalence of byssinotic symptoms in 21 cotton spinning mills in Lancashire. *Ann. Occup. Hyg.* **21**, 239–250

Cinkotai, F.F., Lockwood, M.G. and Rylander, R. (1977) Airborne bacteria and the prevalence of byssinotic symptoms in cotton mills. *Am. Ind. Hyg. Assoc. J.* **38**, 554–559

Cinkotai, F.F. Rigby, A., Pickering, C.A.C., Seaborn, D. and Faragher, E. (1988a) Recent trends in the prevalence of byssinotic symptoms in the Lancashire textile industry. *Br. J. Ind. Med.* **45**, 782–789

Cinkotai, F.F., Seaborn, D., Pickering, C.A.C. and Faragher, E. (1988b) Airborne dust in the personal breathing zone and the prevalence of byssinotic symptoms in the Lancashire textile industry. *Ann Occup. Hyg.* **32**, 103–113

Clarke, P.S. (1979) Immediate respiratory sensitivity to abalone. *Med. J. Aust.* **1**, 623

Cleare, M.J., Hughes, E.G., Jacoby, B. and Pepys, J. (1976) Immediate (type 1) allergic responses to platinum compounds. *Clin. Allergy* **6**, 183–195

Cockcroft D.W., Cartier, A., Jones, G., Tarlo, S.M., Dolovitch J. and Hargreave, F.E. (1980) Asthma caused by occupational exposure to a furan-based binder system. *J. Allergy Clin. Immunol.* **66**, 458–463

Cockcroft, A., Edwards, J., McCarthy, P. and Andersson, N. (1981) Allergy and laboratory animal workers. *Lancet* **2**, 827–830

Collis, E.L. (1915) The occurrence of an unusual cough among weavers of cotton cloth. *Proc. R. Soc. Med.* **8** (Part 2) 108–112

Collis, E.L. (1909) *Annual Report of Chief Inspector of Factories for 1908.* HMSO, London

Colten, H.R., Polikoff, P.L. Weinstein, S.F. and Strieder, D. (1975) Immediate hypersensitivity to hog trypsin resulting from industrial exposure. *J. Allergy Clin. Immunol.* **55**, 130

Corrado, O.J. (1986) Asthma and rhinitis after exposure to glutaraldehyde in endoscopy units. *Human Toxicol.* **5**, 325–327

Cotes, J.E. (1979) *Lung Function. Assessment and Applications in Medicine,* 4th ed, Blackwell, Oxford, Edinburgh

Coutts, I.I., Dally, M.B., Newman Taylor, A.J., Pickering, C.A.C. and Horsfield, N. (1981) Asthma in workers manufacturing cephalosporins. *Br. Med. J.* **283**, 950

Coutts, I.I., Lozewicz, S., Dalley, M.V., Newman Taylor, A.J., Burge, P.S., Flynd, A.C. and Rodgers, D.J.H. (1984) Respiratory symptoms related to work in a factory manufacturing cimetidine tablets. *Br. Med. J.* **288**, 14–18

Dally, M.B., Hunter, J.V., Hughes, E.G., Stewart, M. and Newman Taylor, A.J. (1980) Hypersensitivity to platinum salts: a population study. *Am. Rev. Respir. Dis.* **121**, 230a

Darke, C.S., Knowelden, J., Lacey, J. and Ward, A.M. (1976) Respiratory disease of workers harvesting grain. *Thorax* **31**, 293–302

Davies, B.E. and McArdle, L.A. (1981) Allergy to laboratory animals: A survey by questionnaire. *Int. Archs Allergy Appl. Immun.* **64**, 302–307

Davies, G.E., Thompson, A.V. Niewola, Z., Burrows, G.E., Teasdale, E.L., Bird, D.J. and Philips, D.A. (1983) Allergy to laboratory animals: a retrospective and prospective study. *Br. J. Ind. Med.* **40**, 442–449

Davies, R.J. and Pepys, J. (1975) Asthma due to inhaled chemical agents – the macrolide antibiotic Spiramycin. *Clin. Allergy* **55**, 99–107

Davies, R.J., Green, M. and Schofield, N. McC. (1976) Recurrent nocturnal asthma after exposure to grain dust. *Am. Rev. Respir. Dis.* **114**, 1011–1019

Davies, R.J., Hendrick, D.J. and Pepys, J. (1974) Asthma due to inhaled chemical agents – ampicillin, benzyl penicillin, 6 amino penicillanic acid and related substances. *Clin. Allergy* **4**, 227–247

Davies, R.J., Butcher, B.T., O'Neill, C.E. and Salvaggio, J.E. (1977) The in vitro effect of toluene diisocyanate on lympho-cyte cyclic adenosine monophosphate production by isopro-terenol, prostaglandin and histamine. *J. Allergy Clin. Immunol.* **60**, 223–229

Davison, A.G., Britton, M.G., Forrester, J.A., Davies, R.J. and Hughes, D.T.D. (1983a) Asthma in merchant seamen and laboratory workers caused by allergy to castor oil beans: Analysis of allergens. *Clin. Allergy* **13**, 1353–1361

Davison, A.G., Haslam, P.L., Corrin, B., Coutts II, Dewar, A., Riding D., Studdy, P. and Newman Taylor, A.J. (1983b) Interstitial lung disease and asthma in hard metal workers; bronchoalveolar lavage, ultrastructure, and analytical findings and results of bronchial provocation tests. *Thorax* **38**, 119–128

Davison, A.G., Durham, S., Newman Taylor, A.J. and Schilling, C.J. (1986) Asthma caused by pulverised fuel ash. *Br. Med. J.* **292**, 1561

DeClerk, F.F. and Herman, A.G. (1983) 5-Hydroxytryptamine and platelet aggregation. *Fed. Proc.* **42**, 228–232

Diem, J.E., John, R.N., Hendrick, D.J. et al. (1982) Five year longitudinal study of workers employed in a new toluene diisocyanate manufacturing plant. *Am. Rev. Respir. Dis.* **126**, 420–428

Docker, A., Wattie, J.M., Topping, M.D., Luczynska, C.M., Newman Taylor, A.J., Pickering, C.A.C., Thomas, P. and Gompertz, D. (1987) Clinical and immunological investigations of respiratory disease in workers using reactive dyes. *Br. J. Ind. Med.* **44**, 534–541

Doig, A.T. (1949) Other lung diseases due to dust. *Postgrad. Med. J.* **25**, 639–649

Dolan, T.F. and Myers, A. (1974) Bronchial asthma and allergic rhinitis associated with inhalation of pancreatic extracts. *Am. Rev. Respir. Dis.* **810**, 812–813

doPico, G.A. (1978) Asthma due to dust from redwood (*Sequoia sempervirens*). *Chest* **73**, 424–425

Durham, S.R., Graneek, B.J., Hawkins, R. and Newman Taylor, A.J. (1987) Temporal relationship between increases in airway responsiveness to histamine and late asthmatic responses induced by occupational agents. *J. Allergy Clin. Immunol.* **73**, 398–406

Eaton, K.K. (1973) Respiratory allergy to exotic wood dust. *Clin. Allergy* **3**, 307–310

Editorial (1985) Smoking, occupation and allergic lung disease. *Lancet* **1**, 965

Edwards, C., Macartney, J., Rooke, G. and Ward, F. (1975) The pathology of the lung in byssinotics. *Thorax* **30**, 612–623

Edwards, J.H. and Jones, B.M. (1974) Immunology of byssinosis: a study of the reactions between the isolated byssinosis 'antigen' and human immunoglobulins. *Ann. NY Acad. Sci.* **221**, 59–63

Edwards, J.H., McCarthy, P., McDermott, M., Nicholls, P.J. and Skidmore, J.W. (1970) The acute physiological, pharmacological and immunological effects of inhaled cotton dust in normal subjects. *J. Physiol.* **208**, 63–64

Edwards, J.H., McConnochie, K., Trotman, D.M., Collins, G., Saunders, M.J. and Latham, S.M. (1983) Allergy to inhaled egg material. *Clin. Allergy* **13**, 427–432

Edwards, R.G., Beeson, M.F. and Dewdney, J.M. (1983) Laboratory animal allergy: the measurement of airborne urinary allergens and the effects of different environmental conditions. *Lab. Animals* **17**, 235–239

El-Ansary, E.H., Tee, R.D., Gordon, D.J. and Newman Taylor, A.J. (1987) Respiratory allergy to inhaled bat guano. *Lancet* **1**, 316–318

Elkarim, M.A.A. and Onsa, S.M. (1987) Prevalence of byssinosis and respiratory symptoms among spinners in Sudanese cotton mills. *Am. J. Ind. Med.* **12**, 281–289

Elwood, P.C., Pemberton, J., Merrett, J.D., Carey, G.C.R. and McAulay, I.R. (1965) Byssinosis and other respiratory symptoms in flax workers in Northern Ireland. *Br. Med. J.* **22**, 27–37

Elwood, P.C., Thomas, H.F., Sweetnam, P.M. and Elwood, J.H. (1982) The mortality of flax workers. *Br. J. Ind. Med.* **39**, 18–22

Etkind, P.H., Odell, T.M., Canada, A.T., Shama, M.D., Finn, A.M. and Tuthill, R. (1982) The gypsy moth caterpillar: A significant new occupational and public health problem. *J. Occup. Med.* **24**, 659–662

Evans, E. and Nicholls, P.J. (1974) Histamine release by Western red cedar (*Thuja plicata*) from lung tissue *in vitro*. *Br. J. Ind. Med.* **31**, 28–30

Fabbri, L.M., Boschetto, P., Zocca, E., Milani, G., Pivirotto, F., Plebani, M. et al. (1987) Bronchoalveolar neutrophilia during late asthmatic reactions induced by toluene diisocyanate. *Am. Rev. Respir. Dis.* **136**, 36–42

Fairman, R.P., Hankinson, J., Imbus, H., Lapp, N.L. and Morgan, W.K.C. (1975) Pilot study of closing volume in byssinosis. *Br. J. Ind. Med.* **32**, 235–238

Fawcett, I.W. and Pepys, J. (1976) Allergy to a tetracycline preparation. *Clin Allergy* **6**, 301–303

Fawcett, I.W., Pepys, J. and Erooga, M.A. (1976) Asthma due to glycyl compound powder. An intermediate in production of salbutamol. *Clin. Allergy* **6**, 405–409

Fawcett, I.W., Newman Taylor, A.J. and Pepys, J. (1976) Asthma due to inhaled chemical agents, fumes from 'Multicore' soldering flux and colophony resin. *Clin. Allergy* **6**, 577–585

Fawcett, I.W., Newman Taylor, A.J. and Pepys, J. (1977) Asthma due to inhaled chemical agents – epoxy resin systems containing phthalic anhydride, trimellitic anhydride and triethylene tetramine. *Clin. Allergy* **7**, 1–14

Fawcett, I.W., Merchant, J.A., Simmonds, S.P. and Pepys, J. (1978) The effect of sodium cromoglycate, beclomethasone dipropionate and salbutamol on the ventilatory response to cotton dust in mill workers. *Br. J. Dis. Chest* **72**, 29–38

Field, G.B. and Owen, P. (1979) Respiratory function in an Australian cotton mill. *Bull. Eur. Physiopathol. Respir.* **15**, 455–468

Figley, K.D. and Rawling, F.A. (1950) Castor bean: An industrial hazard as a contaminant of green coffee dust and used burlap bags. *J. Allergy* **21**, 545–553

Fishwick, D., Fletcher, A.M., Pickering, C.A.C., Niven, R.McL. and Faragher, E.B. (1992) Lung function, bronchial reactivity, atopic status, and dust exposure in Lancashire cotton mill operatives. *Am. Rev. Respir. Dis.* **145**, 1103–1108

Flindt, M.L.H. (1969) Pulmonary disease due to inhalation of derivatives of *Bacillus subtilis* containing enzyme. *Lancet* **1**, 1177–1181

Flindt, M.L.H. (1979) Allergy to alpha-amylase and papain. *Lancet* **1**, 1407–1408

Fowler, P.B.S. (1952) Printers' asthma. *Lancet* **2**, 755–757

Fox, A.J., Tombleson, J.B.L., Watt, A. and Wilkie, A.G. (1973) A survey of respiratory disease in cotton operatives. Part II Symptoms, dust estimations and the effect of smoking habit. *Br. J. Ind. Med.* **30**, 48–53

Frankland, A.W. (1953) Locust sensitivity. *Ann. Allergy* **11**, 445–453

Frankland, A.W. and Lunn, J.A. (1965) Asthma caused by the grain weevil. *Br. J. Ind. Med.* **22**, 157–159

Gaddie, J., Legge, J.S., Friend, J.A.R. and Reid, T.M.S. (1980) Pulmonary hypersensitivity in prawn workers. *Lancet* **2**, 1350–1353

Gailhofer, G., Wilders-Truschnig, M., Smolle, J. and Ludvan, M. (1988) Asthma caused by bromelain: an occupational allergy. *Clin. Allergy* **18**, 445–450

Gandevia, B. (1964) Respiratory symptoms and ventilatory capacity in men exposed to isocyanate vapour. *Australas. Ann. Med.* **13**, 157–166

Gandevia, B. and Milne, J. (1965a) Ventilatory capacity changes on exposure to cotton dust and their relevance to byssinosis in Australia. *Br. J. Ind. Med.* **22**, 295–304

Gandevia, B. and Milne, J. (1965b) Ventilatory capacity on exposure to jute dust and the relevance of productive cough and smoking to the response. *Br. J. Ind. Med.* **22**, 187–195

Gandevia, B. and Milne, J. (1970) Occupational asthma and rhinitis due to Western red cedar (*Thuja plicata*) with special reference to bronchial reactivity. *Br. J. Ind. Med.* **27**, 235–244

Gelfand, H.H. (1943) The allergenic properties of vegetable gums. A case of asthma due to tragacanth. *J. Allergy* **14**, 203–217

Gill, C.I. (1947) Byssinosis in the cotton trade. *Br. J. Ind. Med.* **4**, 48–55

Gilson, J.C., Stott, H., Hapwood, B.E.C., Roach, S.A., McKerrow, C.B. and Schilling, R.S.F. (1962) Byssinosis: the acute effect on ventilatory capacity of dusts in cotton ginneries, cotton, sisal and jute mills. *Br. J. Ind. Med.* **19**, 9–18

Gleich, G.J., Welsh, P.W., Yunginger, J.W., Hyatt, R.E. and Catlett, J.B. (1980) Allergy to tobacco: An occupational hazard. *N. Engl. J. Med.* **302**, 607–619

Godnic-Cvar, J. and Gomzi, M. (1990) Case report of occupational asthma due to palisander wood dust and bronchoprovocation challenge by inhalation of pure wood dust from a capsule. *Am. J. Ind. Med.* **18**, 541–545

Gold, B.L., Matthews, K.P. and Burge, H.A. (1985) Occupational asthma caused by sewer flies. *Am. Rev. Respir. Dis.* **131**, 949–952

Gough, J. (1959) Occupational pulmonary disease. In *Modern Trends in Pathology*, Butterworth, London, p. 273

Graneek, B.J. (1988) Serial peak flow records and bronchial challenge tests. *Thorax* **43**, 803

Greenberg, M. (1972) Respiratory symptoms following exposure to Cedar of Lebanon (*Cedra libani*) dust. *Clin. Allergy* **2**, 219–224

Greenberg, M., Milne, J.F. and Watt, J. (1970) Survey of workers exposed to dust containing derivatives of *Bacillus subtilis*. *Br. Med. J.* **2**, 629–633

Greene, S.A. and Freedman, S. (1976) Asthma due to inhaled chemical agents: Amprolium hydrochloride. *Clin. Allergy* **6**, 105–108

Greenhow, H. (1860) Third report of the Medical Officer of the Privy Council, Sir John Simon, p. 152

Gross, M.J. (1980) Allergy to laboratory animals: epidemiologic, clinical and physiologic aspects and a trial of cromolyn in its management. *J. Allergy Clin. Immunol.* **66**, 158–165

Gun, R.T., Janckewicz, G., Esterman, A., Roder, D., Antic, R. McEvoy, R.D. and Thornton, A. (1983). Byssinosis: A cross-sectional study in an Australian textile factory. *J. Soc. Occup. Med.* **33**, 119–125

Haglind, P., Bake, B. and Belin, L. (1983). Is mild byssinosis associated with small airways disease? *Eur. J. Respir. Dis.* **64**, 449–459

Haglind, P., Lundholm, M. and Rylander, R. (1981) Prevalence of byssinosis in Swedish cotton mills. *Br. J. Ind. Med.* **38**, 138–143

Harfi, H.A. (1980) Immediate hypersensitivity to cricket. *Ann. Allergy* **44**, 162–163

Hargreave, F.E. and Pepys, J. (1972) Allergic respiratory reaction in bird fanciers provoked by allergen inhalation tests. *J. Allergy Clin. Immunol.* **50**, 157–173

Harries, M.G. and Cromwell, O. (1982) Occupational asthma caused by allergy to pigs urine. *Br. Med. J.* **284**, 867

Harries, M.G., Burge, P.S., Samson, M., Newman Taylor, J. and Pepys, J. (1979) Isocyanate asthma: respiratory symptoms due to 1,5-naphthylene diisocyanate. *Thorax* **34**, 762–766

Harries, M.G., Lacey, J., Tee, R.D., Cayley, J.R. and Newman Taylor, A.J. (1985) *Didymella exitialis* and late summer asthma. *Lancet* **1**, 1063–1066

Harries, T.R., Merchant, J.A., Kilburn, K.H. and Hamilton, J.D. (1972) Byssinosis and respiratory diseases in cotton mill workers. *J. Occup. Med.* **14**, 199–206

Harvey Gibson, R.J. (1905) Poisonous wood in shuttle making. *Annual Report of the Chief Inspector of Factories and Workshops*, 380. HMSO, London

Hay, J. (1907) Conditions of the workers employed in the manufacture of shuttles from African boxwood. *Annual Report of the Chief Inspector of Factories and Workshops*, pp. 266–268. HMSO, London

Hayes, J.P. and Newman Taylor, A.J. (1991) Bronchial asthma in a paediatric nurse caused by inhaled pancreatic extracts. *Br. J. Ind. Med.* **48**, 355–356

Hendrick, D.J. and Lane, D.J. (1977) Occupational formalin asthma. *Br. J. Ind. Med.* **34**, 11–18

Hendrick, D.J., Davies, R.J. and Pepys, J. (1976) Bakers' asthma. *Clin. Allergy* **6**, 241–250

Hendy, M.S., Beattie, B.E. and Burge, P.S. (1985) Occupational asthma due to an emulsified oil mist. *Br. J. Ind. Med.* **42**, 51–54

Henschler, D., Assman, W. and Meyer, K.O. (1962) The toxicology of toluene di-isocyanate. *Archs Toxicol.* **19**, 364–387

Hill, A.B. (1930) Sickness amongst operatives in Lancashire cotton spinning mills (with special reference to the cardroom). *Report of the Industrial Health Research Board Report*, No. 59. HMSO, London

Hinojosa, M., Moneo, I., Dominguez, J., Delgado, E., Losada, E. and Alcover, R. (1984) Asthma caused by African maple (*Triplochiton scheroxylon*) wood dust. *J. Allergy Clin. Immunol.* **74**, 782–786

Hinojosa, M., Losada, E., Moneo, I., Dominguez, J., Carrillo, T. and Sanchez-Cano, M. (1986) Occupational asthma caused by African maple (Obeche) and Ramin: evidence of cross reactivity between these two woods. *Clin. Allergy* **16**(2), 145–153

Hitchcock, M., Piscitelli, D.M. and Bouhuys, A. (1973) Histamine release from human lung by a component of cotton bracts and by compound 48/80. *Archs Environ. Health* **26**, 177–182

Hodgson, J.T. and Jones, R.D. (1990) Mortality of workers in the British Cotton Industry in 1968–84. *Scand. J. Environ. Health* **16**, 113–120

Holt, P.G., Holt, B.J., Beijer, L. and Rylander, R. (1983) Platelet serotonin release by human polymorphonuclear leukocytes stimulated by cotton dust bacteria. *Clin. Expl Immunol.* **51**, 185–190

Honeybourne, D. and Pickering, C.A.C. (1986) Physiological evidence that emphysema is not a feature of byssinosis but is due to concomitant cigarette smoking. *Thorax* **41**, 6–11

Honeybourne, D., Finnegan, M.J. and Pickering, C.A.C. (1985) Does atopy matter in byssinosis? In *New Light on Byssinosis*, MRC Epidemiology Unit, Cardiff, pp. 57–60

Howe, W., Venables, K.M., Topping, M.D., Dalley, M.B., Hawkins, E.R., Law, S.J. and Newman Taylor, A.J. (1983) Tetrachlorophthalic anhydride asthma: evidence for specific IgE antibody. *J. Allergy Clin. Immunol.* **71**, 5–11

Howie, A.D., Boyd, G., and Moran, F. (1976) Pulmonary hypersensitivity to Ramin (*Gonystylus bancanus*). *Thorax* **31**, 585–587

Hunter, D., Milton, R. and Perry, K.M.A. (1945) Asthma caused by the complex salts of platinum. *Br. J. Ind. Med.* **2**, 92–98

Imbus, H.R. and Suh, M.W. (1973) Byssinosis: a study of 10, 133 textile workers. *Archs. Environ. Health* **26**, 183–191

Imbus, H.R. and Suh, M.W. (1974) Steaming of cotton to prevent byssinosis – a plant study. *Br. J. Ind. Med.* **31**, 209–219

Ingram, C.G., Jeffrey, I.G., Symington, I.S. and Cuthbert, O.D. (1979) Bronchial provocation studies in farmers allergic to storage mites. *Lancet* **2**, 1330–1332

Introna, F. (1966) L'asthma bronchiale allergica comemaletta professionale. *Min. Med.* **86**, 176–181

Iyo, T., Kohmoto, K., Katsutan, T. et al (1980) Hoya (sea squirt) asthma. In *Occupational Asthma* (ed. R.C.A. Frazier) Van Nostrand Reinhold, New York, pp. 209–229

Jamison, J.P. and Lowry, R.C. (1986) Bronchial challege of normal subjects with the endotoxin of *Enterobacter agglomerans* isolated from cotton dust. *Br. J. Ind. Med.* **43**, 327–331

Johnson, A., Chan-Yeung, M., MacLean, L., Atkins, E., Dybuncio, A., Cheng, F. and Enaison, D. (1985) Respiratory abnormalities among workers in an iron and steel foundry. *Br. J. Ind. Med.* **42**, 94–100

Johnston, T.G., Cazort, A.G., Marvin, H.N., Pringle, R.B. and Sheldon, J.M. (1951) Bronchial asthma, urticaria and allergic rhinitis from tannic acid. *J. Allergy* **22**, 494–499

Jones, R.N., Carr, J., Glindmeyer, H., Diem, J. and Weill, H. (1977) Respiratory health and dust levels in cotton-seed mills. *Thorax* **32**, 281–286

Jones, R.N., Diem, J.E., Glindmeyer, H. Dharmarajan, V., Hammad, Y-Y., Carr, J. and Weill, H. (1979) Mill effect and dose–response relationships in byssinosis. *Br. J. Ind. Med.* **36**, 305–313

Jones, R.N., Butcher, B.T., Hammond, Y.Y., Diem, J.E., Glindmeyer III, H.W., Lehrer, S.B., Hughes, J.M. and Weill, H. (1980) Interaction of atopy and exposure to cotton dust in the bronchoconstrictor response. *Br. J. Ind. Med.* **37**, 141–146

Joules, H. (1952) Asthma from sensitisation to chromium. *Lancet* **2**, 182–183

Juniper, C.P., How, M.J., Goodwin, B.F.J. and Kinshott, A.K. (1977) *Bacillus subtilis* enzymes: a seven year clinical epidemiological and immunological study of an industrial allergen. *J. Soc. Occup. Med.* **27**, 32

Kamat, S.R., Tskar, S.P., Tyer, E.R., Naik, M. and Kamat, G.R. (1979) Discrimination between byssinosis and chronic bronchitis in cotton mill workers by serum immunoglobulin patterns. *J. Soc. Occup. Med.* **29**, 102–106

Kammermeyer, J.K. and Mathews, K.P. (1973) Hypersensitivity to phenylglycine acid chloride. *J. Allergy Clin. Immunol.* **52**, 73–84

Kay, J.P. (1831) Observations and experiments concerning molecular irritation of the lungs as one source of tubercular consumption; and on spinner's phthisis. *North Engl. Med. Surg. J.* **1**, 348–363

Kennedy, S.M., Christiani, D.C., Eisen, E.A., Wegman, D.H., Greaves, I.A., Olenchock, S.A., Ye, T-T. and Lu, P-L. (1987) Cotton dust and endotoxin exposure–response relationships in cotton textile workers. *Am. Rev. Respir. Dis.* **135**, 194–200

Kern, R.A. (1939) Asthma and allergic rhinitis due to sensitisation to phthalic anhydride. *J. Allergy* **10**, 164–165

Keskinen, H., Kalliomaki, P-L. and Alanko, K. (1980) Occupational asthma due to stainless steel welding fumes. *Clin. Allergy* **10**, 151–159

Keskinen, H. (1983) Epidemiology of occupational lung diseases: Asthma and allergic alveolitis. In: *The XIth International Congress of Allergology and Clinical Immunology: Proceedings of Invited Symposia* (eds J.W. Kerr and M.A. Ganderton), Macmillan Press, London, pp. 403–447

Kobayashi, S. (1974) Occupational asthma due to inhalation of pharmacological dusts and other chemical agents with some reference to other occupational asthma in Japan. In: *Allergology* (eds Y. Yamamura et al.), Excerpta Medica, Amsterdam, pp. 124–132

Koskela, R.S., Klockars, M. and Jarvinen, E. (1990) Mortality and disability amongst cotton mill workers. *Br. J. Ind. Med.* **48**, 143–144

Lachance, P., Cartier, A., Dolovich, J. and Malo, J.L. (1988) Occupational asthma from reactivity to an alkaline hydrolysis derivative of gluten. *J. Allergy Clin. Immunol.* **81**, 385–390

Lam, S. and Chan-Yeung M. (1980) Ethylenediamine induced asthma. *Am. Rev. Respir. Dis.* **121**, 151–155

Landsteiner, K. and van der Scheer, J. (1936) On cross reactions of immune sera to azoprotein. *J. Expl Med.* **63**, 325

Lehrer, S.B., Kerr, R.M. and Salvaggio, J.E. (1978) Extraction and analysis of coffee bean allergens. *Clin. Allergy* **218**, 217–226

Losada, E., Hinojosa, M., Moneo, I., Dominguez, J., Gomez, M.L.D. and Ibanex, M.D. (1986) Occupational asthma caused by cellulase. *J. Allergy Clin. Immunol.* **77**, 639

Lozewicz, S., Assoufi, B.K., Hawkins, R. and Newman Taylor, A.J. (1987) Outcome of asthma induced by isocyanate. *Br. J. Dis. Chest* **81**, 14–22

Lu, P., Christiani, D.C., Ye, T., Shi, N., Gong, Z., Dai, H., Zhang, W., Huang, J. and Liu, M. (1987) The study of byssinosis in China: A comprehensive report *Am. J. Ind. Med.* **12**, 743–753

Luczynska, C.M. and Topping, M.D. (1986) Specific IgE antibodies to reactive dye–albumin conjugates. *J. Immunol. Methods* **95**, 177–186

Luczynska, C., Marshall, P.E., Scarisbrick, D.A. and Topping, M.D. (1984) Occupational allergy due to inhalation of ipecacuanha dust. *Clin. Allergy* **14**, 169–175

Luo, J.C.J., Nelson, K.G. and Fischbein, A. (1990) Persistent reactive airways dysfunction syndrome after exposure to toluene di-isocyanate. *Br. J. Ind. Med.* **47**, 239–241

Lutsky, I., Teichtahl, H. and Bar-Sela, S. (1984) Occupational asthma due to poultry mites. *J. Allergy Clin. Immunol.* **73**, 56–60

Maccia, C.A., Bernstein, I.L., Emmett, E.A. and Brookes, S.S.M. (1976) In vitro demonstration of specific IgE in phthalic anhydride sensitivity. *Am. Rev. Respir. Dis.* **113**, 701–704

McConnell, L.H., Fink, J.N., Schlueter, D.P. and Schmidt, M.G. (1973) Asthma due to nickel sensitivity. *Ann. Intern. Med.* **78**, 888–890

McDermott, M., Skidmore, J.W. and Edwards, J. (1971) The acute physiological, immunological and pharmacological effects of inhaled cotton dust in normal subjects. In: *International Conference on Respiratory Disease of Textile Workers,* Alicante, Spain, 1968, pp. 133–136

McKerrow, C.B. and Molyneux, M.K.B. (1971) The influence of previous dust exposure on the acute respiratory effects of cotton dust inhalation. In *International Conference on Respiratory Diseases in Textile Workers*, Alicante, Spain, 1968, pp. 95–101

McKerrow, C.B., McDermott, M., Gilson, J.C. and Schilling, R.S.F. (1958) Respiratory function during the day in cotton workers: a study in byssinosis. *Br. J. Ind. Med.* **15**, 75–83

Mackay, R.T. and Brooks, S.M. (1983) Effective toluene diisocyanate on beta-adrenergic receptor function. *Am. Rev. Respir. Dis.* **128**, 150–153

Maestrelli, P., Marcer, G., and Dal Vecchio, L.D. (1987) Occupational asthma due to ebony wood (*Diospyros crassiflora*) dust. *Ann. Allergy* **59**, 347–349

Mair, A., Smith, D.H., Wilson, W.A. and Lockhart, W. (1960) Dust disease in Dundee textile workers. An investigation into chronic respiratory disease in jute and flax industries. *Br. J. Ind. Med.* **17**, 272–278

Malo, J.L. and Cartier, A. (1987) Occupational asthma due to fumes of galvanized metal. *Chest* **92**, 375–377

Malo, J.L. and Cartier, A. (1989) Occupational asthma caused by exposure to ash wood dust (*Fraxinus americana*). *Eur. Respir. J.* **2**, 385–387

Malo, J.L. and Zeiss, C.R. (1982) Occupational hypersensitivity pneumonitis after exposure to diphenylmethane diisocyanate. *Am. Rev. Respir. Dis.* **125**, 113–116

Malo, J.L., Gagnon, G. and Cartier, A. (1984) Occupational asthma due to heated freon. *Thorax* **39**, 628–629

Malo, J.L., Pineau, L. and Cartier, A. (1985) Occupational asthma due to azobisformamide. *Clin. Allergy* **15**, 261–264

Malo, J.L., Cartier, A., Doepner, M., Nieboer, E., Evans, S. and Dolovitch, J. (1982) Occupational asthma caused by nickel sulphate. *J. Allergy Clin. Immunol.* **69**, 55–59

Malo, J.L., Ouimet, G., Cartier, A., Lebitz, D. and Zeiss, C.R. (1983) Combined alveolitis and asthma due to hexamethylene diisocyanate (HDI), with demonstration of crossed respiratory and immunologic reactivities to diphenylmethane (MDI). *J. Allergy Clin. Immunol.* **72**, 413–419

Malo, J.L., Cartier, A., Ghezzo, H., Lefrance, M., McCants, M. and Lehrer, S.B. (1988) Patterns of improvement in spirometry, bronchial hyper-responsiveness, and specific IgE antibody levels after cessation of exposure in occupational asthma caused by snow crab processing. *Am. Rev. Respir. Dis.* **138**, 807–812

Mareska, J. and Heyman, J. (1845). Enquête sur le travail et la condition physique et morale des ouvriers employes dans les manufactures de coton, à Gand. *Ann. Soc. Med. Gand.* **16.11**, 5, 199

Massoud, A. and Taylor, G. (1964) Byssinosis antibody to cotton antigens in normal subjects and in cotton card-room workers. *Lancet* **2**, 607–610

Massoud, A., Taylor, G. and Lucas, F. (1971) Bronchial challenge with cotton plant antigen in byssinosis. *International Conference on Respiratory Diseases in Textile Workers.* Alicante, Spain, 1968, pp. 124–132

Massoud, A.E., Altounyan, R.E.C., Howell, J.B.L. and Lane, R.E. (1967) Effects of histamine aerosol in byssinotic subjects. *Br. J. Ind. Med.* **24**, 38–40

Menon, M.P.S. and Das, A.K. (1977) Tetracycline asthma. *Clin. Allergy* **7**, 285–290

Merchant, J.A. and Ortmeyer, C. (1981) Mortality of employees of two cotton mills in North Carolina. *Chest* **79S**, 6S–11S

Merchant, J.A., Kilburn, K.H., O'Fallon, W.M., Hamilton, J.D., and Lumsden, J.C. (1972) Byssinosis and chronic bronchitis among cotton textile workers. *Ann. Intern. Med.* **76**, 423–433

Merchant, J.A., Lumsden, J.C., Kilburn, K.H., O'Fallon, W.M., Ujda, J.R., Germino, V.H. and Hamilton, J.D. (1973a) An industrial study of the biological effects of cotton dust and cigarette smoke exposure. *J. Occup. Med.* **15**, 212–221

Merchant, J.A., Lumsden, J.C., Kilburn, K.H., Germino, V.H., Hamilton, J.D., Lynn, W.S., Byrd, H. and Baucom, D. (1973b) Pre-processing cotton to prevent byssinosis. *Br. J. Ind. Med.* **30**, 237–247

Merchant, J.A., Halprin, G.M., Hudson, A.R., Kilburn, K.H., McKenzie, W.M., Bermanzohn, P., Hurst, D.J., Hamilton, H.D. and Germino, V.H. (1974a). Evaluation before and after exposure – the pattern of physiological response to cotton dust. *Ann NY Acad. Sci.* **221**, 38–43

Merchant, J.A., Lumsden, J.C., Kilburn, K.H., O'Fallon, W.M., Copeland, K., Germino, V.H., McKenzie, W.N., Baucom, D., Curran, P. and Stilman, J. (1974b) Intervention studies of cotton steaming to reduce biological effects of cotton dust. *Br. J. Ind. Med.* **31**, 261–274

Meredith, S.K., Taylor, V.M. and McDonald, J.C. (1991) Occupational respiratory disease in the United Kingdom 1989: A report by the British Thoracic Society and the Society of Occupational Medicine by the SWORD project group. *Br. J. Ind. Med.* **48**, 292–298

Middleton, D., Logan, J.S., Magennis, B.P. and Nelson, S.D. (1979) HLA frequencies in flax byssinosis patients. *Br. J. Ind. Med.* **36**, 123–126

Milne, J. and Brandt, S. (1975) Occupational asthma after inhalation of dust of the proteolytic enzyme papain. *Br. J. Ind. Med.* **32**, 302–307

Mitchell, C.A. and Gandevia, B. (1971) Respiratory symptoms and skin reactivity in workers exposed to proteolytic enzymes in the detergent industry. *Am. Rev. Respir. Dis.* **104**, 1–12

Moller, D.R., Gallagher, J.S., Bernstein, D.I., Wilcox, T.G., Burroughs, H.E. and Bernstein, I.L. (1985) Detection of IgE mediated respiratory sensitisation in workers exposed to hexahydrophthalic anhydride. *J. Allergy Clin. Immunol.* **75**, 663–672

Morgan, P.G.M. and Ong, S.G. (1981) First report of byssinosis in Hong Kong. *Br. J. Ind. Med.* **38**, 290–292

Molyneux, M.K.B. and Berry, G. (1971) The correlation of cotton dust exposure with prevalence of respiratory symptoms. In: *International Conference of Respiratory Diseases in Textile Workers (Byssinosis)*, Alicante, Spain, 1968, pp. 177–183

Molyneux, M.K.B. and Tombleson, J.B.L. (1970) An epidemiological study of respiratory symptoms in Lancashire mills, 1963–1966. *Br. J. Ind. Med.* **27**, 225–234

Morey, P.R. (1979) Botanically what is raw cotton dust? *Am. Ind. Hyg. Assoc. J.* **40**, 702–708

Mundie, T.G., Boackle, R.J. and Ainsworth, S.K. (1983) In vitro alternative and classical activation of complement by extracts of cotton mill dust: a possible mechanism in the pathogenesis of byssinosis. *Environ. Res.* **32**, 47–56

Mundie, T.G., Pilia, P.A. and Ainsworth, S.K. (1985) Byssinosis: Serum immunoglobulin and complement concentrations in cotton mill workers. *Archs Environ. Health* **40**, 326–329

Mundie, T.G., Whitener, C. and Ainsworth, S.K. (1985) Byssinosis: Release of prostaglandins, thromboxane, and 5-hydroxytryptamine in bronchopulmonary lavage fluid after inhalation of cotton dust extracts. *Am. J. Pathol.* **118**, 123–133

Mundie, T.G., Osguthorpe, J.D., Martin, C. and Ainsworth, S.K. (1985) An investigation of atopy in byssinosis. *Immunol. Allergy Pract.* **2**, 367–372

Musk, A.W., Venables, K.M., Crook, B., Nunn, A.J., Hawkins, R., Crook, G.D.W., Graneek, B.J., Tee, R.D., Farrer, N., Johnson, D.A., Gordon, D.J., Darbyshire, J.H. and Newman Taylor, A.J. (1989) Respiratory symptoms, lung function and sensitisation to flour in a British bakery. *Br. J. Ind. Med.* **46**, 636–642

Mustafa, K.Y., Lakha, A.S., Milla, M.H. and Dahoma, U. (1978) Byssinosis, respiratory symptoms and spirometric lung function tests in Tanzanian sisal workers. *Br. J. Ind. Med.* **35**, 123–128

Nagy, L. and Orosz, M. (1984) Occupational asthma due to hexachlorophene. *Thorax* **39**, 630–631

Neal, P.A., Schneiter, R. and Caminita, B.H. (1942) Report on acute illness among rural mattress makers using low grade stained cotton. *J. Am. Med. Assoc.* **119**, 1074–1082

Newhouse, M.L., Tagg, B., Pocott, S.J. and McEwan, A.C. (1970) An epidemiological study of workers producing enzyme washing powders. *Lancet* **1**, 689–693

Newman Taylor, A.J. and Davies, R.J. (1981) Inhalation challenge testing. In *Occupational Lung Diseases: Research Approach and Methods* (eds H. Weill and M. Turner-Warwick), Marcel Dekker, New York, pp. 143–167

Newman Taylor, A.J., Longbottom, J.L. and Pepys, J. (1977)

Respiratory allergy to urine proteins of rats and mice. *Lancet* **2**, 847–849

Newman Taylor, A.J., Davies, R.J., Hendrick, D.J. and Pepys, J. (1979) Recurrent nocturnal asthmatic reactions to bronchial provocation tests. *Clin. Allergy* **9**, 213–219

Newman Taylor, A.J., Venables, K.M., Durham, S.R., Graneek, B.J. and Topping, M.D. (1987) Acid anhydrides and asthma. *Int. Archs Allergy Appl. Immunol.* **82**, 435–439

Nicholls, P.J. (1976) Release of histamine from lung tissue *in vitro* by dimethylhydantoinformaldehyde resin and polyvinyl pyrrolidone. *Br. J. Ind. Med.* **33**, 127–129

Nicholls, P.J. and Skidmore, J.W. (1975) Comparative study of the smooth muscle contractor activity of airborne dusts and of dustiness in cotton flax and jute mills. *Br. J. Ind. Med.* **32**, 289–296

Nicholls, P.J., Nicholls, G.R. and Bouhuys, A. (1966) Histamine release by compound 48/80 and textile dusts from lung tissue *in vitro*. In *Inhaled Particles and Vapours, II*, Pergamon, Oxford, New York, pp. 69–74

Nordman, H., Keskinen, H. and Tuppuranainen, M. (1985) Formaldehyde asthma – rare or overlooked? *J. Allergy Clin. Immunol.* **75**, 91–99

Novey, J.S., Habib, M. and Wells, I.D. (1983) Asthma and IgE antibodies induced by chromium and nickel salts. *J. Allergy Clin. Immunol.* **72**, 407–412

Noweir, M.H., Abdel-Kader, H.M. and Omran, F. (1984) Role of histamine in the aetiology of byssinosis. Blood histamine concentrations in workers exposed to cotton and flax dusts. *Br. J. Ind. Med.* **41**, 203–208

Noweir, M.H., Amine, E.K. and Osman, H.A. (1975) Epidemiological investigations of the role of family susceptibility and occupational and family histories in the development of byssinosis among workers exposed to flax dusts. *Br. J. Ind. Med.* **32**, 297–301

Noweir, M.H., Noweir, K.H., Osman, H.A. and Moselhi, M. (1984) An environmental and medical study of byssinosis and other respiratory conditions in the cotton textile industry in Egypt. *Am. J. Ind. Med.* **6**, 173–183

O'Brien, I.M., Harries, M.G., Burge, P.S. and Pepys, J. (1979a) Toluene diisocyanate induced asthma. 1. Reactions to TDI, MDI, HDI and histamine. *Clin. Allergy* **9**, 1–6

O'Brien, I.M., Newman Taylor, A.J., Burge, P.S., Harries, M.G., Fawcett, I.A.W. and Pepys, J. (1979b) Toluene diisocyanate induced asthma. 2. Inhalation challenge tests and bronchial reactivity studies. *Clin. Allergy* **9**, 7–15

Oliver, T. (1902) *Dangerous Trades*, Murray, London, p.273

Ordman, B. (1949) Wood dust as an inhalant allergen. Bronchial asthma caused by kejaat wood (*Pterocarpus angolensis*). *S. Afr. Med. J.* **23**, 973–976

Paggiaro, P.L., Cantalupi, R., Filieri, M., Loi, A.M., Parlanti, A., Toma, G. and Baschieri, L. (1981) Bronchial asthma due to inhaled wood dust: *Tanganyika aningre*. *Clin. Allergy* **111**, 605–610

Paggiaro, P.L., Loy, A.M., Rossi, O., Ferrante, B., Pardi, F., Roselli, M.G. and Bascheiri, L. (1984) Follow up study of patients with respiratory disease due to toluene diisocyanate (TDI) *Clin. Allergy* **14**, 463–469

Paggiaro, P., Bacci, E., Paoletti, P., Bernard, P., Dente, F.L., Marchetti, G., Talini, D., Menconi, G.F. and Geantini, C. (1990) Bronchoalveolar lavage and morphology of the airways after cessation of exposure in asthmatic subjects sensitised to toluene diisocyanate. *Chest* **98**, 536–542

Parikh, J.R., Chatterjee, B.B., Mohan Rao, N. and Bhagia, L.J. (1986) The clinical manifestations of byssinosis in Indian textile workers. *J. Soc. Occup. Med.* **36**, 24–28

Patissier, P. (1822) *Traité des Maladies des Artisands*, Paris

Pepys, J. (1973) Immunopathology of allergic lung disease. *Clin. Allergy* **3**, 1–22

Pepys, J. Hutchcroft, B.J. and Breslin, A.B.X. (1976) Asthma due to inhaled chemical agents – persulphate salts and henna in hairdressing. *Clin. Allergy* **2**, 399–404

Pepys, J., Pickering, C.A.C. and Hughes, E.G. (1972) Asthma due to inhaled chemical agents – complex salts of platinum. *Clin. Allergy* **2**, 391–396

Pepys, J., Pickering, C.A.C. and Loudon, H.W.G. (1972) Asthma due to inhaled chemical agents – piperazine dihydrochloride. *Clin. Allergy* **2**, 189–196

Pepys, J., Hargreaves, F.E., Longbottom, J.L. and Faux, J. (1969) Allergic reactions of the lungs to enzymes of *Bacillus subtilis*. *Lancet* **1**, 1181–1184

Pepys, J., Pickering, C.A.C., Breslin, A.B.X. and Terry, D.J. (1972) Asthma due to inhaled chemical agents – toluene diisocyanate. *Clin. Allergy* **2**, 225–236

Pepys, J., Wells, E.D., D'Souza, M. and Greenburg, M. (1973) Clinical and immunological responses to enzymes of *Bacillus subtilis* in factory workers and consumers. *Clin. Allergy* **3**, 143–160

Pepys, J., Parish, W.E., Cromwell, O. and Hughes, E.G. (1979) Passive transfer in man and the monkey of type I allergy due to heat labile and heat stable antibody to complex salts of platinum. *Clin. Allergy* **9**, 99–108

Pepys, J., Mitchell, J., Hawkins, R. and Malo, J.L. (1985) A longitudinal study of possible allergy to detergent enzymes. *Clin. Allergy* **15**, 101–115

Perks, W.H., Burge, P.S., Rehahn, M. and Green, M. (1979) Work related respiratory disease in employees leaving an electronics factory. *Thorax* **34**, 19–22

Pernis, B., Vigliani, E.C., Cavagna, G. and Finulli, M. (1961) The role of bacterial endotoxins in occupational diseases caused by inhaling vegetable dusts. *Br. J. Ind. Med.* **18**, 120–129

Peto, R., Speizer, F.E., Cochrane, A.L., Moore, F., Fletcher, C.M., Tinker, C.M., Higgins, I.T.T., Gray, R.G., Richards, S.M., Gilliland, J. and Norman-Smith, B. (1983) The relevance in adults of airflow obstruction but not of mucus hypersection, to mortality from chronic lung disease: 20 year results from prospective surveys. *Am. Rev. Respir. Dis.* **128**, 491–500

Petronio, L. and Bovenzi, M. (1983) Byssinosis and serum IgE concentrations in textile workers in an Italian cotton mill. *Br. J. Ind. Med.* **40**, 39–44

Pickering, C.A.C. (1989) What is byssinosis? *Proceedings of the Thirteenth Cotton Dust Research Conference*, Beltwide Cotton Research Conference, Nashville, pp. 156–157

Pickering, C.A.C., Batten, J.C. and Pepys, J. (1972) Asthma due to inhaled wood dusts: Western red cedar and iroko. *Clin. Allergy* **2**, 213–218

Pickering, C.A.C., Bainbridge, D., Birtwistle, I.H. and Griffiths, D.L. (1986) Occupational asthma due to methyl methacrylate in an orthopaedic theatre sister. *Br. Med. J.* **292**, 1362–1363

Pilat, L., Popa, V. and Tecoulesco, D. (1967) L'allergie professionelle aux hormone protéiques dans l'industrie pharmaceutique. *Rev. fr. Allergie* **7**, 153–160

Popa, V., Gavrilescu, N., Preda, N., Teculescu, D., Plecias, M. and Cîrstea, M. (1969) An investigation of allergy in byssinosis: sensitisation to cotton, hemp, flax and jute antigens. *Br. J. Ind. Med.* **26**, 101–108

Pratt, P.C., Vollmer, R.T. and Miller, J.A. (1980) Epidemiology of pulmonary lesions in nontextile and cotton textile workers: a retrospective autopsy analysis. *Archs Environ. Med.* **35**, 133–137

Price, J.A. and Longbottom, J.L. (1987) Allergy to mice; 1. Identification of two major mouse allergens (A1 and A3) and investigation of their possible origin. *Clin. Allergy* **17**, 43–53

Price, J.A. and Longbottom, J.L. (1988) ELISA method for measurement of airborne levels of major laboratory animal allergens. *Clin. Allergy* **18**, 95–107

Prichard, M.G., Ryan, G. and Musk, A.W. (1984) Wheat flour sensitisation and airway disease in urban bakers. *Br. J. Ind. Med.* **81**, 450–454

Prichard, M.G., Ryan, G., Walsh, B.J. and Musk, A.W. (1985) Skin test and RAST responses to wheat and common allergens and respiratory disease in bakers. *Clin. Allergy* **15**, 203–210

Promisloff, R.A., Lenchner, G.S. and Cichelli, A.V. (1990) Reactive airways dysfunction syndrome in three police officers following a road side chemical spill. *Chest* **98**, 928–929

Raghuprasad, P.K., Brooks, S.M., Litwin, A., Edwards, J.J., Bernstein, I.L. and Gallagher, J. (1980) Quillaja bark (soap bark)-induced asthma. *J. Allergy Clin. Immunol.* **65**, 285–287

Riedel, F., Kramer, M., Sheibenbogen, C. and Rieger, C.H.L. (1988) Effects of SO_2 exposure on allergic sensitisation in the guinea pig. *J. Allergy Clin. Immunol.* **82**, 527–534

Roach, S.A. and Schilling, R.S.F. (1960) A clinical and environmental study of byssinosis in the Lancashire cotton industry. *Br. J. Ind. Med.* **17**, 1–9

Roberts, A.E. (1951) Platinosis. A five year study of the effects of soluble salts on employees in a platinum laboratory and refinery. *Archs Ind. Hyg.* **4**, 549

Rohrbach, M.S., Rolstad, R.A., Tracy, P.B. and Russell, J.A. (1984) Platelet 5-hydroxytryptamine release and aggregation promoted by cotton bracts tannin. *J. Lab. Clin. Med.* **103**, 152–156

Rooke, G.B. (1981) The pathology of byssinosis. *Chest* **79**(4), 675–715

Rüttner, J.R., Spycher, M.A. and Engeler, M-L. (1968) Pulmonary fibrosis induced by cotton fibre inhalation. *Pathol. Microbiol.* **32**, 1–14

Rylander, R. and Lundholm, M. (1978) Bacterial contamination of cotton and cotton dust and effects on the lung. *Br. J. Ind. Med.* **35**, 204–207

Rylander, R. and Snella, M-C. (1976) Acute inhalation toxicity of cotton plant dusts. *Br. J. Ind. Med.* **33**, 175–180

Schachter, E.N., Buck, M.G., Merrill, W.W., Askenase, P. and Witek, T.J. (1985) Skin testing with an aqueous extract of cotton bract. *J. Allergy Clin. Immunol.* **76**, 481–487

Salvato, G. (1961) Mast cells in bronchial connective tissue of man; their modifications in asthma and after treatment with the histamine liberator 48/80. *Int. Archs Allergy Appl. Immunol.* **18**, 348–358

Schilling, R.S.F. (1950) Byssinosis. *Br. Med. Bull.* **7**, 52–56

Schilling, R.S.F. (1956) Byssinosis in cotton and other textile workers. *Lancet* **2**, 261–265

Schilling, R., Goodman, N. and O'Sullivan, J. (1952) Cardiovascular disease in cotton workers. Part II. A clinical study with special reference to hypertension. *Br. J. Ind. Med.* **9**, 146–156

Schilling, R.S.F., Vigliani, E.C., Lammers, B., Valić, F. and Gilson, J.C. (1963) A report on a Conference on Byssinosis. (14th International Conference on Occupational Health. Madrid, 1963). *International Congress Series.* No. 62. Excepta Medica, Amsterdam, pp. 137–144

Schlueter, D.P., Banaszak, R.F., Fink, G.N. and Barboriak, J. (1978) Occupational asthma due to tetrachlorophthalic anhydride. *J. Occup. Med.* **20**, 183–188

Schumacher, M.J., Tait, B.D. and Holmes, M.C. (1981) Allergy to murine antigens in a biological research institute. *J. Allergy Clin. Immunol.* **68**, 310–318

Sepulveda, M.J., Castellan, R.M., Hankison, J.L. and Cocke, J.B. (1984) Acute lung function response to cotton dust in atopic nonatopic individuals. *Br. J. Ind. Med.* **41**, 487–491

Silberman, D.E. and Sorrell, A.H. (1959) Allergy in fur workers with special refe rence to paraphenylenediamine. *J. Allergy* **30**, 11–18

Sherson, D., Hansen, I. and Sigsgaard, T. (1989) Occupationally related respiratory symptoms in trout-processing workers. *Allergy* **44**, 336–341

Slovak, A.J.M. (1981) Occupational asthma due to plastics blowing agent azodicarbonamide. *Thorax* **36**, 906–909

Slovak, A.J.M. and Hill, R.N. (1981) Laboratory animal allergy: A clinical survey of an exposed population. *Br. J. Ind. Med.* **38**, 38–41

Slovak, A.J.M. and Hill, R.N. (1987) Does atopy have any predictive value for laboratory animal allergy? A comparison of different concepts of atopy. *Br. J. Ind. Med.* **44**, 129–132

Smiley, J.A. (1951) The hazards of rope making. *Br. J. Ind. Med.* **8**, 265–270

Smith, D.H., Lockhart, W., Mair, A. and Wilson, W.A. (1962) Flax workers byssinosis in East Scotland. *Scott. Med. J.* **7**, 201–211

Smith, G.F., Coles, G.V., Schilling, R.S.F. and Walford, J. (1969) A study of rope workers exposed to hemp and flax. *Br. J. Ind. Med.* **26**, 109–114

Sosman, A.J., Schlueter, D.P., Fink, J.N. and Barboriak, A.J. (1969) Hypersensitivity to wood dust. *N. Engl. J. Med.* **281**, 977–980

Spieksma, F.T.M., Vooren, P.H., Kramps, J.A. and Dijkman, J.H. (1986) Respiratory allergy to laboratory fruit flies (*Drosophila melanogaster*). *J. Allergy Clin. Immunol.* **77**, 108–113

Steinberg, D.R., Bernstein, M.D., Gallagher, J.S., Arlian, L. and Bernstein, I.L. (1987) Cockroach sensitization in laboratory workers. *J. Allergy Clin. Immunol.* **80**, 586–590

Sterling, G.M. (1967) Asthma due to aluminium soldering flux. *Thorax* **22**, 533–537

Stimler, N.P., Bach, N.K., Bloor, C.M. and Hugli, T.E. (1982) Release of leukotrienes from guinea pig lung stimulated by C5a anaphylotoxin. *J. Immunol.* **128**, 2247–2252

Swanson, M.C., Agarwal, M.K., Yunginger, J.W. and Reid, C.E. (1984) Guinea pig derived allergens: clinicoimmunologic studies, characterization, airborne quantitation and size distribution. *Am. Rev. Respir. Dis.* **129**, 844–849

Szulc, E.J. (1971) The effect of working conditions in the cotton industry upon the respiratory and circulatory system. *Med. Pract.* **22**, 145–164

Takam, J. and Nemery, B. (1988) Byssinosis in a textile factory in Cameroon: a preliminary study. *Br. J. Ind. Med.* **45**, 803–809

Takiszawa, T. and Thurlbeck, W.M. (1971) Muscle and mucous gland size in the major bronchi of patients with chronic bronchitis, asthma and asthmatic bronchitis. *Am. Rev. Respir. Dis.* **104**, 331–336

Tanser, A.R., Bourke, M.P. and Blandford, A.G. (1973) Isocyanate asthma: respiratory symptoms caused by diphenyl-methane diisocyanate. *Thorax* **28**, 596–600

Taylor, G., Massoud, A.A.E. and Lucas, F. (1971) Studies in aetiology of byssinosis. *Br. J. Ind. Med.* **28**, 141–151

Tee, R.D., Gordon, D.J. and Newman Taylor, A.J. (1987) Cross-reactivity between antigens of fungal extracts studied by RAST inhibition and immunoblots technique. *J. Allergy Clin. Immunol.* **79**, 627–633

Tee, R.D., Gordon, D.J., Lacey, J., Nunn, A.J., Brown, M. and Newman Taylor, A.J (1985) Occupational allergy to the common house fly (*Musca domestica*): use of immunological response to identify atmospheric allergen. *J. Allergy Clin. Immunol.* **76**, 826–831

Tee, R.D., Gordon, D.J., Hawkins, E.R., Nunn, A.J., Lacey, J., Venables, K.M., Cooter, R.J., McCaffery, A.R. and Newman Taylor, A.J. (1988) Occupational allergy to locusts: An investigation of the sources of the allergen. *J. Allergy Clin. Immunol.* **81**, 517–525

Textile Research Institute (1978) Chemical composition of cotton dust and its relation to byssinosis: a review of the literature. Regulatory Technical Information Centre, T.F. Cooke, Director. Report No 1. Textile Research Institute, Box 625, Princeton, New Jersey 08540.

Thomas, H.F., Elwood, J.H. and Elwood, P.C. (1988) Byssinosis in Belfast ropeworkers: an historical note. *Ann. Occup. Hyg.* **32**, 249–251

Thurlbeck, W.M. (1976) *Chronic Airflow Obstruction in Lung Disease*, Vol. V. *Major Problems in Pathology*, W.B. Saunders, Philadelphia, London, Toronto, pp. 54–55

Tiller, J.R. and Schilling, R.S.F. (1958) Respiratory function during the day in rayon workers. *Trans. Assoc. Ind Med. Offrs* **7**, 161–162

Topping, M.D., Venables, K.M., Luczynska, C.M., Howe, W. and Newman Taylor, A.J. (1986) Specificity of the human IgE response to inhaled acid anhydride. *J. Allergy Clin. Immunol.* **77**, 834–842

Tse, K.S., Chan, H. and Chan-Yeung, M. (1982) Specific IgE antibodies in workers with occupational asthma due to western red cedar. *Clin. Allergy* **12**, 249–258

Twiggs, J.T., Agarwal, M.K., Dahlberg, M.J. and Yunginer, J.W. (1982a) Immunochemical measurements of airborne mouse allergens in a laboratory animal facility. *J. Allergy Clin. Immunol.* **69**, 522–526

Twiggs, J.T., Yunginger, J.W., Agarwal, M.K. and Reed, C.E. (1982b) Occupational asthma in a florist caused by the dry plant, 'Baby's breath'. *J. Allergy. Clin. Immunol.* **69**, 474–477

Uragoda, C.G. (1970) Tea makers' asthma. *Br. J. Ind. Med.* **27**, 181–182

Uragoda, C.G. (1975) A clinical and radiographic study of coir workers. *Br. J. Ind. Med.* **32**, 66–71

Uragoda, C.G. (1977) An investigation into the health of kapok workers. *Br. J. Ind. Med.* **34**, 181–185

Valić, F. and Žuškin, E. (1971) A comparative study of respiratory function in female non-smoking cotton and jute workers. *Archs Environ. Health* **23**, 359–364

Valić, F. and Žuškin, E. (1972) Effects of different vegetable dust exposures. *Br. J. Ind. Med.* **29**, 293–297

Vallieres, M., Cockcroft, D.W., Taylor, D.M., Dolovitch, J. and Hargreave, F.E. (1977) Dimethylethanolamine induced asthma. *Am. Rev. Respir. Dis.* **115**, 867–871

van Hage-Hamsten, M., Johansson, S.G.O., Hoglund, S., Ptull, P., Wyren, A. and Zetterström, O. (1985) Storage mite allergy common in a farming population. *Clin. Allergy* **15**, 555–564

Velvart, J. (1971) Respiratory symptoms and changes in lung function workers handling hemp, flax and sisal in Czechoslovakia. In *Proceedings of the International Conference on Respiratory Disease In Textile Workers (Byssinosis)*, Alicante, Spain, 1968, pp. 55–58

Velvart, J. (1972) Schadigung der Atemwege durch Staubeinwirkung von Sisal. *Int. Arch. Arbeitsmed.* **30**, 213–222

Venables, K.M., Topping, M.D., Howe, W., Luczynska, C.M., Hawkins, R. and Newman Taylor, A.J. (1985a) Interaction of smoking and atopy in producing specific IgE antibody against a hapten protein conjugate. *Br. Med. J.* **290**, 201–204

Venables, K.M., Dally, M.B., Burge, P.S., Pickering, C.A.C. and Newman Taylor, A.J. (1985b) Occupational asthma in a steel coating plant. *Br. J. Ind. Med.* **42**, 517–524

Venables, K.M., Topping, M.D., Nunn, A.J., Howe, W. and Newman Taylor, A.J. (1987) Immunologic and functional consequences of chemical (tetrachlorophthalic anhydride) induced asthma after 4 years of avoidance of exposure. *J. Allergy Clin. Immunol.* **80**, 212–218

Venables, K.M., Tee, R.D., Hawkins, E.R., Gordon, D.J., Wale, C.J., Farrer, N.M., Lam, T.H., Baxter, P.J. and Newman Taylor, A.J. (1988) Laboratory animal allergy in a pharmaceutical company. *Br. J. Ind. Med.* **455**, 660–666

Venables, K.M., Dally, M.B., Nunn, A.J., Stevens, J.F., Stephens, S.R., Farrer, N., Hunter, J.V., Stewart, M., Hughes, E.G. and Newman Taylor, A.J. (1989a) Smoking and occupational allergy in workers in a platinum refinery. *Br. Med. J.* **299**, 939–942

Venables, K.M., Davidson, A.G., Browne, K. and Newman Taylor, A.J. (1989b) Pseudo-occupational asthma. *Thorax* **44**, 760–761

Vigliani, E.C., Parmeggiani, I. and Sassi, C. (1954) Studio de un epidemia di bronchite asmatica fra gli operati di una tessitura di cotone. *Med. Lav.* **45**, 349–378

Walsh, B.J., Wrigley, C.W., Musk, A.W. and Baldo, B.A. (1985) A comparison of the binding of IgE in the sera of bakers with bakers' asthma to soluble and insoluble wheat grain proteins. *J. Allergy Clin. Immunol.* **76**, 23-28

Warren, P., Chermick, R.M. and Tse, K.S. (1974) Hypersensitivity reactions to grain dust. *J. Allergy Clin. Immunol.* **53**, 139–149

Weill, H., Waddell, L.C. and Ziskind, M. (1971) A study of workers exposed to detergent enzymes. *J. Am. Med. Assoc.* **217**, 425–433

Weill, H., Butcher, B., Dharmarajan, V., Glindmeyer, H., Jones, R., Carr, J., O'Neill, C. and Salvaggio, J.E. (1981) Respiratory and immunologic evaluation of isocyanate exposure in a new manufacturing plant. *NIOSH Technical Report No. 81-125.* US Government Printing Office, Washington DC

Weiner, A. (1961) Bronchial asthma due to organic phosphate insecticide. *Am. Allergy* **19**, 397–401

Wakelyn, P.J. Greenblatt, G.A., Brown, D.F. and Tripp, V.W. (1976) Chemical properties of cotton dust. *Am. Ind. Hyg. Assoc. J.* **37**, 22–31

Widdicombe, J.G. (1979) Dyspnoea. *Bull. Eur. Physiopathol. Respir.* **15**, 437–440

Williams, H. (1952) Vanadium poisoning from cleaning oil fired boilers. *Br. J. Ind. Med.* **9**, 50–55

Wilson, M.R., Sekul, A., Ory, R., Salvaggio, J.E. and Lehren, S.B. (1980) Activation of the alternative complement pathway by extracts of cotton dust. *Clin. Allergy* **10**, 303–308

WHO (1983) Recommended Health-based Occupational Exposure Limits for Selected Vegetable Dusts. Report of a WHO study group. *Technical Report Series 684*

Zammit-Tabbona, M., Cherkin, M., Kijek, K., Chan, H. and Chan-Yeung, M. (1983) Asthma caused by diphenylmethane diisocyanate in foundry workers: clinical bronchoprovocation and immunologic studies. *Am. Rev. Respir. Dis.* **128**, 226–230

Zaritskala, L.P. (1979) Environmental pollution in relation to occupational lung diseases among workers of a flax mill. *Gig. Tr. Prof. Zuda* **5**, 20–23

Zeiss, C.R., Patterson, R., Pruzansky, J.J., Miller, M.M., Resonberg, M. and Lebitz, D. (1977) Trimellitic anhydride induced airways syndrome: clinical and immunologic studies. *J.*

Allergy Clin. Immunol. **60**, 96–103

Zeiss, C.R., Kanellaks, T.M., Bellone, T.D., Levitz, D., Pruzansky, J.J. and Patterson, R. (1980) Immunoglobulin E mediated asthma and hypersensitivity pneumonitis with precipitating antihapten antibodies due to diphenylmethane diisocyanates (MDI) exposure. *J. Allergy Clin. Immunol.* **65**, 347–352

Zeiss, C.R., Wolkonsky, P., Chacon, R. and Tuntland, P. (1983) Syndromes in workers exposed to trimellitic anhydride ash, a longitudinal, clinical and immunologic study. *Ann. Intern. Med.* **98**, 8–12

Zetterström, O. (1977) Challenge and exposure test reactions to enzyme detergents in subjects sensitised to subtilisin. *Clin. Allergy* **7**, 355–363

Zetterström, O. and Wide, L. (1974) IgE antibodies and skin test reactions to a detergent enzyme in Swedish consumers. *Clin.*

Allergy **4**, 273–280

Zetterström, O., Osterman, K., McHardo, L. and Johansson, S.G.O. (1981) Another smoking hazard: raised serum IgE concentration and increased risk of occupational allergy. *Br. Med. J.* **283**, 1215–1217

Zetterström, O., Nordvall, S.L., Björksten, B., Ahlstedt, S. and Stelander, M. (1985) Increased IgE antibody responses in rats exposed to tobacco smoke. *J. Allergy Clin. Immunol.* **75**, 594–598

Žuškin, E. and Valić, F. (1972) Respiratory symptoms and ventilatory function changes in relation to length of exposure to cotton dust. *Thorax* **27**, 454–458

Žuškin, E., Valić, F. and Bouhuys, A. (1976) Byssinosis and airway responses due to exposure to textile dust. *Lung* **154**, 17–24

Žuškin, E. Valíc, F., Butkovíc, D. and Bouhuys, S. (1975) Lung function in textile workers. *Br. J. Ind. Med.* **32**, 283–288

22

Infectious diseases and zoonoses

Mark Woodhead

These are discussed only briefly with the intention of concentrating on their occupational significance, diagnostic difficulties and prevention. Hence, the clinical, pathological, bacteriological, mycological and treatment details are brief, because this information is fully presented in specialized standard works.

Bacterial infections

Tuberculosis

The unusual susceptibility of patients with silicosis to develop tuberculosis is referred to in Chapter 12.

Although the prevalence of pulmonary tuberculosis has, in general, fallen dramatically since the 1950s, it is an occasional occupational hazard in doctors, nurses, and laboratory and pathology technicians, and is fairly common among seafarers (Oliver, 1979). It is, however, difficult to make an accurate assessment of the population at risk. Guidelines for the protection of health service staff are available (British Thoracic Society, 1990). All tuberculin-negative staff in these categories should be inoculated with BCG (bacillus of Calmette–Guérin). Seafarers under treatment are not normally permitted to serve at sea.

'Opportunist' mycobacteria

These organisms do not appear to cause occupationally related disease in the absence of pre-exist-

ing silicosis, coal pneumoconiosis or other forms of fibrotic pneumoconiosis (see Chapters 5, 12 and 13).

Legionnaires' disease

Legionnaires' disease is the term given to the spectrum of diseases caused by bacteria of the genus *Legionella*. This includes asymptomatic seroconversion, the 'influenza-like' Pontiac fever (Glick et al., 1978) and the classic pneumonic illness (Tsai et al., 1979). More than 25 different species of *Legionella* are now recognized, at least 15 of which have been documented as causing disease in human beings (Woodhead, 1988). The pattern of illness is similar whichever species of *Legionella* is involved. *L. pneumophila* serogroup I accounts for over 90 per cent of human infections. Legionella bacteria are widespread in the environment, in both temperate (Fliermans et al., 1979, 1981) and tropical climates (Ortiz-Roque and Hazen, 1987). Fresh water is essential for the existence of the organism where the presence of blue–green algae (Tison et al., 1980) and amoebae (Rowbotham, 1980; Wadowsky et al., 1988; Fields et al., 1989) may be important for its growth and replication. Optimal growth occurs only over a critical temperature range (25 to 42°C).

About 200 cases of Legionnaires' disease are reported each year in England, Wales and Ireland, of which nearly half are acquired abroad (PHLS, Communicable Disease Surveillance Centre, unpublished data). Pneumonia is most commonly reported with only 8 of 232 cases in 1989 being due to Pontiac fever (PHLS, Communicable Disease Surveillance Centre, unpublished data). Most cases are sporadic and are acquired in the community. Case clusters or epidemics account for only one-quarter of cases in the UK (PHLS, Communicable Disease Surveillance Centre, 1988).

Disease in human beings is a result of the inhalation of an aerosol contaminated by the bacterium. The development of clinical illness relates to the virulence of the particular organism, the inhaled dose of the organism and host factors. The reasons why some individuals develop Pontiac fever and others pneumonia is not known, but both may occur in different individuals following exposure to the same source (Girod et al., 1982; Mitchell et al., 1990). For the majority of cases of sporadic community-acquired Legionnaires' disease, the source of the infection is not known. Inhalation of environmental organisms and possibly contamination of domestic water supplies (Arnow, Weil and Para, 1985; Stout, Yu and Muraca, 1987) are the likely sources.

Buildings and industrial settings that incorporate water-containing systems provide a suitable environment for growth of the organism. Most hotels and hospitals in Britain harbour the organism (Bartlett, Macrae and Macfarlane, 1985). Under appropriate circumstances liberation of the organism from these systems can give rise to a disease epidemic. The circumstances that can give rise to epidemics of Legionnaires' disease are now fairly well understood (Bartlett, Macrae and Macfarlane, 1985). The following have been shown to be potential sources of epidemics of legionellosis (Bartlett, Macrae and Macfarlane, 1985):

1. Domestic hot water systems in large buildings.
2. Cooling water systems used for air conditioning.
3. Cooling water systems used for industrial purposes.
4. Whirlpool spas (jacuzzis).
5. Decorative fountains (Fenstersheib et al., 1990).
6. Industrial coolants used for grinding and machine lubrication.
7. Respiratory therapy equipment.

In each of these circumstances the common factors that give rise to legionella growth are the presence of water temperatures at which the organism grows best and design faults or interruption in supplies which lead to water stagnation and hence a build-up in the concentration of bacteria. The final requirements for an epidemic are that the system is colonized by a strain of *Legionella* that is virulent to human beings (Plouffe et al., 1983), that there is a means of dissemination of the organism (e.g. the plume from a cooling tower) and that susceptible hosts are exposed (Bartlett, Macrae and Macfarlane, 1985).

It is not possible to identify groups of workers at particular risk from legionella infection due to the ubiquitous nature of the potential sources. Hotels and hospitals are the buildings most frequently associated with epidemics, but the risk to staff in these institutions appears to be low (Marrie et al., 1986a).

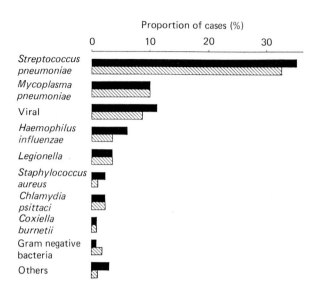

Figure 22.1 Causes of adult community-acquired pneumonia. ■ United Kingdom (six studies); *n* = 1156. ▨ Europe (nine studies); *n* = 2237. (Reproduced from the literature: White et al., 1981; Macfarlane et al., 1982; McNabb et al., 1984; Almirante et al., 1985; Berntsson et al., 1985; Font et al., 1985; Aubertin et al., 1987; British Thoracic Society, 1987; Holmberg, 1987; Solans et al., 1987; Woodhead et al., 1987; Ausina et al., 1988; Levy et al., 1988; Hone et al., 1989; Ruf et al., 1989)

Clinical and laboratory features

Pontiac fever is a mild, self-limiting, influenza-like illness in which radiographic pulmonary consolidation does not occur. The typical features begin within 48 hours of exposure (Herwaldt et al., 1984) and are of malaise, myalgia, fever, chills and headache. Cough, dizziness, neck pain, nausea, chest pain and arthralgia occur less frequently (Glick et al., 1978). The acute illness resolves in 2 to 5 days, but feelings of lassitude, forgetfulness and poor concentration may persist for several months (Glick et al., 1978).

Legionella infection can cause both community- and hospital-acquired pneumonia. Legionella organisms are infrequent, but regular causes of community-acquired pneumonia account for less than 5 per cent of adult cases in most studies of patients admitted to hospital (Figure 22.1) and less than 1 per cent of those managed at home (Woodhead et al., 1987). In occasional studies, a higher frequency of legionella infection has been found (Macfarlane et al., 1982; Aubertin et al., 1987), possibly reflecting unrecognized local sources for epidemic infection or genuine geographical differences in incidence. Men are affected more often than women, but the illness seldom occurs in children. The incubation period is from 2 to 10 days. Despite early suggestions of a specific clinical picture in legionella pneumonia

(Miller, 1979), it is now known that the clinical features of this condition are similar to those of the other common causes of pneumonia (Tsai et al., 1979; Nordstom et al., 1983; Helm et al., 1984; Woodhead and Macfarlane, 1986, 1987). Most patients have been ill for 1 week before hospital admission and present with cough, which is often non-productive, dyspnoea, chest pain and headache. Confusion, diarrhoea and other neurological features may be present in the severely ill. Features on examination are non-specific with pyrexia, tachypnoea, tachycardia and inspiratory crackles on chest auscultation being recorded most frequently. Laboratory investigations usually show a peripheral blood leucocytosis and a raised erythrocyte sedimentation rate (ESR). Abnormal renal and liver function tests occur commonly, and haematuria and proteinuria may occur.

Radiographic appearances

The admission chest radiograph shows consolidation confined to one lobe in two-thirds of cases with pleural effusion and collapse occurring frequently. Lymphadenopathy and cavitation are unusual. Progression of consolidation occurs in up to half of all cases (Figure 22.2) and resolution of these changes is slow, being complete in only 50 per cent of cases by 3 months (Macfarlane et al., 1984).

Diagnosis

The absence of specific clinical, laboratory or radiographic features means that Legionnaires' disease should be suspected in any patient with pneumonia, especially if this is severe (Woodhead et al., 1985), or if occurring at the time of a known outbreak. The diagnosis may be confirmed by demonstration of the organism in respiratory secretions, by *direct fluorescent antibody testing* (DFAT) or culture, or by serological means. The diagnosis is confirmed most rapidly by demonstration of the presence of the organism by DFAT. This may be aided by bronchoscopic aspiration of respiratory specimens (Winter et al., 1987). The *indirect immunofluorescent antibody test* (IFAT) and the *rapid microagglutination test* (RMAT) are the most widely available serological tests and produce comparable results (Harrison, Dournon and Taylor, 1987). A fourfold or greater rise in titre to more than 64 or a single titre of more than 128 for the IFAT, or a fourfold rise in titre to more than 16 or a single titre of more than 32 for the RMAT, confirm the diagnosis (Harrison, Dournon and Taylor, 1987). One-third of serological tests are positive within 48 hours of admission, up to 40 per cent within 1 week and 71 per cent within 4 weeks (Woodhead and

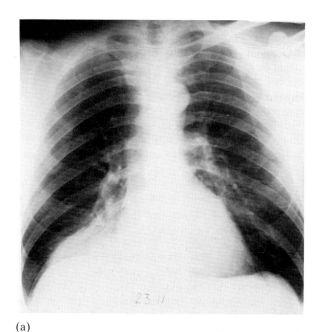

(a)

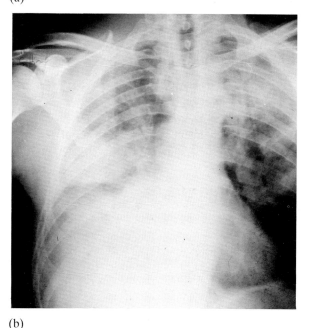

(b)

Figure 22.2 *Legionella pneumophila* pneumonia: (a) admission chest radiograph; (b) film taken 24 hours later showing rapid progression of radiographic shadowing

Macfarlane, 1986; Harrison, Dournon and Taylor, 1987; Harrison and Taylor, 1988). Seroconversion may occur more slowly in older patients and in those with a high alcohol consumption (Monforte et al., 1988). Routine serology may miss infections due to *Legionella* species other than *L. pneumophila* serogroup I, but these represent a small proportion of the total (McIntyre, Kurtz and Selkon, 1990). In the future, antigen detection in urine may offer an alternative rapid method of diagnosis (Kohler, Winn and Wheat, 1986).

Treatment and outcome

Legionella pneumonia is often a severe illness (Woodhead et al., 1985); a wide variety of complications has been recorded (Woodhead and Macfarlane, 1985) and recovery is often slow, with persistence of myalgia, poor memory and fatigue for several months (Nordstrom et al., 1983; Edelstein and Meyer, 1984). Mortality varies from 0 per cent in an epidemic of Legionnaires' disease affecting the community (Nordstom et al., 1983) to 70 per cent in nosocomial infection (Helm et al., 1984). Overall mortality in England, Wales and Ireland is 12 per cent (PHLS, Communicable Disease Surveillance Centre, unpublished data), compared to 6 per cent for community-acquired pneumonia overall (British Thoracic Society, 1987).

Our knowledge of the antibiotic therapy of Legionnaires' disease is based on retrospective analysis of published series and animal studies (Bartlett, Macrae and Macfarlane, 1985). Erythromycin has emerged as the antibiotic therapy of choice for legionella infection. Rifampicin is usually added in cases of severe infection. Continuation of treatment for at least 3 weeks is usually recommended because occasional relapses have been recorded with discontinuation before this time.

Prevention

Owing to the fact that the majority of cases of Legionnaires' disease are sporadic and of unknown source, these are not preventable. Investigation of the features that give rise to an epidemic of Legionnaires' disease has produced guidelines that may prevent future cases (Committee of Inquiry, 1986; Health and Safety Executive, 1987). Design of domestic water systems should avoid the inclusion of areas in which stagnation might occur and should allow water to be maintained at constant temperature. Cold water should be stored at temperatures below 20°C; hot water should be stored above 60°C and distributed at not less than 50°C. Continuous chlorination to levels of 1 to 2 mg/l (p.p.m. or parts per million) is effective.

Where possible, especially in hospitals, air-cooled, rather than wet-cooled, air-conditioning systems should be installed. With wet-cooled air-conditioning systems, cooling towers should be sited where their drift cannot easily enter a ventilation system and drift eliminators should be fitted. Ideally, there should be continuous dosing with biocides to prevent bacterial growth. All systems should be inspected and cleaned regularly. Despite the publicity given to such measures, problems continue to arise in the maintenance and cleaning of cooling towers (Mitchell et al., 1990). Surveillance is important to detect further outbreaks at an early stage, and to allow appropriate investigation and the institution of control measures (Bartlett, Macrae and Macfarlane, 1985). Legionnaires' disease is not a notifiable disease, but because the diagnosis is dependent on laboratory tests, the present voluntary laboratory-based reporting scheme should continue to be effective.

Brucellosis ('undulant fever')

The six species of the genus *Brucella* affect a wide variety of wild and domestic animals, but it is the four species that affect farm animals which usually lead to infection in human beings. Transmission from person to person is unknown, and so each individual case has an animal source. In Britain, and other developed countries, cattle (*B. abortus*) are the most common source of disease in human beings, but sheep and goats (*B. melitensis*), pigs and reindeer (*B. suis*) or dogs (*B. canis*) may be more important in other parts of the world (Alton and Plommet, 1986). Almost complete freedom from brucellosis has been achieved in some countries (for example, Britain and the USA) by eliminating infected animals (Buchanan, Faber and Feldman, 1974; Public Health Laboratory Service (PHLS), Communicable Disease Surveillance Centre, 1984) whilst in others (for example, Kuwait) epidemics in the human population follow uncontrolled expansion of the animal industry associated with difficulties enforcing control measures in a highly mobile population (Manes, 1984; Alton and Plommet, 1986; Lulu et al., 1988). Between 20 and 30 cases are reported each year in England, Wales and Ireland of which two-thirds are due to *Brucella abortus* and one-third to *B. melitensis* (PHLS, Communicable Disease Surveillance Centre, unpublished data). A cow with brucellosis is most infectious in the month after calving. The placenta, membranes and discharges are heavily contaminated with the organism which is also present in the aborted calf and the cow's milk, urine and faeces. Contamination of the environment – for example, farm buildings, abattoirs and knackers' yards – occurs easily. In Britain those most at risk are dairy farmers, cattle breeders and dealers and their families, abattoir workers, knackers, butchers and veterinary surgeons (PHLS, Communicable Disease Surveillance Centre, 1984). In the USA infection is chiefly associated with the slaughter of pigs and the processing of pig meat. Medical laboratory workers may be infected (Harrington, 1975; Olle-Goig and Canela-Solar, 1987; Lulu et al., 1988).

Transmission of infection to human beings is usually via infected, unpasteurized milk (Lulu et al., 1988). In the UK, skin abrasions, the conjunctiva and mucous membranes, and the respiratory tract may be more frequent portals of entry.

Clinical and laboratory features

The disease may be acute, subacute or chronic. The symptoms in each form are similar with fever, sweating, fatigue, chills, low back pain, arthralgia, headache and myalgia occurring most frequently (Lulu et al., 1988). Respiratory symptoms are uncommon occurring in between 0 and 30 per cent of cases (Garcia-Rodrigues et al., 1989), with cough being recorded most frequently.

The white blood cell count is usually normal, although the ESR is high; abnormal liver function tests are a common finding, but clinical hepatitis is rare (Lulu et al., 1988), and arthritis is the most common complication occurring in about one-quarter (Lulu et al., 1988).

Radiographic appearances

Radiographic changes are uncommon, usually being reported in about 1 per cent of cases (Lulu et al., 1988), although studies reporting frequencies of radiographic abnormality as high as 16 per cent have been reported (Patel et al., 1988). Soft miliary mottling occurs most frequently, but hilar and paratracheal lymphadenopathy, parenchymal nodules, consolidation that may cavitate (Garcia-Rodrigues et al., 1989), chronic diffuse changes, pneumothorax (Patel et al., 1988) and pleural effusion (Lulu et al., 1988; Garcia-Rodrigues et al., 1989) may be seen. In chronic disease, sarcoid-type granulomas may be present in lung, liver, spleen and bone marrow (Ganado, 1965) and the chest radiograph may show scattered irregular opacities.

Diagnosis

A high index of suspicion, based on features of the clinical history, is essential for diagnosis. Specific antibodies detected by ELISA (enzyme-linked immunosorbent assay) are the best means of confirming the diagnosis. *Brucella*-specific IgM is usually present in acute disease, IgG or IgA being more reliable for the confirmation of chronic disease. Blood cultures may be positive in 35 per cent of acute, 18 per cent of subacute and 5 per cent of chronic cases of brucella infection (Lulu et al.,

1988). In the investigation of lung shadowing, especially in chronic disease, lung biopsy or pleural biopsy may be performed (Garcia-Rodrigues et al., 1989). The histological appearances could be confused with other granulomatous lung disease. A simple and sensitive spot agglutination test or a skin test can be used for screening flocks of sheep or goats (Alton and Plommet, 1986), animals with positive results then being re-tested with more accurate serological tests.

Treatment

The recommended treatment for brucellosis is rifampicin plus doxycycline, given once daily for 6 weeks (World Health Organization, 1986). In uncomplicated, acute brucellosis either drug alone may produce high cure rates, but in severe disese (for example, neurobacillosis), the addition of streptomycin and steroids should be considered (Lulu et al., 1988).

Prevention

Pasteurization of milk, slaughter of infected animals and vaccination of calves, lambs and goats are the main routes for prevention of the infection (Alton and Plommet, 1986).

Tularaemia

Necrotic pneumonia with abscess formation and, in most cases, septicaemia caused by *Francisella tularensis (Pasteurella tularensis)* may occur among people handling carcasses and skins of infected wild rabbits, hares, squirrels and foxes, and as a laboratory-acquired infection mainly in North America, although cases have been reported in Norway, Sweden and Japan. The infection may also be water borne (Greco et al., 1987) or transmitted by ticks.

Sugar refinery workers in Czechoslovakia have apparently been affected by handling sugar beet imported from endemic areas (Černý, 1976). It appears to be unknown in the UK.

Diagnosis depends on the isolation of the organism or the presence of an increased or rising antibody titre in the blood.

Anthrax

When ingested by cattle, pigs, sheep or goats, the spores of *Bacillus anthracis* germinate and cause disease. The hides, hair and wool of sick animals, and the straw, hay and sacking associated with them, are heavily contaminated by the organism and are thus a source of infection to human beings in a variety of ways. In the UK nowadays anthrax is uncommon in farm animals, but occasional cases are a source of infection to those who handle them. Anthrax is endemic in India, Pakistan, north and east Africa and the Near and Far East. Materials from these areas are potential sources of infection.

Imported materials which may be infected include: (1) hides and skins from endemic areas – those from the Argentine and Australasia are less likely to be affected; (2) hair from China, India and the Near East, and horse hair from China, Siberia and Russia; (3) crushed and dried bone from Pakistan and India; and (4) hooves and horn from endemic areas.

Occupations in which there is a potential risk from these and other sources are the following:

1. Tanning of skins and hides.
2. Manufacture of glue and gelatin from imported bone and hooves.
3. Production of fertilizers and charcoal for sugar and refining from crushed bone.
4. Sorting of goat, camel and alpaca hair.
5. Mechanical opening and cleaning of imported wools.
6. Processing of horse hair for the manufacture of brushes.
7. Agricultural workers, knackers and veterinary surgeons in contact with sick animals.
8. Dockers and transport workers handling infected material (such as hides); medical and veterinary bacteriology laboratory staff may occasionally be at risk.
9. Direct infection of medical and nursing staff by a patient with pulmonary anthrax, and of the pathologist and his or her attendants who perform the autopsy, may occur because, owing to its rarity, the disease is not often diagnosed during life, and thus is frequently fatal.

Contaminated bone meal is currently believed to be the most common source of potential infection in the UK. A fatal case of pulmonary anthrax in London attributed to this source was reported by Enticknap et al. in 1968.

Pulmonary anthrax must be considered in any patient with pneumonia who works in a potential anthrax hazard. Its incidence is related to the number and size of anthrax-containing particles inhaled.

Although cutaneous anthrax is still seen occasionally in Britain, pulmonary disease, which consists of haemorrhagic pneumonia with septicaemia, pleural effusions and recurrent haemoptysis, is now rare, but may be encountered in those areas of the world where anthrax is endemic (Plotkin et al., 1960). This

is due largely to effective preventive measures, but also, to some extent, to the low infectivity of *B. anthracis* for man. In spite of the fact that enormous numbers of anthrax-contaminated particles – many less than 5 μm in diameter – may be present in the workplace air, only very few cases of inhalation anthrax occur (Brachman et al., 1960).

Preventive measures

These consist of the following:

1. Vaccination of susceptible animals.
2. Cremation or deep burying in quicklime (anhydrous calcium oxide) of a diseased animal, preferably at the site of death, and burning of all contaminated materials.
3. Restriction of movement of other animals in or out of the area inhabited by the affected animal.
4. In the UK disinfection of imported skins, hides, hair and wool by factories approved under the Anthrax Prevention Act 1971 before use.
5. Immunization of workers at a substantial risk with alum-precipitated vaccine by three intramuscular injections of 0.5 ml at 3-weekly intervals and a fourth 0.5 ml injection 6 months later.
6. Obligatory exhaust ventilation, protective clothing and proper washing facilities in all factories processing potentially contaminated material.

Education of workers in the mode of transmission of spores, and the control of effluents and trade wastes are also necessary measures.

Anthrax is a notifiable industrial disease in the UK.

Chlamydial infections

The three species of the genus *Chlamydia* may all give rise to pulmonary disease in human beings. *C. trachomatis* is an important cause of pneumonia in infants in the first 3 months of life (Harrison et al., 1986; Brasfield et al., 1987), but does not cause adult pulmonary disease except in the immunocompromised (Tack et al., 1980). Psittacosis, caused by *C. psittaci* and typically acquired from psittacine birds (members of the parrot family), is, perhaps, the best known chlamydial pulmonary infection. Although parrots remain the most important source of psittacosis, this name, or even its alternative ornithosis, is in reality a misnomer because the importance of other avian species, mammals (especially sheep) and even human subjects as a source of human *C. psittaci* infection is being increasingly recognized. The third species, *C. pneumoniae* (formerly 'TWAR' strain of *C. psittaci*), has only recently been identified (Grayston et al., 1986). The importance of this organism as a cause of human pulmonary disease is as yet unclear, but it does not appear to have an animal source, being transmitted from person to person, and giving rise to a spectrum of respiratory disease from pharyngitis to pneumonia (Grayston, 1989). The only occupational importance of *C. pneumoniae* is its propensity to cause epidemics of respiratory illness in closed communities of young adults such as university students (Grayston et al., 1986) or military trainees (Kleemola et al., 1988). The remainder of this section refers to *C. psittaci* infection.

Inhalation of the organism from an infected source is the usual route of transmission of human *C. psittaci* infection. Direct contact by handling or bite wounds may also be responsible.

Epidemiology

At least 130 different species of wild and domestic birds are know to be hosts to *C. psittaci* (Schachter and Dawson, 1978). The most important groups with respect to the transmission of the disease to human beings are parrots (including parakeets, budgerigars, macaws and cockatoos), ducks, geese, chickens, turkeys, pigeons and finches (for example, canaries). More unusual species may be important to the staff of aviaries and zoological gardens – for example, toucans, hummingbirds and penguins (Keymer, 1974); and in isolated communities, as exemplified by fulmar petrels (Haagen and Mauer, 1938).

People with occupations in which there may be a risk of psittacosis include: pet-shop owners and staff (Parry and Mason, 1972; Jernelius et al., 1975), employees in duck, turkey and chicken farms and processing plants especially in the USA (Anderson, Stoesz and Kaufmann, 1978; Andrews, Major and Palmer, 1981; Kuritsky et al., 1984). The highest attack rate of disease is in killing, plucking, eviscerating and packing operations (Dickerson, Bilderback and Pessarra, 1976); railway guards handling crates of pigeons carried in guard's vans and carriers delivering sick birds to dealers (Dew et al., 1960); workers repairing buildings and roofing heavily contaminated with pigeon excreta; veterinary surgeons and pathologists (McKendrick, Davies and Dutta, 1973); laboratory workers handling infected material from patients or birds; rarely medical and nursing staff may be infected directly from patients suffering from the disease (Olsson and Treuting, 1944; Meyer, 1965).

Sheep are the only important mammalian source of human *C. psittaci* infection, but transmission from

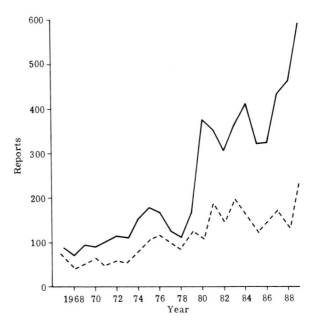

Figure 22.3 Laboratory reports (England, Wales and Ireland) from 1967 to 1989. — *Chlamydia B/Chlamydia psittaci;* ---- *Coxiella burnetii.* (PHLS Communicable Disease Surveillance Centre, unpublished data)

cattle and domestic cats has also been recorded (Johnson, 1983). Mice, ferrets, hamsters and goats may also harbour the organism. Members of the farming community, especially pregnant women, are the groups at risk from ovine *C. psittaci* infection.

Despite detailed knowledge of the possible sources of *C. psittaci* infection, less than 20 per cent of cases in the UK give a history of such exposure (Nagington, 1984) which is a source of continuing mystery. Person-to-person spread may explain some cases (Buttery and Wreghitt, 1987; Huminer et al., 1988), and overlap between the serological tests used for *C. psittaci* and *C. pneumoniae* may explain others (Wreghitt et al., 1990).

The number of cases of human *C. psittaci* infection has been steadily rising in England and Wales (Figure 22.3), Japan (about 330 cases per year – Kawane, 1984) and the USA (about 200 cases per year), but is more variable in other countries such as Finland (Puolakkainen, Ukkonen and Saikku, 1988). Continued importation of exotic birds appears to be an important factor in those countries with a rising incidence of the disease (Reeve, Carter and Taylor, 1988; Wreghitt and Taylor, 1988).

Clinical features in animals and birds

Up to 8 per cent of parakeets may be carriers of *C. psittaci* (Meyer, 1942) which is the most common cause of infectious disease in pet parrots (Keymer, 1972). Overt signs of disease are often absent.

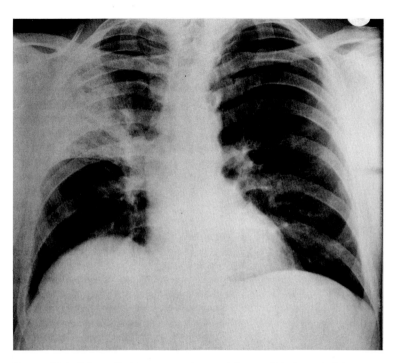

Figure 22.4 Chlamydia B pneumonia: partial consolidation of right upper lobe – from a man aged 52 years with a history of cough, lassitude, diarrhoea and fever for 1 week. No pathogenic organisms were grown from the sputum. Initial chlamydial complement fixation titre was 1 : 160 rising to 1: 132 in 1 month. Complete recovery occurred with tetracycline treatment. He was a pigeon breeder who kept 20 racing birds one of which was sick shortly before he became ill. (Dr J.P. Anderson's case, reproduced with permission)

Exposure to highly virulent strains of *C. psittaci* or periods of stress, such as inappropriate feeding, overcrowding, transportation, breeding or superimposed viral, fungal or bacterial infection, may lead to acute disease with high mortality. Anorexia, lethargy, diarrhoea, and nasal and conjunctival discharge are features of the disease (Johnson, 1983). Transmission between birds and from birds to human beings is via exposure to the organism which may be found in the discharges and faeces, and on contaminated feathers. Asymptomatic birds may continue to excrete the organism.

C. psittaci is widespread throughout flocks of all breeds of sheep in the UK where it is the most common cause of abortion. Occasional live, infected lambs are weak and of poor viability. The ewes usually make an uncomplicated recovery. Transmission to human beings is via exposure to birth products which contain huge numbers of infectious organisms, but transmission between sheep can also occur through asymptomatic faecal carriage (Johnson, 1983). Abortion in cattle due to *C. psittaci* has been recorded, but the importance of this in the UK is not clear. Human infection via this route has not been recorded in the UK (Johnson, 1983).

Human keratoconjunctivitis may be caused by transmission of chlamydial infection from cats, but no cases of pulmonary disease from this source have been documented (Johnson, 1983).

Clinical and laboratory features in man

The incubation period is from 7 to 15 days. The infection is uncommon below the age of 20 years. The illness varies in severity from a mild influenzal illness to a severe pneumonia (Byrom, Walls and Mair, 1979; Wainwright, Beaumont and Kox, 1987). *C. psittaci* infection is an uncommon, but regular, cause of adult community-acquired pneumonia in the UK accounting for up to 5 per cent of cases (see Figure 22.1). The clinical features are similar to those found with other causes of community-acquired pneumonia (CAP), cough being the most frequent symptom. The cough is usually productive, but the sputum is seldom purulent. Haemoptysis may occur; fever, rigors, headache, myalgia, pleuritic chest pain, malaise and anorexia are common, but dyspnoea is often not prominent. Abdominal pain and diarrhoea are less common features (Macfarlane and Macrae, 1983; Coutts, Mackenzie and White, 1985; Yung and Grayson, 1988).

Physical signs on examination are non-specific, with fever and inspiratory crackles on auscultation of the chest being most frequent (Macfarlane and Macrae, 1983; Yung and Grayson, 1988). Less common features have included erythema nodosum (Coutts, Mackenzie and White, 1985), endocarditis (Ward and Ward, 1974; Jariwalla, Davies and White, 1980), myocarditis (Coll and Horner, 1967), pericarditis (Murray and Tuazon, 1980), hepatomegaly (Schaffner et al., 1967; Coutts, Mackenzie and White, 1985; Yung and Grayson, 1988) and splenomegaly (Yung and Grayson, 1988).

Routine laboratory investigations, including the peripheral blood white cell count, which is usually normal (Yung and Grayson, 1988), are unhelpful.

Radiographic appearances

The chest radiograph is abnormal in up to 75 per cent of cases (Coutts, Mackenzie and White, 1985; Yung and Grayson, 1988), but the features are non-specific. Consolidation may be patchy (often unilateral) (Figure 22.4) or homogeneous affecting predominantly the lower lobes, as in other pneumonias. Pleural effusions occur in up to one-fifth of cases and hilar lymphadenopathy has been reported in as many as two-thirds of cases (Macfarlane and Macrae, 1983; Macfarlane et al., 1984). Radiographic resolution occurs at a similar rate to that seen in pneumococcal pneumonia with 50 per cent of chest radiographs returning to normal by 6 weeks (Macfarlane and Macrae, 1983). *C. psittaci* infection of ovine origin usually gives rise to mild respiratory illness (Baker and Cooper, 1983), but the illness occurring in pregnant women in contact with infected sheep is severe. Fever, headache, cough, arthralgia, nausea and vomiting, and lower abdominal pain herald the onset of spontaneous labour, typically leading to abortion (Beer, Bradford and Hart, 1982; Johnson et al., 1985; McGivern et al., 1988; Helm et al., 1989). Hypotension (Johnson et al., 1985; Helm et al., 1987), thrombocytopenia (Beer, Bradford and Hart, 1982; Johnson et al., 1985; Helm et al., 1987, 1989; McGivern et al., 1988), jaundice (McGivern et al., 1988; Helm et al., 1989) and acute renal failure (Johnson et al., 1985; Helm et al., 1987) may follow. Pulmonary changes may be due to pulmonary oedema (Johnson et al., 1985) or consolidation (McGivern et al., 1988). In one case, coincident *C. psittaci* and *Coxiella burnetii* infections have been recorded (McGivern et al., 1988).

Diagnosis

The diagnosis is usually made serologically from a single high titre (≥256) or a fourfold or greater rise in complement fixing antibodies (Macfarlane and Macrae, 1983). This test, although widely available, has drawbacks. It seldom allows the diagnosis to be made early in the course of the patient's illness and the antigen used is genus specific and not species specific, hence *C. pneumoniae*, and sometimes *C. trachomatis*, infection can be confused with that of *C. psittaci*. Newer immunofluorescent tests can differentiate antibody responses to these three organisms (Grayston, 1989). Isolation of the organism from respiratory secretions is possible, but few laboratories offer this service. Recently, application of ELISA and direct immunofluorescence testing to detect the genus-specific antigen in respiratory secretions has been suggested as a fast, sensitive, but non-specific, method of diagnosing respiratory chlamydial infection (Riordan, Lewis and Oliver, 1990; Sillis and White, 1990).

Treatment and outcome

Tetracycline is the antibiotic of choice in the treatment of all *C. psittaci* infections. Erythromycin is an alternative and is the treatment of choice in pregnant women. Recovery from *C. psittaci* infection is usually prompt and uncomplicated (Yung and Grayson, 1988). Radiographic shadowing may persist despite clinical improvement resolving at the same rate as in pneumococcal infections (Macfarlane et al., 1984). Occasional severe complications include acute respiratory failure (Wainwright, Beaumont and Kox, 1987), acute renal failure (Byrom, Walls and Mair, 1979) and endocarditis (Ward and Ward, 1974). A restrictive defect of lung function, which responded to steroids, has been described as a complication of recovery from *C. psittaci* infection (Price and Harrison, 1982).

Infection in pregnant women is a severe illness that usually results in the death of the fetus despite appropriate antibiotics (Beer, Bradford and Hart, 1982; Johnson et al., 1985; Helm et al., 1987, 1989; McGivern et al., 1988). Following abortion the woman recovers.

Prevention

Continuing importation of wild infected birds makes control difficult. All exotic birds imported into the UK are placed in quarantine for 35 days and in the USA all imported birds are treated with tetracycline – neither method is foolproof. When a sick bird is identified the local Divisional Veterinary Officer of the Ministry of Agriculture, Fisheries and Food should be contacted. It is preferable for the bird to be destroyed and the disease confirmed at autopsy (performed with scrupulous precaution – Keymer, 1973).

Pregnant women should avoid all contact with sheep, especially during the lambing season. Segregation of aborting animals from the remainder of the flock and treatment of the ewe with tetracycline is important in preventing spread within the flock (Johnson, 1983).

Rickettsial infection

Q fever

'Query fever' was first described as a febrile illness of unknown cause occurring in abattoir workers in Queensland in 1937 (Derrick, 1937). Q fever is now known to have worldwide distribution and is caused by the rickettsia, *Coxiella burnetii*. The organism is liberated into the environment especially at times of parturition and can survive for prolonged periods. This is one of the most infectious agents known to humankind – the inhalation of a single organism is sufficient to establish infection (Tigertt, Benenson and Gochenour, 1961). Inhalation of an infected aerosol is the usual mode of transmission. Ingestion of unpasteurized milk (Marmion and Stoker, 1958) and entry through skin abrasions (Brown, Colwell and Hooper, 1968) are other sources of the disease. Q fever is nearly always acquired by animal contact, either direct or indirect, although apparent case-to-case transmission has occasionally been reported (Mann et al., 1986).

Epidemiology

A wide variety of wild and domestic animals are the normal host for *C. burnetii*. The organism may be carried by ticks, but this does not appear to be an important transmission route to human beings. Sheep and cattle are the most important sources for human infection in the UK. Farmers, shepherds and their families; veterinary surgeons and their assistants; stockyard workers; abattoir employees; workers manufacturing fertilizer from animal products; medical and veterinary laboratory technicians; and pathologists and post-mortem room technicians are the main 'at-risk' occupations (McCallum, Marmion and Stoker, 1949; Johnson and Kadull, 1966; Hart, 1973; Hall et al., 1982; Mann et al., 1986; Rauch et al., 1987). Examples of indirect animal contact leading to human infection include: handling contaminated laundry (Oliphant et al., 1949); the clearing out of sheds, previously occupied by sheep (Holland et al., 1960); art school students

handling straw from a packing case (Harvey, Forbes and Marmion, 1951); and living in villages through which sheep have travelled (Dupuis et al., 1987). A number of outbreaks have occurred in which a source has not been identified, including an outbreak in Newport, Wales in 1981 (Salmon et al., 1982), an outbreak in Oxford postal workers in 1983 (Winner et al., 1987) and an outbreak in Birmingham affecting 105 adults in 1989 (PHLS, Communicable Disease Surveillance Centre, unpublished data). Each outbreak occurred around the time of lambing and predominantly affected men. The Newport outbreak was attributed to infected straw falling at the roadside from farm vehicles and the other two may have been due to air-borne spread of the organism. Recently attention has been drawn to the possible role of domestic cats (Kosatsky, 1984; Langley et al., 1988; Marrie et al., 1988) and wild rabbits (Marrie et al., 1986b) as sources of Q fever in Canada, but the importance of these observations to other parts of the world is not yet established.

Between 100 and 200 cases of Q fever are reported in England, Wales and Ireland each year (see Figure 22.3), with over one-third occurring in Wales and south-west England (PHLS, Communicable Disease Surveillance Centre, unpublished data). Pneumonia due to *C. burnetii* infection accounts for a constant, but small, proportion of all cases of community-acquired pneumonia in the UK and in most of Europe (see Figure 22.1). In some parts of the world it occurs more frequently accounting for 22 per cent of adult community-acquired pneumonias in rural Nova Scotia, Canada (Marrie et al., 1985) and a similar proportion in the Basque region of Spain, where it is the second most common cause of community-acquired pneumonia (Baranda, Carranceja and Errasti, 1985; Sobradillo et al., 1989).

Clinical features

C. burnetii infection in animals is usually asymptomatic making case detection and effective control difficult.

Human infection is also frequently asymptomatic, giving rise to clinical illness in as few as 50 per cent of cases. Q fever occurs in acute and chronic forms. The acute illness is primarily a respiratory disease, but the clinical features are non-specific. Fever, cough, headache and myalgia are the dominant features with pyrexia and crackles on chest auscultation being the main findings on examination. Laboratory investigations are similarly unhelpful with a normal peripheral blood white cell count and raised ESR being typical findings. Abnormal liver function tests are a common finding, the proportion varying from 45 per cent (Sobradillo et al., 1989) to

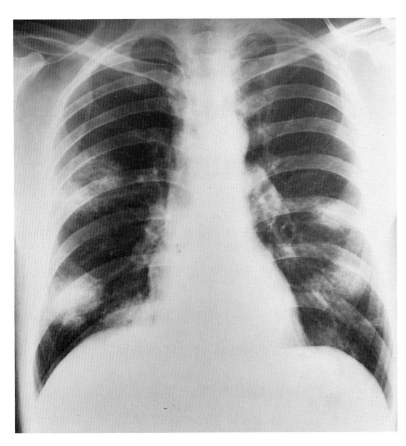

Figure 22.5 Q fever: rounded opacities due to segmental consolidation. (Reproduced, with permission, from Millar, 1978)

85 per cent (Spelman, 1982) of cases. Acute hepatitis may be the presenting illness, but this is unusual (Sawyer, Fishbein and McDade, 1987; PHLS, Communicable Disease Surveillance Centre, unpublished data).

Chronic Q fever is uncommon and occurs 3 to 20 years after the acute illness (Wilson et al., 1976). The reasons for recurrence are not clear, but patients with cardiac valvar abnormalities are likely to be most at risk. Endocarditis is the typical manifestation of chronic Q fever, but osteomyelitis, miscarriages and sudden infant death have been recorded (Ellis, Smith and Moffat, 1983). A case of miscarriage due to concomitant *C. burnetii* and ovine *C. psittaci* infection has been reported (McGivern et al., 1988).

Radiographic appearances

Radiographic evidence of pneumonia is often present in the absence of clinical signs, but the proportion of patients showing radiographic changes varies from less than 10 per cent (Powell, 1960; Spelman, 1982) to 75 per cent (Baranda, Carranceja and Errasti, 1985) of cases. The reasons for this difference are not clear. There are no specific radiographic features of Q fever pneumonia which, like other pneumonias, occurs mainly in the lower lobes. Multiple rounded opacities may be more common in Q fever pneumonia (Figure 22.5) (Millar, 1978; Gordon et al., 1984; Lipton et al, 1987; Pickworth et al., 1991), but no direct comparisons with other causes of pneumonia have been made. Signs of cavity formation are sometimes found in round opacities (Segger, Levin and Schey, 1986) which have been mistaken for bronchial carcinoma (Janigan and Marrie, 1983).

Diagnosis

This should be considered in any febrile patient with an appropriate occupation or with a history of contact with parturient animals, especially sheep. Confirmation of the diagnosis should be sought by serology. Complement fixing and indirect immunofluorescent antibody tests are the most widely available, and may be complementary (Marrie et al., 1985). The detection of antibodies to two surface antigens is used in an attempt to distinguish acute from chronic infection. Antibodies to phase II antigen appear early in acute illness, whereas antibodies to phase I antigen appear late, may not be present within 1 year of acute infection (Dupuis et al., 1985) and, when present, suggest previous acute or current chronic infection. Distinction between IgM, IgA and IgG antibodies by indirect immunofluorescent testing can also help distinguish acute from chronic infection (Peacock et al., 1983). Isolation of the organism is seldom performed because it is difficult and poses a hazard to laboratory workers.

Treatment and outcome

Acute *C. burnetii* infection is frequently mild and self-limiting, but occasionally gives rise to severe illness requiring intensive care (Torres et al., 1987). Treatment is advisable in all cases due to the uncertainty about progression to chronic disease. Tetracycline is the treatment of choice and may be more effective than erythromycin (Sobradillo et al., 1989). In Q-fever endocarditis tetracycline in combination with co-trimoxazole, lincomycin or rifampicin has been shown to be effective (Freeman and Hodson, 1972; Kimbrough et al., 1979; Varma, Adgey and Connolly, 1980; Tobin et al., 1982).

Prevention

Vaccines for use in those with high-risk occupations are under investigation, but as yet are not widely available. The lack of illness in infected animals makes detection and control difficult. Pasteurization of milk should block this route of transmission. Recommendations for preventing infection in the USA include the following:

1. Surveillance of the Q-fever antibody status of researchers.
2. Confining research on sheep to buildings solely dedicated to that purpose.
3. Restriction of those at risk (pregnant women, immunosuppressed and those with valvar heart disease) from high-risk jobs.

Other recommendations that are more difficult to implement are:

1. Surveillance of the Q-fever antibody status of animal flocks used for research.
2. Vaccination of new employees.
3. Vaccination of ewes.

Viral infections

Smallpox handlers' lung

A pneumonic illness with bilateral, patchy, low-density, radiographic opacities has been reported in nurses and others in close contact with smallpox patients (Howat and Arnott, 1944; Morris Evans and Foreman, 1963). As the illness may be followed by multiple, widespread, calcified pulmonary lesions similar to those that may be seen following chickenpox it is more likely to have been a modified smallpox pneumonia than a form of extrinsic allergic alveolitis (Ross et al., 1974). Smallpox has now been eliminated throughout the world.

Mycotic infections

Aspergillosis

Disease due to *Aspergillus* species is related, in the main, either to a lack of resistance in immunologically compromised patients or to an allergic response with asthma in atopic individuals. Occupational pulmonary aspergillosis is uncommon. Extrinsic allergic alveolitis due to *A. clavatus* in malt workers has been referred to already. *Aspergillus* sp. is ubiquitous in nature and is found in decaying vegetation, in grain, hay and straw, and in farm buildings; it is a fairly common cause of disease in many species of birds – it may be present in their droppings. High levels of contamination by the spores may, therefore, be encountered by farmworkers, threshers, millers, pigeon fanciers, poultry tenders, bagasse and aviary workers and hair sorters. Chronic granulomatous disease, which closely resembles cavitary tuberculosis, occasionally occurs in individuals in these fields of activity in the absence of underlying disease or atopy (Hildick-Smith, Blank and Sarkany, 1964).

Diagnosis

This may be difficult as isolation of such ubiquitous organisms as aspergilli from the sputum, even with proper laboratory precautions, does not establish the diagnosis, although repeated isolation makes it likely, and the presence of large numbers of mycelia in mucus sputum 'plugs' or in samples obtained at bronchoscopy makes it almost certain. Serum precipitins to aspergilli are found in the majority of cases of bronchopulmonary aspergillosis. However, histological proof from a lung biopsy may be necessary.

Histoplasmosis

This disease, which is primarily of respiratory origin, is caused by inhalation of the microconidia of the dimorphic fungus *Histoplasma capsulatum* and occurs in temperate and tropical climates – in particular, eastern and central USA, Central and South America, Mexico, South and South-West Africa. However, it is found in at least 60 countries and, although not indigenous to the UK, appears to be endemic in Europe (Ajello, 1971). It is, perhaps, the most important occupational pulmonary mycosis.

H. capsulatum is a soil-inhabiting, filamentous fungus which readily breaks up into minute particles if the soil is disturbed and these may become air borne. Its growth and sporulation are favoured by enrichment of the soil with the droppings or guano of birds and bats so that it has a predilection for their habitats. It is found in soil with substantial accumulation of droppings in and around chicken houses, under the roosts of gregarious birds such as starlings and buildings inhabited by bats. In the USA the term 'blackbird' includes starlings, which are mainly congregated in enormous numbers in the southern States, red-winged blackbirds, cowbirds and grackles – relatives of the mynah bird (Chick et al., 1980). The organism has been shown to survive in known contaminated soil for 4 to 6 years after being first isolated (di Salvo and Johnson, 1979), but it is unusual to find it in guano from a roosting site less than 3 years old (Chick et al., 1980). Interestingly, birds are not infected by the organisms because their body temperature does not favour its reproduction, but the organism may be harboured in the birds' feathers and thus contaminate their nests and other areas. By contrast, bats, which have a lower body temperature, may be infected and their faeces are not only a nutrient for fungal growth, but may be infectious (Goodwin and Des Prez, 1978). Hence, although the distribution of the fungus is predominantly rural, it is found in cities, for example, in the soil of a tree-lined shopping area in Washington DC (Emmons, 1961).

The soil apart, contaminated deposits of bird or bat droppings may occur in chicken houses, silos, barns and attics of old buildings in both town and country; outbreaks of histoplasmosis have followed the cleaning of accumulated droppings from such places and from belfries, towers, civic buildings, the girders and pillars of bridges and the ground beneath (Dean et al., 1978; Goodwin and Des Prez, 1978; Sorley et al., 1979). Large collections of bat guano are particularly common in caves, disused mine shafts, old ruins and hollow trees.

Therefore, occupations in which there is likely to be a risk of histoplasmosis in endemic areas include farm workers and their families, poultry keepers, gardeners and horticulturists using guano as a fertilizer, construction workers, bulldozer drivers, workers demolishing derelict buildings, bridge maintenance workers, ornithologists, geologists, spelaeologists, archaeologists and medical laboratory technicians handling cultures of the organism. Outbreaks of acute histoplasmosis in South Carolina and Louisiana have been associated with the clearing of bamboo cane fields (which were blackbird roosting sites) for pipe laying or construction work (di Salvo and Johnson, 1979; Storch et al., 1980) and with the felling of a giant oak tree (Ward et al., 1979).

More recently, three outbreaks of histoplasmosis, related to cutting and gathering decayed wood as a firewood source, occurred in Minnesota, a state where histoplasmosis was not thought to be prevalent (Pladson, Stiles and Kuritsky, 1984).

Campbell (1980) has pointed out that the demolition and construction work in city areas contaminated by bird or bat droppings may cause extensive outbreaks of disease and sporadic cases of severe pulmonary infection in passers-by who may live elsewhere. Bulldozing of positive bird roost sites is particularly apt to cause epidemics of disease (Chick et al., 1980).

Most reported outbreaks of histoplasmosis have been due to acute pulmonary disease, but an outbreak of chronic disease was observed in southern Kentucky following excavation of a substantial 'blackbird' roosting site (Latham et al., 1980).

Cave-sickness – so named by Washburn, Tuohy and Davies (1948) – has been shown to be caused by *H. capsulatum* from the dust of bat guano in cave explorers in the USA (Lottenberg et al., 1979), Venezuela (Campins et al., 1956), South Africa (Murray et al., 1957) and Zimbabwe (then Rhodesia – Dean, 1957). *H. capsulatum* var. *duboisii*, which is widely distributed between the Sahara and Kalahari deserts, was probably responsible for cases on the African continent. Acute pulmonary disease due to this variant was reported in a white mining engineer in Ghana (Duncan, 1958). Dean (1975) has quite plausibly suggested that the fatal 'Curse of the Pharaohs' suffered by Lord Carnarvon and some others involved in the exploration of the tomb of Tutankhamun in 1923 was in fact histoplasmosis, because, during this period, the entrance to the tomb passages was guarded by a temporary open-grill iron door through which innumerable bats passed freely for temporary domicile.

Pathological features

Pathologically the microscopic appearances are those of epithelioid granulomas similar to tuberculosis but in which *H. capsulatum* can be identified by the periodic acid–Schiff stain, and acid-fast bacilli are absent.

Clinical features

Clinically histoplasmosis may be asymptomatic, a benign or widely disseminated and fatal acute disease, or a chronic lung disease. Its severity appears to depend on intensity of exposure and pre-existing immunosuppression. Disseminated disease occurs predominantly in the elderly and immunosuppressed, and is being increasingly recognized in patients with the acquired immune deficiency syndrome (Huang et al., 1987). Fatal disease is uncommon in the absence of immunodeficiency states.

Acute disease may be a mild illness with cough, chest pain, haemoptysis, fever, night sweats and joint pains. In the more severe cases there may be evidence of localized lung consolidation, and endocarditis and meningitis may occur in disseminated disease. Chronic disease is marked by lassitude, low-grade fever, productive cough and occasional haemoptysis.

Radiographic appearances

Radiographically, the appearances are identical to various stages of tuberculosis. In acute disease, there may be multiple small or blotchy opacities or 'infiltrates', more sharply defined round opacities, scattered linear opacities, and signs of segmental consolidation and bilateral hilar node enlargement. Single or multiple cavitary lesions may also occur in asymptomatic and acute disease (Chick and Bauman, 1974; Bennish, Radkowsky and Ripon, 1983; Davies and Sarosi, 1987). This last appearance may be mistaken for a lung tumour (Goodwin, Owens and Snell, 1976). In reinfection-type acute disease in patients who have retained an active immune response, widespread miliary opacities are more commonly seen (Goodwin and Des Pres, 1978). Acute disease either resolves completely or undergoes fibrosis and calcification resulting in a single dense opacity or in multiple, small, 'buckshot' opacities. Rarely a single opacity enlarges gradually over a few years due to concentric layers of collagen being added to a healed primary focus. This so-called *histoplasmoma* may closely imitate a neoplasm but a central nidus or concentric rings of calcification are often present (Goodwin and Des Prez, 1978).

Chronic disease resembles fibrocavernous tuberculosis.

Diagnosis

This depends on the occupational history and culture of *H. capsulatum* from the sputum samples obtained at bronchoscopy (Prechter and Prakash, 1989) or the histological features on biopsy.

Rising antibody titres, detected by complement fixation or immunodiffusion, in successive sera, strongly suggest active disease. Newer serological tests such as enzyme immunoassay and radio-immunoassay are more sensitive, and likely to be positive earlier in the course of the disease, but may be less specific than established serological tests (Davies and Sarosi, 1987).

Skin testing, to either histoplasmin or the yeast-phase antigen, indicates prior exposure to the organism and is not diagnostic in the acute or chronic illness. Overlap with coccidioidomycosis and especially blastomycosis may occur and histoplasmin may increase serum antibody titres, making interpretation of serological results difficult. Both serological and skin tests may be negative in active disease in immunosuppressed patients. Differentiation from tuberculosis, psittacosis, coccidioidomycosis, tularaemia or tumour of the lung may be necessary according to how the disease presents. In non-endemic areas, especially where tuberculosis is common, the diagnosis is easy to miss (Tong, Tan and Pang, 1983).

In the UK the possibility of an individual having contracted histoplasmosis while working in an occupational hazard in an endemic area should be remembered. Occasional cases have arisen from imported contaminated fomites (Ajello, 1971).

Treatment

Amphotericin B remains the therapy of choice. Ketoconazole may be an alternative in mild disease in the immunocompetent, but treatment is often limited by adverse effects (Saag and Dismukes, 1988).

Prevention

This is difficult. Personal protection in the form of lightweight masks and protective clothing may be of some use when exposure is suspected. Known blackbird and chicken roosting sites should not be disturbed unnecessarily. When an area of soil is known or thought to be contaminated by the fungus it should be thoroughly treated with a 3 per cent solution of formalin before being disturbed (Storch et al., 1980). So far as possible, geologists, spelaeologists, ornithologists and archaeologists who are likely to visit bird- or bat-infested locations in endemic areas should be histoplasmin positive.

Coccidioidomycosis

Similar to histoplasmosis this is a disease of respiratory origin. It has acute primary and chronic forms which may be mild or disseminated and fatal.

It is caused by inhalation of arthrospores of *Coccidioides immitis*, a soil-inhabiting fungus endemic to semi-arid regions of the USA and South America, which varies in virulence and antigenicity. It is apparently restricted to the Western Hemisphere and is unknown in Europe (Drutz and Catanzaro, 1978). Important factors in infection are long, dry summers, mild winters, a light soil productive of much dust which contains the spores, and windy conditions to scatter the dust. A widespread epidemic of coccidioidomycosis occurred in California following air-borne dispersal of arthrospores by a high-velocity dust storm (Flynn et al., 1979).

Persons at risk in endemic areas are agricultural workers (including tractor drivers), cotton pickers, cotton gin and compress operators, grape pickers, road and construction workers, and laboratory technicians. Anthropology, archaeology, geology and civil engineering students – particularly in California – have been affected by minor epidemic disease; museum personnel handling unearthed specimens may also be at risk (Werner et al., 1972; Drutz and Catanzaro, 1978). In addition, it is important to recognize that the transportation of contaminated material (as in the case of a cotton-mill employee working with Californian cotton who had never been near the endemic areas) and laboratory infection may cause isolated cases of disease outside endemic areas (Gehlbach, Hamilton and Conant, 1973).

In the UK the infection is only likely to be encountered in visitors from endemic areas, such as service personnel (PHLS, Communicable Disease Surveillance Centre, unpublished data).

The *histopathology* consists of granulomatous lesions in which the fungus is readily demonstrated by periodic acid–Schiff or Gomori stains.

Clinical and laboratory features

Acute disease

This is usually a benign self-limiting influenza-like illness. Occasional, severe pneumonic disease with intense pleuritic pain, cough, haemoptysis, myalgia and sometimes pleural effusion may occur.

Dissemination may occur early or late in about 0.5 per cent of cases due to haematogenous spread of sporangiospores. Afro-Caribbeans, Mexicans and Fillipinos are particularly susceptible. Lesions develop in skin, bone and visceral organs.

Chronic disease

This follows acute disease in 2 to 9 per cent of cases and is usually symptomless, although cough and haemoptysis may occur. Sometimes, however, it is complicated by pleural effusion, empyema or spontaneous pneumothorax due to rupture of a cavity (Emmons et al., 1977).

Peripheral blood eosinophilia is a common finding and pulmonary eosinophilia may occur (Drutz and Catanzaro, 1978; Lombard, Tazelaar and Krasne, 1987).

Radiographic appearances

The radiographic appearances in acute disease are those of scattered patchy opacities often with bilateral hilar node enlargement. In chronic disease cavities, often single, which are usually thin-walled and may contain fluid, are seen. Occasionally there are miliary shadows.

Diagnosis

This depends on occupational history, isolation of the fungus in culture or its demonstration in sputum, pus or tissue sections.

Rising antibody titres, detected by complement fixation, are the best method of confirming the diagnosis. Skin testing is usually unhelpful. It may be necessary to differentiate the disease from tuberculosis, histoplasmosis or lung tumour.

Treatment

This is usually unnecessary because the vast majority of patients with primary pulmonary coccidioidomycosis recover spontaneously. If the disease progresses, amphotericin B is the therapy of choice. Ketoconazole may offer an alternative in cases of mild disease.

Prevention

In California guidelines have been set out for dealing with potential occupational exposure (Schmelzer and Tabershaw, 1968).

North American blastomycosis

This is a systemic fungal infection which originates in, and may be confined to, the respiratory tract. The causal organism is *Blastomyces dermatitidis*, the origin of which is uncertain but is thought to be from a restricted distribution in soil and organic debris. Infection in both human beings and animals

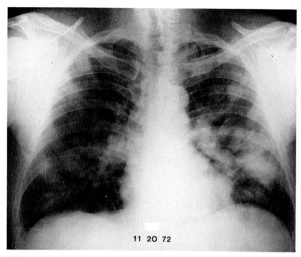

(a)

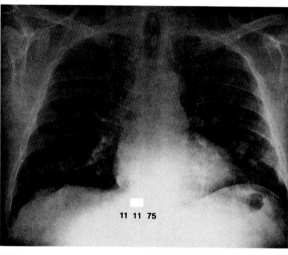

(b)

Figure 22.6 (a) Multiple, ill-defined, round opacities due to acute blastomycotic pneumonia in a 52-year-old man who assisted in building a lakeside log cabin. He developed fever, photophobia, arthralgia and persistent cough with sputum from which, after digestion with 10% KOH, *B. dermatitidis* was cultured. The blastomycin skin test was positive. (b) The radiographic changes resolved spontaneously and, although his health returned to normal within a few weeks, some opacities indicative of healed granulomas were still present in the left lower lung field 7 years later. (Reproduced with personal permission of Dr G.A. Sarosi)

is believed to result from inhalation of conidia in dust (Emmons et al., 1977). Although the disease is most common in the North American continent, a substantial number of cases occur in South America and Africa, and a few in the Middle East and India. It is not believed to occur in Europe but infection due to *B. dermatitidis* has been reported in a French

Tunisian and in an individual in Poland, neither of whom was ever in North America (Drouhet et al., 1968; Kowalska et al., 1976).

It is difficult to prove occupational origin in individual cases but acute blastomycosis in a professional horticulturist was traced to *B. dermatitidis* isolated from pigeon manure which he had used as a fertilizer and subsequently stored in a hot house (Sarosi and Serstock, 1976). The disease is most prevalent in people with occupations involving contact with the soil and wooded areas. These include farmers, farmworkers, labourers, construction workers, gardeners, oil field workers, woodmen, miners and heavy equipment workers. Some affected persons in cities have regularly visited remote rural areas. An outbreak of disease in the members of four families was associated with their co-operative effort to build a cabin on a wooded lake side (Tosh et al., 1974). Laboratory technicians may be infected from agar plate cultures. The highest incidence of blastomycosis in the world is in the Mississippi region of the USA.

As with tuberculosis the disease takes three forms: *acute* or *primary, subacute* or *postprimary* and *chronic* (Sarosi and Davies, 1979). The acute phase consists of proliferative epithelioid granulomas with giant cells and radiographic changes indicative of pulmonary infiltration or consolidation which may take a multiple nodular form (Figure 22.6). This stage may resolve spontaneously or progress to postprimary disease which is occasionally miliary and fatal. However, subacute disease is usually mild and not always preceded by an obvious primary illness. Chronic disease is clinically and radiographically identical to chronic tuberculosis; skin, bones and other organs may be affected (Baum and Schwarz, 1959; Laskey and Sarosi, 1978).

Diagnosis

This rests on occupational history, and identification of *B. dermatitidis* in the sputum digested with 10 per cent KOH or by culture of the organism. It may have to be differentiated from pneumonic and other granulomatous pulmonary disease (including histoplasmosis and coccidioidomycosis), nodular pneumoconiosis and lung tumour.

Treatment

This is not required for most cases of acute illness in immunocompetent individuals because the condition is self-limiting. For severe or acute progressive pulmonary blastomycosis or chronic disease, amphotericin B is still the drug of choice. Ketoconazole may be effective in mild cases.

Cryptococcosis

This mycosis is caused by *Cryptococcus neoformans*. It is primarily a pulmonary infection, but the most frequent clinical presentation is with meningitis, following spread from the lungs. It is an increasingly common complication of the acquired immune deficiency syndrome which now accounts for most cases in the UK (PHLS, Communicable Disease Surveillance Centre, unpublished data). The lung disease is often mild, but may be pneumonic and severe, sometimes with pleural effusion. Occasionally solitary nodules containing the fungus are found in the lungs. Strains of varying virulence are often present in old pigeon nests and in accumulated guano under pigeon roosts, on buildings and on window ledges in cities, and in stables and barns in rural areas. It is probable, therefore, that the disease may occur in people whose occupations involve disturbing these deposits, for example, demolition and farm workers (Emmons et al., 1977).

The chest radiograph shows unilateral, or bilateral, blotchy opacities or, on occasion, a solitary opacity. Hilar lymphadenopathy and pleural effusion are common (Wasser and Talavera, 1987). The fungus can be identified in or cultured from the sputum, and a complement fixation test for antigen is helpful; however, false-negative results are fairly common.

Sporotrichosis

This occurs throughout the world in both temperate and tropical climates and is caused by *Streptothrix schenkii*. Granulomatous and pyogenic lesions are usually confined to the skin and superficial lymph nodes and only rarely affect the lungs, but when they do the disease is clinically and radiographically indistinguishable from tuberculosis.

The fungus grows in soil, vegetation and rotting mine timbers. Hence, lung disease has been reported in farmworkers, nursery men and miners (Baum et al., 1969; Zvetina, Rippon and Daum, 1978).

Helminth infections

Hydatid disease

Hydatid disease has a worldwide distribution, occurring most commonly in countries where sheep and cattle are reared, such as Australia, New Zealand,

the Middle East, Mediterranean countries, East Africa, Russia and South America. It is uncommon in the UK with between 5 and 30 reported cases each year (PHLS, Communicable Disease Surveillance Centre, unpublished data). The highest incidence occurs in Wales with 1.5 cases per million of the population.

Tapeworms of the genus *Echinococcus* are the cause of human hydatid disease. Two species, *E. granulosus* and *E. multilocularis*, can cause human disease. Human beings are an accidental host to the worm in which a life cycle between dogs, which act as definitive hosts, and sheep and other ungulate animals, which are intermediate hosts, is more usual. The adult worms live within the jejunum of the infected dog. Eggs pass to the ground in faeces and are ingested by the sheep on contaminated grass. Human beings are infected at this stage by handling contaminated hair of infected dogs or ingestion of contaminated vegetable matter. The eggs hatch in the duodenum of the intermediate host and the larval stages reach the liver and other organs via the portal veins. Within these organs the larvae develop into parent cysts. The cyst is composed of an elastic membrane and an inner germinal membrane from which daughter cysts bud. The life cycle is completed by the ingestion of infected offal by dogs.

Clinical features

These depend on the location of the cyst and its size. Any organ can be affected, with the lung being involved in about one-third of cases and the liver in up to two-thirds. In only 10 per cent of cases are neither of these organs affected. In up to one-third of cases of pulmonary disease, the presentation is as an incidental finding on the chest radiograph (Dogan et al., 1989). The remainder present with symptoms that relate to compression of thoracic structures by the enlarging cyst (for example, Pancoast's syndrome – Stathatos, Kontaxis and Zafiracopoulos, 1969) or complications of the cyst such as rupture or infection. Rupture may occasionally give rise to anaphylaxis, hepatobiliary, hepato-bronchial and bronchopulmonary fistulae, and pneumothorax can also occur. Cough, classically with expectoration of salty cyst fluid, fever, chest pain and haemoptysis are the typical symptoms (Wolcott et al., 1971; Aytac et al., 1977).

Radiographic appearances

The uncomplicated hydatid cyst is a spherical mass of uniform density with well-defined edges. In endemic areas this is the most common cause of a 'coin lesion' on the chest radiograph. Any part of the lung or mediastinum may be affected, but the

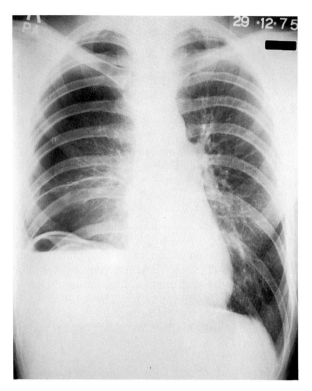

Figure 22.7 Hydatid disease: partially collapsed hydatid cyst at the right lung base showing the 'water lily sign'

lower lobes of the lungs are affected most frequently (Wolcott et al., 1971; Aytac et al., 1977). The lesions are multiple in 40 per cent and bilateral in 20 per cent. Rupture of the cyst may produce the 'water lily sign' (Figure 22.7) which is pathognomonic of hydatid disease. The 'water lily' is the collapsed germinal membrane outlined in an air–fluid level. Other radiographic signs have been described (Xu, 1985). Later in the disease the cysts may calcify. CT scanning demonstrates the lesions well and, together with ultrasound, is the best way of demonstrating hepatic lesions.

Diagnosis

In endemic areas the clinical history and radiographic appearances are sufficient to make the diagnosis. Supportive evidence is most difficult to obtain for the isolated, uncomplicated cyst, because this stimulates little immunological response from the host. The Casoni skin test is neither specific nor sensitive, but widely available. A wide variety of immunological tests is now also available, of which the latex agglutination, immunoelectrophoresis and complement fixation tests are probably the best; however, none is 100 per cent reliable.

Treatment

Surgery is the treatment of choice (Wolcott et al., 1971; Aytac et al., 1977: Dogan et al., 1989) with emphasis on the conservation of as much lung tissue as possible, due to the risk of recurrence. Sterilization of the cyst prior to its removal may be helpful, but anaphylaxis is a risk and some prefer to avoid this. The role of drugs is still limited. Mebendazole, which was initially suggested to be of value, is poorly absorbed, but encouraging reports of the use of albendazole are appearing (Morris et al., 1983, 1985; Saimot et al., 1983).

Prevention

Interruption of the natural life cycle of the worm should produce effective control. The value of this approach has been shown in island communities, such as those in Iceland and Tasmania, with special emphasis on preventing access of dogs to offal (McConnell and Green, 1979). Immunization of dogs and control of stray dogs may be alternative or supplementary approaches.

References

Ajello, L. (1971) Coccidioidomycosis and histoplasmosis. A review of their epidemiology and geographic distribution. *Mycopathol. Mycol. Appl.* **45**, 221–230

Almirante, B., Pahissa, A., Planes, A.M., Martinez Vazquez, J., Guardia, J., de Buen, M.L., Juste, C., Calico, I., Bacardi, R. and Arcalis, Y.L. (1985) Etiologia de las neumonias extrahospitalarias. *Med. Clin. (Barc.)* **85**, 175–178

Alton, G.G. and Plommet, M. (1986) Brucellosis summit in Geneva. *WHO Chron.* **40**, 19–21

American Thoracic Society (1988) Clinical usefulness of skin testing in histoplasmosis, coccidioidomycosis and blastomycosis. *Am. Rev. Respir. Dis.* **138**, 1081–1082

Anderson, D.C., Stoesz P.A. and Kaufmann, P.F. (1978) Psittacosis outbreak in employees of a turkey-processing plant. *Am. J. Epidemiol.* **107**, 140–148

Andrews, B.E., Major, R. and Palmer, S.R. (1981) Ornithosis in poultry workers. *Lancet* **1**, 632–634

Arnow, P.M., Weil, D. and Para M.F. (1985) Prevalence and significance of *Legionella pneumophila* contamination of residential hot water tap systems. *J. Infect.* **152**, 145–151

Aubertin, J., Dabis, F., Fleurette, J., Bornstein, N., Salamon, R., Brottier, E., Brune, J., Vincent, P., Migueres, J., Jover, A. and Boutin, C. (1987) Prevalence of legionellosis among adults: A study of community acquired pneumonia in France. *Infection* **15**, 328–331

Ausina, V., Coll, P., Sambeat, M., Puig, I., Condom, M.J., Luquin, M., Ballester, F. and Prats, G. (1988) Prospective study on the etiology of community-acquired pneumonia in children and adults in Spain. *Eur. J. Clin. Microbiol.* **7**, 342–347

Aytac, A., Yudakul, Y., Ikizler, C., Olga, R. and Saylam, A.

(1977) Pulmonary hydatid disease: report of 100 cases. *Ann. Thorac. Surg.* **23**, 145–151

Baker, C.C. and Cooper, B. (1983) A case of good management. *J. Infect.* **6**, 71–73

Baranda, M.M., Carranceja, J.C. and Errasti, C.A. (1985) Q fever in the Basque country: 1981–1984. *Rev. Infect. Dis.* **7**, 700–701

Bartlett, C.L.R., Macrae, A.D. and Macfarlane, J.T. (1985) *Legionella Infections*, Edward Arnold, London

Baum, G.L. and Schwarz, J. (1959) North American blastomycosis. *Am. J. Med. Sci.* **238**, 661–684

Baum, G.L., Donnerburg, R.L., Stewart, D., Mulligan, W. and Puttnam, L.R. (1969) Pulmonary sporotrichosis. *N. Engl. J. Med.* **280**, 410–413

Beer, R.J.S., Bradford, W.P. and Hart, R.J.C. (1982) Pregnancy complicated by psittacosis acquired from sheep. *Br. Med. J.* **284**, 1156–1157

Bennish, M., Radkowsky, M.A. and Ripon, J.W. (1983) Cavitation in acute histoplasmosis. *Chest* **84**, 496–497

Berntsson, E., Blomberg, J., Lagergard, T. and Trollfors, B. (1985) Etiology of community-acquired pneumonia in patients requiring hospitalisation. *Eur. J. Clin. Microbiol.* **4**, 268–272

Brachman, P.S., Plotkin, S.A., Bumford, R.H. and Atchinson, M.M. (1960) An epidemic of inhalation anthrax; the first in the twentieth century. II epidemiology *Am. J. Hyg.* **72**, 6–23

Brasfield, D.M., Stagno, S., Whitley, R.J., Cloud, G., Cassell, G. and Tiller R.E. (1987) Infant pneumonitis associated with cytomegalovirus, chlamydia, pneumocystis and ureaplasma; follow-up. *Pediatrics* **79**, 76–83

British Thoracic Society. (1987) Community acquired pneumonia in adults in British hospitals in 1982–1983: a survey of aetiology, mortality, prognostic factors and outcome. *Q. J. Med.* **62**, 195–220

British Thoracic Society (1990) Control and prevention of tuberculosis in Britain: an updated code of practice. *Br. Med. J.* **300**, 995–999

Brown, G.L., Colwell, D.C. and Hopper, W.L. (1968) An outbreak of Q fever in Staffordshire. *J. Hyg. (Camb.)* **66**, 649–655

Buchanan, T.M., Faver, L., and Feldman, R.A. (1974) Brucellosis in the United States, 1960–1972. An abattoir-associated disease. *Medicine* **53**, 403–413

Buttery, R.B. and Wreghitt, T.G. (1987) Outbreak of psittacosis associated with a cockatiel. *Lancet* **2**, 742–743

Byrom, N.P., Walls, J. and Mair, H.J. (1979) Fulminant psittacosis. *Lancet* **1**, 353

Campbell, C.C. (1980) Histoplasmosis outbreaks. Recommendations for mandatory treatment of known microfoci of *H. capsulatum* in soils. *Chest* **77**, 6–7

Campins, H., Zubillaga, C., Lopex, L.G. and Dorante, M. (1956) An epidemic of histoplasmosis in Venezuela. *Am J. Trop. Med. Hyg.* **5**, 690–695

Černý, Z. (1976) Tularemia infection rate and evaluation of the risk of the infection being contracted by workers of sugar refineries processing sugar-beet from areas of its endemic incidence. *Cslka. Epidem. Mikrobiol. Immun.* **25**, 39–49. (Abstracts *Hyg.* 1976; 51: 878)

Chick, E.W. and Bauman, D.S. (1974) Acute cavitary histoplasmosis – fact or fiction. *Chest* **65**, 479–480

Chick, E.W., Flanigan, C., Gompton, S.B., Pass III, T., Gayle, C., Hernandez, C., Pitzer, F.R. and Austin Jr, E. (1980) Blackbird roosts and histoplasmosis. An increasing medical problem? *Chest* **77**, 584–585

Committee of Inquiry (1986) First report into the outbreak of Legionnaires' disease in Stafford in April 1985. Cmnd 9772. HMSO, London

Coutts, I.I., Mackenzie S. and White, R.J. (1985) Clinical and radiographic features of psittacosis infection. *Thorax* **40**, 530–532

Coll, R. and Horner, I. (1967) Cardiac involvement in psittacosis. *Br. Med. J.* **4**, 35–36

Davies, S.F. and Sarosi, G.A. (1987) Serodiagnosis of histoplasmosis and blastomycosis. *Am. Rev. Respir. Dis.* **136**, 254–255

Dean, G. (1957) Cave disease. *Centr. Afr. J. Med.* **3**, 79–81

Dean, G. (1975) The curse of the Pharaohs. *World Med.* **10**, 17–21

Dean, A.G., Bates, J.H., Sorrels, C., Correls, T., Germany, W., Ajella, L., Kaufman, L., McGrew, C. and Fitts, A. (1978) An outbreak of histoplasmosis at an Arkansas courthouse with five cases of probable reinfection. *Am. J. Epidemiol.* **108**, 36–46

Derrick, E.H. (1937) 'Q' fever, new fever entity; clinical features, diagnosis and laboratory investigation. *Med. J. Aust.* **2**, 281–299

Dew, J., Mawson, K., Ellman, P. and Brough, D. (1960) Ornithosis in two railway guards: an occupational hazard. *Lancet* **2**, 18–19

Di Salvo, A.F. and Johnson, W.M. (1979) Histoplasmosis in South Carolina; support for the microfocus concept. *Am. J. Epidemiol.* **109**, 480–492

Dickerson, M.S., Bilderback, W.R. and Pessarra, L.W. (1976) Ornithosis (chlamydiosis) outbreaks in Texas. *Texas Med. J.* **72**, 57–61

Dogan, R., Yuksel, M., Cetin, G., Suzer, K., Alp, M., Jaya, S., Unlu, M. and Moldibi, B. (1989) Surgical treatment of hydatid cysts of the lung: report on 1055 patients. *Thorax* **44**, 192–199

Drouhet, E., Enjalbert, L., Planques, J., Bollinelli, R., Moreau, G. and Sabatier, A. (1968) A propos d'un cas de blastomycose a localisations mutiples chez un francais doridine Tunisienne guerison par l'amphotericine B. *Bull. Soc. Pathol. Exot.* **61**, 202–210

Drutz, D.J. and Catanzaro, A. (1978) Coccidioidomycosis. Parts I and II. *Am. Rev. Respir. Dis.* **117**, 559–585, 727–772

Duncan, J.T. (1958) Tropical African histoplasmosis. *Trans. R. Soc. Trop. Med. Hyg.* **52**, 468–474

Dupuis, G., Peter, O., Peacock, M., Burgdorfer, W. and Haller, E. (1985) Immunoglobulin responses in acute Q fever. *J. Clin. Microbiol.* **22**, 484–487

Dupuis, G., Petite, J., Peter, O. and Vouilloz, M. (1987) An important outbreak of human Q fever in a Swiss alpine valley. *Int. J. Epidemiol.* **16**, 282–287

Edelstein, P.H. and Meyer, R.D. (1984) Legionnaires' disease. A review. *Chest* **85**, 114–120

Ellis, M.E., Smith, C.C. and Moffat, M.A.J. (1983) Chronic or fatal Q fever infection: a review of 16 patients seen in North-East Scotland (1967–1980). *Q. J. Med.* **52**, 54–66

Emmons, C.W. (1961) Isolation of *Histoplasma capsulatum* from soil in Washington DC. *Publ. Health Rep.* **76**, 591–596

Emmons, C.W., Binford, C.H., Utz, J.P. and Kwon-Chung, K.J. (1977) *Medical Mycology*, 3rd Ed. Lea and Febiger, Philadelphia

Enticknap, J.B., Galbraith, N.S., Tomlinson, A.J.H. and Elias-Jones, T.F. (1968) Pulmonary anthrax caused by contaminated sacks. *Br. J. Ind. Med.* **25**, 72–74

Fenstersheib, M.D., Miller, M., Diggins, C., Liska, S., Detwiler, L., Werner, S.B., Lindquist, D., Thacker, W.L. and Benson, R.F. (1990) Outbreak of Pontiac fever due to *Legionella anisa*. *Lancet* **336**, 35–37

Fields, B.S., Sanden, G.N., Barbaree, J.M., Morrill, W.E., Wadowsky, R.M., White E.H. and Feeley, J.C. (1989) Intracellular multiplication of *Legionella pneumophila* in amoebae isolated from hospital water tanks. *Curr. Microbiol.* **18**, 131–137

Fliermans, C.B., Cherry, W.B., Orrison, L.H. and Thacker, L. (1979) Isolation of *Legionella pneumophila* from non-epidemic related aquatic habitats. *Appl. Environ. Microbiol.* **37**, 1239–1242

Fliermans, C.B., Cherry, W.B., Orrison, L.H., Smith, S.J., Tison, D.L. and Pope, D.H. (1981) Ecological distribution of *Legionella pneumophila. Appl. Environ. Microbiol.* **41**, 9–16

Flynn, N.M., Hoeprich, P.D., Kawachi, M.M., Less, K.K., Lawrence, R.M. Goldstein, E., Jordan, G.W., Kundargi, R.S. and Wong, G.A. (1979) An unusual outbreak of windborne coccidioidomycosis. *N. Engl. J. Med.* **301**, 358–361

Font, S.C., de Morlius, M.J., Rodriguez, C.S., Martinez, A.C., Sargatal, J.D., Pombo, E.P. and Monty, Y.F.G. (1985) Etiologia de la neumonia extrahospitalaria en un medio urbano. *Med. Clin. (Barc.)* **84**, 4–7

Freeman, R. and Hodson, M.E. (1972) Q fever endocarditis treated with trimethoprim and sulphamethoxazole. *Br. Med. J.* **1**, 419–420

Ganado, W. (1965) Human brucellosis – some clinical observations. *Scott Med. J.* **10**, 451–460

Garcia-Rodrigues, J.A., Garcia-Sanchez, J.E., Bellido, J.L.M., de la Tabla V.O. and Barbero, J.B. (1989) Review of pulmonary brucellosis: a case report on brucella pulmonary empyema. *Diagn. Microbiol. Infect. Dis.* **11**, 53–60

Gehlbach, S.H., Hamilton, J.D. and Conant, N.F. (1973) Coccidioidomycosis. An occupational disease in cotton mill workers. *Archs Intern. Med.* **14**, 254–255

Girod, J.C., Reichman, R.C., Winn, W.C., Klaucke, D.N, Vogt, R.L. and Dolin, R. (1982) Pneumonic and non-pneumonic forms of legionellosis. The result of a common source exposure to *Legionella pneumophila. Archs Intern. Med.* **142**, 545–547

Glick, T.H., Gregg, M.B., Berman, B., Mallison, G., Rhodes, W.W. and Kassanoff, I. (1978) Pontiac Fever: an epidemic of unknown aetiology in a health department: 1. clinical and epidemiological aspects. *Am. J. Epidemiol.* **107**, 149–160

Goodwin, R.A. and Des Prez, R.M. (1978) Histoplasmosis. *Am. Rev. Respir. Dis.* **117**, 929–956

Goodwin, R.A., Owens, F.T. and Snell, J.D. (1976) Chronic pulmonary histoplasmosis. *Medicine* **55**, 413–452

Gordon, J.D., Mackeen, A.D., Marrie, T.J. and Fraser, D.B. (1984) The radiographic features of epidemic and sporadic Q fever pneumonia. *J. Can. Assoc. Radiol.* **35**, 293–296

Grayston, J.T. (1989) *Chlamydia pneumoniae*, strain TWAR. *Chest* **95**, 664–669

Grayston, J.T., Kuo, C-C., Wang, S-P. and Altman, J. (1986) A new *Chlamydia psittaci* strain, TWAR, isolated in acute respiratory tract infections. *N. Engl. J. Med.* **315**, 161–168

Greco, D., Allergrini, G., Tizzi, T., Ninu, E., Lamanna, A. and Luzi, S. (1987) A waterborne tularemia outbreak. *Eur. J. Epidemiol.* **3**, 35–38

Haagan, von E. and Mauer, G. (1938) Ueber eine auf menschen ubertragbare viruskrankheit bei sturmvogeln und ihre beziehung zur psittakose. *Zentralbl. Bacteriol.* Abt. 1 Orig. **143**, 81–88

Hall, C.J., Richmond, S.J., Caul, E.O., Pearce, N.H. and Silver, I.A. (1982) Laboratory outbreak of Q fever acquired from sheep. *Lancet* **1**, 1004–1006

Harrington, J.M. (1975) Some occupational health hazards for hospital staff. *Proc. R. Soc. Med.* **68**, 94–95

Harrison, H.R., Magder, L.S., Boyce, T., Hauler, J., Bicker, T.M., Stewart, J.A. and Humphrey, D.D. (1986) Acute *Chlamydia trachomatis* respiratory infection in childhood. *Am. J. Dis. Child.* **140**, 1068–1071

Harrison, T.G. and Taylor, A.G. (1988) Timing of seroconversion in Legionnaires' disease. *Lancet* **1**, 795

Harrison, T.G., Dournon, E. and Taylor, A.G. (1987) Evaluation of sensitivity of two serological tests for diagnosing pneumonia caused by *Legionella pneumophila* serogroup I. *J. Clin. Pathol.* **40**, 77–82

Hart, R.J.C. (1973) The epidemiology of Q fever. *Postgrad. Med. J.* **49**, 535–538

Harvey, M.S., Forbes, G.B. and Marmion, B.P. (1951) An outbreak of Q fever in East Kent. *Lancet* **2**, 1152–1157

Health and Safety Executive (1987) Legionnaires' disease. Guidance note EH48. HMSO, London

Helm, C.M., Viner, J.P., Weisenberger, D.D., Chiu, L.C., Renner, E.D. and Johnson, W. (1984) Sporadic Legionnaires' disease: clinical observations on 87 nosocomial and community-acquired cases. *Am. J. Med. Sci.* **288**, 2–12

Helm, C.W., Smart, G.E., Gray, J.A., Cumming, A.D., Lambie, A.T., Smith, I.W. and Allan, N.C. (1987) Exposure to *Chlamydia psittaci* in pregnancy. *Lancet* **1**, 1144–1145

Helm, C.W., Smart, G.E., Cumming, A.D., Lambie, A.T., Gray, J.A., Macaulay, A. and Smith I.W. (1989) Sheep-acquired severe *Chlamydia psittaci* infection in pregnancy. *Int. J. Gynaecol. Obstet.*. **28**, 369–372

Herwaldt, L.A., Gorman, G.W., McGarth, T., Toma, S., Brake, B., Hightower, A.W., Jones, J., Reingold, A.L., Boxer, P.A., Tang, P.W., Moss, C.W., Wilkinson, H., Brenner, D.J., Steigerwalt, A.G. and Broome, C.V. (1984) A new *Legionella* species, *Legionella feeleii* species nova, causes pontiac fever in an automobile plant. *Ann. Intern. Med.* **100**, 333–338

Hildick-Smith, G., Blank H. and Sarkany, I. (1964) *Fungus Diseases and Their Treatment.* J. and A. Churchill Ltd, London, pp. 334–339

Holland, W.W., Rowson, K.E.K., Taylor, C.E.D., Allen, A.B., Ffrench-Constant, M. and Smelt C.M.C. (1960) Q fever in the RAF in Great Britain in 1958. *Br. Med. J.* **1**, 387–390

Holmberg, H. (1987) Aetiology of community-acquired pneumonia in hospital treated patients. *Scand. J. Infect. Dis.* **19**, 491–501

Hone, R., Haugh, C., O'Connor, B. and Hollingsworth, J. (1989) Legionella: an infrequent cause of adult community-acquired pneumonia in Dublin. *Irish J. Med. Sci.* **158**, 230–232

Howat, H.T. and Arnott, W.M. (1944) Outbreak of pneumonia in smallpox contacts. *Lancet* **2**, 312

Huang, C.T, McGarry, T., Cooper, S., Saunders, R. and Andavolu, R. (1987) Disseminated histoplasmosis in the acquired immunodeficiency syndrome. Report of five cases from a nonendemic area. *Archs Intern. Med.* **147**, 1181–1184

Huminer, D., Samra, Z., Weisman, Y. and Pitlik, S. (1988) Family outbreaks of psittacosis in Israel. *Lancet* **2**, 615–618

Janigan, D.T. and Marrie, T.J. (1983) An inflammatory pseudo-tumour of the lung in Q fever pneumonia. *N. Engl. J. Med.* **308**, 86–88

Jariwalla, A.G., Davies, B.H. and White, J. (1980) Infective endocarditis complicating psittacosis. *Br. Med. J.* **280**, 155

Jernelius, H., Pettersson, B., Schvarcz, J. and Vahlne, A. (1975) An outbreak of ornithosis. *Scand. J. infect. Dis.* **7**, 91–95

Johnson, F.W.A. (1983) Chlamydiosis. *Br. Vet. J.* **139**, 93–101

Johnson, F.W.A., Matheson, B.A., Williams, H., Laing, A.G., Jandial, V., Davison-Lamb, R., Halliday, G.J., Hobson, D., Wong S.Y., Hadley, K.M., Moffat, M.A.J. and Postlethwaite, R. (1985) Abortion due to infection with *Chlamydia psittaci* in a sheep farmer' wife. *Br. Med. J.* **290**, 592–594

Johnson, N.E. and Kadull, P.J. (1966) Laboratory acquired Q fever: a report of fifty cases. *Am. J. Med.* **41**, 391–403

Kawane, H. (1984) Psittacosis. *Br. Med. J.* **298**, 1543

Keymer, I.F. (1972) The unsuitability of non-domesticated animals as pets. *Vet. Rec.* **91**, 373–381

Keymer, I.F. (1973) Psittacosis. *Lancet* **2**, 1436

Keymer, I.F. (1974) Psittacosis. *Proc. R. Soc. Med.* **67**, 733–735

Kimbrough, R.C., Ormsbee, R.A., Peacock, M., Rogers, W.R., Bennetts, R.W., Raaf J., Krause, A. and Gardner, C. (1979) Q fever endocarditis in the United States *Ann. Intern. Med.* **91**, 400–402

Kleemola, M., Saikku, P., Visakorpi, R., Wang, S.P. and Graston, J.T. (1988) Epidemics of pneumonia caused by TWAR, a new chlamydia organism, in military trainees in Finland. *J. Infect. Dis.* **57**, 230–236

Kohler, R.B., Winn, W.C. and Wheat, L.J. (1986) Onset and duration of antigen excretion in Legionnaires' disease. *J. Clin. Microbiol.* **20**, 605–607

Kosatsky, T. (1984) Household outbreak of Q fever pneumonia related to a parturient cat. *Lancet* **2**, 1447–1449

Kowalska, M., Hanski, W., Bielunska, S. and Gawkowska-Turyczyn, M. (1976) North American blastomycosis and possibilities of its occurrence in Poland. *Przegl. Derm.* **63**, 641–674

Kuritsky, J.N., Schmid, G.P., Potter, M.E,, Anderson, D.C. and Kaufmann, A.F. (1984) Psittacosis: a diagnostic challenge. *J. Occup. Med.* **26**, 731–733

Langley, J.M., Marrie, T.J., Covert, A., Waag, D.M. and Williams, J.C. (1988) Poker players' pneumonia. An urban outbreak of Q fever following exposure to a parturient cat. *N. Engl. J. Med.* **319**, 354–356

Laskey, W. and Sarosi, G.A. (1978) The radiological appearances of pulmonary blastomycosis *Radiology* **126**, 351–357

Latham, R.H., Kaiser, A.B., Dupont, W.D. and Dan, B.B. (1980) Chronic pulmonary histoplasmosis following the excavation of a bird roost *Am. J. Med.* **68**, 504–508

Levy, M., Dromer, F., Brion, N., Leturdu, F. and Carbon, C. (1988) Community-acquired pneumonia. Importance of initial noninvasive bacteriologic and radiographic investigations. *Chest* **92**, 43–48

Lipton, J.H., Fong, T.C., Gill, M.J., Burgess, K. and Elliott, P.D. (1987) Q fever inflammatory pseudotumour of the lung. *Chest* **92**, 756–757

Lombard, C.M., Tazelaar, H.D. and Krasne, D.L. (1987) Pulmonary eosinophilia in coccidioidal infections *Chest* **91**, 734–736

Lottenberg, R., Waldman, R.H., Ajello, L., Hoff, G.L., Bigler, W. and Zellner S.R. (1979) Pulmonary histoplasmosis associated with exploration of a bat cave. *Am. J. Epidemiol.* **110**, 156–161

Lulu, A.R., Araj, G.F., Khateeb, M.I., Mustafa, M.Y., Yusuf, A.R. and Fenech, F.F. (1988) Human brucellosis in Kuwait: a prospective study of 400 cases. *Q. J. Med.* **66**, 39–54

McCallum, F.O., Marmion, B.P. and Stoker, M.G.P. (1949) Q fever in Great Britain: isolation of *Rickettsia burnetii* from an indigenous case. *Lancet* **2**, 1026–1027

McConnell, J.D. and Green, R.J. (1979) The control of hydatid disease in Tasmania. *Aust. Vet. J.* **55**, 140–145

Macfarlane, J.T. and Macrae, A.D. (1983) Psittacosis. *Br. Med. Bull.* **39**, 163–167

Macfarlane, J.T., Finch, R.G., Ward, M.J. and Macrae, A.D. (1982) Hospital study of adult community-acquired pneumonia. *Lancet* **2**, 255–258

Macfarlane, J.T., Miller, A.C., Roderick Smith, W.H., Morris, A.H. and Rose, D.H. (1984) Comparative radiographic features of community-acquired Legionnaires' disease, pneumococcal pneumonia, mycoplasma pneumonia and psittacosis. *Thorax* **39**, 28–33

McGivern, D., White, R., Paul, I.D., Caul, E.O., Roome, A.P.C.H. and Westmoreland, D. (1988) Concomitant zoonotic infections with ovine Chlamydia and Q fever in pregnancy: clinical features, diagnosis, management and public health implications. Case report. *Br. J. Obstet. Gynaecol.* **95**, 294–298

McIntyre, M. Kurtz, J.B. and Selkon, J.B. (1990) Prevalence of antibodies to 15 antigens of Legionellace in patients with community-acquired pneumonia *Epidemiol. Infect.* **104**, 39–45

McKendrick, G.D.W., Davies, J. and Dutta, T. (1973) A small outbreak of psittacosis *Lancet* **2**, 1255

McNabb, W.R., Shanson, D.C., Williams, T.D.M. and Lant, A.F. (1984) Adult community-acquired pneumonia in central London. *J. R. Soc. Med.* **77**, 550–555

Manes, G. (1984) Epidemiological situation of brucellosis in the mediterranean countries. *Dev. Biol. Stand.* **56**, 739–747

Mann, J.S., Douglas, J.G., Inglis, J.M. and Leitch, A.G. (1986) Q fever: person to person transmission within a family. *Thorax* **41**, 974-975

Marmion, B.P. and Stoker, M.G.P. (1958). The epidemiology of Q fever in Great Britain. An analysis of the findings and some conclusions. *Br. Med. J.* **2**, 809–816

Marrie, T.J., Haldane, E.V., Faulkner, R.S., Kwan, C., Grant, B. and Cook, F. (1985) The importance of *Coxiella burnetii* as a cause of pneumonia in Nova Scotia. *Can. J. Publ. Health* **76**, 233–236

Marrie, T.J., George, J., Macdonald, S. and Haase, D. (1986a) Are health care workers at risk of infection during an outbreak of nosocomial Legionnaires' disease? *Am. J. Infect. Control* **14**, 209–213

Marrie, T.J., Schlech, W.F., Williams, J.C. and Yates, L. (1986b) Q fever pneumonia associated with exposure to wild rabbits. *Lancet* **1**, 427–429

Marrie, T.J., Macdonald, A., Durant, H., Yates, L. and McCormick, L. (1988) An outbreak of Q fever probably due to contact with a parturient cat. *Chest* **93**, 98–103

Meyer, K.F. (1942) Ecology of psittacosis and ornithosis. *Medicine* **21**, 175–206

Meyer, K.F. (1965) Psittacosis-lymphogranuloma venereum agents. In *Viral and Rickettsial Infections of Man* (Eds F.L. Horsfall and I. Tamm), Lippincott, Philadelphia, p. 1006

Millar, J.K. (1978) The chest film findings in Q fever – a series of 35 cases. *Clin. Radiol.* **29**, 371–375

Miller, A.C. (1979) Early clinical differentiation between Legionnaires' disease and other sporadic pneumonias. *Ann. Intern. Med.* **90**, 526–528

Mitchell, E., O'Mahony, M., Watson, J.M., Lynch, D., Joseph, C., Quigley, C., Aston, R., Constable, G.N., Farrand, R.J., Maxwell, S., Hutchinson, D.N., Craske, J. and Lee, J.V. (1990) Two outbreaks of legionnaires' disease in Bolton health district *Epidemiol. Infect.* **104**, 159–170

Monforte, R., Estruch, R., Vidal, J., Cervera, R. and Urbano-Marquez, A. (1988) Delayed seroconversion, Legionnaires' disease, and age. *Lancet* **2**, 1190–1191

Morris, D.L., Dykes, P.W., Dickson, B., Marriner, S.E., Bohjan, J.A. and Burrows, F.G.O. (1983) Albendazole in hydatid disease *Br. Med. J.* **286**, 103–104

Morris, D.L., Clarkson, M.J., Stallbaumer, M.F., Pritchard, J., Jones, R.S. and Chinnery, J.B. (1985) Albendazole treatment of pulmonary hydatid cysts in naturally infected sheep; a study with relevance to the treatment of hydatid cysts in man. *Thorax* **40**, 453–458

Morris Evans, W.H. and Foreman, H.M. (1963) Smallpox handlers' lung. *Proc. R. Soc. Med.* **56**, 274–283

Murray, H.W. and Tuaczon, C. (1980) Atypical pneumonias. *Med. Clin. N. Am.* **64**, 507–527

Murray, J.F., Lurie, H.I., Kaye, J.I. Komins, C., Borok, R. and Way, M. (1957) Benign pulmonary histoplasmosis (cave disease) in South Africa. *S. Afr. Med. J.* **31**, 245–253

Nagington, J. (1984) Psittacosis/ornithosis in Cambridgeshire 1975–1983. *J. Hyg. (Camb.)* **92**, 9–19

Nordstrom, K., Kallings, I., Dahnsjo, H. and Clemens, F. (1983) An outbreak of Legionnaires' disease in Sweden: report of sixty-eight cases. *Scand. J. Infect. Dis.* **15**, 43–55

Oliphant, J.W., Gordon, D.A., Meis, A. and Parker, R.R. (1949) Q fever in laundry workers presumably transmitted from contaminated clothing. *Am. J. Hyg.* **49**, 76–82

Oliver, P.O. (1979) Medical hazards at sea. *Br. J. Hosp. Med.* **22**, 615–618

Olle-Goig, J.E. and Canela-Soler, J. (1987) An outbreak of *Brucella melitensis* infction by airborne transmission among laboratory workers. *Am. J. Publ. Health* **77**, 335–338

Olsson, B.J. and Treuting, W.L. (1944) An epidemic of severe pneumonitis in the Bayon region of Lousiana. 1. Epidemiological study. *Publ. Health Rep. (Wash.)* **59**, 1299–1311

Ortiz-Roque, C.M. and Hazen, T.C. (1987) Abundance and distribution of legionellaceae in Puerto Rican waters. *Appl. Environ. Microbiol.* **53**, 2231–2236

Parry, W.H. and Mason, K.D. (1972) Psittacosis in pet shops: an occupational hazard *Commun. Med.* **128**, 209–210

Patel, P.J., Al-Suhaibani, H., Al-Aska, A.K., Kolawole, T.M. and Al-Kassimi, F.A. (1988) The chest radiograph in brucellosis. *Clin. Radiol.* **39**, 39–41

Peacock, M.G., Philip, R.N., Williams, J.C. and Faulkner, R.S. (1983). Serological evaluation of Q fever in humans: enhanced phase I titres of immunoglobulins G and A are diagnostic for Q fever endocarditis. *Infect. Immunol.* **41**, 1089–1098

PHLS, Communicable Disease Surveillance Centre (1984) Brucellosis in Britain. *Br. Med. J.* **289**, 817

PHLS, Communicable Disease Surveillance Centre (1988) Report. *Br. Med. J.* **296**, 778–779

Pickworth, F.E., El-Sousi, M., Wells, I.P., McGavin, C.R. and Reilly, S. (1991) The radiological appearances of 'Q' fever pneumonia. *Clin. Radiol.* **441**, 150–153

Pladson, T.R., Stiles, M.A. and Kuritsky, J.N. (1984) Pulmonary histoplasmosis. A possible risk in people who cut decayed wood. *Chest* **86**, 435–438

Plotkin, S.A., Brachman, P.S., Utel, M., Bumford, F.H. and Atchison, M.M. (1960) An epidemic of inhalation anthrax, the first in the twentieth century. *Am. J. Med.* **29**, 992–1001

Plouffe, J.F., Para, M.F., Maher, W.E., Hackman, B. and Webster, L. (1983) Subtypes of *Legionella pneumophila* serogroup I associated with different attack rates. *Lancet* **2**, 649–650

Powell, O. (1960) Q fever: clinical features in 72 cases. *Australas. Ann. Med.* **9**, 214–223

Prechter, G.C. and Prakash, U.B.S. (1989) Bronchoscopy in the diagnosis of pulmonary histoplasmosis. *Chest* **95**, 1033–1036

Price, M.E. and Harrison, B.D.W. (1982). Restrictive pattern of lung function following psittacosis treated with corticosteroids. *Br. J. Dis. Chest* **76**, 199–201

Puolakkainen, M., Ukkonen, P. and Saikku, P. (1988) Import of psittacine birds and chlamydial infections in Finland. *Lancet* **2**, 287–288

Rauch, A.M., Tanner, M., Pacer, R.E., Barrett, M.J., Brokopp, C.D. and Schonberger, L.B. (1987) Sheep-associated Q fever, Idaho. *Archs Intern. Med.* **147**, 341–344

Reeve, R.V.A., Carter, L.A. and Taylor, N. (1988) Respiratory tract infections and importation of exotic birds. *Lancet* **1**, 829–830

Riordan, T., Lewin, I. and Oliver, M.H. (1990) Rapid diagnosis of psittacosis. *Lancet* **335**, 471

Ross, P.J., Seaton, A., Foreman, H.M. and Morris Evans, W.H. (1974) Pulmonary calcification following smallpox handler's lung. *Thorax* **29**, 659–665

Rowbotham, T.J. (1980) Preliminary report on the pathogenicity of *Legionella pneumophila* for fresh water and soil amoeba. *J. Clin. Pathol.* **33**, 1179–1183

Ruf, B., Schurmann, D., Horback, I., Fehrenbach, F.J. and Pohle, H.D. (1989) Incidence and clinical features of community-acquired legionellosis in hospitalised patients. *Eur. Respir. J.* **2**, 257–262

Saag, M.S. and Dismukes, W.E. (1988) Treatment of histoplasmosis and blastomycosis. *Chest* **93**, 848–851

Saimot, A.G., Meulemans, A., Cremieux, A.C., Giovangeli, M.D., Hay, J.M., Delaitre, B. and Coulaud, J.P. (1983) Albendazole as a potential treatment of human hydatidosis. *Lancet* **1**, 1002–1004

Salmon, M.M., Havells, B., Glencros, E.J.G., Evans, A.D. and Palmer S.R. (1982) Q fever in an urban area. *Lancet* **1**, 1002–1004

Sarosi G.A. and Davies, S.F. (1979) Blastomycosis. *Am. Rev. Respir. Dis.* **120**, 911–938

Sarosi, G.A. and Serstock, D. (1976) Isolation of *Blastomyces dermatitidis* from pigeon manure. *Am. Rev. Respir. Dis.* **114**, 1179–1183

Sawyer, L.A., Fishbein, D.B. and McDade, J.E. (1987) Q fever: current concepts. *Rev. Infect. Dis.* **9**, 935–945

Schachter, J. and Dawson, C.R. (1978) *Human Chlamydial Infections*, PSG, Littleton, MA, pp. 9–43

Schaffner, W., Drutz, D.J., Duncan, G.W. and Koenig, M.G. (1967) The clinical spectrum of endemic psittacosis. *Archs Intern. Med.* **119**, 433–443

Schmelzer, L.L. and Tabershaw, I.R. (1968) Exposure factors in occupational coccidioidomycosis. *Am. J. Publ. Health* **58**, 107–113

Segger, I.S., Levin, S. and Schey, G. (1986) Unusual radiological manifestations of Q fever. *Eur. J. Respir. Dis.* **69**, 120–122

Sillis, M. and White, P.M.B. (1990) Rapid diagnosis of psittacosis. *Lancet* **335**, 726

Sobradillo, V., Ansola, P., Baranda, F. and Corral, C. (1989) Q fever pneumonia: a review of 164 community-acquired cases in the Basque country. *Eur. Respir. J.* **2**, 263–266

Solans, P., Gudiol, F., Ponz, M., Linares, J. and Ariza, Y.K. (1978) Neumonia aguda de adquisicion extrahospitalaria. Distribucion etiologica en 415 casos. *Rev. Clin. Esp.* **148**, 367–371

Sorley, D.L., Levin, M.L., Warren, J.W., Flynn, J.P.G. and Gerstenblith, J. (1979) Bat-associated histoplasmosis in Maryland bridge workers. *Am. J. Med.* **67**, 623–626

Spelman, D.W. (1982) Q fever a study of 111 consecutive cases. *Med. J. Aust.* **67**, 623–626

Stathatos, C., Kontaxis, A.N. and Zafiracopoulos, P. (1969) Pancoast's syndrome due to hydatid cysts of the thoracic outlet. *J. Thorac. Cardiovasc. Surg.* **58**, 764–768

Storch, G., Burford, J.G., George, R.B., Kaufman, L. and Ajello, L. (1980) Acute histoplasmosis. Description of an outbreak in Northern Louisiana. *Chest* **77**, 38–42

Stout, J.E., Yu, V.L. and Muraca, P. (1987) Legionnaires' disease acquired within the homes of two patients. Link to the home water supply. *J. Am. Med. Assoc.* **257**, 1215–1217

Tack, K.J., Peterson, P.K., Rasp, F.L., O'Leary, M., Hanto, D., Simmons, R.L. and Sabath, L.D. (1980) Isolation of *Chlamydia trachomatis* from the lower respiratory tract of adults. *Lancet* **1**, 116–120

Tigertt, W.D., Benenson, A.S. and Gochenour, W.S. (1961) Airborne Q fever. *Bacteriol. Rev.* **25**, 285–293

Tison, D.L., Pope, D.H., Cherry, W.B. and Fliermans, C.B. (1980) Growth of *Legionella pneumophila* in association with blue-green algae (cyanobacteria). *Appl. Environ. Microbiol.* **39**, 456–459

Tobin, M.J., Cahill, N., Gearty, G., Maurer, B., Blake, S., Daly, K. and Hone R. (1982) Q fever endocarditis *Am. J. Med.* **72**, 396–400

Tong, P., Tan, W.C. and Pang, M. (1983) Sporadic disseminated histoplasmosis simulating miliary tuberculosis *Br. Med. J.* **287**, 822–823

Torres, A., de Celis, M.R., Roisin, R.R., Vidal, J. and Vidal, A.A. (1987) Adult respiratory distress syndrome in Q fever. *Eur. J. Respir. Dis.* **70**, 322–325

Tosh, F.E., Hammerman, K.J., Weeks, R.J. and Sarosi, G.A. (1974) A common source epidemic of North American blastomycosis. *Am. Rev. Respir. Dis.* **109**, 525–529

Tsai, T.F., Finn, D.R., Plikaytis, B.D., McCauley, W., Martin, S.M. and Fraser, D.W. (1979) Legionnaires' disease: clinical features of an epidemic in Philadelphia. *Ann. Intern. Med.* **90**, 509–517

Varma, M.P.S., Adgey, A.A.J. and Connolly, J.H. (1980) Chronic Q fever endocarditis. *Br. Heart J.* **43**, 659–672

Wadowsky, R.M., Butler, L.J., Cook, M.K., Verma, S.M., Paul, M.A., Fields, B.S., Keleti, G., Sykora, J.L. and Yee, R.G. (1988) Growth supporting activity for *Legionella pneumophila* in tap water cultures and implication of Hartmannellid amoebae as growth factors. *Appl. Environ. Microbiol.* **54**, 2677–2682

Wainwright, A.P., Beaumont, A.C. and Kox, W.J. (1987) Psittacosis: diagnosis and management of severe pneumonia and multiorgan failure. *Intens. Care Med.* **13**, 419–421

Ward, C. and Ward, A.M. (1974) Acquired valvular heart disease in patients who keep pet birds. *Lancet* **2**, 734–736

Ward, J.I., Weeks, M., Allen, D., Hutchenson, Jr R.H., Anderson, R., Fraser, D.W., Kaufman, L., Ajello, L. and Spickard, A. (1979) Acute histoplasmosis: clinical, epidemiologic and serologic findings of an outbreak associated with exposure to a fallen tree. *Am. J. Med.* **66**, 587–595

Washburn, A.M., Tuohy, J.H. and Davis, E.L. (1948) Cave sickness. A new disease? *Am. J. Publ. Health* **38**, 1521–1526

Wasser, L. and Talavera, W. (1987) Pulmonary cryptococcosis in AIDS. *Chest* **92**, 692–695

Werner, S.B., Pappagianis, D., Heindl, I. and Mickel, A. (1972) An epidemic of coccidioidomycosis among archaeology students in Northern California. *N. Engl. J. Med.* **286**, 507–512

White, R.J., Blainey, A.D., Harrison, K.J. and Clarke, S.K.R. (1981) Causes of pneumonia presenting to a district general hospital. *Thorax* **36**, 566–570

Wilson, H.G., Neilson, G.H., Galea, E.G., Stafford, G. and

O'Brien, M.F. (1976) Q fever endocarditis in Queensland. *Circulation* **53**, 680–684

Winner, S.J., Eglin, R.P., Moore, V.I.M. and Mayon-White, R.T. (1987) An outbreak of Q fever affecting postal workers in Oxfordshire. *J. Infect.* **14**, 255–261

Winter, J.H., McCartney, A.C., Fallon, R.H., Telfer, A.B.M., Drury, J.K., Reece, I.J. and Timbury, M.C. (1987) Rapid diagnosis of an outbreak of Legionnaires' disease at Glasgow Royal Infirmary. *Thorax* **42**, 596–599

Wolcott, M.W., Harris, S.H., Briggs, J.N., Dobell, A.R.C. and Brown, R.K. (1971) Hydatid disease of the lung. *J. Thorac. Cardiovasc. Surg.* **62**, 465–469

Woodhead, M.A. (1988) Atypical infections and legionella. *Curr. Opin. Infect. Dis.* **1**, 548–554

Woodhead, M.A. and Macfarlane, J.T. (1985) The protean manifestations of Legionnaires' disease. *J. R. Coll. Physicians Lond.* **19**, 224–230

Woodhead, M.A. and Macfarlane, J.T (1986) Legionnaires' disease: a review of 79 community-acquired cases in Nottingham. *Thorax* **41**, 635–640

Woodhead, M.A. and Macfarlane, J.T. (1987) Comparative clinical and laboratory features of legionella with pneumococcal and mycoplasma pneumonias. *Br. J. Dis. Chest* **81**, 133–139

Woodhead, M.A., Macfarlane, J.T., Rodgers, F.G., Laverick, A., Pilkington, R. and Macrae, A.D. (1985) Aetiology and outcome of severe community-acquired pneumonia. *J. Infect.* **10**, 204–210

Woodhead, M.A., Macfarlane, J.T., McCracken, J.S., Rose, D.H. and Finch, R.G. (1987) Prospective study of the aetiology and outcome of pneumonia in the community. *Lancet* **1**, 671–674

World Health Organization (1986) Joint FAO/WHO expert committee on brucellosis. *Sixth Report, Technical Report Series.* No 740. WHO, Geneva

Wreghitt, T.G. and Taylor, C.E.D. (1988) Incidence of respiratory tract infections and importation of psittacine birds. *Lancet* **1**, 582

Wreghitt, T.G., Barker, C.E., Treharne, J.D., Phipps, J.M., Robinson, V. and Buttery, R.B. (1990) A study of human respiratory tract chlamydial infections in Cambridgeshire 1986–88. *Epidemiol. Infect.* **104**, 479–488

Xu, M. (1985) Hydatid disease of the lung. *Am. J. Surg.* **150**, 568–573

Yung, A.P. and Grayson, M.L. (1988) Psittacosis – a review of 135 cases. *Med. J. Aust.* **148**, 228–233

Zvetina, J.R., Rippon, J.W. and Daum, V. (1978) Chronic pulmonary sporotrichosis. *Mycopathologia* **64**, 53–57

23

Disorders caused by other organic agents

Mark Woodhead and W. Raymond Parkes

Oil granuloma (lipoid pneumonia)

Oils have some importance as an uncommon cause of occupational lung disease and of pulmonary disease of non-occupational origin, which may give rise to diagnostic difficulty in individuals exposed to a pneumoconiosis risk.

Aspiration of milk, olive oil, cod liver oil and mineral paraffin oil used as a laxative or in nasal drops has been known for years as a cause of lipoid pneumonia in the young, elderly and chronically sick. Oily nose drops are no longer widely used but are still available. Occasionally, the disease has been caused by using poppy seed oil as a bronchography medium.

Mineral oils are the chief cause of lipoid pneumonia in industry. They are used extensively as lubricants and cutting fluids and, in fluid or spray form, for turning, milling and grinding operations. They are employed in drop-forging, metal rolling; in the jute and rope industry; as a base for synthetic fibre finishers; and in high-speed dental drills. Their physical character varies from thin spindle oil to thick, heavy oils according to the purpose for which they are required. Many of these operations are capable of producing a fine oil mist or vapour (see Chapter 3, page 35). Mineral oils have also found use as vehicles for spraying insecticides and other agents.

Lung disease caused by inhalation of mineral oil sprays was described by Pendergrass (1942) in a metal turner and by Proudfit, van Ordstrand and Miller (1950) in a man using a spray to lubricate cash registers. Subsequently, oil granuloma has been reported in workers exposed to mineral oil sprays used for insect extermination (Seidel, 1959), for cleaning aircraft (Foe and Bigham, 1954), and

generated by compressed air jets applied to machine parts for removal of surface oil (Weissman, 1951) and from cutting oil (Skorodin and Chandrasekhar, 1983). More recently, lipoid pneumonia was reported in a commercial diver due to inhalation of aerosolized mineral oil from unfiltered air generated from a surface air compressor (Kizer and Golden, 1987) (see also page 832). Exposure to burning animal and vegetable fats over a prolonged period during the testing of fire extinguishers on flash fires has, apparently, caused the disease (Oldenberger et al., 1972). Lipoid pneumonia or pneumonitis resulting from aspiration of petroleum or kerosene (paraffin) in high concentration has been reported in 'fire eaters' of both sexes ('fire eater's lung'). The liquid, held in the mouth, is blown out against a burning stick and ignites to produce a dramatic jet of flame; for fire eating the burning, liquid-soaked stick is placed in the mouth while the breath is held until the flame is extinguished (Beerman et al., 1984; Iverson and Christensen, 1984; Brander, Taskinen and Stenius-Aarniala, 1992). Oil pneumonitis followed aspiration of diesel oil-contaminated sea water by survivors from torpedoed ships in both World Wars (Weissman, 1952). Increased linear opacities have been described in the chest radiographs of workers exposed to oil mist arising from the cold water reduction of mineral oil-coated, hot-rolled, strip steel, but the significance of this observation is uncertain (Jones, 1961).

Most recent studies of men exposed to oil mists in machine shops have not revealed any attributable respiratory symptoms, impairment of lung function or radiographic abnormality (Hendricks et al., 1962; Ely et al., 1970; Goldstein, Benoit and Tyroler, 1970; Pasternack and Ehrlich, 1972; Welter, 1978). However, Cullen et al. (1981) reported respiratory symptoms in five of nine tandem-mill operators who were exposed to oil mists. Detailed investigation of one case revealed cytological and histological changes consistent with lipoid pneumonitis. Another study of 164 men exposed to oil mists for a mean of 16.2 years found an excess of respiratory symptoms (cough) in this group compared to a control group of non-exposed workers, but no radiographic or pulmonary function abnormalities were detected (Järvholm et al., 1982).

There are a number of possible reasons for these disparities in disease potential, including differing work conditions over the years and the methodology of investigation. The comparative responses of the human respiratory tract to different mineral oils do not seem to be known, so that some may be more harmful than others. Again, oil in work atmospheres may be present either in the droplet phase (mist) or vapour phase. The lifespan of droplets, which usually range from about 1 to 5 µm in diameter, depends largely on the boiling point of the oil. Those having high boiling points (and high molecular weights) persist as a fine aerosol for a long time whereas those with low boiling points have a fleeting existence – a few milliseconds. Furthermore, increase in temperature from 20°C (for example) to 37°C, as may occur between ambient and tidal air, shortens droplet life dramatically. These points have, incidentally, an important bearing on methods of sampling oil in the atmosphere (Muir and Emmet, 1976; Davies 1977). Oils with a very short droplet life (such as kerosene) are unlikely to present a threat to the lungs unless at a very high concentration, but those with higher boiling points and longer life may be potentially harmful. However, little seems to be known about the effect on the lungs of oil in the vapour phase. In principle, therefore, it appears that mineral oils are only likely to cause lung disease if present in the atmosphere in high concentration or if their boiling points are in excess of about 300°C.

Pathology

Droplets averaging 2.5 µm in size have been shown to pass through the nasal passages of mice exposed for up to 4 days to an oil mist, and those which reach the alveoli are quickly taken up by alveolar macrophages and transported to pulmonary connective tissues and lymph nodes (Shoshkes, Banfield and Rosenbaum, 1950).

The gross appearances of human lungs are those of a diffuse interstitial pneumonia or a localized dense fibrotic mass which often occupies the upper part of the lung.

The development of lesions is probably similar whether they are due to mineral, animal or vegetable oils and it has been subdivided into four stages by Wagner, Adler and Fuller (1955).

Stage I

Stage I consists of haemorrhagic bronchopneumonia in which macrophages and giant cells quickly appear and take up oil droplets.

Stage II

Stage II presents as numerous oil-laden macrophages in the alveoli, the walls of which are epithelialized and thickened by infiltration of lymphocytes and plasma cells, and by reticulin proliferation. Oil-bearing macrophages are present in the lymphatics, lymphoid follicles are hyperplasic and there is endarteritis obliterans.

Stage III

This is the development of loose collagenous fibrosis of the alveolar walls, in which globules of oil and oil-containing macrophages are enmeshed, and there is some loss of alveolar pattern. Numerous giant cell granulomas resembling tubercles are present (Figure 23.1). Endarteritis is prominent, and disruption of elastic fibres and bronchiolectasis are usual.

Stage IV

In this normal lung architecture is obliterated by dense fibrosis in which there are areas of hyaline

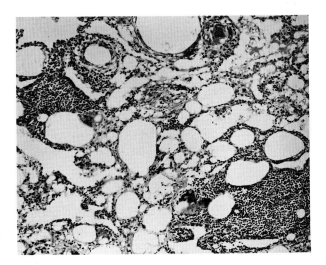

Figure 23.1 Microsection of stage III oil granulomas due to aspiration of mineral oil. Foreign body giant cells are present in some areas and there is some early, loose, collagenous fibrosis. The enlarged alveolar spaces were occupied by oil globules dissolved out during fixing but clearly demonstrated by Sudan in frozen section; osmium tetroxide stain negative. (Magnification × 160)

degeneration and necrosis. Arterioles are completely occluded and bronchioles degenerated and flattened. Globules of oil are pooled in the fibrous tissue but granulomas have disappeared.

Exactly how mineral and other oils cause these changes is not fully understood.

Inhalation of shellac in sprays used in the furniture trade and in hair sprays appears to have caused disease similar to stage III and IV lipoid pneumonia (Hirsh and Russel, 1945; McLaughlin, Bidstrup and Konstam, 1963). This is discussed further in the next section (page 783).

Oil can only be identified in frozen sections because it is dissolved out in formalin-fixed and stained microsections. Vegetable and cod liver oils stain scarlet with Sudan IV and black with osmium tetroxide, whereas mineral oil is paler red with Sudan IV and is *not* stained by osmium tetroxide (Wagner, Adler and Fuller, 1955).

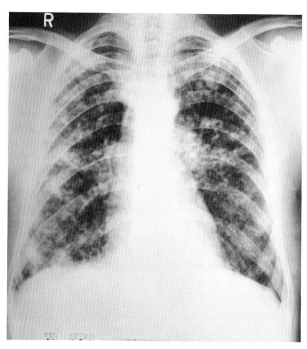

(a)

Clinical features

Symptoms and abnormal physical signs are, as already indicated, absent in many cases, but, in some, cough, sputum, breathlessness on effort, and unilateral or bilateral, basal, coarse, inspiratory crackles may be present, in which case there may be restriction of ventilation, fall in FEV_1 and reduction in $TLCO$ and PaO_2 without airflow obstruction (Weill et al., 1964; Järvolm et al., 1982; Brander, Taskinen and Stenius-Aarniala, 1992). In cases of accidental aspiration of an oil–water mixture, the features may be those of 'shock-lung' with sequelae caused by the oil.

Radiographic appearances

These are disparate. There may be small, multiple, discrete opacities either in groups or widespread throughout both lung fields having, in some cases, a miliary appearance (Figure 23.2). In other cases there are irregular opacities, similar to those of DIPF, in the lower halves of the lung fields; alternatively, there are single or multiple large opacities. A single opacity is usually associated with medicinal oil aspiration (Figure 23.3) and multiple large opacities are most likely to result from massive aspiration of oil-contaminated water (Figure 23.4). Cavitary lesions have been reported in lipoid pneumonia associated with cocaine sniffing (Casademont et al., 1988). In pneumonitis caused by liquid hydrocarbons (for example, 'fire eater's lung'), pneumato-

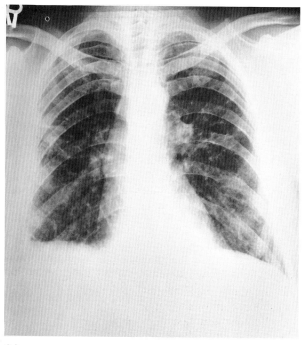

(b)

Figure 23.2 (a) Multiple opacities due to accidental aspiration of diesel oil aerosol. (b) Appearances 7 years later with evidence of residual fibrosis. Radiographs of coal miner exposed underground to a hot oil mist from sudden accidental leakage of a diesel engine. Initially coal pneumoconiosis wrongly diagnosed but lipoid pneumonia later confirmed by biopsy

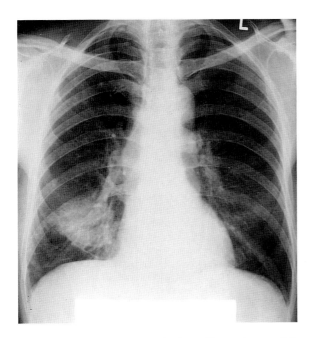

Figure 23.3 Lipoid pneumonia (paraffinoma) resembling, and diagnosed as, lower zone PMF (progressive massive fibrosis) in an aged ex-coal miner addicted to medicinal paraffin oil. Radiographic appearances unchanged for a few years before death. *Post mortem:* moderate numbers of dust macules and occasional small coal pneumoconiosis nodules but no PMF; mass in right lower lobe thought, by naked eye, to be a carcinoma; when frozen and sections stained with H & E, lipoid pneumonia was demonstrated

celes may be seen in areas of the densest infiltrations and are well demonstrated by CT. Usually, they disappear in a few weeks or months (Brander, Taskinen and Stenius-Aarniala, 1992).

Diagnosis

A thorough occupational history and enquiry into the use of oily nasal drops or laxatives are essential. The possibility of aspiration of diesel oil should be considered in any case of pneumonic disease following immersion in the sea or water in ships' holds or factory vessels.

Repeated identification of oil-laden macrophages in sputum stained with Sudan IV or with benzpyrene caffeine, examined by fluorescence microscopy, strongly suggests the diagnosis (Weill et al., 1964). Although oil-containing macrophages are occasionally seen with chronic inflammatory lung disease and histiocytosis X, the history and other features of the disease should readily distinguish them.

The plain radiographic appearances are neither specific nor very helpful: discrete opacities may be mistaken for pneumoconiosis (see Figure 23.2), sarcoidosis, tuberculosis and other causes of such opacities (see Table 7.3). Large opacities are likely to be mistaken for evidence of primary or secondary neoplasia or interpreted as progressive massive fibrosis (PMF) (see Figure 23.3).

CT scanning may assist in establishing the diagnosis by detecting attenuation values of fat density in pulmonary infiltrates which are considered to be specific at densities from –30 to –50 Hounsfield units (Wheeler et al., 1981; Joshi and Cholankeril, 1985; Bréchot et al., 1991) and magnetic resonance imaging may also be useful but is non-specific (Carillon et al., 1988; Bréchot et al., 1991).

The detection of oil-laden macrophages in samples obtained at bronchoscopy, including bronchoalveolar lavage (Spatafora et al., 1987; Silverman et al., 1989), strongly suggests the diagnosis, but lung biopsy may be needed to establish it. Accurate identification of the lipid requires sophisticated procedures, such as infrared spectrophotometry, used to confirm the presence of medicinal liquid paraffin in the lung (Corrin et al., 1987).

In many cases spontaneous resolution of disease is complete, but, in others, it is only partial. Recurrent aspiration – as might occur in fire eaters – could result in localized pulmonary fibrosis or bronchiolitis obliterans (Brander, Taskinen and Stenius-Aarniala, 1992).

Treatment

If still exposed to an oily atmosphere the individual should be removed from it without delay.

Oral prednisolone has been reported to produce a striking resolution of disease: oil-containing macrophages increase in the sputum and oil deposits in the lungs are reduced (Ayvazian et al., 1967) (see Figure 23.4). The value of steroid therapy is, however, disputed (Marks et al., 1972; Steele, Conklin and Mark, 1972).

Prevention

Oil aerosols in machine shops and other factory situations are greatly reduced or eliminated by enclosure of processes, automation and efficient exhaust ventilation systems. These methods usually keep the atmospheric concentrations below the recommended threshold limit values. Periodic medical examinations should be carried out. In other circumstances, however, it is difficult to prevent accidental exposure.

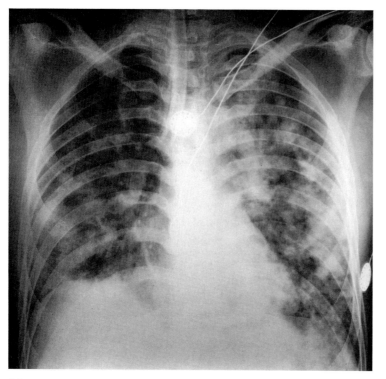

(a)

Figure 23.4 Acute aspiration lipoid pneumonia: the case of a marine engineer who, on entering a ship's ballast tank to investigate a pump failure, was overcome by an oxygen-depleted atmosphere and fell unconscious, face down, into a mixture of sea water and diesel oil. He was quickly rescued and recovered consciousness in a few minutes. After about 4 hours, during which he appeared to suffer little ill-effect, he became acutely ill with fever, cough and severe dyspnoea, and was admitted to intensive care. (a) Radiograph taken in supine position. In spite of clinical improvement, substantial radiograph abnormality persisted, but gradually resolved with prednisolone treatment. (b) Twelve months later (standard film, erect), some abnormal shadows remain in the right cardiophrenic angle and left mid-zone. Lung function at this time: mild decrease in FEV_1, FVC and TLC, with moderate reduction of RV and gas transfer. (Reproduced, with permission, from Dr J.B. Wilkinson)

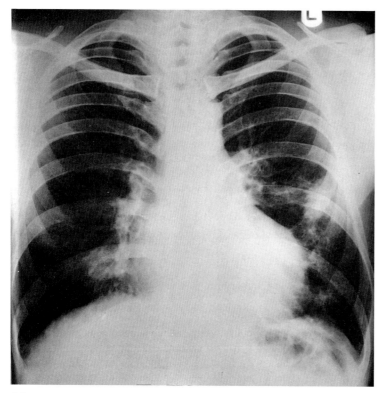

(b)

Lung disease associated with hair sprays

Aerosol hair sprays contain three essential components: the propellant, solvents and other ingredients, and the active agent.

The propellants commonly used are fluorochlorohydrocarbons (trade name Freons) which are gases at room temperature and virtually inert so that they do not react with other materials in the canister. Vinyl chloride is also added in some preparations (Gay et al., 1975) (see page 785).

Solvents and other ingredients include ethyl alcohol, aromatic oils, castor oils and lanolin or its derivatives.

The active agents include:

1. Polyvinylpyrrolidone (PVP).
2. Polyvinyl acetate (PVA) and a co-polymer (PVP–PVA).
3. Shellac: dewaxed shellac is mixed in some preparations with castor oil and aromatic oils. Sometimes it is combined with one of the polyvinyls.
4. Dimethyl hydantoin–formaldehyde resin.
5. Modified polyacrylic acid resin.
6. Lanolin.

The possibility that inhalation of hair sprays may be responsible for lung disease was suggested by Bergmann, Flance and Blumenthal in 1958 and thought to be due to persistence of macromolecules of PVP or its co-polymers in the lungs. It was thus considered to be a 'storage' disorder or 'thesaurosis'. But the existence of a cause-and-effect relationship has been widely disputed on the grounds that other causes of disease have not been satisfactorily excluded in individual cases and that, in general, surveys of exposed populations and animal studies have not confirmed its existence.

Hairdressers, both male and female, and 'beauticians' are occupationally exposed but, in the home, women may fequently use, and children play with, hair sprays. Hence, exposure is very widespread.

The size distribution of the spray aerosols is evidently important with regard to their ability to reach the gas-exchanging region of the lungs, but reported data are widely and remarkably contradictory. At one extreme more than 50 per cent of particles were in excess of 35 µm (Brunner et al., 1963); in between, there are reports of a mass median diameter of 7.8 µm (Swift, Žuškin and Bouhuys, 1976), 50 per cent of particles being smaller than 8.5 µm (Draize et al., 1959) and 20 per cent being less than 3 µm (Ripe et al., 1969). At the other extreme, the majority of particles were under 2 µm in diameter (McLaughlin, Bidstrup and Konstam, 1963).

Undoubtedly, these discrepancies were due to differences in sampling and sizing techniques.

Microscopically, disease attributed to hair sprays has been variously described as DIPF with hilar lymphadenopathy (Bergmann, Flance and Blumenthal, 1958; Bergmann et al., 1962; McLaughlin, Bidstrup and Konstam, 1963), sarcoid-type granulomas (Bergmann et al., 1962) or foreign body granulomas (Gowdy and Wagstaff, 1972; Gebbers et al., 1980). In some cases the features have been those of a desquamative fibrosing alveolitis. Intracytoplasmic, PAS-positive granules observed in macrophages in lung tissue and in lymph nodes were thought to be diagnostic of PVP particles (Bergmann et al., 1962), but similar PAS-staining granules may be seen in sarcoid and other granulomas, and chemical analysis has failed to demonstrate PVP. Brunner et al. (1963) discounted PVP as a cause of lung disease. However, a characteristic infrared absorption spectrum of PVA, not seen in normal lungs, has been reported in a case of alleged 'hairspray lung' by Ripe et al. (1969) who pointed out that, whereas PVP is water soluble, PVA is only slightly so and is precipitated in the presence of water into plastic droplets ranging from 0.1 to 20 µm in diameter. In theory, therefore, PVA is likely to be precipitated on airways' walls and could be more injurious than PVP. PVP and PVA are, apparently, eliminated by the kidney when their molecular weights are less than 20 000 but are retained when these are 60 000 to 70 000 (Gebbers et al., 1980).

It has been argued, however, that many of these cases are, in fact, examples of sarcoidosis (Scheper, 1962; Herrero, Feigelson and Becker, 1965), although this does not appear to be true of them all.

The possibility that oily or fatty substances in PVP and 'mixed' sprays might give rise to granulomatous and fibrotic lesions seems to have received little or no attention. The patient described by McLaughlin, Bidstrup and Konstam (1963), in whom sarcoidosis was apparently excluded, was exposed to shellac-based sprays. Inhalation of shellac in the furniture trade is known to have caused fibrosing lung disease which was presumed to be due to its high fatty acid content and related oils (Hirsch and Russell, 1945) (see previous section). Shellac consists of lac (which is a resinous material obtained from insects of the Coccidae family *Laccifer lacca*) in a solvent which, in hair lacquers, is often an oil as already indicated. Lac itself is highly purified and consists essentially of complex fatty acids, but no insect remains. It seems likely, therefore, that disease associated with shellac inhalation may be an oil granuloma and not, as was suggested in the first edition of this book, a possible example of extrinsic allergic alveolitis due to insect protein.

It is improbable that the relatively inert and insoluble Freons, which resist chemical transformation and absorption of water, are responsible for disease, but some suspicion may attach to vinyl chloride (see next section).

Epidemiology

Radiographic surveys of 2155 hairdressers in the UK, the USA, Italy and Germany revealed only 12 possible cases (Cambridge, 1973). However, a study of 500 students and graduate beauticians in the USA, compared with controls matched for age, smoking habits and geographical locality, is reported to have shown unspecified abnormalities of the chest radiographs, reduced vital capacity (VC) and gas transfer, and atypical cells in the sputum; however, no quantitative or other details are given (Frank, 1975). Nonetheless, the incidence of the disease – if it exists as a specific entity – is evidently very low.

Experimental observations

Following brief exposure to various hair sprays by volunteers, transient changes in their maximal expiratory flow–volume curves were observed by Žuškin and Bouhuys (1974), but the presence of abnormal airways' function was not confirmed by Cohen (1976) and Friedman et al. (1977). Acute exposure of non-smokers to a hair spray aerosol, however, resulted in a short-lived impairment of tracheal mucociliary transport which lasted under 3 hours, whereas similar inhalation of Freon propellant alone had no effect (Friedman et al., 1977).

Exposure of various species of animals to hair spray aerosols has failed to provoke pulmonary disease (Calandra and Kay, 1958; Draize et al., 1959; Giovacchini et al., 1965; Lowsma, Jones and Prendergast, 1966). After almost continuous exposure of guinea-pigs for 5 days a week over 12 months to hair spray particles ranging from 0.6 to 1.2 μm in diameter, there were no histopathological changes other than progressive lymphoid infiltration, although this was also observed in a control group of animals maintained during the same period (Cambridge, 1973). However, the possibility that a granulomatous response can be induced in animals treated previously wih Freund's adjuvant raises the question of hypersensitivity (Gialdroni, Grassi and Clini, 1964) for which, at present, there appears to be no convincing evidence in human beings. Although, in one case, it appears that pulmonary infiltration, which had cleared when exposure ceased, reappeared when use of hair spray was resumed and disappeared yet again when it was stopped (Bergmann, 1973).

Storage of PVP does not seem to have been established in any of the reported cases of 'thesaurosis' but was shown to occur in the reticuloendothelial system following intravenous injection, as was discovered when PVP was used some years ago as an inert plasma substitute.

Clinical features

Affected individuals may complain of cough and breathlessness, sometimes with mild pyrexia, but others are symptomless. Abnormal physical signs are few or absent.

The chest radiograph may show patchy bilateral infiltrates, fine linear opacities, a clear diffuse interstitial pulmonary fibrosis (DIPF) pattern or the appearances of lobar consolidation – the least frequently reported abnormality. After the use of sprays has ceased, the radiographic appearances have returned to normal rapidly, or within 6 months in most cases (suggesting that the sprays might have been the cause); however, in a few, resolution took about 2 years (Ripe et al., 1969; Gowdy and Wagstaff, 1972).

Lung function tests have been described in very few cases and, on the whole, have shown little abnormality, although impairment of gas transfer was reported in cases with radiographic evidence of DIPF (Garibaldi and Caprotti, 1964).

Conclusion

When all the available evidence, much of which is circumstantial, is considered, inhalation of hair sprays has evidently not been proven to be a specific cause of lung pathology although it remains under suspicion. As 'storage' or accumulation of PVP or co-polymers in the lungs has not been demonstrated, the term 'thesaurosis' is distracting and best abandoned.

Lung disease in individuals exposed to hair spray aerosols may be due to the following:

1. Unrelated and coincidental disease – possibly the most common explanation.
2. Lipoid pneumonia, if there has been heavy exposure to oily shellac or lanolin preparations.
3. Some ingredient other than oils or fatty acids which is not the active agent or propellant.
4. Possibly PVA or vinyl chloride.

Hypersensitivity to any particular ingredient has not so far been demonstrated.

In attempting diagnosis, the presence of PAS-positive granules in lung tissue is of no help, but staining for mineral and vegetable oils might be (see page 780).

If, in the individual patient, known causes of lung disease can be confidently excluded, he or she should be advised to avoid further exposure whether at work or in the home.

Finally, as the use of hair sprays is so widespread and there is still a question as to whether they can occasionally cause disease, more detailed and carefully controlled investigations than so far carried out seem desirable to establish once and for all whether we are faced with a rare, but real, disease or an illusion (Bergmann, 1973).

Polyvinyl chloride lung disease

Polyvinyl chloride (PVC) has been used extensively in the plastics industry for some 30 years or more. It is produced by the polymerization of vinyl chloride monomer (VCM) (CH_2CHCl) – a gas at normal temperature – under pressure at 40°C to 70°C. Polymerization does not normally proceed beyond about 95 per cent conversion, so that some 5 to 6 per cent monomer remains and is returned to the gas holders. However, because VCM has a strong affinity for PVC, it is difficult to remove it all. PVC is dried in continuous driers and the resultant powder may contain about 50 parts per million (p.p.m.) VCM (Barnes, 1976). Vinyl chloride monomer is also used as a propellant in some aerosol sprays and as a refrigerant.

An association between prolonged exposure in the PVC production process and acro-osteolysis, Raynaud's disease, scleroderma, hepatomegaly with elevated alkaline phosphatase, and angiosarcoma of the liver is now well known, although only apparent in recent years (Lilis et al., 1975; Sakabe, 1975; Suciu et al., 1975; Laplanche et al., 1987). Vinyl chloride monomer has been regarded as the responsible agent even in workers exposed only to PVC dust. Pulmonary disease has, however, rarely been described.

Uses of PVC

These include manufacture of floor coverings, imitation leather, a wide variety of plastic goods and synthetic fibres.

Sources of exposures

Sources occur during production of VCM and PVC, drying and bagging of PVC and in the initial stages of plastics manufacture in which PVC particles are generally less than 5 µm in diameter. High concentrations of VCM may be produced by hair spray or insecticide canisters in confined spaces (Gay et al., 1975).

Experimental observations

Inhalation of VCM and PVC by animals is reported to cause lung fibrosis (Frongia, Spinazzola and Bucarelli, 1974; Prodan et al., 1975), although PVC is not, apparently, cytotoxic to alveolar and peritoneal macrophages in vitro (Styles and Wilson, 1973).

Clinical features

Studies of workers in the PVC manufacturing industry have shown lung function and radiographic abnormalities related to exposure. Lloyd et al. (1984) described a fall in gas transfer (TLCO) in PVC manufacturers. This abnormality was associated with working in a factory prior to 1975 – a time when VCM levels were much higher than subsequently – suggesting that VCM, or some other unidentified agent, was responsible rather than PVC. However, a PVC worker with low gas transfer, normal lung volumes but minimal VCM exposure has been reported (Antti-Poika et al., 1986). Other workers have reported either no change in lung function (Chivers, Lawrence-Jones and Paddle, 1980) or a small reduction in lung volumes (FEV_1, FVC) related to PVC exposure, but these changes were of little functional significance (Soutar et al., 1980; Soutar and Gauld, 1983).

Airflow obstruction has been reported in PVC processing workers (Miller et al., 1975; Ernst et al., 1988), but these changes may be related to exposure to plasticizers (for example, trimellitic anhydride) rather than to PVC itself.

Lillis et al. (1975) described an increased prevalence of irregular and small, rounded radiographic opacities mainly in the middle and lower lung fields of workers exposed to PVC and VCM. These findings have been confirmed by others (Soutar et al., 1980; Soutar and Gauld, 1983), but again the functional significance of the changes is questionable.

Three cases of pulmonary fibrosis, two of which were associated with granulomatous changes, have been described in workers exposed to PVC dust. One had shovelled PVC powder for a year in a plastics factory; one had worked for 13 years in the bagging area of a polymerization plant; and the third had worked in a PVC factory for 12 years but had an accumulated exposure to PVC dust of only about 750 days. In one, the chest radiograph was normal, but, in the other two, blotchy, irregular opacities or 'diffuse micronodular' opacities were seen. PVC was extracted with a solvent from lung tissue in one case, and electron microscopy showed oval bodies identical to particles of PVC powder in the pulmonary macrophages. X-ray microanalysis in one case showed the presence of chlorine, suggesting that the phagocytosed material was PVC dust (Szende et al., 1970; Arnaud et al., 1978; Antti-Poika et al., 1986).

There is some evidence that disease caused by PVC is an immune complex disorder intitiated by the adsorption of vinyl chloride or a metabolite onto tissue or plasma protein (Ward et al., 1976).

Conclusions

Minor changes in the chest radiograph and lung function may occur in workers exposed to PVC or VCM, or both, but major functional changes are unusual.

Strict hygiene control in VCM polymerization plants, and in the use of PVC powder for the manufacture of plastics, has been in force for the last few years due to the risk of serious extrapulmonary disease, so that the likelihood of new cases of lung disese occurring is now probably small. However, regular medical surveillance with ventilatory function tests and full size chest radiographs, in addition to other screening tests, is essential.

Polymer fume fever

This is an influenza-like disorder, similar in many respects to metal fume fever (see Chapter 18, page 593), caused by pyrolysis products of tetrafluoroethylene (TFE) resins, notably polytetrafluoroethylene (PTFE – trade names Fluon, Teflon and Halon) and polyvinyl fluoride.

PTFE resin is produced by controlled polymerization of TFE emulsion under pressure. It is then moulded in sintering ovens or by pressure processes. Physiologically, it is inert and causes neither irritation nor allergic sensitization of body tissues. However, if heated to between 315°C and 375°C, particles, probably consisting of polymer chain

fragments, are evolved. Above 380°C small amounts of the toxic gases hexafluoropropylene and octafluoroisobutylene are produced and, at temperatures in excess of 500°C (when the rate of pyrolysis increases), perfluoroisobutylene and carbonyl fluoride, which are also toxic, are formed. These toxic compounds can cause pulmonary oedema in animals (Harris, 1951; Okawa and Polakoff, 1974).

PTFE resins are used extensively for most modern plastics products including insulation materials, electrical components, bearings, gaskets, piping, coatings for wires, chemical vessels and nonstick cooking utensils, and in dirt-repellant starch sprays.

There is no hazard to health unless the polymer is subjected to heat in excess of 300°C. This may occur in a variety of circumstances: the operation of moulding and extruding machines, high-speed machining of components, welding of metal coated with PTFE or attached to PTFE resin blocks, ironing clothes sprayed with polymer– starch mixture for prolonged periods, and smoking cigarettes contaminated with the polymer either by direct contact or by particles suspended in the workplace atmosphere. The temperature in the burning zone of a cigarette exceeds 800°C (Touey and Mumpower, 1957; Harris, 1959; Adams, 1963; Lewis and Kerby, 1965; Wiliams and Smith, 1972; doPico et al., 1973; Kuntz and McCord, 1974).

Clinical features

There is always a delay of some hours – often about 3 or 4 – between exposure to the 'fume', or particulate, before symptoms develop.

Usually the first complaint is discomfort or an oppressive sensation in the chest and breathlessness with or without cough. General malaise, joint pains, rigors, sweating, pyrexia up to about 40°C and tachycardia follow. Physical signs in the lungs are either absent or there may be a few scattered inspiratory crackles and the chest radiograph is normal. Recovery is complete in 1 to 2 days.

The illness is frequently regarded as influenza or some other acute infection by both patient and doctor unless there are recurrences. Hence, 'polymer fume fever' should be borne in mind in cases of 'pyrexia of unknown origin'.

The fundamental pathogenesis of the symptoms is not known. Unlike metal fume fever, to which tolerance is quickly acquired on repeated exposures and equally rapidly lost when exposure ceases during weekends or holidays, polymer fume fever seems to occur without regard to previous exposure (Malten and Zielhuis, 1964; Kuntz and McCord, 1974).

However, disease is not always so innocuous and pulmonary oedema may occasionally follow exposure to polymer subjected to high temperatures, for example, during welding. This is marked by respiratory distress and the physical and radiographic signs of oedema of the lungs. Recovery is rapid and no fatalities seem to have been reported (Robbins and Ware, 1964; Evans, 1973). Furthermore, DIPF appears to have followed numerous attacks of polymer fume fever caused by PTFE present on cigarettes contaminated at work (Capodaglio, Monarco and de Vito, 1961; Williams, Atkinson and Patchefsky, 1974). Hence, although polymer fume fever is a benign and transient disorder in most instances, continued observation of workers who have suffered multiple episodes is probably desirable.

It is likely that many cases of polymer fume fever and occasional cases of pulmonary oedema are overlooked.

Prevention

Enclosure and ventilation of the manufacturing processes, good housekeeping and prohibition of smoking where PTFE is cut, machined or processed are now general, and there is little hazard to health. Analysis of soluble fluoride levels in the urine is a helpful index of toxicity in workers who may have mild symptoms of polymer fume fever. The normal range is 0.098 to 2.19 mg/l (Okawa and Polakoff, 1974). Accidental exposure to toxic products of pyrolysis may occur in other circumstances from time to time.

Paraquat poisoning

Paraquat (known in Britain as Gramoxone, which is concentrated, and Weedol which is dilute, and in the USA as Orthoparaquat, Orthodualparaquat and Orthospot) is a bipyridyl herbicide. It is used on a global scale in more than 130 countries and in Europe it is estimated that 5×10^6 hectares are sprayed annually with this agent (Sagar, 1987).

The value of paraquat in food production is due to its ability to destroy weeds on contact with their green parts while becoming harmless in the soil due to adsorption onto clay minerals (Conolly, 1975).

Paraquat is well known as a cause of serious lung disease which is commonly, but not invariably, fatal.

The majority of cases have been due to ingestion of the liquid accidentally from unmarked bottles or with suicidal intent (Bullivant, 1966; Campbell, 1968), and the possibility of absorption by routes other than the gastrointestinal tract has been regarded on the whole as unimportant (Swan, 1969; Fairshter and Wilson, 1975). Certainly, direct inhalation into the lungs from sprays is improbable because the particle size range appears to be too large (Kimbrough, 1974; Levin et al., 1979; Chester and Ward, 1984) and field studies have confirmed the low risk of inhalation exposure to workers involved in hand-held (Chester and Woollen, 1981), vehicle-mounted (Staiff et al., 1975) and aerial (Chester and Ward, 1984) spraying of paraquat. However, paraquat mist drifting into a garden from nearby agricultural spraying operations has, apparently, caused non-fatal lung disease (George and Hedworth-Whitty, 1980). Absorption through intact or abraded skin and entry into the circulation can occur and is facilitated if paraquat is combined with a surface-active 'wetting' agent as is usually the case (McDonagh and Martin, 1970; Jaros, 1978; Levin et al., 1979). Hence, although paraquat has occasionally been drunk accidentally by agricultural or horticultural workers, the chief occupational hazard is percutaneous absorption of spray solution. In fact, human skin provides a very good barrier against penetration by paraquat and, although local skin and nail changes are not uncommon with prolonged exposure, systemic poisoning is unlikely from recommended agricultural use (Swan, 1969; Hearn and Keir, 1971; Howard, 1979, 1980). Systemic poisoning related to agricultural use of paraquat usually relates to misuse of the product.

The severity of the clinical presentation following the ingestion of paraquat depends on the dose taken, 20 to 40 mg/kg probably being fatal (Conolly, 1975). Three degrees of intoxication are recognized: mild poisoning (20 mg paraquat ion/kg body weight); moderate to severe poisoning (20 to 40 mg paraquat ion/kg body weight) and acute fulminant poisoning (>40 mg paraquat ion/kg body weight) (Vale, Meredith and Buckley, 1987). In mild poisoning, which may be asymptomatic or associated with vomiting and diarrhoea, all patients recover fully; the majority of patients in other categories die, usually after 2 to 3 weeks following the development of renal failure and pulmonary fibrosis. In acute fulminant poisoning, multiple organ failure occurs early and death follows within a few hours or days with coma and cardiorespiratory failure. Cough and dyspnoea are the usual respiratory features, although haemoptysis may occur. Pneumothorax and pleural effusion may occur (Vale, Meredith and Buckley, 1987). In milder cases, lung disease with bilateral or unilateral crackles and pneumonic-type or small round radiographic opacities develop in 2 to 5 days. This is often followed by progressive

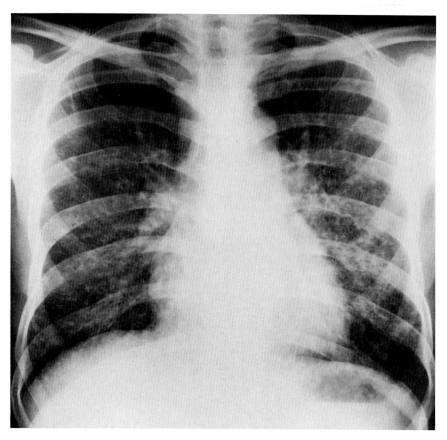

Figure 23.5 Bilateral soft opacities following percutaneous absorption of paraquat from a leaky spray reservoir. The man was in good health 2 weeks earlier. (Reproduced, with permission, from Levin et al., 1979)

fibrosis. In some cases, the disease appears to resolve completely with supportive treatment only (Conolly, 1975; Higenbottom et al., 1979; Hendy, Williams and Ackrill, 1984), whereas, in others, persistent, non-progressive pulmonary fibrosis can occur (Hudson et al., 1991). Disease following percutaneous absorption is likely to be less severe than that following intestinal absorption. The former can be distinguished by a lack of reddening and ulceration of mouth and pharynx, and of gastrointestinal disturbance, and by the presence of erythema and burning of the area of contaminated skin – sometimes with ulceration.

Jaros (1978) described a fatality following exposure of the skin of an agricultural worker to concentrated paraquat which leaked from a container on to his neck, back and legs. Six days later he had respiratory distress which rapidly worsened. The chest radiograph showed multiple, small and occasionally coalescent opacities. Pulmonary oedema and necrotizing alveolitis were present *post mortem*. Levin et al. (1979) have reported the case of 10 workers who sprayed weeds

in a vineyard with Gramoxone. One had balanced a leaky spray reservoir on his shoulder resulting in a burnt area of skin with ulceration, subsequent dyspnoea, cyanosis, inspiratory crackles, bilateral ill-defined opacities in the chest radiograph and rapid deterioration to death in respiratory failure (Figure 23.5). Of the other nine, who were less heavily exposed, but whose trousers were always soaked with spray below the knees with burning and redness of the underlying skin, none had distinctive symptoms, but six had reduced gas transfer. In three of these in whom the reduction was greatest there were increased basal markings in the chest radiograph. Lung biopsy in two men showed medial hypertrophy of pulmonary arteries with evidence of fresh and organized thrombi and, in one, DIPF. The remaining three cases showed no abnormality. It is possible that mild lesions may regress completely.

Patients who survive an episode of paraquat poisoning may not have clinically significant residual pulmonary damage, although, occasionally, there are irreversible fibrotic changes (Fitzgerald et al., 1979; Hudson et al., 1991).

Pathology

Two distinct phases are recognizable. The first, a destructive phase, consists of swelling and fragmentation of the alveolar epithelium followed by alveolar oedema and an acute inflammatory exudate. In the second, which is proliferative, there is a diffuse cellular *intra-alveolar* – not mural – fibrosis. this becomes dense and obliterates the pulmonary architecture. Medial hypertrophy of muscular pulmonary arteries which may contain organizing thrombi is often present (Smith and Heath, 1975; Thurlbeck and Thurlbeck, 1976; Fitzgerald et al., 1979) (Figure 23.6).

Levin et al. (1979) were able to reproduce changes identical to those shown in human lungs in the pulmonary arteries of rats by painting the skin at weekly intervals with a paraquat solution. They attributed these lesions in both human beings and animals not to chronic hypoxia (Smith and Heath, 1975), but to paraquat itself absorbed in low dosage through the skin over a prolonged period; this was in contrast to the extensive alveolar changes caused by high ingested doses.

Diagnosis

This depends upon the clinician being aware that paraquat poisoning may occasionally occur occupationally from percutaneous absorption. A careful history is, therefore, required. The skin of arms, shoulders, legs and feet must be inspected for 'burns' erythema, and ulceration or abrasions; also the mouth and pharynx should be inspected to exclude the possibility of ingestion. Other acute pulmonary disorders must, of course, be excluded.

Measurement of plasma and urine paraquat concentrations may be of value in assessing the severity and predicting the outcome of poisoning (Proudfoot et al., 1979; Schermann et al., 1987).

Treatment

This is directed towards preventing gastrointestinal absorption, enhancing elimination from the body (thereby preventing active accumulation in the lung) and supportive therapy.

Absorption from the gastrointestinal tract is rapid and the use of adsorbents (for example, fuller's earth or activated charcoal) more than 6 hours after ingestion is unlikely to be effective. Similarly, due to the rapid uptake and binding by the lungs, steps

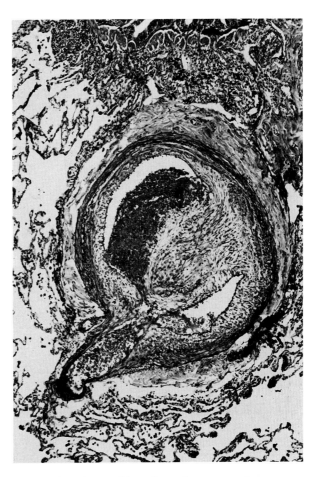

Figure 23.6 Biopsy of lung from the same patient as Figure 23.5 showing a pulmonary artery with muscular hyperplasia and recent organizing thrombus. (Magnification × 30.) (Reproduced, with permission, from Levin et al., 1979)

to eliminate paraquat more than 18 hours after exposure may be unhelpful. Within this 'therapeutic window' fluid losses should be replaced and extracorporeal elimination techniques – for example, haemodialysis, haemoperfusion (Bismuth et al., 1987; Proudfoot, Prescott and Jarvie, 1987) – or continuous arteriovenous haemofiltration (Pond et al., 1987) – may be of value, but there is little evidence that such invasive procedures improve survival.

Although paraquat is thought to damage the lung via reactive oxygen radicals and depletion of reduced nicotinamide adenine dinucleotide phosphate (NADPH) (Smith, 1987), this is insufficiently understood to have therapeutic implications. The value of steroids (Davies and Connolly, 1975), superoxide dismutase (Saltzman and Fridovich, 1973), cyclophosphamide (Addo and Poon-King, 1986; Bateman, 1987) and radiotherapy (Webb et al., 1984; Williams and Webb, 1987) is unproven.

Early assessment of severity, according to plasma and urine paraquat levels, is essential. In those with severe poisoning, efforts should be directed to symptom relief.

Prevention

Used correctly, paraquat should not be an occupational risk. Workers should be educated in the use of paraquat sprays, avoidance of spillage or leakage of concentrated paraquat (for example, when decanting), and wearing of protective clothing and impervious footwear during spraying operations.

Newer formulations, including the use of lower concentrations of paraquat and the use of 'additives' such as 'stenching' agents, to produce an unpleasant smell, a blue colour and an emetic agent, may also help to reduce the chances of accidental intoxication.

Organic insecticides

Chlorinated camphene (toxaphene)

This is a waxy material containing chlorine. When ingested it causes acute stimulation of the central nervous system in human beings and animals. It is used against cotton worms and other pests.

Inhalation may cause bilateral pneumonic disease which ranges radiographically from the appearances of pulmonary oedema to widespread miliary opacities in the middle and lower zones (Warraki, 1963). The underlying cause is not known.

Recovery is usually complete by 8 weeks.

Organophosphates

Chief among these are parathion and malathion, which may be absorbed via the skin, gastrointestinal tract or the lungs. They cause an excessive cholinergic effect by inhibiting the enzyme acetylcholinesterase at nerve endings. This results in excessive sweating and salivation, miosis, bradycardia, increased peristalsis and bronchial secretions and, in some cases, pulmonary oedema of sudden onset which, if not treated promptly, is likely to be fatal (Bledsoe and Seymour, 1972). It is imperative, therefore, to anticipate the possibility of development of lung disease.

Those who are at risk from these chemicals are farm workers during and after spraying crops and, occasionally, employees involved in their manufacture and transport.

Treatment consists primarily in inhibiting excessive cholinergic activity with atropine.

Pyrethrum

This has been referred to already as a possible cause of extrinsic allergic alveolitis in Chapter 20 (page 702).

Dimethyl sulphate $((CH_3)_2SO_4)$

This organic ester is used extensively as a solvent of mineral oils and as a methylating agent in the perfume, dye and pharmaceutical industries. It is highly toxic and vesicant both as a liquid and a vapour; in the presence of water or moisture it hydrolyses readily to sulphuric acid and methyl alcohol. Its effects are comparable to those of phosgene (see page 627).

Exposure is likely to occur as a result of accidental spillage, breakage or leakage of bottles or vessels containing the liquid, or when transferring the liquid from one container to another.

Symptoms are usually delayed for about 6 to 24 hours after exposure. Swelling of the face, eyelids and fauces occurs due to severe oedema and vesication of all exposed or unprotected parts of the body. There is pyrexia up to about 37.8°C (100°F), tachycardia or bradycardia, dysphagia, respiratory distress with severe cough, bronchospasm and, commonly, the clinical and radiographic signs of pulmonary oedema which may be fatal. Hepatitis, nephritis, analgesia, convulsions and coma may also occur (Littler and McConnell, 1955; Haswell, 1960; Fassett, 1963; Browning, 1965).

Speedy application of treatment with oxygen, corticosteroids and antibiotics results in complete recovery in a few days but all drugs that are central nervous system depressants must be avoided. Inhalation of steam is helpful in relieving initial respiratory distress. Before the antibiotic era death from pneumonia was common.

Intermittent exposure to low concentrations of the vapour may be associated with persistent tracheitis.

Preventive measures include: education of employees, good ventilation, closed handling systems, provision of airline respirators and protective clothing when entering a contaminated zone, and decontamination of spillages with a dilute alkali.

References

Adams, W.G.F. (1963) Polymer fume fever due to inhalation of fume from polytetrafluoroethylene. *Trans. Assoc. Ind. Med. Offrs* **13**, 20–21

Addo, E. and Poon-King, T. (1986) Leucocyte suppression in treatment of 72 patients with paraquat poisoning. *Lancet* **1**, 1117–1120

Antti-Poika, M., Nordman, H., Nickels, J., Keskinen, H. and Viljanen, A. (1986) Lung disease after exposure to polyvinyl chloride dust. *Thorax* **41**, 566–567

Arnaud, A., DeSanti, P.P., Garbe, L., Payan, H. and Charpin, J. (1978) Polyvinyl chloride pneumoconiosis. *Thorax* **33**, 19–25

Ayvazian, L.F., Steward, D.S., Merkel, C.G. and Frederick, W.W. (1967) Diffuse lipoid pneumonitis successfully treated with prednisone. *Am. J. Med.* **43**, 930–934

Barnes, A.W. (1976) Vinyl chloride and the production of PVC. *Proc R. Soc. Med.* **69**, 277–280

Bateman, D.N. (1987) Pharmacological treatments of paraquat poisoning. *Human Toxicol.* **6**, 57–62

Beerman, B., Christenson, T., Möller, P. and Stillström, A. (1984) Lipoid pneumonia: an occupational hazard of fire eaters. *Br. Med. J.* **289**, 1728–1729

Bergmann, M. (1973) Thesaurosis: Illness or illusion? *Chest* **64**, 153–154

Bergmann, M., Flance, I.J. and Blumenthal, J.H. (1958) Thesaurosis following inhalation of hair spray. *N. Engl. J. Med.* **258**, 472–476

Bergmann, M., Flance, I.J., Cruz, P.T., Klam, N., Aronson, P.R., Joshi, R.A. and Blumenthal, H.T. (1962) Thesaurosis due to inhalation of hair spray. Report of 12 new cases including 3 autopsies. *N. Engl. J. Med.* **266**, 750–755

Bledsoe, F.H. and Seymour, E.Q. (1972) Acute pulmonary oedema associated with parathion poisoning. *Radiology* **103**, 53–56

Bismuth, C., Scherrmann, J.M., Garnier, R., Band, F.J. and Pontal, P.G. (1987) Elimination of paraquat. *Human Toxicol.* **6**, 63–67

Brander, P.E., Taskinen, E. and Stenius-Aarniala, B. (1992) Fire eater's lung. *Eur. Respir. J.* **5**, 112–114

Bréchot J.M. Buy, J.N., Laaban, J.P. and Rochemaure, J. (1991) Computed tomography and magnetic resonance findings in lipoid pneumonia. *Thorax* **46**, 738–739

Browning, E. (1965) *Toxicity and Metabolism of Industrial Solvents*, Elsevier, Amsterdam, London, New York, pp. 713–717

Brunner, M.J., Giovacchini, R.P., Wyatt, J.P., Dunlap, F.E. and Calandra, J.C. (1963) Pulmonary disease and hair spray polymers: a disputed relationship. *J. Am. Med. Assoc.* **184**, 851–857

Bullivant, C.M. (1966) Accidental poisoning by paraquat: report of two cases in man. *Br. Med. J.* **1**, 1272–1273

Calandra, J. and Kay, J.A. (1958) The effects of aerosol hair sprays on experimental animals. *Proc. Sci. Sect. Toilet Goods Assoc.* **30**, 41–44

Cambridge, G.W. (1973) Inhalation toxicity studies. *Aerosol. Age* **18**, 32–68

Campbell, S. (1968) Death from paraquat in a child. *Lancet* **1**, 144

Capodaglio, E., Monarco, G. and de Vito, G. (1961) Sindrome respiratio da malazione di composi fuori alifatici nella preparazione del politetra-fluoretilene. *Rass. Med. Ind.* **30**, 124–129

Carillon, Y., Tixier, E., Revel, D. and Cordier, J.F. (1988) MR diagnosis of lipoid pneumonia. *J. Comput. Assist. Tomogr.* **12**, 876–877

Casademont, J., Xaubert, A., Lopez-Guillermo, J., Agusti, C. and Ramirez J. (1988) Radiographic bilateral cavitary lesions in lipoid pneumonia. *Eur. Respir. J.* **1**, 93–94

Chester, G. and Ward, R.J. (1984) Occupational exposure and drift hazard during aerial application of paraquat to cotton. *Archs Envir. Contam. Toxicol.* **13**, 551–563

Chester, G. and Woollen, B.H. (1981) A study of the occupational exposure of Malaysian plantation workers to paraquat. *Br. J. Ind. Med.* **38**, 23–33

Chivers, C.P., Lawrence-Jones, C. and Paddle, G.M. (1980) Lung function in workers exposed to polyvinyl chloride dust. *Br. J. Ind. Med.* **37**, 147–151

Cohen, B.M. (1976) Peripheral airway responses to acute hair spray exposure. *Am. Rev. Respir. Dis.* **113** (suppl.), 123

Conolly, M.E. (1975) Paraquat poisoning. *Proc. R. Soci. Med.* **68**, 441

Corrin, B., Crocker, P.R., Hood, B.J., Levison, D.A. and Parkes, W.R. (1987) Paraffinoma confirmed by infrared spectophotometry. *Thorax* **42**, 389–390

Cullen, M.R., Balmes, J.R., Robins, J.M. and Walker Smith, G.J. (1981) Lipoid pneumonia caused by oil mist exposure from a steel rolling tandem mill. *Am. J. Ind. Med.* **2**, 51–58

Davies, C.N. (1977) Atmospheric concentrations of oil mist. *Ann. Occup. Hyg.* **20**, 91–92

Davies, D.S. and Conolly, M.E. (1975) Paraquat poisoning – possible therapeutic approach *Proc. R. Soc. Med.* **68**, 442

doPico, G.A., Layton, Jr, C.R., Clayton, J.W. and Rankin, J. (1973) Acute pulmonary reaction to spray starch with soil repellant. *Am. Rev. Respir. Dis.* **108**, 1212–1215

Draize, J.H., Nelson, A.A., Newburger, S.H. and Kelley, E.A. (1959) Inhalation toxicity studies of six types of aerosol hair sprays. *Proc. Sci. Sect. Toilet Goods Assoc.* **31**, 28–32

Ely, T.S., Pedley, S.F., Hearne, F.T. and Stille, W.T. (1970) A study of mortality, symptoms and respiratory function in humans occupationally exposed to oil mist. *J. Occup. Med.* **12**, 253–261

Ernst, P., de Guire, L., Armstrong, B. and Theriault, G. (1988) Obstructive and restrictive ventilatory impairment in polyvinyl chloride fabrication workers. *Am. J. Ind. Med.* **14**, 273–279

Evans, E.A. (1973) Pulmonary oedema after inhalation of fumes from polytetrafluoroethylene (PTFE). *J. Occup. Med.* **7**, 599–601

Fairshter, R.D. and Wilson, A.F. (1975) Paraquat poisoning: manifestations and therapy. *Am. J. Med.* **59**, 751–753

Fassett, D.W. (1963) Esters. In *Industrial Hygiene and Toxicology, Vol. II* (ed. F.A. Patty), Interscience, New York, London, pp. 1927–1930

Fitzgerald, G.R., Barnville, G., Gibney, R.T.N. and Fitzgerald, M.X. (1979) Clinical, radiological and pulmonary function assessment in 13 long-term survivors of paraquat poisoning. *Thorax* **34**, 414–415

Foe, R.B. and Bigham, Jr, R.S. (1954) Lipoid pneumonia following occupational exposure to oil spray. *J. Am. Med. Assoc.* **155**, 33–34

Frank, R. (1975) Are aerosol sprays hazardous? *Am. Rev. Respir. Dis.* **112**, 485–489

Friedman, M., Dougherty, R., Nelson, S.R., White, R.P., Sackner, M.A. and Wauner, A. (1977) Acute effects of an aerosol hair spray on tracheal mucociliary transport. *Am. Rev. Respir. Dis.* **116**, 281–286

Frongia, N., Spinazzola, A. and Bucarelli, A. (1974) Lesioni polmonari sperimentali da inalazione prolungata di polveri di PVC in ambiente di lavaro. *Med. Lav.* **65**, 321–342

Garibaldi, R. and Caprotti, M. (1964) Ricerche cliniche su un gruppo di soggetti esposti alla inalazione di lacche nebulizzate per capelli. *Med. Lav.* **55**, 424–433

Gay, B.W., Lonneman, W.A., Bridbord, K. and Moran J.B. (1975) Measurements of vinyl chloride from aerosol sprays. *Ann. NY Acad. Sci.* **246**, 286–295

Gebbers, J-O., Burkhardt, A., Tetzner, C., Rudiger, H.W. and Von Wichert, P. (1980) Haarspray-Lunge, Klinische und morphologische Befunde. *Schweiz. Med. Wochenschr.* **110**, 610–615

George, M. and Hedworth-Whitty, R.B. (1980) Non-fatal lung disease due to inhalation of nebulised paraquat. *Br. Med. J.* **280**, 902

Gialdroni, C., Grassi, G. and Clini, V. (1964) Sulla possibilita di indurre sperimentalmente reqzioni sarcoid-simila livello del pulmone *Min. Pneumon.* **3**, 170–175

Giovacchini, R.P., Becker, G., Brunner, M. and Dunlop, F.E. (1965) Pulmonary disease and hair spray polymers: effects of long-term exposure of dogs. *J. Am. Med. Assoc.* **193**, 298–299

Goldstein, D.H., Benoit, J.N. and Tyroler, H.A. (1970) An epidemiological study of oil mist exposure. *Archs Environ. Health* **21**, 600–603

Gowdy, J.M. and Wagstaff, M.J. (1972) Pulmonary infiltration due to aerosol thesaurosis. *Archs Environ. Health* **25**, 101–108

Harris, D.K. (1951) Polymer-fume fever. *Lancet* **2**, 1008–1011

Harris, D.K. (1959) Some hazards in the manufacture and use of plastics. *Br. J. Ind. Med.* **16**, 221–229

Haswell, R.W. (1960) Dimethyl sulfate poisoning by inhalation. *J. Occup. Med.* **2**, 454–455

Hearn, C.E.D. and Keir, W. (1971) Nail damage in spray operators exposed to paraquat. *Br. J. Ind. Med.* **28**, 399–403

Hendricks, N.V.C., Linden, N.J., Collings, G.H., Dooley, A.E., Garrett, J.T. and Rather, J.B. Jr (1962) A review of exposure to oil mist. *Archs Environ. Health* **4**, 139–145

Hendy, M.S., Williams, P.S. and Ackrill, P. (1984) Recovery from severe pulmonary damage due to paraquat administered intravenously and orally. *Thorax* **39**, 874–875

Herrero, E.U., Feigelson, J. and Becker, A. (1965) Sarcoidosis in a beautician *Am. Rev. Respir. Dis.* **92**, 280–283

Higenbottam, T., Crome, P., Parkinson, C. and Nunn, J. (1979) Further clinical observations on the pulmonary effects of paraquat ingestion. *Thorax* **34**, 161–165

Hirsch, E.F. and Russell, H.B. (1945) Chronic exudative and indurative pneumonia due to inhalation of shellac. *Archs Pathol.* **39**, 281–286

Howard, J.K. (1979) A clinical survey of paraquat formulation workers. *Br. J. Ind. Med.* **36**, 220–223

Howard, J.K. (1980) Paraquat: a review of worker exposure in normal usage. *J. Soc. Occup. Med.* **30**, 6–11

Hudson, M., Patel, S.B., Ewen, S.W.B., Smith, C.C. and Friend, J.A.R. (1991) Paraquat induced pulmonary fibrosis in three survivors. *Thorax* **46**, 201–224

Iversen, E. and Christensen, B.E. (1984) Lungekomplikationer hos 'ildsluger'. *Ugeskr. Laeger.* **146**, 26–27

Jaros, F. (1978) Acute percutaneous paraquat poisoning. *Lancet* **1**, 275

Järvholm, B., Bake, B., Lavenius, B., Thiringer, B. and Vokmann, R. (1982) Respiratory symptoms and lung function in oil mist exposed workers. *J. Occup. Med.* **24**, 473–479

Jones, J.G. (1961) An investigation into the effects of exposure to an oil mist on workers in a mill for the cold reduction of steel strip. *Ann. Occup. Hyg.* **3**, 264–271

Joshi, R.R. and Cholankeril, J.V. (1985) Computed tomography in lipoid pneumonia. *J. Comput. Assist. Tomogr.* **9**, 211–213

Kimbrough, R.D. (1974) Toxic effects of the herbicide paraquat. *Chest* **65** (suppl.), 655–675

Kizer, K.W. and Golden, J.A. (1987) Lipoid pneumonitis in a commercial abalone diver *Undersea Biomed. Res.* **14**, 545–552

Kuntz, W.D. and McCord, C.P. (1974) Polymer-fume fever. *J. Occup. Med.* **16**, 480–482

Laplanche, A., Clavel, F., Contassot, J-C. and Lanouzierc, C. (1987) Exposure to vinyl chloride monomer: report on a cohort study. *Br. J. Ind. Med.* **44**, 711–715

Levin, P.J., Klaff, L.J., Rose, A.G. and Feguson, A.D. (1979) Pulmonary effects of contact exposure to paraquat: a clinical and experimental study. *Thorax* **34**, 150–160

Lewis, C.E. and Kerby, G.R. (1965) An epidemic of polymer-fume fever. *J. Am. Med. Assoc.* **191**, 375–378

Lilis, R., Anderson, H., Nicholson, W.J., Daum, S., Fischbein, A.S. and Selikoff, I.J. (1975) Prevalence of disease among vinyl chloride and polyvinyl chloride workers. *Ann. NY Acad. Sci.* **246**, 22–40

Littler, T.R. and McConnell, R.B. (1955) Dimethyl sulphate poisoning. *Br. J. Ind. Med* **12**, 54–56

Lloyd, M.H., Gauld, S., Copland, L. and Soutar, C.A. (1984) Epidemiological study of the lung function of workers at a factory manufacturing polyvinyl chloride. *Br. J. Ind. Med.* **41**, 328–333

Lowsma, H.B., Jones, R. and Prendergast, J. (1966) Effects of respired polyvinyl pyrrolidone aerosols in rats. *Toxicol. Appl. Pharmacol.* **9**, 571–582

McDonagh, B.J. and Martin, J. (1970) Paraquat poisoning in children. *Archs Dis. Child.* **455**, 425–427

McLaughlin, A.I.G., Bidstrup, P.L. and Konstam, M. (1963) The effect of hair lacquer sprays on the lungs. *Food Cosmet. Toxicol.* **1**, 171–188

Malten, K.E. and Zielhuis, R.L. (1964) *Industrial Toxicology and Dermatology in the Production and Processing of Plastics.* Elsevier Monographs

Marks, M.I., Chicoine, L., Legeve, G. and Hillman, E. (1972) Adrenocorticocosteroid treatment of hydrocarbon pneumonia in children: a cooperative study. *J. Pediatr.* **81**, 366–369

Miller, A., Teirstein, AS., Chuang, M., Selikoff, I.J. and Warshaw, R. (1975) Changes in pulmonary function in workers exposed to vinyl chloride and polyvinyl chloride. *Ann. NY Acad. Sci.* **246**, 42–52

Muir, D.C.F. and Emmett, P.C. (1976) Methods for determination of the atmospheric concentrations of oil mist. *Ann. Occup. Hyg.* **19**, 89

Okawa, M.T. and Polakoff, P.L. (1974) Occupational Health Case Reports – No 7 Teflon. *J. Occup. Med* **16**, 350–355

Oldberger, D., Maurer, W.J., Beltaos, E. and Magnin, G.E. (1972) Inhalation lipoid pneumonia from burning fats. A newly recognised industrial hazard. *J. Am. Med. Assoc.* **222**, 1288–1289

Pasternack, B. and Ehrlich, L. (1972) Occupational exposure to an oil mist atmosphere. A 12 year mortality study. *Archs Environ. Health* **25**, 286–294

Pendergrass, E.P. (1942) Some considerations concerning the roentgen diagnosis of pneumoconiosis and silicosis. *Am. J. Roentgenol.* **48**, 571–594

Pond, S.M., Johnston, S.C., Schoof, D.D., Hampson, E.C., Bowles, M., Wright, D.M. and Petric, J.J. (1987) Repeated hemoperfusion and continuous arteriovenous hemofiltration in a paraquat poisoned patient. *Clin. Toxicol.* **25**, 305–316

Prodan, L., Suciu, I., Pislaru, V., Ilea, E. and Pascu, L. (1975) Experimental chronic poisoning with vinyl chloride (monochloroethene). *Ann. NY Acad Sci.* **246**, 159–163

Proudfit, J.P., van Ordstrand, H.S. and Miller, C.W. (1950) Chronic lipid pneumonia following occupational exposure. *Ind. Hyg. Occup. Med.* **1**, 105–111

Proudfoot, A.T., Stewart, M.S., Levitt, T. and Widdop, B. (1979) Paraquat poisoning: significance of plasma-paraquat concentrations. *Lancet* **2**, 330–332

Proudfoot, A.T., Prescott, L.F. and Jarvie, D.R. (1987) Haemodialysis for paraquat poisoning. *Human. Toxicol.* **6**, 69–74

Ripe, E., Hanngren, A., Holmgren, A. and Johansson, I. (1969) Thesaurosis? – Analysis of a case. *Scand. J. Respir. Dis.* **50**, 156–167

Robbins, J.J. and Ware, R.L. (1964) Pulmonary edema from Teflon fumes. *N. Engl. J. Med.* **271**, 360–361

Sagar, G.B. (1987) Uses and usefulness of paraquat. *Human Toxicol.* **6**, 7–12

Sakabe, H. (1975) Bone lesions among polyvinyl chloride production workers in Japan. *Ann. NY Acad. Sci.* **246**, 78–79

Saltzman, H.A. and Fridovich, I. (1973) Oxygen toxicity. Introduction to a protective enzyme: superoxide dismutase. *Circulation* **48**, 921–923

Schepers, G.W.H. (1962) Thesaurosis versus sarcoidosis. *J. Am. Med. Assoc.* **181**, 635–637

Schermann, J.M., Houze, P., Bismuth, C. and Bourdon, R. (1987) Prognostic value of plasma and urine paraquat concentrations. *Human Toxicol.* **6**, 91–93

Seidel, J. (1959) Mucolytic aerosol therapy for lipid pneumonia. *J. Am. Med. Assoc.* **171**, 1810–1813

Shoshkes, M., Banfield, W.G. and Rosenbaum, S.J. (1950) Distribution, effect and fate of oil aerosol particles retained in the lungs of mice. *Archs Ind. Hyg. Occup. Med.* **1**, 20–35

Silverman, J.F., Turner, R.C., West, R.L. and Dillard, T.A. (1989) Bronchoalveolar lavage in the diagnosis of lipoid pneumonia. *Diagn. Cytopathol.* **5**, 3–8

Skorodin, M.S. and Chandrasekhar, A.J. (1983) An occupational cause of exogenous lipoid pneumonia. *Archs Pathol. Lab. Med.* **107**, 610–611

Smith, L.L. (1987) Mechanism of paraquat toxicity in lung and its relevance to treatment. *Human Toxicol.* **6**, 31–36

Smith, P. and Heath, D. (1975) The pathology of the lung in paraquat poisoning. *J. Clin. Pathol.* **28** (suppl. 9), 81–93

Soutar, C.A. and Gauld, S. (1983) Clinical studies of workers exposed to polyvinyl chloride dust. *Thorax* **38**, 834–839

Soutar, C.A., Copland, L.H., Thornley, P.E., Hurley, J.F., Ottery, J., Adams, W.G.F. and Bennett, B. (1980) Epidemiological study of respiratory disease in workers exposed to polyvinyl chloride dust. *Thorax* **35**, 644–652

Spatafora, M., Bellia, V., Ferrara, G. and Genova, G. (1987) Diagnosis of a case of lipoid pneumonia by bronchoalveolar lavage. *Respiration* **52**, 154–156

Staiff, D.C., Comer, S.W., Armstrong, J.S. and Wolfe, H.R. (1975) Exposure to the herbicide paraquat. *Bull. Environ. Contam. Toxicol.* **14**, 334–340

Steele, R.W., Conklin, R.H. and Mark, H.M. (1972) Corticosteroids and antibiotics for treatment of fulminant hydrocarbon aspiration. *J. Am. Med. Assoc.* **219**, 1434–1437

Styles, J.A. and Wilson, J. (1973) Comparison between in vitro toxicity of polymer and mineral dusts and their fibrogenicity. *Ann. Occup. Hyg.* **16**, 241–250

Suciu, I., Prodan, L., Ilea, E., Paduraru, A. and Pascu, L. (1975) Clinical manifestations in vinyl chloride poisoning. *Ann. NY Acad. Sci.* **246**, 53–69

Swan, A.A.B. (1969) Exposure of spray operators to paraquat. *Br. J. Ind. Med.* **26**, 322–329

Swift, D.L., Žuškin, E. and Bouhuys, A. (1976) Respiratory deposition of hair spray aerosol and acute lung function changes. *Am. Rev. Respir. Dis.* **113** (suppl.), 96

Szende, B., Lapis, K., Nemes, A. and Pinter, A. (1970) Pneumoconiosis caused by the inhalation of polyvinyl chloride dust. *Med. Lav.* **61**, 433–436

Thurlbeck, W.M. and Thurlbeck, S.M. (1976) Pulmonary effects of paraquat poisoning. *Chest* **69**, 276–280

Touey, G.P. and Mumpower, R.C. (1957) Measurement of the combustion-zone temperature of cigarettes. *Tobacco NY* **144**, 18–22

Vale, J.A., Meredith, T.J. and Buckley, B.M. (1987) Paraquat poisoning: Clinical features and immediate general management. *Human Toxicol.* **6**, 41–48

Wagner, J.C., Adler, D.I. and Fuller, D.N. (1955) Foreign body granulomata of the lungs due to liquid paraffin. *Thorax* **10**, 157–170

Ward, A.M., Udnoon, S., Watkins, J., Walker, A.E. and Darke, C.S. (1976) Immunological mechanisms in the pathogenesis of vinyl chloride disease. *Br. Med. J.* **1**, 936–938

Warraki, S. (1963) Respiratory hazards of chlorinated camphene. *Archs Environ. Health* **7**, 253–256

Webb, D.B., Williams, M.V., Davies, B.H. and James, K.W. (1984). Resolution after radiotherapy of severe pulmonary damage due to paraquat poisoning. *Br. Med. J.* **288**, 1259–1260.

Weill, H., Ferrans, V.J., Gay, R.M. and Ziskind, M.M. (1964) Early lipoid pneumonia. Roentgenological, anatomic and physiologic characteristics. *Am. J. Med.* **36**, 370–376

Weissman, H. (1951) Lipoid pneumonia: a report of two cases. *Am. Rev. Tuberc.* **64**, 572–576

Welter, E.S., (1978) Manufacturing exposure to coolant-lubricants. *J. Occup. Med.* **20**, 535–538

Wheeler, P.S., Stitik, F.P., Hutchins, G.M., Klinefelter, H.F. and Siegelman, S.S. (1981) Diagnosis of lipoid pneumonia by CT. *J. Am. Med. Assoc.* **245**, 65–66

Williams, M.V. and Webb, D.B. (1987) Paraquat lung: is there a role for radiotherapy. *Human Toxicol.* **6**, 75–81

Williams, N. and Smith, F.K. (1972) Polymer fume fever. An elusive diagnosis. *J. Am. Med. Assoc.* **219**, 1587–1589

Williams, N., Atkinson, W. and Patchefsky, A.S. (1974) Polymer-fume fever: not so benign. *J. Occup. Med.* **16**, 519–522

Žuškin, E. and Bouhuys, A. (1974) Acute airway response to hair spray preparations. *N. Engl. J. Med.* **290**, 660–663

24

The lungs in aerospace and at high altitude

John Ernsting and J.A.C. Hopkirk

Introduction

The major features of the environment of flight which affect the lungs and respiratory gas exchange are the reduction of environmental pressure, the associated fall in the partial pressures of oxygen and nitrogen, and the accelerative forces associated with changes in the speed and direction of flight. The magnitude of the changes in the physical environment to which individuals are exposed in flight varies greatly with the type of aircraft (or space vehicle) and its roles. Thus the modern civil passenger aircraft has a cabin environment which is not far removed from that on the ground whilst the pilot of a military fighter aircraft can be exposed to low environmental pressures and very high accelerative forces. Furthermore, whilst pressurization of the cabin and the delivery of high concentrations of oxygen by breathing equipment are widely employed to reduce the effects of the low pressure

at altitude, these techniques of themselves introduce potential hazards to the lungs. The pulmonary and respiratory changes that are associated with space flight are, with one important exception, those due to microgravity – simply extensions of those that occur in flight within the earth's atmosphere.

This chapter is divided into three parts: the first part considers, in order, the relevant physical characteristics of the flight environment and how the magnitude of the physical hazards is modified by the aircraft or space vehicle; the effects of pressure and gaseous environments on the lungs; and, then, those of accelerative forces and microgravity. The second part is concerned with the impact that physiological stresses during flying may have in the presence of pre-existing respiratory disease. The third part reviews the respiratory effects of chronic hypoxia associated with prolonged exposure to high altitudes that may occur in travel to such altitudes for occupational reasons as well as for touring and mountaineering.

Part I: The aerospace environment and its effects on the lungs

John Ernsting

Physical characteristics of the flight environment

Environmental pressure

The pressure exerted by the atmosphere (P_B) falls progressively with ascent from the surface of the

earth towards outer space. It varies in an approximately exponential manner with vertical distance from the surface of the earth. Departures from an exponential relationship are caused by variations in temperature with altitude due to the heating of the lower layers of the atmosphere (up to 25 000 to 50 000 feet) by the warm earth below and the heat produced by the destruction of ozone in the upper reaches of the atmosphere (at altitudes between

Table 24.1 The ICAO International Standard Atmosphere (1968)

Altitude (feet)	(metres)	Pressure (mmHg)	Temperature (°C)
0	0	760	+15.0
5 000	1 525	632	+5.1
10 000	3 048	523	−4.8
15 000	4 572	429	−14.7
20 000	6 096	349	−24.6
25 000	7 620	282	−34.5
30 000	9 144	226	−44.4
35 000	10 668	179	−54.2
40 000	12 192	141	−56.5
50 000	15 240	87.3	−56.5
60 000	18 288	54.1	−56.6
80 000	24 384	20.7	−52.1
100 000	30 480	8.2	−46.0

oxygen by short wavelength (200 nm) ultraviolet light. The ozone thus formed is dissociated at lower altitudes to molecular oxygen by long wavelength (210 to 300 nm) ultraviolet light. The consequences of these dynamic processes are that the concentration of ozone reaches a peak of 6 to 16 parts per million by volume (p.p.m.v.) at 100 000 feet, depending upon latitude and season. The concentration falls progressively below this altitude, typical concentrations being 1.0 p.p.m.v. at 40 000 feet and 0.03 p.p.m.v. at sea level (see Chapter 18). The marked increase in the intensity and energy of ionizing radiation is of significance for flights in the upper atmosphere (above about 40 000 feet) and beyond the earth's atmosphere, where a vehicle is exposed to galactic and solar cosmic radiation (Harding, 1988a).

Ozone is discussed in detail in Chapter 18, page 626.

40 000 feet and 140 000 feet). A standard internationally recognized description of the relationship between barometric pressure and altitude (the International Civil Aviation Organisation (ICAO) standard atmosphere 1968) is employed in aviation where barometric pressure is used to indicate the height of an aircraft above the ground. In international aviation, altitude is expressed in feet rather than in SI units, and this convention is employed in those parts of this chapter that relate to aviation.

The relationship between atmospheric pressure and altitude as defined by the ICAO standard atmosphere is summarized in Table 24.1. The barometric pressure at 18 000 feet (380 mmHg) is half that at ground level, whilst the pressure is reduced to one-quarter of the ground level value at an altitude of 33 800 feet. The atmospheric pressure at an altitude of 100 000 feet (8.2 mmHg) is approximately one-hundredth of that at ground level. The temperature profile of the ICAO standard atmosphere is also summarized in Table 24.1.

Temperature of the atmosphere

The temperature of the air falls progressively with increasing altitude in the lower parts of the atmosphere at a lapse rate of approximately 2°C per 1000 feet up to an altitude of 25 000 to 60 000 feet (depending upon latitude and season), above which it remains relatively constant up to an altitude of about 150 000 feet. The temperature of the atmosphere even at moderate altitude is such that the heat must be delivered to crew and passenger compartments of an aircraft in order to maintain thermal comfort. Heat generated by the engines is usually used to create an acceptable thermal environment in the cabin. Infrared radiation from the sun is also an important source of heat particularly beyond the earth's atmosphere.

Composition of the atmosphere

The composition of the atmosphere from sea level to very high altitudes (more than 300 000 feet) is remarkably constant, the concentrations (by volume in dry air) of the major components being 21.0 per cent oxygen, 78.1 per cent nitrogen and 0.9 per cent argon. Thus, the partial pressures of oxygen and nitrogen in the atmosphere fall with ascent to altitude in direct proportion to the barometric pressure. The other constituent of the atmosphere of significance in aviation is ozone, the triatomic form of oxygen. Ozone is formed in the upper atmosphere (above 100 000 feet) by irradiation of

Cabin pressurization

As manned balloons and then aircraft began to ascend to the upper atmosphere it became essential to provide a physical barrier to isolate the crew and passengers from the hostile environment and to create, within the crew and passenger cabin, an acceptable pressure and temperature environment. Thus, the cabins of virtually all modern fixed-wing aircraft, both military and civil, are pressurized and ventilated with conditioned air. The jet engine draws in large quantities of air from the atmosphere and compresses it before burning fuel and ejecting the heated air to give forward motion to the aircraft. The process of compression raises the temperature of the air. Hot pressurized air is drawn from the compressor stages of the engine to condition the cabin. In most conditions of flight, this tapped air has to be cooled by passage through heat exchangers and a compressor–expansion turbine unit (cold air unit) prior to distribution within the cabin (Allan, 1988). Relatively high flows of conditioned air are passed through the cabin in order to remove heat, water vapour, carbon dioxide and noxious fumes such as tobacco smoke. The airflow through the cockpit of a two-seat fighter aircraft is typically 15 000 litres (NTP)/minute whilst in large passenger aircraft a flow of 400 litres (NTP)/passenger per minute is commonly employed. The pressure within the cabin, relative to that of the atmosphere in which the aircraft is flying, is controlled by the cabin outlet valves. The degree of opening of the outlet valves is controlled automatically in relation to atmospheric (external) and cabin pressures to maintain the desired absolute pressure within the cabin. There is a wide variety of cabin pressurization schedules, that is, relationships between cabin and aircraft altitudes. The form of schedule is determined by a number of factors including whether or not the occupants will routinely use breathing equipment supplying oxygen-enriched gas, the altitude at which the aircraft will operate, the rates of ascent and descent of the aircraft, the maximum acceptable rates of change of pressure within the cabin (particularly during descent), the structural mass and fatigue of the pressure cabin, and the likelihood of a failure of the pressurized structure, a consideration which should be restricted to military combat aircraft (Macmillan, 1988b). At one extreme of pressurization schedules is that of the modern subsonic passenger aircraft where the cabin altitude, even during flight at an aircraft altitude of 40 000 feet, will not exceed 5000 feet (which will require a pressure differential across the cabin wall of 65.4 kPa or 9.5 lbf/in²) (Figure 24.1). In contrast, the cabin altitude of a modern fighter aircraft, in which the crew will routinely breathe supplemental oxygen, will rise to 20 000 to 22 000 feet when the aircraft is at its ceiling. The much lower differential pressure (of the order of 34.5 kPa or 5.0 lbf/in²) minimizes the consequences of failure of the pressure cabin due to enemy action. The cabin altitudes of some older civil passenger aircraft may rise as high as 8000 feet. The supersonic Concorde has a very high cabin differential pressure so that the cabin altitude at an aircraft altitude of 60 000 feet is 6000 feet.

The relatively high concentration of ozone in the atmosphere at medium and high altitudes is of concern when conditioning the cabins of aircraft operating at these altitudes. Ozone is an irritant gas. Exposure to 1.0 p.p.m.v. ozone for 1 hour at sea level produces soreness of the eyes and throat with coughing. Exposure to 10 p.p.m.v. can cause

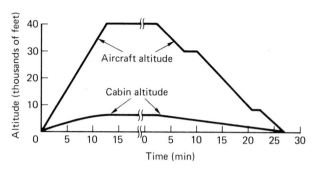

Figure 24.1 The time course of the cabin altitude (lower curve) of a high differential pressure passenger aircraft during a flight (aircraft altitude, upper curve) up to 40 000 feet and back to ground level

pulmonary oedema. Thus, compression of external air at, say, 60 000 feet to condition the pressure cabin could result in a partial pressure of ozone in the cabin atmosphere which would produce significant toxic effects. However, the heat generated in compressing the atmospheric air dissociates the ozone so that, in practice, the concentration of this gas in the cabin atmosphere of an aircraft flying at 60 000 feet does not generally exceed 0.1 to 0.2 p.p.m.v. (Harding, 1988c).

It is impractical to pressurize the pressure cabin with external air when the altitude exceeds 80 000 feet and this technique, which is expensive in terms of energy, is unacceptable for space vehicles. These vehicles employ sealed cabins which have very low leak rates. Carbon dioxide, water vapour and noxious gases are removed from the atmosphere and oxygen added to maintain the desired partial pressure of oxygen. Early American space vehicles such as Mercury and Gemini used 100 per cent oxygen at 259 mmHg (34.5 kPa). Nitrogen was added to the atmosphere of the Apollo vehicles after the fatal fire which occurred during the ground test of Apollo I in 1967. The concentration of oxygen rose progressively from 64 per cent at launch towards 100 per cent during flight. An atmosphere of 70 per cent oxygen and 30 per cent nitrogen at a total pressure of 259 mmHg was maintained throughout flight in the Skylab project. All Russian spacecraft have employed an atmosphere of air at a pressure of 760 mmHg which is also used in the US Shuttle programme.

Accelerations

Human beings live in the gravitational field of the earth. The occupants of aerospace vehicles may be exposed to a variety of different acceleration environments as the speed and direction of motion

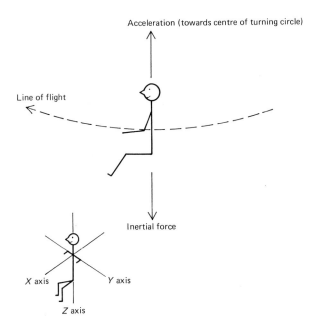

Figure 24.2 Acceleration and inertial forces generated by a turn in flight. The acceleration towards the centre of the turn generates a +**G**z inertial force which tends to displace tissues towards the feet. The insert shows the standard aviation terminology for the axes of the body

towards his head whilst the inertial force that it induces acts in the diametrically opposite direction, that is, footwards. A headward acceleration tends to displace tissues – such as the eyes and the viscera – footward and the resultant force is termed positive **G** (+**G**z) (Figure 24.2). Aerodynamic and aircraft structural considerations make the occurrence of the opposite, negative **G** (–**G**z), a rarity except in aerobatics in specially designed aircraft.

When a body falls freely (in the absence of air resistance) towards the earth it will accelerate at 9.81 m/s² and will have no weight. However, such a condition of weightlessness can only be maintained for very short periods in these circumstances. In space flight, microgravity where the vehicle and its occupants will be exposed to accelerations of the order of 1×10^{-4} to 1×10^{-5} **G**, is the normal gravitational environment (see page 806). The only method whereby microgravity can be experienced on earth, apart from free-fall, is during parabolic flight where the aircraft is flown so that the –**G**z forces created by the outside loop manoeuvre balance exactly the gravitational acceleration, a situation that can only be maintained for 10 to 14 seconds.

(velocity) of the vehicle changes. Of interest in the present context are the prolonged changes in accelerations (defined as accelerations lasting for longer than 2 seconds), produced by changes in the direction of flight of an aircraft and the microgravity associated with space flight. In aerospace, applied accelerations are usually expressed as multiples of the acceleration due to gravity. The latter which is termed the 'gravitational constant' (**G**) has the value of 9.81 m/s². Thus, an applied acceleration of 19.62 m/s² is expressed as 2 **G**. The weight of a body is the product of its mass and the accelerative force acting upon it. Thus, a body which weighs 1 kg at 1 **G** (that is, exposed to earth's gravitational field) will weigh 3 kg at 3 **G**. The increases in accelerations that are sustained in aircraft are virtually always produced by changes in the direction of motion (*radial accelerations*). Passenger aircraft are designed and flown so that the applied radial accelerations are minimal (1.1 to 1.3 **G**), whilst agile military aircraft can maintain very high accelerations of the order of 6 to 9 **G** for many seconds in turning flight. The direction in which the acceleration acts upon the pilot of such an aircraft will be determined by the relationship of the change in direction of the aircraft to the axes of his body. In the vast majority of flight manoeuvres, the increase in acceleration acts along the longitudinal axis (*Z* axis) of the seated pilot with the pilot's head pointing towards the centre of the turn. The accelerative force so generated acts

Effects of pressure change

The changes in the absolute pressure of the environment associated with changes in altitude in flight are transmitted throughout all the tissues of the body, and either directly or indirectly to the gas-containing cavities of the body. The consequent changes in the volume of gas in such cavities as the lungs are governed by a modification of Boyle's law, which takes account of the presence of water vapour. The gas within the lungs is saturated with water vapour at body temperature and the ratio of the moist alveolar surface to the volume of gas within the lungs is such that this condition is maintained, even when the lung gas expands rapidly on a rapid decompression. Thus, the partial pressure of water vapour in lung gas remains at 47 mmHg under all rates of change of the volume of lung gas that occur in aviation. Under these conditions, the relative gas expansion, that is, the ratio of final to initial volume of a given quantity of gas in a gas-containing cavity such as the lungs, is determined by the relationship

$$\text{Relative gas expansion} = \frac{(P_i - 47)}{(P_f - 47)}$$

where P_i = initial pressure of the gas in the cavity (mmHg) and P_f = final pressure of the gas in the cavity (mmHg).

Theoretically, because the barometric pressure (P_B) at 63 000 feet (19 215 m) is 47 mmHg, a decompression to this altitude or higher should result in an infinite expansion of gases in the lungs. In practice, however, the alveolar gas continues under these circumstances to contain oxygen, nitrogen and carbon dioxide which evolve from the blood in the pulmonary capillaries. A physical equilibrium is not reached before death supervenes, large volumes of frothy fluid being expelled from the respiratory tract (Bancroft and Dunn, 1965).

During normal flight, whether or not the cockpit or cabin is pressurized, the rates of ascent and descent are such that the changes in the volume of the gases of the lungs consequent on the change in environmental pressure are readily accommodated by the passage of gas through the conducting airways to the environment. Thus, the lung volumes will not change unless there is a significant obstruction to the exchange of gas between the lung and the environment. Manoeuvres that obstruct this free exchange, such as closure of the glottis during swallowing, speech and straining, are extremely unlikely to be of sufficient duration to give rise to significant additional transthoracic pressure differences. However, pulmonary diseases in which there is partial or complete blockage of the communication of groups of alveoli with the conducting airways may well give rise to significant disturbances (see pages 807 to 810). Disturbances of function produced by the increases in environmental pressure associated with normal aircraft descent rates do, however, occur in other gas-containing cavities, particularly the middle ear (Sharp and Macmillan, 1988). Respiratory manoeuvres such as the Valsalva manoeuvre with the nostrils occluded are frequently necessary to introduce air into the middle ear during descent.

The accidental sudden failure of the pressure cabin of an aircraft can give rise to a very rapid fall of pressure within the cabin which is potentially damaging to the lungs. The rate of fall of cabin pressure is determined principally by the altitude of the aircraft, the pressure in the cabin, the size of the defect in the cabin wall and the volume of the cabin. The loss of the canopy of the small volume cockpit of a fighter aircraft can result in an initial cabin differential pressure of 34.6 kPa (5.0 lbf/in²) falling to 0 in less than 0.1 second. By contrast, an accidental sudden decompression of the larger cabin of a wide-bodied passenger aircraft which does not result in the destruction of the aircraft as a flying machine is unlikely to decompress the cabin in less than 2 seconds, whilst loss of a passenger window in such an aircraft will give a decompression time of greater than 30 seconds (Macmillan, 1988b). The forces created by the very high velocity at which the escaping air travels through the cabin are more likely to produce serious and fatal injuries by hurling the occupants against the internal aircraft structure than is gas expansion within the body which causes damage to, for example, the parenchyma of the lungs.

Pulmonary barotrauma can occur as a result of the rapid decompression of a pressure cabin when the resistance to venting of the expanding lung gas to the environment generates a transthoracic pressure differential that cannot be accommodated by the normal elasticity of the lungs and chest wall. The limiting case is represented by a rapid decompression while the glottis is closed (either due to straining or voluntarily), when no lung gas can escape. Similar circumstances exist when the occupant is using oxygen delivery equipment which prevents the venting of gas from the respiratory tract during a decompression (Ernsting, 1984). The mechanism of lung damage on decompression of an aircraft has close similarities to that which operates during free ascent through water with the breath held (see Chapter 25). If the breath is held at the resting lung volume, then decompression from 8000 feet to 30 000 feet can be accommodated without exceeding the elastic limits of the lung. If, however, the resultant lung expansion exceeds the normal total lung volume there will be excessive stretching of the parenchyma which will eventually tear, and blood vessels will be severed in the process. The transthoracic pressure required to tear the lungs when the thoracic and abdominal muscles are relaxed is 80 to 100 mmHg. When lung tissue tears, alveolar gas passes along tissue planes into the mediastinum, into the neck producing surgical emphysema and into the pleural space producing a pneumothorax which may be of the tension variety. Gas entering the torn blood vessels, which are held open by the expanded lungs, passes through the left side of the heart into the systemic arterial tree. Bubbles will, in the erect individual, pass preferentially into the cerebral vessels.

In practice, lung damage due to a rapid decompression either in flight or in a hypobaric chamber is an extremely rare event. Thus, very large numbers of military aircrew have been decompressed over large pressure differentials in 2 to 3 seconds in hypobaric chambers during training with no adverse effects, and lung damage due to rapid decompression of an aircraft cabin in flight is virtually unknown. The treatment of the condition, should it occur on sudden decompression in a hypobaric chamber, is immediate descent to ground level (1 bar) followed by compression to 4 to 6 bars in a hyperbaric chamber with support as for pulmonary barotrauma caused by ascent through water (see Chapter 25, page 822).

Hypoxia

It is generally recognized that the most serious single hazard of flight at altitude is hypobaric hypoxia. The relatively mild hypoxia induced by breathing air at altitudes above 5000 feet produces significant impairment of certain aspects of mental performance (Denison, Ledwith and Poulton, 1966; Ernsting, 1978), whilst sudden decompression to 50 000 feet will result in loss of consciousness in 12 to 15 seconds and death in 4 to 6 minutes. In the Second World War, many military aircrew were killed by hypoxia in flight (Ernsting and Stewart, 1965) whilst the performance of many more was impaired by the condition. Although the incidence of serious hypoxia in miliary operations is now very low, incidents of hypoxia continue to occur in military and commercial airline operations and in private flying. The principal causes of hypoxia in flight are ascent to altitude without supplemented oxygen, failure of breathing equipment to supply oxygen and decompression of the pressurized cabin at high altitude. The magnitude of the effects of hypoxia and its rate of development vary markedly with the manner in which the condition is induced.

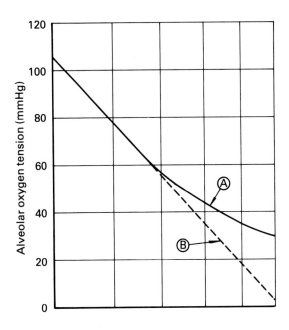

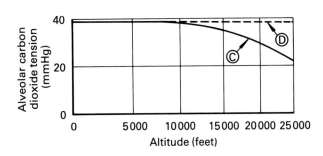

Figure 24.3 The effect of acute exposure (5–20 minutes) to various altitudes, while breathing air, on the alveolar tensions of oxygen (curve A) and carbon dioxide (curve C). The curves describe the mean values for a group of 30 subjects seated at rest. The broken lines indicate the values of alveolar tensions of oxygen (curve B) and carbon dioxide (curve D) which would be obtained if the hypoxia induced by ascent to altitude did not increase pulmonary ventilation

Alveolar gas composition

When air is breathed at altitude, the oxygen tension in the alveolar gas reflects the reduced partial pressure of oxygen in the inspired gas. Indeed as is shown by the alveolar air equation, provided the alveolar carbon dioxide tension (P_{ACO_2}) and the respiratory exchange ratio (R) remain constant, the reduction of the partial pressure of oxygen in the alveolar gas (P_{AO_2}) equals the fall in the partial pressure of oxygen in the inspired gas (P_{IO_2}):

$$P_{IO_2} - P_{AO_2} = P_{ACO_2} \left[F_{IO_2} + \left(\frac{1 - F_{IO_2}}{R} \right) \right]$$

where F_{IO_2} = fractional concentration of oxygen in the inspired gas, that is, 0.21.

The alveolar tensions of oxygen and carbon dioxide of subjects breathing air at various altitudes whilst seated at rest are shown in Figure 24.3, where altitude is depicted on a linear pressure scale. Alveolar carbon dioxide tension remains constant at its sea level between sea level and 10 000 feet. With ascent above 10 000 feet, the carbon dioxide tension is reduced progressively, falling to about 30 mmHg at 20 000 feet and close to 20 mmHg at 25 000 feet (where unconsciousness supervenes in 3 to 7 minutes). This reduction in alveolar carbon dioxide tension is due to the increase in pulmonary

ventilation stimulated by the fall of the oxygen tension of the arterial blood. In acute exposures of individuals at rest, this stimulation does not occur until the alveolar oxygen tension has fallen to below about 60 mmHg. The magnitude of the increase in pulmonary ventilation, at a given altitude above 10 000 feet, is a function of the stimulation of respiration by the low arterial oxygen tension acting through the peripheral chemoreceptors in the carotid and aortic bodies, and the respiratory depressant effect of the concomitant hypocapnia. The increase in pulmonary ventilation, and hence the fall in alveolar carbon dioxide tension, varies considerably from one individual to

Table 24.2 Typical values for arterial blood gases of resting subjects acutely exposed to altitude while breathing air

Altitude (feet)	Arterial blood gases			
	Oxygen tension (mmHg)	*Carbon dioxide tension (mmHg)*	*Oxygen concentration (ml (STPD)/ 100 ml blood)*	*Oxygen saturation of haemoglobin (%) (±s.d.)*
0	95	40	20.5	97
8 000	56	38	18.8	93
12 000	43	35	16.9	84
15 000	37	30	15.7	78 (±3.6)
18 000	32	28	14.5	72 (±6.0)
20 000	29	26	13.2	66

another and with the duration of the exposure. Acute exposure of seated subjects to breathing air at an altitude of 18 000 feet increases pulmonary ventilation by 20 to 50 per cent. The increase in ventilation commences immediately following a fall in the alveolar oxygen tension and the respiratory exchange ratio rises as carbon dioxide is removed from the body stores (Rahn and Otis, 1947). Thus, the respiratory exchange ratio on rapid ascent to an altitude between 16 000 and 22 000 feet rises immediately to 1.1 to 1.2, and after 30 minutes has fallen back to 0.95. Figure 24.3 depicts the mean values of the alveolar gas tensions during the first 5 to 20 minutes of exposure to altitude. The additional changes in these gas tensions when the exposure is prolonged to several days is shown in Figure 24.6 and is discussed later in this chapter. Exercise at altitude produces a greater increase in pulmonary ventilation than the same intensity of exercise at sea level (see page 811). At altitudes between 10 000 and 18 000 feet, moderate exercise (oxygen consumption of 0.75 to 1.0 litre (STPD)/ min) will reduce the alveolar carbon dioxide tension by 3 to 5 mmHg below that seen at rest at the same altitude. The alveolar oxygen tension is consequently some 3 to 5 mmHg higher in moderate exercise than at rest.

Gas exchange in the lungs and the arterial blood gases

The moderate hypoxia induced in resting subjects breathing air at altitudes between 10 000 and 18 000 feet (alveolar oxygen tensions of 35 to 55 mmHg) reduces somewhat the difference between the oxygen tensions of the alveolar gas and the arterial blood (West et al., 1962). This oxygen tension difference is about 5 mmHg at 16 000 feet. Thus, although the difference between the oxygen tension of the alveolar gas and that of the mixed venous blood flowing into the pulmonary capillaries is markedly reduced in moderate hypoxia, falling from the normal sea level value of 60 mmHg to 15 mmHg when breathing air at 16 000 feet, the diffusing capacity of the lungs is adequate to ensure that, at rest, the oxygen tension of the blood leaving the pulmonary capillary is equal to that of the alveolar gas surrounding it. The contributions of unevenness of distribution of ventilation–perfusion ratios and venous admixture to the overall alveolar–arterial oxygen tension difference are reduced in hypoxia. Typical values for the composition of the arterial blood in subjects acutely exposed to breathing air at altitudes up to 20 000 feet are summarized in Table 24.2. The large values of the standard deviations (s.d.) of the values at altitude reflect the very considerable individual variations in the pulmonary ventilatory response to hypoxia.

Even moderate exercise during acute exposures to altitudes above about 15 000 feet produces a very considerable increase in the arterial hypoxaemia. The arterial oxygen tension falls by 6 to 10 mmHg in spite of the increase of alveolar oxygen tension of 3 to 5 mmHg noted earlier (West et al., 1962). The explanation of the large increase in the alveolar–arterial oxygen tension difference in these circumstances lies in the increase in pulmonary blood flow which reduces the time that each red cell is exposed to alveolar gas. The diffusing capacity of the alveolar–capillary membrane is such that the oxygen tension of the blood leaving the pulmonary capillaries is considerably lower than that of the alveolar gas.

Alveolar gases when breathing supplemental oxygen

The fall of the oxygen tension of the alveolar gas associated with ascent to altitude can be combated by increasing the concentration of oxygen in the inspired gas. Where economy in the use of oxygen aboard an aircraft is of importance, it is normal practice to increase the concentration of oxygen in the inspired gas at a given altitude to a level that maintains an alveolar oxygen tension of 103 mmHg (Ernsting, 1984). Where great economy is required (for example, when supplying the passengers of an aircraft in a decompression emergency), a considerably lower standard, such as an alveolar oxygen tension of 55 to 65 mmHg, is often accepted. The concentrations of oxygen in the inspired gas needed to maintain alveolar oxygen tensions of 103 and 65 mmHg are given in Table 24.3.

Breathing 100 per cent oxygen at an altitude of 33 700 feet (P_B = 190 mmHg) produces an alveolar oxygen tension of 103 mmHg. It is generally accepted that, during short duration exposures to altitudes above 33 700 feet, such as may follow decompression of an aircraft, the hypoxia associated with an alveolar oxygen tension of 55 to 60 mmHg is acceptable for aircrew. Above 40 000 feet (P_B = 141 mmHg), however, oxygen must be delivered at a pressure greater than that of the environment, in order to maintain an acceptable level of oxygenation of the arterial blood. Thus, continuous positive pressure breathing with, at higher altitudes (above 45 000 to 50 000 feet), counterpressure applied to the trunk and limbs is employed to prevent significant hypoxia in the emergency of cabin decompression (Ernsting, 1966). When the altitude of exposure is very high, or the duration of the exposure is prolonged, then a full pressure suit is required (Harding, 1988b).

Hypoxia induced by rapid decompression

The sudden fall of the pressure in the cabin which occurs on a rapid decompression produces a virtually simultaneous fall of the tensions of the alveolar gases. Decompression to moderate or high altitude produces very rapid and profound falls of the alveolar tensions of oxygen and carbon dioxide. The magnitude of this effect depends upon the composition of the gas breathed prior to the decompression and upon the ratio of the environmental pressures before and after the decompression. The subsequent changes in the composition of the alveolar gas will

Table 24.3 Concentrations of oxygen required in the inspired gas at altitude to maintain alveolar oxygen tensions of 65 and 103 mmHg

Altitude (feet)	Concentration of oxygen in inspired gas % to maintain alveolar oxygen tension of	
	65 mmHg	*103 mmHg*
10 000	23	31
15 000	29	38
20 000	36	49
25 000	47	63
30 000	60	81
35 000	80	100*
40 000	100*	100*

*Breathing 100% oxygen alveolar oxygen tension will fall below 103 mmHg above 33 700 feet and below 65 mmHg above 39 500 feet.

depend principally upon the final environmental pressure (and whether this is increased by descending the aircraft), the gas being breathed and the respiratory responses to the hypoxia induced by the decompression (Ernsting, 1978). Thus, a decompression from 8000 feet to 40 000 feet in 1.6 seconds while breathing air reduces the alveolar oxygen tension immediately from 65 to 15 mmHg (Figure 24.4). The inspired (tracheal) oxygen tension breathing air at 40 000 feet is only 20 mmHg and the alveolar oxygen tension remains at 15 to 17 mmHg for as long as air is breathed following the decompression. The alveolar oxygen tension will thus be considerably less than the oxygen tension of the mixed venous blood flowing into the lungs so that oxygen will pass from the blood into the alveolar gas. The delivery of 100 per cent oxygen to the respiratory tract will raise the alveolar oxygen tension as nitrogen is washed out of the alveolar gas (Figure 24.4). The alveolar carbon dioxide tension is also reduced, by a rapid decompression, to as low as 8 to 10 mmHg. The markedly increased difference between the carbon dioxide tensions of the mixed venous blood and the alveolar gas causes a large outpouring of carbon dioxide into the alveolar gas, so that, typically, the alveolar carbon dioxide tension rises over the 30 seconds following a decompression to 20 to 30 mmHg. It remains at this level until the hypoxic stimulus is removed and pulmonary ventilation returns to normal.

As is apparent from Figure 24.4, rapid decompression over a large pressure change will produce a profound reduction of the alveolar oxygen tension even when 100 per cent oxygen is breathed immediately following the decompression (oxygen at 2 seconds). Extensive studies have shown that if, in these circumstances, the alveolar oxygen tension is reduced to below 30 mmHg, then the consequent

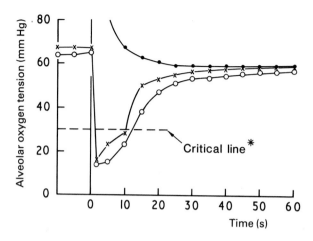

Figure 24.4 Mean alveolar oxygen tensions of four subjects before and after rapid decompression at time 0 from 8000 feet to 40 000 feet in 1.5 seconds. Each subject was decompressed on three occasions: once breathing air before and after the decompression with 100% oxygen delivered to the facemask 8 seconds after time 0 (O_2 late: ○–○), once breathing air before and after the decompression with 100% oxygen delivered to the facemask 2 seconds after time 0 (O_2 early: x-x), and once breathing 100% oxygen throughout (O_2 throughout: ●–●). *Note that if the area described by the alveolar oxygen tension curve below the critical line exceeds 140 mmHg seconds, consciousness will almost certainly be lost

cerebral hypoxia results in significant impairment of mental performance (Ernsting et al., 1973). The further the alveolar oxygen tension is reduced below 30 mmHg, and the longer the time for which it is less than 30 mmHg, the more profound are the effects on the central nervous system. If the area described by the alveolar oxygen tension–time curve below the critical line of 30 mmHg exceeds 140 mmHg seconds then unconsciousness will supervene. The severity of the hypoxia induced by a given rapid decompression to an altitude below 44 000 feet can be reduced by increasing the concentration of oxygen breathed prior to the decompression. The concentrations of oxygen required in the inspired gas to prevent the alveolar oxygen tension falling below 30 mmHg on rapid decompression from 8000 feet to final altitudes of 35 000 feet, 40 000 feet and 44 000 feet are 30, 40 and 60 per cent respectively (Ernsting, 1978).

Rapid decompression to altitudes above 45 000 feet even when 100 per cent oxygen is breathed before, during and after the decompression produce large reductions of the tensions of oxygen and carbon dioxide in the alveolar gas. Thus the alveolar oxygen tension is reduced to 10 mmHg on decompression to 52 000 feet (P_B = 79 mmHg). Prevention of this very severe hypoxia requires the

immediate increase of the total pressure in the respiratory tract by rapid recompression, by the use of positive pressure breathing or by the inflation of a full pressure suit.

The changes in the alveolar gas induced by rapid decompression produce equally profound changes in the gas tensions of the systemic arterial blood. The arterial oxygen tension is reduced to a value between that of the mixed venous blood and that of the alveolar gas. Thus, a rapid decompression while breathing air from 8000 feet to 40 000 feet reduces the arterial oxygen tension to 18 to 20 mmHg and the arterial oxygen saturation to 45 per cent. Changes in cerebral function do not occur until some 15 seconds after such a rapid decompression. This time interval comprises the circulation time from the pulmonary to cerebral capillaries (6 to 8 seconds) and the buffer provided by the oxygen stores of the cerebral tissues.

Oxygen delivery equipment

Supplemental oxygen is required in many circumstances in flight. Oxygen is used by the crews of military aircraft with low differential pressure cabins throughout flight, whilst it is provided to prevent hypoxia in the emergency of cabin decompression in all those aircraft with high differential pressure cabins that operate at altitudes above 10 000 feet. Supplemental oxygen is provided for all the passengers in transport aircraft operating at altitudes above 25 000 feet.

The majority of aircraft carry oxygen either as liquid or compressed gas (Harding, 1988b). A liquid oxygen supply has the advantage of lower mass, but the disadvantage that evaporative losses require frequent replenishment. Liquid oxygen is used extensively in military combat aircraft. Compressed gas is the storage method of choice where mass is less critical and oxygen is only used infrequently during routine flight. Solid chemical storage of oxygen as sodium chlorate (oxygen candles) is increasingly employed as the source of oxygen for passengers. Various methods of generating breathing gas from air on board aircraft have been explored in the last 15 years. The most successful technique employs molecular sieves (synthetic zeolites) and a pressure swing adsorption process to remove nitrogen from bleed air supplied by the engine compressor – producing breathing gas with a high concentration of oxygen (Ernsting, 1984).

All oxygen delivery systems fitted to aircraft are open circuit. Closed or semi-closed systems, where expired gas is processed and rebreathed, are prone to freezing at low temperatures and can lead to the accumulation of nitrogen which will reduce the oxygen tension of the inspired gas. Aircraft oxygen delivery systems, therefore, comprise a regulating device, an oronasal mask and connecting pipework. Virtually all delivery systems for aircrew employ demand regulators. These devices frequently dilute the oxygen from the store with cabin air to provide the required total concentration of oxygen which is adjusted automatically in accordance with the cabin altitude. Pressure-demand oxygen regulators provide oxygen under pressure (pressure breathing) at those altitudes (above 40 000 feet) where it is required. Oxygen delivery systems for passengers (and often for cabin crews) are usually less sophisticated, employing a continuous flow of oxygen, an oxygen reservoir (which may allow a degree of rebreathing) and a means of drawing in cabin air when the pulmonary ventilation exceeds the oxygen flow. The reader is referred to Harding (1988b) for further details of oxygen storage and delivery systems.

Aircraft oxygen systems generally deliver 100 per cent oxygen only when this concentration is required to prevent hypoxia or when the equipment is used to exclude smoke or toxic fumes from the respiratory tract. The major considerations responsible for this approach are economy in the use of the stored gas and, in agile combat aircraft, *acceleration atelectasis*. Appropriate dilution of the oxygen supply with cabin air will, when oxygen is breathed throughout flight, reduce the amount of oxygen used to 20 to 25 per cent of that which would be consumed if 100 per cent oxygen was employed. Oxygen toxicity is not a significant factor in conventional aviation as the duration of exposure to high oxygen tensions is relatively short (Ernsting, 1963). Absence of nitrogen from the alveolar gas on exposure to increased accelerations does, however, give rise to marked *absorption atelectasis* (see page 805). It is standard practice to provide at least 40 per cent nitrogen in the inspired gas (at cabin altitudes below 20 000 feet) to avoid this condition (Ernsting, 1978).

Decompression sickness

The rate at which the cardiorespiratory system can excrete nitrogen from the tissues is slow relative to the rate at which aircraft ascend to low environmental pressures. Supersaturation of the tissues with nitrogen, especially those rich in fat, can, therefore, occur on ascent. The gas bubbles which subsequently form in the tissues and the capillary blood give rise to the syndrome of decompression sickness – although similar to compressed air decompression sickness (Chapter 25, page 822) it has important differences (Fryer, 1969).

The symptoms of altitude decompression sickness are varied. They include pain in a joint or limb ('bends'), respiratory disturbances ('chokes'), disturbances in the central nervous system (hemianopia, anaesthesia, paralysis and fits) and cardiovascular collapse. Providing descent to low altitude is undertaken soon after the appearance of symptoms, recovery occurs rapidly in the vast majority of cases. Very occasionally cardiovascular collapse, secondary to a reduction of circulating blood volume caused by increased capillary permeability, leads to coma and death in spite of treatment (see Chapter 25).

Symptoms of subatmospheric decompression sickness are not seen at altitudes below 18 000 feet unless the individual has breathed air at pressures above 1 bar during the preceding 6 to 12 hours. The widespread participation in subaqua activities for recreational purposes of recent years has given rise to cases of decompression sickness in passenger aircraft at cabin altitudes of 5000 to 8000 feet. Most professional divers are aware of this hazard. The National Astronautics and Space Administration (NASA) and the US Air Force were stimulated to study flying after diving by the need for NASA astronauts to fly immediately following training in underwater simulators (which are used to simulate weightlessness) at depths of 30 to 50 feet of water. The UK Ministry of Defence regulations for flying after diving bar individuals from flying within 12 hours of swimming using compressed air breathing apparatus and within 24 hours if a depth of 30 feet has been exceeded.

The incidence of decompression sickness increases progressively with exposure to altitudes above 22 000 to 24 000 feet, depending not only on the altitude but also on the duration of exposure. Thus, the incidence of incapacitating decompression sickness (bends in two or more limbs, 'chokes' or collapse) in seated subjects exposed to 28 000 feet for 2 hours is 1 per cent, whilst exposure to an altitude of 35 000 feet for 2 hours will produce incapacitating symptoms in 23 per cent of normal resting individuals. Physical exercise greatly increases the incidence of decompression sickness. Incapacitating decompression sickness will occur in 35 to 40 per cent of individuals performing moderate exercise for 2 hours at 35 000 feet. Cardiovascular collapse can occur while the individual is at altitude, but may arise after the return to ground level of an individual who has suffered 'bends' or more serious manifestations of decompression sickness while at altitude. The total number of reported fatal cases of decompression sickness in many hundreds of thousands of exposures to high altitude over the last 40 years is less than 25 (Fryer, 1969; Davis et al., 1977).

Respiratory disturbances ('chokes') are a serious manifestation of decompression sickness, occurring in 2 to 4 per cent of the individuals who develop decompression sickness at altitude. The first symptom is virtually always a sense of constriction around the lower chest, often with a tight feeling in the epigastrium. Attempts to take a deep breath cause an inspiratory snatch which limits inspiration. Retrosternal soreness and pain develop with dyspnoea. There is often a general feeling of malaise and, as the disorder develops, an attempt to take a deep breath causes coughing which frequently becomes paroxysmal. The cough is non-productive. If the exposure to altitude is maintained, cardiovascular collapse almost invariably develops. The symptoms of 'chokes' frequently persist for several hours after descent to ground level, with coughing being precipitated by a deep breath.

The respiratory manifestations of decompression sickness are caused by gas bubbles and aggregations of platelets lodging in the pulmonary vasculature. There is now ample evidence for the presence of gas bubbles in the systemic venous blood even in the absence of any symptoms of decompression sickness on exposure to altitudes above 13 000 to 15 000 feet. The higher the altitude, the longer the duration of the exposure, and the greater the physical activity of the individual, the more profuse and intense are the ultrasonic Doppler signals of gas bubbles in the venous blood flowing into the right ventricle (Dixon, Adams and Harvey, 1986). These bubbles and the associated aggregations of platelets usually accumulate in the lungs without causing any respiratory symptoms. Under certain circumstances, however, when larger quantities of gas bubbles and aggregated blood particles enter the lungs the pulmonary vasculature is compromised and the symptoms of 'chokes' occur. If not terminated by recompression to low altitude which eliminates the bubbles, further changes may occur in the lungs with a rise of pulmonary artery pressure and the opening of arteriovenous connections, so that bubbles and cellular aggregates may pass into the systemic arterial circulation to be carried to other organs of the body.

The treatment of 'chokes' is the treatment of serious decompression sickness. Recompression to ground level together with the administration of 100 per cent oxygen should be carried out as rapidly as possible. If respiratory symptoms are present at ground level, then the patient should be compressed in a hyperbaric chamber, to a pressure of 2.8 bars and given intermittent oxygen therapy (Davis et al., 1977; Macmillan, 1988a). If a hyperbaric chamber is not immediately available, then supportive treatment including the administration of oxygen should be continued and the patient transported as rapidly

as possible to the nearest hyperbaric chamber unit. When a patient is transferred by air the cabin altitude of the aircraft should be kept as low as possible, ideally below 1000 feet (see also Chapter 25, page 828). Subsequent treatment including, if necessary, prolonged compression to pressures greater than 2.8 bars is determined by the clinical response to the initial compression therapy. An individual who has developed severe chokes complicated by any other manifestation of altitude decompression sickness should almost certainly be debarred for life from exposure to altitude in excess of 18 000 feet.

Altitude decompression sickness may be prevented in several ways. The most satisfactory is to avoid exposure to altitudes at which the condition can occur. Thus, ideally aircrew and passengers should not be exposed to altitudes greater than 18 000 feet. In practice, where, as in combat aircraft, it is important to minimize the cabin differential pressure and the duration of exposure to high cabin altitude is of necessity limited, a maximum cabin altitude of 22 000 feet is generally accepted (Macmillan, 1988a). The increased risk of decompression sickness occurring on exposure to altitude after diving may be avoided by not flying within 12 hours of swimming using compressed air breathing apparatus, and within 24 hours if a depth of 30 feet has been exceeded (see Chapter 25, page 828). It is of considerable practical import that the incidence of severe decompression sickness is very low during the first 5 minutes of any exposure to high altitude. Thus, provided that an aircraft can descend rapidly to below 20 000 feet following a decompression at high altitude, no specific measures have to be taken to avoid decompression sickness (Ernsting, 1966). The other important preventive method is to eliminate nitrogen from the tissues by breathing 100 per cent oxygen prior to the ascent to altitude. This technique, which is necessarily tedious, is widely used to avoid altitude decompression sickness during the training of military aircrew in pressure breathing and in the use of pressure suits in hypobaric chambers. Breathing 100 per cent oxygen at ground level for 30 minutes will prevent decompression sickness during a subsequent short duration exposure (less than 5 minutes) to altitudes between 20 000 feet and 45 000 feet. Pre-oxygenation is also used in special missions and in research. Because prolonged exposure to an altitude of 27 000 feet – the cabin altitude employed in US space vehicles prior to the 'Shuttle' – will give rise to a significant incidence of decompression sickness, the US astronauts using those vehicles breathed 100 per cent oxygen for at least 4 hours before flight. Similar breathing of 100 per cent oxygen is required before extravehicular activity in a space suit of internal pressure less than 380 mmHg (50.6 kPa).

Long duration positive acceleration

General effects

The crews of agile aircraft are frequently exposed to sustained positive accerations (+**G**z) in flight, the magnitude of which can be as high as +9 **G** for periods of up to 60 seconds. Such exposures, by increasing the weight of all the tissues of the body, have profound effects upon mobility, the cardiovascular system and the lungs (Glaister, 1988a). The increase in the weight of the blood under +**G**z reduces the arterial and venous pressures in the portions of the systemic and pulmonary circulations above the heart and increases them in the parts below the heart. The reduced arterial pressure at head level, in the relaxed seated subject, causes loss of peripheral vision at 3.5 to 4.0 **G**, complete loss of vision ('blackout') at about 4.5 **G** and loss of consciousness at 5 to 6 **G**, depending upon the duration of the exposure. The increase in cardiovascular pressures below the heart leads to a decrease in peripheral resistance and pooling of blood in the capacity vessels. The circulatory disturbances are often partially combated by the use of **G** trousers which apply counterpressure by bladders to the abdomen and the lower limbs. The bladders of the **G** trousers are inflated automatically on exposure to +**G**z.

Pulmonary function at +**G**z

There are only small changes in pulmonary ventilation on exposure of experienced subjects to positive accelerations up to at least 5 **G**, although the novice will often hyperventilate. Exposure to positive accelerations greater than 3 **G** reduces the vital capacity and the total lung capacity. The diaphragm and abdominal contents descend under +**G**z so that the functional residual capacity is increased.

Positive acceleration accentuates the regional differences in the ventilation of the lung seen in the erect individual at +1 **G**z. The pressure gradient down the pleural space is increased so that, at +5 **G**z, the pleural pressure at the base of the lung is some 30 cmH$_2$O (2.9 kPa) greater than at the apex. The pressure changes produced by exposure to +**G**z increase the distension of the alveoli at the apex of the lung while reducing the size of the basal alveoli. Thus, exposure to +**G**z increases the gradient of alveolar ventilation down the lung. Alveoli at the base of the lung are compressed to their minimal volume and the airways leading to them are closed. The proportion of the lower lung in which there is closure

of the terminal airways increases progressively with the applied acceleration. Inflation of **G** trousers accentuates this effect by raising the level of the diaphragm. Thus, exposure to +5 **G**z when wearing **G** trousers increases the closing capacity of the lung to 50 per cent of the total lung capacity (Glaister, 1988a).

The changes of the pressures in the pulmonary circulation produced by +**G**z have a profound effect upon the regional distribution of blood flow. The height above the hilum of the lung at which the pulmonary artery pressure is 0 is reduced from 20 cm at +1 **G** to 5 cm at +4 **G** so that, at the latter level of acceleration, the upper half of the lung is not perfused. There is a progressive increase in the regional blood flow in lower parts of the lung, except close to the bases where the increase in the pressure in the non-ventilated alveoli increases the resistance to blood flow. The upper part of the lung, which continues to be ventilated but not perfused during exposure to +**G**z, contributes to the respiratory dead space. The changes in the distribution of the regional ventilation/blood flow ratios that occur in the lower ventilated and perfused portion of the lung on exposure to increased +**G**z cause a small but significant increase in the alveolar–arterial oxygen tension difference. However, the continued perfusion of non-ventilated alveoli in the basal parts of the lung is of greater significance. The oxygen tension in the latter falls rapidly until it is close to that of the mixed venous blood, and this non-oxygenated blood forms a right-to-left shunt that produces arterial hypoxaemia. About 50 per cent of the cardiac output is shunted through non-ventilated alveoli at +5 **G**z. Exposure to +5 **G**z while breathing air reduces the arterial oxygen tension to 60 mmHg, and at +7 **G**z, the arterial oxygen tension is reduced to 50 mmHg.

Lung collapse

The terminal airways in the lower parts of the lung are closed by exposure to +**G**z. The greater the level of acceleration, the larger the alveolar volume that is not ventilated. When air is breathed prior to the exposure to +**G**z, the tensions of oxygen and carbon dioxide in this trapped alveolar gas become rapidly (within 2 to 3 seconds) very close to the corresponding values in mixed venous blood. Subsequently, however, the rate of absorption of the trapped gas is relatively very slow because it depends on the removal of nitrogen from the alveolar gas and nitrogen is some 200 times less soluble in blood than oxygen and carbon dioxide at the relevant tensions. Thus, the non-ventilated lung remains filled with gas throughout the exposure to +**G**z, and the airways reopen when the acceleration returns to +1 **G**. Removal of nitrogen from the

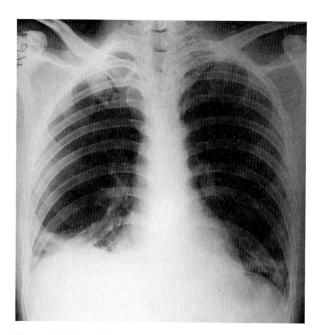

Figure 24.5 Typical areas of basal collapse in a pilot who had just completed a flight in which he performed repeated high +**G**z (5–6 **G**) manoeuvres while wearing **G** trousers and breathing 100% oxygen

alveolar gas by breathing 100 per cent oxygen prior to the exposure leads, however, to gross basal lung collapse on exposure to increased acceleration.

The extensive absorption collapse, which occurs in the lower parts of the lungs when aircrew breathing 100 per cent oxygen are exposed to even moderate +**G**z, was recognized in 1959 (Ernsting, 1960). Aircrew who have been exposed to positive accelerations while breathing 100 per cent oxygen report a post-flight syndrome that consists of difficulty in taking a deep breath, coughing and retrosternal discomfort/pain. Chest radiographs taken immediately after flight reveal marked basal collapse (Figure 24.5) which is associated with a 40 to 50 per cent reduction of the vital capacity. As long as it remains, the lung collapse produces a large right-to-left shunt of blood flowing through the lungs. Lung collapse is accentuated by the use of **G** trousers which, by raising the diaphragm, increase the compression of the lower part of the lungs. This situation can be avoided at cabin altitudes up to 20 000 feet by ensuring that the concentration of nitrogen in the gas breathed prior to exposure to +**G**z is not less than 40 per cent (Ernsting, 1963, 1965).

G protective procedures

Several voluntary manoeuvres are employed by aircrew to increase their tolerance of +**G**z (Glaister,

1988b). These comprise combinations of respiratory manoeuvres which raise the intrathoracic pressure together with tensing of the skeletal musculature which supports the peripheral circulation, increasing peripheral resistance and decreasing venous pooling. Exhaling forcibly against a closed or partially closed glottis raises the arterial pressure. If, however, the raised intrathoracic pressure is maintained beyond 4 to 5 seconds, the arterial pressure falls as venous return to the right side of the heart virtually ceases while the intrathoracic pressure is raised. Thus, the effective anti-**G** straining manoeuvre (AGSM) comprises a strain against a closed glottis for 3 to 4 seconds followed by a rapid expiration and inspiration which are completed in about 1 second. This cycle is repeated in a regular manner. Correctly performed, the AGSM can increase the tolerance of positive acceleration by 3.5 to 4 **G**. The intrathoracic pressure is typically raised to 60 to 70 mmHg during the expiratory strain and this increase in pressure is reflected in the arterial blood pressure. Whilst trained aircrew can maintain full vision at 8 to 9 **G** by performing the AGSM and wearing **G** trousers, they can do so for only relatively short periods (5 to 10 seconds) without experiencing marked fatigue. Continuous positive pressure breathing, with chest counterpressure using a breathing pressure of 60 mmHg at 9 **G**, and **G** trouser inflation, are very effective in maintaining vision using a minimum of muscular strain (Glaister, 1988b). This method is being introduced into modern, highly agile, combat aircraft in which the pilot may experience positive accelerations of 9 **G** for many seconds.

Microgravity

Microgravity is a unique feature of space flight that has many physiological effects of which the most important are those affecting the neurovestibular, the cardiovascular and the musculoskeletal systems (Nicogossian and Parker, 1982; Harding, 1988c). A large proportion of crew members suffer from space motion sickness during the first few days of flight, whilst prolonged exposure to microgravity produces muscle atrophy and bone demineralization. Of direct interest in this chapter are the changes induced in the cardiovascular system which affect the distribution of blood and blood flow throughout the body, including the lungs.

The normal hydrostatic pressure gradients which exist in the cardiovascular system are absent in microgravity. From the instant at which the individual enters microgravity, the removal of the normal hydrostatic pressure gradients leads to a profound redistribution of the circulating blood volume. There is a headward shift of fluid which is complete in 24 to 48 hours. Anthropometric measurements suggest that 1.5 to 2 litres of blood and interstitial fluid are translocated from the lower parts of the body. The increased distension of the capacity vessels in the head gives rise to sensations of fullness and stuffiness (due to engorgement of the nasal mucosa) which, with visible distension of the superficial veins and puffiness of the face, remain throughout the flight.

A large proportion of this headward shift of blood is accommodated within the thorax. The consequent distension of the pulmonary veins and atria gives rise to reflex suppression of the secretion of vasopressin which, in turn, induces a diuresis – the *Gauer–Henry reflex* (Gauer, Henry and Behn,

1970). Some 3 to 4 kg body mass is lost during the first 3 to 4 days of flight, partly by the increased output of urine and partly by a decrease in fluid intake (Nicogossian and Parker, 1982). The reduction in the circulating blood volume, and probably changes in cardiovascular reflexes, result in a decrease in orthostatic tolerance which persists for several days after return to earth.

The removal of the normal hydrostatic gradients in the pulmonary circulation when in microgravity results in a more even distribution of regional blood volume and blood flow. The absence of gravitational force also results in removal of the normal regional differences in the distribution of alveolar ventilation. Indeed, exposure to microgravity should eliminate that component of the alveolar–arterial oxygen tension difference due to the existence of a span of ventilation–blood flow ratios. This predicted change has yet to be demonstrated experimentally.

Part II: Flying with existing respiratory disease

J.A.C. Hopkirk

Introduction

The major physiological stresses in the flying environment, which are of importance if there is underlying respiratory disease, are a lowered inspired oxygen tension, decreased atmospheric pressure and acceleration forces. The magnitude of these stresses is dependent on the type of flying, being much less in passenger and air transport aircraft and much greater in fast jet military aircraft. The importance of the effects of these stresses depends on whether the individual is a passenger or a member of the aircrew. Minor degrees of discomfort or breathlessness will be tolerated by a passenger, but these can be very distracting to an aircrew member and interfere with the safe performance of his or her duty.

When flying as a passenger in a civil airliner or in military transport aircraft these stresses are small. Passengers are not exposed to clinically significant acceleration forces. In normal flight the cabin of an airliner is pressurized to 6000 to 8000 feet. At 6000 feet the atmospheric pressure will have fallen from 760 to 609 mmHg and the inspired oxygen tension will have fallen to 118 mmHg. However, depressurization may occur during flight due to the failure of a compressor, failure of a door seal, blowing out of a window or a more major structural failure. This

depressurization may be slow or rapid and its degree will depend on the altitude of the aircraft and the nature of the structural failure (see pages 796 and 798). In modern passenger aircraft oxygen is provided for passengers by drop-down masks and a rapid descent of the aircraft initiated by the pilot. In normal flight, changes in the cabin pressure and inspired oxygen tension are small and slow. Depressurization is an uncommon, but not rare, event and in most instances it is slow. Reported instances of respiratory symptoms related to decompressions in passenger flying are very rare but, in aircrew, are of more significance because the safety of the aircraft depends on the well-being of the pilot. Sudden incapacitation or distraction due to pain or breathlessness may compromise the safety of the aircraft.

The flying environment in military aviation and fast jet flying is very different. Pilots of fast jet aircraft have to tolerate high acceleration forces. Current and projected fighter aircraft may require a pilot to tolerate 7 to 9 **G** for many seconds at a time. Owing to mass constraints, cockpit sizes are small and are not pressurized to the level of passenger aircraft cabins. Aircrew are, therefore, exposed to much lower atmospheric pressures and may need to breathe supplemental oxygen, often at pressure, to avoid hypoxia. The risk of sudden decompression in these aircraft is much greater and military aircrew are expected to undergo decompression training – often rapid decompression to 40 000 feet. It is also important that fast jet flying is a single pilot operation.

Asthma

Aeromedical hazards

Asthmatics with marked bronchial hyperreactivity are at risk of sudden incapacitation in flight (Rayman, 1973) but this is a rare occurrence. The presence of fumes in the cockpit is not rare in civil and military flying, and is often associated with mechanical malfunction. These fumes may precipitate acute asthma and incapacitate a pilot. More commonly in aircrew, distraction is the major factor, with discomfort and difficulty in breathing interfering significantly with the performance of the flying task. Hypoxia is also a theoretical danger. In asthmatics, even in remission, it is possible to detect abnormalities in gas mixing. This may make aircrew more susceptible to hypoxia and to the effects of acceleration forces occurring in flight. Due to relapses associated with upper respiratory infections, aircrew with asthma may be unfit to fly for significant periods in a year. Importantly, self-assessment in asthmatic patients is notoriously difficult and asthmatic aircrew may fly unaware of the severity of their condition. Ozone induces asthma in dogs but the concentrations that are present in cabin air, even in high flying aircraft, are so small as not to have given rise to symptoms. Pressure breathing is an irritant stimulus and may provoke asthma.

Disposition

Owing to the nature of the task, asthma is a disqualification for fast jet flying. If asthma is very mild, or is well controlled on inhaled corticosteroids or cromoglycate, then air transport flying is permissible in multicrew aircraft. If the aircrew member has been under observation for a prolonged period of time, and has shown only mild bronchial hyperreactivity with no acute exacerbations, single pilot operation may be considered. Mild or moderate asthma which is well controlled is not a bar to

private pilot flying. In general, passengers with asthma cope well with flying. They are at no greater risk from an acute attack than they are on the ground. Pressurized dose inhalers can be safely used in flight and oxygen is available if necessary.

There is now a move to treat even mild asthmatics with prophylactic cromoglycate or inhaled corticosteroids. In conventional doses these drugs have insignificant side effects from the aeromedical standpoint. Importantly, they may reduce bronchial reactivity and are, therefore, most useful in aircrew. Bronchodilators, such as β_2-agonists (salbutamol, terbutaline), do not alter bronchial reactivity and may have undesirable side effects such as muscle tremor. They are acceptable for use with aircrew but should not be used within 2 hours of flying.

Spontaneous pneumothorax

Aeromedical hazards

In flight spontaneous pneumothorax is rare (Cran and Rumball, 1967; Fuchs, 1967). Flying stresses including pressure breathing have not been shown to increase the risk of spontaneous pneumothorax. If an aircrew member or passenger flies with an undiagnosed pneumothorax, the air in the pleural space will, following Boyle's law, expand as the environmental pressure decreases. This will cause progressive compression of the underlying lung and may lead to tension pneumothorax. The pain and breathlessness associated with pneumothorax may cause distraction or, indeed, incapacitation in flight deck aircrew.

Disposition

Aircrew with a pneumothorax should not fly. Due to the high risk of recurrence, and the loss of flying and disruption to a flying programme that this causes, an aircrew member who has had a single spontaneous pneumothorax should have a pleurectomy (Hopkirk, Pullen and Fraser, 1983). No passenger should fly with an untreated pneumothorax. Passengers with pneumothorax can be safely transported with an intercostal tube in place attached to a Heimlich valve.

Bullous lung disease

Aeromedical hazards

Bullous lung disease is most frequently seen in individuals with chronic airways' obstruction and emphysema, but may also be seen in young individuals with no other underlying lung disease. Bullae in young adults tend to be stable or to increase only slowly in size, but there is a risk of rupture and spontaneous pneumothorax. Bullae in those with underlying emphysema tend to be progressive. The risks in aircrew, therefore, are of sudden incapacitation due to either spontaneous rupture of the bulla with consequent pneumothorax or rupture of the bulla occurring during sudden decompression. Because most bullae have only poor communication with the major airways, a sudden reduction in ambient pressure, such as might occur during a structural failure or window 'blow-out' in an airliner, will lead to sudden increase in size. A bulla may rupture with development either of pneumothorax or, more importantly, of peripheral air embolus (see 'Effects of pressure change', page 798).

Disposition

Owing to the risks, bullous lung disease is incompatible with military flying. If associated with underlying chronic airways' obstruction this bar would be permanent. Aircrew with a single bulla, unassociated with underlying lung disease, may be considered fit if full evaluation shows the presence of no other bullae and surgical resection of the bulla is undertaken. In civil flying the situation is similar. The occurrence of decompression in civil airliners is sufficiently common for aircrew with bullous lung disease to be excluded. Limited flying may be allowed following a full assessment which may require altitude chamber testing. The situation as regards passenger flying is more difficult and, although decompression is not uncommon, reported incidences of individuals with chronic airways' obstruction or bullous lung disease having complications during flight are rare. Nevertheless, there are anecdotal reports of passengers with severe bullous emphysema who developed chest pain and breathlessness during ascent as the cabin pressure fell, only to have their symptoms abate on descent. Decisions about the fitness of passengers with bullous lung disease and emphysema to fly will need to be taken individually. Obviously, those with severe bullous lung disease should be advised not to fly.

Chronic airways' obstruction

Aeromedical hazards

With chronic airways' obstruction the risks are broadly similar to those with asthma, except that incapacitation due to acute changes in airways' size is less common. By the time this disorder presents, it is usually well advanced in its natural history and there will be increasing symptoms of cough, production of sputum and breathlessness, and a measurable decrease in lung function. In the absence of bullous lung disease, sudden incapacitation is not common. In patients with anything less than mild disease, increasing dyspnoea and recurrent episodes of acute or chronic bronchitis will compromise the efficiency of the aircrew member.

Disposition

In those aircrew whose disease is mild and uncomplicated by radiographic evidence of bullae and who have only mild impairment of lung function, unlimited flying can be allowed. However, with increasing disturbance of lung function, limitations on flying or grounding will be necessary. As regards passenger flying, in the absence of serious breathlessness on the ground, little disturbance in normal flight can be expected. Supplemental oxygen is available on aircraft if required.

Bronchial carcinoma

The prognosis in lung cancer remains poor, with a 5-year survival in unselected cases of less than 5 per cent. In cases of squamous cell tumour coming to operation the survival is 25 to 30 per cent. Occult metastatic disease is often present.

Disposition

In most instances, therefore, the diagnosis of bronchial carcinoma will be disqualifying from aircrew duties. Passengers flying will not normally cause trouble unless there is widespread pulmonary involvement with subsequent disturbance in respiratory function.

Sarcoidosis

Sarcoidosis is a systemic granulomatous disease of unknown aetiology. The most common presentation of thoracic sarcoidosis is with bilateral hilar lymphadenopathy. Frequently this is asymptomatic, but it may be associated with erythema nodosum and with minor constitutional or respiratory symptoms. The course is usually benign, most cases resolving spontaneously within 2 years. Pulmonary shadowing may occur and this, in turn, may lead to pulmonary fibrosis and a deterioration in respiratory functions. Myocardial sarcoidosis

may occur and is associated with sudden death (Nissen and Berte, 1964; Fleming, 1974). The presence of myocardial sarcoidosis in aircrew is, therefore, obviously of great aeromedical importance.

Disposition

Patients with acute sarcoidosis and systemic symptoms, neurological or ocular manifestations, or pulmonary disease requiring corticosteroid therapy, should not fly as aircrew. Those with asymptomatic hilar adenopathy pose a problem: that of possible occult myocardial sarcoidosis. A reasonable approach is to ground all patients with sarcoidosis until they are clinically and radiologically free of disease. Only those with a normal, non-invasive, cardiac evaluation (which should include gallium–thallium scintigraphy) should be returned to unrestricted flying.

Part III: Prolonged exposure to high altitude

John Ernsting

The effects of exposure to altitude hypoxia beyond a few hours differ in important respects from the acute effects which are of primary interest in aerospace activities. The rate at which hypoxia is induced is slower and duration of the exposure to low oxygen tension is usually much longer in the climber and the worker at moderate and high altitude than in the aviator. The prolonged exposure induces adaptive changes which commence within a few minutes and take several weeks to develop fully. The duration of the sojourn at high altitude can extend from less than a day to a whole lifetime. In general the adaptive changes permit individuals to live and work at altitudes which would produce serious impairment of performance or even unconsciousness in the unacclimatized individual. Some 10 million people worldwide live permanently at altitudes above 3600 m (12 000 feet).

With appropriate training designed to maximize the adaptive processes, certain individuals can climb to heights well above 6000 m (19 685 feet) and, indeed, since 1978, several have successfully climbed without the aid of supplemental oxygen to the

summit of Everest where the inspired (tracheal) partial pressure of oxygen is 43 mmHg. A variable proportion of individuals develop one or more symptoms of acute mountain sickness (see page 812) during the first few days of arriving at altitude above 2500 m (8200 feet). The symptoms generally subside, but occasionally progress to acute pulmonary or cerebral oedema, conditions which necessitate immediate descent to lower altitude. Some individuals, especially those born at high altitude, deteriorate after spending some time at altitude.

Barometric pressure

In comparing the effects of acute hypoxia induced in the aviation environment with that associated with the ascent of mountains, it is important to recognize that the barometric pressure at a given height on a mountain is often considerably higher than that defined by the ICAO standard atmosphere (Pugh, 1957). Above 6000 m this difference can amount to 15 to 17 mmHg. The barometric pressure measured at the summit of Everest (8848 m) in the 1981 American Medical Research Expedition to Everest (West *et al.*, 1983b) was 253 mmHg, whereas the barometric pressure at this altitude in the ICAO standard atmosphere is 236 mmHg.

Alveolar gas composition

When an individual remains at altitude, there is a progressive increase in pulmonary ventilation over the first 4 days of the exposure (Lenfant and Sullivan, 1971). This hyperventilation is maintained for many years both at rest and during exercise. The increased pulmonary ventilation induces the hypocapnia which is an important feature of the individual who has spent more than a few hours at altitude. The consequent changes in the composition of the alveolar gas are clearly demonstrated in the alveolar oxygen–carbon dioxide diagram (Figure 24.6) originally presented by Rahn and Otis (1949) and extended by West *et al.* (1983a).

The increase in pulmonary ventilation is due to the arterial hypoxaemia stimulating respiration by way of the arterial chemoreceptors, particularly those of the carotid bodies. This stimulation of respiration by the hypoxia is initially limited by the concomitant reduction of arterial carbon dioxide tension and consequent respiratory alkalosis. Within a few hours, however, active transport of hydrogen ions and renal excretion of bicarbonate allow ventilation to increase in response to the hypoxia.

Figure 24.6 shows clearly that even the mild hypoxia associated with ascent to 1000 m which has no immediate effect upon pulmonary ventilation will, in a few days, reduce the alveolar carbon dioxide tension by 2 to 3 mmHg. More severe degrees of hypoxia induce marked reductions of alveolar carbon dioxide tension in the acclimatized individual, so that after several days at 6000 m it is reduced to 20 to 25 mmHg. Direct measurements made by West *et al.* (1983a) of the alveolar carbon dioxide tensions of climbers on Everest at a height of 8050 m yielded a mean value of 11 mmHg and measurements on a single climber at an altitude of 8400 m gave a tension of 8 mmHg. It is doubtful if many individuals could maintain the very high pulmonary ventilations required to produce these very low alveolar carbon dioxide tensions.

The increase in pulmonary ventilation limits the fall of alveolar oxygen tension which is produced by the low oxygen tension of the impaired air. The three curves of Figure 24.6 demonstrate the effects

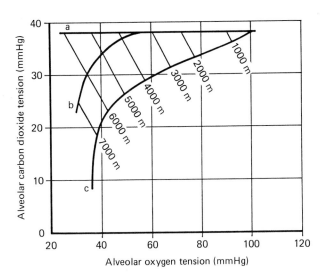

Figure 24.6 Oxygen–carbon dioxide diagram showing the composition of the alveolar gases in (1) seated individuals exposed acutely (0–20 minutes) to breathing air at various altitudes (curve b) and (2) individuals fully acclimatized to various altitude (curve c). Curve a depicts the composition of the alveolar gas at altitude in the absence of any ventilatory response to the hypoxia. Iso-altitude lines for 1000, 2000, 3000, 4000, 5000, 6000 and 7000 metres are also shown. (Data from Rahn and Otis, 1949, and West *et al.*, 1984)

on the alveolar oxygen tension of the immediate (0 to 20 minute) ventilatory response to hypoxia and of that which is fully developed after 4 days' exposure to altitude. Thus, at moderate altitudes (4000 to 6000 m), the alveolar oxygen tension is some 10 mmHg higher in the fully acclimatized individual than it is during the first half hour of exposure to altitude. At altitudes above about 6500 m, the increase in pulmonary ventilation with acclimatization, at least in successful climbers, is very great so that the alveolar oxygen tension at altitudes up to 8050 m does not fall below 35 mmHg.

Gas exchange in the lungs and the arterial blood gases

The changes in the alveolar–arterial oxygen tension difference seen in individuals adapted to moderate altitude when they are at rest are very similar to those seen on acute exposure to these altitudes. Thus, the oxygen tension difference between the alveolar gas and the arterial blood falls in acclimatized individuals from 8 to 10 mmHg at sea level to 3 to 5 mmHg at 4500 to 5000 m. The diffusing capacity of the lungs for oxygen, both at rest and during exercise, is unchanged in individuals acclimatized to high altitude (West, 1962). Exercise in the acclimatized individual results in a marked fall in the arterial oxygen tension due to a large increase in the alveolar–arterial oxygen tension difference, which can rise to 15 to 20 mmHg during moderate exercise (oxygen consumption = 2.0 litres (STPD)/min) at altitudes of 5000 to 6500 m (Sutton et al., 1988). The increase in the alveolar–arterial oxygen tension difference with exercise is primarily due to diffusion limitation (West and Wagner, 1980), although there is evidence of an increase in ventilation–blood flow mismatch in acclimatized individuals, especially during exercise. This effect is probably related to non-uniform pulmonary vasoconstriction and, perhaps, alveolar interstitial oedema produced by the raised pulmonary arterial pressure.

The oxygen tension and oxygen saturation of the arterial blood of individuals acclimatized to altitude are significantly higher than in those acutely exposed to the same altitude. Thus, at medium altitudes (4500 to 6000 m) the process of adaptation raises the arterial oxygen tension by 10 to 12 mmHg and the arterial oxygen saturation by 9 to 11 per cent (in resting subjects). These changes are associated with a reduction of the arterial carbon dioxide tension due to acclimatization of 5 to 7 mmHg. The renal compensation of the respiratory alkalosis produced by the increase in pulmonary ventilation returns the pH of the arterial blood to within normal sea level limits in the individual acclimatized to high altitude. These changes are of the greatest importance because they allow a large increase in the pulmonary ventilation which limits the fall of alveolar oxygen tension.

Another important feature of the acclimatization to high altitude is the increase in the concentrations of red cells and haemoglobin in the blood. Thus, the haemoglobin concentration of individuals acclimatized to 4500 m is typically 20 g/dl. The increased concentration of haemoglobin at altitude tends to maintain the concentration of oxygen in arterial blood, in spite of the fall in the oxygen tension and oxygen saturation, which in turn limits the fall of the oxygen tension of the venous blood. The hypoxia induced at moderate altitudes shifts the oxygen dissociation curve to the right as a result of an increase in the concentration of 2,3-diphosphoglycerate in the red cells. This shift aids unloading of oxygen in the tissue capillaries. The marked uncompensated respiratory alkalosis which occurs at higher altitudes tends to return the oxygen dissociation curve towards it sea level position.

Maximal oxygen uptake

Exposure to altitude, even when the individual is fully acclimatized, reduces markedly the maximal

oxygen uptake in exercise. Thus, the maximal oxygen uptake at 3000 m is reduced to 90 per cent of that at sea level whilst at 6000 m it is 60 per cent of the sea level value. The major factor limiting oxygen uptake in these circumstances is the rate at which oxygen diffuses across the alveolar–capillary membrane into the blood. Breathing air at the summit of Everest (8848 m), where the inspired oxygen tension is 43 mmHg, limits the maximal oxygen uptake to about 1.0 litre (STPD)/minute (West, 1984).

Acute mountain sickness

Individuals exposed to hypoxia at altitude may develop a variety of clinical conditions varying from a relative benign transient sickness to life-threatening pulmonary or cerebral disease. Benign acute mountain sickness which occurs in about half of those climbing to altitudes above about 4000 m (13 200 feet) comprises some or all of the following symptoms: headache, nausea, anorexia, vomiting, insomnia and poor climbing performance (Dickinson, 1982; Ward, Milledge and West, 1989). This condition, depending upon the rate of ascent and individual susceptibility, typically commences within a few hours and generally lasts between 2 and 5 days. These disturbances are related to retention of body water and an increase in the extracellular fluid induced by the hypoxia. They are accentuated by physical exercise.

Benign acute mountain sickness usually resolves over 2 to 5 days but it can, particularly if the sufferer continues to ascend or to indulge in exercise, become more severe and develop into malignant acute mountain sickness. The latter can comprise pulmonary or cerebral disorders or a mixture of the two (Dickinson, 1982; Heath and Williams, 1989). If untreated, these conditions can be fatal. The pulmonary form of malignant acute mountain sickness occurs in 0.5 to 1.5 per cent of individuals ascending to altitudes of 3000 to 6000 m. The incidence of the cerebral form of the condition is somewhat lower, and it is frequently associated with the pulmonary form. The cerebral condition is characterized by disturbed consciousness, ataxia, paresis and abnormal reflex responses (Dickinson, 1979). There is almost always cerebral oedema, and this may be complicated by haemorrhages into the brain and thrombosis in the cerebral venous sinuses (Heath and Williams, 1989).

Acute mountain sickness, both benign and malignant, can normally be avoided by climbing slowly enough to allow adaptive changes to occur. Thus, the climber should be advised to 'hasten slowly', to 'climb high, sleep low' and not to ascend any further if any symptoms of mountain sickness develop (Milledge, 1985). There is a wide individual variation in *susceptibility* to acute mountain sickness, so that it is difficult to lay down a practical safe rate of ascent. The altitude at which the climber sleeps is crucial and a good rule is that above an altitude of 3000 m, each night should be spent not more than 300 m above the last with a rest day, that is two nights, at the same altitude, every 2 or 3 days (Milledge, 1985). Acetazolamide provides effective prophylaxis although ideally it should not replace a slow rate of ascent. Acetazolamide (250 mg every 8 hours or 500 mg slow-release tablet per day) reduces the incidence of acute mountain sickness (Birmingham Study Group, 1981). The drug probably acts by increasing the excretion of bicarbonate by the kidney producing a metabolic acidosis which produces a further fall of alveolar carbon dioxide tension allowing the alveolar oxygen tension to rise.

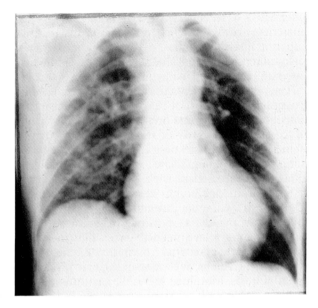

Figure 24.7 High-altitude pulmonary oedema (largely unilateral) in a 52-year-old female who developed typical mixed cerebral and pulmonary mountain sickness at 12 700 feet (3810 m). The lung fields were normal in a film taken 5 days later following removal to lower altitude. (Courtesy of Dr John Dickinson)

High-altitude pulmonary oedema

The pulmonary form of malignant acute mountain sickness, or high-altitude pulmonary oedema, is characterized by the sudden onset of severe oedema of the lung. It may or may not be preceded by the benign form of acute mountain sickness. It can occur at altitudes as low as 2500 m but it commonly occurs at altitudes above 3000 m. The disorder may be precipitated by rapid ascent, for example, by aircraft and by strenuous exercise (Singh et al., 1965). Some individuals are predisposed to developing it each time they return to altitude after a period at sea level. It predominantly affects the young adult. The initial symptoms are dry cough, breathlessness and tachypnoea even at rest. The cough then becomes productive with white frothy sputum which may later be tinged with blood, and severe dyspnoea develops (Heath and Williams, 1989). Clinical examination reveals widespread fine to medium inspiratory crackles throughout the lungs, often with 'bubbling' sounds. If untreated, the patient develops central cyanosis and coma, with haemoptysis occurring in about a fifth of the severe cases. Symptoms are frequently worse at night, and confusion and delirium may occur. Descent to lower altitude rapidly relieves the illness which otherwise can be fatal.

The chest radiograph shows multiple large, soft, frequently confluent, and usually bilateral, opacities which are generally prominent in the hilar regions. The changes may, however, be confined largely to one lung (Figure 24.7). The pulmonary conus is usually prominent and the hilar and major pulmonary arteries are generally dilated (Singh et al., 1965; Heath and Williams, 1989). The shadowing of the lung fields disappears fairly rapidly as the patient recovers. However, exudates may persist for days after clinical recovery.

The mechanism underlying high-altitude pulmonary oedema remains uncertain. Although the clinical picture is similar to that of left ventricular failure, measurements of pulmonary capillary wedge pressure and of left arterial pressure have shown that the left atrial pressure is not raised (Roy et al., 1969). The pulmonary arterial pressure, which is usually increased in individuals exposed to altitudes above 3000 m (Cruz-Jibaja et al., 1964), is often markedly raised in those individuals who develop altitude pulmonary oedema (Roy et al., 1969). The pulmonary hypertension is further accentuated by exercise. The oedema fluid is rich in high-molecular-weight proteins (Schoene et al., 1986), which indicates that the disorder is a high-protein, high-permeability type of pulmonary oedema. The probable mechanism is that the high intravascular pressures induced by non-uniform hypoxic vasoconstriction lead to increased permeability in some pulmonary vessels, particularly those fed by less constricted arterioles. There is also evidence to support thrombosis as a basis for both the pulmonary hypertension and the pulmonary oedema (Heath and Williams, 1989).

The prompt recognition of high altitude pulmonary oedema at an early stage is vital. Repeated coughing and breathlessness, either alone or combined with any of the symptoms of benign acute mountain sickness, should be regarded seriously and immediate descent and oxygen therapy initiated. Increasing the oxygen tension in the inspired gas is the keystone of treatment. Descent to as low an altitude as possible, at least 2400 m, as rapidly as possible is indicated. High flows of oxygen are needed, especially in severe cases. A diuretic such as frusemide or bumetanide should be given in sufficient dosage to produce a good diuresis. Morphine probably has little place in treatment. Virtually all cases respond well to oxygen therapy, rest and immediate descent.

Ascent to moderate altitudes

Numerous occupational groups other than amateur or professional climbers travel to, and live for shorter or longer periods at, moderate altitudes. Business executives, technicians, civil engineers, geologists, astronomers and sports personnel, to name but a few, may ascend to moderate altitudes to work or play. They may well travel from low altitude to the high terrain rapidly by aircraft, or relatively rapidly by motor vehicle or train taking only a few hours to ascend to considerable heights. The disturbances induced by the reduction of the oxygen tension in the inspired air become noticeable at an altitude of 2500 m and become progressively more intrusive at altitudes above 3000 m. The incidence and severity of the disturbances are related to the final altitude, to the rate of ascent, to the physical activity and to the fitness of the individual.

Rapid ascent to an altitude of the order of 3000 m followed by normal physical activity will induce mild symptoms of benign acute mountain sickness in 50 per cent of individuals who remain at altitude for longer than 12 hours. The symptoms typically comprise light-headedness, headache, irritability and nausea. There is dyspnoea on exertion. Individuals also experience lassitude and objective tests show minor but significant impairment of higher mental performance and interpersonality relationships. The disturbances generally reach a maximum after 24 to 48 hours at altitude and then decline as the individual adapts to the hypoxia.

Ascent to altitudes of the order of 4500 m without preceding acclimatization produces severe dyspnoea, weakness and fatigue. There is marked lassitude and many suffer severe headaches, nausea, vomiting and loss of appetite. These symptoms are typically made worse by physical exertion and partially relieved by rest. Sleep is very disturbed as is respiration during sleep. There is periodic breathing with spells of apnoea which may be associated with arousals. There is difficulty in falling asleep and in sustaining sleep, awakenings occurring throughout the night. Higher mental function is impaired. The symptoms of acute mountain sickness, the dyspnoea on exertion and the impairment of mental performance decrease after 2 to 3 days at altitude as acclimatization occurs. Marked physical exertion is to be avoided because it not only increases the severity of the symptoms but also increases the likelihood of the occurrence of malignant acute mountain sickness. Special studies have been made of telescope operators in the observatories at the summit of the high-altitude volcano, Mauna Kea (4200 m) in Hawaii (Forster, 1986). They live in a coastal town and travel by car to the summit – a journey of 90 minutes. Daily travellers have a break of 30 minutes at 2750 m at the acclimatization lodge during the ascent. Shift workers do four shifts each of 5 days, preceded by an initial night in the lodge. Eighty per cent of shift workers developed symptoms of acute mountain sickness on the first day at the summit; this fell to 40 per cent after 5 days. Symptoms included significantly impaired memory and concentration. By contrast, only 40 per cent of the daily travellers had any symptoms on their first day. Their seemingly better acclimatization is, of course, spurious because they leave the hypoxic environment within 9 hours which is the 'lag' period before acute mountain sickness develops. The cost of this is their failure to develop the full acclimatization acquired by long residence at high altitude. However, it has to be remembered that the facility of rapid 'escape' by these workers from the altitude of Mauna Kea, which pre-empts serious medical emergencies, is exceptional and may not be available to others planning short-term working visits to high altitude elsewhere (Heath and Williams, 1989). Forster's (1986) studies demonstrated significant impairment of mental performance at this altitude.

Where slow ascent permitting acclimatization to develop is not possible then severe acute mountain sickness may be avoided by limiting the duration of the exposure. If more than one day is to be spent above 3000 to 3500 m the feasibility of descending to below 3000 m at night to sleep should be explored because this procedure will reduce the severity of the symptoms. When the altitude exceeds 3500 to 4000 m, then the use of prophylactic acetazolamide should be considered. Performance, both physical and mental, is improved and the incidence of benign acute mountain sickness reduced when acetazolamide (250 mg every 8 hours or a 500-mg slow-release tablet per day) is taken immediately before and during the exposure to altitude. The drug also improves sleep at altitude (Nicholson et al., 1988), partly due to its respiratory effects and partly due to its action as a hypnotic. The side effects of acetazolamide include a mild diuresis and paraesthesiae of the hands and feet which almost always diminish with time. The headache of acute mountain sickness is relatively resistant to aspirin or paracetamol, but voluntary hyperventilation often reduces the intensity of the symptoms and probably promotes adaptation (Ward, Milledge and West, 1989).

The evidence with respect to the effects of smoking as such, rather than the respiratory and cardiovascular diseases it may induce upon tolerance to altitude, is somewhat controversial. Whereas earlier studies had suggested that the 10 per cent carboxyhaemoglobinaemia associated with moderate cigarette smoking produced a significant intensification of the mental and physical performance effects of acute hypoxia at 3000 to 4000 m, some modern studies do not support these findings. It is doubtful if cessation of smoking by a smoker on ascent to altitude will ameliorate the effects of the hypoxia or the incidence and severity of benign mountain sickness. The mental and performance effects of alcohol and those of acute hypoxia are additive and, thus, it is wise to avoid the intake of more than small quantities of alcohol on ascent to altitude.

The compatibility of lung disease, such as chronic bronchitis and emphysema, with ascent to moderate altitude depends essentially on the degree of impairment of pulmonary gas exchange produced by the disease process. If lung function is such that the patient has a reasonable exercise tolerance at sea level, then ascent to moderate altitudes is unlikely to produce incapacitation, provided that only moderate exercise is taken. Similarly, those individuals who have a good exercise tolerance after lung surgery will have a good tolerance of ascent to altitude.

Moderate or severe anaemia is a contraindication to exposure to altitudes above 2500 m. Considerable controversy still surrounds the risk of exposure to altitude precipitating a cerebral, splenic or visceral infarct in an individual with sickle-cell trait. There have been a few documented cases of splenic infarctions associated with flight or climbing mountains in patients with sickle-cell trait proven by electrophoresis (Diggs, 1984). The experience of the United States Air Force and other air forces is, however, that the risk of exposure to altitude precipitating a sickling crisis in individuals with the trait is extremely small (Rayman, 1990).

Chronic mountain sickness (Monge's disease)

This is a disorder that develops in some native highlanders after many years of residence at altitudes above 4000 m (Heath and Williams, 1989). The patient, who is usually a young or middle-aged man, exhibits excessive fatigue, decreased exercise tolerance and marked central cyanosis. The cyanosis combined with excessive polycythaemia gives the lips and mucous membranes an almost black colour. There is moderate pulmonary hypertension with hypertrophy of the right ventricle, but right ventricular failure is seldom seen. The haemoglobin concentration exceeds 23 g/dl and the arterial oxygen tension and oxygen saturation are severely depressed (Penaloza, Sime and Ruiz, 1971). The underlying dysfunction is one of chronic alveolar hypoventilation due to the loss of long-established acclimatization. The normal ventilatory responses to hypoxia are lost. The increased arterial hypoxaemia gives rise to a marked increase in the concentration of haemoglobin and to a very high haematocrit (73 to 83 per cent).

The treatment of Monge's disease is descent to a lower altitude. The symptoms and the blood and circulatory disturbances improve rapidly on descent to sea level, but usually recur if the patient returns to high altitude.

References

Allan, J.R. (1988) Thermal protection. In *Aviation Medicine*, 2nd edn (eds J. Ernsting and P. King), London, Butterworths, pp. 247–251

Bancroft, R.W. and Dunn, J.E. (1965) Experimental animal decompressions to a near vacuum environment. *Aerospace Med.* **36**, 720–725

Birmingham Medical Research Expeditionary Society Mountain Sickness Study Group (1981) Acetazolamide in control of acute mountain sickness. *Lancet* **1**, 180–183

Cran, I.R. and Rumball, C.A. (1967) Survey of spontaneous pneumothoraces in the Royal Air Force. *Thorax* **22**, 462–465

Cruz-Jibaja, J., Banchero, N., Sime, F., Penaloza, D., Gamboa, R. and Marticorena, E. (1964) Correlation between pulmonary artery pressure and level of altitude. *Dis. Chest* **46**, 446–451

Davis, J.C., Sheffield, P.J., Schucknecht, L., Heimbach, R.D., Dunn, J.M., Douglas, G. and Anderson, G.K. (1977) Altitude decompression sickness: hyperbaric therapy results in 145 cases. *Aviat. Space Environ. Med.* **48**, 722–730

Denison, D.M., Ledwith, F. and Poulton, E.C. (1966) Complex reaction times at simulated cabin altitudes of 5,000 feet and 8,000 feet. *Aerospace Med.* **37**, 1010–1013

Dickinson, J.G. (1979) Severe acute mountain sickness. *Postgrad. Med. J.* **55**, 454–458

Dickinson, J.G. (1982) Terminology and classification of acute mountain sickness. *Br. Med. J.* **285**, 720–721

Diggs, L.W. (1984) The sickle cell trait in relation to the training and assignment of duties in the Armed Forces: I Policies, Observations and Studies. *Aviat. Space Environ. Med.* **55**, 180–185

Dixon, G.A., Adams, J.D. and Harvey, W.T. (1986) Decompression sickness and intravenous bubble formation using a 7.8 psia simulated pressure-suit environment. *Aviat. Space Environ. Med.* **57**, 223–228

Ernsting, J. (1960) Some effects of oxygen-breathing on man. *Proc. R. Soc. Med.* **53**, 96–98

Ernsting, J. (1963) The ideal relationship between inspired oxygen concentration and cabin altitude. *Aerospace Med.* **34**, 991–997

Ernsting, J. (1965) Influence of alveolar nitrogen concentration and environmental pressure upon the rate of gas absorption from non-ventilated lung. *Aerospace Med.* **36**, 948–955

Ernsting, J. (1966) Some effects of raised intrapulmonary pressure in man. *AGARDograph* 106, Technivision Ltd, Maidenhead, UK

Ernsting, J. (1978) Prevention of hypoxia – acceptable compromises. *Aviat. Space Environ. Med.* **49**, 495–502

Ernsting, J. (1984) Operational and physiological requirement for aircraft oxygen systems. *AGARD Report No 697.* AGARD/NATO, Neuilly sur Seine, pp. 1-1 to 1-9

Ernsting, J. and Stewart, W.K. (1965) Introduction to oxygen deprivation at reduced barometric pressure. In *A Textbook of Aviation Physiology* (ed. J.A. Gillies), Pergamon Press, Oxford, pp. 209–213

Ernsting, J., Byford, G.H., Denison, D.M. and Fryer, D.I. (1973) Hypoxia induced by rapid decompression from 8,000 feet to 40,000 feet – the influence of rate of decompression. Flying Personnel Research Committee *Report No 1324.* Ministry of Defence, London

Fleming, H.A. (1974) Myocardial sarcoidosis. *Br. Heart J.* **36**, 54–68

Forster, P. (1986) Telescopes in high places. In: *Aspects of Hypoxia* (ed. D. Heath), Liverpool University Press, Liverpool, pp. 221–229

Fryer, D.I. (1969) Subatmospheric decompression sickness in man. *AGARDograph* 125, Technivision Ltd, Maidenhead, UK

Fuchs, H.S. (1967) Idiopathic spontaneous pneumothorax and flying. *Aerospace Med.* **38**, 1283–1285

Gauer, O.H., Henry, R.P. and Behn, C. (1970) The regulation of extracellular fluid volume. *Ann. Rev. Physiol.* **32**, 547–595

Glaister, D.H. (1988a) The effects of long duration acceleration. In: *Aviation Medicine,* 2nd edn (eds J. Ernsting and P. King), Butterworths, London, pp. 139–158

Glaister, D.H. (1988b) Protection against long duration acceleration. In: *Aviation Medicine* 2nd edn (eds J. Ernsting and P. King), Butterworths, London, pp. 159–165

Harding, R.M. (1988a) The earth's atmosphere. In: *Aviation Medicine,* 2nd edn (eds J. Ernsting and P. King), Butterworths, London, pp. 3–12

Harding, R.M. (1988b) Oxygen equipment and pressure clothing. In: *Aviation Medicine,* 2nd edn (eds J. Ernsting and P. King), London, Butterworths, pp. 72–111

Harding, R.M. (1988c) Medical aspects of special types of flight. In: *Aviation Medicine,* 2nd edn (eds J. Ernsting and P. King), Butterworths, London, pp. 479–489

Heath, D. and Williams, D.R. (1989) *High Altitude Medicine and Pathology,* London, Butterworths

Hopkirk, J.A.C., Pullen, M.J. and Fraser, J.R. (1983) Pleurodesis: The results of treatment of spontaneous pneumothorax in the Royal Air Force. *Aviat. Space Environ. Med.* **54**, 158–160

Lenfant, C. and Sullivan, K. (1971) Adaptation to high altitude. *N. Engl. J. Med.* **284**, 1298–1309

Macmillan, A.J.F. (1988a) Decompression sickness. In: *Aviation Medicine,* 2nd edn (eds J. Ernsting and P. King), Butterworths, London, pp. 19–26

Macmillan, A.J.F. (1988b) The pressure cabin. In: *Aviation Medicine,* 2nd edn (eds J. Ernsting and P. King), Butterworths, London, pp. 112–126

Milledge, J.S. (1985) Acute mountain sickness: pulmonary and cerebral oedema of high altitude. *Intens. Care Med.* **11**, 110–114

Nicogossian, A.E. and Parker, J.F. (1982) *Space Physiology and Medicine.* Washington DC, NASA SP-477

Nicholson, A.N., Smith, P.A., Stone, B.M., Bradwell, A.R. and Coote, J.H. (1988) Altitude insomnia: studies during an expedition to the Himalayas. *Sleep* **11**, 354–361

Nissen, A.W. and Berte, J.B. (1964) Cardiac arrhythmias in sarcoidosis. *Archs Intern. Med.* **113**, 275

Penaloza, D., Sime, F. and Ruiz, L. (1971) Cor pulmonale in chronic mountain sickness: present concept of Monge's disease. In: *High Altitude Physiology: Cardiac and Respiratory Aspects.* Ciba Foundation Symposium (eds R. Porter and J. Knight), Churchill Livingstone, Edinburgh, pp. 41–60

Pugh, L.G.C.E. (1957) Resting ventilation and alveolar air on Mount Everest: with remarks on the relation of barometric pressure to altitude in mountains. *J. Physiol.* **135**, 590–610

Rahn, H. and Otis, A.B. (1947) Alveolar air during simulated flights to high altitude. *Am. J. Physiol.* **150**, 202–222

Rahn, H. and Otis, A.B. (1949) Man's respiratory response during and after acclimatization to high altitude. *Am. J. Physiol.* **157**, 445–449

Rayman, R.B. (1973) Sudden incapacities in flight 1 Jan 1966 – 30 Nov 1971. *Aerospace Med.* **44**, 953–955

Rayman, R.B. (1990) *Clinical Aviation Medicine,* Lea and Febiger, London, pp. 41–43

Roy, S.B., Guleria, J.S., Khanna, P.K., Manchanda, S.C., Pande, J.N. and Subba, P.S. (1969) Haemodynamic studies in high altitude pulmonary oedema. *Br. Heart J.* **31**, 52–58

Schoene, R.B., Hackett, P.H., Henderson, W.R., Sage, H., Chow, H., Roach, R.C., Mills, W.J. and Martin, T.R. (1986) High altitude pulmonary edema. Characteristics of lung lavage fluid. *J. Am. Med. Assoc.* **256**, 63–69

Sharp, G.R. and Macmillan, A.J.F. (1988) The effects of pressure change. In: *Aviation Medicine,* 2nd edn (eds J. Ernsting and P. King), Butterworths, London, pp. 13–18

Singh, I., Kapila, C.C., Khanna, P.K., Nanda, B.B. and Rao, B.D.P. (1965) High altitude pulmonary oedema. *Lancet* **1**, 229–234

Sutton, J.R., Reeves, J.T., Wagner, P.D., Groves, B.M., Cymerman, A., Malconian, M.K., Rock, P.B., Young, P.M., Walter, S.D. and Houston, C.S. (1988) Operation Everest II: oxygen transport during exercise at extreme simulated altitude. *J. Appl. Physiol.* **64**, 1309–1321

Ward, M.P., Milledge, J.S. and West, J.B. (1989) *High Altitude Medicine and Physiology,* Chapman and Hall, London

West, J.B. (1962) Diffusing capacity of the lung for carbon monoxide at high altitude. *J. Appl. Physiol.* **17**, 421–426

West, J.B. (1984) Man on the summit of Mount Everest. In: *High Altitude and Man* (eds J.B. West, and S. Lahiri) Williams and Wilkins, Baltimore, pp. 15–17

West, J.B. and Wagner, P.D. (1980) Predicted gas exchange on the summit of Mount Everest. *Respir. Physiol.* **42**, 1–16

West, J.B., Lahiri, S., Gill, M.B., Milledge, J.S., Pugh, L.G.C.E. and Ward, M.P. (1962) Arterial oxygen saturation during exercise at high altitude. *J. Appl. Physiol.* **17**, 617–621

West, J.B., Hackett, P.H., Maret, K.H., Milledge, J.S., Peters Jr, R.M., Pizzo, C.J. and Winslow, R.M. (1983a) Pulmonary gas exchange on the summit of Mount Everest. *J. Appl. Physiol.: Respir. Environ. Exercise Physiol.* **55**, 678–687

West, J.B., Lahiri, S., Maret, K.H., Peters Jr, R.M. and Pizzo, C.J. (1983b) Barometric pressures at extreme altitudes on Mount Everest: physiological significance. *J. Appl. Physiol.: Respir. Environ. Exercise Physiol.* **54**, 1188–1194

25

The lungs and diving

Ramsay R. Pearson

The ocean: a body of water occupying two thirds of a world made for man – who has no gills.

Ambrose Bierce

Whatever one may think of the conceit of Ambrose Bierce, a notable American 'curmudgeon', in imagining that the world was made for mankind, he highlights the fundamental inadequacy which, in one way or another, limits all human attempts to venture under water. The earliest recorded underwater activity dates back to 6000 BC although it is certain that diving as a curious or purposeful activity must have occurred much earlier. However, such diving, then and until the early eighteenth century when divers were able to make excursions from diving bells using primitive helmets supplied with air from the bell, depended on breath-hold diving, an activity for which human beings are singularly ill-equipped. The advent of underwater breathing apparatus, of which the first truly practical and reliable variety was the 1819 copper helmet and leather jacket of Augustus Siebe, in which the diver was supplied with compressed air from a force-pump on the surface, provided divers with a totally new freedom and endurance under water. In 1837, Siebe replaced the jacket with a full canvas oversuit and this type of equipment, which came to be known as 'standard' or 'hard hat', became the mainstay of professional diving until the Second World War when closed-circuit oxygen breathing sets, albeit mostly very primitive and often hazardous, became widely used for military purposes. From these early examples of *self-contained underwater breathing apparatus* (SCUBA) came the truly enormous variety of breathing equipment in current use, a process which was also accelerated greatly in 1946 by the development of a simple and reliable demand valve that automatically provided the diver with a supply of breathing mixture at a pressure equal to that of the surrounding water. This simple device led to a veritable explosion in recreational diving as well as changing dramatically the type of diving used for military and commercial activities. However, despite the enormous advances made in breathing equipment, human beings remain relatively poorly adapted to the multiple stresses and challenges of the underwater environment. To understand the scale of the problem, it is necessary to look first at the fundamental responses to the common denominators of all diving, namely immersion and submersion with their inevitable accompaniment of increased pressure on the body.

Effects of immersion

The general effects of immersion on human beings have been researched widely over many decades and the effect on the respiratory system in particular must be seen as only part of a wide-ranging and complex cardiovascular–respiratory response. Equally, it is important to recognize that these responses may be modified dramatically by the other environmental stresses inherent in diving of which cold is by far the most important. Much of the research into these responses has been with erect subjects immersed up to the neck, in contrast to the fully submerged diver who is also frequently prone in the water. However, many of the responses noted in 'head-out' immersion are representative of the fully submerged condition and the general effects of immersion on the respiratory system are summarized as follows:

1. Reduced vital capacity (approximately 5 per cent in head-out immersion).
2. Reduction in static lung compliance.
3. Increased closing volumes leading to:
   (a) increase in 'physiological' (functional) degree of air trapping;
   (b) increase in diffusing capacity;
   (c) increased flow resistance in airways (due to increased gas density);
   (d) altered ventilation distribution (bias moving to apical regions);
   (e) reduction in functional residual capacity.

These effects are mainly due to the hydrostatic pressure exerted by water which gives a redistribution of blood into the large intrathoracic blood vessels and, to a lesser extent, into the pulmonary microcirculation. This redistribution results from a hydrostatic pressure gradient over the immersed body which, in the upright position, is greater over the lower part of the body.

The cardiovascular effects of immersion are equally complex and are summarised as follows:

1. Increased stroke volume with increased cardiac output.
2. Increased peripheral perfusion.
3. Increased central blood volume (hydrostatic gradient effect).
4. Extrasystoles during early phase of immersion (due to cardiac distension).
5. 'Hyperbaric bradycardia' (approximately 10 beats/min).

If other factors such as cold are discounted, the cardiovascular changes are, in common with the respiratory responses, due largely to the hydrostatic pressure gradient over the body and the associated redistribution of blood. Worthy of separate mention is the so-called *hyperbaric bradycardia* which is a phenomenon quite distinct from the bradycardia associated with the *diving reflex* seen in diving mammals and, to a lesser degree, in human subjects in whom it is associated particularly with facial immersion. Hyperbaric bradycardia has been observed in all types of non-breath-hold diving, including the prolonged exposures to pressure associated with saturation diving. Usually of the order of 10 beats/minute, it is not nearly as dramatic as that seen in the diving reflex and is due to a combination of factors, of which the increased partial pressure of oxygen in breathing mixtures supplied to divers is said to be the most important. Other factors probably involved are increased gas density, increased hydrostatic pressure and, possibly, the narcotic effect of an increased partial pressure of inert gas such as the nitrogen found in compressed air or oxygen–nitrogen breathing mixtures.

Gas density and underwater breathing apparatus

If any sustained activity is to be carried out under water, divers must be supplied with a respirable breathing mixture from some form of underwater breathing apparatus of which many varieties exist, although all fall into three basic categories in which the breathing mixture is supplied to the diver: from the surface, from a diving bell, or carried by the diver himself as in the case of SCUBA. The pressure at which the breathing mixture is supplied to the diver must be the same as that of the surrounding water which increases by 1 bar (1 atmosphere or 1 ATA) for every 10 metres (33 feet) of depth. Whatever the breathing mixture used by the diver, the effect of increased gas density is the cause of difficulties common to all types of diving. The breathing mixture can range from pure oxygen, through compressed air, to the various inert gases used as diluents or 'carrier gases' for the essential oxygen supplied to divers at depths in excess of the limits for pure oxygen and compressed air breathing. The diluent gas in almost universal use for deep diving (over 50 m) is helium although a number of alternatives such as neon–helium or hydrogen–helium mixtures have been, or are being, considered in an effort to provide a cheaper alternative. However, such mixtures have a number of drawbacks when compared to helium. For instance, the relative density of neon is an important limiting factor for very deep diving and the narcotic and explosive properties of hydrogen when mixed with oxygen tend to offset its value as the lightest of gases. The density of a typical helium–oxygen (Heliox) mixture supplied to a diver at 300 m (975 feet) will only be equivalent to that of compressed air at a little over 30 m. The most profound effect of increasing gas density is to reduce the maximum ventilatory volume (MVV) and maximum expiratory flow rate (MEFR). This reduced breathing efficiency leads to increasing levels of alveolar carbon dioxide although, fortunately for the diver, the reductions in MVV and MEFR occur more or less exponentially and divers breathing Heliox in experimental compression chamber dives to pressures equivalent to depths in excess of 600 m have been shown to be capable ot MVVs of 40 to 50 l/min – approximately 25 per cent of their surface values. Inevitably, therefore, there is a dramatic reduction in the capacity to work at these extreme pressures. The increased density of breathing mixtures becomes even more critical when the diver uses underwater breathing apparatus and the inherent breathing resistance of the set, which also increases with gas density, is added to the diver's own respiratory resistance.

In summary, therefore, the work of breathing increases with depth and ventilation is impaired to such an extent that the limit to muscular effort under water is respiratory rather than the cardio-vascular limitations that apply at sea level.

A final factor to be considered is the pressure gradient that exists between the regulator and the pressure centroid of the lung and that controls the pressure of the breathing mixture supplied to the diver, which is either combined with the diver's mouth piece or mounted on his or her breathing apparatus. This pressure, usually referred to as *static lung loading* (SLL), depends on the attitude of the diver in the water and can lead to the diver breathing at either positive or negative pressures (Figure 25.1). The pressures involved may be equivalent to as much as 20 cmH₂O and can lead to significant dyspnoea when negative pressures occur, whereas positive pressures can be beneficial in reducing dyspnoea (Lundgren, 1984). SLL can also lead to a significant and detrimental lowering of the functional reserve capacity (FRC) in the erect diver. The ideal breathing apparatus has yet to be designed that, whatever the attitude of the diver, can deliver the breathing mixture at a pressure equal to *eupnoeic pressure*, which is the pressure subjectively most acceptable.

Eupnoeic pressure has been shown to be equivalent to 7 cmH₂O above the lung pressure centroid (Thalmann, Sponholtz and Lundgren, 1979), thus confirming the observations concerning the subjective effects of negative pressure SLL. The range of scientific literature dealing with these various aspects of the effects of immersion and diving on the lung is truly vast, but amplified comment and excellent sources of reference exist in a number of textbooks dealing with diving physiology and medicine.

Breath-hold ('skin') diving

In comparison with the diving mammals which have very compliant chest walls, thick pleura, large airspaces, lungs without lobes and airways that allow high flow rates at low lung volumes, human beings have a relatively rigid chest wall which does not accommodate well to the increased ambient pressures encountered under water. This rigidity of the chest wall combines with other poorly adapted features of the human lung to produce a number of major difficulties which become increasingly severe with depth. The main difficulty occurs with increasingly negative intrathoracic pressures which, among other things, will lead to 'compression' pulmonary *barotrauma* once the lung volume, which must diminish in accordance with Boyle's law, reaches and then falls below residual volume (RV). Compression barotrauma gives rise, in turn, to

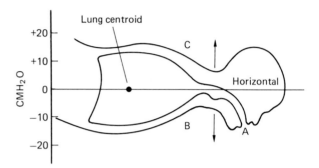

Figure 25.1 Static lung loading levels for three commonly used sites for pressure regulators (A, B and C)

widespread atelectasis, pulmonary vascular damage, haemorrhage and pulmonary oedema. Because RV is normally about 20 to 25 per cent of total lung capacity (TLC), it follows that the limit for human breath-hold diving should occur at about 30 to 40 m assuming that the diver left the surface following a maximum inspiration with lungs inflated to TLC. Almost inevitably, there are individuals who are able to carry out breath-hold dives to much greater depths, and the current world record is held by Jacques Mayol, a Frenchman who achieved an astonishing depth of 103 m using weights to assist his descent and a balloon inflated at depth to provide buoyancy and enable a rapid return to the surface with the minimum of effort. This depth is, nevertheless, somewhat meagre in comparison to the depths achieved by the deeper diving mammals such as the Weddell seal and sperm whale which have been recorded at depths of approximately 600 m and 1000 m respectively. The answer to the apparent impossibility of Mayol's dive is probably a combination of a compensatory increase in the volume of the pulmonary venous bed (Schaefer et al., 1968) which displaces some of the air in the lungs thereby reducing effectively the RV and allowing greater compression, an unusually large TLC and concomitant large FVC, and the conditioning effects of repeated breath-hold diving.

Such feats are, however, extremely dangerous and are further complicated by the other fundamental hazard of breath-holding – *hypoxia*. In the case of breath-hold diving, alveolar gases are governed by Dalton's law of partial pressures and air-breathing breath-hold diving, after a period at depth during which the diver has depleted the available oxygen in the lungs, will, nevertheless, be quite comfortable with an alveolar oxygen level of 5 per cent at 30 m because the alveolar oxygen partial pressure (P_{AO_2}) will still be about 100 mmHg which is the normal value when breathing air at the surface. Once the breath-hold diver in this condition starts to ascend, the alveolar gases expand and the diver will become hypoxic as the P_{AO_2} falls to an unacceptable level and may result in a loss of consciousness. Such loss of consciousness is particularly hazardous in that the diver has no premonitory signs and could not, in any case, take practical preventive action even if aware of imminent loss of consciousness. This process, which can also happen in closed-circuit underwater breathing apparatus if divers forget to recharge the counter-lung of the set with fresh breathing mixture before ascent, is known as *dilution hypoxia*.

A final hazard for the breath-hold diver is the extremely dangerous practice of *hyperventilation* immediately prior to the dive in an attempt to improve breath-hold times by delaying the onset of the 'break-point' when the voluntary effort to resist breathing is overcome by a rising arterial carbon dioxide tension (Pa_{CO_2}). A prolongation of breath-hold time in this way may, however, take the unwitting diver to the point at which the alveolar oxygen level has fallen to a potentially dangerous level if any degree of dilution hypoxia occurs during ascent. For this reason, far too many breath-hold dives end up in loss of consciousness and drowning, and deep breath-hold diving, particularly when combined with pre-dive hyperventilation, must be regarded as highly dangerous.

The use of breath-hold diving for commercial activities is now virtually exclusive to the Far East where women divers of Japan and Korea, known as the Ama, have been diving for shellfish, sea urchins, seaweeds and other marine organisms since at least the third century BC. These women divers have been studied most extensively both in terms of their respiratory adaptation (Hong and Rahn, 1967; Park et al., 1983) and of their adaptation to the cold waters in which they dive (Rennie et al., 1962; Kang et al., 1963; Hong, 1981), although the relatively recent introduction of 'wet' diving suits, affording much better thermal protection than their traditional cotton suits, has led to a radical change in their diving habits because the onset of limiting hypothermia is delayed. A notable feature of their respiratory adaptation is the way in which they dive after inhaling only to about 85 per cent or less of their TLC, a feature generally ascribed to the avoidance of excessive intrapulmonary pressure and also to a reduction in unwanted buoyancy. However, the introduction of the extra buoyancy conferred by wet suits did not change this adaptation (Park et al., 1983) and it makes an interesting comparison with the diving mammals which generally dive after full exhalation – an adaptation that reduces the amount of nitrogen available to the tissues during the dive by about 80 per cent and minimizes the possibility of decompression sickness (DCS; see page 826). Although DCS has occasionally been reported as a consequence of repeated breath-hold diving (Moretti, 1968), it has never been described in the Ama women divers. The Ama also have a number of other adaptations which have been noted in submarine escape training instructors – an occupation involving a great deal of breath-hold diving. This group has also been very fully investigated (Carey, Schaefer and Alvis, 1955; Schaefer, 1961). These adaptations include decreased ventilatory responses to a raised Pa_{CO_2}, better tolerance of a larger than normal oxygen debt and a significant increase in inspiratory reserve volumes, tidal volumes, VC and TLC. All these features may be considered as adaptive responses which demonstrate that breath-hold diving efficiency in human beings, although poor, may be improved by practice.

Adaptive and other responses in divers

Experienced divers may develop a number of characteristic changes in their pattern of ventilation and tend to use very large tidal volumes (TV) when exercising as well as having reduced respiratory rates (Schaefer, 1963). This habit seems to be acquired by most divers but is also taught, sometimes in combination with end-expiratory breath-holding ('skip' or 'pendulum' breathing), as a means of maximizing the efficiency of pulmonary gas exchange and economizing on the use of breathing mixture from SCUBA sets. A further related adaptation, which also occurs in experienced breath-hold divers, is the development of a lowered ventilatory response to carbon dioxide (Morrison, Florio and Butt, 1981), and very high end-tidal carbon dioxide levels can occur in exercising divers. Such degrees of carbon dioxide retention, which may be of an order that indicates a reduction in alveolar ventilation by as much as 45 per cent, may even be the cause of major problems for divers carrying out hard work.

A number of studies have been done to evaluate various aspects of respiratory function in commercial divers in an attempt to identify what, if any, changes could be attributed to diving and whether any of these changes could be assessed as harmful, or potentially so, in the long term. One such study of 404 commercial divers (Crosbie et al., 1977; Crosbie, Reed and Clarke, 1979) showed that they had larger than normal lungs with a rise in forced vital capacity (FVC) which, up to the age of 30 years, correlated positively with the number of years of diving experience. There was no such change seen in forced expiratory volume at 1 second (FEV$_1$) and the FEV$_1$/FVC ratio, a measurement widely used in the assessment of respiratory fitness to dive, was, therefore, affected adversely. For those divers over 30 years old, this group showed a declining FVC and the inference was that, up to the age of 30 years, they were capable of an adaptive enlargement in response to the respiratory challenges of frequent diving, but that this particular response was lost thereafter. Additionally, most of the indices measuring expiratory flow rates suggested a degree of airflow obstruction despite the fact that they were able to move large quantities of air in and out of the lung in response to increasing work loads. This latter finding reflected their unusually large tidal volumes even though they were also found to have reduced respiratory rates when exercising. Finally, this group showed an increased value for gas transfer using the single breath carbon monoxide test ($TLCO$) although gas transfer per unit volume (TL/VA) was decreased. It was concluded that, with time, there was a diving-induced loss of elastic recoil tissue in the lung or possibly even a bronchial hypertrophy to account for the degree of airways' obstruction.

A later study of the records of pulmonary function tests for 858 commercial divers (Davey, Cotes and Reed, 1984), which attempted to assess the effects of diving on FVC and FEV_1 independent of age, height and smoking habits, confirmed the finding that FVC increased with diving exposure and was also correlated with the maximum depth of dives carried out. There was a similar negative correlation between these factors and the FEV_1/FVC ratio, but the increase in FVC with age did not appear to be confined to divers under 30 years old in a group that had a mean age of 29.8 years (range 20 to 47 years).

In studies of single deep saturation dives (Cotes et al., 1987; Suzuki et al., 1989), it was found that transfer factor ($TLCO$) was significantly reduced after the dive. Where it was possible to re-test the divers, these changes returned to normal within 7 weeks (Suzuki, 1989) and 8 months (Cotes et al., 1987). Otherwise, these studies gave somewhat conflicting evidence for other changes which were, in any case, of a minor degree. Until investigated further, the inference must be that the change in $TLCO$ is evidence of a minor degree of pulmonary oxygen toxicity secondary to prolonged exposure to the raised partial pressures of oxygen used in this type of diving. The long-term significance of this finding remains to be determined.

Decompression pulmonary barotrauma

Reference has already been made to compression barotrauma of the lung and the reverse process,

decompression pulmonary barotrauma, sometimes known as the *pulmonary over-inflation syndrome*, is a common hazard in diving. It can occur if there is any degree of gas trapping in the lungs during ascent because entrapped gas expands in accordance with Boyle's law. Gas trapping may be localized due to a variety of pathological features, or generally due to inadequate exhalation during ascent. The more commonly found pre-existing pathological features which may give rise to decompression barotrauma are as follows:

1. Emphysematous bullae.
2. Connecting lung cysts.
3. Obstructive airways' disease.
4. Bronchial obstruction (infective or neoplastic).
5. Fibrotic lung disease (inflammatory or traumatic).
6. Atelectasis (infective or obstructive).
7. Local or general alterations in compliance.

The importance of adequate screening of respiratory function in assessment of fitness to dive will be obvious from this list and this subject will be discussed separately. Breath-holding or failure to exhale adequately during ascent is a particular hazard in emergency ascents, particularly those resulting from a loss of breathing mixture supply – an occasion when the diver needs considerable presence of mind to remember to exhale during ascent. Free ascents with buoyancy aids are one means of escape from sunken submarines and the technique has been taught for many years by various navies. This form of escape commences with a full inhalation and requires vigorous exhalation throughout ascent. Although this technique is not generally recommended for ascents from below 20 m (65 feet), an ascent from such a depth will mean a threefold expansion of gas in the lung as the ambient water pressure goes from 3 bars (3 ATA) to 1 bar at the surface. The terminal stages of any ascent involving gas trapping are critical because the rate of expansion of gas is exponential and the greatest over-pressures are generated immediately before the surface is reached. Many of the data on decompression pulmonary barotrauma have been collected from submarine escape training which has also been the stimulus for much of the basic research into this problem.

The exact pathology involved in decompression pulmonary barotrauma is partly conjectural but the initial event is alveolar rupture with escape of gas into the extra-alveolar tissues. The alveoli involved are the so-called 'marginal' or 'non-partitional' alveoli whose bases rest on bronchioles, connective tissue septa, pleural tissue or blood vessels. 'Partitional' alveoli, in contrast, have intercommunicating pores (pores of Kohn) and are less at risk from over-pressure (see Chapter 1, page 6).

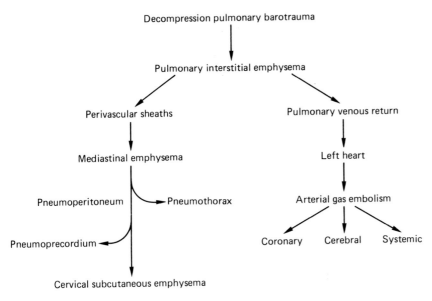

Figure 25.2 Routes taken by extra-alveolar gas following decompression barotrauma

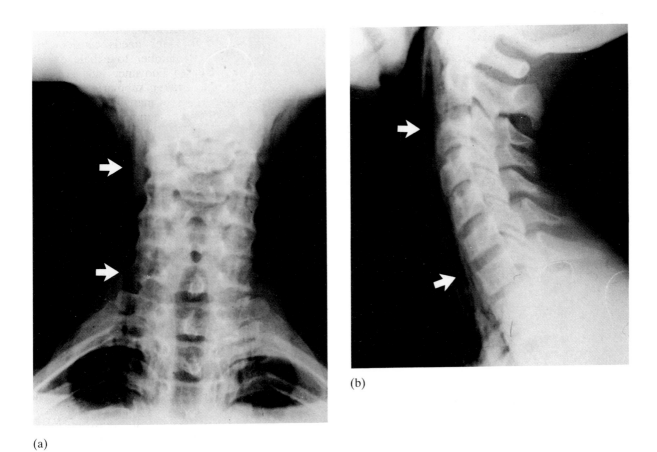

(b)

(a)

Figure 25.3 Posteroanterior and lateral radiographs showing cervical subcutaneous and submucous emphysema (arrowed) secondary to decompression barotrauma

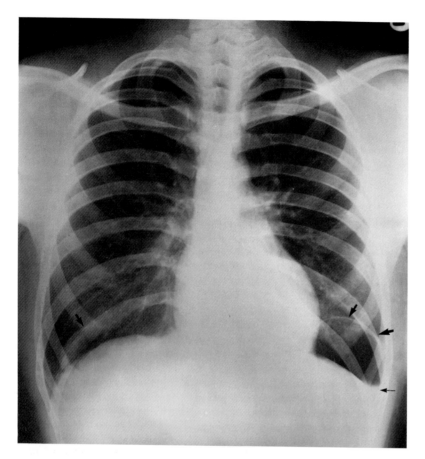

Figure 25.4 Bilateral basal thin-walled cysts following barotrauma of ascent in a diver. He complained of chest tightness during buoyant ascent from 6 bars (4560 mmHg) and became unconscious shortly after surfacing but recovered rapidly on recompression. Initially, his chest radiograph showed bilateral pneumothoraces, basal thin-walled cysts and possible pneumoprecordium. Re-expansion and complete recovery occurred in approximately 2 weeks with bed rest. But the cysts were still present another 2 weeks later (this film), although subsequently they disappeared. Heavy arrows = thin-walled cysts; light arrow = remnant of pleural effusion. (Reproduced by permission of Surgeon Vice-Admiral Sir John Harrison, Ministry of Defence)

The degree of over-pressure necessary to cause decompression barotrauma has been the subject of animal research as well as experiments with human cadavers (Schaefer et al., 1958; Malhotra and Wright, 1959, 1961). Although the results of these various experiments need to be interpreted with some caution, they suggested that an over-pressure of as little as 80 mmHg could cause alveolar rupture. Even allowing for the modifying effects of anaesthesia on the compliance of the lungs of the animals used in these experiments, it is easy to see why decompression pulmonary barotrauma has resulted from breath-hold ascents from depths as shallow as 2 m.

Figure 25.2 shows the two principal routes that are available to gas after alveolar rupture. In the case of mediastinal emphysema, sometimes referred to as 'pneumomediastinum', the driving force for transfer of gas is the pressure difference between intratracheal and intrapleural pressures, whereas intravascular rupture into the pulmonary venous return to the left heart is driven by the pressure gradient between intratracheal and pulmonary venous pressure. The gas is thought to reach the mediastinum by tracking along perivascular sheaths to the hilum of the lung from where it may take the various routes shown in Figure 25.2. By far the most common route taken by mediastinal gas in decompression-related mediastinal emphysema is for it to track up into the tissues of the neck to give subcutaneous cervical emphysema with typical 'crackles' on palpation (Figure 25.3). Occasionally, the amount of gas involved is such that the tissues of the face and upper anterior chest wall are involved. More rarely, the gas involved deeper tissue planes and involvement of the larynx by so-called 'submucous emphysema' gives rise to a peculiar and characteristic brassy voice. Pulmonary barotrauma due to other causes may give rise to interstitial emphysema of the lungs of such severity that a condition known as 'splinting' occurs with predictably profound effects on ventilation. Equally, mediastinal emphysema may be of sufficient severity to cause interference with cardiac function and flow in the major intrathoracic blood vessels. Such dramatic sequelae are extremely rare in decompression accidents but have been described in a number of other clinical situations (Macklin and Macklin, 1944).

Pneumothorax is a relatively common complication of decompression barotrauma and is thought to be due to gas that has escaped into the pleural cavity from the hilum of the lung. Subpleural bullae or 'blebs' have been found in fatal diving accidents involving pneumothoraces (Calder, 1985), although it was not entirely clear what part decompression stress had to play in these accidents. Further, the pneumothoraces associated with decompression barotrauma are often a chance finding on a radiograph and are rarely severe enough to give rise to symptoms or major complications. However, when the lungs have expanded, intrapulmonary air cysts may be visible for a few weeks (Figure 25.4). The not uncommon finding of an asymptomatic bilateral pneumothorax is further support for the belief that the gas has come from the hilum of the lung as an extension of the mediastinal emphysema.

The various symptoms and clinical signs seen in cases of decompression pulmonary barotrauma are listed in Table 25.1. It is worthy of note that haemoptysis, in itself virtually diagnostic, is relatively rare and the most common presenting symptom is chest pain which is rarely severe, often ill-defined and frequently not lateralized. Nevertheless, any post-dive chest pain, particularly after a rapid ascent, should raise the possibility of barotrauma.

The symptoms of pulmonary barotrauma are often delayed and it may be as long as 6 hours before subcutaneous cervical or submucous emphysema is noticed. In the absence of other complications, decompression pulmonary barotrauma rarely needs recompression therapy and any degree of pneumothorax sufficient to give respiratory embarrassment can be treated conventionally. This does not obviate the requirement to be absolutely certain that there is no evidence for arterial gas embolism – a major complication of decompression pulmonary barotrauma.

Table 25.1 Distribution of symptoms and signs in 199 cases of decompression pulmonary barotrauma with or without the complication of arterial gas embolism (AGE)

	Pulmonary barotrauma without AGE (n=20)	*Pulmonary barotrauma with AGE* (n=179)
Symptoms		
Chest pain	19	30
Dyspnoea	4	11
Haemoptysis	3	9
Cough	3	6
Cervical emphysema	5	4
Voice change	2	–
Signs and radiographic findings		
Interstitial emphysema	1	4
Mediastinal emphysema	8	31
Unilateral pneumothorax	2	6
Bilateral pneumothorax	–	5
Pneumoperitoneum	–	3

From Pearson (1981b).

The degree of over-pressure generated during decompression appears to have a determining role in the distribution of extra-alveolar gas and transfer of gas to the left heart with arterialization is by far the most common sequel to decompression barotrauma. Conversely, the most common cause of uncomplicated mediastinal emphysema in divers is a faulty demand valve which does not shut off completely at the end of exhalation and gives a sustained low over-pressure similar to the positive end-expiratory pressure (PEEP) ventilation used in clinical situations. PEEP itself is a well-recognized potential cause of pulmonary barotrauma. One study of 382 decompression accidents in divers and submarine escape trainees (Pearson, 1984) showed that arterial gas embolism occurred in 85 per cent of cases involving pulmonary barotrauma.

Although a seemingly over-simple explanation, the very buoyancy of gas bubbles has a major part to play in their distribution once in the arteries (Van Allen and Hrdina, 1929) and it is, therefore, not surprising that by far the most common route taken by gas entering the arteries of divers and submarine escapers, who are upright as they ascend through the water, is via the carotid arteries to the anterior and middle cerebral arteries of the brain to give the dramatic and life-threatening manifestations of *cerebral arterial gas embolism* (CAGE). Numerous studies with appropriate animal models have shown that the distribution of gas emboli in the cerebral circulation is to the cortical areas supplied by the anterior and middle cerebral arteries with the 'watershed' areas between the regions supplied by those arteries being particularly vulnerable. The effects of the embolic gas are dramatic and complex

Table 25.2 Major presenting symptoms and signs in 179 cases of cerebral arterial gas embolism

Symptom/sign	Number
Coma with convulsions	25
Coma without convulsions	51
Collapse with stupor/confusion	50
Vertigo	22
Visual disturbance	15
Headache	3
Unilateral motor/sensory disturbance	56
Bilateral motor/sensory disturbance	11

From Pearson (1981b).

but the emboli tend to be arrested in precapillary arterioles and cause multifocal ischaemia as well as damage to the blood–brain barrier.

Death from CAGE is recognized widely as the most common single cause of death in recreational divers, even though many fatal diving accidents involving CAGE are incorrectly attributed to drowning due to ignorance or inadequate post-mortem techniques. The presentation of CAGE is usually dramatic and the initial occurrence of the symptoms and signs listed in Table 25.2 is almost unknown more than 10 minutes after the causative decompression. Indeed, the great majority of the serious and dramatic presentations occur immediately on, or within seconds of, surfacing.

Evidence for involvement of other organs and tissues by arterial gas emboli arising as a result of decompression accidents is, somewhat surprisingly, very rare and only one confirmed case of coronary artery embolism has been described (Harveyson, Hirschfield and Tonge, 1956). Presumptive evidence of coronary artery involvement in the form of transient ischaemic ECG changes seen in cases of CAGE has, however, been described more frequently (Pearson, 1981b), and a small number of cases of spinal cord involvement in decompression accidents have been attributed to arterial gas emboli secondary to pulmonary barotrauma rather than decompression sickness, although the distinction, as will be seen, is becoming increasingly academic. The definitive treatment of CAGE is recompression, and formal treatment tables exist to allow use of various combinations of pressure and hyperbaric oxygen. Such treatment is very much a matter for experts and it is sufficient to state that specialist advice should be taken as a matter of urgency if any diver has symptoms or signs, or both, suggestive of pulmonary barotrauma and CAGE.

The main cause of mortality arising from CAGE is thought to be due to cardiac arrest or arrhythmias secondary to brain-stem embolism (Greene, 1978). It also appears to be the case that, provided the initial impact of the embolism is survived, early recompression treatment is very successful, often dramatically so.

The *first aid treatment of CAGE* should include breathing oxygen as soon as possible and during transport to a compression chamber facility. The use of adjuvant drug therapy, particularly as a first aid measure, is more controversial. However, the Royal Navy routinely uses 12 to 16 mg intravenous dexamethasone as part of the immediate treatment of CAGE occurring in submarine escape training. Dexamethasone is given primarily to counteract the effects of arrested arterial gas emboli on the blood–brain barrier and to prevent secondary deterioration due to vasogenic cerebral oedema which, in turn, is thought to have been a major factor in the secondary deterioration formerly seen in at least 30 per cent of the cases of CAGE arising from Royal Navy submarine escape training.

Decompression sickness

Decompression sickness (DCS), first described in the mid-nineteenth century as an illness related to exposure to increased ambient pressure, continues to be a major hazard to compressed air workers and divers, particularly recreational divers. In the UK alone, over 150 cases of DCS are treated each year, the majority of them being 'serious' by definition and resulting, all too frequently, in permanent neurological sequelae.

The lungs have an important part to play in the aetiology and evolution of DCS which is fundamentally different to their causative role in arterial gas embolism resulting from pulmonary barotrauma. By definition, DCS is a chain of reactive events stemming from the nucleation (bubble formation) of inert gas released during or after decompression from a hyperbaric exposure. It may also occur as a result of decompression from ground level to altitude and may arise in pilots of high flying, rapidly climbing aircraft or simulated exposure to altitude in decompression chambers (see Chapter 24, page 803). In the case of diving, inert gas taken up by the tissues of the body during the dive is released as the diver returns to the surface and pressure returns to normal. If the diver breathes compressed air, the inert gas taken up during the dive is nitrogen, whereas DCS arising in divers using Heliox mixtures is caused by helium. The amount of inert gas taken up by tissues varies between different tissues, being a function of both the perfusion of that particular tissue and, to a lesser extent, diffusion of the inert gas through and into tissues. A further important factor is the varying solubility of inert gases in different tissues and the solubility of nitrogen in fatty tissues is very relevant to spinal cord involvement in DCS arising from compressed air diving. In contrast, helium is much less soluble in fatty tissues and spinal cord involvement in DCS arising from Heliox diving is comparatively rare.

'Bounce' and 'saturation' diving

Other than breath-hold diving, only two basic techniques are used to deploy divers under water. The most commonly used technique is 'bounce' or 'intervention' diving where the diver is deployed from the surface and is governed by decompression tables which indicate how much decompression is required for any given depth/time increment. Such diving is generally limited to 50 m on compressed air (due to nitrogen narcosis and gas density) and about 150 m using Heliox. For dives deeper than 50 m requiring prolonged diving activity, a technique known as 'saturation' diving is used. Exclusive to commercial, military and scientific diving, this technique involves compressing divers in a surface compression chamber (usually ship-borne or mounted on an off-shore platform) to a pressure equal to that at which they will be working under water and then transferring them under pressure to the work site using a diving bell. Providing the pressure to which the divers are exposed remains constant, an equilibrium is reached between the inert gas in the body and that in the compression chamber atmosphere. At this point, the tissues of the body are effectively 'saturated' with inert gas. The time taken to reach this equilibrium varies quite markedly for different tissues and also different inert gases, but is generally regarded as being at least 24 hours for certain poorly perfused tissues. Any change in pressure will require a new equilibrium to be established. In theory, the divers can then live and work at pressure for an indefinite period although saturation dives rarely exceed 4 weeks for obvious psychological and social reasons. Decompression from 'saturation' dives is lengthy compared to 'bounce' diving and a dive to 300 m using Heliox takes between 10 and 11 days to decompress safely. The great majority of operational saturation diving occurs shallower than 300 m, although techniques and equipment have been developed for 450 m. Despite the differences between these two types of diving, both lead to release of inert gas during decompression and both can give rise to DCS if decompression is inadequate.

Numerous efforts have been made to produce mathematical models or formulae to explain and predict the uptake and elimination of inert gases in an effort to provide safe decompression procedures

for divers but the majority of current diving tables are, by definition, stochastic. In view of the complexity of the processes involved, the individual variations of the divers and even the puzzling variable susceptibility of individual divers over quite short periods of time, it is small wonder that diving tables are not infallible, particularly when challenging or repeated dives are undertaken. The problem of repetitive diving is especially difficult in that the elimination of inert gas may continue for a significant period after a dive and a diver may commence another dive with sufficient residual inert gas from his or her previous dive to give rise to DCS in what would otherwise have been a safe dive.

Although a variable and, as yet, unquantified amount of inert gas may be lost through the skin during decompression, the majority of the elimination of inert gas is by transport in solution in venous blood to the lungs and exhalation. This process is driven by the gradient between the inert gas partial pressure in the relatively supersaturated tissues and that in the ambient atmosphere. However, the degree of supersaturation may be extreme enough to cause inert gas nucleation which results in both extravascular and intravascular inert gas bubbles. As with decompression to altitude, numerous studies using Doppler-based transducers have shown venous gas emboli (VGE) in decompressing divers. In the case of such divers who are, and remain, asymptomatic, it is assumed that there is a tolerable degree of venous gas embolism with which the lungs can deal effectively. Indeed, a variety of experimental animals has been shown to tolerate surprisingly large amounts of intravenous gas, providing it is given as an infusion at a steady rate rather than as a sudden bolus. However, overloading of the pulmonary vascular bed with venous gas emboli can occur and will give rise to a number of major, sometimes life-threatening, disorders.

It has been estimated that some 10 per cent of the pulmonary vascular bed requires occlusion before ventilation is affected (Bernthal, Horres and Taylor, 1961) and increasing occlusion inevitably leads to the condition known as the 'chokes' – a descriptive term for the manifestation described in detail in the previous chapter. Severe 'chokes' are only rarely seen in divers but are deserving of the most energetic treatment and it is not surprising that they have been described as another variety of 'adult respiratory distress syndrome' (Ence and Gong, 1979). Given that venous inert gas emboli are common to decompression from increased pressure and decompression to altitude, it is interesting that the 'chokes' is seen more commonly as a result of altitude exposure, especially in view of the much more modest pressure changes involved. Animal research suggests that a critical factor may be the increasing hypoxia which accompanies exposure to altitude (Lehner et al., 1984) (see Chapter 24, page 804).

It has been clear for some time that it is possible for VGE to migrate through the pulmonary microcirculation (Butler and Hills, 1979, 1985), a process which is facilitated both by the rising pulmonary artery pressure that accompanies any significant degree of venous gas embolism and by the deformable nature of gas emboli. It has been shown in dogs that the pulmonary vascular pressure gradient (pulmonary artery pressure–pulmonary venous pressure) at which spill-over of detectable bubbles into the arterial circulation occurs is about 35 mmHg (Butler and Katz, 1988). A further factor which no doubt assists such a process is the acquisition of pulmonary surfactant by gas emboli (Butler and Hills, 1983). Once within the arteries, the microbubbles of gas assume a much greater significance and their precise role in the aetiology of central nervous system DCS is a topic of much current research and debate.

Traditionally, 'serious', or type II, DCS has been classified as involving mainly the vestibular, respiratory ('chokes'), cardiovascular and central nervous systems. In contrast, type I, or 'mild', DCS is a classification that covers a group of less serious symptoms and signs including skin itching and rashes, unusual fatigue and the characteristic joint pain which was responsible for the widely used term the 'bends'. Type I DCS is generally considered to result from formation of extravascular inert gas bubbles in periarticular and subcutaneous tissues and the lungs have no obvious part to play in this particular type of DCS. The presenting symptoms and signs of DCS involving the central nervous system have led to the traditional beliefs that the spinal cord was much more frequently involved than the brain and that arterial gas emboli have little part to play in spinal cord damage. Recent research with an animal model has shown that so-called 'autochthonous' bubbles arising in the cord itself are almost certainly responsible for early onset (<15 min) DCS (Francis et al., 1988). Earlier research using a similar animal model (Hallenbeck, Bove and Elliott, 1975) suggested that blockage of the paravertebral venous plexus by inert gas bubbles was also a factor and it may well be that this process occurs at a later stage in very serious decompression insults. It has also been pointed out that the much greater perfusion of the brain in comparison to the spinal cord would lead to many more cases of cerebral involvement if arterial gas emboli were a major factor in the aetiology of DCS (Hallenbeck, Bove and Elliott, 1975). However, this latter theory and the concept that the spinal cord is mainly involved in DCS affecting the central nervous system will certainly need major revision in view of recent evidence which shows that cerebral perfusion deficits in the frontal and parietal cortex appear to be an inevitable accompaniment of cases of DCS with any symptoms or signs indicative of involvement of the central nervous system (CNS) (Macleod

et al., 1988; Adkisson et al., 1989). This new evidence is strongly suggestive that arterial gas emboli do indeed have a major part to play in the aetiology of DCS and, although a patent foramen ovale has been incriminated in a number of cases of serious DCS as the cause of VGE entering the arterial system (Moon, Camporesi and Kisslo, 1989), there is no doubt that migration of VGE through the lungs is an important factor in at least some of the manifestations of DCS. Apart from the amount, nature and origin of the gas, cerebral gas embolism is a process common to both pulmonary barotrauma and DCS. The precise role of arterial gas emboli in the aetiology of spinal cord DCS is the subject of current research by the author which indicates that arterial gas emboli produce spinal cord pathology limited to the grey matter (Pearson et al., 1990); this is quite different from the characteristic lesions of the white matter which result from DCS.

The definitive treatment of DCS remains recompression and delay in treatment almost invariably has an adverse effect on the success of therapy. Delays in transfer of divers with DCS to treatment facilities may be minimized by the use of helicopters or other aircraft although strict rules govern the height at which the aircraft may fly or what cabin pressures must be maintained in order to avoid an exacerbation of the DCS by the additional decompression that accompanies exposure to altitude. For this reason, pilots of helicopters and aircraft used to transfer DCS cases are advised to fly as low as possible and not to fly above 300 metres (approximately 1000 feet) except in the gravest of emergencies where no other choice exists. Whenever possible, the patient should be given oxygen to breathe during transit (see also Chapter 24, page 804).

In the case of asymptomatic divers, post-dive flying or exposure to altitude in mountainous country may provoke DCS and explicit post-dive restrictions exist to avoid such a possibility. The most extreme limitations apply after saturation diving and the Royal Navy rule of a 48-hour embargo on flying in commercial aircraft after a saturation dive is representative of the majority of commercial practice.

Pulmonary oxygen toxicity

The lung, in common with most other organs and tissues in the body, is sensitive to raised pressures of oxygen whether they are the result of breathing pure oxygen or elevated partial pressures of oxygen in breathing mixtures used by divers. The use of pure oxygen as a diving breathing gas is most attractive in a number of ways, not the least of which is the immunity from DCS which results from the lack of inert gas. However, the toxic effect of oxygen on the CNS (originally described by the famous nineteenth century French physiologist, Paul Bert, and sometimes called the 'Paul Bert' effect), is a major limiting factor and diving on pure oxygen remains almost exclusively a military technique limited to 8 m to avoid the risk of convulsions. As with all other tissues affected by oxygen toxicity, the effect on the CNS is of a time/dose nature and susceptibility has quite marked individual variations.

The lungs are somewhat less sensitive in the short term to raised oxygen pressures than the CNS, but pulmonary toxicity (first described by Lorraine Smith in 1897–1899 and, in deference to such an important discovery, frequently called the 'Lorraine Smith' effect) is of great importance in diving, particularly in saturation diving where divers are exposed to hyperoxic mixtures for long periods, and in the therapy of decompression illnesses where pure oxygen at a pressure of 2.8 bars is routinely breathed interspersed with periods of air breathing to avoid the acute manifestations of CNS toxicity.

The significance of the time/dose effect in the case of pulmonary oxygen toxicity is that the rate of development of the characteristic symptoms and signs is proportional both to the degree of elevation of the oxygen pressure (Po_2) and time. For practical diving purposes, the threshold level at which evidence of pulmonary oxygen toxicity occurs in time is generally regarded as 0.5 bar which is the equivalent of 50 per cent oxygen in a mixture breathed at normal atmospheric pressure (1 bar).

It is customary to divide the symptoms and signs of pulmonary oxygen toxicity into 'acute' and 'chronic' and, to a large extent, these definitions are related to the type of exposure involved. It is, however, better to think of the presentation and progression of pulmonary oxygen toxicity as a process that ranges from very minor reversible symptoms to rapidly progressive deterioration which may result in death. Much of the description of the pathology thought to be involved in human beings has in fact been derived from a multitude of animal models and must be qualified in light of the marked variation in the response of various species. What follows is a condensed overview of the manifestations of pulmonary oxygen toxicity.

Symptomatology

The earliest manifestations of pulmonary oxygen toxicity are those of a tracheobronchitis. Carinal irritation, substernal burning discomfort and cough become increasingly severe and distressing with continued exposure and dyspnoea becomes disabling even at rest. Return to partial pressures of oxygen below 0.5 bar brings relief which, in the milder cases, is relatively rapid, and typically within a few hours. Severe symptoms may take much longer to clear up and it is not unusual to find that some months elapse before subjective normality returns, especially in terms of dyspnoea in response to exercise.

Extreme degrees of pulmonary oxygen toxicity give rise to a form of adult respiratory distress syndrome (ARDS) with acute pulmonary oedema, atelectasis and a falling Pao_2. The inability to correct a falling Pao_2 by giving more oxygen means that the condition can easily become irreversible and death will ensue from anoxia and acidosis. Pulmonary oxygen toxicity of this severity should never happen in relation to diving activities or the treatment of diving accidents and it generally arises in intensive care situations.

Pathology

The earliest changes are described as a 'proliferative phase' which is characterized by a perivascular and interstitial inflammatory response with pulmonary endothelial cell damage, alveolar haemorrhage and interstitial oedema. Type I alveolar cells are affected and damaged at a relatively early stage whereas type II alveolar cells are more resistant and are usually only affected by more chronic exposure when they show a modest degree of proliferation. With increasing exposure, the 'proliferative phase' develops with increased interstitial cellularity, destruction of capillaries and embolism of arterioles. At this stage, the architecture of the lung may be seriously and irreversibly damaged and the impaired gas exchange leads to the critical situation described earlier.

A further distinctive series of pathological changes may ensue from repeated exposure to oxygen levels below those required to give acute manifestations such as ARDS. In this case, the reaction has been described as 'bronchopulmonary dysplasia' and is characterized by a marked cellular proliferation with the development of widespread fibrosis which may be rapidly progressive. This response has been termed 'chronic pulmonary oxygen toxicity' in an attempt to distinguish it from the more acute changes but it is debatable whether it warrants such distinction, and it is probably better to view it as a cumulative effect of repeated subacute pathological reactions. Inevitably, these various pathological responses have a major effect on lung function and, in general, mechanical function is affected to a greater degree and at an earlier stage than gas-exchange function (Clark, 1987). Further, the changes seen in mechanical function, namely decrements in VC and MEFR, are the result of changes in small airways' resistance rather than large airways' involvement.

The toxic effects of oxygen on lung tissue are complex indeed but the biochemical events are collectively the result of oxidative reactions following the generation of increased amounts of toxic free radicals (superoxide anion, hydrogen peroxide, hydroxyl radical and singlet oxygen) which would normally be dealt with by protective scavenging enzymes such as superoxide dismutase, catalase and glutathionine peroxidase (Fisher, Bassett and Forman, 1979).

Comprehensive reviews of the causative mechanisms, morphology and pathology of pulmonary oxygen toxicity are available (Clark and Lambertsen, 1971; Small, 1984; Crapo, 1986), and it is a field that continues to generate a great deal of research, particularly attempts to develop an understanding as to how the responses to breathing hyperoxic mixtures might be modified favourably.

Assessment of pulmonary oxygen toxicity

Apart from the subjective symptomatology already described, a number of attempts have been made to quantify the degree of toxicity related to various degrees of exposure with the aim of producing predictive formulae which will allow the beneficial effects of oxygen to be exploited without the accompanying penalty of pulmonary toxicity. The most frequently used quantitative index has been based on decrements in VC (Clark and Lambertsen, 1971b; Wright, 1972). Such decrements can be plotted as a series of dose–time curves which, in effect, represent the rate of development of pulmonary oxygen toxicity for 50 per cent of normal individuals exposed to increasing time–pressure 'doses' of oxygen.

Although quite modest decrements in VC may be associated with severe symptoms, a formula derived from such decrements was developed for predictive purposes (Wright, 1972). It was based on a notional *unit pulmonary toxicity dose* (UPTD) which was defined as *the degree of pulmonary oxygen toxicity resulting from breathing 100 per cent oxygen at a pressure of 1 bar for 1 min*. It assumes that pulmonary oxygen toxicity occurs at partial pressures of oxygen in excess of 0.5 bar, that the same degree of toxicity may be achieved by various time–pressure exposures and that the effect of such

exposures is, in the short term, additive. The formula

$$UPTD = t \left. ^{-1.2} \middle/ \sqrt{\frac{0.5}{P - 0.5}} \right.$$

where t = time of exposure in minutes and P is the ambient pressure to which the subject is exposed, may be simplified for practical use. If, for any given PO_2, P remains constant, as is usually the case in diving situations where such a formula might be of use, the equation reduces to:

$$UPTD = kt$$

Therefore, at any constant PO_2, there is a factor (k) that can be multiplied by time of exposure to give the UPTD for that exposure. Tables exist for k values for any PO_2 likely to be encountered in a diving or therapeutic situation and the UPTD may be rapidly calculated.

Limits for UPTD exposure have been recommended for practical use in various diving situations (Wright, 1972) and a UPTD of 615 has been recommended as the limit for non-critical therapeutic situations with an upper limit of 1425 for the treatment of serious or non-responding decompression illnesses and those that are both. The UPTD concept applies mainly to continuous exposure to a raised PO_2 and is less applicable to intermittent exposure. Further investigation of VC changes following hyperoxic exposure (Harabin et al., 1987) suggested that the decrements were subject to such wide individual variation that a simplified expression:

$$\text{Percentage VC} = -0.011(PO_2 - 0.5)t$$

(PO_2 in bars and time in min) would give an acceptable prediction of a median response without an unacceptable loss in reliability. However, no single measure of pulmonary function is, as yet, entirely satisfactory for use in predicting individual responses to hyperoxic exposure or rate of recovery once so exposed.

Other methods of assessing the early changes of pulmonary oxygen toxicity have been proposed as an alternative to decrements in VC which is a good deal less precise than desirable. Measurement of lung tissue volume (Winsborough and McKenzie, 1977; Miller, Miller and Coggin, 1978) has been claimed to be a better and much earlier reflection of the underlying pathology in that a rise will reflect the accumulation of water in the lung parenchyma which is said to be an early manifestation of pulmonary oxygen toxicity.

Much effort has also been devoted to the effects of intermittent hyperoxic exposure although the problem is essentially related to how fully the lung recovers between each episode of hyperoxic breathing. The margin between tolerable intermittent exposure and the initiation of the changes leading to pulmonary fibrosis may be very fine indeed.

In terms of pulmonary oxygen toxicity, the most prolonged degrees of hyperoxic exposure tend to occur in 'saturation' diving where a common partial pressure of oxygen in Heliox mixtures tends to be between 0.4 and 0.5 bar. However, during excursions in and from the diving bell, levels of 1.2 to 1.4 bars are used and these excursions may last as long as 6 hours. Also, a raised P_{O_2} is frequently used in commercial 'saturation' diving to shorten decompression times and P_{O_2} values as high as 0.6 bar are in current use for quite prolonged periods during decompression. Although there is no evidence of any serious manifestations of pulmonary oxygen toxicity arising from these procedures, there is apocryphal evidence to suggest that divers frequently exhibit minor symptomatic evidence of toxicity towards the end of decompression. The temporary reduction in transfer factor ($T_{L}CO$) found after saturation dives using up to 0.5 bar P_{O_2} for decompression tends to support the evidence for minor reversible degrees of pulmonary toxicity occurring during such dives (see page 822). More florid problems are rare during saturation diving although one such case has been reported (Crosbie, Cumming and Thomas, 1982) which arose from repeated exposure to a P_{O_2} of 1.4 bars during a period of 55 hours with return to an ambient chamber pressure of 0.6 bar in between the working periods at 1.4 bars. Full function and subjective recovery took 12 weeks in this case and, although it was concluded that the condition was reversible, the ambient chamber P_{O_2} was clearly too high to allow any recovery in between the exposures to 1.4 bars. In general, the P_{O_2} of the chamber atmosphere during saturation diving should not exceed 0.45 bar during the working period of the dive and 0.5 bar during decompression. The majority of commercial and military diving operations are carried out within these limits.

In order to avoid the hazard of acute central nervous system oxygen toxicity, diving on pure oxygen is too limited in both time and depth to represent a particular hazard in terms of pulmonary oxygen toxicity, unless such diving is carried out repetitively for prolonged periods. Military organizations using pure oxygen diving are well aware of this potential hazard and regulations exist to avoid any possibility of such an occurrence. Of greater potential significance is the marked reduction in VC which may occur in divers using closed-circuit oxygen breathing apparatus where a back-mounted counterlung leads to a negative SLL (Dahlback and Balldin, 1985) (see page 820). Although this phenomenon was observed in a limited study of four divers, it has been seen also in negative pressure breathing of pure oxygen during head-out immersion and is due to airways' closure consequent upon reduced lung volumes. A similar effect is not seen with compressed air breathing and it is postulated that there is a real risk of localized areas of pulmonary absorption atelectasis due to the gas distal to the point of closure being pure oxygen. However, in a study of six divers who had been diving on pure oxygen at least twice weekly for up to 10 years (Moselhi, Abadallah and Azab, 1980), no unusual decrements in pulmonary function were found.

Perhaps the diving situation most responsible for the generation of pulmonary oxygen toxicity is the treatment of decompression illnesses. P_{O_2} values as high as 2.8 bars are used routinely and, although the tables used for recompression therapy have been designed to avoid acute pulmonary oxygen toxicity, occasions have arisen, albeit infrequently, where, due to over-enthusiasm or ignorance, it has resulted in major incidents. If the patient is severely affected at a pressure where no early relief is possible by decompression to a chamber atmosphere with a P_{O_2} of 0.5 bar or less, the chamber atmosphere may have to be diluted by nitrogen or helium to bring the P_{O_2} down to 0.5 bar or less. The maximum UPTD recommended for routine therapeutic purposes is 1425, although the previously mentioned variability in response makes this a less precise guideline than is desirable. However, the average VC decrement for a UPTD of 1425 is 9 per cent and all patients exposed to this degree of hyperoxia will be symptomatic even allowing for the variability in individual response; some will have severe symptoms. All Royal Navy therapeutic recompression tables, used routinely for the treatment of decompression illnesses, rarely exceed a UPTD of 1000 even with the maximum permissible extensions. However, both very serious and non-responding cases may require difficult decisions to be made about the potential benefits of extending oxygen breathing when compared to the possible complications of pulmonary oxygen toxicity. It is not uncommon to allow minor symptomatic evidence for pulmonary oxygen toxicity to occur if the beneficial effects of continuing oxygen breathing are felt to warrant it. Under no circumstances, however, should a well-managed hyperbaric therapy result in a major or life-threatening degree of pulmonary oxygen toxicity.

Complications associated with breathing mixtures used in diving

Every effort is made to ensure that the breathing mixtures used for diving comply with rigorous

Table 25.3 Representative maximum allowable levels of contaminants in compressed air used for diving

Contaminant	Maximum allowable limit
Carbon monoxide (p.p.m.)	5
Carbon dioxide (p.p.m.)	500
Total volatile non-substituted hydrocarbons (vapours or gas) in methane equivalent (p.p.m.)	25
Oil (condensed or mist) and particulate matter (mg/m)	1
Maximum particle size supplied at pressures >200 lb/in² (μm)	50 (diameter or maximum dimension)
Water vapour supplied at pressures >200 lb/in² (p.p.m.)	25 (20 mg/m)
Odours	Must be free from detectable odours

standards of purity and quality, and, in the case of the UK, these standards are common to both commercial and military diving. Poorly maintained or designed equipment, particularly compressors, may result in contamination of breathing gas. The UK limits for the contaminants most commonly encountered in compressed air are given in Table 25.3 although the range of potential contaminants is considerably wider.

All breathing mixtures prepared for and supplied to commercial and military diving operations must be checked regularly, and extreme care is applied to all phases of manufacture, compression and storage. This degree of control is clearly beyond the scope of recreational diving although well-established rules for the care and maintenance of compressors should avoid any major complications, and it is fortunate that the most common form of contamination of compressed air, namely oil, will lead to a distinctive odour and taste. Strangely enough, in view of the wide range of potential contaminants, reported cases of disease are few. Most of those that occur are connected with carbon monoxide or with pollution of compressed air by oil; extreme pathology, such as the lipoid pneumonitis reported in a Californian commercial abalone diver (abalones are edible molluscs – genus *Haliotis*) who had been repeatedly exposed to compressed air heavily contaminated with oil, appears to be very rare (Kizer and Golden, 1987).

Chest infections due to bacteriological or viral contamination of breathing gas have also been reported occasionally, even though it is difficult to relate cause and effect. However, poor cleaning of the hoses and regulators of SCUBA equipment has been incriminated as the cause of so-called *SCUBA disease* (Kavanagh et al., 1963; Edmonds, 1976;

Bradley and Bornmann, 1984). This is a self-limiting respiratory infection associated with diving in tropical or subtropical waters and is attributed to aspiration of Gram-negative organisms, particularly *Pseudomonas* sp., which accumulate in the equipment. The proper care and cleaning of equipment is of special importance to saturation diving where the warm humid environment of the chambers encourages bacterial growth and antiseptic solutions capable of dealing with *Pseudomonas* sp. are used routinely to disinfect diving equipment. The closed and confined environment of saturation diving chambers is conducive to transmission of upper respiratory infections during the early stages of dives, although every effort is made to ensure that divers commence dives in the fittest possible state.

The inhalation of cold breathing gas, such as might occur in diving in very cold water, has been incriminated in cases of bronchorrhoea and bronchospasm resulting from such diving. Pulmonary oedema as a complication of diving in cold water has also been described (Wilmshurst et al., 1989), although this is said to result from pathological degrees of vasoconstriction with associated cardiac decompensation following the combined challenge of cold water and raised ambient pressure.

Of particular relevance to deep diving is the fact that cold Heliox breathing mixtures have been shown to have a much greater potential than compressed air for stimulating bronchomotor responses and producing a rise in lung resistance (Jammes et al., 1988). Also, the thermal conductivity of representative Heliox mixtures used in deep diving can be as much as seven times that of air, and it is essential that Heliox mixtures supplied to deep divers are heated to prevent the development of a negative thermal balance due to respiratory heat loss (Hoke et al., 1976). In deep diving, unheated breathing mixtures can lead to potentially dangerous degrees of hypothermia, a process that may be surprisingly rapid. Legislation exists in the UK and many other countries to ensure heating of breathing gas for all in-water saturation divers breathing Heliox and non-saturation divers breathing Heliox at depths in excess of 150 m.

Fitness to dive

Initial screening

The importance of the lungs in diving, particularly their role in decompression pulmonary barotrauma with its potentially lethal outcome, makes it essential that all candidates for diving should be subject to assessment of respiratory fitness for diving. The Diving Operations at Work Regulations 1981 (HMSO, 1981) make such screening obligatory for all commercial and military divers, and it is also insisted upon by the various bodies responsible for sports diving in the UK. However, it remains possible for individuals to commence sports diving without any form of medical screening or examination.

In the UK, the criteria for initial and continuing assessment of fitness for diving are virtually identical for commercial and military divers and are contained in Form MA1 issued by the Employment Medical Advisory Service (EMAS) of the Health and Safety Executive. Much of the emphasis on the significance of events in the past medical history, clinical examination and results of lung function testing is related to the need to exclude, as far as possible, any condition which may predispose to air trapping.

Medical history

A careful medical history is essential to exclude all candidates with an admitted and verifiable history of any form of obstructive airways' disease. Obviously, major difficulties arise due to the loose use of the term 'asthma' to describe a number of childhood disorders associated with non-recurring bronchospasm and candidates with a history of childhood wheezing need careful evaluation (see Chapter 6, page 141 and Chapter 9, page 224). It can only be said that childhood wheezing, if not recurrent, is not necessarily a contraindication to diving. Absolute contraindications to diving include a history of spontaneous pneumothorax, emphysema, penetrating chest injuries, chronic and repeated lung infections, granulomatous lung diseases such as sarcoidosis, tuberculosis, and fungal infections, chronic bronchitis and bronchiectasis. Inevitably, many of the features of the past medical history will be less than clear cut and many of the foregoing conditions will need further investigation before a final decision can be made.

Radiographic features

Chest radiographs for diving candidates should always be standard size, posteroanterior (PA) views in inspiration *and* expiration (see Chapter 7). The significance of an expiratory view is that some bullae and cysts capable of trapping air actually increase in size and become visible during expiration (Fraser and Paré, 1970; Ting, Klopstock and Lyons, 1970). In general, all candidates should be excluded if evidence is found of bullae, cysts, fibrotic lesions or any other pathology capable of causing air trapping or localized or general loss of compliance. Although multiple calcified tuberculous lesions in the lung

parenchyma or hilar regions present little difficulty using such criteria, the significance of a single, discrete, calcified primary lymph node (Gohn focus) is debatable. Royal Navy policy was changed in 1985 to allow candidates with such lesions to dive and undergo submarine escape training. The decision was based on a complete lack of evidence that such lesions have ever been found to be, or cited as, the cause of pulmonary over-inflation accidents, even though they were much more common in submarine escape trainees and divers in times before pre-training screening was as thorough as it is today and predisposing factors for decompression pulmonary barotrauma became a cause for concern.

Pulmonary function

Pulmonary function tests for diving candidates tend to have adopted the ratio between FEV_1 and the FVC as a yardstick for determining fitness. The FEV_1/FVC ratio was introduced by the Royal Navy in 1976 as an appropriate screening test for the large numbers of men undergoing submarine escape training. Arbitrary lower limits of 75 and 70 per cent were set for initial trainees and requalifiers respectively. The FEV_1/FVC ratio then became used for screening divers, and similar limits were adopted in 1981 as the EMAS standards for candidates for commercial diving (75 per cent) and trained divers (70 per cent). It must be stressed that these criteria were introduced as a screening test and failure led to full respiratory function testing. However, the use of the FEV_1/FVC ratio has the disadvantage of relating more to the function of large rather than small airways, although it will obviously identify candidates with obstructive disease involving large airways. Clearly, the values obtained for FEV_1 and FVC also need to be compared to predicted age/height related values for individual candidates and the normally used predicted values may not be entirely appropriate for use in divers. Certainly, the Royal Navy has established its own predicted values for FEV_1 and FVC to apply to spirometry carried out on submarine escape trainees and divers (Brooks, Pethybridge and Pearson, 1988). In time, other spirometric criteria have been added by various authorities who set standards for commercial divers and these are summarized in Table 25.4.

Reliance on spirometry for screening purposes must include training of those carrying out the tests and standardization of the techniques used. Fortunately, in the case of divers, motivation to produce optimum results is rarely, if ever, in question.

It is impossible to say how effective these largely empirical spirometric criteria are in preventing decompression pulmonary barotrauma. About 50 per cent of the ascents in submarine escape trainees that result in pulmonary barotrauma do not involve

Table 25.4 Standards applied to pulmonary function tests carried out on divers

Pulmonary function tests:
1. Annual spirometry is required for all commercial divers subject to the requirements of 1981 Diving Operations at Work Regulations (HMSO, 1981) and all UK military divers. The following standards apply:
   FVC must be >3.5 litres
   FEV_1/FVC ratio must be >75% for fitness to commence diving
   FEV_1/FVC ratio must be >70% for continuing fitness to dive
   Failure to meet the above criteria requires full pulmonary function testing
2. Other national standards include the following requirements for commercial and/or military divers:
   MVV must be >70% of predicted (USA)
   FVC must be >50 ml/kg body weight (Norway)
   PEF must be >500 ml/min (Norway)

any obvious causative factors and occur in personnel who have satisfied the prescribed health screening criteria (Pearson, 1981a). A similar situation exists with divers who not infrequently suffer pulmonary barotrauma during apparently normal ascents during which no breath-holding has occurred. This suggests that other, as yet unidentified, predisposing anatomical or physiological factors may be involved. One study of an admittedly limited number of divers who had sustained decompression pulmonary barotrauma found that the six individuals concerned had significantly higher maximum transpulmonary pressures and lowered 'static' pulmonary compliance when compared to a control group of divers (Colebatch, Smith and Ng, 1973). A continuation of this study has apparently confirmed these findings in a larger group of divers who had suffered pulmonary barotrauma from normal decompressions (H.J.H. Colebatch, 1988, personal communication) and the conclusion was that this group had less distensible lungs and airways than average.

In a study of the spirometry carried out on 3788 Royal Navy submarine escape trainees (Brooks, Pethybridge and Pearson, 1988), which was intended to examine the value of forced expiratory flow rates between 75 and 85 per cent of FVC (FEF_{75-85}) as an alternative screening criterion, it was found that, in the 34 accidents that occurred in this group, there was a significant ($P<0.01$) correlation with a low (>2 standard deviations (s.d.) below predicted) FVC. This somewhat surprising finding may simply be connected with the fact that a low FVC may be associated with decreased distensibility due to airspaces that are smaller than normal and have inherently increased surface forces. Candidates for submarine escape training with low FVC values are now being studied in detail to evaluate the use of this single parameter for screening purposes. It is also significant that the study

referred to did not show any correlation between accidents and any other spirometric value and this study underlines the difficulty inherent in using empirical criteria such as FEV_1/FVC ratio values for such specialized applications.

An earlier study of Royal and Swedish Navy submarine escape training accidents (Goad et al., 1982) found a slight but significant correlation with chest dimensions and that individuals with long, thin chests, who are known to have a higher risk of spontaneous pneumothorax (Peters et al., 1978), appear to have a very slightly increased risk of barotrauma during submarine escape training. However, the correlation was of such a low order of significance that it was impractical to recommend chest measurement as a form of screening until considerably more accidents had been studied. The investigation is continuing.

Full pulmonary function testing is generally reserved for divers who fail any aspect of screening spirometry and interpretation of such tests may be extremely difficult in terms of assessment of risk factors. Flow rates, particularly during exhalation, will be of special significance although the available predicted values for certain expiratory flow rates leave something to be desired. A final assessment of value in difficult cases, particularly those where there is any suggestion of a possibility of gas trapping from whatever cause, is CT scanning which has been shown to be of value in determining whether areas of lung are emptying fully (Denison, Morgan and Millars, 1986). The definition available with this technique allows adequately small areas of the lungs to be studied.

Summary

The foregoing comments apply equally to trained divers when their continuing fitness to dive is being considered. Annual medical examinations are almost universally obligatory for commercial and military divers. The requirement for an annual chest radiograph has, however, recently been reduced by the Royal Navy to every 3 years. The reduced FEV_1/FVC ratio of 70 per cent allowed by some authorities for trained divers has no true scientific validity and a number of divers with FVC values that are larger than predicted, and a normal FEV_1, will have a ratio below 70 per cent. Interpretation of such cases requires knowledge of the previously described effects of diving on lung function.

Screening after dysbaric incidents

Perhaps the most controversial question over fitness to dive is that relating to a return to diving after proven decompression pulmonary barotrauma. The only study of recurring pulmonary barotrauma (Leitch and Green, 1985) supported Royal Navy policy that divers who have had decompression pulmonary barotrauma should not dive again. This view is not universally held and there are those who would make the distinction between 'unstressed barotrauma' arising from normal ascents without apparent breath-holding and 'stressed barotrauma' due to abnormal ascents, breath-holding or equipment failure. It is argued that there may be a greater risk of recurrent barotrauma in cases where there is no obvious causative factor, although this is probably a tacit admission of the existence of as yet unknown predisposing factors. In view of the limited evidence upon which such decisions must be based, it is probably wisest to remember the potentially disastrous outcome of any episode of decompression pulmonary barotrauma if arterial gas embolism occurs and advise against further diving. Any other decision should be, at the very least, supported by the most thorough investigation which must include CT scanning. As with any other aspect of fitness to dive, there is no room for sympathy in such matters and possible loss of livelihood in the case of commercial divers should not influence any decision on fitness to dive.

In addition to published health standards for commercial and military divers, much useful comment exists on the application of health standards to divers in general and sports divers in particular (Hamilton and Schilling, 1976; Bove, 1983; Knight, 1983; Hickey, 1984).

References

Adkisson, G.H., Macleod, M.A., Hodgson, M., Sykes, J.J.W., Smith, F., Strack, C., Torok, Z. and Pearson, R.R. (1989) Cerebral perfusion deficits in dysbaric illness. *Lancet* 2, 119–122

Bernthal, T., Horres, A.D. and Taylor, J.T. (1961) Pulmonary vascular obstruction in graded tachypneugenic diffuse embolisation. *Am. J. Physiol.* 200, 279–280

Bove, A.A. (1983) An approach to medical evaluation of the sport diver. *SPUMS J.* 2, 3–17

Bradley, M.E. and Bornmann, R.C. (1984) Scuba disease revisited? In: *Underwater Physiology VIII. Proceedings of Eighth Symposium on Underwater Physiology* (eds A.J. Bachrach and M.A. Matzen), Bethesda, Maryland, Undersea Medical Society, pp. 173–180

Brooks, G.J., Pethybridge, R.J. and Pearson, R.R. (1988) Lung function reference values for FEV$_1$, FVC, FEV$_1$/FVC ratio and FEF$_{75-85}$ derived from the results of screening 3788 Royal Navy submariners and submariner candidates by spirometry. *Report 17/87*, Institute of Naval Medicine, Alverstoke, Hants

Butler, B.D. and Hills, B.A. (1979) The lung as a filter for microbubbles. *J. Appl. Physiol.* 47, 537–543

Butler, B.D. and Hills, B.A. (1983) Role of lung surfactant in cerebral decompression sickness. *Aviat. Spac. Environ. Med.* 54, 11–15

Butler, B.D. and Hills, B.A. (1985) Transpulmonary passage of venous air emboli. *J. Appl. Physiol.* 59, 543–547

Butler, B.D. and Katz, J. (1988) Vascular pressures and passage of gas emboli through the pulmonary circulation. *Undersea Biomed. Res.* 15, 203–209

Calder, I.M. (1985) Autopsy and experimental observations on factors leading to barotrauma in man. *Undersea Biomed. Res.* 12, 165–182

Carey, C.R., Schaefer, K.E. and Alvis, H.J. (1955) Effect of skin diving on lung volumes. *J. Appl. Physiol.* 8, 519–523

Clark, J.M. (1987) Pulmonary limits of oxygen tolerance in man. In: *Proceedings of Symposium on Extension of Oxygen Tolerance.* University of Pennsylvania Medical Center, Philadelphia, PA

Clark, J.M. and Lambertsen, C.J. (1971a) Pulmonary oxygen toxicity – a review. *Pharmacol. Rev.* 23, 37–133

Clark, J.M. and Lambertsen, C.J. (1971b) Rate of development of pulmonary O$_2$ toxicity in man during O$_2$ breathing at 2.0 ATA. *J. Appl. Physiol.* 30, 739–752

Colebatch, H.J.H., Smith, M.M. and Ng, C.K.Y. (1973) Increased elastic recoil as a determinant of pulmonary barotrauma in divers. *Respir. Physiol.* 26, 55–64

Cotes, J.E., Davey, I.S., Reed, J.W. and Rooks M. (1987) Respiratory effects of a single saturation dive to 300 m. *Br. J. Ind. Med.* 44(2), 76–82

Crapo, J.D. (1986) Morphologic changes in pulmonary oxygen toxicity. *Am. Rev. Physiol.* 48, 721–731

Crosbie, W.A., Clarke, M.C., Cox, R.A.F., McIver, N.K.I., Anderson, I.K., Evans, H.A., Liddle, G.C., Cowan, J.L., Brookings, C.H. and Watson, D.G. (1977) Physical characteristics and ventilatory function of 404 commercial divers working in the North Sea. *Br. J. Ind. Med.* 35, 19–25

Crosbie, W.A., Cumming, G. and Thomas, I.R. (1982) Acute oxygen toxicity in a saturation diver working in the North Sea. *Undersea Biomed. Res.* 9, 315–320

Crosbie, W.A., Reed, J.W. and Clarke, M.C. (1979) Functional characteristics of the large lungs found in commercial divers. *J. Appl. Physiol.* 46, 639–645

Dahlback, G.O. and Balldin, U.I. (1985) Pulmonary atelectasis formation during diving with closed-circuit oxygen breathing apparatus. *Undersea Biomed. Res.* 12, 129–138

Davey, I.S., Cotes, J.E. and Reed, J.W. (1984) Relationship of ventilatory capacity to hyperbaric exposure in divers. *J. Appl. Physiol.* 56, 1655–1658

Denison, D.M., Morgan, M.D.L. and Millar, A.B. (1986) Estimation of regional gas and tissue volumes of the lung in supine man, using computed tomography. *Thorax* 41, 620–628

Diving Operations at Work Regulations (1981). *Statutory Instruments. Health and Safety*, No. 399. London: HMSO

Edmonds, C. (1976) A salt water aspiration syndrome. *Milit. Med.* 141, 779–785

Ence, T.J. and Gong, H. Jr (1979) Adult respiratory distress syndrome after venous air embolism. *Am. Rev. Respir. Dis.* 119, 1033–1037

Fisher, A.B., Bassett, D.J.P. and Forman, H.J. (1979) Oxygen toxicity of the lung: biochemical aspects. In: *Pulmonary Edema* (eds A.P. Fishman and E.M. Rankin), American Physiological Society, Bethesda, MD, pp. 207–216

Francis, T.J.R., Pezeshkpour, G.H., Dutka, A.J., Hallenbeck, J.M. and Flynn, E.T. (1988) Is there a role for the autochthonous bubble in the pathogenesis of spinal cord decompression sickness? *J. Neuropathol. Expl Neurol.* **47**, 475–487

Fraser, R.G. and Paré, J.A. (1970) In: *Diagnosis of Diseases of the Chest*, W.B. Saunders, London, p.1024

Goad, R.F., Pethybridge, R.J., Robinson, E.G. and Lindemark, C. (1982) Chest dimensions of men incurring pulmonary barotrauma in the submarine escape training environment. *Report 10/82.* Institute of Naval Medicine, Alverstoke, Hants

Greene, K.M. (1978) Causes of death in submarine escape training casualties: analysis of cases and review of the literature. *AMTE(E) Report R78–402.* Admiralty Research Establishment, Alverstoke, Hants

Hallenbeck, J.M., Bove, A.A. and Elliott, D.H. (1975) Mechanisms underlying spinal cord damage in decompression sickness. *Neurology* **25**, 308–316

Hamilton, R.W. and Schilling, C.W. (Eds) (1976) *Recommended Medical and Operating Standards for Divers.* Contract No. 210-76-0104. National Institute for Occupational Safety and Health, Washington DC

Harabin, A.L., Homer, L.D., Weathersby, P.K. and Flynn, E.T. (1987) An analysis of decrements of vital capacity as an index of pulmonary oxygen toxicity. *J. Appl. Physiol.* **63**, 1130–1135

Harveyson, K.B., Hirschfeld, B.E.E. and Tonge, J.I. (1956) Fatal air embolism resulting from the use of a compressed air diving unit. *Med. J. Austr.* **1**, 658–660

Hickey, D.D. (1984) Outline of medical standards for divers. *Undersea Biomed. Res.* **11**, 407–432

Hoke, B., Jackson, D.L., Alexander, J.M. and Flynn, E.T. (1976) Respiratory heat loss and pulmonary function during cold gas breathing at high pressure. In: *Underwater Physiology V. Proceedings of Fifth Symposium on Underwater Physiology* (ed. C.J. Lambertsen), Federation of the American Society for Experimental Biology, Bethesda, MD

Hong, S.K. (1981) Pattern of cold adaptation in women divers of Korea (ama). *Fed. Proc.* **32**, 1614–1622

Hong, S.K. and Rahn, H. (1967) The diving women of Korea and Japan. *Sci. Am.* **216**, 34–43

Jammes, Y., Burnet, H., Cosson, P. and Luciano, M. (1988) Bronchomotor responses to cold air or helium–oxygen at normal and high ambient pressures. *Undersea Biomed. Res.* **15**, 179–182

Kang, B.S., Song, S.H., Suh, C.S. and Hong, S.K. (1963) Changes in body temperature and basal metabolic rate of the ama. *J. Appl. Physiol.* **18**, 483–488

Kavanagh, A.J., Halverson, C.W., Jordan, C.J., Lachapelle, N.C., Sanborn, W.R., Emmons, C.W. and Siess, E.R. (1963) A scuba syndrome. *Connecticut Med.* **27**(6), 315–318

Kizer, K.W. and Golden, J.A. (1987) Lipoid pneumonitis in a commercial abalone diver. *Undersea Biomed. Res.* **14**, 545–552

Knight, J. (1983) What should we ask for in a sports diver medical? *SPUMS J.* **2**, 17–22

Lehner, C.E., Will, J.A., Lightfoot, E.N. and Lanphier, E.H. (1984) Decompression sickness in sheep: fatal chokes after 24 hour dives with altitude provocation. In: *Underwater Physiology VIII. Proceedings of Eighth Symposium on Underwater Physiology* (eds A.J. Bachrach and M.M. Matzen), Undersea Medical Society, Bethesda, MA, pp. 191–200

Leitch, D.R. and Green, R.D. (1985) *Recurrent pulmonary barotrauma. Report 5/85.* Institute of Naval Medicine, Alverstoke, Hants

Lundgren, C.E.G. (1984) Respiratory function during simulated wet dives. *Undersea Biomed. Res.* **11**, 139–147

Macklin, M.T. and Macklin, C.T. (1944) Malignant interstitial emphysema of the lungs and mediastinum as an important occult complication in many respiratory diseases and condi-

tions: an interpretation of the literature in light of laboratory experiments. *Medicine* **23**, 281–358

Macleod, M.A., Adkisson, G.H., Fox, M.J. and Pearson, R.R. (1988) ^{99m}Tc-HMPAO single photon emission tomography in the diagnosis of cerebral barotrauma. *Br. J. Radiol.* **61**, 1106–1109

Malhotra, M.S. and Wright, H.C. (1959) Air embolism during decompression and its prevention. *Admiralty Report, RNPL 9/59.* Ministry of Defence, London

Malhotra, M.S. and Wright, H.C. (1961) The effects of a raised intrapulmonary pressure on the lungs of fresh unchilled cadavers. *J. Pathol. Bacteriol.* **82**, 198–202

Miller, J.N., Miller, C. and Coggin, R. (1978) Pulmonary tissue volume and vital capacity in early pulmonary oxygen toxicity. *Undersea Biomed. Res.* **5** (suppl.), 16

Moon, R.E., Camporesi, E.M. and Kisslo, J.A. (1989) Patent foramen ovale and decompression sickness. *Lancet* **1**, 513–514

Moretti, G. (1968) Decompression sickness as a result of repeated breath-hold diving. *Ann. Nav. Med. (Roma)* **73**, 509–522

Morrison, J.B., Florio, J.T. and Butt, W.S. (1981) Effects of CO_2 sensitivity and respiratory pattern on respiration in divers. *Undersea Biomed. Res.* **8**, 209–218

Moselhi, M., Abadallah, S.M. and Azab, Y.M. (1980) Pulmonary function in men with intermittent exposure to hyperbaric oxygen. *Undersea Biomed. Res.* **7**, 149–157

Park, Y.S., Rahn, H., Lee, I.S., Lee, S.I., Kang, D.H., Hong, S.Y. and Hong, S.K. (1983) Patterns of wet suit diving in Korean women breath-hold divers. *Undersea Biomed. Res.* **10**, 203–216

Pearson, R.R. (1981a) A review of submarine escape training accidents with reference to the use of slowed or interrupted training ascents. *Report No. 15/81.* Institute of Naval Medicine, Alverstoke, Hants

Pearson, R.R. (1981b) The aetiology, pathophysiology, presentation and therapy of pulmonary barotrauma and arterial gas embolism resulting from submarine escape training and diving. MD Thesis, University of Newcastle upon Tyne

Pearson, R.R. (1984) Diagnosis and treatment of gas embolism. In: *The Physicians Guide to Diving Medicine* (eds C.W. Shilling and R.A. Mathias), Plenum Press, London, pp. 333–367

Pearson, R.R., Francis, T.J.R., Peneshkpour, G.H. and Dutka, A.J. (1990) Spinal cord dysfunction and pathology following afterial gas embolism. *Undersea Biomed. Res.* **17** (suppl.), 32–33

Peters, R.M., Peters, W.A., Benirschke, S.K. and Friedman, P.J. (1978) Chest dimensions in young adults with spontaneous pneumothorax. *Ann. Thor. Surg.* **25**, 193–196

Rennie, D.W., Cevino, B.G., Howell, B.J., Hong, S.H., Kang, B.S. and Hong, S.K. (1962) Physical insulation and Korean diving women. *J. Appl. Physiol.* **17**, 961–966

Schaefer, K.E., McNulty, W.P., Carey, C.R. and Liebow, A.A. (1958) Mechanisms in development of interstitial emphysema and air embolism in decompression from depth. *J. Appl. Physiol.* **13**, 15–29

Schaefer, K.E. (1961) Adaptation to skin diving. *Fed. Proc.* **20**, 215–220

Schaefer, K.E. (1963) Effect of prolonged diver training. In: *Proceedings of Second Symposium on Underwater Physiology* (eds C.J. Lambertsen and L.J. Greenbaum), National Academy of Science/National Research Council, Washington DC, pp. 271–275

Schaefer, K.E., Allison, R.D., Dougherty, J.H. Jr, Carey, C.R., Walker, R., Yost, F. and Parker, D. (1968) Pulmonary and circulatory adjustment determining the limits of depths in breath-hold diving. *Science* **162**, 1020–1025

Small, A. (1984) New perspectives on hyperoxic pulmonary toxicity – a review. *Undersea Biomed. Res.* **11**, 1–24

Suzuki, S., Ikeda, T., Hashimoto, A. and Hamada, K. (1989) Decrease in single breath diffusing capacity of the lung after 300 and 320 msw saturation dives. *Undersea Biomed. Res.* **16** (suppl.), 34

Thalmann, E.D., Sponholtz, D.K. and Lundgren, C.E.G. (1979) Effects of immersion and static lung loading on submerged exercise at depth. *Undersea Biomed. Res.* **6**, 259–290

Ting, I.Y., Klopstock, R. and Lyons, H.A. (1963) Mechanical properties of pulmonary cysts and bullae. *Am. Rev. Respir. Dis.* **87**, 538

Van Allen, C.M. and Hrdina, L.S. (1929) Air embolism from the pulmonary vein. *Archs Surg.* **19**, 567–599

Wilmshurst, P.T., Nuri, M., Crowther, A. and Webb-Price, M.M. (1989) Cold induced pulmonary oedema in SCUBA divers and swimmers and subsequent development of hypertension. *Lancet* **1**, 62–65

Winsborough, M.M. and McKenzie, R.S. (1977) Pulmonary oxygen toxicity and the pre-oedematous lung. *Med. Aeronaut. Spat. Med. Subaquatique Hyperbare* **16**(63), 254–256

Wright, W.B. (1972) Use of the University of Pennsylvania, Institute of Environmental Medicine procedure for calculation of cumulative pulmonary oxygen toxicity. *US Navy Experimental Diving Unit Report 2-72*. US Government Printing Office, Washington, DC

Appendices

W. Raymond Parkes

Appendix I

Elements of geology and mineralogy

Introduction

A basic knowledge of geology and mineralogy is useful, if not essential, to an informed understanding and recognition of the nature and composition of particular rocks and minerals that are encountered in widely differing circumstances in mining operations and in their use or incidental occurrence in industrial processes. Though not a comprehensive account, it is hoped that this section may offer some guidance in this respect.

The Earth consists of a superficial crust a few miles thick which rests on a denser mass, the mantle, nearly 2000 miles thick, and a central core which is probably solid, but behaves in some respects as if in a molten state. Molten rock material, or magma, which contains gases and steam also exists as pockets within the crust and mantle. As a consequence of abnormally high temperatures, often with earth movements, magma is forced up into the crust. If it cools and solidifies before reaching the surface, the resulting rocks are termed 'igneous rocks'; because they invade the surrounding rocks – referred to as *country rocks* – they are called *intrusive*. But some of the magma may, periodically, reach and pour out, or explode, onto its surface. Rocks formed in this way are styled as *extrusive* or *volcanic*. Thus, igneous rocks are divided into two broad groups: *intrusive* and *extrusive*.

Rock means 'any mass or aggregate of one or more kinds of mineral or of organic matter, whether hard and consolidated or soft and incoherent, which owes its origin to the operation of natural causes. Thus, granite, basalt, limestone, clay, sand, silt and peat are all equally termed rocks' (Geikie, 1908).

Chemically, the average composition of the crust consists of about 27.7 per cent silicon, 46.6 per cent oxygen, 8 per cent aluminium and 16.2 per cent in aggregate of calcium, iron, magnesium, potassium and sodium. This gives a total of 98.5 per cent, the remainder consisting of all the other elements.

The ingredients available for formation of rocks are known as minerals. A *mineral* is *a naturally occurring, inorganic, homogeneous substance of distinct chemical composition, atomic structure and physical properties*. Minerals fall into two broad categories:

1. *Primary minerals*, that is, rock constituents which crystallized out of the magma. These are of two kinds: *essential minerals* which determine the species of rocks, and *accessory minerals* which are accidental ingredients (usually in small quantity) in igneous, sedimentary and metamorphic rocks, and whose presence or absence does not affect the general character of the rock.
2. *Secondary minerals*: these are formed by chemical alterations of essential and accessory minerals.

Minerals crystallize in different habits, or forms, under different physical conditions. The term 'habit' denotes the characteristic shapes of crystals caused by variations in the number, size and shape of their faces: for example, prismatic, acicular and platy for single crystals, and columnar, radiating granular, asbestiform (or fibrous), massive and foliated for crystalline aggregates (Zoltai and Wylie, 1979).

Silicon (Si) and oxygen are the two most predominant elements in the crust. However, silicon does not exist in a free state in nature, although its compounds, which are ubiquitous as oxides and as a large group of silicates, constitute the most important rock-forming minerals.

Silica

Silicon and oxygen form a fundamental silicon tetraoxide (SiO_4) tetrahedral unit consisting of a central silicon ion with oxygen ions attached three dimensionally at the four 'corners' of a tetrahedron. All forms of silica, that is, silicon dioxide $(SiO_2)_x$, are composed of a three-dimensional network of tetrahedra joined by common oxygen atoms, so that each crystal consists of a giant molecule with an average stoicheiometric formula of SiO_2. As they are uncombined they are referred to as *free silica*. The tetrahedra are linked in various ways by –Si–O–Si– chains, and the manner in which metallic cations are included in this linkage controls their form and characteristics.

The distinction between free and combined silica is important. *Free (uncombined) silica* (SiO_2) is by far the major component of the Earth's crust; *combined silica* is SiO_2 in combination with various cations as silicates. Free silica occurs in three main forms: crystalline, cryptocrystalline (microcrystalline) and amorphous (non-crystalline).

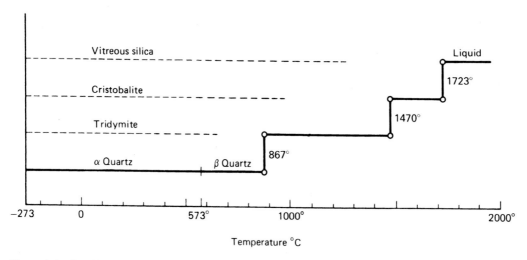

Figure A.1 Graphic classification of the better-known phases (polymorphs) of silica in stable states at 1 atmosphere pressure, as controlled by temperature. (Reproduced, with permission, from Sosman, 1965. Copyright 1965, Rutgers University Press, New Brunswick, NJ)

Most of the following section owes much to the classic work of Sosman (1965).

The principal phases (polymorphs) of silica

Crystalline silica

In nature, crystalline silica occurs in six different polymorphic phases: *quartz, tridymite* and *cristobalite*, and *keatite, coesite* and *stishovite*; the last three are formed only under conditions of high temperature and pressure – usually in the craters of meteorites.

Quartz

This is the most common polymorph found in nature, and is the main constituent of igneous rocks and sandstones formed from the breakdown of igneous rocks; it is a common constituent of many metamorphic rocks. It also occurs in varying amounts, by detrital deposition, at different stages in the development of sedimentary rocks – including carbonaceous rocks.

Tridymite

This is only found in nature in acid volcanic rocks.

Cristobalite

This occurs as minute crystals in some lavas, and as small globules (spherulites) in acid lavas and glasses. However, it is frequently present in bentonite clays in the western USA.

Under certain industrial and laboratory conditions reversible transformation, or inversion, of these phases occurs at different temperatures at atmospheric pressure (Figure A.1). Thus:

$$\text{Quartz} \underset{}{\overset{867°C}{\rightleftharpoons}} \text{Tridymite} \underset{}{\overset{1470°C}{\rightleftharpoons}} \text{Cristobalite} \underset{}{\overset{1723°C}{\rightleftharpoons}} \text{Vitreous silica}$$

They are interconvertible at the points of inversion. Inversions, by which one polymorph of silica changes into another, are of two kinds: (1) a *slow change* that requires a moderate amount of energy, less than that needed for melting; (2) a *rapid and reversible change* requiring much less energy.

Quartz exists in two reversible temperature modifications at constant pressure: α-quartz, which is stable from absolute zero up to 573°C, and β-quartz which is stable at temperatures between 573°C and 867°C. Below 867°C, therefore, under atmospheric pressure and if the temperature is constant and uniform, quartz remains stable no matter how long heating continues, and it does not change into any other phase (Figure A.1).

Between 867°C and 1470°C, over a brief period, pure quartz almost invariably converts to cristobalite, not to tridymite. But if heating is continued below 1470°C the stable form of tridymite is ultimately formed. However, in the presence of fluxing oxides (such as CaO and Al_2O_3) conversion is accelerated and crystalline tridymite may then form at temperatures as low as 950°C. Thus, excellent samples of stable tridymite are found in silica brick from open-hearth furnace roofs where temperatures may be held at 867° to 1470°C for several weeks or longer. Similarly, silica brick from by-product coke ovens maintained at high temperatures, often for years, are an equally rich source.

Cristobalite is the stable polymorph of silica at atmospheric pressure between about 1470°C and 1723°C, its melting point. If the temperature remains uniform and constant, it does not convert permanently to any other crystalline phase. However, cristobalite may also form at temperatures below 1470°C, in which case it is in a metastable state; between 867°C and 1470°C, whether alone or in contact with a melt, it inverts first to the metastable, and then to the stable, form of tridymite. Thus, with repeated firings of silica brick below 1470°C, quartz gradually disappears and cristobalite forms and then decreases steadily as the formation of tridymite increases and replaces it; however, for a time, both cristobalite and tridymite may be present.

The *rate of conversion of quartz to cristobalite* is important and strongly influenced by two factors:

1. The degree of subdivision of quartz: at the same temperature large homogeneous crystals convert extremely slowly, whereas similar crystals reduced to a fine powder are transformed much more rapidly.
2. Temperature: the rate of conversion is not appreciable at temperatures of less than 1000°C and does not become rapid until they exceed 1470°C. At 1160°C complete conversion takes 6 days whereas at 1570°C it takes 1 hour. These rates of change are in line with the usual exponential increase in speed of a chemical reaction with temperature, but the presence of foreign substances may have accelerating or delaying effects on conversion.

Thus, whether heated alone or with added substances, quartz may be expected to transform into cristobalite at any temperature over 1000°C, but the change is only stable and permanent above 1470°C (Figure A.1).

In summary, if given appropriate conditions of temperature and time, conversion of quartz to cristobalite or tridymite may occur in a variety of industrial processes. Examples of possible sources are fired silica (refractory) bricks and other highly siliceous ceramic products, fired insulation bricks, used refractory bricks and foundry sands, and straight and flux calcined diatomite (see Chapter 12).

The occurrence of these polymorphs of silica under such industrial conditions is important in so far as cristobalite and tridymite are at least as fibrogenic as quartz, if not more so. Indeed, King et al. (1953) showed that, in rats exposed to fused (amorphous) silica, quartz, cristobalite and tridymite of high purity and equal particle size, the rate of development and the severity of fibrosis were least with fused silica, greater in ascending order with quartz and cristobalite, and greatest with tridymite, the effect of which was described as 'spectacular' (see page 112).

Cristobalite is specifically manufactured for a variety of refractory purposes, including investment castings, to increase dimensional accuracy and to compensate for shrinkage of the metal being cast.

At this juncture it should be noted that stable phases of well-crystallized cristobalite, together with mullite, may be produced, in the absence of quartz, from aluminium silicates such as kaolinite and andalusite, kyanite and sillimanite at high temperatures (see page 862 and Chapter 16).

Crypto(micro)crystalline silica

This polymorph of silica, also referred to as *chalcedonic silica*, originates from silica derived from the skeletons of a variety of marine animals including sponges – so-called biogenic silica. Densely packed, interlocking microscopic crystals are cemented together by amorphous silica. Its three main varieties are *flint, chalcedony* and *jasper*. Flint and *chert*, which is closely similar to flint but normally exhibits less microcrystalline quartz, occur in calcareous rocks in the form of nodules, layers and irregular concretions. Chalcedony occurs in a large number of subvarieties distinguished chiefly by colour, in particular, *agate, cornelian, bloodstone* and *onyx*. Jasper is a mixture of microcrystalline silica with clay and iron oxides.

Like quartz, all these varieties undergo inversion to cristobalite with heat but, between 1200°C and 1400°C, the rate of change of flint and chert is, in general, greater than that of pure, crystalline quartz.

Amorphous (non-crystalline) silica

Diatomaceous silica or *kieselguhr* is the form of amorphous silica most relevant to pulmonary disease. It, too, is of biogenic origin, being formed mainly of the siliceous skeletons of diatoms, but various stages of transformation to microcrystallization are found in some older deposits (see 'Siliceous deposits'). It converts to cristobalite at all temperatures between 1000°C and 1723°C. In a pure, dry state its conversion to tridymite does not seem to occur between 867°C and 1470°C but it does so in the presence of a flux or water. A flux also facilitates formation of stable cristobalite at significantly lower temperatures than in its absence (see Chapter 12, page 326).

Vitreous (fused) silica is formed when any of the other polymorphs are melted (that is, at temperatures over 1723°C) and quickly cooled. It then remains stable but, if heated for a prolonged period at temperatures over 1150°C (common in many refractories), it devitrifies (recrystallizes) to cristobalite (see Chapter 12, page 331).

The optical properties of crystalline and microcrystalline silica as seen by the medical microscope are discussed briefly in Appendix IV.

Types of rock defined

Because free silica is the principal rock-forming constituent, the proportions in which it is present determine the nature of many rocks.

There are three great classes of rocks:

1. Igneous.
2. Sedimentary.
3. Metamorphic.

Igneous rocks

These are the primary rocks of the crust which were formed from magma either by rapid extrusion of magma on to the Earth's surface or by intrusion of magma within the crust; in the first case, cooling occurred quickly and, in the second, slowly. The rate of cooling determined the size of the rock crystals: the quicker the cooling, the smaller the crystals; the slower the process, the larger the crystals. Granite is an important example that varies in texture from microcrystalline to very coarsely crystalline.

Sedimentary rocks

Sedimentary rocks are formed in two ways:

1. By the gradual breakdown of pre-existing igneous or older sedimentary and metamorphic rocks (see next section) by the action of wind, sun, water, frost and ice in weathering and corrosion processes to form deposits of debris such as sand and mud. The resulting material, in most cases, is transported as solid particles or in solution and deposited at a distance from its origin. Hard and persistent minerals, such as quartz and cristobalite, remain unchanged whereas less stable feldspars and ferromagnesian minerals decompose to produce clay minerals

(hydrous aluminosilicates), iron and manganese hydroxides, and solutions containing calcium, magnesium, sodium and potassium ions which are essential in the formation of non-silicate, rock-forming minerals (see page 847).
2. By the deposition in former seas or swamps of the shells of marine organisms, rotting vegetation and chemical substances.

As a rule, sedimentary rocks are laid down in layers, or strata, which differ significantly in composition and grain size. Slow or cataclysmic earth movements alter the levels of these accumulations and new sediments are deposited on top of them squeezing out their water and compressing them into rocks such as sandstone, limestone and coal.

Metamorphic rocks

Metamorphism implies change of form, structure and constitution in already existing igneous and sedimentary rocks. This change is brought about in four ways:

1. By a local and substantial rise in temperature caused by the intrusion of magma which bakes the neighbouring rocks (*thermal metamorphism*).
2. By movement of the crust which applies shearing or thrusting forces to the rocks and so distorts them that the formation of new minerals results (*dynamic metamorphism*).
3. By percolation of hot water through rocks, and steam and gases through the magma which causes important chemical changes (*hydrothermal metamorphism*).
4. By a combination of thermal and dynamic metamorphism (*regional metamorphism*).

Composition

For the most part all such rocks are composed of *silicate minerals*, that is, silicon dioxide in various combinations with the oxides of other elements such as aluminium, calcium, iron, magnesium and potassium.

The proportion of silica which was available in the original magma determined the form which igneous rocks were to take and it varied from approximately 30 to 75 per cent.

Where the percentage of silicon dioxide was very low, iron and magnesium, which have a strong affinity for it, combined with all that was available, especially if they were predominant among the cations. This gave rise to the 'ferromagnesian' group of minerals (such as the *olivine group*). When a large quantity of uncombined iron remained, this

Table A.1 A classification of the igneous rocks

Mode of occurrence	Proportion of combined silica (SiO$_2$)				
	Over 66% (acid)	52–66% (intermediate)		45–52% (basic)	Under 45% (ultrabasic)
Volcanic lavas	Rhyolite Obsidian Pitchstone	Trachyte	Andesite	Basalt	
Minor intrusions	Microgranite Quartz–porphyry	Microsyenite	Microdiorite	Dolerite	
Major intrusions	Granite	Syenite	Diorite	Gabbro	Periodotite Dunite Serpentinite
Essential minerals	Quartz; hornblende and/or mica; feldspar (orthoclase or sodium-rich plagioclase)	Hornblende or augite; feldspar (orthoclase or sodium-rich plagioclase)	Augite or hornblende; feldspar (calcium-rich plagioclase)	Olivine; augite; feldspar (plagioclase)	Olivine; augite; hornblende

From Bradshaw (1968) with permission of Hodder & Stoughton Ltd.

was deposited as iron ore; when the percentage of silica was of intermediate order, iron and magnesium again combined with it, but, if their concentration was low, aluminium, potassium, sodium and calcium combined with the available remaining silica to produce the *feldspar group* of minerals. Where the percentage of silicon was high, all available cations were absorbed and an excess of silica left which crystallized as quartz.

Acid and basic rocks

Silica-rich magmas are termed 'acid' and those that contain little silica but large quantities of bases, such as aluminium, iron and magnesium, are termed 'basic'. Four magma types are distinguished according to their content, or percentage, of *combined* silica. Thus:

Acid	more than about 66 per cent silica
Intermediate	from about 52 to 66 per cent silica
Basic	from about 45 to 52 per cent silica
Ultrabasic	less than about 45 per cent silica

The more acid the rock, therefore, the more free silica it contains. The proportions of free silica in any rock can only be expressed in general terms. Among the igneous rocks the quartz content of the acid group (chiefly the granite family) may be as much as 30 per cent. In rocks of the intermediate group it may be negligible in some, but as much as 5 per cent in others, and in basic and ultrabasic rocks it is usually very low or absent (see Table A.1).

Classification of igneous rock-forming minerals

According to the ways in which magma penetrated or invaded all kinds of rocks these fall into two main divisions – *intrusive* and *extrusive* – which can be classified according to the minerals they contain. All, apart from quartz and small amounts of iron oxides, are silicates formed in magma during its gradual cooling. The most important and characteristic are the following (Table A.1).

Intrusive rocks

Quartz group

As has been pointed out already, when silica is present in abundance and all other substances have entered into combination with it, a variable amount remains and crystallizes as quartz. This, almost pure, free silica is found in such important igneous rocks as *quartz porphory*, *rhyolite* and *granite*. Hence, the sedimentary and metamorphic rocks which were subsequently formed from them also have a high content of silica.

Feldspar group

Members of this group are the most common of all the rock-forming minerals, and the most important constituents of igneous rocks. They are anhydrous potassium, sodium and calcium aluminiumsilicates or various combinations of all three; they may comprise as much as 75 per cent of granite.

There are two main varieties.

1. *Orthoclase feldspars* which are rich in potassium and usually occur in acid rocks with a high percentage of quartz.
2. *Plagioclase feldspars* which contain variable proportions of sodium and calcium. Sodium plagioclases occur in more acid rocks and are, therefore, frequently associated with orthoclase, whereas calcium plagioclases are found in basic rocks.

Thus, at the acid end of the series, feldspars contain significant amounts of quartz and, at the basic end, they contain little or none.

As the feldspar minerals that are employed in the ceramic industries are silica rich, they have been an important cause of silicosis. However, feldspars that contain no quartz have not been found to be fibrogenic in the lungs of experimental animals (Mohanty et al., 1953; Goldstein and Rendall, 1970).

Feldspathoid group

Members of this group are composed of the same elements as feldspars, but in different proportions, and they play a similar, though subordinate, role in rock formation. Primary quartz and feldspathoid do not occur together in the same rock. If free silica had been present during formation, it would have combined with feldspathoid to form feldspar.

Micas and clay group

This group is generally associated with acid rocks such as granite. The structure of micas is of the sheet lattice type which gives them their well-known characteristic of cleavage into layers. Important members of the group are *biotite*, a complex silicate of magnesium, aluminium, potassium and iron found in many igneous and metamorphic rocks, and *muscovite* (potassium aluminium silicate), the common white mica. *Sericite*, once thought to be important in the pathogenesis of coal pneumoconiosis, is a secondary muscovite which may be produced by the alteration of orthoclase feldspar. And *vermiculite*, which possesses important industrial properties, is a natural alteration product of biotite and phlogopite (magnesium) micas (see Chapter 16, page 558).

The clay minerals are related to the micas and are hydrous aluminium silicates of sheet lattice type formed by the breakdown of feldspars and ferro-magnesian minerals. *Kaolinite*, the chief constituent of *china clay*, is one of the most important of these (see page 861).

Pyroxene group

The pyroxenes are a large group of rock-forming minerals found in intermediate basic and ultrabasic rocks. *Augite*, a silicate of calcium, magnesium, iron and aluminium, is the most common member.

Amphibole group

This group, like the pyroxenes, includes a number of important rock-forming minerals, the physical and chemical character of which link them together as one family. All possess the double chain-type silicate structure (Si_4O_{11}). *Hornblende*, a complex aluminium, calcium, magnesium, iron and sodium silicate, is the most common member of the group. It occurs as a primary mineral in acid and intermediate igneous rocks such as granites and syenites, and in many metamorphic rocks derived from igneous rocks – for example, hornblende–schists and hornblende–gneisses (see page 863). The asbestos minerals *actinolite*, *tremolite*, *amosite* and *crocidolite* are members of this group (see page 856).

Olivine group

Olivines are magnesium iron silicates in which magnesium is in excess of iron in most varieties. Of all the groups they have the lowest proportion of combined silica and quartz is either absent or present in very small amounts. Thus, they are generally confined to basic and ultrabasic rocks.

Extrusive rocks

These are formed from lava flows or from magmatic and rocky material forcibly blown from volcanoes to considerable distances to produce beds of pyroclastic rock. They include basalts, dolerites, pumice, pumicite and perlite.

Basalts are the most common, constituting about 80 per cent of lava rocks. They consist, in essence, of calcium-rich plagioclase feldspar and augite with or without olivine, and they are divided into two major groups according to the proportion of olivine they contain: up to 20 per cent in the one that contains no quartz, and little or none in the other which may contain small quantities of quartz. Basalts are also abundant as intrusive rocks.

Dolerites are similar to basalts but more coarse grained, and occur more in the form of minor intrusions as *olivine–dolerite* without quartz and as *quartz–dolerites*.

Both basalt and quartz–dolerites are quarried extensively in central Scotland for dimension stone, asphalt roofing material, road setts, roadstone chips, as concrete aggregate and for tiles and flooring.

Pumice and *pumicite* consist of frothy, silicic glass which may contain varying amounts of crystalline silica; *perlite* is a volcanic glass of rhyolitic composition. They are discussed in more detail later (page 864).

Crystalline structure

The order of crystallization of rocks depended primarily on the composition of the magma, for example, in a magma rich in silicon dioxide, quartz tended to crystallize first – hence, quartz–porphyries. Similarly, in basic rocks, feldspar often crystallized before pyroxene. Within the ferromagnesian and feldspar groups, therefore, fairly well-defined sequences are observed. For example:

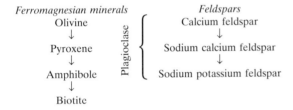

It is worth noting, as a general principle, that some minerals cannot occur together in rocks. In particular, quartz is not present either in rocks of the olivine group (other than those which are almost pure iron-olivine) or in the feldspathoid group. Rocks which contain quartz are often classified as 'oversaturated', those with little or no quartz, but which contain olivine and feldspathoids, as 'undersaturated'.

Non-silicate rock-forming minerals

Non-silicate minerals are important constituents of certain sedimentary and metamorphic rock types. They fall into the following groups.

Carbonates

These are the predominant non-silicates and they consist of *calcite* ($CaCO_3$ – the chief constituent of limestone), *dolomite* ($MgCO_3 \cdot CaCO_3$ – which constitutes dolomite limestone) and *siderite* ($FeCO_3$). *Marbles* are metamorphosed calcite or dolomite. Siderite occurs in some coal measures.

Halides and sulphates

Rock salt (NaCl), *anhydrite* ($CaSO_4$) and *gypsum* ($CaSO_4 \cdot 2H_2O$), which were deposited by evaporation of lakes and land-locked seas, and *fluorspar* (CaF_2) contain no free silica unless by detrital deposition.

Oxides and sulphides

These are chiefly iron minerals. The most important of the oxides are *magnetite* (Fe_3O_4), *hematite* (Fe_2O_3) and *goethite* ($Fe_2O_3 \cdot H_2O$). Magnetite, one of the most valuable iron ores, is an accessory mineral in most igneous rocks and in metamorphic deposits in limestones. Hematite occurs in igneous, hydrothermal metamorphic and volcanic rocks. It is found in limestone beds owing to replacement of the limestone by hematite from overlying ferruginous sandstones in various locations, for example, north Lancashire. The largest deposits in the world, in the Lake Superior district of Minnesota, were formed by alteration and concentration of iron silicates of sedimentary origin (see page 855).

Types of rock described

Igneous rocks

The rate at which the original magma cooled determined the degree and form of its crystallization and, therefore, the 'texture' or fundamental structure of the igneous rock.

Intrusive rocks are subdivided into *minor intrusions* which are fairly near the surface of the crust, and *major intrusions* which lie deep below the surface. More than 600 varieties of igneous rocks have been described but they can all be placed in a few large groups as shown in Table A.1.

Intrusive rocks reach the surface of the crust through the action of earth movements (see page 863) and the erosion and disruption of overlying rocks.

Sedimentary rocks

Sedimentary rocks fall broadly into three categories, according to their origin: fragmental (mechanical)

Table A.2 Classification of some common sedimentary rocks

Group character	Type	Main features of composition
Fragmental (mechanical) origin — Rudaceous	Conglomerate	Quartz content similar to parent rock; iron oxides (e.g. limonite, hematite); sometimes calcite or dolomite
	Breccia	Mixed rock fragments; calcite and limonite with fine silt or mud in matrix
Arenaceous	Sandstone	Quartz, muscovite, and feldspar rock particles cemented by siliceous, ferruginous, calcareous, argillaceous and carbonaceous matter
	Gritstone	Similar to sandstone. Particle slightly different in shape
	Arkose	Sandstone or gritstone subjected to contact metamorphism and about 25% feldspars of various sorts. Siliceous and ferruginous content
	Quartzite	Sandstone or gritstone subjected to contact metamorphism, and detrital quartz cemented by secondary silica
	Ganister	Highly siliceous. Quartz, cherts, orthoclase, feldspar, clay minerals such as kaolinite [$Al_2Si_2O_5(OH)_4$]. Hematite and limonite are accessory minerals
	Siltstone	Fine-grained, compact detritus from rivers, lakes and glacial action. Quartz, muscovite, feldspars and iron ores with siliceous, ferruginous and calcareous cementing material
Argillaceous	Clay	Fine-grained, earthy material, plastic when wet; hard when dry. Consists of orthoclase and plagioclase feldspars, muscovite and occasionally a little quartz (see note)
	Fuller's earth	Mainly montmorillonite [$(Mg \cdot Ca)O \cdot Al_2O_3 \cdot 5SiO_2(5–8)H_2O$] – calcium smectite – but also small amounts of feldspar, mica, glauconite and apatite may be present. Quartz rare except in intercalated sand layers
	Volcanic clay	Bentonite: sodium montmorillonite (sodium smectite) with quartz, cristobalite, feldspar, mica, apatite and ferromagnesian minerals
	Residual clay	Formed in situ from rock decomposition. Very finely divided: for example, bauxite (hydrous aluminium oxides) and china clay (kaolin) (see note)
	Mudstone	Consolidated, non-fissile clay with similar constituents. Usually from beneath coal seams ('seatearths'). Content of quartz variable, often secondary
	Fireclay	Contains quartz, feldspars, mica, secondary silica and iron compounds. Quartz content high
	Shale	Indurated, laminated, fine-grained clay mineral matter; contains quartz, mica, iron ores, secondary silica, calcite and iron oxides. Quartz content up to 30%
Calcareo-argillaceous	Marl	Unconsolidated, non-laminated calcareous clay. Composition as clays but more calcareous materials as matrix. Quartz content small and variable
	Calcareous shale	Consolidated, laminated clay with such calcareous material, i.e. consolidated marl with similar composition
Organic origin — Calcareous	Limestone	$CaCO_3$ mainly of organic origin (e.g. corals, crustacea, molluscs, algae, foraminifera), occasionally iron ores. Very small quantities of free silica may be present
	Dolomite	Limestone with large quantity of $Ca \cdot Mg(CO_3)_2$, much of organic origin; also variable hematite
	Oolitic and pisolitic limestone	Limestone, more chemical than sedimentary in origin, with large characteristic grains of $CaCO_3$ found in successive layers round nucleus of shell fragments or quartz grains. ('Grains' resemble fishroe or peas.) Small and variable amounts of free silica
	Chalk	Almost pure $CaCO_3$. No free silica, but nodules of flint in some chalk deposits
Siliceous	Chert and flint	Crystalline and cryptocrystalline silica (microcrystalline quartz) often aggregated into 'nodules' in chalk. Very high free silica content with traces of limonite
	Siliceous deposits	Mainly organic in origin. Diatomite: amorphous silica content 60–90%; cristobalite and quartz integrated from volcanic ash in some deposits. Sinter: chemical precipitation of amorphous and cryptocrystalline silica from solution
Carbonaceous	Carbonaceous rocks	Peat, lignite, bituminous and anthracite coals. Variable amounts of quartz, iron minerals ore (pyrite, siderite, limonite) and clays (e.g. kaolinite) and illite. Oil shale: combination of essentially sedimentary shale and varying amounts of carbonaceous matter. Contains abundant quartz, and mica; 'kerogen' and, sometimes, feldspar and rutile Asphalt, asphaltic bitumen and bituminous impregnations. Mixtures of different hydrocarbons usually as black or brown, pitchy material; impregnations mainly in limestones in certain locations, also in sandstones and shales. Thus, quartz either absent or abundant according to origin

Continued

Table A.2 continued

Group character		Type	Main features of composition
Chemical origin	Calcareous	Calcium carbonate (calcite)	CaCO₃ but some impurity such as limonite. Traces of free silica, detrital and rare
		Dolomite (partly)	Occurring as mineral, not limestone replacement. Ca·Mg(CO₃)₂ with some iron impurities
	Ferrugineous	Bedded iron ores	From aqueous solutions in mudstones, limestones, primary hematite, magnesite. Variable quartz content
		Bog iron ores	Small amounts of detrital quartz
	Saline	Chlorides	Mainly rock salt (NaCl) with various impurities but no quartz. Carnellite (KMgCl₃·6H₂O) – used as fertilizer and source of potash; quartz absent
		Sulphates	Barytes (BaSO₄), celestine (SrSO₄), anhydrite (CaSO₄), alunite [KAl₃(SO₄)₂(OH)₆], apatite [Ca₅(F,Cl)(PO₄)₃], and gypsum (CaSO₄·2H₂O). Rarely free of some mineral impurity from sands, marls, clays, shales and limestones; thus, small quantities of quartz may be present, but are more substantial in some gypsum formations

Note: the majority of true clays contain very little free silica and what there is depends upon the nature of the parent rock. Clays with particle size greater than 2 μm may contain a small quantity (occasionally up to 10 per cent) but those of smaller particle size contain an insignificant quantity.
'Free silica' refers to crystalline or cryptocrystalline forms unless otherwise stated.
Table freely adapted, by permission of the publishers, from Milner, H.B. (1962) *Sedimentary Petrography*, Vol. 2. London: Allen and Unwin.

origin, non-fragmental organic origin and non-fragmented chemical origin (Table A.2).

Fragmental rocks

As the chief ingredients of these were produced mechanically by attrition and erosion they are classed according to the nature and size of the fragments.

Rudaceous (rubbly) rocks

These are composed of granules, pebbles or boulders which, when rounded by wear produce *conglomerates*; but if angular, they are called *breccias*. The fragments are cemented together by a mineral such as secondary silica, leached out from elsewhere, or by mud.

Arenaceous (sandy) rocks

The raw materials of these are sands and silts cemented by siliceous and clay substances. The chief members of this group are the *sandstones* and they are composed predominantly of quartz grains.

Argillaceous (clayey) rocks

These consist essentially of naturally plastic clay minerals but they may also contain significant quantities of free silica derived from older quartz-bearing rocks (detrital quartz). They are laid down as clays and, when consolidated, become rocks known as mudstones and shales. Clays or a mixture of clay and non-clay minerals have considerable commercial importance. They can be considered under two broad headings: clays and mudstones.

Clays These are composed of single clay minerals the most important of which, industrially, are *china clay* (known internationally as kaolin), *fuller's earth* and *bentonite*. The significant amount of quartz often present in raw china clay and kaolin is an undesirable impurity in most industrial processes (for example, manufacture of paper) and is, therefore, removed principally by washing with water. The quantity of quartz present in fuller's earth and bentonite varies but, for the most part, is small.

Although most deposits of china clay world-wide are sedimentary in origin, the deeper deposits in Cornwall and Devon are of hydrothermal metamorphic origin from granite and, thus, have different physical characteristics and composition (see page 861 and Chapter 16, page 550).

Mudstones These are indurated, massive argillaceous sediments that have the texture and composition of shales (see page 851) but lack their fine lamination and fissility. Both mudstones and shales may contain substantial amounts of quartz.

Unbedded mudstones associated with coal-bearing (carbonaceous) strata are sometimes called *fireclays* which have been widely exploited in the past for their refractory properties. In British geological terminology these mudstones, in general, are referred to as *seatearths*, the composition of which varies widely from almost pure clay rocks (that is, *seatclays*), through silty and sandy sediments, to quartz-rich sandstones which, until recently, were also valued as refractory materials

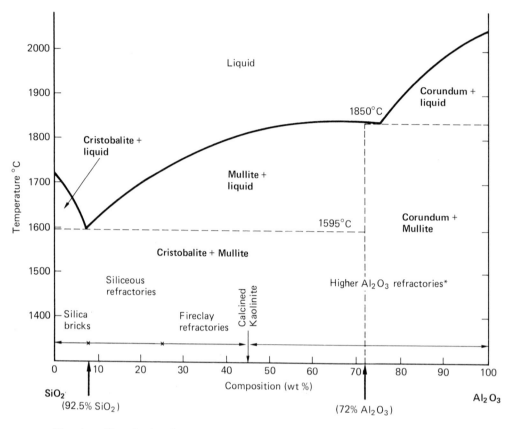

*Based on sillimanite, kyanite, bauxite and alumina

Figure A.2   Phase diagram for the $Al_2O_3:SiO_2$ binary system, broadly illustrating the behaviour of refractory aluminium silicates according to temperature and relative content of Al_2O_3 and SiO_2. *Based on sillimanite, kyanite, bauxite and alumina. (Reproduced, with permission, from Highley (1982) and the HMSO, after Aramaki and Roy (1959) *J. Am. Ceram. Soc.* **42**, 644–645)

(the so-called *ganisters*). In North America the term 'underclay' is used to describe clay-rich seatearths. Today the term 'fireclay', in general, describes seatclays that are of economic interest. They consist of kaolinite, mica and quartz, in varying proportions, with some impurities such as ironstone nodules and carbonaceous matter. Because of their physicochemical properties, fireclays have commercial value for both refractory and non-refractory applications. An essential constituent of fireclays is *kaolinite*. It is predominant in refractory fireclays but present in approximately equal proportions with mica and quartz in non-refractory fireclays. Thus, it is kaolinite that confers the valuable refractory properties whereas clays that contain higher proportions of quartz and mica have important non-refractory applications, for example, in the manufacture of vitrified clay pipes, facing bricks, stoneware, sanitary ware and floor and wall tiles (Highley, 1982).

It is convenient, at this point, to consider the effects of heating fireclays and the resultant mineralogical changes that occur. These are also a paradigm for some other aluminium silicates. The overall chemical equation for the stable phases when kaolinite is heated at temperatures of about 1550°C is

$$3[Al_2(SiO_5)(OH)_4] \rightarrow 3Al_2O_3 \cdot 2SiO_2 + 4SiO_2 + 6H_2O$$
Kaolinite   Mullite   Cristobalite

The refractoriness of fireclays is mainly determined by the $Al_2O_3:SiO_2$ ratio. The effects of differences or changes in this ratio and the temperatures applied are shown in Figure A.2 which is also relevant to other aluminium silicate minerals (see 'Anhydrous aluminium silicates', page 862). The lowest temperatures, 1595°C, at which complete melting occurs (that is, the *eutectic*) corresponds to a composition of 92.5 per cent by weight SiO_2 and 7.5 per cent by weight Al_2O_3. With increasing alumina and silica refractoriness increases. Calcined kaolinite containing a maximum of approximately 45 per cent Al_2O_3 is the chief source of alumina in fireclay. For aluminium silicates in general, containing between 7.5 and 72 per cent Al_2O_3, pure mullite is formed between 1595°C and 1850°C (the melting point of mullite) and its needle-shaped crystals occur in a viscous liquid. As the content of alumina falls and temperature increases, more of the liquid phase is formed. Because the crystals of mullite are hard and elongated, their presence in a refractory product denotes a well-fired body: the more it contains, the greater the density and strength of the body, and the better its refractory properties. However, this simple relationship between alumina content and refractoriness is complicated by the presence of alkalis (K_2O, Na_2O), alkaline earths (CaO, MgO) and iron oxide (FeO) which can significantly lower the temperature of the initial formation of the liquid phase and, thus, greatly reduce the refractoriness of the fireclay. Formation of the liquid phase, for example, begins at 985°C in a mix of K_2O–Al_2O_3–SiO_2. Therefore, a simple model based solely on the content of alumina is not valid when fluxes are present (Highley, 1982).

Cristobalite is seldom present in structural clay products and does not form from the kaolinite of Cornish clay heated to high temperatures because of its high alkali content which produces a glass phase instead.

The importance of the aluminium silicate clay materials in the combustion of coal is discussed in Chapter 13 (page 343).

The term 'fuller's earth' refers to clay that has been extracted in Britain since Roman times and used primarily for cleaning and adsorbing natural oils from woollen cloth (that is, 'fulling') until the latter part of the nineteenth century. Many clays, and sometimes silts, were used for this purpose and, thus, became known as 'fuller's earths'. However, modern analytical methods for identification of clay minerals have shown that the most effective fuller's earths are those that contain a high proportion of clay minerals of the *smectite group* (that is, layered silicate clay minerals distinct from the mica group), the most commonly occurring member of which is *montmorillonite* – the essential constituent of fuller's earth in Britain (see page 861).

There are additional reasons for terminological confusion. The most effective fulling clays are those that are rich in montmorillonite which contains loosely bonded exchangeable cations, usually calcium, magnesium and sodium. Depending upon the dominant cation present, the clay, either as calcium smectite or sodium smectite, has markedly different properties and, thus, different, industrial applications. In Britain clay consisting mainly of calcium montmorillonite is known as fuller's earth, and sodium montmorillonite as bentonite. There are two geological formations in Britain in which clays consist essentially of calcium smectite (more than 60 per cent) and are referred to as fuller's earth: the Jurassic Fuller's Earth Formation and the Lower Greensand. The former, which is generally of lower quality, was worked by underground mining near Bath (Somerset) until 1979 and the latter is currently worked in Surrey (Redhill), Bedfordshire and Oxfordshire by open pit methods. Outside Britain, the term 'bentonite' is used to describe montmorillonite-rich clays irrespective of the dominant cation present. Sodium montmorillonite is comparatively rare world-wide, although large deposits occur in the western USA. Fortunately, however, calcium montmorillonite can easily be converted to sodium montmorillonite by a simple sodium-exchange process. Montmorillonite-rich clays are the alteration products of volcanic ash. In countries other than Britain, particularly the USA, the term 'fuller's earth' applies to any clay that has the capacity to decolorize oil, and may consist of either montmorillonite or *attapulgite* (*palygorskite*) – another clay mineral so named because it was found at Attapulgus, in Georgia, USA (see page 861). Originally these clays were developed as a substitute for fuller's earth imported from England. Both attapulgite and its magnesian analogue, *sepiolite*, are imported into Britain for use as granular adsorbents (Moorlock and Highley, 1991).

Differences and misunderstandings of the nomenclature undoubtedly help to explain the disparity in reports as to whether or not fuller's earth can cause pulmonary fibrosis. It is important, therefore, to recognize that fuller's earths of comparable grade, but from different localities, may exhibit appreciably different properties. The applied properties of an individual clay are dependent on the crystal structure of the clay mineral, itself a function of the geological history of the deposit, and on the nature and amount of impurities present (Moorlock and Highley, 1991). The presence of such impurities, which include quartz, varies widely in different deposits. They are, as a rule, removed by beneficiation from the final products.

Ball clays also consist of kaolinite, mica and quartz, and have similar mixed, mineral assemblages to fireclays. They are more plastic than fireclays and are white, or near-white, on firing due to their low iron content which makes them suitable for the manufacture of whiteware ceramics – their major application.

Shales are indurated clay rocks, which are characterized by a poorly laminated structure parallel to the beading planes along which they split. They represent a further stage in consolidation of clay, mud and organic remains, and include black, carbonaceous shales, associated with coal measures, and oil shales which contain bitumen and a rubbery hydrocarbon called 'kerogen' derived from deposits of aquatic organisms and small plants. When heated to about 500°C kerogen decomposes to produce shale oil, light hydrocarbon gases and a coke-like carbon residue.

All shales contain varying, and sometimes large, quantities of detrital quartz. For example, in some coal measure shales it may exceed 20 per cent; in the Green River Formation oil shales in Colorado, Utah and Wyoming, it is reported to range from 10 to 20 per cent, and in shales used for the manufacture of bricks, pipes and similar materials may be as much as 60 per cent.

The clay minerals are discussed in Chapter 16.

Non-fragmental rocks of organic origin

Limestones

These are chiefly of organic origin and consist mostly of calcium carbonate. Small amounts of magnesium carbonate are often present but when this reaches significant proportions the rock is referred to as dolomitic limestone or *dolomite*. Many different types of organism have contributed to their formation including among others corals, crustacea, foraminifera, molluscs and algae. The calcium carbonate of some limestones, however, is entirely of chemical origin. In general they do not contain any free silica but small amounts are sometimes present as an impurity. However, flint also occurs as nodules in some chalk deposits, and chert in some limestone deposits (see page 843).

Tripoli, rottenstone and wollastonite are found in association with limestones and have a wide variety of applications in industry.

Tripoli is a microcrystalline, very finely grained, particulate form of silica (more than 89 per cent silica) that results from the leaching and weathering of siliceous limestone or calcareous chert. Particles commonly range from 1 to 10 µm in diameter. It should be noted that, commercially, it has sometimes been wrongly referred to as 'amorphous silica' although none has been detected by X-ray or scanning electron microscope analysis (Bradbury and Ehrlinger, 1975).

Either underground or open-cast methods of mining are used for extraction, according to the type and location of the deposit.

Tripoli has many uses: as an abrasive in soaps and cleaning powders; in polishing compounds; as a filler and extender in paints, plastics and rubber; for refractories, ceramic glazes and foundry facings; and as a filler in wallboards and plastic wood.

Rottenstone is a siliceous–argillaceous limestone from which calcium carbonate has been removed in solution. It contains up to 15 per cent quartz and 85 per cent alumina, and has been used in industry as a refractory material and filler.

Wollastonite is a naturally occurring calcium metasilicate ($CaSiO_3$) formed mainly by contact metamorphism of quartz-bearing limestone and by silica-bearing emanations from igneous intrusions

(often granite) reacting with pure or impure limestone. It is used in some countries as a substitute for flint, quartz, sand, feldspar and china clay in ceramic-bonded abrasives, and in other industries (see page 560).

Carbonaceous rocks

Coal Coal is an extremely heterogeneous substance, consisting largely of carbon, hydrogen, oxygen and nitrogen, which is difficult to characterize. In essence it is composed of a number of distinct organic entities, known as 'macerals', and smaller, but important, amounts of minerals. These occur in distinct associations known as *lithotypes*. The basic units, *coal seams*, in which coal is found consist of layers of coal lithotypes; individual seams often have a unique set of physical and chemical properties. Even if two coal seams have a similar composition of macerals and minerals, the seams may have significantly different properties if the lithotypes in the two seams differ (Crelling, 1989). Coal seams comprise a small proportion (1 to 2 per cent) of the Upper Carboniferous rocks and are known as *coal measures*.

Coals are the products of progressive change ('coalification') in accumulations of rotting vegetation (trees, ferns, giant club mosses) in swampy conditions. These are subsequently overlaid by deposits of sediment from inundation from rivers, lakes or seas, resulting in layers of sandstones, clays, shales and limestones. Accumulated sediment consolidates the vegetable debris and squeezes out water to form coal of progressively increasing maturity as depth increases. The organic-rich petrographic components produced by progressive rotting of macerated vegetation – the *macerals* just referred to – can be regarded as the organic counterparts of the mineral matter in coal. A large number of macerals have been defined. They are derived from different parts of plants and trees degraded under critical conditions and are optically homogeneous aggregates with distinctive physical and chemical properties. There are, however, three main groups: *vitrinites*, *liptinites* and *inertines*. Most of these contain between 73 and 85 per cent carbon with more widely differing quantities of hydrogen and oxygen.

The degree of maturity of coal is referred to, and classified, as *rank*. All coal begins as peat which is then changed into progressively higher ranks – *lignite, sub-bituminous, bituminous* and *anthracite* coals. This transformation occurs in two phases: the first at the peat stage when most of the plant material in the peat is biochemically altered (*diagenesis*), although spores and pollens survive without much change; the second, during which altered peat is buried and subjected to the geological forces of temperature, pressure and time. Temperature, which rises with increasing depth and pressure, is the chief factor in coalification which takes place between 50°C and 150°C and results in devolatization and the formation of bituminous and higher rank coals.

As rank of coal increases most of its properties change: moisture, volatile matter and ultimate oxygen decrease; fixed and ultimate carbon, calorific value and reflectance increase. *Reflectance of coal* is a characteristic based upon the amount of light that is reflected from vitrinite macerals in the coal under examination, compared with a glass standard of known refractive index and reflectance. All of these properties have been used as a measure of rank but reflectance is the most reliable because, unlike the others, it changes uniformly across most of the coal-rank range (Crelling, 1989). However, in medical research, the definition of rank normally used is the ratio of carbon to volatile matter in the coal – the so-called *fuel ratio*. In high-rank anthracite, the content of carbon is high (approximately 92 to 95 per cent), and that of volatile substances very low; at the other end of the scale, low-rank lignite contains much less carbon (65 to 75 per cent) but a greater quantity of volatile substances (Table A.3).

Although spore cases, either empty or filled with mineral matter, may have survived intact in some coals, organic matter with immunogenic potential does not appear to exist in bituminous or anthracite coals.

Coal contains considerable quantities of important minerals which decrease as rank increases, due to leaching, *but are never absent even in coal of the highest rank*. They are deposited both during its formation in peat swamps by influx of mineral-containing waters and, in some regions, by fall-out of volcanic ash, and after it has been formed also as a result of seepage of mineral-containing waters from a distance. The amounts present vary widely but commercial coal, in general, must contain less than 10 per cent mineral matter as ash. The most common accessory minerals are clays, quartz, pyrite and calcite; trace metals are also usually present but with great variability in their nature and amount in different coal seams and in the same seam. The clay minerals and quartz account for between 60 and 90 per cent of the total non-coal mineral matter in coals; the most common species of clay minerals are muscovite–illites (potassium aluminium silicates), kaolinites (aluminium silicates) and mixed-layer illite–montmorillonites of variable composition (Raask, 1985).

There appears to be no clear correlation between the inorganic content of coals and their maceral composition which indicates that most minerals were introduced by detrition rather than accumulating as a result of peat degradation. Where a transport mechanism for detritus existed, detrital

Table A.3 Carbon content of coals

Coal type	Rank	Composition (%) (dry mineral matter-free basis)		
		Carbon	Hydrogen	Oxygen
Peat		50–65	5–7	30–40
Lignite	(Low)	65–75	5–6	20–30
Sub-bituminous	↓	75–80	5–6	13–20
Bituminous	(Intermediate)	80–90	4.9–5.7	5–15
Semi-bituminous	↓	90–92	4.5–4.9	4–5
Anthracite	(High)	92–95	2–4	2–4

material occurs in the peat in considerable amounts and, thus, in varying quantity in the subsequent ranks of coal (Davis et al., 1984). Silica usually occurs in coal seams in the form of discrete, fine grains of quartz and, sometimes, cristobalite from ash fall-out in volcanic regions or chalcedony formed by weathering of feldspar and mica (Mackowsky, 1968). The clay minerals originated from deposited detritus, transformation of other clay minerals and precipitation of a gel or solution (Davis et al., 1984).

The great variability in the distribution of mineral species in different coal strata is exemplified in coal fields in the east Midlands of the UK. Examination of more than 50 seams showed that: quartz, kaolin and mica were the principal non-coal minerals in all seam-profiles; quartz was more abundant in roof and floor strata and least in the coal layers and interseam strata; the highest concentrations of kaolin occurred in the coal and some interseam dirt bands; and 20 to 90 per cent of mineral matter in the coal seam consisted of non-silicate minerals (Raask, 1985). The majority of US coals have a quartz content of between 1 and 20 per cent of the total mineral matter, and some coal ashes have over 30 per cent quartz (Raask, 1985).

Accessory minerals in coal, including quartz, are disseminated as discrete particles ranging from submicrometre to more than 1 mm in size, but their mean grain size is about 5 μm, so that most of them are near, or below, the resolution of the optical microscope, and they are intimately intermixed with maceral material (Finkelman, 1988). In their identification it is difficult to recognize fine-grained minerals that are intimately mixed with the coal matter by the petrological microscope. Therefore, carefully controlled low-temperature ashing (LTA), which has the advantage of providing a relatively unchanged sample for the identification of its constituent minerals, is employed to prepare samples that are substantially free of organic matter. However, the yield of ash is slightly lower than the mineral matter in the coal chiefly because of losses of water and gaseous products of decomposition of some minerals, depending on the temperature of the ashing (Swaine, 1990). A variety of methods for identification is employed. These include scanning electron microscopy (SEM), energy dispersive X-ray analysis (EDXA), combined SEM–EDXA and infrared spectrophotometry (see Appendix V). The SEM–EDXA system appears to be the best for studying accessory minerals and their relationships with macerals in situ (Finkelman, 1988). But it is important to stress that, although the minerals in coal are readily identified by these techniques, accurate determination of their quantities has not yet been achieved (Crelling, 1989).

Beneficiation of coal To improve the quality of coal for commercial purposes, removal or lessening of unwanted run-of-mine, non-coal constituents is required, that is, beneficiation. The processes involved are often referred to as 'coal cleaning' or 'coal washing'. It is important to understand exactly what this means because, in medical literature, it is commonly supposed that washing with water frees coal of all non-coal minerals producing, in effect, 'pure coal' (see Chapter 13, page 342). The facts are otherwise.

Extraneous run-of-mine dirt and relatively large mineral particles or clusters of minerals are readily removed by washing, but finely divided particles, especially when embedded in coaly matter, are impossible to remove by the methods normally used for large-scale beneficiation based on density separations in water (Swaine, 1990). This is due to the fact that the vast majority of mineral matter in coal is insoluble in water as well as being so intimately mixed with macerals and other coal material that, unless the coal is finely ground (which is generally impractical in industry), most of the mineral matter is inaccessible to water (J.W. Patrick, 1992, personal communication). But such grinding fails to remove fine-grained particles that are encapsulated in organic coaly matter. For the same reasons, methods of beneficiation that depend on separation by differences in specific gravity are unpredictable (Finkelman and Gluskoter, 1983).

Thus, industrial beneficiation has little, if any, effect in removing small particles of quartz (or other polymorphs of silica) and clay silicates from within coals (J.W. Patrick, 1992, personal communication); trace elements, many of which are associated with the clay minerals, are only partially freed (Swaine, 1990) (see Chapter 13, 'Coal trimming'). The definitive separation of coal into coal and non-coal minerals that is often implied in medical literature is, therefore, an over-simplification that overlooks this intimate relationship.

In laboratory conditions coal can be very finely milled and treated with hydrochloric and hydrofluoric acids. This 'demineralized' coal has been widely used in coal laboratories for experiments in which

mineral matter would interfere significantly (J.W. Patrick, 1992, personal communication). However, such techniques for the production of samples of coal dust for animal experiments do not seem to have been described in the medical literature, although finely ground anthracite ('pulverized coal') has been used in some reported inhalation experiments.

Compositional changes caused by the combustion (complete or incomplete) and carbonization of coal – namely, fuel ash and fly ash, pitches, cokes and polycyclic hydrocarbons – are discussed in Chapters 13 and 19.

The close association of some coal measures with mudstones (fireclays and ganisters) and shales has been discussed earlier (see 'Argillaceous rocks').

Bitumens These, in essence, are hydrocarbons of the paraffin and naphthalene series, different proportions of which occur in different bitumens. They include members ranging from a very liquid, light yellow oil through gradations to solid bitumens.

Natural petroleum and crude oil These are usually found in sandstones and dolomites and seldom in relation to coal measures. They were probably formed from the remains of minute marine organisms in deep muddy seas. Oil shales have been referred to earlier.

Asphalt or mineral pitch This is a mixture of different hydrocarbons that occurs as a black semisolid or solid substance at or near the surface of the earth. It may occur as lakes (notably in Trinidad) or impregnations of sandstones or dolomites (*rock asphalt*) in which as much as 15 per cent of asphalt may be present. Asphaltic rocks have, until recently, been worked for extraction of asphalt or for natural paving, flooring and roofing material especially in the USA, France, Germany and Italy. It is possible that the working of impregnated sandstones (blasting, crushing and grading) may have presented a silica hazard. Synthetic mastic asphalt is discussed in Chapter 12, page 290.

Siliceous deposits

Diatomite

Also referred to as *diatomaceous earth* and *kieselguhr*, diatomite is the most important member of the group. It consists principally of the fossilized skeletal remains of diatoms, unicellular aquatic plants of the class Bacillariophyceae, related to the algae. It is, in fact, a rock formed by induration of diatomaceous silica, a biogenic *amorphous silica* closely resembling opal or hydrous silica ($SiO_2 \cdot nH_2O$), secreted by the walls of the cells of living diatoms. Diatomaceous silica is, however, not entirely pure hydrous silica. Particles of rock-forming minerals may be integrated as part of diatomite rock, sand, feldspar, clay and volcanic ash being some of the typical contaminants. Indeed, diatomites that are richest in silica are associated with vulcanism. Analysis of quarry samples (source not stated) by Vorwald et al. (1949) revealed 75 per cent diatomite, 2 to 3 per cent crystalline free silica of which 2 per cent was quartz and 0.3 per cent cristobalite, and 14 per cent feldspar and clay silicates. Thus, these polymorphs of silica may be present in some natural diatomite deposits. In addition, commercial diatomite may contain fossilized fragments and particles of organisms such as Radiolaria and siliceous sponges (Kadey, 1975).

Diatomite forms in fresh-water and marine conditions and is deposited in beds in large, shallow ponds and lakes, and in proximity to collections of volcanic ash. It is usually extracted by quarrying or open pit mining, though underground methods are used in some small operations.

Cryptocrystalline silica

Layers of cryptocrystalline silica formed by chemical precipitation are exemplified by some forms of chalcedonic silica, flint and chert, in which remnants of tests of Radiolaria or sponge spicules are sometimes found (see page 843); and by *sinter* that is formed around the mouths of volcanic geysers and some hot springs.

Non-fragmental rocks of chemical origin

Saline deposits

These were formed by precipitation in dried-up, enclosed bodies of salt water from seas and lakes, and they include *calcite*, *rock salt*, *apatite* [$Ca_5F(PO_4)_3$ and $Ca_5Cl(PO_4)_3$], *anhydrite* ($CaSO_4$), gypsum, *carnallite* ($KMgCl_3 \cdot 6H_2O$) and a form of calcium carbonate known as *aragonite*.

Gypsum needs further comment. It was formed in three ways:

1. As pure saline residues caused by the evaporation of enclosed basins of sea water, notably in Germany and the USA.
2. In association with alteration of limestones to dolomite.
3. As a result of the action of sulphuric acid generated by decomposition of pyrite on $CaCO_3$ in clays such as mudstones and shales which, as stated earlier, contain variable amounts of fine-grained quartz – 30 per cent being fairly common. Deposits of this type occur in the UK in Sussex and Nottingham but the associated silica is higher in the former than the latter (see Chapters 11 and 12).

Gypsum occurs mainly in tabular, prismatic or acicular habit but a variety called *satin spar* has a silky, fibrous form.

Ferruginous deposits

Iron from aqueous solutions or iron-storing bacteria is found in two forms.

Bedded ironstones These are deposits in which iron was deposited in mudstones and limestones as *glauconite* (hydrous silicate of iron and potassium), *hematite* (Fe_2O_3) and *limonite* ($Fe_2O_3 \cdot H_2O$).

Hematite from overlying ferruginous sandstones replaces the limestone in limestone beds in various geological locations – for example, in Cumbria and north Lancashire – and, thus, contains quartz which may become air-borne during underground mining operations. The largest of the world's deposits, in Lake Superior District of Minnesota, was formed by the alteration and concentration of iron silicates of sedimentary origin. The term 'taconite' was used originally to refer to a hard, fine-grained, banded, iron-bearing rock (not a mineral) in this region which contains magnetite and hematite or both, either banded or disseminated with cherty rocks. But, in recent years, it has been applied more generally to low-grade, iron–quartz, iron ores that can be beneficiated and agglomerated to produce high-grade, iron-containing pellets. Hence, mining and beneficiation of hematite and taconite rock may be associated with exposure to dust containing quartz or chert. (But see page 287 in regard to taconite.)

Bog iron ore This consists of an impure ferruginous deposit formed in swampy ground and associated with clay which often underlies it. The mineral composition includes limonite, siderite ($FeCO_3$), iron sulphate and iron silicate. Quartz is usually absent. Limonite and siderite are found in many bituminous coals throughout the world. Siderite forms the clay ironstones that are associated with some coal measures in Britain, notably South Wales, Staffordshire and Durham.

The optical properties of limonite and siderite are mentioned briefly in Appendix IV ('Polarized light microscopy').

Metamorphic rocks

Only examples of these rocks that are important in industry are considered. They differ widely in type and origin.

Table A.4 Asbestiform and non-asbestiform varieties of asbestos

Asbestiform variety	Chemical composition	Non-asbestiform variety
Serpentine group		
Chrysotile	$3MgO, 2SiO_2, 2H_2O$	Antigorite, lizardite
Amphibole group		
Crocidolite	$Na_2O, Fe_2O_3, 3FeO, 8SiO_2, H_2O$	Riebeckite
Grunerite asbestos (amosite)	$5.5FeO, 1.5MgO, 8SiO_2, H_2O$	Cummingtonite–grunerite
Anthophyllite asbestos	$7MgO, 8SiO_2, H_2O$	Anthophyllite
Tremolite asbestos	$2CaO, 5MgO, 8SiO_2, H_2O$	Tremolite
Actinolite asbestos	$2CaO, 4MgO, FeO, 8SiO_2, H_2O$	Actinolite

Reproduced, with modifications, from Kelse and Thompson (1989) by permission of the American Hygiene Association.

The asbestos group

'Asbestos' is a collective term that refers to two large, but different, groups of rock-forming minerals and not to one family, nor to a particular type of rock. It is, rather, a commercial term applied to two groups of silicate minerals – *serpentines* and *amphiboles* – that are capable of separating readily into long, thin, strong fibres which have many invaluable properties and industrial applications (Figures A.3 and A.4, and see Figure 14.1). The non-fibrous variants of these minerals are not equated with asbestos.

Serpentines

Chrysotile, the sole fibrous variety of the group, has a growth form that is readily distinguishable from the non-asbestos serpentines such as antigorite and lizardite (Table A.4). It is the most abundant type of asbestos. Most chrysotiles formed in ultrabasic rocks in which olivines and pyroxenes were altered to serpentine by hydrothermal action – a process completed by intrusion of acid magma and subsequent further hydrothermal action. Talc and magnetite are common impurities and, in some geological regions (for example, Québec, Canada and the Xeros-Troodos area in Cyprus), intergrowths of the amphiboles tremolite and actinolite occur in the ore body. Although tremolite occurs in commercial chrysotile in only small quantities (less than 1 per cent), unlike chrysotile, it is apt to resist leaching and decomposition in biological systems for very long periods of time (Hodgson, 1986).

Amphiboles

The paragenesis of amphibole asbestos (*crocidolite, amosite, anthophyllite, tremolite* and *actinolite*) occurred at a higher metamorphic grade than that of chrysotile, thus forming minerals with a lower content of water of crystallization. Bulk formations of tremolite and anthophyllite, and some actinolite, are derived from direct metamorphism of pyroxenites with associated silica by igneous activity, but, at the same time, there are localized transitions, particularly to tremolite, in chrysotile-bearing serpentine rocks. Amosite and crocidolite formed in banded ironstones by chemical reaction and crystallization from original iron hydroxides and colloidal silica under conditions of very high hydrostatic compression and shear. Some actinolite fibre formed in similar conditions.

To mineralogists, the term 'asbestos' implies a pattern of fibrous crystal growth described as the 'asbestiform' or *fibrous habit* although these minerals also occur in nature in non-asbestiform (nonfibrous) habit. Whereas chrysotile has a growth and internal crystal structure that is readily distinguishable from non-asbestos, rock-forming serpentines (Zussman, 1957), both the asbestiform and nonasbestiform rock-forming analogues of the amphiboles have the same composition and internal crystal structure; in the case of tremolite, anthophylite and actinolite, they have the same names (Table A.4). This, undoubtedly, has sometimes been, and may still be, a source of misinterpretation and error in mineralogical analyses of samples of

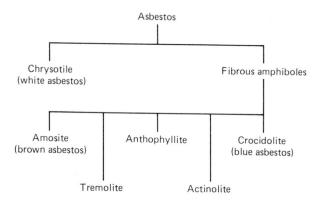

Figure A.3 Classification chart of the asbestos minerals

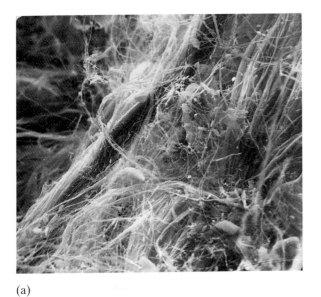

(a)

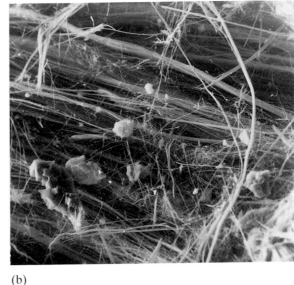

(b)

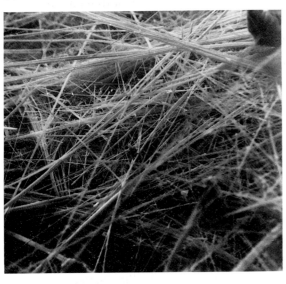

(c)

Figure A.4 Stereoscan electron micrographs of chrysotile (a), crocidolite (b) and amosite (c). Magnification × 550. Compare with electron micrographs in Figure 14.1a–c. (By courtesy of Cape Asbestos Fibres Ltd)

dust both in the workplace and in the lungs. The basic differences between the two patterns of crystal growth are summarized graphically in Figure A.5, and two examples of microscopic differences are seen in Figure A.6. Rock-forming, non-asbestiform tremolite, anthophyllite and actinolite are of more common occurrence than their asbestiform counterparts.

Asbestos fibres are characterized by high length-to-breadth ratios (*aspect ratios*), by flexibility and often, being curved with splayed ends, by a higher tensile strength than the non-asbestiform habits of the same material, and by aggregation in parallel or radiating bundles from which the fibres can easily be separated (Zoltai and Wylie, 1979). A variety of habits occurs in the non-asbestos amphiboles, the

growth-forms ranging from blocked, straight-edged laths to acicular (needle-like) particles. As for other rock-forming silicates, they all exhibit prismatic cleavage, the microscopic fragments of which have parallel edges after comminution by grinding. At times it may be difficult to distinguish these particles from small, short fibres (less than 1 μm in diameter or 5 μm in length) – which also have parallel edges – by optical microscopy, although they are readily differentiated by scanning electron microscopy (SEM) and transmission electron microscopy (TEM), which renders the fibrils making up each fibre visible (see Appendix V).

As pointed out in Chapter 14 (page 411), the morphological definition of a fibre given by mineralogists rests on the aspect ratio of the particle being

(a)

Asbestiform

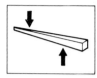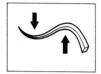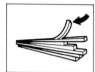

(b)

Nonasbestiform

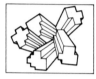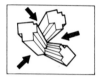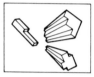

Figure A.5 Graphic representation of the distinction between the (a) asbestiform and (b) non-asbestiform habits. (a) In the asbestiform habit, mineral crystals grow in a single dimension, in a straight line, until they form long, thread-like fibres with aspect ratios of 20:1 to 1000:1 and higher. When pressure is applied, the fibres do not shatter but simply bend much like a wire. Fibrils of a smaller diameter are produced as bundles of fibres are pulled apart. This bundling effect is referred to as polyfilamentous. Milling breaks longer into shorter fibres and reduces their diameter. (b) In the non-asbestiform variety, crystal growth is random, forming multidimensional prismatic patterns. When pressure is applied, the crystal fractures easily, fragmenting to prismatic particles. Some of the particles or cleavage fragments are acicular or needle-shaped as a result of the tendency of amphibole minerals to cleave along the two dimensions, but not along the third. Stair-step cleavage along the edges of some particles is common, and oblique extinction is exhibited under the microscope. Cleavage fragments never show curvature. (Reproduced from Kelse and Thompson (1989) by permission of the American Hygiene Association)

10:1 or more. The American Society for Testing and Materials, in fact, proposed that mineral particles 'are not demonstrated to be asbestos, in the absence of further analysis, if their length-to-width ratio is less than 20:1' (Ross, Kuntze and Clifton, 1984); indeed, populations of fibres of asbestiform minerals generally have aspect ratios ranging from 20:1 to 100:1 or higher, and lengths in excess of 5 μm (Kelse and Thompson, 1989). However, differentiation between asbestiform and non-asbestiform amphiboles (cleavage fragments) tends to be blurred when, due to comminution, most of the particles in a sample are less than 1 μm in diameter and 5 μm in length. Even so, cleavage fragments of these minerals are entirely distinct from a similar sized group of asbestos particles (Pooley, 1987; Langer, Nolan and Pooley, 1990; Schenk, Gobb and Kolmer, 1990). They can, for example, be differentiated by a systematic approach to the analysis of particles using electron microscopy with selected area electron diffraction (SAED) (Lee and Fisher,

1979) or high-resolution TEM. If, using such methods, a specimen contains elongated cleavage fragments some of which have the same widths and lengths as asbestos fibres, 'elongated cleavage fragments will have a greater variation in diameter as a function of length than asbestos, tending to have lower aspect ratios' (Langer, Nolan and Addison, 1990) (Table A.5).

The morphological difference between asbestiform and non-asbestiform particles is of capital importance in the pathogenesis of disease (see Chapter 14). But, unfortunately, it has been confused and obscured by a recent redefinition of 'asbestos', for regulatory health purposes (chiefly air-borne particles), by the US Occupational Safety and Health Administration (OSHA) (1986) and the National Institute for Occupational Safety and Health (NIOSH), and supported, particularly in relation to tremolite, by the American Thoracic Society (1990). It defines asbestos as mineral fibres of crystalline hydrated silicates that are 5 μm or more in length and with an aspect ratio greater than 3:1; although the OSHA statement recognizes the difference between asbestiform and non-asbestiform habits, it does not specify methods for their differentiation. Thus, elongated, cleavage fragments with these dimensions become 'asbestos fibres'; indeed, the new rule states that the non-asbestiform variants of tremolite, anthophyllite and actinolite are to be treated *as if* they were asbestos. Apart from this redefinition being a frank departure from established mineralogical taxonomy, it implies that both variants have similar biological effects, although there is no evidence that non-asbestiform amphiboles have the same pathogenic properties as asbestos (McDonald et al., 1978; Cooper, Otto Wong and Graebner, 1988) (see Chapter 14). In this respect it is pertinent to note that most elongated (acicular) amphibole cleavage fragments have aspect ratios less than 10:1 and are small enough to be completely ingested by alveolar macrophages (see Chapter 1, page 14 and Chapter 14).

Detailed size distribution of particles obtained by counting from SEM observations can distinguish one type of asbestos from another (Campbell, Huggins and Wylie, 1980). Table A.5 shows that, as aspect ratio increases, the length of particles increases up to 6 μm. It will also be observed that the aspect ratio for non-fibrous tremolite (cleavage fragments) is substantially less than 3:1. In general, this investigation 'gives considerable weight to the extension of aspect ratios well above the currently acceptable 3:1 ratio for purposes of counting by optical microscopy' (Hodgson, 1986). In fact, it has been categorically asserted that a particle with an aspect ratio of 3:1 cannot be considered to be a fibre (Kelse and Thompson, 1989; Langer, Nolan and Addison, 1991). Figure A.7 shows, in a graphic form, a clear distinction between the aspect ratios of

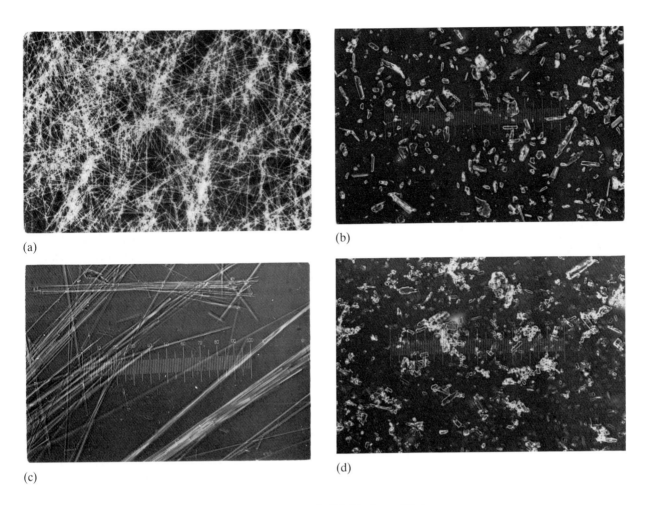

Figure A.6 Examples of asbestiform (a,c) and non-asbestiform (b,d) habits in amphiboles with different names (a,b) and the same name (c,d). (a) Amosite; (b) cummingtonite–grunerite; (c) tremolite; (d) tremolite. Magnification × 265; 2.75 μm per division. (Reproduced from Kelse and Thompson (1989) by permission of the American Hygiene Association)

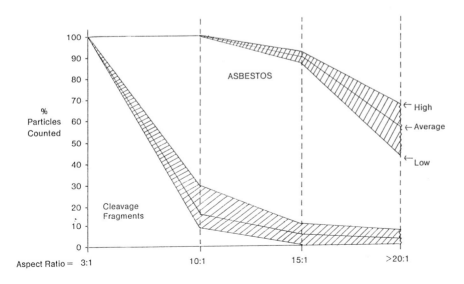

Figure A.7 Air-borne asbestos versus cleavage fragment aspect ratio comparison (particles with an aspect ratio of 3:1 or greater, >5 μm length, >0.25 μm width). Note that the majority of cleavage fragments do not fall into this range (most reflect lengths of <5 μm). The 100 per cent value therefore represents the starting point for 3:1 aspect ratio particles counting and not the total percentage of air-borne cleavage fragments. (Reproduced from Kelse and Thompson (1989) by permission of the American Hygiene Association)

Table A.5 Particle size distributions by SEM

Length range (µm)	Percentage particles by aspect ratio				
	1:1 to 3:1	3:1 to 5:1	5:1 to 10:1	10:1 to 20:1	20:1 to 50:1
Chrysotile					
0–1	25	18	50	7	
1–2	2	4	24	52	16
2–3		1	5	34	50
3–4			2	22	60
4–5				5	71
5–6				6	47
Representing 55% of all particles					
Amosite					
0–2	12	34	43	11	
2–4		10	52	34	4
4–6		6	23	52	18
Representing 26% of all particles					
Crocidolite					
0–1	12	64	24		
1–2	2	15	60	23	
2–3		2	25	57	15
3–4			21	64	15
4–5			2	51	46
5–6			3	36	58
Representing 60% of all particles					
Tremolite (non-fibrous)					
0–1	100				
1–2	92	8			
2–3	75	22	3		
3–4	67	29	4		
4–5	76	18	6		
5–6	67	30	3		
>10	35	37	18	4	
Representing 85% of all particles, below 6 µm					

From Hodgson (1986) after Campbell, Huggins and Wylie (1980) with permission.

asbestiform particles and cleavage fragments. Unfortunately, the criterion of a 3:1 aspect ratio has been widely employed for some years by pathologists for interpreting the significance of mineral particles in human lungs, often with erroneous conclusions.

Commercial asbestos, in general, is subjected to some form or other of processing to increase its degree of 'fiberization' before it is applied in industry. This results in some reduction in the proportion of long fibres, an increase in that of short fibres, and decrease in the upper limit of the diameter of fibres (Hodgson, 1986). Nonetheless, a significant number of fibres longer than 10 µm, with aspect ratios greater than 10:1, are present in all commercial grades of asbestos, and it is these that are of biological importance. For this reason, and because the presence of a substantial number of short particles or of a few large particles in a sample has a disproportionate distorting effect, in opposite directions, on particle distribution data, the necessity for careful measurement of size distribution in samples used for biological research has been emphasized. It is neces-sary to correlate the number of particles in any size range to the weight of the sample; any method used for analysing fibre size must be capable of measuring both long and short fibres (Campbell, Higgins and Wylie, 1980) (see Appendix V, 'Bulk or microanalysis'). This has to be borne in mind when evaluating reports in the medical literature.

Thus, strict mineralogical definitions and criteria of asbestiform and non-asbestiform habits and of fibres (aspect ratio in excess of 10:1) must always be observed when studying (or interpreting) the biological effects of minerals and their presence in the lungs, both animal and human.

Hydrous magnesium silicates

Talc (french chalk)

This is a hydrated magnesium silicate which was formed by regional metamorphic processes applied to dolomitic limestones and ultrabasic igneous rocks. It may take the form of flat, polygonal, flaky plates, granules or short 'fibres'. These are not true fibres, however, but rolled up, flat, talc plates – an example of pseudomorphism. The formation of talc was closely akin to that of the production of asbestos minerals and, in fact, the amphiboles actinolite, anthophyllite and tremolite may be present as accessory minerals with talc which is then often referred to as *asbestine*; in addition, chlorites, calcite, dolomite, magnesite, magnetite, pyrite, pyrophyllite (see next section) and quartz may be present. The amount of quartz varies from negligible to about 20 per cent in some deposits (Weiss and Boettner, 1967). Talc and serpentine share a common origin from metamorphosed ultrabasic rocks but, in the majority of talc deposits, talc has replaced serpentine; hence, chrysotile is rarely found as an accessory mineral.

Analysis of bulk talc samples imported into the UK has shown that quartz is a fairly common contaminant in minor amounts (1 to 2 per cent by weight), although it exceeded 5 per cent in one sample; an asbestiform tremolite was an uncommon finding, but chrysotile was absent. No other varieties of asbestos minerals were detected (Pooley and Rowlands, 1977).

Hence, most commercial talc is not a pure mineral. Some examples of 'talc' may contain substantial quantities of quartz and others may consist to a large extent of tremolite (in both asbestiform and non-asbestiform habits) or talcose anthophyllite. This wide variation in the identity and quantity of accessory minerals which depends upon the source of the talc deposits is undoubtedly an important determinant of the pathogenesis and variable characteristics of 'talc' pneumoconiosis (see Chapter 16). The term 'asbestiform talc' is sometimes found in medical literature. It is misleading and inaccurate, and should not be used.

Talc has a low refractive index and is strongly birefringent. Its plate-like habit is not destroyed by grinding.

For industrial use, talcs which are virtually free of all impurities are known as 'high grade' and those in which impurities may be as much as 50 per cent, as 'low grade'. The term 'steatite' (*soapstone*) has long been applied to an impure, massive form of talc which can be quarried in large blocks, but it is now often used to designate especially pure forms of talc for industry.

Palygorskite (attapulgite) and sepiolite

These are clay materials derived by metamorphism, often hydrothermal, from montmorillonites, amphiboles and pyroxenes. Large deposits exist in the USA. They occur as lath-like particles and fine, very short, intertwined fibres. The compact variety of sepiolite is known as *meerschaum* (see page 557).

Vermiculite

Although a hydrous magnesium silicate, it contains varying amounts of iron and aluminium. It is derived from biotite and phlogopite mica (see page 846) by hydrothermal metamorphism but, probably more often from chlorite, an altered product of biotite, itself altered by surface waters and weathering. It occurs as thin plates, similar to talc, and granules, and is often classed with clay minerals when, in very fine particulate form, it has some of the appearance of the montmorillonite group.

Hydrous aluminium silicates (see Chapter 16)

China clay (kaolin)

This finely divided aluminium silicate (kaolinite) is formed by hydrothermal and pneumatolytic attack on the feldspars of granites in some regions, notably Cornwall and Devon in the UK, but otherwise results from ordinary weathering and sedimentation of the feldspar. Thus, most of the commercial china clay in the USA is not metamorphic in origin. In advanced stages of the hydrothermal metamorphism, only quartz may remain unaltered in powdery feldspar so that it is present in significant, although variable, quantities. This is the form of china clay most suitable to the ceramic industry. The content of quartz in Cornish china clay is under 1 per cent and that of ball clays up to 25 per cent.

It is relevant to point out here that *china stone* is a largely kaolinized granite composed principally of feldspar and quartz in which the relative absence of iron-bearing minerals makes it suitable for use as a flux in ceramic manufacture. It occurs in general association with metamorphic china clay but is worked separately. Its content of quartz is that of granite – about 25 per cent.

The smectite group

The term 'smectite' is used, for convenience, as a group name for montmorillonite (by far the most common) and other hydrous aluminium silicates – beidelite, saponite, hectorite and sauconite – because of confusion concerning the meaning of montmorillonite and the difficulty in distinguishing mineralogically between the other species.

All montmorillonites are essentially volcanic in origin and are altered either by weathering of airborne deposits of ash at considerable distances from their origin (for example, bentonites in England and Wyoming, USA) or by decomposition in situ, often under marine conditions. Thus, cristobalite and some poorly ordered forms of silica, and other minerals, are present in many deposits – as in western USA.

Pyrophyllite ('fire-stone')

This is closely similar in origin, structure and properties and is commercially included with, and defines as, 'talc'. However, aluminium replaces the magnesium of talc in its composition and, unlike talc, it does not fuse when fired and, thus, is valuable for refractory purposes; it is also used as a ceramic raw material and paint extender. It undergoes dehydroxylation at about 800°C to give a metastable phase which, on heating in excess of 1100°C, forms a felted mass of cristobalite and mullite needles.

Pyrophyllite is found in metamorphosed volcanic rocks of acid composition. Quartz and sericite are the chief impurities. It occurs as fine-grained, foliated lamellae with platy cleavage, as compact masses of small crystals and, less often, as aggregates of radiating needle-like crystals. All have a low refractive index and are strongly birefringent.

It is mined by open-cast and underground methods.

Anhydrous aluminium silicates (see Chapter 16)

These comprise a trio of metamorphic minerals – *kyanite*, *sillimanite* and *andalusite* – all of which have the same composition ($Al_2O_3 \cdot SiO_2$), and *mullite*. Industrially, kyanite is the most important of the trio because it is available in large, easily accessible deposits.

Kyanite, which was formed by regional and hydrothermal metamorphism in granite and pegmatite intrusions, occurs as long, thin, bladed crystals. Large deposits are exploited in India where it is found in schist associated with quartz and pegmanites. In the USA it is disseminated in quartzite.

Sillimanite, also known as *fibrolite*, occurs in argillaceous rocks, schists and slates as long, acicular crystals that shatter readily, as slender prismatic crystals and as wispy, fibrous aggregates.

Andalusite occurs as nearly square prismatic crystals in metamorphosed clayey rocks, in some slates and as an accessory mineral in granite.

All are used, either raw or calcined, in heavy duty, refractory materials. The low electrical conductivity of sillimanite is exploited in porcelain for electrical equipment.

When any of these minerals is heated to temperatures of about 1300°C to 1600°C they are converted to mullite and cristobalite (see Figure A.2). (See Chapter 16 and 'Argillaceous (clayey) rocks' later.)

The presence of stable cristobalite probably explains pulmonary fibrosis that has been attributed to sillimanite in some reports in the past (for example, Jötten and Eickhoff, 1944).

Mullite ($3Al_2O_3 \cdot 2SiO_2$)

This is of exceptionally rare occurrence in nature being found originally in shales fused by immersion in basic magma in the Isle of Mull, Scotland. However, in synthetic form (the basis of a large industry), it is greatly valued as a 'superduty' refractory with irreversible expansion characteristics which compensate for shrinkage of other mineral components after firing, and for electrical and chemical porcelain. It is stable at temperatures up to 1800°C. It occurs as weakly birefringent crystals of long prismatic habit, laths or needles, but not in fibrous form.

Most calcined kaolins (china clay) such as those used in paper, paints and plastics, however, do not contain mullite because the temperatures to which they are subjected are too low.

Mullite in pulverized fuel ash is discussed in Chapter 13 and in Chapter 16 (page 554).

The consequences of heating aluminium silicates in various circumstances is described earlier (see 'Argillaceous (clayey) rocks', page 849).

Quartzites

These are formed either by thermal, contact metamorphism of sandstones which recrystallizes their quartz grains into an interlocking mosaic of quartz crystals or by regional metamorphism of detrital sandy rocks, which consist of small grains of quartz cemented by a scanty bond of silica and other minerals such as calcium carbonate and iron oxide. The content of quartz in both is very high, especially in the sedimentary type. Sands formed from these rocks are often called 'quartzite sands'.

Slates

Shales and mudstones containing quartz grains and clay minerals were compressed and flattened by considerable lateral forces (low-grade regional metamorphism) resulting in a re-orientation of their crystalline structure to form a rock with well-developed and fine cleavage. The quartz content of all slates is usually high, being about 30 to 45 per cent by weight. The production of commercial slate powders results in a slight loss; thus, for example, powdered Cornish slate contains about 25 per cent quartz, and powdered slate from North Wales, eastern Pennsylvania and eastern New York State about 30 per cent.

Schists

These rocks are composed largely of flaky minerals such as mica, chlorite and talc or prismatic minerals such as hornblende, characterized by parallel lamellation, which were subjected to medium-grade regional metamorphism. This process greatly altered the structure of sedimentary and igneous rocks rendering them more plastic. Some sedimentary rocks formed mica–schists and igneous rocks recrystallized to form hornblende–schists or amphiboles.

Gneisses

The most intense metamorphism – high-grade metamorphism – completely transformed various existing rocks into these coarse-grained, roughly banded rocks which are composed essentially of pyroxenes, feldspar, quartz, biotite mica and hornblende in varying proportions. Quartzo-feldspathic layers alternate with mica-rich layers.

Marbles

These are the results of thorough recrystallization of limestone by thermal and regional metamorphism which obliterated their sedimentary and fossiliferous features. Pure limestone (more than 99 per cent calcium carbonate) yielded white marble – such as Italian Carra Marble. But, if the parent rock was impure limestone or a dolomitic limestone (a mixture of calcium carbonate and calcium magnesium carbonate), prominent, streaky colouring resulted. Most marbles contain several per cent of other minerals. Chief among the non-silicate impurities are quartz, graphite, limonite, hematite and pyrite, and among the silicates, mica chlorite, non-asbestiform tremolite, hornblende, diopside and wollastonite. Thus, most marbles, other than those that contain quartz, are unlikely to present a hazard.

It is important, however, to note that, commercially, 'marble' is usually any stone other than granite, and mostly sedimentary, which is of attractive appearance and takes a polish. Geologically, it is not marble (see Chapter 11, page 280).

Mineral ores

These originated in a number of ways: by early crystallization from magma and then separation – for example, *chromite* ($FeCr_2O_4$); by percolation and subsequent solidification of magmatic gas or liquid in pockets within native rock which was often of igneous type (for example, *beryl, copper, gold, lead, silver, tin, zinc*); and by subterranean, volcanic waters dissolving scattered minerals and depositing them elsewhere in increased concentration. Decay and weathering of aluminium-bearing rocks – igneous rocks high in aluminium silicates and clayey limestones – resulted in the formation of *bauxite* (see page 594). Hence, it contains a variety of mineral impurities. Silica, iron oxides and titanium minerals are always present, with the silica usually as quartz but, in some deposits, as cristobalite. Others include clay minerals such as kaolinite and chlorite.

Thus, mineral ores are apt to be found deposited in 'pockets' and 'veins' in rocks of widely differing type and composition.

Graphite

This is a soft black form of carbon disseminated mostly in mica–schists, micaceous quartzites and, occasionally, in some igneous rocks. Accordingly it may contain a variety of impurities, especially in the mined material. These include feldspars, pyrites, iron oxides, muscovite and quartz. (See Chapter 13, page 345, for more detailed discussion.)

Earth movements

The various rock types have not remained in the order in which they were formed. The effects of weathering and enormous pressures due to earth movements caused by earthquakes and volcanic activity folded, dislocated and fractured the crust. The effects of movements are exemplified by simple folds, overfolds, faults and thrusts of sedimentary rocks, the original strata of which were thereby extensively displaced and intermingled.

This means that in tunnelling and mining or quarrying for a mineral in a particular stratum, a variety of different and unrelated materials will be encountered. Thus, the composition of dusts produced by these processes will vary from locality to locality.

Products of active volcanic eruptions

Particular interest in the possibility of a hazard to the lungs of human beings in the vicinity of active volcanoes was aroused by the dramatic eruption of

Mount St Helens in Washington State, USA, in March 1980. It offered an unprecedented opportunity to evaluate the products of volcanic eruptions from this standpoint.

Violent eruptions are characterized by forceful ejection of a variety of pyroclastic fragments, hot toxic gases, superheated steam, radiation and lava flows. Thus, apart from physical injury (as may be caused by high velocity blast waves), the potential hazards to be considered are respirable dust, toxic gases and radiation.

Pyroclastic fragments consist of the following:

1. *Ash*: pulverized lava composed of crystals, glass or rock fragments, or a mixture of all three, less than 4 mm in diameter. The finest particles are dusts.
2. *Lapilli*: small stones.
3. *Blocks and bombs*: larger rocks up to boulder size.

These fragments are formed from erupting fluid magma and the fracture and ejection of old rocks and lava in the walls of the volcano's conduit by the force of the eruption. But it is the composition of ash and dust that is relevant here.

As noted earlier, magmas consist of various gradations of molten basalts, andesites and rhyolites. Free silica may be present in volcanic ash as cristobalite as well as quartz even though the temperature within the conduits and at the vents of volcanoes is believed to be no more than about 1200°C, that is, below the temperature range (1470°C to 1723°C) at which cristobalite is normally stable at atmospheric pressure. This is probably explained by a high ambient water vapour pressure in the conduit facilitating inversion of quartz to cristobalite at lower temperatures. The surface temperatures of some lavas may be higher due to burning of hydrogen and other volcanic gases escaping from the lava. Thus, cristobalite is typically a mineral of volcanic rocks and not of igneous (plutonic) rocks formed at depth. However, much of the silica is converted to glass, usually as minute spheroids, during the rapid cooling of magma as it is ejected from the vent.

Ash

The average size of air-fall ash deposit fragments at any point decreases exponentially with the distance from the vent, the largest and heaviest thus being nearest. The distances at which ash-falls occur depend upon the severity of the eruption. When very violent the ash cloud is projected miles into the air and fall-out occurs over enormously large areas (often hundreds of miles) and is most concentrated down-wind. The finest and furthest travelled ash derived from siliceous magmas (rhyolites and andesites) commonly consists largely of glass shards; some rock minerals such as feldspar may be present as well as substantial amounts of cristobalite. Long, flexible fibrous particles or threads are a feature of the air-fall dust and ash of some eruptions often at very great distances. These are formed of basaltic glass and are known as Pelée's hair – after the legendary goddess of Hawaiian volcanoes.

Analysis of Mount St Helens' ash – in which 90 per cent of particles were less than 10 µm in diameter – showed that crystalline silica ranged from 2.8 to 6.6 per cent by weight of ash and consisted of quartz and approximately two-thirds cristobalite, but there was considerable interlaboratory variability in the values of cristobalite (Green et al., 1983). Although these concentrations are fairly low the theoretical possibility exists that exposure to high concentrations of ash particles for a short period could cause 'acute silicosis' or silico-lipoproteinosis, but this does not seem to have been observed. A radiographic study of survivors of a Japanese eruption in 1977 did not reveal any pulmonary disease related to ash exposure. No fibrous particles were identified in the Mount St Helens' ash (Green et al., 1983).

Thus, exposure to air-fall ash – which is usually short-lived and only a matter of days – is unlikely to be a pneumoconiosis hazard, although, as mentioned later, near the source of an eruption it may cause acute respiratory distress or asphyxia in unprotected individuals. But when the eruption has ceased, personnel in various occupations (in particular, bulldozer and truck drivers; forestry, agricultural and vinicultural workers; geologists and vulcanologists) may be subjected to more prolonged exposure from ash resuspended by their activities and by the wind. However, subsequent rainfall transforms the ash into a cement-like texture. It is worth noting that, experimentally, Mount St Helens' ash appears to be less toxic than quartz, and some studies have suggested that it behaves more like an inert dust; however, this requires confirmation (Martin, Wehner and Butler, 1983).

Pumice and pumicite are lavas full of gas bubbles, produced by rapid frothing of viscous lava due to a sudden fall in pressure. They consist of silicic glasses, the composition of which varies according to the conditions of their formation. They may be simply a frothy glass, sometimes with streaks of non-cellular glass, or they may contain quartz, cristobalite and feldspars. Thus, crystalline silica is either absent or present in varying and sometimes substantial amounts in different deposits; consequently prolonged occupational exposure may result in nodular silicosis or 'mixed dust fibrosis'. Pumice usually forms near the vent of a volcano but pumicite (being composed of small particles) is carried great distances by winds before settling as accumulations of fine-grained 'ash'.

Perlite, a volcanic glass of rhyolitic composition, has a concentric structure consisting of minute spheroids a few millimetres in diameter. It often contains inclusions of quartz, feldspar and biotite and, sometimes, of cristobalite. Because of its content of combined water it possesses the valuable commercial property of sudden expansion on rapid heating.

Pumice and perlite are discussed in Chapter 12.

Toxic gases

Another danger of volcanic activity which is not confined to the immediate vicinity of an eruption is the presence of toxic gases (see Chapter 18). These include sulphur dioxide, sulphur trioxide, hydrogen sulphide, chlorine and hydrogen chloride in varying proportions, and also carbon dioxide. They are present in ash clouds, and unexpected jets of gas may be expelled from innocent-looking cooling lava flows distant from the centre of the eruption. The predominant gas in the early stages of an eruption is sulphur dioxide but hydrogen sulphide is more common later. Not all eruptions are short and violent; some grumble on for years with episodic emissions of these and other gases. Steam vents (*fumaroles*) which may be found in the vicinity of both active and dormant volcanoes often produce high concentrations of carbon dioxide and sulphur dioxide.

Sulphur dioxide, hydrogen sulphide and carbon dioxide are potentially the most hazardous of volcanic gases because, being heavier than air, they hug the ground and accumulate in hollows and can thus cause acute respiratory disease or asphyxia in human beings and animals. Carbon dioxide is especially dangerous as it is odourless and non-irritant and its presence is likely to be unsuspected.

Ionizing radiation

The plume from Mount St Helens was estimated to contain about 3 million curies of radon gas which, in view of the rapid decay of radon, is unlikely to have presented a hazard. Radioactivity of longer-lived radioactive isotopes – ^{232}Th, ^{226}Ra and ^{40}K – was similar to that present in the Earth's crust. It was computed, from all the available data, that, over the period of a lifetime, the radiation effect of exposure to the ash would be a negligible threat to human populations (Soldat, Kathren and Corley, 1981; Green et al., 1983).

Clinicopathological effects

Most acute respiratory complaints associated with the Mount St Helens' eruption were cough, wheeze and shortness of breath – symptoms similar to those recorded in other eruptions at different geographical locations: the USU volcano in Japan in 1977, Irazu

volcano in Costa Rica in 1963 and Mount Katmai, Alaska in 1913 (Green et al., 1983). Among individuals who had been fairly close to the eruption and were overtaken by ash clouds projected at high speed near ground level, the most common cause of death was asphyxia from inhalation of ash which, with mucus, formed occlusive plugs in the upper thoracic airways – in particular the larynx and trachea. In those further afield (chiefly loggers), who survived longer, the ash extended to the peripheral bronchi but not as far as the bronchioles (Eisele et al., 1981). The findings in two individuals who did not die of asphyxia and survived for 10 and 16 days respectively revealed a combination of thermal burns of the large airways, acute alveolar injury and respiratory failure. In the first case there was alveolar oedema, interstitial infiltration of inflammatory cells with accumulations of ash-containing macrophages in the alveoli, and desquamation of type 1 cells; in the second, bronchiolitis obliterans and organizing intra-alveolar exudates with occasional granulomas. There was little or no evidence that toxic gases played any part in the pathology (Green et al., 1981; Parshley et al., 1982).

Conclusion

The products of volcanic activity can cause potentially lethal, acute pulmonary disease due to inhalation of large amounts of ash or toxic gases; and it is possible that survivors of heavy exposure to ash may develop chronic bronchiolitis obliterans. Transient bronchoconstriction (possibly severe in some cases) may be provoked in asthmatic subjects and others with hyperactive bronchial airways exposed to lower levels of ash or toxic gas.

Although the size distribution of air-borne ash particles is well within 'respirable' range, and crystalline silica is usually present, a silicosis risk is highly improbable because the duration and intensity of exposure, even if repeated as a result of episodic resuspension of ash, are too short-lived (days or weeks rather than years), and the percentage of silica is low. Apart from prolonged occupational exposure to pumice (which is a different matter), pneumoconiosis has not been observed.

Ionizing radiation from volcanic eruptions does not appear to present any hazard to the lungs.

Ionizing radiation from rocks

Uranium-238 and thorium-232 are present in most igneous rocks and in minute amounts in all rocks and soils.

Uranium gives rise to decay chain products of which uranium-238 is the first member through a series of solid elements to radium-226 which decays to the gas radon-222 which, in turn, when in air, rapidly gives rise to other isotopes – radon 'daughters'. The important members of the series in the present context are those which emit α-particles, namely, radon-222 (half-life 3.8 days) and the three radon daughters, polonium-218 (half-life 3.05 minutes), polonium-214 (half-life 26.8 minutes) and polonium-210 (half-life 19.4 years). Radon-222 leaks from rocks, fallen ore and soil and escapes into the air although concentrations at ground level are very low (Morgan, 1970). But in enclosed areas, such as mines, shafts, underground chambers and tunnels – especially if poorly ventilated – concentrations may be high because the gas has less chance to diffuse away. It may also be carried into mine-workings by waters from a distant source.

Thorium, also fairly abundant in the Earth's crust, is usually found in association with uranium. It decays into thoron gas (radon-220), thorium A (polonium-216), thorium B (lead-212) and thorium C (bismuth-212). Of these thoron, thorium B and thorium C are α emitters.

The amount of radiation that escapes into the atmosphere varies greatly in different areas for three reasons: differing concentrations or uranium and thorium in the bedrock; the nature of their mineralization; and the permeability of the bedrock. Thus, only a proportion of either gas becomes airborne, and although high levels of radon are associated with granites, this is not always the case. Because of differences in the style of mineralization of uranium, some granites in which its levels are comparable may have low radon levels. And many basic igneous rocks have low contents of uranium with no production of radon. But, in some regions, other rocks – such as limestones and black shales – may yield high radon levels. Hence, there is considerable global and local variation in doses of radiation received from this source.

When first formed, the decay products are single ionized atoms but they readily attach themselves to molecules of water vapour or to dust particles as 'cluster ions'. It has been calculated that their mean radioactivity diameter is about 0.25 μm in non-operational mines and about 0.4 μm diameter in operational mines (Davies, 1967). In this aerosol state, therefore, they can, on inhalation, penetrate to the trachea, bronchi and peripheral airways, and be retained in the lungs.

α-Particles are positively charged helium nuclei with two protons and neutrons which have a greater mass than other radiation particles and great kinetic energy but, owing to their large mass and positive charge, have only feeble penetrating power. β-Particles, being electrons, have greater penetrating capacity but less ionizing power. It is believed that ionization is the cause of malignant change in living cells.

For this reason inhaled α-particles are more important than β-particles – although high doses of the latter may induce lung tumours in experimental animals – and there is strong evidence that exposure of human beings to radon-222 and α-emitting radon daughters is responsible for a significantly increased risk of developing carcinoma of the lung. The radiation dose to the lungs of radon and thoron appears to be approximately similar (Albert, 1966) (see also Chapter 19, page 656).

References

Albert, R.E. (1966) *Thorium and its Industrial Hygiene Aspects.* Academic Press, New York and London

American Thoracic Society (1990) Official Statement. Health effects of Tremolite. *Am. Rev. Respir. Dis.* **142**, 1453–1458

Andrews, R.W. (1970) *Wollastonite.* Institute of Geological Science. HMSO, London

Bradbury, J.C. and Ehrlinger III, H.P. (1975) Tripoli. In *Industrial Minerals and Rocks* (ed.-in-chief S.J. Lefond) American Institute of Mining, Metallurgical and Petroleum Engineers, Inc., New York, pp. 1209–1218

Bradshaw, M.J. (1968) *A New Geology.* The English Universities Press, London

Campbell, W.J., Huggins, C.W. and Wylie, A.G. (1980) Chemical and physical characterization of amosite, chrysotile, crocidolite and non-fibrous tremolite for oral ingestion studies by the National Institute of Environmental Health Sciences. *Bureau of Mines Report of Investigations*, R I 8452, US Department of the Interior

Cooper, W.C., Otto Wong and Graebner, R. (1968) Mortality of workers in two Minnesota taconite mining and milling operations. *J. Occup. Med.* **30**, 506–511

Crelling, J.C. (1989) Coal as a material. In *Introduction to Carbon Science* (ed. H. Marsh) Butterworths, London, Boston, Sydney, pp. 260–284

Davies, C.N. (1967) In *Assessment of Airborne Radioactivity.* International Atomic Energy Agency, Vienna, pp. 3–20

Davis, A., Russell, S.J., Rimmer, S.M. and Yeakel, D. (1984) Some genetic implications of silica and aluminosilicates in peat and coal. *Int. J. Coal Geol.* **3**, 293–314

Dorling, M. and Zussman, J. (1980) Comparative studies of asbestiform and non-asbestiform calcium-rich amphiboles. 4th International Asbestos Conference, Torino

Eisele, J.W., O'Halloran, R.L., Reay, D.T., Lindholm G.R., Lewman, L.V. and Brady, W.J. (1981) Deaths during the May 18, 1980, eruption of Mount St Helens. *N. Engl. J. Med.* **305**, 931–936

Finkelman, R.B. (1988) The inorganic chemistry of coal: a scanning electron microscopy view. *Scan. Microsc.* **2**, 97–105

Finkelman, R.B. and Gluskoter, H.J. (1983) Characterization of minerals in coal: problems and promises. In *Fouling and Slagging Resulting from Impurities in Combustion Gases* (ed. R.W. Bryers) *Proceedings of the 1981 Engineers Foundation Conference*, New York, pp. 299–318

Geikie, J. (1908) *Structural and Field Geology*, 2nd edn. Oliver and Boyd, London, p. 32

Goldstein, B. and Rendall, R.E.G. (1970) The relative toxicities of the main classes of minerals. In *Pneumoconiosis, Proceedings of International Conference*, Johannesburg, 1969 (ed. H.A. Shapiro), Oxford University Press, Cape Town, South Africa, pp. 429–434

Green, F.H.Y., Vallyathan, V., Mentnech, M.S., Tucker, J.H., Merchant, J.A., Keissling, P.J., Antonius, J.A. and Parshley, P. (1981) Is volcanic ash a pneumoconiosis risk? *Nature* **293**, 216–217

Green, F.H.Y., Dollberg, D., Tucker, J.H. and Keissling, P. (1983) Toxicity of Mount St Helens' volcanic ash and relevance to mining populations. In *Health Issues Related to Metal and Nonmetallic Mining* (eds W.L. Wagner, W.N. Rom and J.A. Merchant), Butterworths, Boston, London, pp. 105–120

Highley, D.E. (1972) Fuller's earth. *Mineral Dossier No. 3.* Mineral Resources Consultative Committee. HMSO, London

Highley D.E. (1982) Fireclay. *Mineral Dossier No. 24.* HMSO, London

Hodgson, A.A. (1977) Nature and paragenesis of asbestos minerals. *Phil. Trans. R. Soc. London* **A286**, 611–624

Hodgson, A.A. (1986) *Scientific Advances in Asbestos, 1967–1985.* Anjalena Publications, Jupiter Press, Croydon, Surrey, UK

Jötten, K.W. and Eickoff, W. (1944). Lungenveränderungen durch Sillimanistaub. *Arch. Gewerbepath. Gewerbehyg.* **12**, 223–232

Kadey, Jr, F.L. (1975) Diatomite. In *Industrial Minerals and Rocks* (ed.-in-chief S.J. Lefond) American Institute of Mining Engineers, New York, pp. 605–635

Kelse, J.W. and Thompson, C.S. (1989) The regulatory and mineralogical definitions of asbestos and their impact on amphibole dust analysis. *Am. Ind. Hyg. Assoc. J.* **50**, 613–622

King, E.J., Mohanty, G.P., Harrison, C.V. and Nagelschmidt, G. (1953) The action of different forms of pure silica on the lungs of rats. *Br. J. Ind. Med.* **10**, 9–17

Langer, A.M., Nolan, R.P. and Pooley, F.D. (1990) Phyllosilicates: associated fibrous minerals. In *Health-related Effects of Phyllosilicates* (ed. J. Bignon), Springer Verlag, Berlin, Paris, pp. 59–61

Langer, A.M., Nolan, R.P. and Addison, J. (1991) On talc, tremolite and tergiversation. *Br. J. Ind. Med.* **48**, 359–360

Lee, R.J. and Fisher, R.M. (1979) Identification of fibrous minerals. *Ann. NY Acad. Sci.* **330**, 645–660

McDonald, J.C., Gibbs, G.W., Liddell, F.K.W. and McDonald, A.D. (1978) Mortality after exposure to cummingtonite–grunerite. *Am. Rev. Respir. Dis.* **118**, 271–277

Mackowsky, M-Th. (1968) Mineral matter in coal. In *Coal and Coal-bearing Strata* (eds D.G. Murchison and T.S. Westoll), Oliver and Boyd, London, pp. 309–321

Martin, T.R., Wehner, A.P. and Butler, J. (1983) Pulmonary toxicity of Mt St Helens' volcanic ash. *Am. Rev. Respir. Dis.* **128**, 158–162

Mohanty, G.P., Roberts, D.C., King, E.J. and Harrison, C.V.

(1953) The effect of feldspar, slate and quartz on the lungs of rats. *J. Pathol. Bacteriol.* **65**, 501–512

Moorlock, B.S.P. and Highley, D.E. (1991) An appraisal of fuller's earth resources in England and Wales. British Geological Survey. *Technical Report*, WA/91/75

Morgan, A. (1970) Physical behaviour of radon and its daughters with particular reference to monitoring methods. In *Pneumoconiosis: Proceedings of the International Conference*, Johannesburg, 1969 (ed. H.A. Shapiro), Oxford University Press, Cape Town, pp. 540–543

Parshley, P.F., Kiessling, P.J., Antonius, J.A., Connell, R.S., Miller, S.H. and Green, F.H.Y. (1982) Pyroclastic flow injury, Mount St Helens', May 18, 1980. *Am. J. Surg.* **143**, 565–568

Pooley, F.D. (1987) Asbestos mineralogy. In *Asbestos-related Malignancy* (eds K. Antman and J.E. Aisner), Grune and Stratton, Orlando, FL, p. 21

Pooley, F.D. and Rowlands, N. (1977) Chemical and physical properties of British talc powders. In *Inhaled Particles IV* (ed. W.H. Walton and B. McGovern), Pergamon Press, Oxford, New York, pp. 639–646

Raask, E. (1985) *Mineral Impurities in Coal Combustion – Behaviour, Problems and Remedial Measures.* Hemisphere, Washington

Ross, M., Kuntze, R.A. and Clifton, R.A. (1984) A definition of asbestos. *A.S.T.M. Special Technical Publication* **834**, 139–147. American Society for Testing and Materials, Philadelphia, USA

Schenk, W.M., Gobb, P. and Kolmer, H.A. (1990) A morphological study of mesomorphs. In *Health-related Effects of Phyllosilicates* (ed. J. Bignon), Springer Verlag, Berlin, Paris, pp. 85–86

Soldat, J.K., Kathren, R.L., Corley, J.P. and Strange, D.L. (1981) Radiation doses from Mount St Helens, May 1980 eruption. *Science* **213**, 585

Sosman, R.B. (1965) *The Phases of Silica.* Rutgers University Press, New Brunswick, NJ

Swaine, D.J. (1990) *Trace Elements in Coal.* Butterworths, London, Boston, Singapore, Sydney

United States Department of Labor, Occupational Safety and Health Administration (1986) Occupational exposure to asbestos, tremolite, anthophyllite and actinolite: final rules. *Federal Register 51* (NO 119): 22612–22790 (29 CFR parts 1910 and 1926)

Vorwald, A.J., Durkan, T.M., Pratt, P.C. and Delahant, A.B. (1949) Diatomaceous earth pneumoconiosis. In *Proceedings of the IXth International Congress on Industrial Medicine*, Wright, Bristol, pp. 726–741

Weiss, B. and Boettner, E.A. (1967) Commercial talc and talcosis. *Archs Environ. Health* **14**, 304–308

Zoltai, T. and Wylie, A.G. (1979) Definitions of asbestos-related mineralogical terminology. *Ann. NY Acad. Sci.* **330**, 707–709

Zussman, J. (1957) Electron diffraction studies of the serpentine minerals. *Am. Mineralogist* **42**, 133–153

Appendix II

Stokes' law

This states that the fluid resistance experienced by a small sphere of radius 'r' moving at a uniform velocity 'v' through a fluid of viscosity 'η' is $6\pi r\eta v$. On being released a small sphere rapidly attains a constant (terminal) velocity and, when falling at this speed, the fluid resistance equals the gravitational force 'g'. Thus:

$$\tfrac{4}{3}\pi r^3(\sigma - \rho)g = 6\pi r\eta v$$

where σ is the density of the spheres and ρ, the density of the fluid. Hence:

$$v = \tfrac{2}{9}\frac{r^2(\sigma - \rho)g}{\eta}$$

In air $\sigma \approx \sigma/800$ and is neglected. The formula fails in air if the spheres are so small as to be comparable with the mean free path of the air molecules. It also fails in air and in liquids if the spheres are too large, since the rate of fall then rises to such an extent that the velocities communicated to the fluid become large enough to introduce a fluid inertia effect. This results in the lines of fluid flow failing to close up on the lee side of the sphere as they do in viscous (Stokes) flow, so raising the fluid resistance. Therefore, larger spheres fall more slowly than is given by Stokes' law.

The law is valid within 10 per cent for particles between 1 and 40 μm diameter but can be extended to particles from 0.001 to 200 μm diameter by applying shape correction factors (Brain and Valberg, 1978). It applies mainly to the deposition of particles by impaction and sedimentation.

Reference

Brain, J.D. and Valberg, P.A. (1978) Deposition of aerosol in the respiratory tract. *Am. Rev. Respir. Dis.* **120**, 1325–1373

Appendix III

Post-mortem preparation of lungs

Formaldehyde fixation methods

After removal of the intact lungs, main bronchi and trachea formol acetate solution (10 per cent formalin in 4 per cent sodium acetate) is run through a cannula into both main bronchi from a reservoir placed at a height of about 120 cm, or delivered at this pressure by an electric pump. When perfusion is complete the lungs are placed in a large vessel containing the same solution for at least 48 hours. This is the method of Gough and Wentworth (1960).

Another method, employing formalin vapour, is used for research purposes especially where quantitative studies of the lung or examination of bronchial mucus (which is unaffected) is to be made; but it is not appropriate for routine use and also tends to cause some shrinkage of the lungs.

Silverton (1964) made a detailed survey and comparison of these and similar methods which should be referred to.

Lungs prepared by these methods are best examined by cutting serial slices 1 to 3 cm thick in the sagittal plane (in some cases the coronal plane may be preferable). The slices can then be studied in order and the observations recorded in writing and diagrammatically or photographically. When the lung is inspected in this way, discrete, non-fibrotic dust macules are indistinguishable to touch from the surrounding lung and are not raised above the surface; by contrast, discrete, fibrotic dust lesions are firm, hard and 'nodular' to touch and are raised above the cut surface.

A *whole lung section* mounted on paper for permanent record is prepared by cutting 300 to 500 μm sections from slices about 4-cm thick and, after special processing which preserves the natural colours of the lung, attaching them to paper (Gough and Wentworth, 1960; Silverton, 1964). They are then covered with Cellophane or a layer of methacrylic resin. A modification of this method which permits more rapid preparation of sections has been described by Whimster (1969).

Impregnation of lung slices with barium sulphate

This simple technique, introduced by Heard, greatly improves the macroscopic clarity and detail of emphysema and DIPF, and does not mask dust pigmentation. It provides good specimens for demonstration and photography. The technique is as follows:

> A selected slice from the middle of the lung is lightly squeezed free of excess water and placed flat in a tray (25 × 30 cm) containing saturated aqueous barium nitrate at room temperature for one minute. It is pressed with the fingertips intermittently to encourage the solution to enter the depths of the slice. After squeezing, it is transferred to a tray of saturated aqueous sodium sulphate for one minute; a cloud of precipitated barium sulphate appears at this stage and the slice quickly whitens. It is then squeezed and washed briefly in running tap water to remove excess barium sulphate. One impregnation is sufficient as a rule. The reagents are used for several weeks and the supernatant is selected each time. The precipitate is retained to strengthen the solution when it is returned to the bottle.
>
> (Heard, 1969)

Preparation for electron microscopy

An effective, practical method of injecting a fixative solution into the periphery of the lung within 30 minutes after death without opening the thorax, described by Bachofen, Weibel and Roos (1975), achieves good preservation for at least 8 hours. The solution consists of an isomolar mixture of 5 per cent glutaraldehyde and 0.025 g indocyanine green in 19 ml distilled water and 1 ml pasteurized plasma protein.

References

Bachofen, M., Weibel, E.R. and Roos, B. (1975) Postmortem fixation of human lungs for electron microscopy. *Am. Rev. Respir. Dis.* **111**, 247–256

Gough, J. and Wentworth, J.E. (1960) Thin sections of entire organs mounted on paper. In *Recent Advances in Pathology*, 7th edn (ed. C.V. Harrison), Churchill, London

Heard, B.E. (1969). *Pathology of Chronic Bronchitis and Emphysema*. J. and A. Churchill Ltd, London, p. 9

Silverton, R.E. (1964) A comparison of formaldehyde fixation methods used in the study of pulmonary emphysema. *J. Med. Lab. Technol.* **21**, 187–217

Whimster, W.F. (1969) Rapid giant paper sections. *Thorax* **24**, 737–741

Appendix IV

Routine optical microscopy

Routine examination of lung tissue requires sections about 6 to 7 μm thick and standard staining practice should include haematoxylin and eosin and van Giesen methods. The use of other stains is referred to in relevant places in the text. Search for asbestos and other ferruginous bodies is greatly facilitated by 30-μm sections.

During fixation of tissue it is important to avoid contamination by particulate matter, such as starch, talc and asbestos.

Most mineral particles deposited in the lungs are less than 5 μm in diameter so that many are at, or below, the limits of resolution of light microscopy.

Because invalid deductions are often made concerning mineral particles in sections examined by polarized light brief discussion of this subject is appropriate.

Polarized light microscopy

Microscopes in pathology laboratories are invariably fitted with two polaroid filters: a *polarizer* and an *analyser*. As the polarizer (below the stage) is rarely removed, the beam of light reaching specimens during routine histopathological examinations is said to be 'plane polarized', that is, confined to one plane of vibration. Almost all mineral particles appear brighter than the pulmonary tissue in which they are found. This is because the *refractive index* (RI) of all, apart from a few rare exceptions, is higher than that of the tissue. The RI-related relief ('luminosity') of light passing through contrasting media or crystals is generally determined in plane-polarized light (PPL). The relief, or brightness, of an individual particle varies according to its optical crystallography. In isotropic substances (crystals of the cubic system), light is transmitted with the same velocity in all directions because the RI has a constant value irrespective of the crystallographic direction that the light is following; in anisotropic substances (all other crystals) it varies with the crystallographic direction of the transmitted light. Thus, the relief of different minerals seen by plane-polarized light varies considerably according to their RIs.

Accurate measurement of RI by special petrological techniques can be used to identify particles by the relationship of their indices to crystal symmetry. But such methods are not available in the medical microscope. Hence, mineral particles in microsections of pulmonary tissue cannot be identified with any certainty by their degree of brightness.

The other optical property of minerals often referred to in histopathology is that of *birefringence* (Table A.6). This is the difference between the wave paths of two light rays transmitted through anisotropic minerals possessing two or more RIs (or vibration directions). Isotropic minerals are not birefringent because they possess only one RI (or vibration direction). The birefringence of any particular mineral particle depends upon its orientation in relation to its optic axes. To determine birefringence accurately a three- or five-axis universal stage is required for orienting the mineral with respect to the incident light beam, together with a knowledge of optical crystallography. Neither commodity is normally available in the pathology laboratory. However, rotation of the analyser of a medical microscope with respect to the specimen will show whether a particle is birefringent, and the intensity of the birefringence. The intensity of birefringence (and brightness) of a particle depends on its mineral species and its optical orientation; the more colourful and greater the intensity, the stronger the birefringence. Birefringent colours and brightness from a mineral particle extinguish and reappear four times during a complete revolution of the analyser or of the stage of a petrological microscope. But it is important to note that, in Sosman's (1965) words, 'the phenomena as seen are strongly influenced by the chance orientation of the fragment, for a flat

Table A.6 Levels of refractive index and birefringence of some commonly encountered minerals

	Refractive index	*Birefringence*
Quartz	Low	Weak
Tridymite	Low	Very weak
Cristobalite	Low	Almost absent
Vitreous silica	Low	Absent
Kaolinite	Low	Weak
Sericite mica	Low	Strong
Siderite* ⎫		
Limonite ⎭	Very high	Extreme
Talc	Low	Strong

*Exhibits the phenomenon of 'twinkling' on rotation of the analyser.

piece of any birefringent substance can be taken in one or more special positions in which it does not show the phenomena of double refraction at all, while in other positions it will show effects intermediate between zero and the maximum which is characteristic of the substance. The appearances are also influenced by twinning and by the overlapping of crystals in fine-grained material'.

For many years, however, birefringence of mineral particles in lung tissue has frequently been taken, in the medical literature, to identify them as quartz, and lack of birefringence to indicate its absence. This 'rule of thumb' has undoubtedly been responsible for errors of interpretation of pathogenesis and diagnosis. It is still a common practice in many routine pathological reports.

Quartz is weakly, though distinctly, birefringent, lighting up and darkening with rotation of the analyser, but, as the luminosity of its particles is low, it may be wholly or partly obscured by deposits of coal or carbon dust. Furthermore, as just stated, like other minerals, if the particles are oriented with their optic axes parallel to the light beam they will show no birefringence although they will still appear brighter than adjacent pulmonary tissue in PPL. Statements in some medical papers over the last 40 years or more asserting that, if there is 'little or no evidence' of birefringent particles in lung tissue, then quartz is absent are erroneous. On the one hand, particles of quartz (and other polymorphs of silica) are often too small to be detected by optical methods (see 'Carbonaceous rocks: coal') and, on the other, carbonaceous dust may obscure their birefringent luminosity. In addition, the birefringence of tridymite is weaker than that of quartz, and that of cristobalite is weaker still (Sosman, 1965). Thus, should cristobalite be the predominant phase of silica in the lungs, 'little or no' birefringence will be seen. However, the 'rule of thumb' has frequently been relied upon in studies and reports of the pathology of coal and carbon pneumoconiosis, 'mixed dust fibrosis' and various other occupational disorders of the lungs.

Particles of kaolinite, the mica group of minerals and siderite are often present in the lungs of coal miners and workers in other dust hazards. The birefringence of kaolinite is weak but that of the micas (for example, sericite) and of siderite is strong, and, thus, much brighter than the luminosity of quartz which is feeble. It seems likely that these or other more strongly birefringent minerals are often misinterpreted as quartz in routine histopathological reports.

Talc, which is associated with a variety of occupational hazards, is strongly birefringent.

The refractive indices and birefringence of a few examples of minerals encountered in 'occupational' dust are compared in Table A.6.

The following conclusions regarding the application of these optical phenomena in medical microscopy can be made:

1. The luminosity of mineral particles compared with surrounding lung tissue by PPL does not establish their identity.
2. The birefringent luminosity of quartz and other polymorphs of silica is low, or negligible, compared with a variety of other minerals that may be found in the lungs, such as the micas, siderite and talc. Although particles cannot be positively identified by their birefringence, it is sometimes possible, if they are large enough for their morphology to be discerned, to reach a tentative identification. Thus, a strongly birefringent, polygonal, platy particle may suggest talc (see Figure 16.4c). This, however, is not possible in the case of small silica particles in the lungs.
3. Failure to find birefringent particles in specimens of lung tissue does not exclude the presence of quartz or other polymorphs of silica.
4. The identity of minerals in the lungs can, at best, only be suspected by these optical properties; accurate identification requires more definitive techniques, such as X-ray diffraction analysis.

The term 'refractile' is often found in medical texts on occupational pulmonary disease in regard to luminosity of mineral particles, although its meaning is obscure; it may refer to RI or birefringence, possibly interchangeably. The expression is not known to mineralogists or petrologists. On either count, therefore, it should not be used.

Reference

Sosman, R.B. (1965) *The Phases of Silica*. Rutgers University Press, New Brunswick, NJ, pp. 125–127

Appendix V

Identification of minerals in the lungs

Systemic analysis of particulate matter in the lungs is a well-established and advancing discipline that provides important quantitative and qualitative information about particulate matter in the lungs of individuals in both occupational and non-occupational populations. Although detailed discussion of this essentially specialized subject is clearly beyond the scope of this book, some general understanding of the methodology by the non-expert is desirable.

In brief, the reasons for analysing particles are the following: uncertainty as to the identity of the minerals in lung tissue; no indication of the presence of mineral particles by light microscopy when occupational history suggests a possible dust hazard; characterization of the size and morphology of particles; and quantification of the burden of dust in the lungs. Quantitative analysis of this burden has three important applications:

1. Correlation with other measurements – physiological, radiological and pathological.
2. Investigation of dose–response and clearance of particles.
3. Comparison of interlaboratory techniques for purposes of standardization (Abraham, 1984).

To identify a mineral species, or a variety of a species, a number of its characteristics have to be determined. These fall into three categories: *chemical composition*, *crystallography* and *morphology*. But, because most mineral particles deposited in the lungs are less than 5 μm in diameter, and thus below the limits of resolution by light microscopy, and also cannot be accurately identified by conventional electron microscopy, more sensitive techniques are required. A large number of these, in which production of X-rays forms the basis of the majority of 'microprobe analysis' investigations, are available but, apart from research purposes, only a few are needed in practice. Brief mention of instrumentation techniques, their application and analytical procedures commonly used for clinical and histopathological investigation will, it is hoped, provide the 'bare bones' of the principles involved. But for detailed discussion, including validation and limitation of the various techniques, the reader should consult the texts of Abraham and Burnett (1983), Abraham (1984), Ingram, Shelburne and LeFurgey (1989) and Churg (1991) from which most of what follows is drawn.

The criteria for appropriate selection of lung tissue for biopsy and at autopsy, and the various methods of its preparation for analytical techniques, are described by Gaensler (1981), Abraham and Burnett (1983) and Stettler et al. (1989).

Instrumentation
(Ingram, Shelburne and LeFurgey, 1989)

Scanning electron microscopy (SEM)

A general term indicating any instrument in which the electron beam is scanned over the sample.

Transmission electron microscopy (TEM)

Electrons of the primary beam are transmitted through the specimen. It enables high resolution of morphology.

Scanning transmission electron microscopy (STEM)

Same as TEM apart from scanning of the sample. It finds and analyses particles in intact lung tissue and in ashed or digested tissue.

Back-scattered electron imaging (BEI)

Electrons of the primary beam are scattered back from, and not transmitted through, the specimen. It detects particles of medium-to-high atomic number in tissue, and produces topographic contrast.

Energy-dispersive X-ray analysis (EDXA)

Sometimes called energy-dispersive spectrometry. It detects and measures simultaneously most elements of atomic number greater than about 9; below this it yields no identifying data. It does not provide exact molecular or crystallographic data.

Selected area electron diffraction (SAED)

This defines crystalline structure of inorganic particles and organic crystals.

Secondary ion mass spectrometry (SIMS)

This analyses and provides three-dimensional delineation of elements in particles, cells and tissues. The sample is destroyed.

Secondary electron imaging (SEI)

The image is produced by secondary electrons ejected from the sample and gives three-dimensional detail of surface images with moderate resolution and good depth of field.

X-ray fluorescence (XRF)

This identifies and quantifies inorganic particles and is valuable for bulk analysis. It can be used in scanning electron microscopes.

Infrared spectrophotometry (IRS)

This relatively simple technique detects, quantifies and distinguishes the various polymorphs of silica as well as microgram quantities of other dusts. The results are in good agreement with those of EDXA, and, for chalcedonic silica, superior.

There are two approaches to the elemental analysis of particles in the lungs: (1) bulk or macroanalysis and (2) microanalysis.

Bulk or macroanalysis

A known quantity of tissue (usually 1 g), obtained from selected sites for biopsy or at necropsy, is ashed at low temperature and the residue extracted and weighed (gravimetric sampling). IRS or EDXA are most commonly used for identification.

Alternatively, SEM and EDXA provide more detailed information about the size of individual particles, their morphology and composition. An automated SEM–EDXA procedure enables the analysis to be carried out more speedily and eliminates potential observer-bias in the choice of particles for analysis (Stettler et al., 1989). For the determination of the burden of fibrous particles the organic parts of the lung are digested away by one of a number of methods, usually sodium hypochlorite (common bleach) which has the advantage of not damaging fibres or affecting their mineral chemistry (Churg, 1991).

This mode of analysis has the disadvantage of making correlation of the locations and concentrations of dust with histopathology impossible.

Microanalysis

This involves particle-by-particle analysis in situ in intact lung tissue for which standard 5 μm paraffin-mounted sections can be used, but resolution of EDXA is improved by thinner sections. Particles are found by BEI and their composition identified by EDXA or, occasionally, SIMS. Their location and morphology are displayed by TEM, STEM and SEI. Elements of atomic weight below 9 (for example, beryllium) call for other analytical techniques such as SIMS. The particulate burden can also be quantified using a point-counting, morphometric technique the results of which compare well with bulk analysis (Abraham, 1984) (see Chapter 17, page 583).

SAED is an invaluable complementary technique to EDXA for the identification of inorganic crystals especially in asbestos fibres. By combining EDXA and TEM in searching for these fibres, it is possible to achieve good spatial resolution together with chemical analysis (Churg, 1991).

For the analysis of coal-mine dust from ashed lungs and in respirable samples of dust from the mines, IRS has a considerable advantage over EDXA for a number of reasons: measurements of quartz are relatively unaffected by the presence of the mica minerals; it is highly sensitive and can distinguish the different polymorphs of silica; and is cheaper (Dodgson and Whittaker, 1973).

The advantages of establishing comprehensive *databases* which contain individuals' occupational and social history, the identity and burden of inorganic particles in the lungs, the accompanying pathology and the diagnosis have been described by Abraham, Burnett and Hunt (1991). As individuals who have been exposed only to dust in the ambient air (urban or rural), as well as those with occupational exposure to dusts or fumes, are included, comparative information from both groups is provided. Virtually any combination of items of the data can be extracted for statistical analysis. Dust

levels in the lungs of persons with no occupational exposure are orders of magnitude lower than those in occupationally exposed individuals with, say, a fibrotic pneumoconiosis.

Conclusion

There is no question about the great value of the analysis of mineral particles in lung tissue in diagnosis or about its contribution to the aetiology of occupational disease. However, interpretation of the data needs to be careful and balanced. Unfortunately, in recent years there has been a tendency for an uncritical, but often confident, attribution of pulmonary disease to a variety of minerals identified in individual cases. Therefore, it must be emphasized that the presence of an exogenous mineral in the lungs is *not necessarily proof* of a pathogenic relationship to existing disease *even if* the mineral is of a type known to be capable of fibrogenic or other pathogenic potential (see Appendix VI). Nonetheless, the association of mineral matter with a specific lesion may indicate the need for detailed investigation.

References

Abraham, J.L. (1984) Identification and quantities analysis of tissue particulate burden. *Ann. NY Acad. Sci.* **428**, 60–66

Abraham, J.L. and Burnett, B.R. (1983) Quantitative analysis of inorganic particulate burden *in situ* in tissue sections. *Scanning Electron Microsc.* **11**, 681–696

Abraham, J.L., Burnett, B.R. and Hunt, A. (1991) Development and use of a pneumoconiosis database of human pulmonary inorganic particulate burden in over 400 lungs. *Scanning Microsc.* **5**, 95–108

Churg, A. (1991) Mineral analysis of the lung parenchyma. In *The Lung* (eds R.G. Crystal et al.), Scientific Foundations, Raven Press, New York, pp. 1869–1883

Dodgson, J. and Whittaker, W. (1973) The determination of quartz in respirable dust samples by infrared spectrophotometry – 1. *Ann. occup. Hyg.* **16**, 373–387

Gaensler, E.A. (1981) Open and closed lung biopsy. In *Diagnostic Techniques in Pulmonary Disease*, Part II (ed. M.A. Sackner), *Lung Biology in Health and Disease* series (ed. C. Lenfant), Marcel Decker, New York, pp. 579–622

Ingram, P., Shelburne, J.D. and LeFurgey, A. (1989) Principles and instrumentation. In *Microprobe Analysis in Medicine* (eds P. Ingram, J.D. Shelburne and V.I. Roggli), Hemisphere Publishing, New York, Washington, Philadelphia, pp. 1–31

Stettler, L.E., Groth, D.H., Platek, S.F. and Burg, J.R. (1989) Particulate concentrations in urban lungs. In *Microprobe Analysis in Medicine* (eds P. Ingram, J. Shelburne and V.I. Roggli), Hemisphere Publishing, New York, Washington, Philadelphia, pp. 133–146

Appendix VI

Proof of a causal relationship between a specific exogenous agent (inorganic or organic) and disease

By modifying the principle of the postulates originally enunciated by Henlé and Koch a number of criteria for testing the validity of a suggested relationship can be applied. In the main, these rely on the identification of a specific suspect substance or agency, its consistent presence in the lungs (or in the lesions) in associated disease, thorough epidemiological investigation of the disease, and, where possible, production of similar disease in animals by the substance. For example, some support for a causal relationship is provided if the mineral in question can be *consistently* shown to produce the same pathological response in a dose-dependent manner in animal or human subjects. However, additional influences – genetic, immunological or physiological – may be involved and extrapolation of animal experiments to human beings can lead to dubious, even inadmissible, conclusions.

A group of basic criteria for causation of chronic disease which require to be satisfied is as follows (Surgeon General, Advisory Committee of the USPHS, 1964):

1. The consistency of the association.
2. The strength of the association.
3. The specificity of the association.
4. The temporal relationship of the association.
5. The coherence of the association.

In some circumstances particular difficulty may be encountered in that the same clinical and pathological state may be produced by a variety of causal agencies. The fact that workers in any industry are not exempt from developing disorders of the lung or pleura which occur in the general population should always be kept in mind. Thus, in spite of their having had appropriate occupational exposure, lung disease in some individuals is not necessarily of occupational origin. Other factors may also have to be accounted for. For example: a single agent may produce different clinical and pathological responses in different circumstances; and two or more agents or co-factors acting in conjunction may be required to cause disease (Evans, 1976).

This important question is also discussed, in the light of Sir Bradford Hill's (1965) nine criteria, in Chapter 8 (page 219).

References

Evans, A.S. (1976) Causation and disease: the Henlé–Koch postulates revisited. *Yale J. Biol. Med.* **49**, 175–195
Hill, A.B. (1965) The environment and disease: association and causation. *Proc. R. Soc. Med.* **58**, 295–300
Surgeon General, Advisory Committee of the USPHS (1964) *Smoking and Health.* PHS Pub. No. 1103, Washington DC, Supt. of Doc. (Quoted by Evans, 1976)

Index

Note: DIPF = Diffuse interstitial
pulmonary fibrosis

Abdominal wall, vital capacity and, 21
Abrasive(s):
    manufacture of, 288–9, 595–6
    polishes, 255, 258, 270, 288–9, 295
    sandblasting:
        'finishing off' by, 289, 293
        mixed-dust exposure from, 294
        silicosis and, 297–8, 313
        zircon, 261, 289
Abscess, tuberculous bronchial, 398
Absolute lung volumes, 27
Absorption atelectasis, 22, 23, 803, 831
Acceleration, 41, 796–7, 805–6
    atelectasis, 803
Acetaldehyde, 615–16
Acetazolamide, 813, 815
Acetic acid, 616
Acetylcholinesterase, 627
Acetylcysteine, 615
Achalasia of the cardia, 140
Acid anhydrides, 716, 718, 722, 726, 729
Acid mists, 658
Acinus (acini):
    airways of, 4–6
        intersegmental bronchiolar
            communications, 5–6
    blood vessels of, 10–11
    connective tissue of, 6, 10–11
    definition of, 4
    emphysema and, 227
    morphology of, 4–6
    particle deposition in, 41
    particle elimination from, 44–5
    see also Alveolus
Acrolein, 616
Acrylonitrite, 656
Actinolite, 412–13, 414, 856–60
Actinomycetes, thermophilic:
    conditions for growth of, 684
    farmers' lung and associated species of,
        683
    in sputum, 685
    spores of, dimensions, 668
    Thermoactinomycete species, 683
        air conditioner lung disease and, 699
        bagassosis and, 692–3, 684

Actinomycetes, thermophilic (*cont.*)
    in baled cotton, 739
    mushroom worker's lung and, 695–6
Activated carbons, 348
    pneumoconiosis and, 353, 381
β_2–Adrenoceptor, 92, 717
Aerodynamic diameter of particle, 36
Aerosol(s), 35–46
    aerodynamic properties of, 35–6
    bronchodilator, therapeutic, 144, 618
    characteristics of, 35, 51
    definition of, 35
    deposition in lung airways of, 36–41
    elimination from airways of, 41–5, 52–3
    host responses to, 50–1
    see also Particle *and also individual*
        substances
Aerospace, *see* Aircraft; Space flight
Agate, 289, 843
AIDS (Acquired Immunodeficiency
        Syndrome):
    bronchoalveolar lavage and, 85
    cryptococcosis and, 771
    Pneumocystis carinii pneumonia and,
        175, 179, 201
    tumours and, 69
Air-conditioning:
    extrinsic allergic alveolitis and, 698–700
    Legionnaires' disease and, 756, 758
Aircraft:
    altitude decompression sickness in,
        803–4
    cabin decompression of, 798, 801–2
    cabin pressurization of, 795–6
    fitness to fly in, 807–10
    oxygen delivery equipment in, 802–3
    ozone exposure in, 626, 627, 796
Airway(s):
    asymmetrical dichotomy of, 3–4
    blood vessels of, 10–11
    branching patterns of, 2–4, 7, 20, 41
    breath sounds and, 146–55
    cells of, 7–10
    gas solubility and, 26
    morphology of, 1–6, 41
    nerve supply of, 2, 12
    particle deposition in, 36–41, *see also*
        Aerosol; Particle
    reactivity of, 31

Airway(s) (*cont.*)
    respiratory physiology and, 20
    surface area of, 8
    see also individual structures
Albendazole, 772
Alcalase (*B.subtilis*)
    skin responses to, 717, 718, 720
    specific IgE antibody to, 726
Alcohol:
    ascent to altitude and, 815
    mucociliary transport and, 44
Allergic reaction(s), 51
    classification of, 72–4
    epidemiological studies of, 211, 214
    latent interval of, 211
    treatment of, 92
    see also Atopy; Hypersensitivity
        reactions; *and also individual*
        allergens and disorders
α-Amylase, fungal, 720, 721
α_1-Antitrypsin, 232–3
Altitude, 794–815
    air travel and, 626, 627, 794–810
    moderate, 814–15
    ozone exposure at, 626, 627, 796
    prolonged exposure to, 810–15
Aluminium, 594–7
    abrasives, 595–6
    bronchoalveolar lavage detection of, 87
    hypersensitivity granulomas and, 589
    lung cancer and, 655
    metal fume fever, 593–4
    powder, 596–7
    quartz pneumoconiosis and, 109,
        112–13, 317–18, 371
    welding with, 630
'Aluminium lung', 596–7
Aluminium phosphide, 628
Aluminosilicates, 850–1
    anhydrous, 559–60, 862–3
    deposits in coal-fired boilers of, 293
    hydrous, 861–2
    refractories, 292–3
    see also individual minerals
Alunite, 554
    in production of potassium sulphate,
        554
    mineralogy of, 554
Alveolar duct(s), 4, 6